LOVELL AND WINTER'S
PEDIATRIC ORTHOPAEDICS

SEVENTH EDITION

LOVELL AND WINTER'S

PEDIATRIC ORTHOPAEDICS

SEVENTH EDITION

VOLUME 1

EDITORS

Stuart L. Weinstein, MD

Ignacio V. Ponseti Chair and Professor
  of Orthopaedic Surgery
Professor of Pediatrics
University of Iowa Hospitals and Clinics
Iowa City, Iowa

John M. (Jack) Flynn, MD

Professor of Orthopaedic Surgery
University of Pennsylvania
Associate Chief of Orthopaedic Surgery
The Children's Hospital of Philadelphia
Philadelphia, Pennsylvania

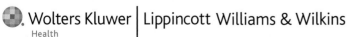
Wolters Kluwer | Lippincott Williams & Wilkins
Health

Philadelphia • Baltimore • New York • London
Buenos Aires • Hong Kong • Sydney • Tokyo

Acquisitions Editor: Brian Brown
Product Development Editor: David Murphy
Production Project Manager: David Orzechowski
Senior Manufacturing Coordinator: Beth Welsh
Marketing Manager: Dan Dressler
Senior Design Coordinator: Teresa Mallon
Production Service: SPi Global

Printed in China

Library of Congress Cataloging-in-Publication Data
    Lovell and Winter's pediatric orthopaedics. — 7th ed. / editors, Stuart L. Weinstein, John M. Flynn.
       p. ; cm.
    Pediatric orthopaedics
    Includes bibliographical references and index.
      ISBN 978-1-60547-814-2 (hardback)
    I. Lovell, Wood W., 1915- II. Weinstein, Stuart L. III. Flynn, John M.. IV. Title: Pediatric orthopaedics.
    [DNLM: 1. Orthopedics. 2. Adolescent. 3. Child. 4. Infant. WS 270]
    616.70083—dc23

                               2012017197

To purchase additional copies of this book, call our customer service department at (800) 638-3030 or fax orders to (301) 223-2320. International customers should call (301) 223-2300.

Visit Lippincott Williams & Wilkins on the Internet: at LWW.com. Lippincott Williams & Wilkins customer service representatives are available from 8:30 am to 6 pm, EST.

10 9 8 7 6 5 4 3 2 1

CONTRIBUTORS

Michael C. Ain, MD
Associate Professor
Department of Orthopaedic and Neurosurgery
Johns Hopkins Hospital
Baltimore, Maryland

Benjamin A. Alman, MD, FRCSC
Distinguished James R. Urbaniak Professor
Chair, Department of Orthopaedic Surgery
Duke University
Durham, North Carolina

Alexandre Arkader, MD
Assistant Professor of Clinical Orthopaedic Surgery
University of Southern California Keck School
    of Medicine
Director, Bone and Soft Tissue Tumor Program
Children's Orthopaedic Center
Children's Hospital Los Angeles
Los Angeles, California

David D. Aronsson, MD
Professor
Department of Orthopaedics and Rehabilitation and
    Department of Pediatrics
University of Vermont College of Medicine
Burlington, Vermont

Donald S. Bae, MD
Associate Professor
Department of Orthopaedic Surgery
Harvard Medical School
Associate in Orthopaedic Surgery
Department of Orthopaedic Surgery
Boston Children's Hospital
Boston, Massachusetts

Frank R. Berenson, MD
Pediatric and Adolescent NeuroDevelopmental
    Associates and Atlanta Headache Specialists
Atlanta, Georgia

Richard E. Bowen, MD
Clinical Professor
Department of Orthopaedic Surgery
Geffen School of Medicine at UCLA
Orthopaedic Institute for Children
Los Angeles, California

Michael T. Busch, MD
Chief Executive Officer, Children's Orthopaedics of Atlanta
Orthopaedic Surgery Fellowship Director, Children's
    Healthcare of Atlanta
Surgical Director of Sports Medicine, Children's Healthcare
    of Atlanta
Atlanta, Georgia

Haemish Crawford, FRACS
Pediatric Orthopaedic Surgeon
Department of Orthopaedics
Starship Children's Hospital
Auckland, New Zealand

Luciano Dias, MD
Professor
Department of Orthopaedic Surgery
Feinberg School of Medicine
Northwestern University
Attending Physician
Department of Pediatric Orthopaedic Surgery
Medical Director
Motion Analysis Center
Children's Memorial Hospital
Chicago, Illinois

Matthew B. Dobbs, MD
Professor
Department of Orthopaedic Surgery
Washington University School of Medicine
St. Louis Children's Hospital and Shriners Hospital
    for Children – St. Louis
St. Louis, Missouri

John P. Dormans, MD
The Richard M. Armstrong Jr. Endowed Chair in Pediatric
    Orthopaedic Surgery
Professor of Orthopaedic Surgery at the University of
    Pennsylvania School of Medicine
Chief of Orthopaedic Surgery
The Children's Hospital of Philadelphia
Division of Orthopaedic Surgery
Philadelphia, Pennsylvania

Amy L. Dunn, MD
Associate Professor of Pediatrics
Emory University/Children's Healthcare of Atlanta
Aflac Cancer and Blood Disorders Service
Atlanta, Georgia

Georges Y. El-Khoury, MD
Professor
Department of Radiology and Orthopaedics
University of Iowa Carver College of Medicine
Director, Musculoskeletal Section
Department of Radiology and Orthopaedics
University of Iowa Hospitals and Clinics
Iowa City, Iowa

John M. Flynn, MD
Professor of Orthopaedic Surgery
University of Pennsylvania
Associate Chief of Orthopaedic Surgery
The Children's Hospital of Philadelphia
Philadelphia, Pennsylvania

Steven Frick, MD
Professor
Department of Orthopaedic Surgery
University of Florida College of Medicine
Chair
Department of Orthopaedic Surgery
Nemours Children's Hospital
Orlando, Florida

Theodore J. Ganley, MD
Director of Sports Medicine
The Children's Hospital of Philadelphia
Associate Professor of Orthopaedic Surgery
The University of Pennsylvania School of Medicine
Philadelphia, Pennsylvania

Mark C. Gebhardt, MD
Frederick W. and Jane M. Ilfeld Professor of Orthopaedics
Departmeny of Orthopaedic Surgery
Harvard Medical School
Orthopaedic Surgeon-in-Chief
Department of Orthopaedic Surgery
Beth Israel Deaconess Medical Center
Boston, Massachusetts

Michael J. Goldberg, MD
Director, Skeletal Health Program
Chief
Skeletal Dysplasia Clinics
Orthopaedic Surgeon
Department of Orthopaedics
Seattle Children's Hospital
Seattle, Washington

J. Eric Gordon, MD
Professor
Department of Orthopaedics
Washington University in St. Louis
School of Medicine
St. Louis, Missouri

H. Kerr Graham, MD, FRCS(Ed), FRACS
Professor of Orthopaedic Surgery
The University of Melbourne
Consultant Orthopaedic Surgeon/Director of Hugh
    Williamson Gait Analysis Laboratory
The Royal Children's Hospital
Murdoch Childrens Research Institute
Parkville, Victoria, Australia

Matthew A. Halanski, MD
Associate Professor, Pediatric Orthopedics
Department of Orthopedics and Rehabilitation
University of Wisconsin
Madison, Wisconsin

Martin J. Herman, MD
Associate Professor of Orthopaedic Surgery and Pediatrics
Drexel University College of Medicine
St. Christopher's Hospital for Children
Philadelphia, Pennsylvania

Andrew W. Howard, MD, MSc, FRCSC
Director, Office of International Surgery
Medical Director, Trauma Program
Associate Professor
Departments of Surgery and Health Policy,
    Management, and Evaluation
University of Toronto
The Hospital for Sick Children
Toronto, Ontario, Canada

Robert M. Kay, MD
Professor of Orthopaedic Surgery
Keck University of Southern California School of Medicine
Vice Chief
Children's Orthopaedic Center
Children's Hospital – Los Angeles
Los Angeles, California

Geetika Khanna, MD
Associate Professor, Radiology
St. Louis Children's Hospital
Mallinckrodt Institute for Radiology
Washington University School of Medicine
St. Louis, Missouri

Young-Jo Kim, MD, PhD
Associate Professor
Department of Orthopaedic Surgery
Harvard Medical School
Director
Child and Adult Hip Program
Boston Children's Hospital
Boston, Massachusetts

Mininder S. Kocher, MD, MPH
Professor
Department of Orthopaedic Surgery
Harvard Medical School
Associate Director
Division of Sports Medicine
Children's Hospital – Boston
Boston, Massachusetts

Lawrence G. Lenke, MD
Jerome J. Gilden Distinguished Professor of
    Orthopaedic Surgery
Professor of Neurosurgery
Chief of Spinal Surgery
Department of Orthopaedic Surgery
Washington University
St. Louis, Missouri

Jennifer W. Lisle, MD
Assistant Professor
Department of Orthopaedics and
    Rehabilitation
The University of Vermont College of
    Medicine
Chief, Pediatric Orthopaedics
Orthopaedics and Rehabilitation Health Care Service
Fletcher Allen Health Care
Burlington, Vermont

Randall T. Loder, MD
George J. Garceau Professor of Orthopaedic Surgery
Department of Orthopaedic Surgery
Indiana University
Director of Pediatric Orthopaedics
James Whitcomb Riley Children's Hospital
Indianapolis, Indiana

Scott J. Luhmann, MD
Associate Professor
Department of Orthopaedics
Washington University School of
    Medicine
Chief of Spine Surgery
Department of Orthopaedics
Shriner's Hospital for Children – St. Louis
St. Louis, Missouri

James J. McCarthy, MD
Associate Professor
Department of Orthopaedic Surgery
Cincinnati Children's Hospital
Director
Department of Orthopaedic Surgery
Cincinnati Children's Hospital Medical Center
Cincinnati, Ohio

Yusuf Menda, MD
Associate Professor
Clinical Director, PET Center
Department of Radiology
University of Iowa Hospitals and Clinics
Iowa City, Iowa

José A. Morcuende, MD, PhD
Professor
Department of Orthopaedic Surgery and
    Rehabilitation and Department of Pediatrics
University of Iowa
Iowa City, Iowa

Vincent S. Mosca, MD
Professor of Orthopaedics
Department of Orthopaedics and Sports Medicine
University of Washington School of Medicine
Pediatric Orthopaedic Surgeon
Director, Pediatric Orthopaedic Fellowship
Seattle Children's Hospital
Seattle, Washington

Peter O. Newton, MD
Clinical Professor
Department of Orthopaedics
University of California at San Diego
Chief of Orthopedics, Medical Practice
    Foundation
Rady Children's Hospital
San Diego, California

Kenneth J. Noonan, MD
Chief, Pediatric Orthopaedics
University of Wisconsin
Madison, Wisconsin

Tom F. Novacheck, MD
Adjunct Associate Professor of Orthopaedic Surgery
University of Minnesota
Director, Jarmes R Gage Center for Gait and Motion
    Analysis
Gillette Children's Specialty Healthcare
St. Paul, Minnesota

Norman Y. Otsuka, MD
Joseph E. Milgram Professor
Department of Orthopaedic Surgery
New York University
Director, Center for Children
NYU Langone Hospital for Joint Diseases
New York, New York

Alexander K. Powers, MD
Assistant Professor
Department of Neurosurgery, Orthopaedics,
    and Pediatrics
Wake Forest University School of Medicine
Winston-Salem, North Carolina

Margaret M. Rich, MD
Orthopaedic Surgeon
Shriners Hospital for Children – St. Louis
St. Louis, Missouri

James O. Sanders, MD
Professor of Orthopaedics and Pediatrics
Department of Orthopaedics and Rehabilitation
University of Rochester
Chief, Division of Pediatrics
Golisano Children's Hospital at Strong
Rochester, New York

Jeffrey R. Sawyer, MD
Associate Professor
Department of Orthopaedic Surgery
University of Tennessee
Campbell Clinic
Le Bonheur Children's Hospital
Memphis, Tennessee

Perry L. Schoenecker, MD
Professor
Department of Orthopaedic Surgery
Chief
Department of Pediatric Orthopaedics
Shriners Hospital for Children – St. Louis
St. Louis, Missouri

Suken A. Shah, MD
Division Chief, Spine and Scoliosis Service
Clinical Fellowship Director
Attending Pediatric Orthopaedic Surgeon
Nemours/Alfred I. duPont Hospital for Children
Wilmington, Delaware
Associate Professor
Department of Orthopaedic Surgery
Jefferson Medical College of Thomas
    Jefferson University
Philadelphia, Pennsylvania

Ernest L. Sink, MD
Associate Professor
Department of Orthopaedic Surgery
Weil Cornell Medical School
Hospital for Special surgery
New York, New York

Kit Song, MD, MHA
Clinical Professor
Department of Orthopedic Surgery
UCLA School of Medicine
Chief of Staff
Shriners Hospitals for Children – Los Angeles
Los Angeles, California

David L. Skaggs, MD, MMM
Professor and Chief of Orthopaedic Surgery
Children's Hospital Los Angeles
University of Southern California Keck School of Medicine
Children's Hospital Chair of Pediatric Spinal Disorders
Los Angeles, California

Paul D. Sponseller, MD, MBA
Sponseller Professor and Head, Pediatric Orthopaedics
Johns Hopkins Bloomberg Children's Center
Baltimore, Maryland

Anthony A. Stans, MD
Consultant
Department of Orthopaedic Surgery
Mayo Clinic
Rochester, Minnesota

Vineeta T. Swaroop, MD
Instructor of Orthopaedic Surgery
Northwestern University
Feinberg School of Medicine
Children's Memorial Hospital
Chicago, Illinois

Pam Thomason, BPhty, M Physio
Senior Physiotherapist and Manager
Hugh Williamson Gait Analysis Laboratory
The Royal Children's Hospital – Melbourne
Parkville, Victoria, Australia

George H. Thompson, MD
Professor of Orthopaedic Surgery and Pediatrics
Case Western Reserve University
Director, Pediatric Orthopaedics
Rainbow Babies & Children's Hospital
Vice-Chairman, Department of Orthopaedics
University Hospitals Case Medical Center
Cleveland, Ohio

William C. Warner Jr, MD
Professor of Orthopaedics
Department of Orthopaedic Surgery
University of Tennessee
Campbell Clinic
Le Bonheur Children's Hospital
Memphis, Tennessee

Peter M. Waters, MD
Orthopedic Surgeon in Chief
Children's Hospital Boston
John E. Hall Professor of Orthopaedic Surgery
Harvard Medical School
Boston, Massachusetts

Stuart L. Weinstein, MD
Ignacio V. Ponseti Chair and Professor of Orthopaedic
    Surgery
Professor of Pediatrics
University of Iowa Hospitals and Clinics
Iowa City, Iowa

Pamela F. Weiss, MD, MSCE
Attending Physician
Division of Rheumatology
Children's Hospital of Philadelphia
Assistant Professor
Department of Pediatrics
University of Pennsylvania
Philadelphia, Pennsylvania

Dennis R. Wenger, MD
Clinical Professor
Department of Orthopaedic Surgery
University of California San Diego
Director, Pediatric Orthopedic Training Program
Rady Children's Hospital San Diego
San Diego, California

R. Baxter Willis, MD
Head, Department of Surgery
Children's Hospital of Eastern Ontario
Professor of Surgery (Orthopaedics)
University of Ottawa
Ottawa, Ontario, Canada

Burt Yaszay, MD
Assistant Clinical Professor
Department of Orthopaedics
University of California at San Diego
Orthopaedic Surgeon
Rady Children's Hospital
San Diego, California

This seventh edition of *Pediatric Orthopaedics* represents a complete renovation and reorganization of the central textbook of pediatric orthopaedics. The editors and publishers have worked to incorporate into the main textbook the atlas material (which in the past stood as a separate volume) so that the surgeon can move seamlessly from background and indications to surgical technique and outcomes. The science of pediatric orthopaedics has now been married to its art, to create a comprehensive source for those who care for children and adolescents with musculoskeletal problems and injuries. Incorporating the atlas has been an immense task, relying on the hard work and patience of many: authors, editors, the artist, and production personnel. We are gratified to see that the final product accomplished our vision to meet the needs of the modern pediatric orthopaedist.

Since the last edition, the field of pediatric orthopaedics has moved forward at a rapid pace and grown substantially in the number of orthopaedists who make caring for children the central part of their practice. Basic science work in molecular biology, genetics, and embryology continues to inform our understanding of etiology, but there is still much mystery and very little therapeutic intervention at this time. There have been innumerable advances and changes in standard of care in many areas in the last few years: clubfoot, hip dysplasia, limb deformity, slipped capital femoral epiphysis, pediatric sports medicine, spinal deformity, musculoskeletal oncology and infection, and upper extremity disorders. Meanwhile, trauma care has become more operative, achieving better results with more rapid mobilization. One clear trend in

pediatric orthopaedics is subspecialization. To give readers the most evidence-based and cutting-edge information, we have enlisted the expertise of a large number of new authorities in many different pediatric orthopaedic subspecialties. We have asked these experts to synthesize the literature, provide the best indications for surgery, describe the best procedures in careful detail, and warn the reader about potential pitfalls in care.

One unique strength that sets this pediatric orthopaedic textbook apart is the tremendous diversity of expertise from around the world. The authors of this edition hail from 28 different centers of excellence and several countries from around the world. By inviting such a wide range of authors from so many different institutions, we have avoided a narrow, parochial approach to solving orthopaedic problems for children. In many cases, the chapters are coauthored by experts from different centers, so that each can critique the other when necessary.

We live in an age where parents can learn more about a condition in twenty minutes on the Internet than most clinicians could learn years ago sorting through textbooks and journals for hours. We also live in an age where families and payers are demanding increased attention to quality and value. In this seventh edition of *Pediatric Orthopedics*, we have worked to assemble a single source of information so the pediatric orthopaedist can deliver the highest quality and highest value care and satisfy the information needs of the most informed and sophisticated families they encounter.

SLW and JMF

ACKNOWLEDGMENTS

The editors would like to acknowledge the hard work and dedication of the authors, the skill of our medical illustrator, and the commitment of our publisher to complete this important project.

Stuart Weinstein would like to thank his wife Lynn and son Will for their support and encouragement over the years and his former collaborator Ray Morrissy for his guidance and inspiration on previous editions of *Pediatric Orthopaedics* and most importantly his friendship.

Jack Flynn would like to acknowledge the patience and understanding of his wife Mary and children Erin, Colleen, John, and Kelly as he dedicated many hours to the project. They understand that Dad has homework too.

CONTENTS

LOVELL AND WINTER'S

PEDIATRIC ORTHOPAEDICS

SEVENTH EDITION

CHAPTER 1

José A. Morcuende
James O. Sanders

Embryology and Development of the Neuromuscular Apparatus

INTRODUCTION

The development of an adult organism from a single cell is an unparalleled example of integrated cell behavior. The single cell divides many times to produce the trillions of cells of the human organism, which form structures as complex and varied as the eyes, limbs, heart, or the brain. This amazing achievement raises multitude of questions. How the body's tissues and organs are formed? How do the different patterns form in the embryo that tells different parts what to become? How individual cells become committed to particular development fates? Increased knowledge in developmental biology comes from the understanding of how genes direct those developmental processes. In fact, developmental biology is one of the most exciting and fast-growing fields of biology and has become essential for understanding many other areas of biology and medicine.

Embryology at the level of gross anatomy and microscopic anatomy is fairly well described. Manipulation of experimental animals, mainly the chick and mouse, has provided insights into the relationship of tissues involved in normal growth and differentiation. Molecular mechanisms underlying developmental events are being discovered. An integration of the approaches of genetics, molecular biology, developmental biology, and evolutionary biology is taking place, resulting in an explosion in our understanding of the importance of individual genes and interactions of cells and tissues in specifying development of complex organisms from single cells. One of the major reasons for the synthesis and complementariness of these varying disciplines is the existence of homology, both within organisms and between species. It turns out that genes and their gene products are often very similar in structure and function in fruit flies, chickens, mice, and men. In complex organisms, the same gene is often used at different times in development and in different areas of the body to perform similar functions.

This chapter describes the early stages of embryonic development, followed by the descriptive anatomy of limb development and the formation of the vertebral column. It also examines bone formation and growth and emphasizes the progress in the understanding of the cellular and molecular mechanisms involved in these aspects of development. Concluding each section are observations that relate developmental anatomy to the clinical problems faced by orthopaedic surgeons. Finally, a section on growth in pediatric orthopaedics will provide a framework of understanding growth and development's effects on the musculoskeletal system.

DEVELOPMENTAL ANATOMY OF EARLY EMBRYOGENESIS AND ORGANOGENESIS

Embryogenesis has been traditionally divided into the embryonic period and the fetal period. The embryonic period is considered from fertilization to the end of the first trimester. During this period, the body plan is completed and all major organs are established. The stages of the embryonic period include fecundation, cleavage, gastrulation, neurulation, and organogenesis. By the 12th week of gestation, the organism shape is fully formed and the remaining of the gestation will involve the growth and the maturation of the organ functions.

Creating Multicellularity.
The first stage of development after fertilization is a series of cleavage divisions in which the zygote divides in an ordered pattern to produce a ball of much smaller cells, called blastula, and this starts the production of a multicellular organism. Cleavage is a very well-coordinated process under genetic regulation. The specific type of cleavage depends upon the evolutionary history of the species and on the mechanism used to support the nutritional requirements to the embryo. The pattern and symmetry of cell cleavage particular to a species is determined by the amount and distribution of the cytoplasm (yolk), and by those factors in the cytoplasm influencing the angle of the mitotic spindle and the timing of its formation. In most species (mammals being the exception), the rate of cell division and the placement of the blastomeres with respect to one another is completely under

the control of proteins and mRNA stored in the mother oocyte. The zygote DNA is not used in early cleavage embryos. In addition, the differential cellular cleavage provides the embryo with axis information, dividing the cell in an animal pole (where the nucleus is frequently found) and a vegetal pole.

In mammals, the protected uterine environment permits an unusual process of early development. It does not have the same need as the embryos of most other species to complete the early stages rapidly. Moreover, the development of the placenta provides for nutrition from the mother, so that the zygote does not have to contain large stores of material such as yolk. Thus, cleavage has several specific characteristics. First, it is a relatively slow process. Each division is about 12 to 24 hours apart. A frog egg, for example, can divide into 37,000 cells in just 43 hours. Second, there is a unique orientation of the cells with relation to one another. The first cleavage is a meridional division, but in the second division, one pair of cells divides meridionally and the other equatorially (Fig. 1-1). This type of cleavage is called rotational cleavage (1). Third, there is an asynchrony in the early divisions. Cells do not divide at the same time. Therefore, embryos do not increase evenly from 2- to 4- to 8-cell stages but frequently contain odd number of cells. Fourth, the zygotic genome is activated early during cleavage divisions to produce the proteins needed for the process to occur (2). Finally, the most crucial difference with other species is the phenomenon of compaction. At 8-cell stage, blastomeres form a loose arrangement of cells, but after the third division, the cells cluster together and form a compact ball with the outside cells stabilized by tight junctions and the inner cells developing gap junctions which enables the passing of small molecules and ions between cells (Fig. 1-2).

Up to the 8-cell stage, the embryo is remarkably adaptable, and each of its cells can form any part of the later embryo or adult. One example is seen in the development of a pair

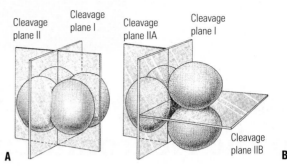

FIGURE 1-1. Comparison of early cleavage divisions in the sea urchin and in mammals. **A:** The plane of cell division in the sea urchin is perpendicular to the cells whereas in mammals **(B)**, in the second division, one of the two blastomeres divides meridionally and the other divides equatorially. Early cell division in mammals is asynchronous—not all cells divide at the same time. (Reproduced from Gilbert SF. *Developmental biology*, 4th ed. Sunderland, MA: Sinauer Associates, Inc. Publishers,1994:178, with permission.)

of identical twins from a single fertilized egg. Similarly, this embryonic cell potential can be demonstrated experimentally by using chimeras. These are animals made by combining individual cells from early embryos of genetically different strains of animals and then the reaggregated cells implanted in foster mothers. Analysis of the genetic composition of the tissues of the developed animal shows that the single cells from the four-cell stage can participate in forming many different parts of the animal; they are said to be totipotent (3, 4).

In mammals, the next stage in development is the generation of the cells that will form the placenta and the membranes that surround the developing embryo. The cells of the compacted embryo divide to produce a 16-cell morula. This morula consists of a small group (one or two) of internal cells surrounded by a larger group of external cells (Fig. 1-2D) (5). The

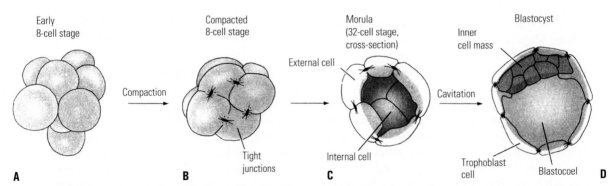

FIGURE 1-2. The cleavage of a mouse embryo up to blastocyst. **A:** Early 8-cell stages with loose cell arrangement. **B:** Compacted 8-cell stage. During the process of compaction, cells suddenly huddle together, maximizing their contacts. Tight junctions, sealing off the inside of the sphere, stabilize outside cells. The inner cells develop gap junctions, thereby enabling the passing of small molecules and ions. **C:** Morula with differentiation between the external cells and the inner cell mass. **D:** Blastocyst before implantation. (Reproduced from Gilbert SF. *Developmental biology*, 4th ed. Sunderland, MA: Sinauer Associates, Inc. Publishers,1994:179, with permission.)

position of a cell at this stage determines whether it will form extraembryonic structures or contribute to the embryo proper. Inner cells will form the embryo and most of the external cells the trophoblast. This structure will enable the embryo to get oxygen and nourishment from the mother and will secrete hormones and regulators of the immune response so that the mother will not reject the embryo. Experimentally, this separation of cell activities has been shown also with chimeras. Cells from different strains of mouse can be arranged so that the cells of one strain surround the cells of the other strain. The development of such cell aggregates shows that only the cells on the inside contribute to the mouse development (6). By the 64-cell stage, the inner cell mass and the trophoblast have become separate cell layers, neither of which contributes cells to the other group. Thus, the distinction between these two cell types represents the first differentiation event in mammalian development.

Organizing the Embryonic Cells to Form Tissues and Organs.

In human beings, implantation begins 1 or 2 days after the blastocyst enters the uterus, approximately on day 9 (Fig. 1-3A). At the time of implantation, the exposed surface of the uterine lining, the endometrium, is a single-layered epithelial sheet, which forms numerous tubular glands. Having adhered to the epithelium, the trophoblastic cells penetrate it and erode it (Fig. 1-3B). The endometrium responds by a dramatic increase in vascularity and capillary permeability, the so-called decidual reaction (Fig. 1-4). These processes are apparently mediated by estrogens produced by the blastocyst and estrogen receptors in the wall of the uterus. In addition, the trophoblast initiates the secretion of chorionic gonadotropin, which will maintain the production of progesterone by the ovaries, which is essential for the maintenance of the pregnancy. HCG is detectable in the blood and urine and serves as the basis of pregnancy tests.

The next phase of development—the gastrulation—involves a remarkable process in which the ball of cells of the blastula turns itself into a multilayered structure and rearranges to form the three embryonic tissue layers known as endoderm, ectoderm, and mesoderm. In addition, during gastrulation, the body plan of the organism is also established. Gastrulation thus involves dramatic changes in the overall structure of the embryo, converting it into a complex three-dimensional structure.

The mechanics of gastrulation in mammals are not well understood. In sea urchins and insects, the phenomenon of gastrulation is like what happens if a ball is punctured and then kicked: the ball collapses and the inner surface on one

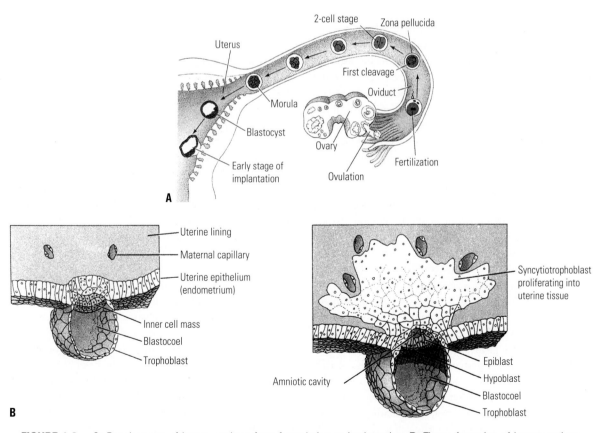

FIGURE 1-3.   **A:** Development of human embryo from fecundation to implantation. **B:** Tissue formation of human embryo between days 7 and 8. The inner cell mass will give rise to the embryo proper and the trophoblast to the placenta. The distinction between those two groups of cells represents the first differentiation event in embryonic development. (Reproduced from Gilbert SF. *Developmental biology*, 4th ed. Sunderland, MA: Sinauer Associates, Inc. Publishers,1994:177 and 235, with permission.)

FIGURE 1-4. Placenta development in human embryo at the end of the 3rd week of gestation. The trophoblast cells forming the placenta are coming into contact with the blood vessels of the uterus. The endometrium responds by a dramatic increase in vascularity and capillary permeability, the so-called decidual reaction. The trophoblast divides into the cytotrophoblast, which will form the villi, and the syncytiotrophoblast, which will ingress into the uterine cavity. The actual embryo forms from the cells of the epiblast. (Reproduced from Gilbert SF. *Developmental biology*, 3rd ed. Sunderland, MA: Sinauer Associates, Inc. Publishers,1991:149, with permission.)

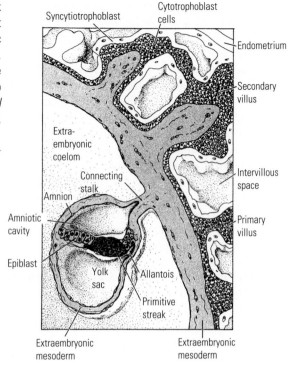

side makes contact with the other side, making a large dimple. In the embryo, by a complicated invagination, a large area of cells on the outside of the embryo is brought to lie inside it. Subsequent development depends on the interactions of the outer ectoderm, middle mesoderm, and inner endoderm layers of cells. The ectoderm will give rise to the epidermis of the skin and the nervous system; the mesoderm will give rise to connective tissues including the bones, muscle, and blood; and the endoderm will give rise to the lung and the lining of the gut and associated organs.

In addition, during gastrulation, the cells are positioned according to the body plan appropriate to the species, and there is a process of differentiation of the functional characteristics required of each part of the body plan. Specification of the axes in mammals does not involve any maternal component. The dorsoventral (DV) axis is established by the interaction between the inner cell mass and the trophectoderm, while the anterior–posterior (AP) axis may be set only at implantation. The generation of the left–right asymmetry is under genetic control. This vertebrate body plan will be maintained thereafter as the embryo grows.

The movements of gastrulation involve the entire embryo. Cell migration in one part of the embryo must be intimately coordinated with other cell movements occurring simultaneously elsewhere. However, gastrulation depends on a relatively simple repetition of basic cell activities. Cells can change their shape by extending or contracting. They can group or separate by forming or breaking their adhesions to neighboring cells or to the extracellular matrix. They can secrete extracellular matrix that constrains or guides their location or movement. These activities, together to

cell proliferation, underlie almost all-morphogenetic activities during gastrulation. The special problem posed in early embryonic development is to understand how these and other elementary cell activities are coordinated in space and time.

Interestingly, recent experiments have suggested that the maternal and paternal genomes (imprinting) have different roles during mammalian gastrulation. Mouse zygotes can be created that have only sperm-derived or oocyte-derived chromosomes. The male-derived embryos die without embryo proper structures but with well-formed chorionic structures. Conversely, the female-derived embryos develop normally but without chorionic structures (7–9). Therefore, the maternal and paternal genomic information may serve distinct functions during early development.

Early Organogenesis in Vertebrate Development: Neurulation and Mesoderm Segmentation. During gastrulation, the germ layers—ectoderm, mesoderm, and endoderm—move to the positions in which they develop into the structures of the adult organism. The AP body axis of the vertebrate embryo emerges, with the head at one end and the future tail at the other. During the next stage of development, the main organs of the body begin to emerge gradually (10). A major set of interactions takes place between the mesodermal cells and the ectoderm in the dorsal midline (Hensen's node) so that the ectoderm cells layer will form the nervous system (Fig. 1-5). At the same time, the mesoderm on either side of the middle breaks up into blocks of cell to form the somites, a series of repeated segments along the axis of the embryo (Fig. 1-6) (11). The interactions between the dorsal

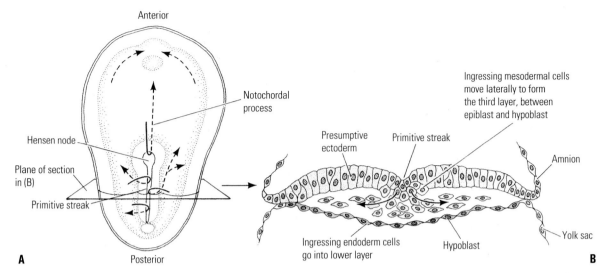

FIGURE 1-5. Cell movements during the gastrulation stage. **A:** Cells migrating through Hensen's node travel anteriorly to form the notochord. Cells traveling through the primitive streak will become the precursors of mesoderm and endoderm. **B:** Transverse section of the embryo. (Reproduced from Gilbert SF. *Developmental biology*, 3rd ed. Sunderland, MA: Sinauer Associates, Inc. Publishers, 1991:148, with permission.)

mesoderm and its overlying ectoderm are one of the most important interactions of all development. The action by which the flat layer of ectodermal cells is transformed into a hollow tube is called neurulation (Fig. 1-7). The first indication of neurulation is a change in cell shape in the ectoderm.

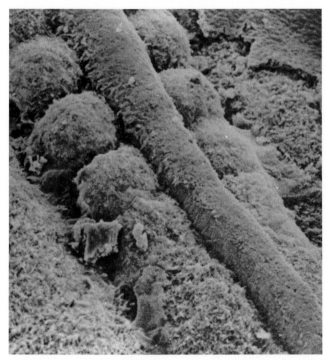

FIGURE 1-6. Scanning electron microscopy showing the neural tube and the well-formed somites with paraxial mesoderm that has not yet separated into distinct somites. (Courtesy of KW Tosney.)

Midline ectodermal cells become elongated, whereas cells destined to form the epidermis become flattened. The elongation of the cells causes this region to rise above the surrounding ectoderm, thus creating the neural plate. Shortly thereafter, the edges of the neural plate thicken and move upward to form the neural folds that subsequently will fuse to form the neural tube beneath the overlying ectoderm. The formation of the neural tube does not occur simultaneously. It starts near the anterior end of the embryo and proceeds in both directions—anteriorly and posteriorly. The two open ends are called anterior and posterior neuropores (Fig. 1-8). In mammals, failure to close the anterior neuropore results in anencephalia, and the posterior neuropore in spina bifida. Neural tube defects (NTDs) can now be detected during pregnancy by ultrasonography and chemical analysis of the amniotic fluid.

The process of neurulation is intimately linked to changes in cell shape generated by the cytoskeleton (microtubules and microfilaments). Differential cell division seen in different regions of the neural plate would also contribute to the size and shape of this region. In addition, those cells directly adjacent to the notochord and those cells at the hinges of the neural groove will also help to mold the neural tube. Separation of the neural tube from the ectoderm that will form the skin requires changes in cell adhesiveness. While molecules that can induce neural tissue, such as noggin protein, have been identified, induction of neurulation is due to inhibition of bone morphogenetic protein (BMP) activity. Positional identity of cells along the AP axis is encoded by the combinatorial expression of genes of the four Hox complexes.

The cells at the dorsal-most portion of the neural tube become the neural crest. These cells will migrate throughout the embryo and will give rise to several cell populations.

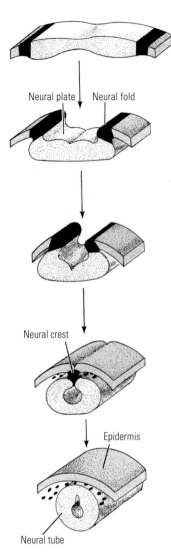

FIGURE 1-7. Diagrammatic representation of neural tube formation. The ectoderm folds in at the most dorsal point, forming a neural tube that is connected by neural crest cells, and an outer epidermis. (Reproduced from Gilbert SF. *Developmental biology*, 3rd ed. Sunderland, MA: Sinauer Associates, Inc. Publishers,1991:158, with permission.)

Although derived from the ectoderm, the neural crest has sometimes been called the fourth germ layer because of its importance. It gives rise to the neurons and supporting glial cells of the sensory, sympathetic, and parasympathetic nervous systems; the melanocytes of the epidermis; and the cartilage and connective tissue components of the head. Although not well understood, the mechanisms of neural crest migration are not random but rather follow precise pathways specified by the extracellular matrix. Differences in adhesiveness between the anterior and posterior halves of the somites result in neural crest being prevented from migrating over the posterior halves. Thus, presumptive dorsal ganglia cells collect adjacent to anterior halves, giving them a segmental arrangement.

The formation of mesodermal structures is not subsequent to the neural tube but occurs simultaneously. The brain and spinal cord must develop in the correct relationship with other body structures, particularly the mesoderm. Five regions of mesoderm can be identified at the neurula-stage embryo (Fig. 1-9). The chordamesoderm will generate the notochord, a transient organ whose functions include inducing neural tube formation and establishing the body axis. The dorsal (somitic) mesoderm will produce many of the connective tissues of the body. The intermediate mesoderm will form the urinary system and genital ducts. The lateral plate mesoderm will give rise to the heart, blood vessels, and blood cells, and the body lining cavities. Lastly, the head mesoderm will contribute to the connective tissues and muscles of the face.

At the neural stage, the body plan has been established and the regions of the embryo that will form limbs, eyes, heart, and the other organs have been determined. But although the positions of various organs are fixed, there is no overt sign yet of differentiation. The potential to form a given organ is now confined to specific regions. Each region has, however, considerable capacity for regulation, so that if a part of the region is removed a normal structure can still form. In later sections, limb and axial skeleton formation will be discussed in more detail.

Conceptual Insights of Embryogenesis and Early Organogenesis. Development is essentially the emergence of organized and specialized structures from an initially very simple group of cells. Thus, the cells of the body, as a rule, are genetically alike (they all have the same DNA content) but phenotypically different—some are specialized as muscle, others as neurons, and so on. During development, differences are generated between cells in the embryo that lead to spatial organization, changes in form, and the generation of different cell types. All these features are ultimately determined by the DNA sequence of the genome. Each cell must act according to the same genetic instructions, but it must interpret them with regard to time and space.

Multicellular organisms are very complex, but they are generated by a limited repertoire of cell activities. As an artist moves from one part of a sculpture to another to achieve first the overall's figure shape, and then the specific anatomic features using a selected number of instruments over and over again, nature also displays a comparable economy in choosing the processes and molecular tools. The key to understanding development lies in cell biology, in the processes of signal transduction, and in the control of gene expression that result in changes of cell state, movement, and growth. The single most important fact in development is based on the surprising finding that the developmental control genes are maintained through evolution. Thus, for many genes discovered in the invertebrate systems, homologue genes have been identified in vertebrates and they have similar developmental roles in species ranging from the fruit fly to fish to mouse to human.

It is convenient to distinguish three main developmental processes, even though they overlap with, and influence, one another considerably. These are the emergence of pattern, cell differentiation, and change in form or morphogenesis.

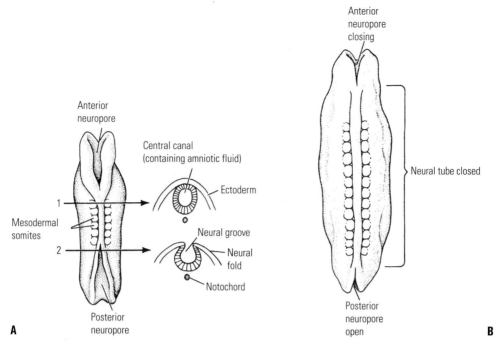

FIGURE 1-8. Neural tube formation in human embryos does not occur simultaneously throughout the ectoderm. **A:** At the initial stages, both anterior and posterior neuropores are open. **B:** Closing of the neural tube proceeds both cranially and caudally. Failure to close the posterior neuropore at day 27 results in spina bifida, the severity of which depends upon how much of the spinal cord remains open. Failure to close the anterior neuropore results in the lethal anencephaly. (Reproduced from Gilbert SF. *Developmental biology*, 3rd ed. Sunderland, MA: Sinauer Associates, Inc. Publishers, 1991:162, with permission.)

Pattern Formation.   Pattern formation is the process by which spatial and temporal arrangements of cell activities are organized within the embryo so that a well-defined structure develops. Pattern formation is critical for the proper development of every part of the organism. In the developing limb, for example, pattern formation enables the cells to know whether to make the upper arm or the fingers, and where the muscles should form.

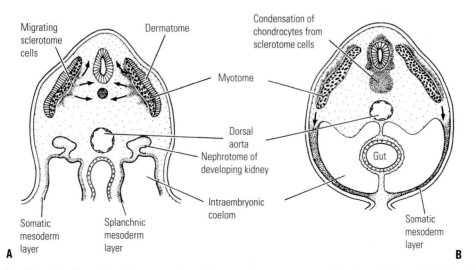

FIGURE 1-9. Mesoderm formation in human embryo. Diagram of a transverse section through the trunk of an early 4-week **(A)** and late 4-week embryo **(B)**. Sclerotome cells migrate from the somite, and these cells ultimately become chondrocytes. The remaining dermatome cells will form the dermis. The myotome will give rise to the striated muscle of both the back and limbs. (Reproduced from Gilbert SF. *Developmental biology*, 3rd ed. Sunderland, MA: Sinauer Associates, Inc. Publishers, 1991:205, with permission.)

Pattern formation in many animals is based on a mechanism where the cells first acquire a positional identity, which determines their future behavior. The ability of cells to sense their relative positions within a limited population of cells and to differentiate according to this position has been the subject of intense research. Interestingly, pattern formation in many systems has similar principles, and more striking similar genes. Many of the so-called homeotic genes that determine segment identity in *Drosophila* have turned up in vertebrates and appear to play similar roles in segmentation of structures such as the brain or the vertebral column.

Homeotic genes are like embryonic switches, analogous to switches of railroad yards that directed trains into one path rather than another. Homeotic genes are involved in specifying regional identity along the AP axis. The name comes from the fact that mutations in some of these genes result in what is called a homeotic transformation, in which one body structure replaces another. For example, in mice in whom Hoxd11 is mutated, anterior sacral vertebrae are transformed into lumbar vertebrae. Homeotic genes in all systems work similarly: they code for proteins called transcription factors that control gene expression. In vertebrates and *Drosophila*, the order of homeotic genes on the chromosome corresponds to their temporal and spatial expression on the AP axis of the embryo.

Cell Differentiation. Cell differentiation is the process in which cells become structurally and functionally different from each other, ending up as distinct types as muscle, bone, or cartilage. Since each cell of the organism has the same genetic material, the achievement and persistence of the differentiation state depends on a series of signals that ultimately control the transcription of specific genes. In humans, the zygote gives rise to about 250 clearly distinguishable types of cells. One of the major goals of developmental biology is to discover how these differences emerge from the fertilized oocyte.

In any organism, differentiation leads to the production of a finite number of discrete kinds of cells, each with its peculiar repertory of biochemical activities and possible morphological configurations. When cells achieve a distinctive state of differentiation, they do not transform into cells of another type. Differentiation leads to a stable, irreversible set of cellular activities. At the organ level, once an embryonic part is capable of realizing its prospective fate in the absence of the conditions that established that capability, it is said to be determined. Determination is thus a step that limits the subsequent development of the part to a specific tissue and cellular differentiation.

Pattern formation and cell differentiation are very closely interrelated as we can see by considering the difference between the upper and lower extremities. Both contain the same tissues—muscle, cartilage, bone, and so on—yet the pattern in which they are arranged are different. It is essentially pattern formation that makes human beings different from rabbits or chimpanzees.

Morphogenesis. Although vertebrate morphogenesis—change in form—is far from completely understood, developmental biology findings support that the same family of molecules and pathways that guide the earliest stages of embryogenesis—setting up such basic elements of body pattern as the head-to-tail and DV axis—also help out in morphogenesis. What is more, these molecules and pathways have been conserved over the course of evolution. Morphogenesis relies on a rather restricted number of cellular activities and encompasses the formation of all tissues and organs from the first embryonic tissue layers to the finished limb, spine, or brain. However, before any tissue or organ can form, earlier steps must occur, steps that tell cells who they are and what tissues they should form. Those early steps take place in the "control room" for development, and morphogenesis is then what happens on the "factory floor"—the actual assembly of the tissues and organs that make up the organism. In addition, spatial patterns of cell proliferation, folding of cell groups, rearrangement of cells, and cell migration make important contributions to morphogenesis, the process that shapes the embryo. Finally, as the embryo develops, cells become different, and this process culminates in the specialization of cells for particular functions. Therefore, during development, morphogenesis give rise to structures appropriate to their position within the embryo and, within these structures, the differentiation of individual cells and their interactions are spatially ordered.

Clinical Significance. Broadly defined, birth defects or congenital abnormalities occur in 6% of all live births. Twenty percent of infant deaths are due to congenital anomalies. About 3% of newborns have significant structural abnormalities. At present, the cause of approximately 50% to 60% of birth defects is unknown. Six to seven percent are due to chromosomal abnormalities. Specific gene mutations cause 7% to 8%. Environmental teratogens are responsible for 7% to 10% of defects. Combined genetic predisposition with environmental factors causes the remaining 20% to 25% of congenital abnormalities.

Starting from a single cell, the embryo can spawn all the new cells and tissues needed to provide an organism with its correct complement of organs. Many of the molecules and pathways known to control cell differentiation and growth during organ formation in the embryo do not become obsolete in the adult. They do help maintain and repair tissues and regulate their response to external environment signals. Some of these proteins are or will soon be in clinical use such as erythropoietin, which trigger red blood cell production, platelet-derived growth factor (PDGF) for diabetic skin ulcers, or BMPs for bone and cartilage regeneration. Finally, in malignant disease, the control of cell activities such as proliferation, differentiation, and migration appears to break down. An understanding of the way in which cell behavior is coordinated in embryos could therefore give insights into bone and cartilage regeneration and cancer biology.

DEVELOPMENTAL ANATOMY OF THE LIMB

At 26 days after fertilization, the upper limb is evident as a slight elevation on the ventrolateral body wall at the level of the pericardial swelling. The lower limb elevation appears 2 days later just caudal to the level of the umbilical cord and develops similarly, but slightly later than the upper limb (Fig. 1-10). At this time the neural tube is closed, all somites are present, and the anlage of the vertebrae and intervertebral discs are present. The limb bud initially consists of loose mesenchymal tissue enclosed in an epithelial ectodermal sheath. The limb bud is formed from mesenchymal cells of the lateral plate and then augmented by cells from the adjacent somites. The skeletal elements and tendons develop from the lateral plate mesenchyme, while limb muscle arises from somitic mesenchymal cells that migrate into the limb bud.

This mesenchymal swelling is covered by ectoderm, the tip of which thickens and becomes the apical ectodermal ridge (AER) (Fig. 1-11). Underlying the AER are rapidly proliferating, undifferentiated mesenchymal cells which are called the progress zone (PZ). Proliferation of these cells causes limb outgrowth. Cells begin to differentiate only after leaving the PZ. The interaction between the AER and the undifferentiated mesenchymal cells underlying it is crucial for limb development. Experimental procedures on chick embryos reveal the following about the limb bud mesenchyme: (a) if removed, no limb develops; (b) when grafted under the ectoderm at a location other than the normal limb area, an AER is induced and a limb will develop; and (c) lower limb mesoderm will induce leg formation, when placed under an upper limb AER. Grafting experiments with the AER reveal that: (a) AER removal aborts further limb development. The later in limb development the AER is removed the less severe is the resulting limb truncation (limb elements develop from proximal to distal); (b) An extra AER will induce a limb bud to form supernumerary limb structures; (c) Nonlimb mesenchymal cells placed beneath the AER will not result in limb development and the AER withers (12).

The implications of these experiments are that the AER is necessary for the growth and development of the limb, while the limb bud mesenchyme induces, sustains, and instructs the AER. In addition to biochemical influence on the PZ, the tightly packed columnar cells of the AER perform a mechanical function directing limb shape by containing these undifferentiated cells in a dorsoventrally flattened shape. The length of the AER controls the width of the limb as well. When all limb elements are differentiated, the AER disappears.

INITIAL APPEARANCE OF VARIOUS FEATURES OF THE LIMBS

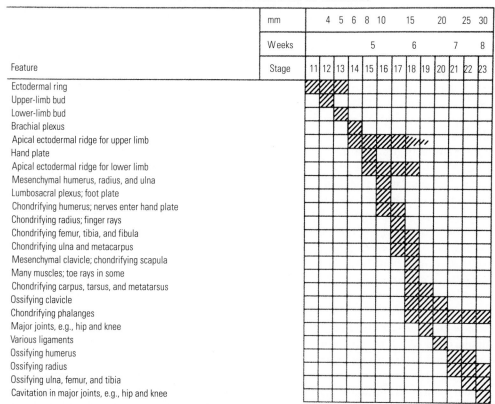

FIGURE 1-10. Timing of the appearance of limb features. (Reproduced from Thorogood P. *Embryos, genes and birth defects.* West Sussex, UK: John Wiley & Sons, Ltd, 1997:350, with permission.)

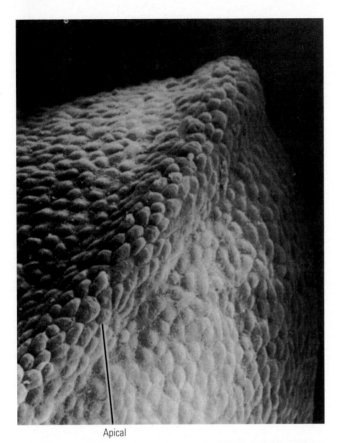

Apical

FIGURE 1-11. Scanning electron photomicrograph of an early chick forelimb bud with the AER at the tip of the limb bud. (Courtesy of KW Tosney.)

The three axes of limbs—AP (thumb to small finger), DV (back of hand to palm), and proximal–distal—are specified very early in limb development. The AP and DV axes are fixed before morphological differentiation of limb components occurs. The PD axis is determined as the limb grows out. The AP axis is set first, followed by the DV axis and then the PD axis. This has been shown by rotation of transplanted limb buds' from their normal position and finding, at different stages, that the limb bud retained the axis orientation of its original limb position or developed the orientation of the host bud (9, 13, 14).

AP axis determination is under the control of an area of tissue in the posterior aspect of the limb bud called the zone of polarizing activity (ZPA) or polarizing region. If this tissue is grafted onto the anterior aspect of a limb bud, a duplication of digits in a mirror image to the normally present digits occurs (15). Cells for the new digits are recruited from the underlying mesoderm and the distal part of the limb widens, as does the AER. If less tissue from the polarizing region is grafted, fewer new digits develop (16). This and other experiments suggest a morphogenic gradient of a diffusible signal originating from the ZPA determines AP axis. This will be discussed in the section on the molecular biology of limb development.

The DV axis is under the control of both the mesoderm and ectoderm of the limb bud at different stages of development. The mesoderm specifies the axis initially, but very early after limb bud formation the ectodermal orientation becomes preeminent. If the ectoderm of right limb bud is transplanted onto the mesenchyme of a left limb bud, the distal limb that develops will be that of a right limb with respect to muscle pattern and joint orientation (13, 14).

The PD axis seems to be determined by the length of time a mesodermal cell remains at the tip of the limb bud in the PZ under the influence of the AER. Once a cell leaves the tip, its position in the limb is fixed. Young tips grafted on older limb buds will duplicate existing limb elements, whereas older tips grafted on young buds will only form distal elements. The best hypothesis as to how this information is passed is that the number of rounds of cell division that occurs while under the influence of the AER determines the PD fate of a cell. Support for this hypothesis comes from experiments in which the limb bud is irradiated. The surviving cells of the irradiated tip have to undergo several extra rounds of mitosis before they can escape the influence of the AER and, thereby, gain positional determination. In these experiments, intermediate limb elements are not formed, just the preexisting proximal elements and newly formed distal elements (17).

Cellular differentiation of the homogenous, undifferentiated appearing mesenchymal cells in the limb bud results from different signals than those conveying the axis/positional information as described above. The center of the limb bud develops a condensation of cells that prefigures the skeletal elements, the chondrogenic core, which begins at the body wall and progresses distally with limb elongation. A rich vascular bed surrounds the chondrogenic core. Immediately adjacent to the vascular bed is a thick avascular zone that extends to the ectodermal sheath of the limb bud. Although the signaling mechanism has not been discovered, the ectoderm appears to control initial mesodermal differentiation by maintaining the adjacent mesenchymal cells in a flattened configuration, which prevents differentiation into chondrogenic cells. The central mesenchymal cells assume a rounded shape and form the chondrogenic core (16, 18). This process of differentiation occurs from proximal to distal. Early in the 7th week, cartilage anlage of the entire upper limb skeletal elements except the distal phalanges are present. Paddle-shaped hand plates have formed by the end of the 6th week and condensations of cells have formed identifiable digital rays in the hand. The same is true of the foot 1 week later. The cells between the digital rays are a loose mesenchyme that undergoes programmed cell death (apoptosis) to create the separated fingers and toes.

After the chondrogenic anlagen of the future skeletal structures and the vascular bed develop comes the ingrowth of nerves, which is immediately followed by the development of muscle tissue. All bones are prefigured in mesenchyme, followed by cartilage, then bone. Actual bone appears toward the end of the embryonic period, first in the clavicle, mandible, and maxilla between the 6th and 7th weeks. Ossific centers appear soon after in the humerus, then radius, then femur, then tibia, and then ulna. Just prior to birth, ossific centers appear in the calcaneus, talus, cuboid, distal femoral epiphysis, and proximal tibial epiphysis.

The mechanisms controlling the development and patterning of the vasculature are not well worked out. Vascular cells are believed to have an intrinsic capacity to form vessels and branch that is controlled by inhibitory signals extrinsic to the angiotrophic tissues. Well-developed veins develop on the postaxial border of the limb buds and persist as the fibular and saphenous veins, permitting identification of the embryonic postaxial border even in mature organisms. The early preaxial veins, the cephalic and great saphenous veins, develop secondarily. The initial arterial supply to the limb bud organizes into a single axial artery. In the arm, this artery becomes the subclavian/axillary/brachial/anterior interosseous arteries. In the leg, the axial artery comes from the umbilical artery and becomes the inferior gluteal artery/sciatic artery/the proximal popliteal and the distal peroneal artery. The femoral and tibial arteries develop secondarily.

The brachial and lumbosacral plexuses and the major peripheral nerves are present by the 5th week. They progressively invade their target tissues and by the 7th week have innervated muscles and cutaneous tissues in the adult pattern. Each dermatome represents a single dorsal root's sensory fibers. From cranial to caudal, the dermatomes of the limbs descend along the preaxial border and ascend along the postaxial border of the limb. Overlapping and variability amongst individuals make assessment of dermatomal sensation nonspecific for single nerves (Fig. 1-12).

Mesenchymal cells that are to become limb muscles migrate from the somatic layer of the lateral mesoderm during the 5th week and surround the chondrogenic core of the limb bud. They develop into dorsal and ventral groups from an undifferentiated mass and individual muscles gradually become distinct, again in a proximal/distal sequence. Most

anatomically distinct adult muscles are identifiable in the 8th week. Mesenchymal cells develop into myoblasts which then elongate, form parallel bundles, and fuse into myotubes. Muscle-specific contractile proteins, actin and myosin, are synthesized and the myotubes form sarcomeres. By the 8th week, both myotube development and innervation are sufficiently advanced for movement to begin. By 12 weeks, the cross-striations of the myofibrils are apparent in myotube cytoplasm. Most muscle cells are formed prior to birth, with the remaining cells developing in the first year of life. Enlargement of muscles results from an increase in diameter with the creation of more myofilaments and elongation with the growth of the skeleton. Ultimate muscle size results from genetic programming, exercise, and the hormonal milieu.

Development of the synovial joints commences in the 6th week of development. A condensation of cells where the joint develops is called the interzone. The interzone cells differentiate into chondrogenic cells, synovial cells, and central cells. The chondrogenic cells are adjacent to the mesenchymal cells and form the articular cartilage. The central cells form the intra-articular structures. The synovial cells differentiate into both the tough fibrous capsule and the loose, vascular synovium. Programmed cell death (apoptosis) results in the cavitation that produces the joint per se. Motion is necessary for normal joint development as the host of conditions causing arthrogryposis demonstrate as well as animal experiments that create joint anomalies by paralyzing the developing fetus.

During the embryonic period, all four limbs are similar with parallel axes. The preaxial borders are cephalad and the postaxial borders are caudad. The thumb and hallux are preaxial; the radius/tibia and ulna/fibula are homologous bones occupying the same positions in the limb bud. The longitudinal axis at this stage passes through the long finger and

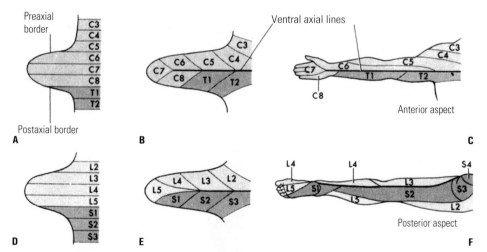

FIGURE 1-12. Development of the dermatome pattern in the limb. **A and D**: Diagram of the segmental arrangement of dermatomes in the 5th embryonic week. **B and E:** The pattern is shown 1 week later as the limb bud grows. **C and F**: The mature dermatome pattern is shown. The original ventral surface becomes posterior in the mature leg and anterior in the mature arm due to the normal rotation of the limbs. (Reproduced from Moore KI, Persaud TVN. *Before we are born. Essentials of embryology and birth defects*, 4th ed. Philadelphia, PA: W.B. Saunders Company, 1993:266, with permission.)

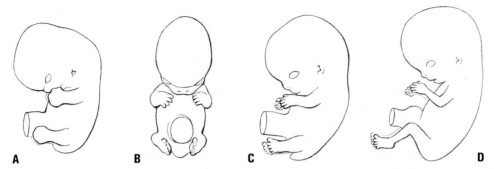

FIGURE 1-13. Normal limb rotation is depicted. **A:** 48 days, the hand-and-foot plates face each other. **B:** 51 days, elbows are bent laterally. **C:** 54 days, the soles of the feet face each other. **D:** lateral rotation of the arms and medial rotation of the legs result in caudally facing elbows and cranially facing knees. (Reproduced from Moore KI, Persaud TVN. *Before we are born. Essentials of embryology and birth defects*, 4th ed. Philadelphia, PA: W.B. Saunders Company, 1993:265, with permission.)

the second toe. During the fetal period, the upper limb rotates 90 degrees externally (laterally) and the lower limb rotates 90 degrees internally (medially). The forearm flexors come to lie medially and the forearm extensors laterally. The leg extensors lie ventrally and the leg flexors dorsally (Fig. 1-13).

Thus, by the 8th week, the task of tissue differentiation is largely completed and growth is the major task ahead.

Molecular Insights of Limb Development.

The explosion in molecular biology and molecular genetic techniques has revealed much about how individual gene's activation at specific moments in development causes the events that create complex organisms from single cells. The story is incomplete, and this section will highlight presently known or suspected molecular mechanisms that underlie development. The development of organs employs similar mechanisms of cell growth, differentiation, and patterning as occur in earlier development of the basic body plan. The mechanisms for differentiation and patterning are remarkably conserved from fruit flies to chicks to mice and to men.

The limb is one of the best studied body structures, and much information is available from the study of nonhuman animals, especially chicks, mice, and fruit flies. Much knowledge is inferential from the observations that certain genes and gene products are present at crucial moments in development. Often, many different genes and molecules are expressed simultaneously or in a closely overlapping sequence, and the complex interactions that control development are not fully worked out. The information presented in this section is based on the study of limb development in the chick except where noted. Most other information comes from gene "knockout" experiments in mice, wherein a specific gene is rendered nonfunctional and the effects on development are noted.

Limb Bud Outgrowth and Proximal–Distal Patterning.

As discussed previously, the AER is required for limb bud outgrowth (Fig. 1-14). The AER is a band of cells at the limb bud tip, lying between the dorsal and ventral limb ectoderm. Although the stimulus for AER formation, which resides in the mesoderm, is unknown, some of the molecular signals which are important

FIGURE 1-14. A diagram of the tip of the limb bud showing the AER and PZ and some of the molecules that are expressed in these tissues. (Reproduced from Thorogood P. *Embryos, genes and birth defects*. West Sussex, UK: John Wiley & Sons, Ltd, 1997:109, with permission.)

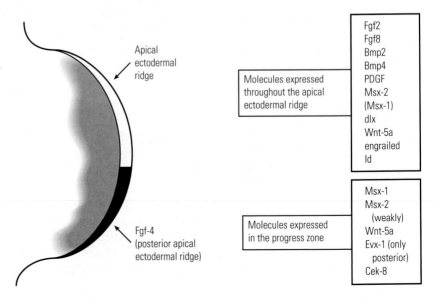

in specifying the location of the AER have been identified. Engrailed-1 (En-1) is a homeobox containing transcription factor whose expression is limited to the ventral limb ectoderm (19). Radical fringe (r-Fng) is a secreted factor that modulates signaling that is expressed only in the dorsal ectoderm (20). Radical fringe is a homolog of the *Drosophila* gene fringe, which helps specify DV boundaries in the fruit fly (21, 22).

Excision of the AER results in truncation of the limb. The earlier the excision, the more proximal is the truncation. Limb bud outgrowth can be sustained after excision of the AER by insertion of beads carrying fibroblast growth factors. Fibroblast growth factors are a group of similar proteins that affect cell proliferation, differentiation, and motility. During development, they have in common a role in mediating mesenchymal–epithelial tissue interaction. To obtain the most normal limb development, two fibroblast growth factor (FGF)-soaked beads must be placed so that the polarizing region is mimicked as well as the AER (23). The absence of the mechanical flattening of the limb bud by the AER results in a bulbous limb bud and bunching of the digits. Nevertheless, fully differentiated limb skeletal structures can be produced.

FGF-2, -4, and -8 are expressed in the AER, and each is able by itself to sustain limb bud outgrowth (probably because of the ability of different FGFs to activate the same receptors) (24–26). *In vivo* FGF-8 is found in the entire AER, while FGF-4 expression is limited to the posterior portion of the AER. FGF-10 and -8 are the critical FGFs expressed during the initiation of limb bud outgrowth. FGF-10 is expressed first in the lateral plate mesoderm at the site of the future limb bud. FGF-10 induces FGF-8 expression in ectodermal cells that will become the AER. Some experiments suggest that FGF-8 and -10 act in a positive feedback loop, that is, the expression of each supports and promotes the expression of the other. Mice in whom FGF-10 function is eliminated develop normally except for the complete absence of limbs and failure of normal pulmonary development (27).

Proximal–distal positional information is engraved upon individual cells in the PZ based on the length of time (number of mitoses?) the cell spends in the PZ as discussed earlier in this chapter (28, 29). Some experimental work suggests that transforming growth factor β (TGFβ) act in a gradient from the AER to increase cell adhesion by activating integrins—mediators of cell adhesion. Perhaps, the longer a cell is in the PZ, the more TGFβ it sees, and the more integrins are activated the greater the cell adhesion, and ultimately, the more distal is the limb positional information programmed into the cell.

Anterior–Posterior Axis Determination/Zone of Polarizing Activity (Fig. 1-15).

The ability of a small piece of tissue excised from the posterior and proximal limb bud to induce duplication of digits when grafted to an anterior position on another limb bud suggested that this region of polarizing activity synthesized a morphogen acting by a gradient to specify AP limb elements (15). If acting through a morphogenic gradient, the ZPA should give different digit patterns when transplanted to different areas of the limb bud, which it does (30). Furthermore, if a physical barrier is placed between the anterior and posterior parts of the limb bud, a normal number and order of digits is formed in the posterior portion of the limb bud, and no digits are formed anteriorly (31).

By serendipity, retinoic acid was found to cause reduplication of limbs in amputated salamanders (32). Subsequently, retinoic acid was identified in the limb bud with a high concentration posteriorly and a low concentration anteriorly. Retinoic acid on filter paper, placed anteriorly, induces mirror image digits to those formed from the natural posterior gradient (33). Nevertheless, retinoic acid is not a simple morphogen acting through a gradient. Bathing an entire limb bud in retinoic acid should eliminate the gradient, but instead mirror image reduplication occurs. Also, when retinoic acid concentration is at a minimum, the polarizing activity of the ZPA is

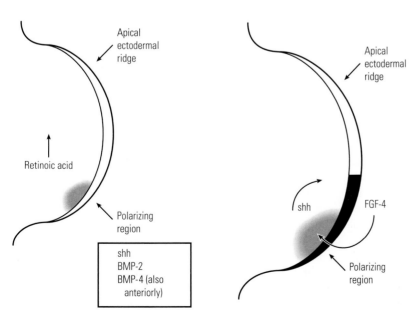

FIGURE 1-15. The two diagrams of the tip of the limb bud illustrate some of the molecules involved in the interaction between the polarizing region and mesenchyme of the PZ which specify the AP axis of the limb. On the left, the arrow shows the direction of the decreasing concentration of retinoic acid. Retinoic acid acts by regulating cell production of sonic hedgehog (shh). Sonic hedgehog, in turn, stimulates BMP-2, which is a homolog of a *Drosophila* segment polarity specifying gene. BMP-4 expression overlaps that of BMP-2 and is, therefore, probably involved in AP axis determination as well. The diagram on the right shows the feedback loop between shh and FGF-4, an ectodermally expressed protein, that appears to maintain the AER. (Reproduced from Thorogood P. *Embryos, genes and birth defects.* West Sussex, UK: John Wiley & Sons, Ltd, 1997:111, with permission.)

maximum. The action of retinoic acid is complex and includes several classes of nuclear retinoic acid receptors and retinoic-binding proteins in the cytoplasm. These different receptors and binding proteins are present in different amounts in various parts of the developing limb, suggesting a very complex role for retinoic acid. If retinoic acid synthesis is blocked, limb bud outgrowth does not occur or is severely stunted. At present, it appears that retinoic acid acts by regulating the cells that can express a protein called sonic hedgehog (34). It is likely that a Hox gene is an intermediate that is stimulated by retinoic acid and the Hox gene expression specifies the sonic hedgehog-expressing cells. If retinoic acid receptors are blocked after sonic hedgehog expression has been established, limb malformations still occur, suggesting some additional role in limb patterning, perhaps through its affect on Hox genes (34). Retinoic acid is interesting and important, not only for its role in normal development, but because it is a powerful teratogen. Various retinoids, which are derivatives of vitamin A, have been used in pharmacological doses mainly to treat dermatologic conditions such as types of acne, psoriasis, exfoliative dermatitis, and disorders of keratinization. The retinoids have been associated in animal and humans with multiple different birth defects, and the systemic usage of retinoids is not recommended for 2 years after discontinuing systemic retinoids, because of the prolonged elimination half-life of these compounds (35).

Liver and central nervous system toxicity, as well as anemia and hyperlipidemia, may occur with systemic retinoid use. These problems usually resolve with the discontinuation of retinoid therapy. Rheumatologic complications of retinoid use include hyperostosis, arthritis, myopathy, vasculitis, and a condition mimicking seronegative spondyloarthropathy (36).

The sonic hedgehog gene is expressed in the ZPA. Activation of this gene, through cell transfection, in anomalous locations in the limb bud will cause digit duplication in the same manner as transplantation of the ZPA tissue (37). It appears that sonic hedgehog stimulates the gene for BMP-2 (38). The gene activation of both occurs in the same cells with sonic hedgehog preceding that of BMP-2. The bone morphogenic proteins are members of the TGFβ superfamily and BMP-2 is, specifically, a homolog of a fruit fly gene that specifies segment polarity—making it a good candidate for an axis determining gene. BMP-2 is secreted from cells and, therefore, its action extends over a larger area than just the cells in which it is produced. BMP-4 expression overlaps that of BMP-2, and it is probably involved in AP axis specification as well. Sonic hedgehog in the mesenchyme also appears to participate in a positive feedback loop with FGF-4 in the ectoderm which may be important in maintaining the AER and supporting continued limb outgrowth and patterning (39). BMP-2 and BMP-4 also function in regulating the size and shape of long bones. Overexpression of these genes appears to cause and increase in the quantity of mesenchymal cells that differentiate into the chondrogenic precursors of the skeleton.

It appears that BMP-2 and BMP-4 are involved, as well, in the molecular mechanisms of joint formation. If noggin, a BMP inhibitor, is not present, joints do not form. Present evidence suggests that members of the Hox A and Hox D families are regulators of BMP and GDF-5 (growth and differentiation factor-5). GDF-5 (a BMP-related protein) is expressed specifically in the prospective joint region. If noggin is not present, GDF-5 is not expressed, and BMP-2 and BMP-4 are not inhibited resulting in a continuous, jointless skeleton. A balance of activating and inhibiting signals seems to be necessary for normal joint cavitation (40, 41).

Some experimental work suggests that cell–extra cellular matrix interactions are involved in the mechanism of joint cavitation. Specifically, CD44s, an isoform of a cell surface receptor that interacts with hyaluronan, is found in a single layer of cells outlying the presumptive joint cavity in rats (42). One hypothesis is that the creation of a hyaluronan-rich, but proteoglycan- and collagen II-poor, extracellular matrix results in a loss of cell adhesion and allows joint cavity formation (42).

Dorsal–Ventral Axis Patterning/Ectodermally Controlled Patterning. Experiments in which limb bud ectoderm is transplanted onto mesoderm with reversal of its DV axis reveal that digits, muscles, and tendons conform to the axis of the overlying ectoderm (13). Several genes involved in DV specification have been identified. Evidence suggests that Wnt-7A, a secreted signaling protein, confers the dorsal character to the ectoderm and it stimulates Lmx-1 (43). Lmx-1 is a homeobox gene that encodes a transcription factor that dorsalizes mesoderm. The ventral limb expresses the homeobox-containing transcription factor engrailed (En-1). En-1 appears to suppress Wnt-7A expression, thereby limiting the activity of Lmx-1 to the dorsal mesenchyme (44).

The actions of several genes are important in determining more than a single axis. For example, Wnt-7A expression is necessary for normal AP digit formation and sonic hedgehog is necessary for limb outgrowth, proximal-distally, in addition to AP patterning. The coordinated development of all three axes is believed to be regulated by interactions of several signaling genes. Wnt-7A, sonic hedgehog, and FGF-4 are promising candidates for this role (45, 46).

Both the AER and the ZPA activate HOX A and HOX D genes. HOX genes are the vertebrate homologs of the fruit fly homeogenes which specify body segment identity. HOX D genes are expressed in an overlapping, nested fashion in the AP axis of the developing limb (47) (Fig. 1-16). HOX D gene can also be activated by sonic hedgehog alone. HOX A genes have an overlapping expression along the dorsal axis, suggesting a role in specifying limb components. HOX genes have specifically been shown to affect the growth of cartilage and precartilaginous condensations (48, 49). They may be important in determining the length, segmentation, and branching of limb elements. HOX genes are not expressed strictly along AP or DV axes, and their position of expression differs in various areas of the limb. Human limb malformations caused by mutations in Hox genes have been identified and are discussed in the section on clinical correlates. Hox genes' activity overlaps and is sufficiently redundant that a mutation of a single Hox gene generally results in a minor limb anomaly.

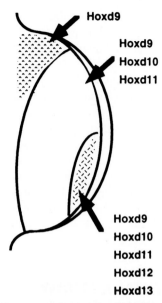

FIGURE 1-16. The pattern of expression of the Hox-d genes is shown. The overall Hox-d expression is sequential from the anterior to posterior aspect of the limb bud; however, several individual Hox-d genes have clustered expression patterns. The pattern of Hox-d gene expression can be altered by polarizing signals, implicating the Hox-d genes in limb pattern determination. (Reproduced from Thorogood P. *Embryos, genes and birth defects*. West Sussex, UK: John Wiley & Sons, Ltd, 1997:111, with permission.)

The specific signals and mechanisms that control muscle, ligament, and tendon development have not been identified. Exploration of these mechanisms may ultimately be of great clinical utility.

Clinical Significance. Limbs are extremely susceptible to anomalies, probably due to their complex developmental biology and their exposed position outside of the body wall. Nearly all teratogens and chromosomal anomalies have ill effects on limb development. A large number of single gene mutations disturb the normal development of limbs as well. Rapid advances in molecular genetics are resulting in the identification of the gene(s) responsible for many Mendelian disorders. Developmental molecular biologists are identifying genes that create limb deformities in animals, whose homologous human genes may be responsible for other specific limb defects.

Limb deficiencies occur in 3 to 8 per 1000 live births (50). One-half of limb deficiencies occur as isolated defects and the other half occur with associated malformations (50). These associated malformations may be life threatening. The most common associated malformations are musculoskeletal, head and neck, cardiovascular, gastrointestinal, and genitourinary.

As discussed previously, destruction of the AER, the PZ, or failure of expression of critical signaling molecules can result in truncation or absence of limb development. Although specific defects have not been identified in humans, there are several inherited disorders with limb deficiencies that may well have a mutation in a specific signaling molecule. These include Roberts syndrome with phocomelia; Acheiropodia (Brazil Type) with absent hands and feet; "Buttiens: distal limb deficiencies syndrome"; and CHILD syndrome with variable transverse and longitudinal deficiencies. A mouse mutant with a single digit has been found to have a mutation in the Hoxa-13 gene (51). Human split hand/split foot deformity (lobster claw deformity) is characterized by a failure of central ray formation, and at least one causative gene has been localized, but not yet identified (52).

Vascular anomalies or accidents probably cause some limb deficiencies by prohibiting limb outgrowth or by causing necrosis of already differentiated limbs (53, 54). Amniotic bands result in amputation by interfering with vascular supply (50).

Intercalary limb deficiencies, with absence of proximal structures, may result from a temporary injury to the PZ as discussed in the section *Developmental Anatomy of the Limb*.

Synostoses are failures of joint formation or separation of adjacent bone, such as the radius and ulna, with a single exception. That exception is distal syndactyly caused by amniotic bands (55). The vast majority of synostoses are inherited, but only a few of the mutated genes have been identified. Identification of the causative genes is likely in the near future and will shed much light on the mechanisms of normal joint formation and of normal bone modeling from the mass of undifferentiated mesenchymal cells that prefigure the skeletal elements. Nearly 100 disorders have synostosis as a feature. The mouse mutant limb deformity gives a flavor for the kind of causation of these deformities. Limb deformity mice are characterized by fusion of adjacent bones such as the radius and ulna. The limb bud is narrow and the AER is patchy (56). A decrease in sonic hedgehog expression and an absence of FGF-4 expression has been found (57).

Teratogens such as thalidomide and alcohol can cause synostoses in humans. Retinoic acid creates synostoses in animals when applied during chondrogenesis of developing limbs (58).

Failure of programmed cell death may be an important factor in causing some disorders with synostosis as a feature. A failure of aphotic cell death in the interdigital mesenchyme is presumed to be the cause of some syndactyly.

Excessive partitioning of skeletal elements are usually inherited conditions. Triphalangeal thumb is the most common of these disorders. Several affected families' abnormality has been linked to a region on chromosome 7, but the gene has not been identified (59, 60). Other families do not link to this locus, implying that more than one gene mutation causes triphalangeal thumb.

Polydactyly, whether isolated or associated with other anomalies, is usually an inherited condition. Given the complex interactions that occur in limb pattern specification, it is not surprising that a number of causes of this condition are being found.

Grieg cephalopolysyndactyly is an autosomal dominant disorder characterized by postaxial polysyndactyly of the hands and preaxial polysyndactyly of the feet and dysmorphic facies.

A DNA-binding transcription factor, named GLI 3, is the cause of this disorder (61). GLI 3 expression is restricted to the interdigital mesenchyme and joint-forming regions of the digits. A mouse mutant with a defect in the homologous gene has ectopic expression of both sonic hedgehog and FGF-4 in the anterior limb bud (62). Another mutation causing human polydactyly is in the Hox D cluster of homeobox genes that has been implicated in digit specification. Synpolydactyly is caused by a mutation of Hox D-13 (63). Smith-Lemli-Opitz syndrome is characterized by a variety of birth defects including postaxial polydactyly and brachydactyly. Cholesterol synthesis is defective in children with this syndrome and sonic hedgehop utilizes cholesterol as a transport molecule. It is possible that the limb anomalies in this syndrome result from a distortion of the normal sonic hedgehog gradient due to cholesterol insufficiency.

Skeletal dysplasias are a heterogeneous group of disorders whose genetic causes are rapidly being discovered, giving insight into the mechanisms of normal and disordered skeletal development (see Chapter 7).

Many single and groups of congenital anomalies that occur sporadically are believed to result from vascular disturbances in the embryo or fetus. The best developed of the vascular causation hypotheses is the subclavian artery disruption sequence, which seeks to explain Klippel-Feil syndrome, Poland anomaly, Möbius syndrome, absence of the pectoralis major, terminal transverse limb deficiencies, and Sprengel deformity. A disruption occurs when a normal embryo suffers a destructive process with cascading consequences. Since all the tissues affected in these various disorders receive their major blood supply from the subclavian artery, it is hypothesized that a defect of arterial formation or an injury to existing arteries causes these defects. The location and extent of tissue abnormality is determined by the extent, location, and timing of the interruption of normal blood supply. The observation underlying this hypothesis is that the disorders listed above often occur together in various combinations.

Possible mechanisms resulting in arterial ischemia include vessel occlusion from edema, thrombus, or embolus; extrinsic vessel compression due to surrounding tissue edema, hemorrhage, cervical ribs, aberrant muscles, amniotic bands, or uterine compression; abnormal embryologic events, including delayed or abnormal vessel formation and disruption of newly formed vessels; and environmental factors such as infection, hyperthermia, hypoxia, vasculitis, or drug effects. It is possible that some fetuses suffer ischemia due to normal embryologic events that are idiosyncratically not well tolerated, such as the rapid descent of the heart and great vessels.

The vascular accident hypothesis is attractive in explaining combinations of congenital anomalies and their, usually, sporadic occurrence. However, there are often combinations of anomalies that are difficult to relate to a single vascular event and the question of whether the anomalies resulted in, rather than being caused by, vascular abnormalities is not easily resolved.

Amniotic bands or constriction rings cause a large portion of nonhereditary congenital limb anomalies. Constriction rings are diagnosed by the occurrence of soft-tissue depression encircling a limb or injured from amputations or disruptions. Constriction rings are commonly multiple and may be broad or narrow. The depth of the ring determines whether the limb distal to the ring is normal, hypoplastic, engorged (from venous or lymphatic obstruction), or amputated (from vascular insufficiency). Syndactyly, clubfoot, and clubhand have also been associated with constriction rings.

The origin of constriction rings is uncertain. The mechanisms by which amniotic strands might form are disputed (64–67). One hypothesis holds that amnion adheres to areas of preoccurring hemorrhage and by itself is not pathogenic (68). Nonetheless, the syndrome is common, affecting 1 in 5000 to 15,000 births. Recurrence risks of this syndrome are low (50).

DEVELOPMENTAL ANATOMY OF THE VERTEBRAL COLUMN

The vertebral column, be it cartilage or bone, defines the species of the subphylum of "vertebrates." Evolution of a vertebral column to replace the notochord allows a strength, flexibility, and protection to the neural tube that conferred many advantages to vertebrate species. Minor and even major anomalies of the vertebral column are compatible with life and good function. Vertebral column development depends on the appropriate prior development of the notochord and somites.

While the mesoderm is forming during gastrulation, a mass of ectodermal cells proliferates and forms the archenteron—a tube that migrates cranially in the midline between the ectoderm and the endoderm. The floor of the archenteron forms the notochordal plate. For a short time, there is a direct connection between the primitive gut and the amniotic cavity since the endodermal floor is not continuous and the blastopore (the opening of the archenteron) communicates with the amniotic cavity. This connection is obliterated by the end of the 3rd week, and remnants of this connection are presumed to be responsible for diastematomyelia.

The notochord arises from cells in the primitive streak which come from the ingress of cells from the epiblast during gastrulation and, later, from the caudal eminence. This ingress of cells forms the endoderm as well as the notochord and the paraxial mesoderm (segmental plate). The notochord develops from cranial to caudal by adding cells as it develops. It is initially a solid rod in which a small central canal develops. The notochord induces the formation of the neural groove, which gradually closes to form a tube with a central canal. By the 23rd day, the neural groove is closed except at its most cranial and caudal ends. These openings are termed the neuropores, which close by the end of the 4th week. Closure of the neural tube progresses from cranially to caudally. Failure to close properly is hypothesized to be the cause of NTDs such as myelomeningocele.

The somites also develop from cells that are internalized through the primitive streak. These cells form the paraxial mesoderm that will become the somites and ultimately become the vertebrae. Pre-somitic cells cluster by increased adhesion into distinct balls of epithelial cells surrounding mesenchymal cell giving the embryo its first segmental organization. Positional information is programmed into the somites by the time they are morphologically distinct. For example, a thoracic somite will still form a rib when transplanted into the cervical region. The positional information is imparted during gastrulation (69, 70). Somites do not depend on interaction with the neural tube or notochord for development and fated cells will develop into somites *in vitro*.

Four occipital, 8 cervical, 12 thoracic, 5 lumbar, 5 sacral, and 4 or 5 coccygeal pairs of somites will develop. The first somites are evident at three and a half weeks and 30 pairs are present at four and a half weeks. Not all of the somites are visible simultaneously. Somites develop a complex internal organization. The somite begins as a ball of pseudostratified epithelium surrounding a central cavity, the somitocoel. The central cavity becomes filled with mesenchymal cells. Some of these cells, along with cells in the medioventral portion of the somite become the sclerotome. Cell from the sclerotome will form the vertebral bodies and vertebral arches and emerge without the epithelial portion of the sclerotome to surround the neural tube. In addition to contributing to the sclerotome, cells from the central cavity migrate to become the intervertebral discs and contribute to rib formation. The dorsolateral wall of the somite is called the dermomyotome. It separates into the dermatome laterally and the myotome lying between the dermatome and the sclerotome. The dermatome gives rise to the dermis of the skin and the myotome supplies cells for muscle, tendons, and fascia (Fig. 1-17).

The sclerotomal cells from the paired somites migrate medially, meeting around the notochord and separating it from the dorsal neural tube and the ventral gut. The continuous perichordal sheath is distinct from the more lateral, segmented sclerotomes. Between the adjacent somites lie the transverse intersegmental arteries. The segmental spinal nerves originally exit at the midportion of the somitic sclerotomal mass. Resegmentation of the sclerotomic tissues occurs at four and a half weeks (Fig. 1-18). This process of resegmentation occurs by variable rate mitosis, the results in each somitic sclerotome's thinning cranially and condensing caudally. The transverse intersegmental arteries and spinal nerves traverse the cellularly loose cranial portion of the sclerotome. The dense caudal portion of each sclerotome unites with the cranial, less condensed part of the next sclerotome to form the primordium of the vertebrae. Thus, the skeletal portions of the somites no longer correspond to the original segmentation. The segmental spinal nerves that originally were in midsomite now lie at the level of the disc. The intersegmental arteries located between somites come to lie at the midportion of the vertebral bodies and the myotomes bridge the vertebrae. The densely cellular, caudal portion of the sclerotome gives rise to the vertebral arch. The initially continuous notochordal sheath segments into loosely cellular cranial and densely cellular caudal portions. The cranial portion becomes the vertebral centrum and the dense caudal portion becomes the intervertebral disc. The vertebral centrum surrounds the notochord and forms the vertebral body. Notochordal cells in the vertebral centra degenerate, although some remnants of the notochord may remain. Rests of notochordal cells persisting in the sacral or cervical areas may give rise to chordomas in later life. The neural arches develop from ventral to dorsal, enclosing the neural tube, and unite in the fetal period. The spinal nerves and the dorsal root ganglia arise at the level of the somite and enter the myotome at the beginning of the 6th week. The presence of ganglia is necessary for normal neural arch segmentation. Although somites form from cranial to caudal, resegmentation progresses from midspine cranially and caudally.

Neural crest cells (a specialized region of neuroectoderm) accumulate just before closure of the neural tube cranially and are situated between the neural tube and somites. These cells become the peripheral nervous system sensory cells and nerve fibers as well as the Schwann cells and melanocytes. Peripheral nerve afferents and preganglionic fibers of the autonomic nervous system develop from the neural tube, as do the brain and spinal cord. At each cervical, thoracic and lumbar somite, a corresponding ganglion develops.

Molecular Insights of Vertebral Column Development.
Hox genes are expressed in an overlapping fashion in the developing spinal column, and evidence suggests that they specify individual vertebrae's morphology (71). Transgenic mice with out-of-sequence activation of certain Hox genes can be created that transform the atlas into a cervical vertebra with a body, and lumbar vertebrae can become like thoracic vertebrae with rib formation (72, 73). Conversely, Hox gene inactivation can transform the axis into and atlas-appearing vertebra (74). Overlapping, redundant expression of Hox genes occurs and inactivation of more than one adjacent Hox gene has been found necessary to alter vertebral morphology in some regions of the vertebral column (75). Retinoic acid application can alter the normal expression patterns of Hox genes, and it can create varying morphologic abnormalities depending on the timing and location of its application. A particular retinoic acid receptor (the gamma receptor) is expressed only in prebone tissue, and its inactivation causes transformation of the axis to an atlas and c7 to c6 (76).

PAX genes are a family of genes containing a DNA-binding domain and are expressed in the sclerotome at high levels during sclerotome condensation. Some evidence suggests that a defect in specific PAX genes or genes they modify may result in failure of formation of vertebral elements (77). The homeobox gene MSX2 is necessary for spinous process development in mice (78). Clearly, the interactions of genes and tissues involved in vertebral column formation are complex.

Clinical Significance.
The vertebral column represents the central, characteristic skeletal structure of vertebrates, and

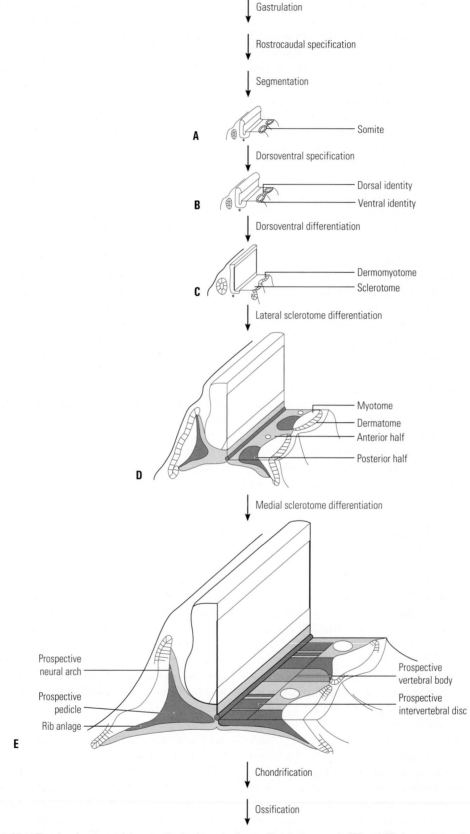

FIGURE 1-17. The development of the vertebral column is shown. The dark areas in (**D**) and (**E**) demonstrate the portion of the sclerotome that develops into the neural arch, the vertebral body, rib anlage, and the intervertebral disc. (Reproduced from Thorogood P. *Embryos, genes and birth defects.* West Sussex, UK: John Wiley & Sons, Ltd, 1997:282, with permission.)

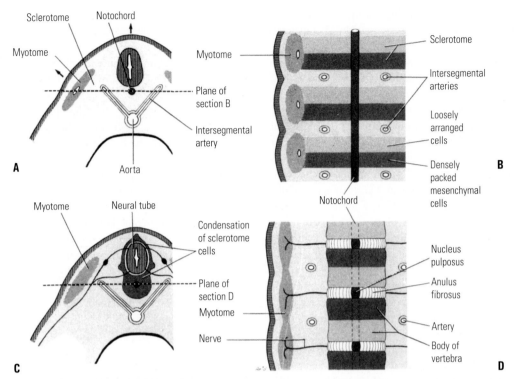

FIGURE 1-18. **A:** Transverse section through a 4-week embryo. The *top arrow* shows the direction of the growth of the neural tube and the *side arrow* shows the dorsolateral growth of the somite remnant. **B:** Coronal section of the same stage embryo showing the condensation of sclerotomal cells around the notochord with loosely packed cells cranially and densely packed cells caudally. **C:** A transverse section through a 5-week embryo depicting the condensation of sclerotome cells around the notochord and neural tube. **D:** Coronal section illustrating the formation of the vertebral body from cranial and caudal halves of adjacent sclerotomes resulting in the segmental arteries' crossing the bodies of the vertebrae and the spinal nerves' lying between the vertebrae. (Reproduced from Moore KI, Persaud TVN. *Before we are born. Essentials of embryology and birth defects*, 4th ed. Philadelphia, PA: W.B. Saunders Company, 1993:257, with permission.)

it is remarkable how even severe vertebral abnormalities are so well tolerated by the organisms. Since vertebral column development has been highly conserved during evolution, most if not all the vertebral abnormalities seen in vertebrates can also be found in humans. In fact, mouse genetics had led to the identification of probably all types of vertebral abnormalities (79, 80).

Defects at different stages of embryo development will result in different vertebral malformations. In general, the earlier the disruption in the developmental process, the more severe will be the phenotype. The developmental processes that can be affected include mesoderm formation during gastrulation, axial patterning, notochordal mesoderm induction, somite formation, sclerotome condensation, neural tube closure, and axial identity specification. While disorders in pattern formation result in specific prevertebral phenotypes, general disorders of mesenchyme condensation, cartilage, or bone formation affect composition and therefore morphology of the skeleton. Misspecifications of vertebral identity, called homeotic transformations, are characterized by the presence of all vertebral components but with shape characteristic of usually the adjacent vertebra.

Disruption of the allocation of the mesodermal cells during gastrulation leads to a block in the whole vertebral column formation. Since gastrulation also generates the other two germ layers, the embryo will have multiple congenital abnormalities and will not survive (81). Defects during sclerotome formation are compatible with life and typically results in segmental vertebral agenesis. Since sclerotome formation depends on the inductive activity of the notochord, it is mainly notochord mutants that are found within this category. In the affected region, somite ventralization is hindered, and the corresponding vertebrae appear to be deleted.

While disruptions of gastrulation and sclerotome formation lead to the absence, truncation, or interruption of vertebral column formation, disorders of somatogenesis are compatible with vertebral development. However, multiple vertebral components can be lacking or fused. Variations on number, shape, and position of vertebrae are common developmental anomalies. Most columns have 24 segments including 7 cervical, 12 thoracic, and 5 lumbar vertebrae. However, columns with 23 or 25 elements are commonly seen, and they are most likely related with differences in the number of elements of the lumbar spine. This number difference may be due to the last lumbar vertebra being incorporated into the sacrum (sacralization) or the first sacral vertebra being freed (lumbarization).

Developmental anomalies that affect vertebral shape are varied. The most common conditions are spina bifida, hemivertebra and wedge vertebrae, and vertebral bars. Spina bifida occulta is a failure in the completion of the neural arch but without neurological compromise. Failure of the neural arch to fuse in the cervical spine and sometimes in the upper thoracic spine is seen shortly after birth, but spina bifida is most commonly seen at the level of the lumbosacral spine. This is a normal finding in children at 2 years of age, in 50% at 10 years, and in approximately 20% of adults. NTD can be subdivided into four subgroups. First, a cyst that involves only the meninges but not the neural elements is a meningocele. Second, a myelomeningocele included the abnormal elements as part of the sac. Third, a lipomeningocele is a deformity in which there is a sac containing a lipoma that is intimately involved with the sacral nerves. Finally, rachischisis is a complete absence of skin and sac, with exposure of the muscle and dysplastic spinal cord.

Closure of the neural tube progresses from cranially to caudally. Failure to close properly is widely believed to be the cause of most causes of myelomeningocele (82). This hypothesis is supported by observations of early fetuses with myelomeningocele and is consistent with animal models of NTDs (83). The competing hypothesis, championed by Gardner, suggests that overdistension and rupture of a closed neural tube causes NTDs (84, 85). Myelomeningocele has multiple causes resulting in a common phenotype. An inherited predisposition to NTDs appears to be present in some cases based on an increased incidence of NTDs in some families and a variation in prevalence in different ethnic groups (86). Furthermore, a mouse model of NTD has been shown to result from a mutation in the gene Pax-3. Pax-3 is a homeobox gene that has been shown to be involved in the fusion of the dorsal neural tube as well as in neutral crest cell migration and dermomyotome development (83). Environmental factors are responsible for some proportion of NTDs and multiple teratogens have been identified that interfere with neurulation. Examples include vinblastine, which disrupts actin microfilaments, and calcium channel blockers, which interfere with microfilament contraction (87, 88). Retinoic acid, hydroxyurea, and mitomycin C interfere with the timing of neuroepithelial development and cause NTDs in animal models (89). Folate supplements during pregnancy decrease the risk of NTD in subsequent children when a prior child has been affected, as well as decreasing the incidence of NTDs in pregnancies without a prior history of NTD (82). The mechanism of folate's effect on NTDs is unknown. The interaction of genes and environment that act to cause myelomeningoceles as well as the molecular pathology is under active investigation (83).

Defects of vertebrae formation or segmentation include hemivertebra and vertebral bars. Hemivertebra appears as wedge, usually situated laterally between two other vertebrae.

As a consequence, a lateral curvature of the spine develops. Vertebral bars are due to localized defects in segmentation and are observed most frequently in the posterolateral side of the column, resulting in the absence of growth in that side. The outcome is a progressive lordosis and scoliosis. When located anteriorly, vertebral bars lead to progressive kyphosis. Klippel-Feil sequence is regarded as a defect in cervical segmentation. Clinically, there is a short, broad neck; low hairline; limited range of motion of the head and neck; and multiple vertebral abnormalities.

Finally, other congenital abnormalities may be observed. Diastematomyelia is a longitudinal splitting of the spinal cord associated with a bony or fibrocartilaginous spicule or septum arising from the vertebral body which is believed to result from remnants of the early connection between the primitive gut and the amniotic cavity. It is commonly associated with skin changes and abnormalities of the lower extremities. A chordoma is a neoplasm that arises from notochordal rests and is found especially in the sacrococcygeal region. Sacrococcygeal teratoma is a neoplasm composed of multiple embryonic tissues that can undergo malignant transformation.

DEVELOPMENTAL ANATOMY OF THE NERVOUS SYSTEM

The neural tube is pivotal in development and has been discussed on pages 16 to 20. The neural tube becomes the central nervous system (the brain and spinal cord) and the neural crest develops into most of the peripheral nervous system. The spinal cord develops from the portion of the neural tube that is caudal to the four occipital somites. The neural tube forms from the folding of the neural groove and begins at the brain/spinal cord junction. As the neural groove fuses, so does the neural fold. Neural crest cells begin their migration from neural fold tissue just after neural tube closure occurs in the spinal regions. Neural crest cells migrate either beneath the surface ectoderm or between the neural tube and the somite. Migration occurs through extracellular matrix along relatively cell-free paths. Neural crest cells from the pia matter, the spinal ganglia, and the sympathetic trunks and ganglia.

As the neural tube closes, the dorsal region, called the alar laminae is separated from the ventral basal laminae by a shallow groove—the sulcus limitans. A thin bridge of tissue persists to connect the two halves of the alar and basal laminae named the roof and floor plates. The alar plate develops into the sensory pathways (dorsal columns) and the basal plate develops into the motor pathways (ventral horns). The notochord is necessary for floor plate induction and the floor plate appears to specify the DV organization of cell types in the developing spinal cord.

The ventral horn neurons develop axons which form the ventral roots. The dorsal root ganglia develop from neural crest cells. The ganglion cells' axons form central processes which become the dorsal roots and peripheral processes that end in sensory organelles.

Spinal cord development proceeds in a rostral–caudal direction, and motor neurons develop neural capabilities before sensory nerves. Autonomic nerve function is established last (42). Movement is visible by ultrasound five and a half weeks postfertilization. The spinal cord extends the entire length of the vertebral column during the embryonic period. During fetal development, the vertebral column grows more rapidly than the spinal cord. Coupled with some loss of caudal spinal cord tissue, the caudal tip of the spinal cord ends at the 2nd or 3rd lumbar vertebra in newborns. In the adult, the spinal cord terminates at the inferior portion of the first lumbar vertebra. Thus, the lumbar and sacral nerve roots have an oblique course below the conus medullaris before their exit from their intervertebral foraminae resulting in the formation of the cauda equina (Fig. 1-19).

Myelination of peripheral nerve axons begins in the fetal period and continues during the first year after birth. Schwann cells myelinate peripheral nerves, whereas oligodendrocytes myelinate the axons within the spinal cord.

Molecular Insights of Nervous System Development.

The molecular basis of nervous system formation is not well understood, but probably will be in the next decade. There is an intimate relationship between the notochord and the neural plate and tube that is necessary for differentiation of the floor plate or the spinal cord and for specification of ventral structures in the developing spinal cord. Hepatocyte nuclear factor-3 appears to regulate sonic hedgehog (an important axis specifying gene in the limb as well), which can induce ventral structures (90). PAX genes have dorsoventrally restricted expression in the developing spinal cord. Dorsal structures can develop without the notochord, but specific molecules may be necessary for complete dorsal specification. For example, dorsalin-1, a TGFβ family member, can induce neural crest

cell differentiation (91). The transcription factor genes Pax-3 and Gli-3 are necessary for neural tube closure (92). The large number of NTDs suggests that neural tube closure does not have a large redundancy in developmental regulation.

Clinical Significance. Multiple anomalies of the brain occur and have orthopaedic implications due to disordered control of limbs, but are not discussed here. Failure of closure of the caudal neuropore may result in myelomeningocele. Other evidence suggests that increased CSF pressure causes rupture of an already close neural tube at its weakest point, where it closed last. At least 10 genes have been identified in mutant animals that result in NTDs. Multiple teratogens, such as valproic acid and vitamin A, or exposure to hypothermia, can cause NTDs. Although the mechanism is unknown, perifertilization folic acid decreases the incidence of NTDs in humans.

Myeloschisis is a rare condition in which the neural groove fails to form a neural tube. Myelomeningocele has uncovered neural tissue that has herniated into the dysraphic area of the spine. Meningocele, in which the neural elements remain in their normal location, is probably a primary defect of the vertebral column development, rather than a primary neural defect. Ten percent of people have spina bifida occulta in which the vertebral neural arch fails to fully develop and fuse, usually at L5 or S1.

BONE FORMATION AND GROWTH

An examination of the human skeleton reveals the numerous sizes and shapes of bones, which have precise functions of locomotion, protection of vital organs, are major sites for hematopoiesis, and participate in calcium hemostasis and store of phosphate,

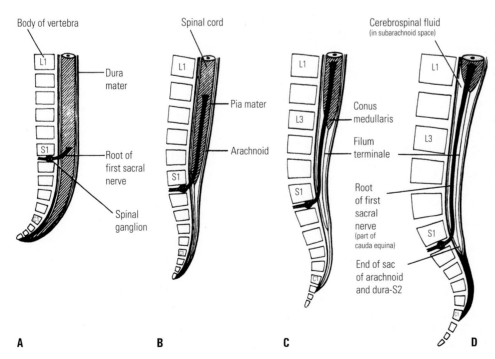

FIGURE 1-19. Illustration of the position of the spinal cord and meninges in relation to the vertebral column at **(A)** 8 weeks, **(B)** 24 weeks, **(C)** birth, and **(D)** adult. (Reproduced from Moore KI, Persaud TVN. *Before we are born. Essentials of embryology and birth defects*, 4th ed. Philadelphia, PA: W.B. Saunders Company, 1993:283, with permission.)

A   B   C   D

magnesium, potassium, and bicarbonate. Interestingly, the molecular composition of the bone is remarkably constant. Regardless of the animal species or the bone considered, bone is always a two-phase composite substance made up of two very different materials. The two major components of bone are the organic matrix, or osteoid, and the inorganic matrix. Various calcium salts, primarily hydroxyapatite, are deposited in crystals within and between the matrix. These inorganic crystals give bone its rigidity, hardness, and strength to compression.

Connective tissue, cartilage, and bone all differentiate from that type of diffuse mesoderm known as mesenchyme. Mesenchyme arises primarily from the primitive streak and secondarily from mesodermal segments and the lateral somatic and splanchnic mesodermal layers (Fig. 1-9). In early embryos, the mesenchyme acts as a unspecialized "packing" material but soon differentiates into various tissues and organs.

There are two mechanisms of bone formation (osteogenesis), and both involve the transformation of a preexisting connective tissue into bone tissue. The transformation of fibrous primitive connective tissue into bone is called intramembranous ossification. The replacement of cartilage by bone is called endochondral ossification. Except the clavicle and the flat bones of the skull, all bones of the appendicular and axial skeleton form by endochondral ossification.

Intramembranous Ossification.
Intramembranous ossification occurs by mesenchymal cells derived from the neural crest that interact with the extracellular matrix secreted by the epithelia cells arising from the head. If the mesenchymal cells do not contact this matrix, no bone will be developed (93, 94). The mechanism responsible for the conversion of mesenchymal cells to bone is still unknown. However, BMPs may play a significant role in this process.

During intramembranous ossification, the mesenchymal cells proliferate and condense into packed nodules. Some of these cells differentiate into capillaries and others change their shape to become osteoblasts. These cells are capable of secreting osteoid, the organic extracellular matrix that subsequently will become mineralized. High levels of alkaline phosphatase and the appearance of matrix vesicles mark the commencement of ossification. The cells will eventually be surrounded by calcified matrix and become osteocytes.

Endochondral Ossification.
By far, the most common mechanism of ossification is cartilaginous (or endochondral). The process begins with the formation of a cartilage precursor or template. Mesenchyme cells condense and proliferate but instead of turning into osteoblasts, like in intramembranous ossification, they become chondroblasts. These cells will then secrete the cartilage extracellular matrix. Soon after the cartilaginous model is formed, the cells in the center become hypertrophic and secrete a matrix that will subsequently be invaded by capillaries. As this matrix is degraded and the chondrocytes die, osteoblasts carried by the blood vessels begin to secrete bone matrix. Eventually, all cartilage is replaced by bone (Fig. 1-20). This process appears to be dependent on the mineralization of the extracellular matrix. Interestingly, a special, condensed mesenchymal tissue, the perichondrium, surrounds the cartilage model. This tissue is essentially the same as that surrounding the intramembranous centers of ossification, but in the perichondrium the osteoprogenitor cells remain dormant for a time, while the cartilage model is enlarged by the chondrocytes.

Ossification begins at the primary center, within the shaft, and proceeds outward from the medullary cavity and inward from the periosteum in a repetitive sequence. As the cartilage model is replaced by bone, extensive remodeling occurs.

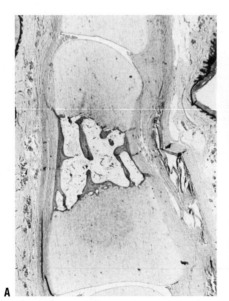 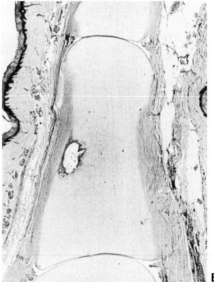

FIGURE 1-20. **A:** Formation of the primary ossification center of a phalanx. Note the central location with bone and bone marrow formation. **B:** Delayed ossification center formation in a case of digital duplication. (Reproduced from Ogden JA. *Pediatric orthopaedics*, 3rd ed. Philadelphia, PA: JB Lippincott, 1990:2, with permission.)

First, the medullary cavity is created and enlarged by resorption of the bony struts and spicules. Second, the developing bone continues to enlarge by both interstitial and appositional growth. The same repetitive sequence of events occurs in the epiphyseal centers of ossification. Once the shaft and epiphyses are ossified, leaving the cartilage physeal plates between them, each skeletal segment increases in size until maturity. The initiation of the endochondral ossification process, as well as the highly ordered progression of the chondrocytes through the growth plate, must be under strict spatial and temporal control. In view of the complexity of the process, it is remarkable that the human bones in the limbs can growth for some 15 years independently of each other, and yet eventually match to an accuracy of 0.2%.

Growth Plate Structure and Development. Growth of the different parts of the body is not uniform, and different bones grow at different rates. Patterning of the embryo occurs while the organs are still very small. For example, the limb has its basic structure established when its size is about 1 cm long. Yet, it will grow to be hundred times longer. How is this growth controlled? Most of the evidence suggests that the cartilaginous elements in the limb have their own individual growth program. These growth programs are specified when the elements are initially patterned and involve both cell proliferation and extracellular matrix secretion. An understanding of the processes of bone formation, growth, and remodeling is fundamental in pediatric orthopaedics.

The process of endochondral ossification, which occurs in all growth plates, is unique to the immature skeleton. Once the growth plates have been formed, longitudinal growth of the bones occurs by appositional growth of cells and extracellular matrix from within the growth plate, and new bone formation on the metaphyseal side. The rate of increase in the length of a long bone is equal to the rate of new cell production per column multiplied by the mean height of the enlarged cell. The rate of proliferation depends on the time the cells take to complete a cell cycle in the proliferative zone, and the size of this zone. Generally, the greater the number of chondrocytes and the higher the plate, the faster the growth rate of the bone (Fig. 1-21). In addition, total longitudinal growth for the life span of the growth plate depends on the total number of

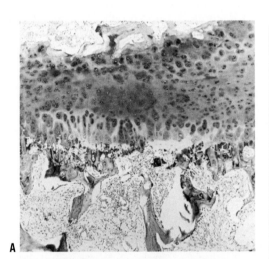

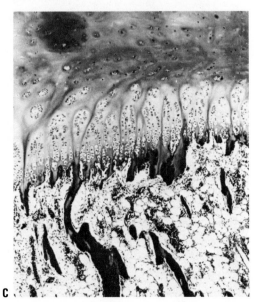

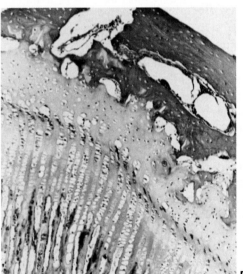

FIGURE 1-21. Variations on growth plate morphology. **A:** Limited column formation in a slow-growing physis. **B:** Elongated cell columns in a fast-growing physis (distal femur). **C:** Some physis form cluster-like groups divided by longitudinal cartilaginous columns. (Reproduced from Ogden JA. *Pediatric orthopaedics*, 3rd ed. Philadelphia, PA: JB Lippincott, 1990:17, with permission.)

progenitor cell divisions and the number of divisions of each daughter cell. The number of cell divisions is genetically determined, but the rate is influenced by hormonal and metabolic factors.

The function of the growth plate is related to its structure as an organ, which depends on the integrated function of three distinct components. The first component is the physeal cartilage, which is divided into three histologically recognizable zones: resting, proliferative, and hypertrophic. The second component is the metaphysis, which is the region where calcified cartilage is replaced by bone. The third component is the circumferential structures known as the perichondrial ring of LaCroix and the groove of Ranvier. Each of these components has its unique cellular architecture and extracellular matrix biochemistry; their integrated functioning results in longitudinal and latitudinal bone growth. Interestingly, although cartilage lacks blood vessels, to a large extent, the metabolic activity of each zone depends on the blood supply system around the physis.

PHYSEAL CARTILAGE

Resting Zone.
The resting zone, located just below the secondary center of ossification, contains chondrocytes that are widely dispersed in an abundant matrix. The cells contain abundant endoplasmic reticulum characteristic of protein synthesis, but low intracellular and ionized calcium content. The function of these cells is not well understood, but data indicate that the resting zone is relatively inactive in cell or matrix turnover, although it may be a source for the continuous supply of chondrocytes to the proliferative zone.

Proliferative Zone.
The proliferative zone is characterized histologically by longitudinal columns of flattened cells parallel to the long axis of the bone. The cells contain glycogen stores and significant amounts of endoplasmic reticulum. The total calcium is similar to the resting zone, but the ionized calcium is significantly greater. The oxygen tension is high in this zone (57 mm Hg) and together with the presence of glycogen suggests an aerobic metabolism. Of the three zones, it has the highest rate of extracellular matrix synthesis and turnover (95–97).

Hypertrophic Zone.
The hypertrophic zone is characterized by enlargement of the cells to five to seven times their original size in the proliferative zone. Electron microscopy studies suggest that these cells maintain cellular morphology compatible with active metabolic activity (98). Biochemical studies have demonstrated that mitochondria of the hypertrophic chondrocyte is used primarily to accumulate and release calcium rather than for ATP production. In addition, the cells have the highest concentration of glycolytic enzymes and synthesize alkaline phosphatase, neutral proteases, and type X collagen, thereby participating in mineralization (99). Because the growth plate is radially constrained by the ring of LaCroix, its volume changes are expressed primarily in the longitudinal

direction. In the last part of this zone, there is a provisional calcification of the cartilage.

Metaphysis.
The metaphysis functions in the removal of the mineralized cartilage of the hypertrophic zone and in the formation of the primary spongiosa. Bone formation begins with the invasion of the hypertrophic lacunae by vascular loops, bringing with them osteoblasts that begin the synthesis of bone (100). The osteoblasts progressively lay down bone on the cartilage template. Subsequently, the initial woven bone and cartilage of the primary trabeculae are resorbed by osteoblasts and replaced by lamellar bone to produce the secondary spongiosa.

Perichondrial Ring of LaCroix and Groove of Ranvier.
Surrounding the periphery of the physis there are a wedge-shape structure, the groove of Ranvier, and a ring of fibrous tissue, the ring of LaCroix. The groove of Ranvier are active proliferative cells that contribute to the increase in diameter, or latitudinal, of the growth plate. The ring of LaCroix contains a thin extension of the metaphyseal cortex and fibrous portion of the groove of Ranvier and periosteum that provides it with a peripheral supporting girdle around the growth plate (101, 102) (Fig. 1-22).

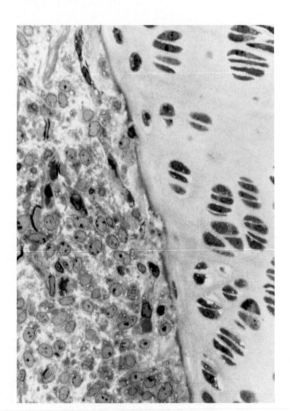

FIGURE 1-22. Photomicrograph of the zone of Ranvier demonstrating the demarcation between the cells of the growth plate and the mesenchymal cells of the zone of Ranvier. (Reproduced from Ogden JA. *Pediatric orthopaedics*, 3rd ed. Philadelphia, PA: JB Lippincott, 1990:19, with permission.)

Vascular Anatomy of the Growth Plate   There are three major vascular systems that supply the growth plate. The epiphyseal arteries enter the secondary ossification center and the terminal branches pass through the resting zone and terminate at the uppermost cell of the proliferative cells. The nutrient artery of the diaphysis supplies the extensive capillary loop network at the junction of the metaphysis and growth plate. Finally, the perichondral arteries supply the ring of LaCroix and the groove of Ranvier. Capillaries from this system communicate with the epiphyseal and metaphyseal systems in addition to the vessels of the joint capsule (100).

Bone grows in thickness in addition to length. Because the metaphysis is larger than the diaphysis, some of it must to be trimmed during the process of remodeling. This process is called funnelization. In the area termed the cutback zone, osteoclasts resorb the peripheral bone of the metaphysis. In this way, the metaphysis gradually narrows to the width of the diaphysis. The epiphysis also grows in circumference by a process called hemispheration, which is a process similar to the growth plate. Thus, the bone acquires its final shape by a combination of intramembranous ossification at the diaphyseal level and endochondral ossification at the epiphysis and growth plate with process of elongation, funnelization, hemispherization, and cylinderization (Fig. 1-23).

GROWTH IN PEDIATRIC ORTHOPAEDICS

Pediatric orthopaedics is inherently connected with growth, whether through disorders caused by abnormal growth from Blount's disease or skeletal dysplasias or from growth's effects

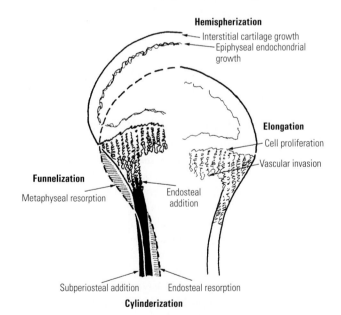

FIGURE 1-23. Diagrammatic representation of the remodeling process of bone during growth. Bone resorption and deposition result in longitudinal growth and shape changes of the epiphysis, metaphysis, and diaphysis. (Adapted from Ham AW. Some histophysiologic problems peculiar to calcified tissue. *J Bone Joint Surg (Am)* 1952;34:701.)

such as fracture remodeling. Other disorders are innately tied to the adolescent growth spurt such as slipped capital femoral epiphysis or scoliosis. Changes in skeletal mass and bone density during growth can affect the strength of skeletal fixation and determine fixation possibilities. The purpose of this section is to provide a framework of understanding growth and developmental effects on the musculoskeletal system.

Although overstating the case, it is helpful to consider the physis as the primary generator of musculoskeletal growth. Muscles, ligaments, nerves, and blood vessels all have their own mechanisms of longitudinal growth, but each grows in response to the skeletal stimulus resulting in well-coordinated growth of the limb, chest, and spine. Although, occasionally, skeletal growth can is inhibited by abnormalities of these other structures like muscle contractures or nerve palsies, more often abnormal growth is intrinsic to the physis or its affecters.

An Overview of Growth and Maturity.   Normal growth is a marvelously coordinated affair from the single-celled zygote to a normal adult. It follows predictable multidimensional patterns with increases in height and weight, development of reproductive and secondary sexual characteristics, changes in muscle and fat mass and distribution, and changes in bony structure. Growth is very rapid during the initial years of life, and then gradually slows until reaching a steady velocity of about 5 cm/year at the age of 4 to 5 with a small mid-childhood growth spurt around age 8. This low, constant rate continues until puberty, when there is a very rapid acceleration of growth followed by a decrease in the rate of growth until maturity. The adolescent growth spurt typically begins around age 10 for girls, age 12 for boys, and spans about 4 years, beginning about 2 years before and extending 2 years beyond the growth peak (see Fig. 1-24). In children with similar environments, normal pubertal timing can vary as much as 4 years (103).

Hormonal Mechanisms of Growth.   Humans have two basic pubertal stages, adrenarche and gonadarche, which are regulated by separate but related systems, the hypothalamic–pituitary–gonadal axis (HPG), and the hypothalamic–pituitary–adrenal axis (HPA) (104). Both growth hormone (GH) and the sex steroids, particularly estrogen, are necessary for the normal adolescent growth spurt in both boys and girls. Between ages 6 and 8 years in both boys and girls, the HPA becomes active in an event called adrenarche. In adrenarche, the hypothalamus releases corticotropin-releasing hormone (CRH) which in turn stimulates ACTH production from the pituitary. This release stimulates the adrenal cortex to produce the adrenal androgens androstenedione, dehydroepiandrostenedione (DHEA), and dihydroepiandrostenedione sulfate (DHEA-S), which in turn causes pubarche, the initial development of pubic and axillary hair and early sebaceous gland secretions causing acne, and body odor though not as substantial as during puberty. This early hair is usually fine and light unlike the

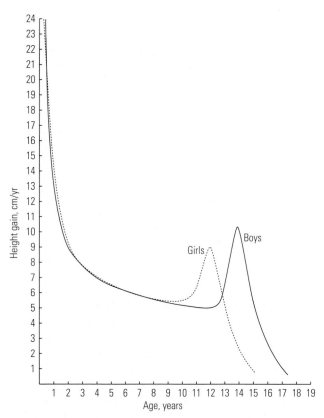

FIGURE 1-24. Typical individual growth velocities in boys and girls over time. (Adapted from Tanner JM, Whitehouse RH, Takaishi M. *Arch Dis Child* 1966;41(220):613–635.)

courser and darker hair occurring later in puberty. While the onset mechanism of adrenal cortical maturation remains unknown, abnormal adrenarche timing does not seem to influence normal puberty (105, 106) but do forewarn of the growth spurt. The major events of the growth spurt are mediated by the hypothalamic-pituitary-adrenal axis (HPA). GnRH (gonadotropin-releasing hormone which is the same as LHRH) release is suppressed between infancy and puberty. The mechanism of GnRH suppression and its subsequent release are only partially understood but include both environmental and CNS-mediated mechanisms. Environmental factors include various diseases or high levels of exercise affecting the amount of body fat and subsequent leptin levels, and possibly some environmental chemical causing either premature or delayed puberty (106–111). The CNS-mediated events seem to be linked to chromosome 2 (112). With GnRH resuming its pulsatile release at the beginning of the adolescent growth spurt[4], estrogen secretion is stimulated from the ovaries in girls and from the testicular testosterone's peripheral aromatization in boys. Estrogen is the critical stimulus of the physis causing the linear growth spurt (110, 113–117). The estrogen

increase causes initial breast development in girls and rapid foot growth in both boys and girls, the first physical signs of the adolescent growth spurt. The initial estrogen increase stimulates further GH release (110, 118–120), although, there is some experimental evidence from rhesus monkeys, one of the few animals having an adolescent growth spurt like humans, that the GH increase can start without sex steroid initiation (120). GH acts both directly and indirectly through production of insulin-like growth factor-1 (IGF-1) to stimulate physeal growth. The growth rate then peaks about 2 years later and then slows to cessation after another 2 years. The two standard deviation range for North American girls' growth peak is 9.7 to 13.3 years (121). Estrogen appears to be the primary factor causing physeal closure at the end of skeletal growth in both males and females. Lower doses of estrogen during early puberty stimulate growth, whereas higher doses in later puberty lead to growth cessation.

The Growth Spurt and the Peak Height Velocity.

The maximum growth rate is called the peak height velocity (PHV). Chronological timing of the PHV has been called both the age at peak height velocity (APHV) and the peak growth age (PGA). For simplicity, we use the term PHV to indicate the timing of the PHV. Maturity may be measured in time intervals from the PHV such that PHV + 0.5 year represents 6 months after the PHV, and PHV – 1.0 year represents 1 year before the PHV. The PHV and its timing are under tight genetic and lesser environmental control (122). Most studies show peak velocities in girls of about 8 cm/year with a standard deviation of 1 cm/year and in boys of about 9 cm/year with a slightly larger standard deviation (122–126). Standard reference curves have been developed (121, 123, 125–127). Because the PHV is the major marker of growth, we spend some time noting other events and their relationship to it.

Muscle, Fat, and Skeletal Mass Development.

The development of normal muscle mass and strength, bone density and strength, and fat mass distribution is under hormonal and genetic influence (128, 129). Muscle, fat, and skeletal mass accretion differ between boys and girls and are strongly related to physical activity with increasing exercise, increasing bone and muscle mass, and decreasing fat mass (130–138). Higher impact sports also create higher bone mineral densities in the areas undergoing the impact (139, 140) but also create higher bone mineral density in general. In general, these tissues have similar accretion velocity curves to height for both boys and girls (141), decelerating rapidly from birth through age 5 with a small spurt at age 6 to 7, a larger growth spurt near the PHV, and then a decrease until maturity.

Secondary Sexual Characteristics. Secondary sexual characteristics are tightly connected with their growth spurt particularly in girls since estrogen is the common cause of both the growth spurt and secondary sexual characteristics. In boys, dependent upon testosterone for their secondary sexual characteristics, there is less association between sexual maturity and height velocity. Boys' secondary sexual characteristics develop earlier in their growth spurt from testosterone with a relative delay in the height velocity from the need for peripheral aromatization explaining why boys are more sexually mature at their growth spurt than girls.

Maturity Determination. Maturity is a multidimensional continuum which, despite often being at the heart of pediatric orthopaedics, makes accurate maturity determination historically both inexact and difficult. The most definitive way to determine PHV is by measuring the height velocity at sequential visits. Accurate height measurement is an exacting task. Ideally, height should be measured at the same time of day for every visit because of diurnal variation of up to 1.4 cm (142). The patient should be stretched by applying gentle manual upward pressure on the mastoids while assuring the feet remain flat on the floor. Sitting height has the potential of looking more closely at spinal growth, but we have found it quite difficult to obtain reliable sitting measurements. Obtaining accurate serial height measurements for maturity determination is often impractical. Short-term growth is nonlinear and has periods of both rapid and of little activity (143) creating strange velocity calculations, and a single misreported height can make PHV assessment difficult (144). Adolescents arriving for evaluation and treatment rarely have prior serial accurate height measurements available, and other maturity indicators are needed.

Secondary Sexual Characteristics. Tanner divided secondary sexual characteristic development into clinically useful stages for breasts and pubic hair development in girl and the scrotum and pubic hair in boys (115, 117, 145). It is helpful to be familiar with these stages (see Fig. 1-25). The pubertal or Tanner stages are highly though not exactly correlated with the growth spurt and the PHV (127, 146, 147). Girls' rapid breast development tends to coincide with the acceleration of growth (126). Girls typically reach their PHV between stages 2 and 3 for breast development and stages 2 to 3 for pubic hair development while boys reach theirs between stages 3 and 5 for testicular and pubic hair growth. Most North American orthopaedists are uncomfortable evaluating patients' secondary sex characteristics in the context of a musculoskeletal examination, and patient self-assessment is unlikely to provide accurate information (148, 149), making secondary sexual characteristic determination problematic in practice. Other secondary characteristics not included in Tanner's staging but helpful in identifying advancing maturity include sweat gland maturation, menarche, voice change, axillary hair, and course facial hair.

Menarche is a readily identifiable maturity indicator associated with beginning the cyclic estrogen—progesterone production in females. While menarche is usually a reliable sign that growth velocity is decreasing (126, 127), the early menstrual periods are often irregular, and menarche's timing relative to the PVH is much too variable for accurate assessments.

Skeletal Maturity. Skeletal age has been the prime maturity measurement for most specialists. Skeletal age is based on bones growing and physis maturing in orderly sequences. It is useful to consider skeletal age as a developmental stage or maturity level rather than a linear "age." The radiographic appearance of the skeleton is dependent upon both the overall hormonal maturation state and the inherent genetic control of each local physis. Any skeletal region with consistent physeal markers is amenable to determining a skeletal age. Just like in linear growth, the physeal appearances are highly dependent upon estrogen levels in both boys and girls. Several longitudinal studies of children's growth were initiated in the early twentieth century which obtained serial radiographs and anthropomorphic measurements throughout growth. The most important of these for orthopaedists is the Bolton-Brush collection started by T. Wingate Todd of Western Reserve University in Cleveland, Ohio. In addition to growth data, the study collected longitudinal radiographs on upper middle class children, many children of university faculty, from the Cleveland area in the 1930s and 1940s. Skeletal ages were determined by correlating the children's hand radiographs with their ages and taking the middle (mode) radiograph as represented in the Greulich and Pyle atlas (150). The study itself and the original atlas by Todd had only the yearly radiographs during adolescence while the later Greulich and Pyle atlas picked some intermediate stages for the "six-month" intervals during adolescence. Other sources of estimating skeletal maturity including the foot, knee (151), and cervical spine (152–163) from the same collection are much less accessible currently. Spinal deformity surgeons commonly use the Risser sign (164–166) of iliac apophyseal ossification.

The Greulich and Pyle atlas is an example of the "atlas method" of determining skeletal maturity. "The individual bone method," which includes the Oxford score (167) of the hip and pelvis, the Tanner-Whitehouse method using the hand and wrist, and the Sauvegrain method (168, 169) using the elbow develop scores from individual ossification center appearances which are then totaled for a maturity score. These can then be correlated via a table or graph with the "skeletal age." These other methods are derived from healthy European children.

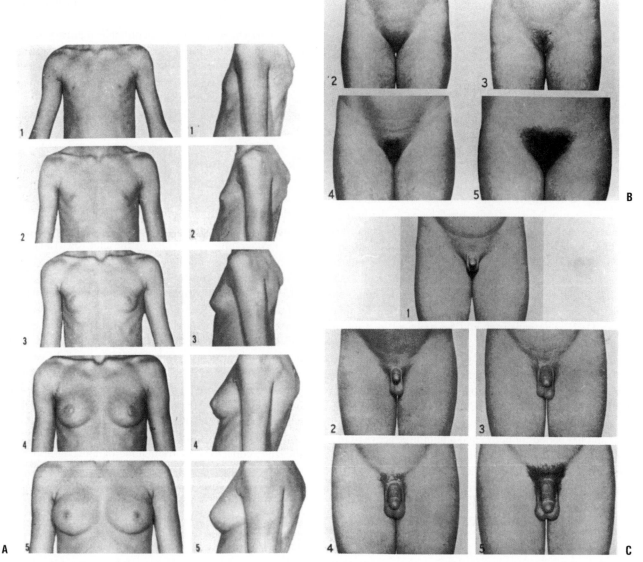

FIGURE 1-25. **A–C:** Tanner's stages of secondary sexual characteristic development in both boys and girls. (Reproduced from Tanner JM. Growth and endocrinology of the adolescent. In: Gardner L, ed. *Endocrine and genetic diseases of childhood.* Philadelphia, PA: W.B. Saunders; 1974, with permission).

Important Skeletal Maturity Nuances for Orthopaedists.

Skeletal ages are derived from healthy children, so their use in children with illness or skeletal dysplasia can be misleading. The most common error in skeletal age determination is malpositioning. In the hand, a slight flexion of any digits making interpretation difficult and rotation can cause the same problem in the elbow.

The Hand: Knowing the various stages of hand's changes is not difficult and is important for accurate maturity determination regardless of which system is used. The various stages of the digits during adolescence are shown in Figure 1-26 going from uncovered, to covered, to capped, to

fusing, to fused. The ulnar side of the hand (the fourth and fifth digits) is the last to have fully covered epiphyses, the proximal epiphyses cap their respective metaphyses slightly before the distal epiphyses, the distal phalanges close before the proximal and middle phalanges, the digits close before the metacarpals, and the distal radius closes last of all. We have developed a reliable classification system based upon this shown in the figures (Fig. 1-27) and table which correspond closely to the PHV.

The Risser sign is commonly used as a maturity indicator in scoliosis based on the radiographic excursion of iliac apophyseal ossification (164–166). The Risser sign's

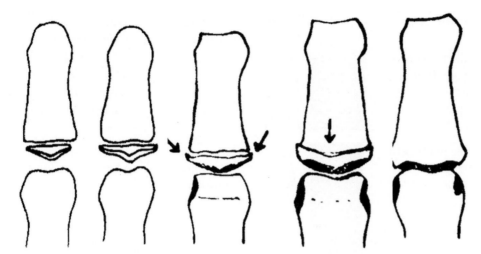

FIGURE 1-26. Stages of digital epiphyseal coverage going sequentially left to right as: uncovered, covered, capped, fusing, and fused. (Adapted from Tanner JM, Healey MJR, Goldstein H, et al. *Assessment of skeletal maturity and prediction of adult height (TW3 method).* 2001, with permission.)

advantages are its ready appearance on standard AP views of the spine and that it typically proceeds in an orderly fashion. However, because of concerns of breast irradiation, most scoliosis films are now PA rather than AP. Unfortunately, because of radiographic parallax, it is much less visible on PA radiographs. If the patient also has a lateral radiograph, then the ossification can sometimes be more clearly seen on the lateral. The Risser sign appears after the PHV (170), does not correlate well with skeletal age, and correlates differently in boys than in girls. Girls typically have little remaining growth at Risser 4 while boys still have significant growth and may continue to have significant curve progression between Risser 4 and 5. The utility of the Risser sign can be improved by including the pelvis, which has a large number of physeal and apophyseal ossification centers, on the radiographs. However, this utility must be balanced with the increased gonadal irradiation. The triradiate cartilage is currently the most useful of these as it typically fuses before initial iliac apophyseal ossification begins and also correlates closely with the PHV (147, 171, 172) (Fig. 1-28).

The elbow has a number of ossification centers visible during the adolescent growth spurt making it useful during puberty (168, 169, 173). DiMeglio and colleagues have looked at the Sauvegrain method (168, 169) during puberty and found it reliable with potential advantages to the Greulich and Pyle with more potential stages during adolescence. Charles et al. (174) have developed a system based on just the olecranon which has reliable stages during adolescence. We (175) compared Sauvegrain scores in both boys and girls and found it highly related to their PHV (Figs. 1-29 and 1-30).

Other Skeletal Markers. Obviously, there are other potentially useful skeletal sites besides the hand, elbow, and pelvis including the spine with a number of markers particularly ossification of the rib heads and the ring apophysis

(176), the cervical spine's appearance (152–163), the knee (151, 177, 178), the foot (179–181), and the shoulder which are rarely used for accurate maturity determination.

Relationship of Skeletal Maturity to the PHV. The PHV was unrecognized as such an important maturity marker when the Greulich and Pyle atlas was completed. A number of investigations (146, 153, 162, 163, 172, 175, 182–190) find a tight collection between skeletal maturity and the PHV. In terms of appearance, phalangeal capping (182–184, 191) and closure of the lateral condyle of the elbow are both closely related to the PHV (146, 186). While evidence is limited, it appears there is less coupling of the pregrowth spurt skeletal maturity than skeletal maturity once the growth spurt has stopped. This has been interpreted in the adolescent growth spurt being able to start at any level of skeletal maturity, but once the growth spurt starts, skeletal maturity quickly becomes tied to peripheral hormonal levels (185). Overall, particularly for orthopaedists, skeletal maturity appears the best reliable and readily available method of maturity determination compared to hormonal and skeletal metabolic markers and secondary sexual characteristics. Recently developed systems for the elbow and hand provide reliability, which was formerly lacking. We concur with Tanner that the concept of skeletal maturity is more appropriate than a skeletal age and prefer a system which does not have a specific "age" attached to the radiograph. Bones do not have a different age than patients, but their maturities differ just as children's do. Skeletal age determinations are based upon normal children. Therefore, for clinicians facing a child with other medical or developmental issues, the skeletal age may not be accurate (192, 193). A number of investigators have questioned the validity of using skeletal age atlases in children of varying cultures, diseases, and epochs without substantial revisions for each particular group (188, 194–217). However, if the concept of skeletal

Stage	Key features	Quick Reference	Radiograph	Related maturity signs	Greulich and Pyle reference
1.	Not all digits are not covered.	Middle phalanx of 5th finger (not as wide as metaphysis)	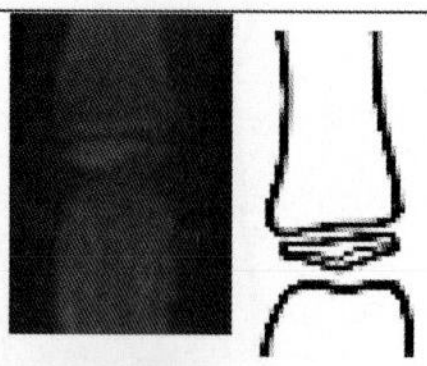	Tanner 1	Female 8+10 Male 12+6 (note 5th middle phalanx)
2.	All digits are covered	Middle phalanx of 5th finger (as wide as metaphysis)	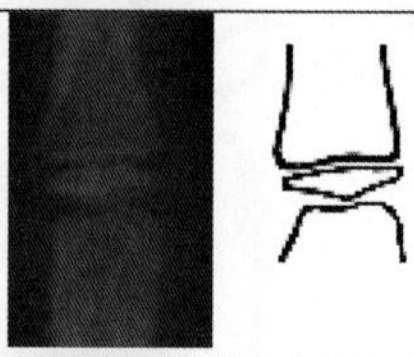	Tanner 2 Starting growth spurt	Female 10 Male 13
3.	All digits are capped. Metacarpal 2-5 epiphyses are wider than their metaphyses.	All fingers (the epiphyses curl over the metaphysis edge)	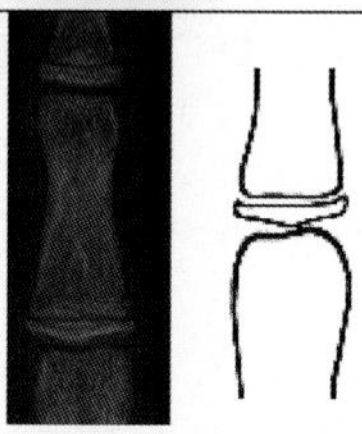	Peak Height Velocity (PHV) Risser 0 Open pelvic triradiate cartilage (TRC)	Female 11 and 12 Male 13+6 and 14
4.	Any of distal phalanges are *beginning* to close	Distal Phalanges digits 2-5 (starting to fuse but not complete)	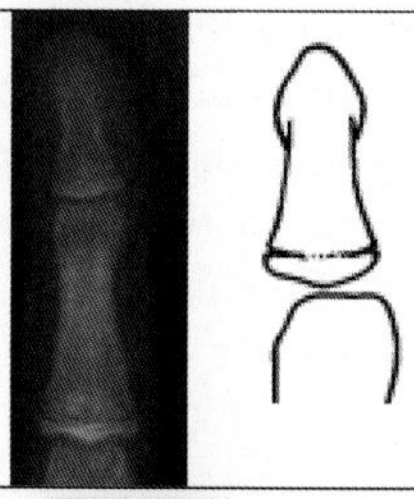	Girls typically Tanner 3 Risser 0 Open TRC	Female 13 (digits 2, 3, and 4) Male 15 (digits 4 and 5)
5.	All Distal phalanges are closed. Others are open.	Distal phalange compared with other digits (fusion is complete)	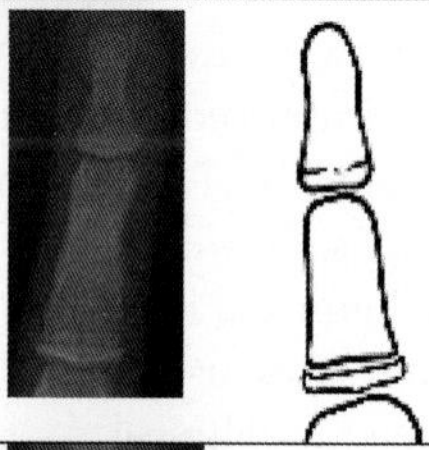	Risser 0 TRC closed Menarche only occasionally starts earlier than this.	Female 13+6 Male 15 + 6
6.	Middle or proximal phalanges are closing.	Distal and middle phalanges	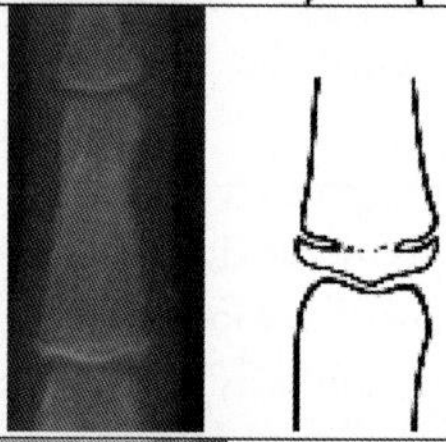	Risser positive (1 or more)	Female 14 Male 16 (late)
7.	**Only** distal radius open. May have metacarpal physeal scars.	Digits and distal radius	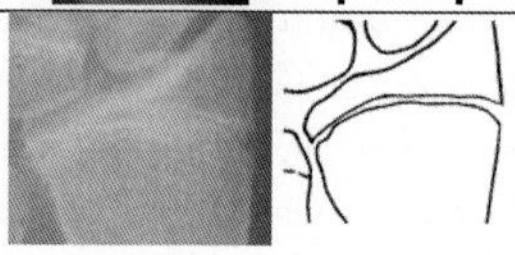	Risser 4	Female 15 Male 17
8.	All closed	Distal Radius	All Closed	Risser 5	Female 17 Male 19

FIGURE 1-27.   This table demonstrates the hand skeletal radiographic system of Sanders et al. (Adapted from Sanders JO, Khour JG, Kishan S, et al. Predicting scoliosis progression from skeletal maturity: reliability and validity of a simplified Tanner-Whitehouse classification system in girls with idiopathic scoliosis. *J Bone Joint Surg Am* 2008;90(3):540–553.) (238)

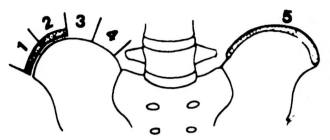

FIGURE 1-28. The Risser sign of iliac apophyseal ossification using the American system. (Reproduced from Urbaniak JR, Schaefer WW, Stelling FH, III. Iliac apophyses. Prognostic value in idiopathic scoliosis. ClinOrthop. 1976;116:80–85, with permission.)

maturity is used rather than skeletal age, most of these differences disappear.

Individual Segment Growth.

Most studies looking at the various segment date from early in the 20th century, though a few are later. Despite a strong relationship between the various body segments, the individual body areas have their own specific growth patterns. Even in the extremities, patterns vary for each physis. The overall pattern is of rapid spine and extremity growth from birth to age 5 and more rapid extremity growth between 5 and adolescence. The spine gains about 10 cm in length between birth and age 5 (146, 218), which probably accounts for the often rapid progression of congenital and infantile curves during this time, but then only gains about 5 cm in length between ages 5 and adolescence. During the adolescent growth spurt, the spine

is the primary location of accelerated growth (146) gaining about 10 cm during this period and accounting for 80% of the growth during that phase (146, 219). The lower extremities have a more constant rate of growth and less conspicuous growth spurt. But, it is a mistake to assume the limbs do not have a growth acceleration and deceleration phase. The growth spurt of the limbs is slightly prior to the spine's growth spurt (220–222) (see Fig. 1-31), and the percentage of segment growth from each physis changes over time. Once extremity growth ceases, the spine still has significant growth remaining (see Fig. 1-31). As the longitudinal growth of the spine slows, there is an increase in iliac crest width, biacromial distance (221), and lastly chest depth and diameter (219, 223).

Pritchet examined the growth of the extremities and found 85% of overall ulnar growth from the distal growth plate, but more exact figures are 90% of growth is from the distal physis at age 5 years and 95% after the age of 8. Similarly for the radius, overall 80% of growth occurs distally increasing to 85% by age of 5 and 90% by the age of 8 years (Pritchett JPO 1991, see Fig. 1-32). In the upper arm, the proximal physis overall accounts for 80% of the growth, but before age 2, <75% of growth is proximal, increasing to 85% by age 8 and constant at 90% after age 11 (224, 225). In the lower extremity, the femur accounts for 55% of the limb's growth and the tibia 45%. About 70% of femoral growth is from the distal growth plate with the proportion of growth occurring at the distal femoral growth plate varying in girls from 60% at 7 years of age to 90% at age 14, and in boys from 55% at 7 years of age to 90% at age 16. The proximal tibial growth plate contributes approximately 57% of the tibia varying in girls from 50% at 7 years of age to 80% at age

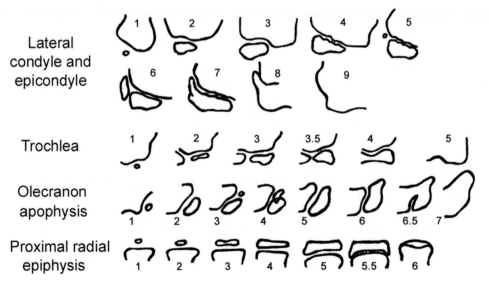

FIGURE 1-29. The Sauvegrain system of estimating elbow maturity. (Reproduced from Sauvegrain J, Nahum H, Bronstein H. Study of bone maturation of the elbow. Ann Radiol (Paris) 1962;5:542–550, with permission.) (239)

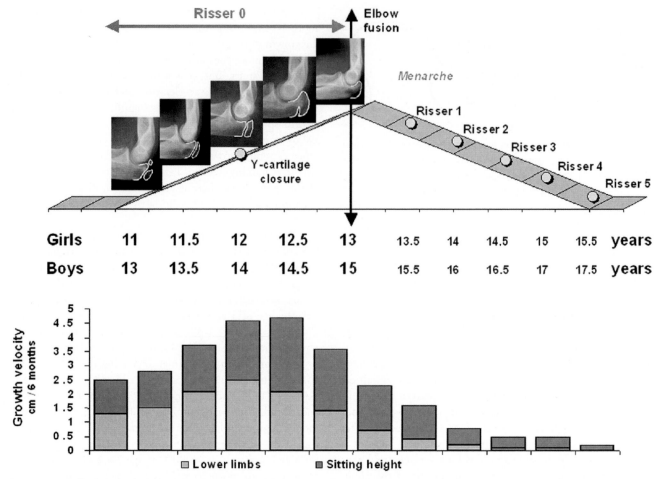

FIGURE 1-30. Olecranon maturity as a simplified Sauvegrain scale relative to the adolescent growth spurt. (Reproduced from Charles et al. Skeletal age assessment from the olecranon for idiopathic scoliosis at Risser grade 0. *J Bone Joint Surg Am* 2007;89:2737–2744, with permission.)

14 and in boys from 50% at 7 years of age to 80% at age 16 (226). Pritchet's figures are similar to Anderson's figures of 71% of the femur growth distally and 51% of the tibia growing proximally (227). Paley has popularized the concept of the multiplier to identify extremity lengths at specific chronological ages (228–237). However, the variation in growth is substantially larger when chronological age is used during the adolescent growth spurt (227) than skeletal age, likely due to the large variation in PHV timing between otherwise normal children.

Much of our knowledge of spine and chest growth comes from studies at Montpellier. These studies are particularly important for spinal and chest wall deformities. DiMeglio notes that from age 5 to puberty, two-thirds of the height growth is from the lower extremities (sub-ischial) with one-third from the spine, but that this ratio is reversed during the adolescent growth spurt (146, 219). Thoracic length and circumference do not grow simultaneously, especially during puberty. At the age of 10 years, the thoracic circumference is at 74% of its final size, whereas the sitting height is almost at 80% of its final length. Globally, the volume of the thorax triples from the age of 4 years until the end of puberty in girls and until 16 years in boys with a doubling between ages of 10 years and skeletal maturity (174, 235, 236) (see Fig. 1-33). The development of the male thorax continues after the age of 16 years. This results in a relative elongation of the rib cage until the end of growth in young men.

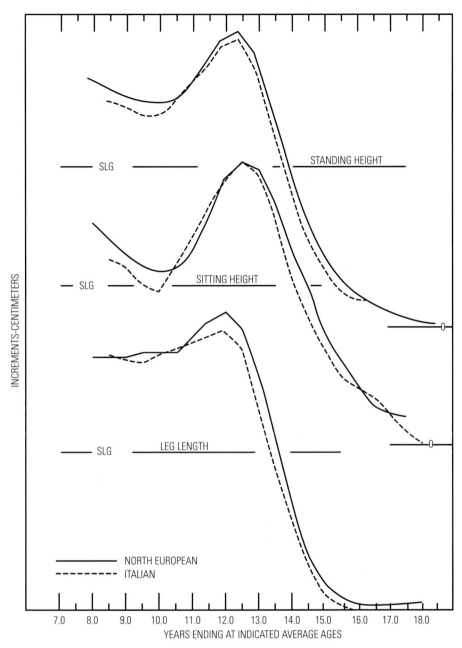

FIGURE 1-31. The lower extremities have a growth spurt slightly before and smaller than the spinal growth spurt. (Reproduced from Shuttleworth FK. Sexual maturation and the physical growth of girls age six to nineteen. *Monogr Soc Res Child Dev* 1937;II(4):253, with permission.)

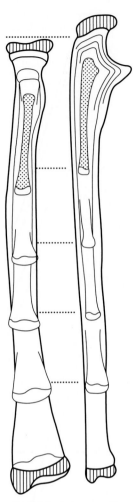

FIGURE 1-32. Growth of the limbs is not equally distributed among the various physis. This schematic by Pritchett demonstrates the difference in rates between the physis of the forearm. (Reproduced from Pritchett JW. Growth and development of the distal radius and ulna. *J Pediatr Orthop.* 1996;Sep–Oct;16(5):575–577, with permission.)

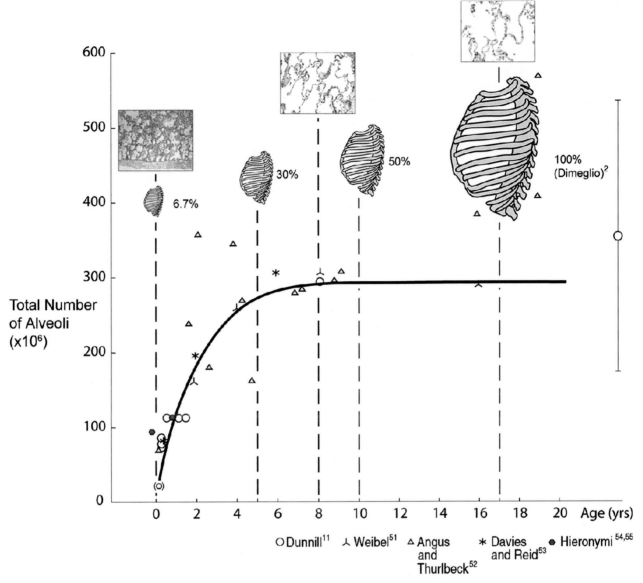

FIGURE 1-33. Growth of the alveoli relative to age and chest volume. (Reproduced from DiMeglio A. In: Campbell RM, Smith MD. *J Bone Joint Surg* 2007:89:108–122, with permission. Redrawn from Murray JF. *The normal lung: the basis for diagnosis and treatment of pulmonary diseases*, 2nd ed. Philadelphia, PA: Saunders, 1986:47; with permission from Elsevier (240).)

SUMMARY

While this chapter can only touch on the many aspects of human growth and development, these issues remain central to properly assessing and treating pediatric orthopaedic conditions. Further work in skeletal maturity assessment and growth modification will likely make these issues more important in the future as well.

REFERENCES

1. Gulyas BJ. A reexamination of the cleavage pattern in eutherian mammalian eggs: rotation of the blastomere pairs during second cleavage in the rabbit. *J Exp Zool* 1975;193:235–248.
2. Piko L, Clegg KB. Quantitative changes in total RNA, total poly(A), and ribosomes in early mouse embryos. *Dev Biol* 1982;89:362–378.
3. McLaren A. *Mammalian chimeras.* Cambridge, UK: Cambridge University Press, 1976.
4. Kelly SJ. Studies of the developmental potential of 4- and 8- cell stage mouse blastomeres. *J Exp Zool* 1977;200:365–376.
5. Barlow P, Owen DA, Graham C. DNA synthesis in the preimplantation mouse embryo. *J Embryol Exp Morphol* 1972;27:432–445.
6. Hillman N, Sherman MI, Graham CF. The effect of spatial arrangement of cell determination during mouse development. *J Embryol Exp Morphol* 1972;28:263–278.
7. McGrath J, Solter D. Completion of mouse embryogenesis requires both maternal and paternal genomes. *Cell* 1984;37:179–183.
8. Surani MAH, Barton SC, Norris ML. Development of reconstituted mouse eggs suggests imprinting of the genome during gametogenesis. *Nature* 1984;308:548–550.
9. Saunders JF, Errick J. Inductive activity and enduring cellular constitution of a supernumerary apical ectodermal ridge grafted to the limb bud of the chick embryo. *Dev Biol* 1976;50:16–25.
10. Gilbert SF. *Developmental biology*, 3rd ed. Sunderland, MA: Sinauer Associates, 1991.
11. Keynes RJ, Stern CD. Mechanisms of vertebrate segmentation. *Development* 1988;103:413–429.
12. Saunders JF. The experimental analysis of chick limb bud development. In: Ede DA, Hinchliffe JR, Balls M, eds. *Vertebrate limb and somite morphogenesis.* Cambridge, UK: Cambridge University Press, 1977:1–24.
13. MacCabe JA, Errick J, Saunders JW. Ectodermal control of the dorsoventral axis in the leg bud of the chick embryo. *Dev Biol* 1974;39:69–82.
14. Akita K. The effect of the ectoderm on the dorsoventral pattern of epidermis, muscles and joints in the developing chick leg: a new model. *Anat Embryol* 1996;193:377–386.
15. Saunders JW, Gasseling MT. Ectoderm–mesenchymal interactions in the origin of the wing symmetry. In: Fleischmajer R, Billingham RE, eds. *Epithelial-mesenchymal interactions.* Baltimore, MD: Williams & Wilkins, 1968:78–97.
16. Solursh M, Singley CT, Reiter RS. The influence of epithelia on cartilage and loose connective tissue formation by limb mesenchyme cultures. *Dev Biol* 1981;86:471–482.
17. Wolpert L, Tickle C, Sampford M. The effect of cell killing by X-irradiation on pattern formation in the chick limb. *J Embryol Exp Morphol* 1979;50:175–198.
18. Zanetti N, Solursh M. Control of chondrogenic differentiation by the cytoskeleton. *J Cell Biol* 1984;99:115–123.
19. Davis CA, Holmyard DP, Millen KJ, et al. Examining pattern formation in mouse, chicken and frog embryos with an En-specific antiserum. *Development* 1991;111:287–298.
20. Johnston SH, Rauskolb C, Wilson R, et al. A family of mammalian Fringe genes implicated in boundary determination and the Notch pathway. *Development* 1997;124:2245–2254.
21. Wu JY, Wen L, Zhang WJ, et al. The secreted product of Xenopus gene lunatic Fringe, a vertebrate signaling molecule. *Science* 1976;273:355–358.
22. Cohen B, Bashirullah A, Dagnino L, et al. Fringe boundaries coincide with Notch-dependent patterning centers in mammals and alter Notch-dependent development in *Drosophila. Nat Genet* 1997;16:283–288.
23. Niswander L, Tickle C, Vogel A, et al. FGF-4 replaces the apical ectodermal ridge and directs outgrowth and patterning of the limb. *Cell* 1993;75:579–587.
24. Ohuchi H, Nakagawa T, Yamamoto A, et al. The mesenchymal factor, FGF10, initiates and maintains the outgrowth of the chick limb bud through interaction with FGF8, an apical ectodermal factor. *Development* 1997;124:2235–2244.
25. Ohuchi HTN, Yamauchi T, Ohata T, et al. An additional limb can be induced from the flank of the chick embryo by FGF-4. *Biochem Biophys Res Commun* 1995;209:809–816.
26. Cohn MJ, Izpisua-Belmonte JC, Abud H, et al. Fibroblast growth factors induce additional limb development from the flank of chick embryos. *Cell* 1995;80:739–746.
27. Min H, Danilenko DM, Scully SA, et al. Fgf-10 is required for both limb and lung development and exhibits striking functional similarity to *Drosophila* branchless. *Genes Dev* 1998;12:3156–3161.
28. Summerbell D, Lewis JH, Wolpert L. Positional information in chick limb morphogenesis. *Nature (Lond.)* 1973;244:492–496.
29. Summerbell D, Lewis JH. Time, place, and positional value in the chick limb-bud. *J Embryol Exp Morphol* 1975;33:621–643.
30. Tickle C, Summerbell D, Wolpert L. Positional signalling and specification of digits in chick limb morphogenesis. *Nature (Lond.)* 1975;254:199–202.
31. Summerbell D. The zone of polarizing activity: evidence for a role in normal chick limb morphogenesis. *J Embryol Exp Morphol* 1979;50:217–233.
32. Maden M. Vitamin A and pattern formation in the regenerating limb. *Nature (Lond.)* 1982;295:672–675.
33. Summerbell D. The effect of local application of retinoic acid to the anterior margin of the developing chick limb. *J Embryol Exp Morphol* 1983;78:269–289.
34. Thaller C, Eichele G. Retinoid signaling in vertebrate limb development. In: Crombrugghe B, Horton WA, Olsen BR, et al., eds. *Molecular and developmental biology.* New York, NY: Annals of the New York Academy of Sciences, 1996;785:1–11.
35. Monga M. Vitamin A and its congeners. *Semin Perinatol* 1997;21(2) (April):135–142.
36. Nester G, Zuckner J. Rheumatologic complications of Vitamin A and retinoids. *Semin Arthritis Rheum* 1995;24(4) (February):291–296.
37. Riddle R, Johnson R, Laufer E, et al. Sonic hedgehog mediates the polarizing activity of the ZPA. *Cell* 1993;75:1401–1416.
38. Francis P, Richardson M, Brickell P, et al. Bone morphogenetic proteins and a signalling pathway that controls patterning in the chick limb. *Development* 1994;120:209–218.
39. Niswander L, Jeffrey S, Martin GR, et al. A positive feedback loop coordinates growth and patterning in the vertebrate limb. *Nature* 1994;371:609–612.
40. Brunet LJ, McMahon JA, McMahon AP, et al. Noggin, cartilage morphogenesis, and joint formation in the mammalian skeleton. *Science* 1998;280:1455–1457.
41. Dickman S. Growing joints use their noggins. *Science* 1998;280:1350.
42. Noonan KJ, Reiter RS, Kurriger GL, et al. Spatial and temporal expression of CD44 isoforms in the developing and growing joints of the rat limb. *J Orthop Res* 1998;16:100–103.
43. Dealy CN, Roth A, Ferrari D, et al. Wnt-5a and Wnt-7a are expressed in the developing chick limb bud in a manner suggesting roles in pattern formation along the proximodistal and dorsoventral axes. *Mech Dev* 1993;43:175–186.
44. Riddle RD, Ensini M, Nelson C, et al. Induction of the LIM homeobox gene Lmxl by Wnt7a establishes dorsoventral pattern in the vertebrate limb. *Cell* 1995;83:631–640.
45. Parr BA, McMahon AP. Dorsalizing signal Wnt-7a required for normal polarity of D-V and A-P axes of mouse limb. *Nature* 1995; 374:350–353.

46. Yang Y, Niswander L. Interaction between the signaling molecules Wnt7a and SHH during vertebrate limb development: dorsal signals regulate anteroposterior patterning. *Cell* 1995;80:939–947.

47. Izpisua-Belmonte JC, Ede DA, Tickle C, et al. Mixexpression of posterior Hox-4 genes in Talpid (ta³) mutant wings correlates with the absence of anteroposterior polarity. *Development* 1922;114:959–963.

48. Duboule D. Vertebrate Hox genes and proliferation: an alternative pathway to homeosis? *Curr Opin Genet Dev* 1995;5:525–528.

49. Goff DJ, Tabin CJ. Analysis of HoxD-13 and HoxD-11 misexpression in chick limb buds reveals that Hox genes affect both bone condensation and growth. *Development* 1997;124:627–636.

50. Stevenson RE, Hall JG, Godoman RM. Human malformations and related anomalies vol II. In: *Oxford monographs on medical genetics*, No. 27. New York, NY: Oxford University Press, 1993.

51. Mortlock DP, Post LC, Innis JW. The molecular basis of hypodactyly (Hd): a deletion in Hoxa -13 leads to arrest of digital arch formation. *Nat Genetics* 1996;13:284–289.

52. Raas-Rothschild A, Manouvrier S, Gonzales M, et al. Refined mapping of a gene for split hand-split foot malformation (SHFM3) on chromosome 10q25. *J Med Genet* 1996;33(12):996–1001.

53. Hoyme HE, van Allen MI, Benirschke K. Vascular pathogenesis of transverse limb reduction defects. *Pediatrics* 1982;101:839.

54. Van Allen MI, Hoyme HE, Jones KL. Vascular pathogenesis of limb defects. I. Radial artery anatomy in radial aplasia. *Pediatrics* 1982;101:832.

55. Torpin R. *Fetal malformation caused by amnion rupture during gestation.* Springfield, IL: Charles C. Thomas Publisher, 1968.

56. Zeller R, Jackson-Grusby L, Leder P. The limb deformity gene is required for apical ectodermal ridge differentiation and antero-posterior limb pattern formation. *Genes Dev* 1989;3:1481–1492.

57. Chan DC, Wynshaw-Boris A, Leder P. Formin isoforms are differentially expressed in the mouse embryo and are required for normal expression of Fgf-4 and shh in the limb bud. *Development* 1995;121:3151–3162.

58. Kochhar DM. Cellular basis of congenital limb deformity induced in mice by vitamin A. In: Bergsma D, Lenz W, eds. *Morphogenesis and malformation of the limb birth.* Defects Original Article Series. Vol. 13. New York, NY: Liss, 1977:111–154.

59. Heutink P, Zguricas J, van Oosterhout L, et al. The gene for triphangeal thumb maps to the subtelomeric region of chromosome 7q. *Nat Genet* 1994;6:287–292.

60. Radhakrishna U, Blouin J-L, Solanki JV, et al. An autosomal dominant triphalangeal thumb: polysyndactyly syndrome with variable expression in a large Indian family maps to 7q36. *Am J Med Genet* 1996;66:209–215.

61. Hui CC, Joyner AL. A mouse model of Greig cephalopolysyndactyly syndrome: the extra-toes mutation contains an intragenic deletion of the Gli3 gene. *Nat Genet* 1993;3:241–246.

62. Masuya H, Sagai T, Wakana S, et al. A duplicated zone of polarizing activity in polydactylous mouse mutants. *Genes Dev* 1995;9:1645–1653.

63. Muragaki Y, Mondlos S, Upton J, et al. Altered growth and branching patterns in synpolydactyly caused by mutations in HOXD 13. *Science* 1996;272:548–551.

64. Lockwood C, Ghidini A, Romero R, et al. Amniotic band syndrome: reevaluation of its pathogenesis. *Am J Obstet Gynecol* 1989;160:1030.

65. Patterson TS. Congenital ring construction. *Br J Plast Surg* 1961;14:1.

66. Streeter GL. Focal deficiencies in fetal tissues and the relation to intra-uterine amputation. *Contrib Embryol* 1930;22:41.

67. Van Allen MI, Curry C, Gallagher L. Limb body wall complex: I. Pathogenesis. *Am J Med Genet* 1987;28:529.

68. Houben JJ. Immediate and delayed effects of oligohydramnios on limb development in the rat: chronology and specificity. *Teratology* 1984;30:403.

69. Chevallier A. Role due mesoderme somitique dans le developpement de la cage thoracique de l'embryon d'oiseau. *J Embryol Exp Morphol* 1975;33:291–311.

70. Chevallier A, Kieny M, Mauger A, et al. Developmental fate of the somitic mesoderm in the chick embryo. In: Ede DA, Hinchliffe JR, Balls M, eds. *Vertebrate limb and somite morphogenesis.* Cambridge, UK: Cambridge University Press, 1977:421–432.

71. Kessel M, Gruss P. Homeotic transformations of murine vertebrae and concomitant alteration of Hox codes induced by retinoic acid. *Cell* 1991;67:89–104.

72. Kessel M, Balling R, Gruss P. Variations of cervical vertebrae after expression of a Hox-1.1 transgene in mice. *Cell* 1990;61:301–308.

73. Pollock RA. Altering the boundaries of Hox-3.1 expression: evidence for antipodal gene regulation. *Cell* 1992;71:911–923.

74. Ramirez-S R. Hoxb-4 (Hox-2.6) mutant mice show homeotic transformation of a cervical vertebra and defects in the closure of the sternal rudiments. *Cell* 1993;73:279–294.

75. Chisaka O, Capecchi MR. Regionally restricted developmental defects resulting from targeted disruption of the mouse homeobox gene hox-1.5. *Nature* 1991;350:473–479.

76. Kessel M. Reversal of axonal pathways from rhombomere 3 correlates with extra Hox expression domains. *Neuron* 1993;10:379–393.

77. Dietrich S, Gruss P. Undulated phenotypes suggest a role of Pax-1 for the development of vertebral and extravertebral structures. *Dev Biol* 1995;167:529–548.

78. Takahashi Y, Monsoro-Burq A-H, Bontoux M, et al. A role for Qhox-8 in the establishment of the dorsoventral pattern during vertebrate development. *Proc Natl Acad Sci U S A* 1992;89:10237–10241.

79. Gruneberg H. *The pathology of development.* Oxford, UK: Blackwell Scientific, 1963.

80. Lyon MF, Seale AG. *Genetic variations and strains of the laboratory mouse.* Oxford, UK: Oxford University Press, 1989.

81. Dietrich S, Kessel M. The vertebral column. In: Thorogood P, ed. *Embryos, genes and birth defects.* Hoboken, NJ: John Wiley & Sons Ltd., 1997.

82. Dias MS. Myelomeningocele. In: Choux M, DiRocco C, Hockley AD, et al., eds. *Pediatric neurosurgery.* London, UK: Churchill Livingstone, 1997:32–59.

83. George TM, McLone. Mechanisms of mutant genes in spina bifida: a review of implications from animal models. *Pediatr Neurosurg* 1995;23:236–245.

84. Gardner WJ. Diastematomyelia and the Klipper–Feil syndrome. Relationship to hydrocephalus, syringomyelia, meningocele, meningomyelocele, and iniencephalus. *Clev Clin Q* 1964;31:19–44.

85. Gardner WJ. *The dysraphic states from syringomyelia to anencephaly.* Amsterdam, the Netherlands: Excerpta Medica, 1973.

86. Partington MD, McLone DG. Hereditary factors in the etiology of neural tube defects. *Pediatr Neurosurg* 1995;23:311–316.

87. Papalopula N, Kintner CR. Molecular genetics of neurulation. In: Bock G, Marsh J, eds. *Neural tube defects.* Ciba Foundation Symposium No. 181. Chickester, UK: John Wiley, 1994:299.

88. Schoenwolf GC, Smith JL. Mechanisms of neurulation: traditional viewpoint and recent advances. *Development* 1990;109:243–270.

89. Copp AJ, Brook FA, Estibeiro P, et al. The embryonic development of mammalian neural tube defects. *Prog Neurobiol* 1990;35:363–403.

90. Echelard Y, Epstein DJ, St-J B, et al. Sonic hedgehog, a member of a family of putative signaling molecules, is implicated in the regulation of CNS polarity. *Cell* 1993;75:1417–1430.

91. Basler K, Edlund T, Jessell TM, et al. Control of cell pattern in the neural tube: regulation of cell differential by dorsalin-1, a novel TGFβ family member. *Cell* 1993;73:687–702.

92. Copp AJ, Bernfield M. Etiology and pathogenesis of human neural tube defects insights from mouse models. *Curr Opin Pediatr* 1994;6:624–631.

93. Tyler MS, Hall BK. Epithelial influence on skeletogenesis in the mandible of the embryonic chick. *Anat Rec* 1977;206:61–70.

94. Hall BK. The embryonic development of bone. *Am Sci* 1988;76:174–181.

95. Bi W, Deng JM, Zhang Z, et al. Sox9 is required for cartilage formation. *Nat Genet* 1999;22:85–89.

96. Vortkamp A, Lee K, Lanske B, et al. Regulation of rate of cartilage differentiation by Indian hedgehog and PTH-related protein. *Science* 1996;273:613–622.

97. Wilsman NJ, Farnum CE, Leiferman EM, et al. Differential growth by growth plates as a function of multiple parameters of chondrocytic kinetics. *J Ortho Res* 1996;14:927–936.

98. Hunziker EB, Schenk RK, Cruz-Orive LM. Quantitation of chondrocyte performance in growth-plate cartilage during longitudinal bone growth. *J Bone Joint Surg Am* 1987;69:162–173.

99. Ballock RT, Heydemann A, Wakefield LM, et al. TGF-B1 prevents hypertrophy of epiphyseal chondrocytes: regulation of gene expression for cartilage matrix proteins and metalloproteases. *Dev Biol* 1993;158:414–429.

100. Gerber HP, Vu TH, Ryan AM, et al. VEGF couples hypertrophic cartilage remodeling, ossification and angiogenesis during endochondral bone formation. *Nat Med* 1999;5:623–628.

101. Alvarez J, Horton J, Sohn P, et al. The perichondrium plays an important role in mediating the effects of TGF-B1 on endochondral bone formation. *Dev Dyn* 2001;221:311–321.

102. Shapiro F, Holtrop ME, Glimcher MJ. Organization and cellular biology of the perichondrial ossification groove of Ranvier: a morphological study in rabbits. *J Bone Joint Surg Am* 1977;59:703–723.

103. Parent AS, Teilmann G, Juul A, et al. The timing of normal puberty and the age limits of sexual precocity: variations around the world, secular trends, and changes after migration. *Endocr Rev* 2003;24:668–693.

104. Buck Louis GM, Gray LE Jr, Marcus M, et al. Environmental factors and puberty timing: expert panel research needs. *Pediatrics* 2008;121(Suppl 3):S192–S207.

105. Saenger P, Dimartino-Nardi J. Premature adrenarche. *J Endocrinol Invest* 2001;24:724–733.

106. Plant TM, Barker-Gibb ML. Neurobiological mechanisms of puberty in higher primates. *Hum Reprod Update* 2004;10:67–77.

107. Tena-Sempere M. Ghrelin and reproduction: ghrelin as novel regulator of the gonadotropic axis. *Vitam Horm* 2008;77:285–300.

108. Barb CR, Barrett JB, Kraeling RR. Role of leptin in modulating the hypothalamic-pituitary axis and luteinizing hormone secretion in the prepuberal gilt. *Domest Anim Endocrinol* 2004;26:201–214.

109. Apter D. The role of leptin in female adolescence. *Ann N Y Acad Sci* 2003;997:64–76.

110. Styne DM. The regulation of pubertal growth. *Horm Res* 2003;60: 22–26.

111. Grumbach MM. The neuroendocrinology of human puberty revisited. *Horm Res* 2002;57(Suppl 2):2–14.

112. Wehkalampi K, Silventoinen K, Kaprio J, et al. Genetic and environmental influences on pubertal timing assessed by height growth. *Am J Hum.Biol* 2008;20:417–423.

113. Nilsson O, Chrysis D, Pajulo O, et al. Localization of estrogen receptors-alpha and -beta and androgen receptor in the human growth plate at different pubertal stages. *J Endocrinol* 2003;177:319–326.

114. Cutler GB Jr. The role of estrogen in bone growth and maturation during childhood and adolescence. *J Steroid Biochem Mol Biol* 1997;61:141–144.

115. Grumbach MM. Estrogen, bone, growth and sex: a sea change in conventional wisdom. *J Pediatr Endocrinol Metab* 2000;13(Suppl 6):1439–1455.

116. Lee PA, Witchel SF. The influence of estrogen on growth. *Curr Opin Pediatr* 1997;9:431–436.

117. Grumbach MM. The role of estrogen in the male and female: evidence from mutations in synthesis and action. *Horm Res* 2000;53 Suppl 3:23–24.

118. Delemarre-van de Waal HA, van Coeverden SC, Rotteveel J. Hormonal determinants of pubertal growth. *J Pediatr Endocrinol Metab* 2001;14(Suppl 6):1521–1526.

119. Rotteveel. Modifications of growth hormone secretion during female puberty. *Ann N Y Acad Sci* 1997;816:60–75.

120. Suter KJ. The ontogeny of pulsatile growth hormone secretion and its temporal relationship to the onset of puberty in the agonadal male rhesus monkey (*Macaca mulatta*). *J Clin Endocrinol Metab* 2004;89:2275–2280.

121. Tanner JM, Davies PS. Clinical longitudinal standards for height and height velocity for North American children. *J Pediatr* 1985;107:317–329.

122. Beunen G, Thomis M, Maes HH, et al. Genetic variance of adolescent growth in stature. *Ann Hum Biol* 2000;27:173–186.

123. Loncar-Dusek M, Pecina M, Prebeg Z. A longitudinal study of growth velocity and development of secondary gender characteristics versus onset of idiopathic scoliosis. *Clin Orthop Relat Res* 1991;(270):278–282.

124. Tanaka T, Suwa S, Yokoya S, et al. Analysis of linear growth during puberty. *Acta Paediatr Scand Suppl* 1988;347:25–29.

125. Buckler JMH, Wild RH. Longitudinal study of height and weight at adolescence. *Arch Dis Child* 1987;62:1224–1232.

126. Buckler JMH. *A longitudinal study of adolescent growth*, 1st ed. New York, NY: Springer-Verlag, 1990.

127. Tanner JM, Whitehouse RH. Clinical longitudinal standards for height, weight, height velocity, weight velocity, and stages of puberty. *Arch Dis Child* 1976;51:170–179.

128. Czerwinski SA, Lee M, Choh AC, et al. Genetic factors in physical growth and development and their relationship to subsequent health outcomes. *Am J Hum Biol* 2007;19:684–691.

129. Hulthen L, Bengtsson BA, Sunnerhagen KS, et al. GH is needed for the maturation of muscle mass and strength in adolescents. *J Clin Endocrinol Metab* 2001;86:4765–4770.

130. Vicente-Rodriguez G, Urzanqui A, Mesana MI, et al. Physical fitness effect on bone mass is mediated by the independent association between lean mass and bone mass through adolescence: a cross-sectional study. *J Bone Miner Metab* 2008;26:288–294.

131. Weeks BK, Young CM, Beck BR. Eight months of regular in-school jumping improves indices of bone strength in adolescent boys and Girls: the POWER PE study. *J Bone Miner Res* 2008;23:1002–1011.

132. Foo LH, Zhang Q, Zhu K, et al. Influence of body composition, muscle strength, diet and physical activity on total body and forearm bone mass in Chinese adolescent girls. *Br J Nutr* 2007;98:1281–1287.

133. Gil SM, Gil J, Ruiz F, et al. Physiological and anthropometric characteristics of young soccer players according to their playing position: relevance for the selection process. *J Strength Cond Res* 2007;21:438–445.

134. Nickols-Richardson SM, Miller LE, Wootten DF, et al. Concentric and eccentric isokinetic resistance training similarly increases muscular strength, fat-free soft tissue mass, and specific bone mineral measurements in young women. *Osteoporos Int* 2007;18:789–796.

135. Wang Q, Alen M, Nicholson P, et al. Weight-bearing, muscle loading and bone mineral accrual in pubertal girls—a 2-year longitudinal study. *Bone* 2007;40:1196–1202.

136. Vicente-Rodriguez G, Ara I, Perez-Gomez J, et al. Muscular development and physical activity as major determinants of femoral bone mass acquisition during growth. *Br J Sports Med* 2005;39:611–616.

137. Greene DA, Naughton GA, Briody JN, et al. Musculoskeletal health in elite male adolescent middle-distance runners. *J Sci Med Sport* 2004;7:373–383.

138. Vicente-Rodriguez G, Jimenez-Ramirez J, Ara I, et al. Enhanced bone mass and physical fitness in prepubescent footballers. *Bone* 2003;33:853–859.

139. Pettersson U, Nordstrom P, Alfredson H, et al. Effect of high impact activity on bone mass and size in adolescent females: a comparative study between two different types of sports. *Calcif Tissue Int* 2000;67:207–214.

140. Pettersson U, Alfredson H, Nordstrom P, et al. Bone mass in female cross-country skiers: relationship between muscle strength and different BMD sites. *Calcif Tissue Int* 2000;67:199–206.

141. Braillon PM. Annual changes in bone mineral content and body composition during growth. *Horm Res* 2003;60:284–290.

142. Tillmann V, Clayton PE. Diurnal variation in height and the reliability of height measurements using stretched and unstretched techniques in the evaluation of short-term growth. *Ann Hum Biol* 2001;28:195–206.

143. Caino S, Kelmansky D, Lejarraga H, et al. Short-term growth at adolescence in healthy girls. *Ann Hum Biol* 2004;31:182–195.

144. Coste J, Ecosse E, Lesage C, et al. Evaluation of adolescent statural growth in health and disease: reliability of assessment from height measurement series and development of an automated algorithm. *Horm Res* 2002;58:105–114.

145. Tanner JM. Normal growth and techniques of growth assessment. *Clin Endocrinol Metab* 1986;15:411–451.

146. Dimeglio A, Bonnel F. *Le rachis en croissance*. Paris, France: Springer-Verlag, 1990.

147. Sanders JO, Herring JA, Browne RH. Posterior arthrodesis and instrumentation in the immature (Risser-grade-0) spine in idiopathic scoliosis. *JBJS A* 1995;77:39–45.

148. Wu Y, Schreiber GB, Klementowicz V, et al. Racial differences in accuracy of self-assessment of sexual maturation among young black and white girls. *J Adolesc Health* 2001;28:197–203.

149. Coleman L, Coleman J. The measurement of puberty: a review. *J Adolesc* 2002;25:535–550.

150. Greulich WW, Pyle SI. *Radiographic atlas of skeletal development of the hand and wrist,* 2nd ed. Palo Alto, CA: Stanford University Press, 1959.

151. Pyle SI, Hoerr NL. *Radiographic atlas of skeletal development of the knee: a standard of reference.* Springfield, IL: Charles C. Thomas, 1955.

152. Chang HP, Liao CH, Yang YH, et al. Correlation of cervical vertebra maturation with hand-wrist maturation in children. *Kaohsiung J Med Sci* 2001;17:29–35.

153. Hassel B, Farman AG. Skeletal maturation evaluation using cervical vertebrae. *Am J Orthod Dentofacial Orthop* 1995;107:58–66.

154. Kamal M, Goyal S. Comparative evaluation of hand wrist radiographs with cervical vertebrae for skeletal maturation in 10–12 years old children. *J Indian Soc Pedod Prev Dent* 2006;24:127–135.

155. Minars M, Burch J, Masella R, et al. Predicting skeletal maturation using cervical vertebrae. *Todays FDA* 2003;15:17–19.

156. Mito T, Sato K, Mitani H. Cervical vertebral bone age in girls. *Am J Orthod Dentofacial Orthop* 2002;122:380–385.

157. San RP, Palma JC, Oteo MD, et al. Skeletal maturation determined by cervical vertebrae development. *Eur J Orthod* 2002;24:303–311.

158. Seedat AK, Forsberg CD. An evaluation of the third cervical vertebra (C3) as a growth indicator in Black subjects. *SADJ* 2005;60:156, 158–160.

159. Uysal T, Ramoglu SI, Basciftci FA, et al. Chronologic age and skeletal maturation of the cervical vertebrae and hand-wrist: is there a relationship? *Am J Orthod Dentofacial Orthop* 2006;130:622–628.

160. Wang JC, Nuccion SL, Feighan JE, et al. Growth and development of the pediatric cervical spine documented radiographically. *J Bone Joint Surg Am* 2001;83-A:1212–1218.

161. Grave K, Townsend G. Hand-wrist and cervical vertebral maturation indicators: how can these events be used to time Class II treatments? *Aust Orthod J* 2003;19:33–45.

162. Grave K, Townsend G. Cervical vertebral maturation as a predictor of the adolescent growth spurt. *Aust Orthod J* 2003;19:25–32.

163. Grave K. The use of the hand and wrist radiograph in skeletal age assessment; and why skeletal age assessment is important. *Aust Orthod J* 1994;13:196.

164. Risser JC. The iliac apophysis: an invaluable sign in the management of scoliosis. *CORR* 1958;11:111–120.

165. Urbaniak JR, Schaefer WW, Stelling FH3. Iliac apophyses. Prognostic value in idiopathic schliosis. *Clin Orthop* 1976;(116):80–85.

166. Zaoussis AL, James JIP. The iliac apophysis and the evolution of curves in scoliosis. *J Bone Joint Surg Br* 1958;40:442–453.

167. Acheson Roy M. The Oxford method of assessing skeletal maturity. *Clin Orthop* 1957;10:19–39.

168. Chaumoitre K, Colavolpe N, Sayegh-Martin Y, et al. Reliability of the Sauvegrain and Nahum method to assess bone age in a contemporary population. *J Radiol* 2006;87:1679–1682.

169. Dimeglio A, Charles YP, Daures JP, et al. Accuracy of the Sauvegrain method in determining skeletal age during puberty. *J Bone Joint Surg Am* 2005;87:1689–1696.

170. Little DG, Song KM, Katz D, et al. Relationship of peak height velocity to other maturity indicators in idiopathic scoliosis in girls. *J Bone Joint Surg Am* 2000;82:685–693.

171. Dimeglio A. Pubertal peak triradiate cartilage and apophysi of the greater trochanter. *Pediatr Orthop Soc North Am* 2000.

172. Sanders JO, Little DG, Richards BS. Prediction of the crankshaft phenomenon by the peak height velocity. *Spine* 1997;22:1352–1356.

173. Schedewie H, Braselman A, Willich E, et al. The determination of bone age in the elbow as compared to the hand. A study in 390 children. *Rev Interam Radiol* 1979;4:11–17.

174. Charles YP, Dimeglio A, Canavese F, et al. Skeletal age assessment from the olecranon for idiopathic scoliosis at Risser grade 0. *J Bone Joint Surg Am* 2007;89:2737–2744.

175. Hans S, Sanders J, Cooperman D. Using the Sauvegrain method to predict peak growth velocity in boys and girls. *J Pediatr Orthop* 2008;28:836–839.

176. Hoppenfeld S, Lonner B, Murthy V, et al. The rib epiphysis and other growth centers as indicators of the end of spinal growth. *Spine* 2004;29:47–50.

177. Roche AF, French NY. Differences in skeletal maturity levels between the knee and hand. *Am J Roentgenol Radium Ther Nucl Med* 1970;109:307–312.

178. Vignolo M, Milani S, DiBattista E, et al. Modified Greulich-Pyle, Tanner-Whitehouse, and Roche-Wainer-Thissen (knee) methods for skeletal age assessment in a group of Italian children and adolescents. *Eur J Pediatr* 1990;149:314–317.

179. Dhamija SC, Agarwal KN, Gupta SK, et al. Evaluation of hand and foot ossification centres for assessment of bone age. *Indian Pediatr* 1976;13:201–208.

180. Hernandez M, Sanchez E, Sobradillo B, et al. A new method for assessment of skeletal maturity in the first 2 years of life. *Pediatr Radiol* 1988;18:484–489.

181. Whitaker JM, Rousseau L, Williams T, et al. Scoring system for estimating age in the foot skeleton. *Am J Phys Anthropol* 2002;118:385–392.

182. Sanders JO. Maturity indicators in spinal deformity. *J Bone Joint Surg Am* 2007;89(Suppl 1):14–20.

183. Sanders JO, Browne RH, Sanders JO, et al. Correlates of the peak height velocity (PHV) in girls with idiopathic scoliosis. *Spine* 2006;31:2289–2295.

184. Sanders JO, Browne RH, McConnell SL, et al. Maturity assessment and curve progression in girls with idiopathic scoliosis. *J Bone Joint Surg Am* 2007;89:64–73.

185. Hauspie R, Bielicki T, Koniarek J. Skeletal maturity at onset of the adolescent growth spurt and at peak velocity for growth in height: a threshold effect? *Ann Hum Biol* 1991;18:23–29.

186. Deming J. Application of the Gompertz curve to the observed pattern of growth in length of 48 individual boys and girls during the adolescent cycle of growth. *Hum Biol* 1957;29:83.

187. Hagg U, Taranger J. Skeletal stages of the hand and wrist as indicators of the pubertal growth spurt. *Acta Odontol Scand* 1980;38:187–200.

188. Kristmundsdottir F, Burwell RG, Marshall WA, et al. Cross-sectional study of skeletal maturation in normal children from Nottingham and London. *Ann Hum Biol* 1984;11:133–139.

189. Marshall WA, Limongi Y. Skeletal maturity and the prediction of age at menarche. *Ann Hum Biol* 1976;3:235–243.

190. Marshall WA. Interrelationships of skeletal maturation, sexual development and somatic growth in man. *Ann Hum Biol* 1974;1:29–40.

191. Sanders J, Khoury J, Kishan S, et al. Predicting scoliosis progression from skeletal maturity: reliability and validity of a simplified Tanner-Whitehouse classification system in girls with idiopathic scoliosis. *J Bone Joint Surg Am* 2008;90:540–553.

192. Parfitt AM. Misconceptions (1): epiphyseal fusion causes cessation of growth. *Bone* 2002;30:337–339.

193. Cox LA. Tanner–Whitehouse method of assessing skeletal maturity: problems and common errors. *Horm Res* 1996;45 (Suppl 2):53–55.

194. Ashizawa K, Kumakura C, Zhou X, et al. RUS skeletal maturity of children in Beijing. *Ann Hum Biol* 2005;32:316–25.

195. Ashizawa K, Asami T, Anzo M, et al. Standard RUS skeletal maturation of Tokyo children. *Ann Hum Biol* 1996;23:457–469.

196. Baughan B, Demirjian A, Levesque GY. Skeletal maturity standards for French-Canadian children of school-age with a discussion of the reliability and validity of such measures. *Hum Biol* 1979;51:353–370.

197. Beunen G, Lefevre J, Ostyn M, et al. Skeletal maturity in Belgian youths assessed by the Tanner-Whitehouse method (TW2). *Ann Hum Biol* 1990;17:355–376.

198. Dreizen S, Spirakis CN, Stone RE. A comparison of skeletal growth and maturation in undernourished and well-nourished girls before and after menarche. *J Pediatr* 1967;70:256–263.

199. Feeley BT, Ip TC, Otsuka NY. Skeletal maturity in myelomeningocele. *J Pediatr Orthop* 2003;23:718–721.

200. Freitas D, Maia J, Beunen G, et al. Skeletal maturity and socio-economic status in Portuguese children and youths: the Madeira growth study. *Ann Hum Biol* 2004;31:408–420.

201. Haavikko K, Kilpinen E. Skeletal development of Finnish children in the light of hand-wrist roentgenograms. *Proc Finn Dent Soc* 1973;69:182–190.

202. Helm S. Skeletal maturity in Danish schoolchildren assessed by the TW2 method. *Am J Phys Anthropol* 1979;51:345–352.

203. Kimura K. Skeletal maturity of the hand and wrist in Japanese children in Sapporo by the TW2 method. *Ann Hum Biol* 1977;4:449–453.

204. Lejarraga H, Guimarey L, Orazi V. Skeletal maturity of the hand and wrist of healthy Argentinian children aged 4–12 years, assessed by the TWII method. *Ann Hum Biol* 1997;24:257–261.

205. Loder RT, Estle DT, Morrison K, et al. Applicability of the Greulich and Pyle skeletal age standards to black and white children of today. *Am J Dis Child* 1993;147:1329–1333.

206. Magnusson TE. Skeletal maturation of the hand in Iceland. *Acta Odontol Scand* 1979;37:21–28.

207. Malina RM, Pena Reyes ME, Eisenmann JC, et al. Height, mass and skeletal maturity of elite Portuguese soccer players aged 11–16 years. *J Sports Sci* 2000;18:685–693.

208. Malina RM, Himes JH, Stepick CD. Skeletal maturity of the hand and wrist in Oaxaca school children. *Ann Hum Biol* 1976;3:211–219.

209. Mora S, Boechat MI, Pietka E, et al. Skeletal age determinations in children of European and African descent: applicability of the Greulich and Pyle standards. *Pediatr Res* 2001;50:624–628.

210. Prakash S, Cameron N. Skeletal maturity of well-off children in Chandigarh, North India. *Ann Hum Biol* 1981;8:175–180.

211. Rikhasor RM, Qureshi AM, Rathi SL, et al. Skeletal maturity in Pakistani children. *J Anat* 1999;195:305–308.

212. Takai S, Akiyoshi T. Skeletal maturity of Japanese children in Western Kyushu. *Am J Phys Anthropol* 1983;62:199–204.

213. Vignolo M, Naselli A, Magliano P, et al. Use of the new US90 standards for TW-RUS skeletal maturity scores in youths from the Italian population. *Horm Res* 1999;51:168–172.

214. Waldmann E, Baber FM, Field CE, et al. Skeletal maturation of Hong Kong Chinese children in the first five years of life. *Ann Hum Biol* 1977;4:343–352.

215. Weil WB Jr. Skeletal maturation in juvenile diabetes mellitus. *Pediatr Res* 1967;1:470–478.

216. Ye YY, Wang CX, Cao LZ. Skeletal maturity of the hand and wrist in Chinese children in Changsha assessed by TW2 method. *Ann Hum Biol* 1992;19:427–430.

217. Zhen OY, Baolin L. Skeletal maturity of the hand and wrist in Chinese school children in Harbin assessed by the TW2 method. *Ann Hum Biol* 1986;13:183–187.

218. Dimeglio A. Growth of the spine before age 5 years. *JPO* 1993;1: 102–107.

219. Dimeglio A. Growth in pediatric orthopaedics. *J Pediatr Orthop* 2001;21:549–555.

220. Knudtzon J, Johannessen TM. The "Large Foot" association. The size of the foot, height and age at menarche. *Tidsskr Nor Laegeforen* 1991;111:3638–3639.

221. Rao S, Joshi S, Kanade A. Growth in some physical dimensions in relation to adolescent growth spurt among rural Indian children. *Ann Hum Biol* 2000;27:127–138.

222. Ulijaszek SJ. Serum insulin-like growth factor-I, insulin-like growth factor binding protein-3, and the pubertal growth spurt in the female rhesus monkey. *Am J Phys Anthropol* 2002;118:77–85.

223. Shuttleworth FK. Sexual maturation and the physical growth of girls age six to nineteen. *Monogr Soc Res Child Dev* 1937;II, No. 4:253.

224. Bortel DT, Pritchett JW. Straight-line graphs for the prediction of growth of the upper extremities. *J Bone Joint Surg Am* 1993;75: 885–892.

225. Pritchett JW. Growth and predictions of growth in the upper extremity. *J.Bone Joint Surg Am* 1988;70:520–525.

226. Pritchett JW. Longitudinal growth and growth-plate activity in the lower extremity. *Clin Orthop Relat Res* 1992;274–279.

227. Anderson M, Green WT, Messner MB. Growth and predictions of growth in the lower extremities. *J Bone Joint Surg Am* 1963;45-A:1–14.

228. Paley D, Gelman A, Shualy MB, et al. Multiplier method for limb-length prediction in the upper extremity. *J Hand Surg (Am)* 2008;33: 385–391.

229. Lamm BM, Paley D, Kurland DB, et al. Multiplier method for predicting adult foot length. *J Pediatr Orthop* 2006;26:444–448.

230. Aguilar JA, Paley D, Paley J, et al. Clinical validation of the multiplier method for predicting limb length discrepancy and outcome of epiphysiodesis, part II. *J Pediatr Orthop* 2005;25:192–196.

231. Aguilar JA, Paley D, Paley J, et al. Clinical validation of the multiplier method for predicting limb length at maturity, part I. *J Pediatr Orthop* 2005;25:186–191.

232. Paley J, Gelman A, Paley D, et al. The prenatal multiplier method for prediction of limb length discrepancy. *Prenat Diagn* 2005;25: 435–438.

233. Paley J, Talor J, Levin A, et al. The multiplier method for prediction of adult height. *J Pediatr Orthop* 2004;24:732–737.

234. Paley D, Bhave A, Herzenberg JE, et al. Multiplier method for predicting limb-length discrepancy. *J Bone Joint Surg Am* 2000;82-A:1432–1446.

235. Charles YP, Dimeglio A, Marcoul M, et al. Volumetric thoracic growth in children with moderate and severe scoliosis compared to subjects without spinal deformity. *Stud Health Technol Inform* 2008;140: 22–28.

236. Charles YP, Dimeglio A, Marcoul M, et al. Influence of idiopathic scoliosis on three-dimensional thoracic growth. *Spine* 2008;33:1209–1218.

237. Pritchett JW. Growth and development of the distal radius and ulna. *J Pediatr Orthop* 1996;(Sep–Oct);16(5):575–577.

238. Sanders JO, Khour JG, Kishan S, et al. Predicting scoliosis progression from skeletal maturity: reliability and validity of a simplified Tanner-Whitehouse classification system in girls with idiopathic scoliosis. *J Bone Joint Surg Am* 2008;90(3):540–553.

239. Sauvegrain J, Nahum H, Bronstein H. Study of bone maturation of the elbow. *Ann Radiol (Paris)* 1962;5:542–550.

240. Campbell RM Jr, Smith MD. Thoracic insufficiency syndrome and exotic scoliosis. *J Bone Joint Surg Am* 2007;89(Suppl 1):108–122.

CHAPTER 2

José A. Morcuende
Benjamin A. Alman

Genetic Aspects of Orthopaedic Conditions

A genetic and molecular revolution is happening in medicine. Led by the Human Genome Project, genetic information and concepts are changing the way disease is defined, diagnosis is made, and treatment strategies are developed. The profound implications of actually understanding the molecular abnormalities of many clinical problems are affecting virtually all medical and surgical disciplines. Importantly, genetic technologies will increasingly drive biomedical research and the practice of medicine in the near future.

It is important for those interested in the musculoskeletal system to be aware of the genetic cause of its inherited disorders in order to make appropriate referrals for genetic counseling and to refine the prognosis and natural history in each individual patient. Current management revolves around treatment to prevent or minimize medical complications, psychosocial support of patients and their families, and modification of the environment where appropriate. Gene discoveries will allow the development of tests to detect disease or to quantify the risk of disease. Furthermore, applying this knowledge is the best hope for developing strategies to modify the pathologic effect of the gene (drug therapy) or repair the gene (gene therapy) or for approaches to restore lost or affected tissue (tissue engineering). Instead of an empiric trial-and-error approach to therapy, it may become feasible to tailor treatment to the specific molecular malfunction. No case demonstrates better this evolution than Marfan syndrome where the discovery of the mutated gene (fibrillin-1) led to a search for the pathophysiologic involvement of transforming growth factor β (TGF-β) signaling (abnormal levels of activation) and ways to treat it (with angiotensin II receptor blockers), now in clinical trials (1–3).

Given the large number of inherited musculoskeletal abnormalities and the power and speed of current genetic and developmental biology information, a few selected disorders are discussed in this chapter to illustrate specific concepts on the basic genetic concepts. It also discusses current classifications and clinical evaluation and provides a perspective about genetic counseling.

MOLECULAR BASIS OF INHERITANCE

It is estimated that there are more than 10 million living species on Earth today. Each species is different, and each reproduces itself faithfully: parent organisms hand down information specifying, in extraordinary detail, the characteristics that the offspring shall have. This phenomenon of heredity is central to the definition of life. Hereditary phenomena have been of interest to humans long before biology or genetics existed as a scientific discipline. Ancient peoples improved crops and domesticated animals by selecting desirable individuals for breeding. However, the prevailing notion at the time was that the spermatozoon and the egg contained sampling of essences from the various parts of the parental bodies and at conception, they blended together. But there were many instances in which this mode of inheritance could not explain many of the observations on heredity. As a modern discipline, genetics began in the 1860s with the work of Gregor Mendel who performed a set of experiments that pointed to the existence of biological elements that we now call genes.

Genetics is the study of genes at all levels, from molecules to populations. The discovery of genes and the understanding of their molecular structure and function have been a source of profound insight into two of the biggest mysteries of biology: what makes a species what it is and what causes variation within a species? In addition, it has exploded our understanding of human diseases, specifically genetic disorders. Genetics took a major step forward with the notion that the genes, as characterized by Mendel, are part of specific cellular structures, the chromosomes. This major concept has become known as the chromosome theory of heredity. This fusion between genetics and cell biology is still an essential part of genetic analysis today and has tremendous implications in many fields including medical genetics (4–6).

Genes encode for the amino acid sequence of the proteins that are the main determinants of the properties of an organism (and also for single catalytic or structural RNAs that do not code for proteins but are essential for RNA metabolism). Importantly, any one gene can exist in several forms (called alleles) that differ from each other, generally in small ways. Allelic variation causes hereditary variation within a species. Three fundamental properties are required of genes: (a) replication—hereditary molecules must be capable of being copied to ensure the continuation of a species from one generation to the next; (b) information storage—genes have the essential coding specifications to be translated to proteins and their by-products which constitute the building blocks of the organism; and (c) mutation—genes can change over time and this is the basis for variation within species and for evolution.

Chromosomes.

A cell's basic complement of DNA is called its genome, and it carries the information for all the proteins the organism will ever synthesize. The body cells of most animals contain two genomes, that is, they are diploid. The cells of most bacteria, algae, and fungi contain just one genome, that is, they are haploid. Interestingly, even closely related species with similar genome sizes can have very different numbers and sizes of chromosomes. Thus, there is no simple relationship between chromosome number, species complexity, and total genome size.

The genome itself is made up of extremely long molecules of DNA that are organized into chromosomes. Karyotype refers to the complement of chromosomes as visualized by cytogenetic analysis at mitosis. Human somatic cells contain two sets of 23 chromosomes, for a total of 46, referred to as euploidy. The maternal and paternal chromosomes of a pair are called homologous chromosomes (homologs). The only non-homologous chromosome pair is the sex chromosomes, where Y is inherited from the father and X from the mother (Fig. 2-1).

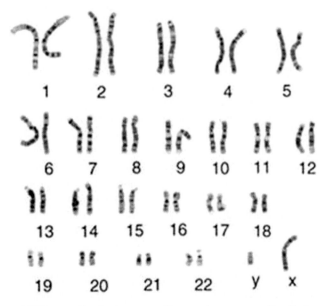

FIGURE 2-1. Banding patterns of human chromosomes. The display of the 46 human chromosomes at mitosis is called the human karyotype. Chromosomes 1 to 22 are numbered in approximate order of size. A typical human somatic cell contains two of each of these chromosomes, plus two sex chromosomes—two X chromosomes in a female and one X and one Y in a male.

Each chromosome carries a different array of genes linearly arranged along the chromosome (each gene occupies a particular position or locus); therefore, genes are present twice (one allele coming from the mother and one from the father). Alleles are truly different versions of the same basic gene. Looked at another way, gene is the generic term and allele is the specific. Allelic variation is the basis for hereditary variation and genetic disorders (7) (Fig. 2-2).

Somatic cells divide by the process of mitosis. When a cell divides, all chromosomes are replicated and each daughter cell contains the full complement of chromosomes. When a chromosome is replicated, all the genes in that chromosome are automatically copied along with it. In contrast, germ-line cells undergo meiosis during which the diploid number of 46 chromosomes is reduced to the haploid number of 23, including one of each of the autosomes and either the sex chromosome X or Y. Therefore, gametes are haploid, containing one chromosome set.

The highly programmed chromosomal movements in meiosis cause the equal segregation of alleles into the gametes. For instance, during meiosis in a heterozygote *A/a*, the chromosome carrying *A* is pulled in the opposite direction from the chromosome carrying *a*, so half the resulting gametes carry *A* and the other half carry *a*. The random assortment of each of the chromosome pairs during meiosis is central to the inheritance pattern of single-gene disorders and some forms of chromosomal derangements. In addition, gene pairs on separated chromosome assort independently at meiosis.

The force pulling the chromosomes to cell poles is generated by the nuclear spindle, a series of microtubules made of the protein tubulin. Microtubules attach to the centromeres of chromosomes by interacting with another specific set of proteins located in this area. The orchestration of these molecular interactions is complex, yet constitutes the basis of the laws of hereditary transmission in eukaryotes.

Gene Structure and DNA Replication.

We have discussed how genes are arranged in chromosomes, but to form a functional chromosome, a DNA molecule must be able to replicate and the copies must be separated and reliably partitioned into daughter cells at each cell division. This process occurs through an ordered series of stages, collectively known as cell cycle.

Approximately 30,000 genes are present in the human genome. Genes are made of linearly aligned nucleotides along the DNA molecules. DNA is a linear, double-helical structure looking rather like a molecular spiral staircase. It is composed of two intertwined chains of building blocks called nucleotides. Each of the four nucleotides is usually designated by the first letter of the base that it contains: A (adenine), G (guanine), C (cytosine), or T (thymine). The nucleotides are connected to each other at the 3' and 5' position; hence each DNA chain is said to have a polarity and each chain runs in the opposite direction, that is, the chains are said to be antiparallel. The two nucleotide chains are held together by hydrogen bonds between the nucleotide bases. The bases that form base pairs (A-T and G-C) are said to be complementary.

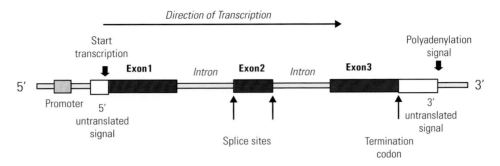

FIGURE 2-2. Generalized structure of a human gene. This example has three exons (coding sequences) and two introns. Note the promoter as the regulatory site for initiation of transcription, the splice sites and termination codon used for mRNA processing. RNA splicing regulation can generate different versions of a protein in different cell types.

The biological role of most genes is to carry or encode information on the composition of proteins. The protein composition, together with the timing and amount of production of each protein, is an extremely important determinant of the structure and physiology of the organism. Each gene is responsible for coding for one specific protein or a part of a protein. In all cells, the expression of individual genes is regulated: instead if manufacturing its full repertoire of possible proteins at full tilt all the time, the cell adjusts the rate of individual gene transcription and translation independently, according to need and the environment (Fig. 2-3). Regulation of gene expression determines the unique biologic qualities of each cell or its phenotype.

Structurally, a typical gene, defined as a segment of DNA that specifies a functional RNA, is composed of (a) a regulatory region called promoter to which various proteins bind, causing the gene to be transcribed at the right time and in the right amount; (b) a region at the end containing sequences encoding the termination of transcription; and (c) the coding region, which is divided into smaller pieces called exons that are separated by noncoding regions called introns (whose function is still unclear). Each set of three nucleotides in the coding region of the exons is called a codon, and the sequence of codons specifies the amino acid composition and order in the protein.

Transcription and Ribonucleic Acid Processing.
The first step taken by the cell to make a protein is to copy, or transcribe, the information encoded in the DNA of the gene as a related but single-stranded molecule called RNA. This primary RNA copy made from the gene is called a primary transcript and represents a "working copy" of the gene. Whereas the cell's genetic information archive in the form of DNA is fixed and sacrosanct, the RNA transcripts are mass-produced and disposable. Thus, the primary role of the transcripts is to serve as intermediaries in the transfer of genetic information: they serve as messenger RNA (mRNA) to guide the synthesis of proteins according to the genetic instructions stored in the DNA.

The primary RNA contains both introns and exons; therefore, to make it functional, it needs to be further processed. After the introns are spliced out (RNA splicing), the remaining exons form the protein-encoding continuous sequence called mRNA. This mRNA molecule is transposed

from the nucleus to the cytoplasm where it will be translated to protein by the ribosome machinery. These processing steps can critically change the "meaning" of an RNA molecule and are therefore crucial for understanding how eukaryotic cells read the genome. Interestingly, a cell can splice the primary RNA in different ways and thereby make different chains for the same gene—a process called alternative RNA splicing. It is estimated that at least one-third of the human genes produce multiple proteins this way. When different splicing possibilities exist at several positions in the transcript, a single gene can produce dozens of different proteins. Furthermore, the regulation of RNA splicing can generate different versions of a protein in different cell types, according to needs of the cell. Finally, there is also the mechanism of RNA editing which alters the nucleotide sequences of mRNA transcripts once they are transcribed.

Some protein-encoding genes are transcribed more or less constantly; they are the "housekeeping" genes that are always needed for basic cellular functions. Other genes may be rendered unreadable or readable to suit the cellular functions at particular moments and under particular external conditions. Regulation of gene expression is thought to be at multiple levels, although control of the initiation of transcription

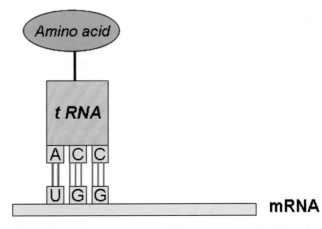

FIGURE 2-3. The process of translation converts genetic information into amino acid sequence. This process takes place on the ribosomes, and each amino acid is brought to the ribosome by a specific tRNA molecule docking at a specific codon of the mRNA.

(transcriptional control) usually predominates. Some genes, however, are transcribed at constant level and turned on and off solely by posttranscriptional regulatory processes. Most of these control process require the recognition of specific sequences or structures in the RNA molecule being regulated. This recognition is accomplished by either a regulatory protein or a regulatory RNA molecule.

Translation. The process of reading the genetic information of the mRNA sequence and converting it into an amino acid sequence is called translation (rather like converting one language (genotype) into another (phenotype). This process takes place on the ribosomes and each amino acid is brought to the ribosome by a specific transfer RNA (tRNA) molecule that docks at a specific codon of the mRNA. The ribosome is a giant multimolecular machine formed of two main chains of RNA, called ribosomal RNA (rRNA), and more than 50 different proteins. Mechanistically, a ribosome attaches to the 5' end of an mRNA molecule and moves along the mRNA, catalyzing the assembly of the string of amino acids that will constitute the primary structure of the protein. The first codon of the coding sequence is methionine, and the primary chain is called a polypeptide. At the end of the mRNA, a termination codon causes the ribosome to detach and recycle to another mRNA. Trains of ribosomes pass along an mRNA molecule, each member making the same type of polypeptide.

Protein Assembly. There are four levels of organization in the structure of a protein. The amino acid sequence is known as the primary structure of the protein. Stretches of polypeptide chain that form α helices and β sheets constitute the secondary structure. The full tridimensional organization is referred as the tertiary structure. Finally, when a protein is formed as a complex of more than one polypeptide chain, the complete structure is designated the quaternary structure (with each polypeptide chain called a protein subunit).

Studies of the conformation, function, and evolution of proteins have revealed a unit of central importance distinct from the previously described organization. This is the protein domain. This is a substructure produced by any part of a polypeptide chain that folds independently into a compact, stable structure. The different protein domains are often associated with different functions.

Proteins are important either as structural components—such as collagen for bone and cartilage—or as active agents in cellular processes, for example, enzymes and active transport proteins. In addition, many proteins undergo numerous posttranslational modifications such as terminal excisions or enzymatic modifications adding sugars, or are assembled into complex polymers.

Interestingly, the synthesis of proteins encoded by genes on the mitochondria takes place on ribosomes inside the organelles themselves. Therefore, the proteins in mitochondria are of two different origins: either encoded in the nucleus and imported into the organelle or encoded in the organelle and synthesized within the organelle compartment. This fact

is important since some genetic disorders are now recognized originating in mutations of these mitochondrial genes.

MOLECULAR BASIS OF MUTATIONS

As discussed before, the mechanisms that maintain DNA sequences are remarkably precise, but they are not perfect. With a few exceptions, cells do not have specialized mechanisms for creating changes in the structures of their genomes: changes depend instead on accidents and mistakes. Errors in DNA replication, DNA recombination, or DNA repair can lead to either simple changes in DNA sequence or to large-scale genome rearrangements.

In medical genetics, mutation is the process whereby genes change from one allelic form to another. Mutations can lead to loss of function or to a new function of the gene. Genes mutate randomly, at any time and in any cell of an organism. Mutations in germ-line cells can be transmitted to progeny, but somatic mutations cannot. Mutations can be passed from generation to generation, following mendelian inheritance, or they can represent new mutations (sporadic mutations) that occur in the sperm or egg of the parents or in the embryo.

Geneticists recognize two different levels at which mutation takes place. In gene mutation, an allele of a gene changes, becoming a different allele. Nowadays, point mutations typically refer to alterations of single base pairs of DNA or to a small number of adjacent base pairs. At the other level of hereditary change—chromosomal mutation—segments of chromosomes, whole chromosomes, or even entire sets of chromosomes change. The effects of chromosome mutations are due to the new arrangements of chromosomes and of the genes that they contain.

Single-Gene Mutations. Point mutations are classified in molecular terms, and these nucleotide substitutions can result in several molecular outcomes. Although point mutations are often considered to occur randomly, there are mutational hot spots in the genome, commonly at CG dinucleotides, and mutations tend to recur at such sites. *Transitions*, which exchange one pyrimidine for the other or one purine for the other, are more common than *transversions*, which exchange one pyrimidine for a purine or vice versa. These substitutions can result in several molecular outcomes:

- Missense mutations occur when a single nucleotide substitution alters the sense of a codon and a different amino acid is added during protein synthesis.
- Nonsense mutations occur when a single nucleotide substitution convert a codon for an amino acid into a termination codon. This change results in the premature termination of translation and a truncated polypeptide.
- Promoter mutations alter the transcription of the gene or generate instability of the mRNA, thereby reducing the production of the relevant protein.
- mRNA splicing mutations occur in the consensus sequences at the exon–intron boundaries resulting in the adjacent

exon to be spliced out and therefore, a shortened protein chain. In addition, abnormal splicing can also occur when a point mutation create a new or cryptic splice site with complex consequences because splicing may remove part of an exon and include intron sequences.

- Frame-shift mutations result from any addition or deletion of base pairs that is not a multiple of 3 changing the reading frame of the DNA resulting in different amino acids from that point on and frequently chain termination.

Finally, it is important to mention *single nucleotide polymorphisms* (SNPs). These are simply points in the genome sequence where one large fraction of the population has one nucleotide, while the other has another. While most of the SNPs and other common variations in the human genome sequence are thought to have no effect on phenotype, a subset of them must be responsible for nearly all of the heritable aspects of human individuality. A major challenge in human genetics is to learn to recognize those relatively few variations that are functionally important (i.e., contribute to genetic disorders) against the large background of neutral variation that distinguishes the genomes of any two human beings. Genome-wide associations studies (GWAS) looking at millions of SNPs are designed to assess these contributions.

Chromosomal Mutations. Chromosomal abnormalities are more frequent than all the single disorders together and result from disruptions in the normal number or the structure of the chromosomes (7, 8). An abnormal chromosome number, called aneuploidy, occurs in approximately 4% of pregnancies. Tetraploidy refers to four copies of the full set of chromosomes (for a total of 92), triploidy to three copies (69 chromosomes), trisomy to one chromosome pair having an extra chromosome (47 chromosomes), and monosomy to one chromosome of one pair being absent (45 chromosomes). Finally, unipaternal disomy refers to the concept that individuals have cells that contain two chromosomes of a particular type that have been inherited from only one parent. Isodisomy exists when one chromosome is duplicated, and heterodisomy when both homologs have been inherited form one parent.

Abnormalities in the chromosomal structure occur less frequently than numerical abnormalities. These abnormalities are called balanced if the chromosome set has the normal complement of DNA and unbalanced if there is additional or missing DNA. Balanced rearrangements do not usually have a phenotypic effect because all of the genetic information is present, but arranged differently. However, these rearrangements can disrupt a gene at the site of the break resulting in that specific gene dysfunction. Unbalanced rearrangements alter the normal amount of genetic information and commonly result in an abnormal phenotype. The basic molecular mechanisms resulting in structural chromosomal abnormalities include *deletion* (a section of the chromosome is absent); *duplication* (an extra section of the chromosome is present); *translocation* (a portion of a chromosome is exchanged with a portion of another chromosome); and *inversion* (a broken portion of a chromosome reattaches to the same chromosome in the same location, but in a reverse direction).

PATTERNS OF INHERITANCE IN MEDICAL GENETICS

In the study of genetic disorders, four mendelian patterns of inheritance are distinguishable by pedigree analysis: autosomal dominant, autosomal recessive, X-linked dominant, and X-linked recessive (9, 10). In addition, there are several other forms of inheritance that do not follow the inheritance laws of Mendel. These include mutations in mitochondrial DNA, trinucleotide repeats, mosaicism, genomic imprinting, and uniparental disomy.

Autosomal Disorders

Autosomal Dominant. In these conditions, the gene mutation is located in one of the autosomal chromosomes. The affected phenotype of an autosomal dominant disorder is determined by a dominant allele, that is, the mutation in one of the alleles is sufficient to express the phenotype. In pedigree analysis, the main clues are that the phenotype tends to appear in every generation and that affected fathers and mothers transmit the phenotype to both sons and daughters. This equal representation of both sexes among the affected individuals rules out X-linked inheritance. People bearing one copy of the A allele (*A/a*) are much more common than those bearing two copies (*A/A*) (which could be lethal in some cases), so most affected individuals are heterozygous. The homozygotes are usually much more severely affected than heterozygotes, often resulting in perinatal death (Fig. 2-4).

These disorders appear in every generation because the abnormal allele of the affected individual must have come from one of the parents in the preceding generation. However, abnormal alleles can arise *de novo* by the process of spontaneous mutation, so this fact has to be kept in mind when analyzing the type of inheritance in that family and for genetic counseling.

Many autosomal dominant disorders have major musculoskeletal anomalies. These disorders include many chondrodysplasias, osteogenesis imperfecta, Marfan syndrome, Ehlers-Danlos syndrome, Charcot-Marie-Tooth disease types IA and IB, and neurofibromatosis 1.

Autosomal Recessive. The affected phenotype of an autosomal recessive disorder is determined by a recessive allele, and the corresponding unaffected phenotype is determined by a dominant allele. For the phenotype to be expressed, the individual has to have both alleles mutated (*a/a*). The presence of an A allele is enough for not expressing the phenotype. The two key points for an autosomal recessive disorder are that (a) generally the disease appears in the progeny of unaffected parents and (b) the affected progeny include both males and females. When we know that both male and female children are affected, we can assume that we are dealing with simple mendelian inheritance, not sex-linked inheritance.

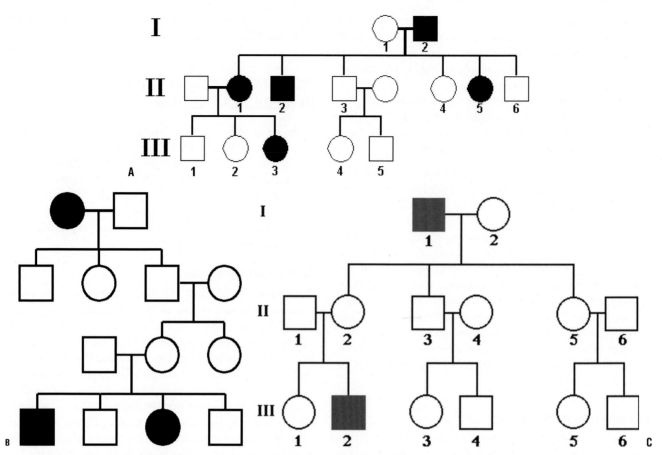

FIGURE 2-4. Pedigree of an autosomal dominant disorder. **A:** Note affected individuals in every generation and both males and females transmit the disorder to both sons and daughters. **B:** Note the disorder appears in the progeny of unaffected parents and the affected progeny include both males and females. **C:** Note that none of the male offspring of an affected male are affected, nor will they pass the condition to their offspring (lack of male-to-male transmission). This is due to the fact that a son obtains his Y chromosome from his father, so he cannot normally inherit the father's X chromosome. On the other hand, all the daughters of an affected male are "carriers" bearing the recessive allele masked in the heterozygous condition (X/x), so half of their sons will be affected.

The pedigrees of autosomal recessive disorders tend to look rather bare, with few black symbols representing affected individuals. In general, a recessive condition shows up in groups of affected siblings, and the people in earlier and later generations tend not to be affected. This is due to the fact that if the condition is rare, most people do not carry the abnormal allele, and those who do are heterozygous (A/a for example) for it rather than homozygous (A/A). The basic reason that heterozygous are much more common than homozygous is that, to be recessive homozygote, both parents must have had the a allele, but, to be heterozygote, only one parent must carry the a allele. The clinically normal parents are called *carriers*. Carrier frequency varies considerably but, for common autosomal recessive disorders, it is approximately 1 in 45 individuals. Autosomal recessive traits are more frequent in consanguineous marriages, particularly if the mutant gene is rare.

X-Linked Disorders. These disorders are readily identified by their characteristic pattern of inheritance. Men have

only one X chromosome, so they are hemizygous. Women (who have two X chromosomes) can be homozygous affected or unaffected, or heterozygous. But importantly, heterozygous women show variable expression of X-linked disorders because of the normal, random inactivation of one of the X chromosomes in the somatic cells (therefore, silencing all the genes in that chromosome). This phenomenon occurs very early in development (16- to 64-cell stage embryogenesis) and either the paternal or maternal X chromosome is inactivated. This specific X chromosomal inactivation will be then transmitted to all of the daughter cells from each inactivated cell. As a result, the somatic cells of women are *mosaic*, with some cells expressing the paternal X chromosome and others the maternal X chromosome. X-linked disorders are classified as dominant, recessive, and atypical form of inheritance.

X-Linked Dominant. Since males are hemizygous for X-linked genes (they only have one X chromosome), affected males pass the condition to all their daughters, but none of their sons. Affected women transmit the mutation in a manner similar to an autosomal dominant trait because they have a pair of X chromosomes. As a result, affected women transmit the mutation to half of their children, regardless of gender. Importantly, affected women demonstrate less severe phenotype because of the random X chromosome inactivation; therefore, the expression depends upon the ratio of cells that express the mutant allele.

X-Linked Recessive.
In these disorders, none of the male offspring of an affected male are affected, nor will they pass the condition to their offspring (lack of male-to-male transmission). This is due to the fact that a son obtains his Y chromosome from his father, so he cannot normally inherit the father's X chromosome. On the other hand, all the daughters of an affected male are "carriers" bearing the recessive allele masked in the heterozygous condition (*X/x*), so half of their sons will be affected.

Atypical X-Linked Disorders.
An example of such a disorder is Fragile X Syndrome. This disorder is characterized by learning disabilities or mild mental retardation. It is also characterized by marfanoid appearance, lax joints, and macroorchidism. Females can be affected, but the phenotype is usually milder. The characteristic molecular abnormality is a failure of condensation of the chromatin during mitosis at position Xq27.3. This defect is attributable to an amplification of a region containing a variable CGG trinucleotide repeat in the 5′ untranslated region of the FMR1 gene (11). Expression of the FMR1 gene is deficient in affected men. More importantly, expansion of permutation to full mutations occurs only after passage through the maternal germ line where expansion of the repeats occurs.

Modifiers of Single-Gene Inheritance.
Although it is possible by genetic analysis to isolate a single gene whose alleles dictate alternative phenotypes for one character, this gene does not control that character by itself; the gene must interact with many other genes in the genome. For many genetic diseases, no matter the type of inheritance as described above, there is little detailed knowledge of the critical factors that link genotype to phenotype. Thus, some affected individuals show minimal abnormalities and others show severe changes. Therefore, other genetic and/or environmental factors must modify the expression of the genotype.

Several definitions are important when analyzing a genetic disorder. *Incomplete dominance* describes the general situation in which the phenotype of a heterozygote is intermediate between the two homozygotes on some quantitative scale of measurement. *Penetrance* of a gene can be defined as the proportion of individuals in which the mutation is appropriately expressed, that is, the gene defect has a phenotypic expression. *Expressivity* refers to the severity of the phenotype among individuals who have the same genotype. For example, patients with Marfan syndrome may have few or all the classic features of the condition. *Pleiotropy* refers to the diverse phenotypic effects of a mutated gene in different tissues.

Other Patterns of Single-Gene Inheritance.
Most single-gene disorders are inherited in accordance to the mendelian laws. However, alternative modes of inheritance have been identified in humans (11–13). These modes include mutations in mitochondrial DNA, trinucleotide repeats, mosaicism, genomic imprinting, and uniparental disomy.

Some neuromuscular and ocular diseases are caused by mutations in the mitochondrial, rather than in the nuclear DNA. In a human cell, the mitochondrial genome consists of 16,569 nucleotide pairs that code for 13 proteins, 2 ribosomal RNA components, and 22 tRNAs. They are inherited from the mother because mitochondria are transmitted in the ovum, not in the sperm. As a result, women transmit their mitochondrial DNA to all their children, but men do not.

Trinucleotide repeats refer to the concept of a molecular mutation characterized based upon the presence of unstable and abnormal expansions of DNA triplets (trinucleotides). This repeats can affect the protein-coding or no-coding regions and result in translation of a series of uninterrupted residues that affect protein function. Importantly, trinucleotide repeat disorders generally show genetic *anticipation*, where their severity increases with each successive generation that inherits them, likely explained by the addition of further repeats in the gene of the progeny of affected individuals.

Mosaicism refers to mutations that result in cell clones that are genetically different from the original zygote. Such individuals are said to be mosaic. Mosaicism can be somatic, gonadal, or both. Because the members of a clone tend to stay close to one another during development, an observable outcome of a somatic mutation is often a patch of phenotypically mutant cells called a mutant sector. The earlier the mutation event in development, the larger the mutant sector will be.

Genomic imprinting refers to the concept that certain genes are marked, or imprinted, in such a way that they are expressed differently when they are inherited from the father than when they are inherited from the mother. Imprinting often involves differences in DNA methylation that alters the transcriptional regulation of the derived genes.

GENETIC BASIS OF ORTHOPAEDIC DISORDERS

The vertebrate skeleton is a fascinating and complex organ system, composed of 206 bones with many different shapes and sizes. Like every other organ system, the skeleton has specific developmental and functional characteristics that define its identity in biologic and pathologic terms. For normal skeletogenesis to take place, the coordination of temporal and spatial gene expression patterns is a crucial prerequisite. Any disturbances in these processes will lead to abnormalities of the skeleton.

The vertebrate skeleton is formed by mesenchymal cells condensing into tissue elements outlining the pattern of future bones (the patterning phase). Shortly thereafter, cells within these condensations differentiate along the chondrocytic pathway. Subsequent growth generates cartilage models (anlagen) of the future bones. The cartilage anlagen will be replaced by bone and bone marrow in a process called endochondral ossification. Finally, a process of growth and remodeling will result in a skeleton that is well adapted to its function as an organ not only for movement and internal organ protection, but also for blood cell production and regulation of calcium homeostasis (discussed in depth in Chapter 1).

Mutations in early patterning genes cause disorders called dysostoses: these affect only specific skeletal elements, leaving the rest of the skeleton largely unaffected. In contrast, mutations in genes that are involved primarily in cell differentiation cause disorders called osteochondrodysplasias, which affect the development and growth of most skeletal elements in a generalized fashion. Many genes have important functions in both of these processes so that some inherited disorders can display features of both dysostoses and osteochondrodysplasias. Genes used during skeletal development may also be important in other organs, so when mutated, the resulting skeletal defects are part of a syndrome.

Disease-Gene Detection Strategies.

There have been tremendous advances in the past 50 years identifying the causative genetic defect for many of the disorders that are treated by pediatric orthopaedists. These efforts utilize several approaches. At the chromosomal level, the region of the chromosome containing the disease gene may be revealed by cytogenetic analysis. Translocations may disrupt a gene and can therefore produce the disease, and a microdeletion may indicate loss of contiguous genes. Translocations, which are common in many tumors, may interrupt and inactivate a gene or may result in the fusion of two genes, which then produce a new fusion protein. The study of contiguous gene deletion syndromes has enabled researchers to associate these genes with specific phenotypes. An example is the deletion of the *EXT1* gene that produces multiple exostoses in children with the contiguous gene deletion Langer-Giedion syndrome.

In some diseases, candidate genes are selected and tested for their association with the disease. For example, the type I collagen genes were the candidate genes in osteogenesis imperfecta because type I collagen is found in all of the major tissues affected by the disease. Mutational analyses can then be undertaken to determine the genotypes and the genotype/phenotype relations.

Genetic linkage analysis is the traditional approach used for identifying a disease gene in humans when no likely candidate genes can be postulated or where candidate gene screening has not revealed any anomalies. Linkage analysis is based on determining whether genetic markers or polymorphisms, either within or flanking the candidate gene, are coinherited with the disease phenotype in families. Large families are usually needed for such studies, and careful evaluation is needed in classifying individuals as phenotypically affected or unaffected. Phenotypic ascertainment can be straightforward, as in classical Ehlers-Danlos syndrome type I, in which symptoms

include skin scars, skin laxity, and generalized joint instability. The syndrome is fully penetrant, in that all individuals bearing the mutant allele show the clinical phenotype. The skin and joints are obviously abnormal at all ages and in both sexes although the severity of the skin scarring worsens with age. In contrast, it may be difficult in the case of other genetic disorders to clinically determine whether asymptomatic individuals bear the mutant allele or not. This difficulty may be due to low penetrance, variable expressivity, age, and gender. Such difficulties are likely to account for the lack of progress in identifying genes for common conditions such as idiopathic scoliosis, clubfoot, and developmental dysplasia of the hip (14, 15).

Microarrays, or "DNA chips," contain arrays of short DNA sequences from all human genes that can also be used to narrow the list of candidate genes that are expressed in the tissues of interest. Also, newer generation sequencing techniques are in development that makes it possible to do whole genome sequencing, providing a high-throughput method to identify genetic abnormalities (16).

Mouse genetic studies are an integral part of the successful identification of disease genes and their function in humans. There are many examples of mouse models of human diseases and even fruit fly models of human diseases. Some of these models were the result of spontaneous mutations, whereas others were produced by targeted mutations or inactivation of genes of interest. Genetic studies of mice are valuable in establishing whether a putative missense mutation identified in humans is a cause of a given phenotype.

Significant progress is being made in identifying the genes involved in multigene or multifactorial disorders of the musculoskeletal system, for example, in degenerative arthritis, intervertebral disk disease, and osteoporosis. The latter studies provide new insights into the etiologies of these disorders and show that some of the multifactorial disorders are part of larger disease families. For example, some mutations of the type IX collagen genes cause multiple epiphyseal dysplasia, whereas other sequence variants predispose adults to the development of degenerative intervertebral disk disease. It is likely that close links will be established between many of the rare single-gene disorders and the common multigene disorders of the musculoskeletal system.

Classification of Musculoskeletal Disorders.

Broadly defined, birth defects or congenital abnormalities occur in 6% of all live births. Twenty percent of infant deaths are due to congenital anomalies. About 3% of newborns have significant structural abnormalities. At present, the cause of approximately 50% to 60% of birth defects is unknown. Chromosomal abnormalities account for 6% to 7% of the abnormalities. Specific gene mutations cause 7% to 8%. Environmental teratogens are responsible for 7% to 10% of defects. Combined genetic predisposition with environmental factors causes the remaining 20% to 25% of congenital abnormalities (7–9).

Genetic disorders of the skeleton comprise a large group of clinically distinct and genetically heterogeneous conditions comprising more than 150 forms. Although individually rare, the different forms add to produce a significant number of affected individuals, with significant morbidity. Clinical manifestations range from neonatal lethality to congenital malformations of the spine and limbs, to only mild growth retardation. Importantly, secondary complications such as early degenerative joint disease and extra-skeletal organ involvement add to the burden of the disease.

Their clinical diversity makes these disorders often difficult to diagnose, and many attempts have been made to delineate single entities or groups of diseases to facilitate the diagnosis. Traditionally, skeletal disorders have been subdivided into dysostoses, defined as malformations of individual bones or groups of bones, and osteochondrodysplasias, defined as developmental disorders of cartilage and bone. The criteria used for their distinction has been based on a combination of clinical, radiographic, morphologic, and, in a few instances, biochemical characteristics. The modes of genetic inheritance and extra skeletal abnormalities have also been used.

Over the past 10 years, we have progressed from this initial broad clinical classification to the present reconsideration and regrouping of the disorders according to their genetic molecular pathogenesis. The International Working Group on the Classification of Constitutional Disorders of Bone updated the classification in 2001 (17). The major change was the addition of genetically determined dysostoses to the skeletal dysplasias. However, it is now becoming increasingly clear that several distinctive classifications are needed that reflect, on the one hand, the molecular pathology, and, on the other, the clinical signs and symptoms. Several reviews of the rapidly changing molecular basis of the skeletal dysplasias have been published, focusing on a molecular-pathogenetic classification, on more specific aspects such as transcriptional deregulation, or on a combination of molecular pathology and developmental biology of the musculoskeletal system. These new concepts directly link the clinical phenotype to key cellular processes of skeletal biology, and should assist in providing a framework accessible to clinicians as well as basic scientists for future understanding of these disorders. It is likely that future insights will lead to reclassification.

With this regard, the "Nomenclature and Classification of the Osteochondrodysplasias," now called "Nosology," has been recently revised to reflect the molecular and pathogenetic abnormalities underlying these disorders. This classification uses similar criteria to those of the functional classification proposed in the 8th edition of *The Metabolic and Molecular Bases of Inherited Disease* (18).

There are numerous online services that allow access to public information and services relevant to the genetics of musculoskeletal disorders. One database that contains a wealth of clinical and genetic data is the Online mendelian Inheritance in Man (OMIM) (10). It provides free text overviews of genetic disorders and gene loci, with the correspondent mouse correlate. In general, congenital abnormalities of non-mendelian inheritance, chromosomal abnormalities, single case reports are not included. The total number of entries exceeds 11,000, but most importantly, it is linked to a wealth of other genetic databases allowing the users to obtain information on gene structure, map location, function, phenotype, literature references, etc. It is found at http://www3.ncbi.nlm.nih.gov/omim/ (10).

The logical extension of the recent success in the field of skeletal dysplasias is to establish precisely what the products of the affected genes do during skeletal development and how mutations disturb these functions to produce the characteristic phenotype. Despite the many hypotheses generated from the work in human genetics and the knowledge that has been gained from animal models, there remains a relatively poor understanding of how these genes interfere with skeletal development. Unraveling this mysteries and defining it in molecular and cellular terms will be the challenge for the near future.

Prenatal and Postnatal Clinical Evaluation. With the increased availability of ultrasonographic prenatal screening, more patients with skeletal dysplasias are being diagnosed before birth. When there is suspicion of a skeletal dysplasia on ultrasound, the femoral length is the best biometric parameter. Further testing may be performed, if indicated, by chorionic villous sampling and mutation analysis.

Most skeletal dysplasias result in short stature, defined as height more than two standard deviations below the mean for the population at a given age. The resultant growth disproportion is commonly referred to as "short trunk" or "short limb." The short-limb types are further subdivided into categories based on the segment of the limb that is affected. Rhizomelic refers to shortening of the proximal part of the limb, mesomelic to the middle segment, and acromelic to the distal segment.

In evaluating a patient with short stature or abnormal bone development, several aspects of the medical history and the physical exam should be investigated. A history of heart disease, respiratory difficulty, immune deficiency, precocious puberty, and malabsorption should be sought since they are associated with some of these disorders. Birth length, head circumference, and weight should be recorded, and pertinent family history of short stature or dimorphism should be sought. The height and weight percentile should be determined using standard charts. The physical examination should include careful characterization of the patient faces, and presence of cleft palate, abnormal teeth, position of the ears, and extremity malformations. A thorough neurological evaluation is needed because of the frequent incidence of spinal compromise in many of these syndromes.

Following the history and physical examination, radiographs are used to identify the area of bone involvement. The so-called skeletal survey may vary from institution to institution, but it should include the following views: skull

(AP and lateral); thoracolumbar spine (AP and lateral); chest; pelvis; one upper limb; one lower limb; and left hand. Flexion–extension views of the cervical spine should be ordered if instability is suspected. In some instances, imaging of other family members suspected of having the same condition may be helpful.

Laboratory tests may include calcium, phosphate, alkaline phosphatase, serum thyroxin, and protein to rule out metabolic disorders. Urine should be checked for storage products if a progressive disorder is found. Referral to a pediatric geneticist is often very helpful in reaching a diagnosis in complex cases, in providing genetic counseling to the family, and in managing the many medical problems associated with these disorders.

Genetic Counseling. The care of children with genetic disorder involves multiple specialists, including genetic specialists. Discussions about the risk of subsequent pregnancies are in the realm of the genetic counselor (19, 20). While parents often assume that if the condition has a name, it is treatable or curable, this sadly is not the case. The importance of understanding the genetic etiology is in recognizing associated medical abnormalities that may be life threatening, adversely influence orthopaedic outcomes, or influence surgical timing and management. Importantly, patients can come to significant harm if an orthopaedist misses recognizing a syndrome. For instance, in the case of Marfan syndrome, starting a child on beta-blockers can prevent a catastrophic cardiovascular event. Even if parents are not planning subsequent pregnancies, and if there are no plans for their child to undergo surgery in the near future, genetic evaluation is still important for proper diagnosis. Correct diagnoses are essential for research into syndrome etiology and treatment. Patients should be given the opportunity to participate in such research, especially in cases of relatively rare syndromes. For instance, recent work on better classifying congenital spinal abnormalities has led the way to the determination of underlying genetic causes (21).

Indications for Genetic Counseling. Whenever there is thought to be an increased risk of a child being born with a birth defect, formal genetic counseling is called for. An orthopaedists should not be ordering genetic tests on their own, but with the help of a geneticist. Indeed, such genetic tests are relatively expensive, and as such should only be ordered to confirm one of a handful of conditions in a differential diagnosis, and at the present time, such tests are generally confirmatory (22). Appropriate genetic counseling requires diagnostic precision and knowledge of the recurrence risk, the burden of the disorder, and the reproductive options. There are several indications for genetic counseling:

- The couple has had a stillbirth or multiple miscarriages.
- The couple already has a child with a birth defect.
- The couple already has a child with mental retardation.
- There is a family history of any of the problems mentioned in preceding text.

- The couple has relatives with known genetically transmittable diseases, such as muscular dystrophy.
- The mother has been exposed to radiation, drugs, or infections during pregnancy.
- The mother is of an advanced age.
- The parents are consanguineously related.
- There are chromosomal translocations.

Diagnostic Precision. The most important element in counseling is establishing the correct diagnosis. A precise diagnosis cannot be made for about half of children who present with mental retardation or dysmorphic features. However, there is a large amount of empiric data that can be used for counseling in this group.

Estimation of Recurrence Risk. After diagnostic evaluation, an estimate of the recurrence risk is made. This is a numeric estimate of the likelihood of a particular disorder occurring in subsequent children, such as a one in four risk of an autosomal recessive disorder and a one in two risk of an autosomal dominant disorder. The recurrence risk for multifactorial disorders, after a single affected child, is approximately 3% to 5%.

Another aspect of risk is the background level of risk for major birth defects. Approximately 1 in 25 children is born with a major defect. In this setting, risks of 1 in 2 and 1 in 4 are high, and risks of 1 in 100 are low.

Burden of Genetic Diseases. The burden of genetic diseases is important in genetic counseling. Clinodactyly is a common autosomal dominant condition with a high recurrence risk of one in two, although it has minimal or no burden to those who have the condition. Clubfeet and congenital dislocation of the hip are multifactorial diseases with lower risks of recurrence. The potential burden of these conditions is minimized by early diagnosis and treatment. In contrast, the burden of additional children with Duchenne muscular dystrophy, severe osteogenesis imperfecta, or severe chondrodysplasia is considerable because there are no curative treatments available.

Prenatal Diagnosis. Prenatal diagnosis is used more selectively but is being offered to an increasing number of families as the number of diseases that can be detected in early pregnancy increases. The most common indication is a maternal age of 35 years or older. The indications for prenatal diagnosis are shown in the following list (19, 20):

- The mother is of advanced age (older than 35 years).
- There is a known chromosomal anomaly in one parent or in a previous pregnancy.
- There has previously been a neural tube defect, or there is a high serum level of α-fetoprotein or a neural tube defect is suspected from ultrasound results.
- There is a family history of disorders detectable by biochemical or DNA technology; these include Duchenne

and Becker muscular dystrophy, myotonic dystrophy, hemoglobinopathies, hemophilia A or B, Huntington disease, cystic fibrosis, and other rare detectable genetic diseases.

In most instances, prenatal diagnosis does not reveal an abnormality, thereby providing reassurance to the parents. Because of the availability of prenatal diagnosis, more families are willing to have children, instead of refraining from having them for fear of birth defects.

Serum α-Fetoprotein Screening. A fetal protein produced by the yolk sac and liver, α-fetoprotein reaches a peak in fetal serum at approximately 13 weeks of gestation and decreases thereafter. Amniotic levels of this protein are high in the fetus with a lesion that is not covered by skin, such as open spina bifida, anencephaly, and exomphalos. The protein leaks into the amniotic fluid and into the maternal circulation. An increased maternal serum level of α-fetoprotein is not diagnostic of open spina bifida but is an indication for further investigation. Abnormally high levels also occur in cases of fetal death, cystic hygroma, polycystic kidneys, and Turner syndrome.

Ultrasound Screening. Real-time ultrasonography is used for visualizing the fetus and fetal movements. Ultrasonography is commonly undertaken to determine gestational age. However, more extensive studies by experienced ultrasonographers are required when examining for fetal abnormalities in at-risk pregnancies. Such examinations are increasingly being undertaken as screening investigations in all pregnancies, but they have an error rate for detecting skeletal abnormalities of roughly 20% (27).

Amniocentesis and Chorionic Villus Sampling. Ultrasound-guided amniocentesis is a relatively safe procedure when undertaken at 16 weeks of gestation. The risk of fetal loss is approximately 0.5% to 1%. The amniotic fluid is most often used for determination of α-fetoprotein levels. The amniotic cells are used for karyotype analysis for the determination of enzyme levels in cases of inborn errors of metabolism and for DNA diagnosis using direct detection of a previously defined mutation, or indirect detection using polymorphisms. Chorionic villus sampling can be undertaken between 9 and 11 weeks of gestation; it allows earlier diagnosis of many genetic diseases and offers the option of first-trimester termination of pregnancy. The risk of fetal loss because of the procedure itself is approximately 4%.

Counseling. Families at risk for genetic diseases and birth defects should seek counseling before the mother becomes pregnant. This approach ensures that there is sufficient time to establish the diagnosis, recurrence risk, burden of the disorder, reproductive alternatives, and suitability for prenatal diagnosis. These options may be limited when counseling is sought during the pregnancy. Parents must be fully informed about the risks of investigational procedures and anticipated

delays in receiving test results, and they must be given all test results and appropriate explanations about the implications of those results. Although genetic testing may reveal that the fetus bears a disease mutation, it is difficult to predict the severity of the phenotype. Parents require much support at this difficult time, and they alone are responsible for the decision about whether to terminate a pregnancy. Parents may not wish to terminate a pregnancy but may use the prenatal diagnostic results to plan the most appropriate method of delivery of the baby. For example, prenatal diagnosis of mild osteogenesis imperfecta (type IA) may be sought in order to determine whether to use vaginal or cesarean delivery. If the fetus is affected, the parents may choose cesarean delivery in order to reduce the likelihood of a birth fracture from a vaginal delivery.

It is increasingly common that parents will come to see an orthopaedic surgeon during this process. They usually come to discuss the implications and treatment options of a potential condition. It is important that accurate information be given to the parent, both about the range of problems a child with such an abnormality might have, and about issues related to diagnostic accuracy and treatment. For instance, ultrasound alone may have an up to 20% error in making a diagnosis of a limb abnormality (19, 20).

Teratologic Disorders. Teratogenic agents affect the fetus by blocking normal cell functions during development. The effects of known teratogens on the fetus are determined by the timing of exposure and the dosage (23, 24). During blastocyst formation, teratogen exposure may be incompatible with life, and this often results in fetal death and spontaneous abortion. During the period of organogenesis, 18 to 60 days after conception, the fetus is quite vulnerable to the effects of teratogens, while later in the pregnancy, the effects are often more subtle (25). Most teratogens act by interfering with metabolic processes. These teratogens may act on cell membranes or on the metabolic machinery of cells. The final common pathway of these various levels of action is cell death or a failure of replication, migration, or fusion of cells. These changes often involve specific organs, but can produce more general changes in the fetus.

Most known teratogenic agents in humans have been identified from clinical observations of unexpected outbreaks of malformations. In most instances, however, unexpected clusters of cases result from natural fluctuations in the frequency of specific birth defects, as shown by birth defect registers. Epidemiologists who deal with birth defect registers play an important role in assessing whether apparent outbreaks of malformations are potentially significant. Animal models are not always the best way to predict if an agent will be a teratogen, since an agent teratogenic effect is species dependent (26). Interestingly, since teratogenic agents often block normal developmental pathways, and have little side effects in adults, many of these agents are starting to be studied as therapeutic approaches to various disorders in which these pathways are activated. For instance, thalidomide is currently being used as an anticancer drug because of its neovascular effects, but this can create problems during pregnancy.

Teratogenic Agents. The items in the following list are some of the drugs and environmental chemicals that can act as teratogenic agents in humans (23):

- Androgens
- Aminopterin
- Chlorobiphenyls
- Warfarin (Coumadin)
- Cyclophosphamide
- Diethylstilbestrol
- D-Penicillamine
- Goitrogens and antithyroid drugs
- Isoretinoin
- Methyl mercury
- Phenytoin
- Tetracyclines
- Thalidomide
- Valproic acid
- Infections
- Cytomegalovirus
- Rubella
- Syphilis
- Toxoplasmosis
- Maternal metabolic imbalance
- Alcoholism
- Diabetes mellitus
- Phenylketonuria
- Virilizing tumors
- Ionizing radiation

While there is continuing concern about the possible adverse effects of drugs and environmental factors on the developing fetus, and there are medicolegal issues regarding prescribing drugs to pregnant women (25), relatively few agents are actually proven to be teratogenic.

Thalidomide. There is an increased frequency of limb-deficient babies born to mothers who used thalidomide as a sedative during pregnancy. In clinical studies, the agent was shown to produce its major effects during the period of limb formation, by blocking vascular development.

Warfarin. Teratogenic effects occur on exposure of the fetus to warfarin between 6 and 9 weeks of gestation. Stippling of the epiphyses is one of the characteristic changes. Exposure during the second and third trimesters produces severe neural anomalies.

Retinoic Acid. Retinoic acid has been used in the treatment of severe cystic acne, and it produces craniofacial, cardiac, thymic, and central nervous system defects. High of vitamin A is also teratogenic. Vitamin A, retinoic acid, and its analogs should be avoided during pregnancy.

Alcohol. Alcohol is the most common teratogen to which a pregnancy is likely to be exposed. It is not known what the threshold safe level of alcohol consumption during pregnancy is, and as such, the mother should avoid alcohol during pregnancy. Despite this recommendation, studies suggest that alcohol exposure during the early stages of pregnancy, before a mother knows she is pregnant, is common (27).

Radiation. Pregnant women should avoid unnecessary exposure to radiographs and isotopes. Doses in excess of 10 Gy will cause microcephaly, growth retardation, and mental retardation, but lower doses may have long-term implications for cancer development (28, 29). A woman of childbearing age should not be exposed to unnecessary radiation if she is pregnant or if there is a possibility that she is pregnant, as the lifetime effect of radiation is greater the younger the individual is at the time of exposure.

Infections. Syphilis was the first known infectious teratogen. Its deleterious effects on the fetus can be prevented by routine testing of pregnant women and by providing treatment when necessary. The virus that causes acquired immunodeficiency syndrome (AIDS) has emerged as a major teratogen. Rubella embryopathy is preventable by vaccination of young girls. When the fetus is exposed to the virus in the first trimester, blindness, deafness, cataracts, microphthalmos, congenital heart disease, limb deficiencies, and mental retardation may occur. Cytomegalovirus infection and toxoplasmosis also produce birth defects.

Diabetes Mellitus. Abnormal embryogenesis occurs more often in babies of mothers with diabetes, particularly if their diabetes is poorly controlled in the first trimester of the pregnancy. For example, cardiac malformations occur three to four times more often in babies of mothers with diabetes than of healthy mothers, and anencephaly and myelomeningocele occur in 1% to 10% of babies born to mothers with diabetes. Caudal regression syndrome, with sacral hypoplasia and fusion of the legs, is a rare disorder, but it is more common in babies of mothers with diabetes.

Online Genetic Educational Resources. A diverse collection of educational resources exist on the Internet for both consumers (e.g., patients/pregnancy and newborn audience) and professionals (e.g., researchers or those working in health care). Many institutions' Web sites present their own content, whether it is a slide set, a case study, or a fact sheet, and will usually include a "Resource" page with links to other organizations. A few Web sites serve as portals by compiling and organizing the myriad of existing resources on the Internet. Tables 2-1 to 2-3 show a selection of Web sites grouped by objective with a notation indicating who the intended audience is along with a brief sampling of the site's educational pieces. Unless noted by an asterisk, most of the organizations listed are government agencies and thus the materials found on these sites are within the public domain.

TABLE 2-1   General Web Sites—Selected Portals to Additional Educational Resources

Organization	URL	Sample Content	Consumer or Professional Audience?
Centers for Disease Control and Prevention's (CDC) National Office of Public Health Genomics Case Studies	www.cdc.gov/genomics/hugenet/casestudies.htm	Case studies to help professionals critically evaluate gene disease association literature	Professionals
Centers for Disease Control and Prevention's National Office of Public Health Genomics: Training	www.cdc.gov/genomics/training/resources.htm	Public health genomics and family history resources, case studies and tools; some Spanish content	Both
Genetic Resources on the Web (GROW)	www.geneticsresources.org/	Search engine crawling various National Coalition for Health Professionals Education in Genetics (NCHPEG) organizations; available in Spanish	Both
Human Genome Project Education Resources	www.ornl.gov/sci/techresources/Human_Genome/education/educations.html	Videos, web casts, graphics, downloadable teaching aids; available in Spanish	Consumers
NCHPEG	www.nchpeg.org/	Flash animation curriculums	Professionals
National Human Genome Research Initiative online genetics education resources	www.genome.gov/10000464	Links to web-based education modules; available in Spanish	Mainly consumers
National Network of Libraries of Medicine	www.nnlm.gov/training/genetics/resources.html	"ABCs of DNA" web resources	Consumers
University of Kansas Genetics Education Center[a]	www.kumc.edu/gec/	Links organized by projects, organizations	Both
University of Utah—Genetic Science Learning Center	www.gslc.genetics.utah.edu/	Podcasts, flash animation; available in Spanish	Consumers

[a]Not in public domain.

TABLE 2-2   Selected "Genetics 101" Web Sites—Learn the Basics About Genes and Implications for Medicine and Public Health

Organization	URL	Sample Content	Consumer or Professional Audience?
Human Genome Project Web site and online publication	http://www.ornl.gov/sci/techresources/Human_Genome/project/infos.html http://www.ornl.gov/sci/techresources/Human_Genome/publicat/primer2001/1s.html	Science behind Human Genome Project series; available in Spanish	Consumers
MD Anderson Center: Genes and Cancer[a]	http://www3.mdanderson.org/depts/hcc/summer99/gen101.htm	"Just the basics" part of 8-part series	Consumers
Public Broadcasting Service NOVA online: Cracking the Code of Life[a]	http://www.pbs.org/wgbh/nova/genome/program.html	2-h video program divided into 16 chapters	Consumers

[a]Not in public domain.

TABLE 2-3 **Selected Web Sites Focused on Genetic Testing Issues (Including Newborn Screening, Prenatal Testing) or Gene–Disease Reviews**

Title	URL	Sample Content	Consumer or Professional Audience?
CDC National Office of Public Health Genomics: Genetic Testing	http://www.cdc.gov/genomics/gTesting.htm	Project descriptions and resource	Professionals
CDC National Office of Public Health Genomics: Public Health Perspectives	http://www.cdc.gov/genomics/training/perspectives/series.htm	Comprehensive series on obesity, family history, asthma plus more	Both
GeneTests	http://www.genetests.org/	Disease reviews, laboratory listings	Professionals
Genetics Home Reference	http://ghr.nlm.nih.gov/ghr/	Fact sheets with links and glossary	Consumers
MedlinePlus: Genetic Testing	http://www.nlm.nih.gov/medlineplus/genetictesting.html	Fact sheet with links; available in Spanish	Consumers
MedlinePlus: Newborn Screening	http://www.nlm.nih.gov/medlineplus/newbornscreening.html	Fact sheet with links; available in Spanish	Consumers
MedlinePlus: Prenatal Testing	http://www.nlm.nih.gov/medlineplus/prenataltesting.html	Fact sheet with links; available in Spanish	Consumers
MedlinePlus: Diagnostic Tests	http://www.nlm.nih.gov/medlineplus/diagnostictests.html	Fact sheet with links; available in Spanish	Consumers
National Health Museum[a]	http://www.accessexcellence.org/AE/AEPC/NIH/	Understanding gene testing module	Consumers

[a]Not in public domain.

REFERENCES

1. Dietz HC, Cutting GR, Pyeritz RE, et al. Marfan syndrome caused by a recurrent de novo missense mutation in the fibrillin gene. *Nature* 1991;352:337–339.
2. Dietz HC, Loeys BL, Carta L, et al. Recent progress towards a molecular understanding of Marfan syndrome. *Am J Med Genet* 2005;139C:4–9.
3. Keane MG, Pyeritz RE. Medical management of Marfan syndrome. *Circulation* 2008;117:2802–2813.
4. Alberts B, Johnson A, Lewis J, et al. *Molecular biology of the cell,* 4th ed. New York, NY: Garland Science, Taylor & Francis Group, 2002.
5. Griffiths AJF, Miller JH, Suzuki DT, et al. *An introduction to genetic analysis,* 7th ed. New York, NY: W.H. Freeman & Company, 2000.
6. Nussbaum RL, McInnes RR, Willard HF. *Thompson and Thompson genetics in medicine,* 7th ed. Philadelphia, PA: Saunders, 2004.
7. Borgaonkar DS. *Chromosomal variation in aman: a catalog of chromosomal variants and anomalies,* 8th ed. Hoboken, NJ: John Wiley & Sons Inc., 1994.
8. Epstein CJ. *The consequences of chromosome imbalance. Principles, mechanisms, and models.* New York, NY: Cambridge University Press, 1986.
9. McKusick VA. *Mendelian inheritance in man: a catalog of human genes and genetic disorders,* 12th ed. Baltimore, MD: The Johns Hopkins University Press, 1998.
10. OMIM–Online. Mendelian Inheritance in Man. http://www.ncbi.nlm.nih.gov/omim
11. Fu Y, Kuhl DP, Pizzuti A, et al. Variation of the CGG repeat at the fragile X site results in genetic instability: resolution of the Sherman paradox. *Cell* 1991;67:1047.
12. Redman JB, Fenwick SK, Fu TH, et al. Relationship between parental trinucleotide GCT repeat and severity of myotonic dystrophy in offspring. *JAMA* 1993;269:1960.
13. Driscoll DJ. Genomic imprinting in humans. *Mol Genet Med* 1994;4:37.
14. Korf BR. Overview of molecular genetic diagnosis. *Curr Protoc Hum Genet* 2006;Chapter 9:Unit 9 1.
15. Cooper DN, Schmidtke J. Molecular genetic approaches to the analysis and diagnosis of human inherited disease: an overview. *Ann Med* 1992;24(1):29–42.
16. Mefford HC. Genotype to phenotype-discovery and characterization of novel genomic disorders in a "genotype-first" era. *Genet Med* 2009;11(12):836–42.
17. Hall CM. International nosology and classification of constitutional disorders of bone (2001). *Am J Med genet* 2002;113:65–77.
18. Scriver CR, Beaudet AL, Sly WS, et al. *Metabolic and molecular bases of inherited disease,* 8th ed. www.ommbid.com. New York, NY: McGraw-Hill, 2004
19. Keret D, Bronshtein M, Weintroub S. Prenatal diagnosis of musculoskeletal anomalies. *Clin Orthop Relat Res* 2005;434:8–15.
20. Crombleholme TM, D'Alton M, Cendron M, et al. Prenatal diagnosis and the pediatric surgeon: the impact of prenatal consultation on perinatal management. *J Pediatr Surg* 1996;31(1):156–162; discussion 62–63.
21. Giampietro PF, Dunwoodie SL, Kusumi K, et al. Progress in the understanding of the genetic etiology of vertebral segmentation disorders in humans. *Ann N Y Acad Sci* 2009;1151:38–67.
22. Alman BA. Genetic etiology does not supplant the need to understand orthopaedic disorders. *Clin Orthop Relat Res* 2002;401:2–3.
23. Brent RL. Environmental causes of human congenital malformations: the pediatrician's role in dealing with these complex clinical problems caused by a multiplicity of environmental and genetic factors. *Pediatrics* 2004;113(4 Suppl):957–968.
24. Brent RL, Beckman DA, Landel CP. Clinical teratology. *Curr Opin Pediatr* 1993;5-2:201–211.
25. Brent RL. How does a physician avoid prescribing drugs and medical procedures that have reproductive and developmental risks? *Clin Perinatol* 2007;34(2):233–262.

26. Brent RL. Utilization of animal studies to determine the effects and human risks of environmental toxicants (drugs, chemicals, and physical agents). *Pediatrics* 2004;113(4 Suppl):984–995.

27. Floyd RL, Weber MK, Denny C, et al. Prevention of fetal alcohol spectrum disorders. *Dev Disabil Res Rev* 2009;15(3):193–199.

28. Fazel R, Krumholz HM, Wang Y, et al. Exposure to low-dose ionizing radiation from medical imaging procedures. *N Engl J Med* 2009;361(9):849–857.

29. Brenner DJ, Hall EJ. Computed tomography–an increasing source of radiation exposure. *N Engl J Med* 2007;357(22):2277–2284.

CHAPTER 3

Geetika Khanna
Georges Y. El-Khoury
Yusuf Menda

Imaging in Pediatric Orthopaedics

Imaging modalities have been in constant evolution since the discovery of x-rays more than a century ago. However, most of the important advances have occurred in the last 30 years. It is now hard to imagine the practice of clinical medicine or research without imaging studies. This intertwined relationship between clinical practice and imaging is very evident in orthopaedics. Radiography accounts for more than 80% of all the imaging studies performed, and it is almost always the first imaging examination that is requested before embarking on more complex studies. Other imaging modalities include fluoroscopy, magnetic resonance imaging (MRI), multidetector row computed tomography (MDCT), ultrasonography, and nuclear medicine. Radiography, fluoroscopy, and MDCT utilize x-rays generated in vacuum tubes. Nuclear medicine utilizes a form of x-rays generated by the decay of radioactive nuclei called γ rays. MRI utilizes radio waves, whereas ultrasonography utilizes sound waves. Under proper and predetermined conditions, x-rays, radio waves, and sound waves can penetrate the human body and carry useful information that can be captured by appropriate detectors and be displayed either on film or on TV monitors for viewing by physicians. Within the diagnostic range, radio waves and sound waves have not been shown to produce harmful effects in humans; however, this is not the case with x-rays, especially when they are used on infants and young children (1). Because x-rays are so central to our ability to perform diagnostic work, it is essential that every physician who performs or requests imaging studies becomes familiar with the nature of this form of electromagnetic energy, understands its interaction with living tissue, and learns how to use it safely.

X-RAY TECHNIQUES

Physical Principles of X-Ray Generation.
Wilhelm Conrad Roentgen discovered x-rays in 1895 and won the Nobel Prize for Physics in 1901 for this discovery. x-Rays and visible light both belong to the electromagnetic spectrum, which has a wide range of wavelengths and frequencies. Less energetic electromagnetic waves have longer wavelengths and lower frequencies and carry radiant heat from its source. More energetic electromagnetic waves have shorter wavelengths and higher frequencies (Fig. 3-1). As the wavelength decreases, the energy of the waves increases until these waves become capable of ejecting electrons from the shells of atoms they come in contact with; this is described by the term *ionizing radiation* (2). By this process, electromagnetic radiation imparts energy to the tissues it interacts with. The energy dose to the tissue is defined in terms of the energy absorbed. In the past, the unit used for measuring dose was the *rad* (radiation absorbed dose), but now the *gray* (Gy) is the unit of choice; 1 Gy = 100 rad.

Electromagnetic radiation has a dual nature, exhibiting the properties of a wave as well as those of particles or bundles of energy called *photons*. These concepts have been postulated to explain a variety of physical characteristics of electromagnetic radiation. In contrast to sound waves, electromagnetic radiation can travel in vacuum and does not require a medium to transport it.

The X-Ray Tube.
In the x-ray tube, x-rays are generated when a fast and energetic stream of electrons strike a metal target, or anode. The electrons originate at the negative terminal of the tube, which is called the *cathode* or *filament* (Fig. 3-2). Electrons are decelerated by the positively charged nuclei in the target or anode, which cause the electrons to change their path and lose their kinetic energy in the form of x-rays of different wavelengths. In order to maximize the process of x-ray production, it is desirable to select a target material with a high atomic number; the nuclei of the material will have a large positive charge, capable of attracting and decelerating electrons. x-Ray tubes are typically equipped with two filaments, one large and one small, which liberate electrons when heated. The large filament is used for large exposures such as thick body parts and large or overweight patients. The area on the target

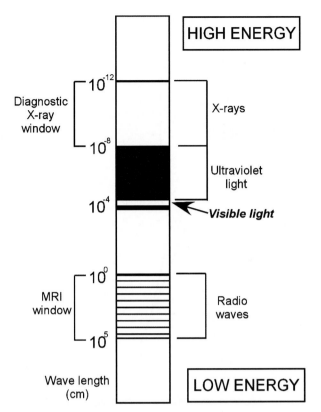

FIGURE 3-1. Diagram of the electromagnetic spectrum. Radio waves have low energy and long wavelength; x-rays have much more energy and shorter wavelength.

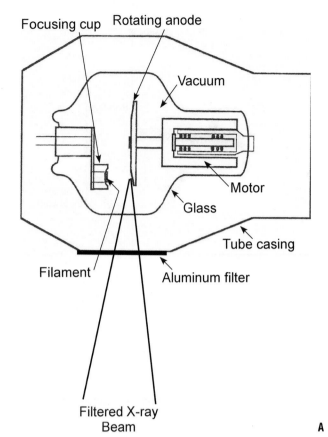

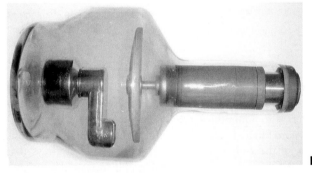

FIGURE 3-2. **A:** The components of the x-ray tube. **B:** Photograph of an x-ray tube. The glass casing maintains absolute vacuum within the tube. All the components of the tube are designed to withstand high temperatures, especially the anode.

that is bombarded by electrons is referred to as the *focal spot*, which, in orthopaedics, should ideally be as small as possible (0.3 to 0.6 mm) in order to produce sharper images (Fig. 3-3). The energy spectrum of the emitted x-rays is determined by the voltage between the cathode and the anode.

The process of converting kinetic energy into x-rays is not an efficient one, and only 1% of the kinetic energy in the electron stream is converted to x-rays; the rest dissipates as heat. The ability of the x-ray tube to achieve high x-ray output is limited by the enormous amount of heat generated at the target or anode. To overcome this problem, the rotating anode was developed so that electrons do not strike the same location on the anode. This allows the x-ray tube to withstand larger amounts of heat generated during large exposures. Both the filament and the target are made of tungsten, which has a high melting point of 3370°C as well as a high atomic number (3).

In every exposure, the emitted x-ray beam consists of a wide spectrum of energies (2). The quantity of x-rays in each exposure is proportional to the number of electrons flowing from the cathode to the anode; this is measured in milliamperes. The quality, or penetrating capability, of the x-ray beam is determined by the kinetic energy of the electrons striking the target or kilovoltage setting between the cathode and anode. Electrons with high kinetic energy produce a preponderance of energetic x-rays with high penetrating power (2). Such x-rays

have shorter wavelengths, higher frequencies, and more penetrating power (2).

Improving the Quality of the X-Ray Beam and Images.

With any milliampere and kilovolt setting, the x-ray beam emerges from the x-ray tube with a variety of x-rays of different wavelengths and frequencies. The interaction of x-rays with living tissue is dependent on the energy of the x-rays emitted (4). Low-energy x-rays are not diagnostically useful and are actually harmful to the patient because they are totally absorbed by the tissues and therefore fail to reach the

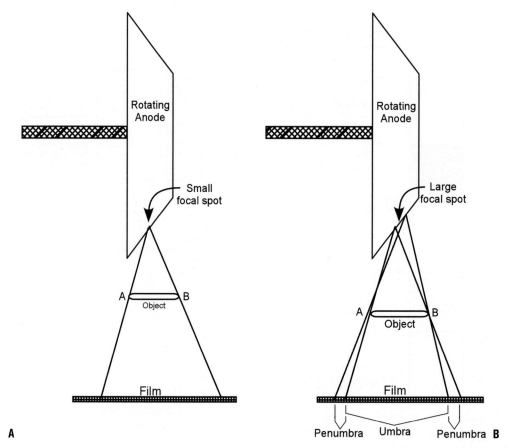

FIGURE 3-3. The effect of the focal spot size on image sharpness. **A:** A small focal spot produces sharp images. **B:** A large focal spot produces unsharp images with significant penumbra.

film or detector. To rectify this problem, x-ray tube casings are designed with filters to remove low-energy x-rays. Aluminum filters, 1 to 3 mm thick, are the most commonly used general-purpose filters. Filtration is useful for changing the composition of the x-ray beam by increasing the ratio of x-rays that are useful for imaging to x-rays that only increase the patient's radiation dose. This process is known as *beam hardening*. By filtering out low-energy radiation and by allowing high-energy x-rays to pass through, a higher proportion of the beam is capable of penetrating the patient, and carrying diagnostically useful information to the film or detector (4).

High-energy diagnostic x-rays are usually favored because the patient absorbs less radiation; however, such x-rays generate significant scattered radiation, resulting in foggy images and diminished tissue contrast on radiographs. x-Rays interacting with tissues bounce off the atoms in the tissue and are deflected from their straight path, giving rise to the scattered radiation. To control scatter and improve image quality, radiographic grids are used. The grid is the most common method for controlling scatter in medical radiography. Grids consist of thin lead strips separated by x-ray–transparent spacers (Fig. 3-4) (5). The amount of scatter is directly proportional to the thickness of the body part, and also to the field size (i.e., the area exposed). Thicker body parts produce more scatter than thinner parts.

Larger field sizes also result in scatter and poorer tissue contrast on images. Thin body parts such as hands, feet, and cervical spine produce little scattered radiation and can be radiographed without a grid. Limiting the field size to the area of interest achieves two important objectives: it reduces scatter and limits the radiation to the body part of clinical interest (Fig. 3-5).

The grid is positioned between the patient and the image receptor. x-Rays traveling in a straight line carry useful information and, for the most part, pass through the transparent spacers in the grid and reach the film or detector. Scattered or deflected rays are absorbed by the lead strips and are therefore prevented from reaching the detector, where they degrade image quality (Fig. 3-4) (5).

FLUOROSCOPY

An important function of fluoroscopy is to visualize human anatomy in real time, especially during surgical or diagnostic intervention. Modern fluoroscopy systems include an image intensifier and a television monitor, but, apart from that, fluoroscopy and radiography share the same imaging components. Because physicians operate the fluoroscopic equipment, it is important that they understand the physical principles that govern the safe use

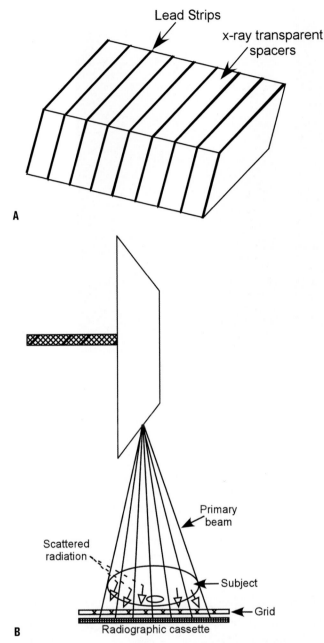

A

B

FIGURE 3-4. A: Diagram demonstrating a cross section of a radiographic grid. **B:** The mechanism by which a radiographic grid absorbs scattered radiation while allowing the primary beam to pass through and reach the radiographic cassette.

of such equipments (6). The difference between fluoroscopy and radiography is that fluoroscopy puts out a low rate of radiation exposure. However, the total radiation exposure from fluoroscopy is more than radiography. Fluoroscopic equipment is available in many different configurations for use in a wide variety of clinical applications. Mobile C-arm units are ideal for orthopaedic work. They provide a compact design, image chain angulation, and image recording devices. Mini C-arm systems are fairly inexpensive. They are designed for imaging the extremities where

only low exposures are needed (6). Physicians using fluoroscopy should be cognizant of techniques that decrease radiation exposure such as pulse fluoroscopy and the "last image hold" feature that modern fluoroscopic units have.

IMAGE FORMATION AND TRANSMISSION

Photons from the x-ray source interact with tissues and pass through the patient's body to reach the film or detector. Variations in tissue composition give rise to differences in attenuation and spatial variations in the x-ray beam exiting the patient's body. For air-containing organs such as the lung, x-rays pass through with only minimal attenuation, whereas most x-rays are absorbed or markedly attenuated as they pass through cortical bone. Fat attenuates x-rays more than air does, whereas water and soft tissues attenuate x-rays more than fat but less than bone. These alterations in the x-ray beam produce different responses on the film or detector. The diagnostic information on a radiograph or fluoroscopic image is obtained from the x-rays that emerge after the incident x-ray beam passes through the body (4).

IMAGING AND IMAGE TRANSMISSION IN THE DIGITAL AGE

In the last two decades, filmless imaging technologies have started to take hold, and at this time almost all imaging in the developed countries is filmless. The advances that brought about this change include faster and cheaper computers along with reasonably priced memory storage devices. In addition, the modern digital equipment manufactured by different companies can communicate information easily using a standard digital protocol called *Digital Imaging and Communication in Medicine* (*DICOM*) standard. There are several factors that may motivate radiologists and hospitals to switch to digital radiography, but the main factor is the ability to acquire high-quality images and to store and distribute them efficiently using a *picture archiving and communications system* (*PACS*). What is also important in a busy orthopaedic practice is the ability of digital radiography to accelerate patient throughput (7, 8).

Large-area flat-panel radiography detectors have been introduced during the last decade. They are now the technology of choice for acquiring high-quality images and distributing them throughout the medical enterprise rapidly and efficiently. Some studies have reported an approximate 50% reduction in the radiation dose required for skeletal imaging. There is also a large ergonomic advantage over the screen/film and computed radiography systems because there is no need for cassette handling (Fig. 3-6).

The advantages of time saving by switching to digital technology will not be fully realized unless there is improved efficiency in image management and reading. Ideally, digital images should be viewed on modern flat-panel monitors using liquid crystal display (LCD) screens with 3 million pixels (2000 × 1500).

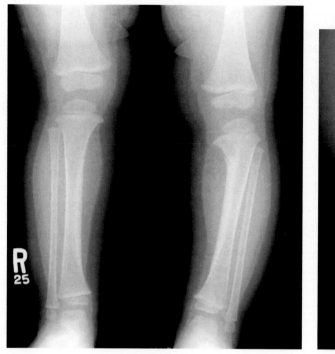
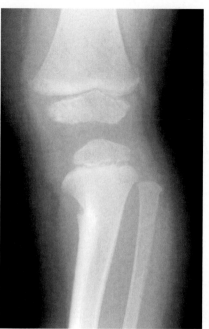

FIGURE 3-5.   Improved resolution resulting from coning down the x-ray beam to the area of interest. The patient is a 4-year-old child who presented with bowing of the left lower extremity. **A:** AP view of both lower extremities demonstrates the bowing in the left lower extremity. An abnormality was noted in the proximal tibial metaphysis medially, but it was difficult to tell what the abnormality was. **B:** A coned-down view of the left knee shows fibrocartilaginous dysplasia of the proximal tibia.

MULTIDETECTOR ROW COMPUTED TOMOGRAPHY AND ITS APPLICATIONS

With the advent of MDCT in 1992, computed tomography (CT) witnessed a significant evolutionary advance in technology. The newer MDCT machines have rows of detectors aligned along the longitudinal axis of the patient (z axis) as well as along the transverse or axial plane (x–y axis). The advantages of this technology include unprecedented speed, increased coverage, isotropic imaging, ability to image structures that have metal hardware, and ease of interpretation. The high speed has reduced the scanning time to a few seconds.

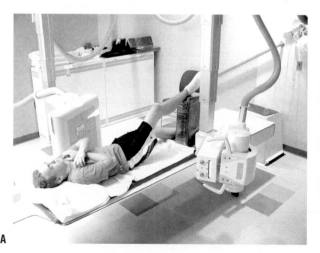
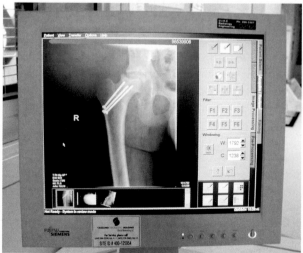

FIGURE 3-6.   Direct digital radiography equipment. **A:** The film–screen combination is substituted with a flat-panel detector. **B:** The image appears on a TV monitor a few seconds after the exposure.

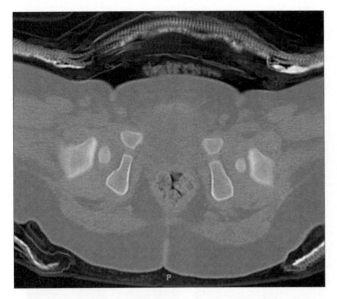

FIGURE 3-7.   MDCT for evaluation of DDH. MDCT was obtained after reduction of a congenitally dislocated left hip. The ossification center of the left femoral head is smaller than the right; however, it is well reduced and well centered within the shallow left acetabulum.

This resulted in better temporal resolution and therefore less motion blur, less need for sedation in children (Fig. 3-7), and considerable time saving in emergency situations (9).

Isotropic imaging provides improved spatial resolution, the ability to obtain two-dimensional (2D) reformatted images

in any arbitrary plane, and high-quality three-dimensional (3D) images (Fig. 3-8). This includes not only images in the standard sagittal and coronal planes but also curved planar reformations, which allow straightening of curved structures such as a scoliotic spine (Fig. 3-9) (10, 11). 3D surface and volume rendering are used to display anatomic relations, which are sometimes essential for surgical planning (Figs. 3-9 and 3-10).

RADIATION SAFETY IN PEDIATRIC ORTHOPAEDICS

Infants and children constitute a special subpopulation for radiation safety considerations because they are the most susceptible to radiation effects. Radiation risk is several fold higher in infants and children than in adults. It is estimated that about 7 million CT scans were obtained on children in 2007, and this number is growing by approximately 10% every year. There has been an almost 400% increase in number of cervical spine CTs obtained on children in the emergency room setting, over the period 2000 to 2006 (12). Although CT remains an extremely valuable diagnostic tool, the radiation exposure from CT has become a public health concern. The Image Gently Campaign is a recent national initiative introduced by the Alliance for Radiation Safety in Pediatric Imaging. The goal of this campaign is to change our practice by increasing our awareness to lower the radiation dose in children. The four main guiding principles issued by the Image Gently Campaign to reduce radiation exposure in children are as follows:

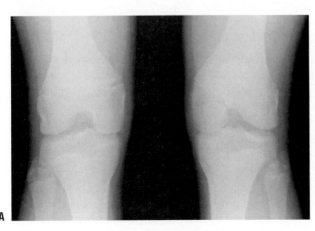

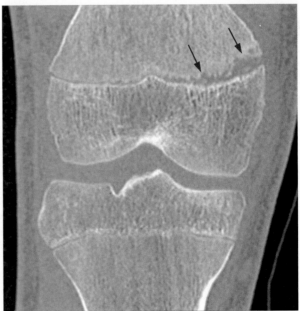

FIGURE 3-8.   MDCT used for studying a stress epiphyseal fracture in a 14-year-old boy who is an athlete. Patient presented with pain on medial aspect of the right knee. **A:** Anteroposterior view of both knees shows widening of the epiphyseal plate in the distal right femur. **B:** Coronal reformatted CT image illustrating the extent of the abnormality (*arrows*) that involves only the medial half of epiphyseal plate.

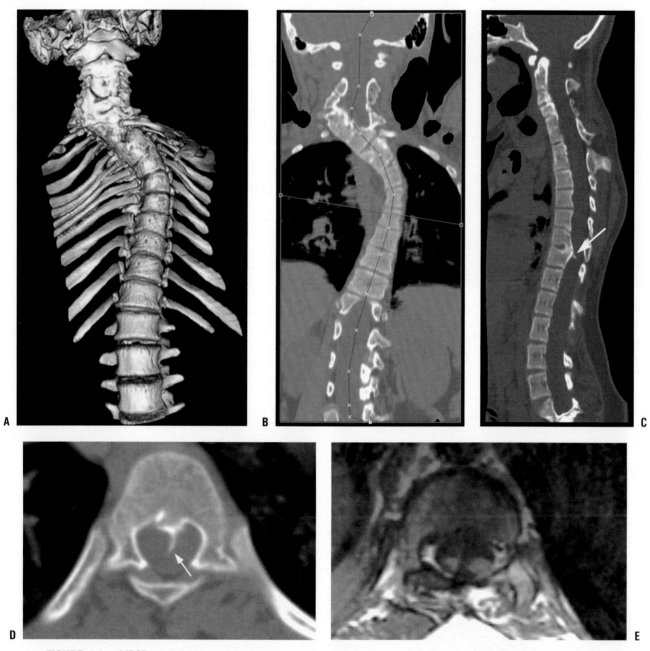

FIGURE 3-9. MDCT used for the evaluation of a 12-year-old patient with congenital scoliosis and diastematomyelia. **A:** 3D image demonstrating severe cervical and thoracic scoliosis caused by congenital segmentation anomalies. **B:** Coronal reformatted image used in planning the curved planar reformation in order to straighten the spine. **C:** Curved planar reformation in the sagittal plane shows the segmentation anomalies in the cervical and thoracic spine. At the level of T12, a spike of bone (*arrow*) is seen arising from the posterior body of T12; this represents diastematomyelia. **D:** Axial section through T12 shows the bony spike (*arrow*) to better advantage. **E:** T1-w magnetic resonance image (MRI) through T12 demonstrates the bony spike splitting the spinal cord into two.

1. Reduce or "child size" the amount of radiation used. The imaging parameters such as kilovoltage and milliamperes should be adjusted to patient size when imaging children. This conforms to the *ALARA principle* (*as low as reasonably achievable*).
2. Scan only when necessary. If the clinical question can be answered using a modality that does not require exposure to radiation, such as ultrasound or MRI, CT should be avoided.
3. Scan only the area indicated. Exposure should be limited to those parts of the body that are absolutely essential to arrive at a diagnosis. When using fluoroscopy, radiation exposure can be limited by using electronic collimators to limit exposure to the area of interest only.
4. Scan once only. Multiphasic scans such as precontrast and postcontrast imaging should be avoided.

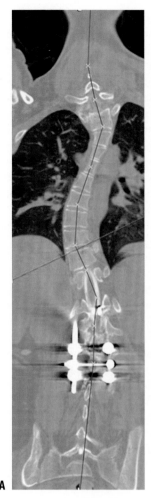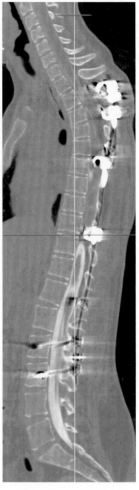

FIGURE 3-10. Multiplanar reconstruction of an isotropic dataset obtained with MDCT. This 13-year-old girl presented with signs of cord compression several months after posterior spinal fusion for scoliosis. A CT myelogram was performed as MRI was limited by metal artifact. Multiplanar reconstruction was performed along the scoliosis **(A)** resulting in a straight sagittal image **(B)** which shows the displaced laminar hooks causing cord compression in the midthoracic spine.

ULTRASONOGRAPHY

Ultrasonography is a valuable imaging technique in infants and children. The high ratio of cartilage to bone in a child's skeleton makes ultrasonography an ideal tool for the pediatric musculoskeletal (MSK) system as compared to radiography or CT. With the increasing awareness of the deleterious effects of radiation on the growing child, ultrasonography has become an even more valuable tool. Other advantages of ultrasonography include the ability to perform real-time imaging with multiplanar capability, no need for sedation, easy portability, wide availability, and relatively low cost.

Physics. Diagnostic sonography typically operates at frequencies between 1 and 20 MHz. The average velocity of sound in soft tissues is 1540 m/s, being higher in tissues with

higher density, such as bone, and lower in tissues of lower density, such as fat. As the sound waves travel through tissues, they become attenuated because of reflection, refraction, absorption, and scattering. The reflected component gives the echo, which forms the image. The brightness of the image is directly proportional to the echo strength and produces what is called the *gray-scale* image. The amount of reflection that occurs at the interface between two tissues is directly proportional to the difference in their acoustic impedance. An interface that reflects most of the sound beam, such as bone, is termed *highly echogenic* and appears bright on the screen. In contrast, sound-transmitting structures, such as cysts, do not reflect the sound waves and appear dark or anechoic. Skeletal muscle is hypoechoic compared to adjacent fat and bone. The perimysial septae, which separate the primary fascicles within muscles, appear as parallel echogenic lines against the hypoechoic background of the muscle on longitudinal scans. Normal tendons are echogenic and exhibit a fibrillar echotexture, corresponding to the interfaces between the densely packed collagen bundles and the surrounding septa. The display of the fibrillar echotexture requires that the ultrasound beam be perpendicular to the axis of the tendon (13). If the ultrasound beam is oblique to the tendon, false hypoechogenicity is produced, which may mimic a tear. Nonossified cartilaginous epiphyses appear hypoechoic relative to the adjacent soft tissues, and usually contain fine-speckled echoes. Ossification centers within cartilage appear hyperechoic. Articular cartilage appears as a smooth, anechoic, 1- to 2-mm-thick layer.

Doppler imaging is based on the principle that when sound waves hit a moving particle, the reflected sound undergoes a frequency change (Doppler shift), which is directly proportional to the velocity of the moving object. In color Doppler imaging, the frequency change or velocity is depicted in different shades (higher frequencies being assigned lighter colors), whereas the direction, according to convention, is denoted in red for flow toward the transducer and in blue for flow away from the transducer. Power Doppler sonography is more sensitive to slow flow but lacks directional information.

Applications

Developmental Abnormalities. Developmental dysplasia of the hip (DDH) is the most common indication for MSK ultrasonography in neonates (14). In the first 6 months of life, sonography offers many advantages over radiographs as it can directly visualize the cartilaginous femoral head and surrounding soft-tissue structures such as the labrum. Though clinical hip screening detects the great majority of cases, the problem of late emergence of developmental hip dysplasia has led to the widespread use of hip sonography for the early diagnosis of this condition. A study of 7236 infants in the Netherlands showed that hip sonography had a sensitivity of 88.5%, specificity of 96.7%, a positive predictive value of 61.6%, and a negative predictive value of 99.4% (15). This study also showed that selective use of neonatal hip sonography in babies with risk factors results in a trend toward a lower rate of emergence of late DDH cases (15). Although universal sonographic screening for DDH would detect cases that are missed clinically, the drawbacks of universal screening include cost, the potential for overtreatment, and complications such as avascular necrosis of the femoral head. In North America, neither the US nor the Canadian government believes that current evidence supports universal screening of the general population with hip sonography (16). Sonography is recommended for neonates in whom the physical examination of the hip is equivocal and for infants with risk factors for DDH. These risk factors include a positive family history, breech birth position, and conditions that can be caused by intrauterine crowding such as neonatal clubfoot and torticollis (17). The current available evidence does not recommend the routine use of hip sonography for infants with an abnormal clinical examination after 2 weeks of age (18). These infants should be referred directly to orthopaedists for treatment. Screening sonography for DDH is optimally performed when the infant is 4 to 6 weeks old. This approach reduces the rate of false-positive cases, which may be seen in the neonatal period due to physiologic immaturity of the hips.

There are two major sonographic methods for evaluating the hip: the static Graf method, which emphasizes morphology, and the dynamic Harcke technique, which emphasizes stability of the femoral head (19, 20). In the static method, coronal plane imaging is performed with the infant in the supine or decubitus position, and the hip is assessed qualitatively and quantitatively (Fig. 3-11A,B). The α angle represents the bony roof, and the β angle represents the cartilaginous roof of the acetabulum. However, these angles have been shown to have poor reproducibility between examiners (21). Dynamic

assessment of the hip subjects the hip to stress maneuvers to determine its stability. With the infant relaxed, the examiner can assess for ligamentous laxity and dislocatability by performing adduction with gentle stress or, for positioning and relocatability, by performing abduction (Fig. 3-12A,B). Based on the sonographic appearance of the hip, the four main classifications used are normal, immature, mild dysplasia, and more severe dysplasia with femoral head displacement (18). Once a child with hip dysplasia has been placed in a harness, sonography can be used to assess the relation of the femoral head to the acetabulum. Color Doppler imaging can determine the adequacy of blood supply to the femoral head and can identify patients at risk for avascular necrosis (22).

Ultrasonography can also be used to evaluate the non-ossified structures in congenital limb abnormalities such as proximal focal femoral deficiency (PFFD), congenital dislocated or hypoplastic patella, and clubfoot (23, 24). PFFD is characterized by a variable degree of deficiency in the proximal femur. Because of its ability to identify the cartilaginous femoral head and the unossified portion of the femur, ultrasonography can be used for determining the severity of PFFD. It is particularly useful for differentiating between type A and type B PFFD, by demonstrating the presence or absence of a cartilaginous connection between the femoral head and femoral shaft. The largely cartilaginous bones of babies' feet allow ultrasound imaging to depict them and also to determine and describe their malalignment in clubfoot and congenital vertical talus. Despite the ability to provide diagnostic information, sonography of infant feet has not become mainstream in evaluation of the foot.

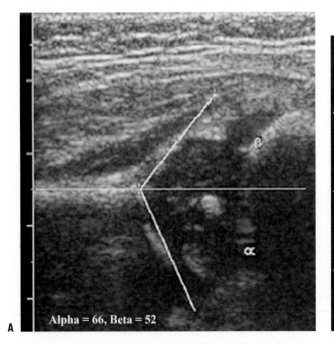

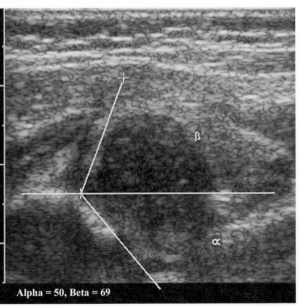

FIGURE 3-11. Static hip ultrasound for hip dysplasia. **A:** Coronal view of a normal hip shows good covering of the femoral head, with normal α and β angles. **B:** Coronal view of a dysplastic acetabulum. The femoral head is uncovered laterally by the shallow acetabulum. The α angle is abnormal (50 degrees), and the labrum is lifted laterally, with an abnormal β angle.

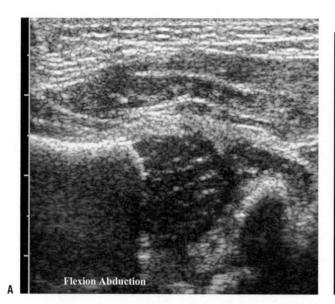
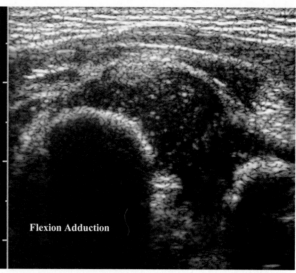

FIGURE 3-12. Dynamic hip ultrasound for hip dysplasia. **A:** In abduction, the femoral head is normally positioned with respect to the acetabulum. **B:** In adduction, the femoral head is situated along the posterolateral aspect of the ischium, at the posterior margin of the acetabulum, consistent with hip dysplasia.

Ultrasonography is a fast and inexpensive method for ruling out the presence of a tethered cord in a child born with a sacral dimple or hairy patch, thereby avoiding an MRI that requires sedation. In the first 6 months of life, the cartilaginous elements of the posterior spinous processes permit sound waves to reach the spinal canal, thereby enabling visualization of the cord. In the newborn, the conus ends at the L2-3 level. Ultrasound can be used to evaluate the appearance and position of the conus and surrounding nerve roots in the thecal sac (Fig. 3-13). Sonographic features of a tethered cord include low-lying conus, dorsally displaced nerve roots (which may be adherent to a posterior wall of the thecal sac), echogenic fat tissue in the thecal sac distally, and lack of normal motion of the cauda equine. A normal ultrasound precludes the need for further evaluation with MRI.

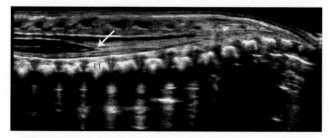

FIGURE 3-13. Ultrasound for evaluation of tethered cord. Longitudinal image of the spine shows a normal conus medullaris tapering to an end at L1 level in a newborn. The surrounding cauda equina has a normal configuration.

Infection and Inflammation. A major application of ultrasonography in pediatric MSK imaging is the evaluation of the painful hip. Ultrasonography is a safe, noninvasive, and sensitive technique for the detection of a joint effusion. Anterior parasagittal images with the foot pointed anteriorly show the normal echogenic capsule and synovium closely applied to and following the concavity of the femoral neck. Fluid that fills the hip joint causes a convex outward shape of the joint capsule, providing a confident diagnosis of joint effusion. Allowing the infant to assume a more comfortable frog-leg posture should be avoided because it allows fluid to pool posteriorly and can lead to a false-negative study. (Fig. 3-14A,B). The asymptomatic, contralateral side offers an excellent comparison. As little as 1 mL of fluid can be detected (25, 26); however, the appearance of fluid on ultrasound is nonspecific and cannot be used to differentiate a septic hip from toxic synovitis (27). Although the detection of increased blood flow on Doppler evaluation suggests septic arthritis, a normal Doppler result does not exclude the possibility of infection. Once the presence of fluid is detected, sonography can be used to guide percutaneous aspiration, in order to distinguish between toxic synovitis and a septic joint.

Ultrasonography is also the preferred diagnostic test for the evaluation of a possible foreign body, especially when the foreign body is small and radiolucent, like a wood splinter (Fig. 3-15). Wood produces posterior acoustic shadowing, whereas metal and glass demonstrate posterior reverberation artifacts. Sonography has been shown to have a sensitivity above 95% in the detection of foreign bodies (28).

In inflammatory arthropathies, such as juvenile idiopathic arthritis (JIA), ultrasonography can be used for monitoring

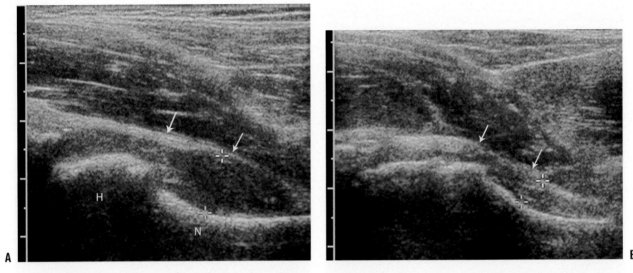

FIGURE 3-14. Ultrasound for detection of hip joint effusion. Three-year-old child with hip pain. **A:** Longitudinal evaluation of the symptomatic hip from an anterior parasagittal approach demonstrates capsular distension (calipers) with anterior bulging of the joint capsule (*arrows*). **B:** The contralateral normal side shows concave configuration of the capsule (*arrows*). (H, femoral head; N, femoral neck).

the inflammatory process by quantifying synovial thickening, suprapatellar effusion, and cartilage thickness (29).

Soft-Tissue Masses. Although MRI is more accurate in characterizing and delineating the extent of soft-tissue masses, ultrasonography is a simple, noninvasive modality that can be used to evaluate suspected soft-tissue lesions and to differentiate between cystic and solid masses (Fig. 3-16). Sonographic evaluation of a soft-tissue mass is best performed with a

high-resolution linear-array transducer. When evaluating a mass, the use of an acoustic standoff pad helps to improve visualization of superficial lesions. Ultrasonography can diagnose soft-tissue masses that have typical imaging features, such as cysts, fibromatosis coli, lymphangiomas, lymphadenopathy with abscess formation, and vascular malformations (Fig. 3-17) (30). When soft-tissue tumors have a nonspecific sonographic appearance, ultrasonography can be used to localize the mass and to provide guidance for needle biopsy.

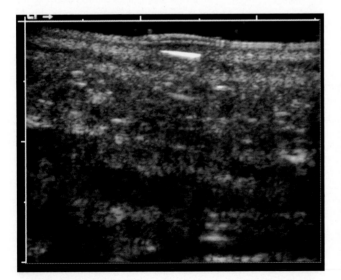

FIGURE 3-15. Ultrasound for detection of foreign body. Ultrasound shows a linear echogenic focus just deep to the subcutaneous tissues in the heel of a child who had stepped on broken glass. A 5-mm fragment of glass was removed at surgical debridement.

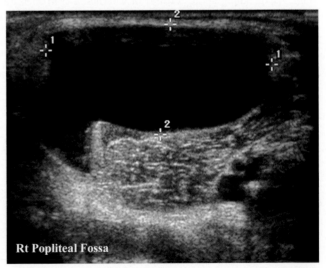

FIGURE 3-16. Ultrasound for evaluation of a palpable mass. Five-year-old child presented with a popliteal mass. Ultrasound shows an anechoic lesion, with a tail extending toward the joint. Findings are consistent with a popliteal cyst.

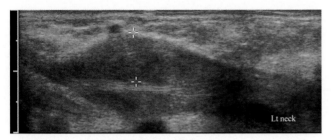

FIGURE 3-17. Ultrasound for evaluation of a palpable mass. Thirty-six-day-old infant with left neck mass. Longitudinal scan of the left side of the neck demonstrates fusiform enlargement of the sternocleidomastoid muscle, consistent with fibromatosis coli.

MAGNETIC RESONANCE IMAGING IN THE EVALUATION OF PEDIATRIC MUSCULOSKELETAL DISEASE

Due to its excellent soft-tissue contrast MRI has become the modality of choice in the evaluation of the bone marrow, cartilage, joints, and soft tissues. The absence of ionizing radiation makes MRI particularly advantageous in the imaging of children. Its primary limitation is the relatively long scan time and the need for sedation in most children under 5 years of age.

MRI Physics. Several excellent texts addressing the physics of MRI are available. We briefly discuss the concept of T1 and T2 weighting in the following paragraphs. The hydrogen nucleus is the most commonly imaged nucleus in clinical MRI because of its abundance in biologic tissues and its favorable magnetic properties. The spinning protons act as small magnets, and when placed in a large external magnetic field, they align themselves parallel with the magnetic field (Fig. 3-18). In conventional spin-echo imaging, a radio frequency (RF) pulse is applied, which causes the protons in the tissue to flip by 90 degrees. When the RF pulse is removed, the protons realign themselves parallel with the external magnetic field. The rate at which the protons realign with the external magnetic field is called *T1 relaxation* (Fig. 3-19A,B). This is a tissue-specific time constant. The time required for 63% of the deflected nuclei to realign with the external magnetic field after the termination of the 90-degree RF pulse is the T1 relaxation time of that tissue. The T1 relaxation time of fat is shorter than that of water; so, on T1-weighted (T1-w) images, fat has high signal intensity, whereas water has relatively low signal intensity. T1-w images are excellent for depicting anatomic detail (Table 3-1).

T2 decay refers to loss of magnetization in the transverse plane. Immediately following the 90-degree RF pulse, all the deflected nuclei lie in the transverse plane and spin in phase; however, soon thereafter, because of interactions with neighboring nuclei, they slip out of phase. As a result, transverse magnetization decreases, and this is called *T2 relaxation* or *decay*. T2 decay is faster for fat than for water, and therefore water has a higher signal than fat on T2-weighted (T2-w) images (Fig. 3-20).

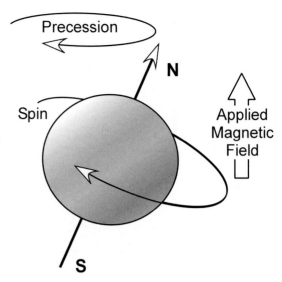

FIGURE 3-18. The spinning proton acts like a small magnetic dipole. When placed in a magnetic field, it aligns itself parallel with the external magnetic field and precesses about the applied field.

Commonly Used Pulse Sequences. The primary imaging sequences used in MSK MRI are T1-w, T2-w, proton density, fat-saturated T2-w, or STIR (short tau inversion recovery) images and postcontrast T1-w images with fat saturation.

T1-w images are excellent for anatomic detail. They also have the highest specificity in detecting marrow pathology and posttraumatic abnormalities such as nondisplaced fractures (Fig. 3-21). Most abnormalities have a low signal intensity on T1-w sequences. A few exceptions include lesions that contain blood products, fat, high protein content, and calcifications (Fig. 3-21). Fat saturated T1-w sequences after intravenous administration of gadolinium (Gd) are used to differentiate tumor from cyst and to assess the presence of fluid collections (abscesses) in cases where osteomyelitis or soft-tissue infections are suspected.

T2-w images are most sensitive for the detection of pathology. Most lesions have high signal intensity on T2-w images, and therefore, T2-w images have higher sensitivity in the detection of pathology. Lesions that have a low T2 signal are relatively few and include mineralized tissue, fibrosis, blood products (e.g., hemosiderin), and high concentrations of Gd. Due to the normal high signal of fat on T2-w images, T2-w sequences should be performed with fat saturation. This is especially true when imaging bone marrow, where edema is much more conspicuous on fat-suppressed T2 fast spin-echo (FSE) images. Fat suppression can be achieved by applying a frequency-selective presaturation pulse, or by using an inversion recovery sequence (STIR). Inversion recovery sequences, however, have less signal-to-noise ratio than the fat-suppressed T2-w images (31). While STIR images are generally used to cover a large area in the coronal or sagittal planes, fat-saturated T2-w images are excellent for numerous thin slices in the axial plane. In the presence of metallic hardware, STIR sequences can be very helpful in reducing the metal artifacts.

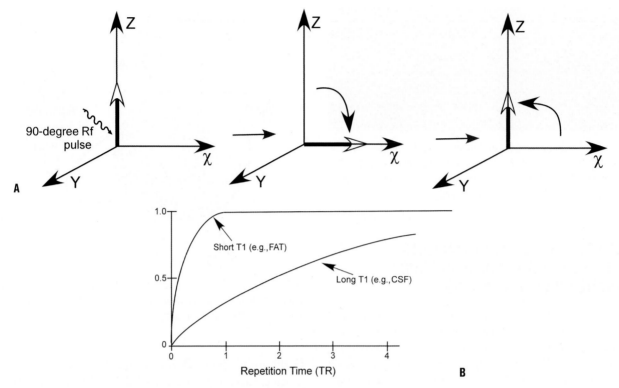

FIGURE 3-19.   T1 relaxation time. **A:** Sequence of events when a 90-degree RF pulse is applied. The magnetized proton tips 90 degrees from the axis of the external field. The tipped protons then start to relax or realign with the external magnetic field at a rate defined by the T1 relaxation time of the tissue. **B:** Tissues with short T1 relaxation times (e.g., fat) appear bright on T1-w images, as compared with tissues with long T1 relaxation times, such as cerebrospinal fluid (CSF).

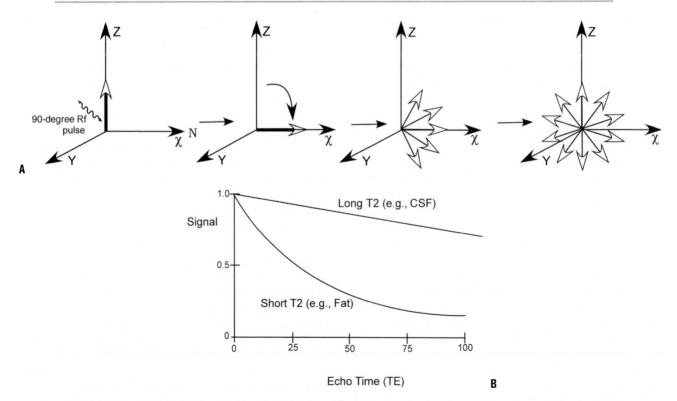

FIGURE 3-20.   T2 relaxation time. **A:** After the application of the 90-degree RF pulse, the transverse magnetization decreases because of the interaction of the tipped protons with the adjacent nuclei. This is called "T2 relaxation." **B:** On a T2-w image, tissues with long T2 relaxation times (e.g., CSF) produce bright signals.

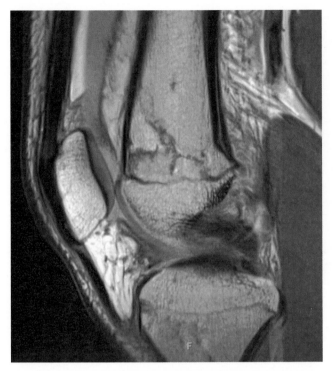

FIGURE 3-21.   T1-w image for detection of fracture. Fourteen-year-old boy with knee pain after trauma. The radiograph was normal. Sagittal T1-w image shows a metaphyseal nondisplaced fracture. In addition, a layering effusion is present with the nondependent portion being brighter consistent with a lipohemarthrosis.

The proton density sequence provides excellent anatomic detail of soft-tissue structures such as muscles, tendons, articular cartilage, and menisci, due to its high spatial resolution and enhanced signal to noise ratio.

The above commonly used sequences can be supplemented with gradient echo images (GRE) for evaluating cartilage and when looking for blood products. Isotropic 3D GRE techniques allow the creation of high-resolution reconstructions in any arbitrary plane. The main disadvantage of GRE sequences is that they are much more prone to magnetic susceptibility, which exaggerates metal artifact. On the other hand, the advantage of GRE sequences lies in its more sensitivity in detecting blood and blood products, such as hemosiderin (Table 3-1 and Fig. 3-22) (32).

Use of Contrast Agents.   Gd chelates are the most commonly used agents in MRI for contrast enhancement. Gd is used intravenously for evaluating inflammation, vascular lesions, neoplasms, and revascularization in the presence of avascular necrosis. The recommended intravenous dose is 0.1 mmol per kg. Gd should be avoided in patients with an estimated glomerular filtration rate of <60 mL/min/1.73 m^2 due to the risk of developing nephrogenic systemic fibrosis (33). Diluted Gd (1:100) can also be injected intra-articularly to obtain MR arthographic images. The intra-articular contrast distends the joint and aids in outlining abnormalities. MR arthrography is the imaging modality of choice for evaluating the labrum in the shoulder and hip and for evaluating stability

TABLE 3-1	Pulse Sequences: Clinical Applications	
Sequence	**Strengths**	**Limitations**
T1 SE	• Anatomy delineation • Sensitive technique for detection of fat, subacute hemorrhage, and proteinaceous fluid • Meniscal pathology • Fracture lines	• Less sensitive to detection of edema and marrow pathology, as compared with T2-w techniques
T2 SE Proton density	• Detection of edema, marrow pathology • Meniscal pathology • Anatomic detail	• Long imaging time • Not sensitive for detection of edema, marrow pathology
T2 FSE	• Less susceptibility artifact, therefore good for imaging patients with hardware • Faster imaging time than T2 SE • Fat-saturated images good for detecting marrow and soft-tissue edema, tumors, infection, and inflammation	• Fat brighter than conventional T2 SE images
STIR	• Sensitive for detection of marrow and soft-tissue edema, tumors, infection, and inflammation	
Gradient echo	• Prone to susceptibility artifact, therefore good for detecting hemorrhage, hemosiderin, and loose bodies • Evaluation of articular cartilage, ligaments, tendons • 3D imaging	• Prone to susceptibility effects; artifacts from metallic hardware more pronounced • Less sensitive to marrow edema

SE, spin echo; FSE, fast spin echo; STIR, short tau inversion recovery; 3D, three-dimensional.

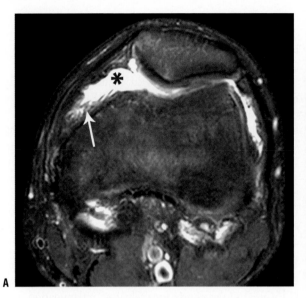 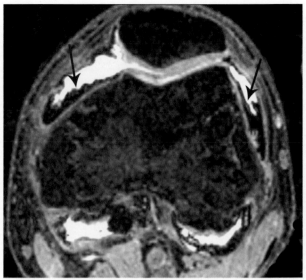

FIGURE 3-22. Detection of hemosiderin in a 13-year-old boy with a history of hemophilia. **A:** Axial T2-w image through the knee demonstrates a joint effusion (∗), with a hypointense synovial lining (*arrow*). **B:** The hypointensity of the synovium is more pronounced on the gradient-echo image, secondary to magnetic susceptibility of hemosiderin (*arrows*).

of osteochondral lesions (Figs. 3-23 and 3.24). MRI should be started within 30 minutes from the injection of the contrast to minimize absorption of the contrast and loss of capsular distension.

APPLICATIONS

Magnetic Resonance Imaging of Bone Marrow.
MRI is the modality of choice for imaging bone marrow abnormalities (34). Normal bone marrow can have a variable

appearance on MRI, depending upon the imaging sequence used and the age of the patient (35, 36). The signal characteristics of fatty marrow are similar to those of subcutaneous fat because of its high lipid content (Table 3-2). Hematopoietically active marrow or red marrow has signal intensity equal to or higher than muscle on T1-w images and essentially isointense to slightly hyperintense to muscle on fat-saturated T2-w images. Although, there are no absolute values, a marrow with very low signal intensity on T1-w images and increased signal intensity on fat-saturated T2-w images is suspicious for

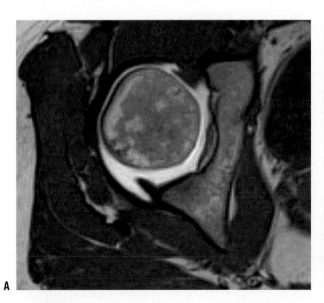 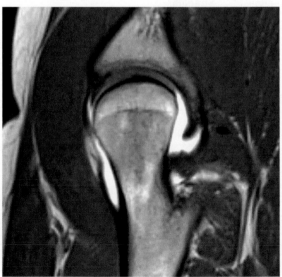

FIGURE 3-23. MR arthrogram for evaluation of labrum in a 13-year-old girl with history of hip dysplasia. Axial **(A)** and sagittal **(B)** T1-w images demonstrate a hypertrophied labrum in the setting of a dysplastic hip. No labral tear was identified.

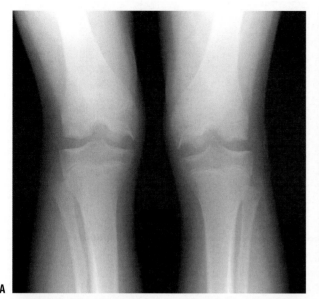
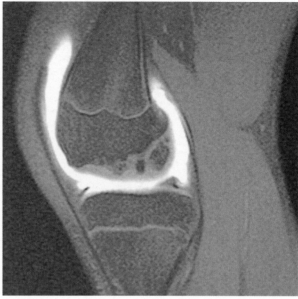
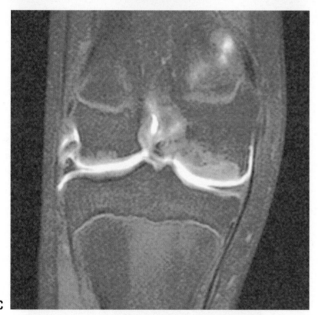

FIGURE 3-24. Magnetic resonance (MR) arthrography in a child with abnormal-looking epiphyses. **A:** Plain radiographs of both knees demonstrate marked irregularity of the epiphysis and fragmentation. **B:** Sagittal image. **C:** Coronal image. MR arthrogram using fat suppressed T1-w sequence demonstrates intact overlying cartilage suggesting the presence of multiple ossification centers of the epiphyses.

TABLE 3-2   Tissue Signal Characteristics on Various Sequences

Sequence	Parameters	Weighting	Fluid	Fat	Muscle	Disk
Proton density	Long TR Short TE	Spin density	Gray	Bright	Isointense	Gray
T1 spin echo	Short TR Short TE	T1	Dark	Bright	Isointense	Isointense
T2 spin echo	Long TR Long TE	T2	Bright	Gray	Gray	Bright
Inversion recovery	Long TE	T2	Bright	Gray	Gray	Bright
Gradient echo	Flip angle <20 degrees Long TE	T2	Bright	Gray	Isointense	Isointense
Gradient echo	Flip angle >45 degrees Short TE	T1	Dark	Bright	Gray	Bright

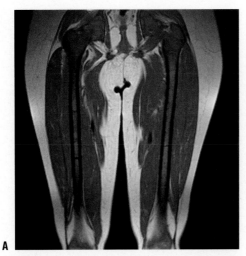 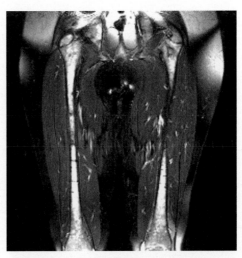

FIGURE 3-25. Diffuse marrow replacement with metastatic neuroblastoma. **A:** Coronal T1-w image of both femurs demonstrates diffuse loss of normal T1 hyperintensity of fatty marrow. Note that the epiphyses also demonstrate replacement of the fatty marrow. **B:** The marrow infiltration, caused by metastatic neuroblastoma, appears diffusely hyperintense on the fat-suppressed T2-w FSE image.

marrow disease (Fig. 3-25). Reduction of fat signal either by fat suppression or by STIR sequences helps increase the conspicuity of marrow lesions, especially when using FSE T2-w sequences.

Because the signal characteristics of diseased marrow closely approximate those of hematopoietic marrow, knowledge of the normal distribution pattern of hematopoietic marrow at different ages becomes important (34). In the neonate, the marrow is entirely hematopoietic and therefore of low signal on T1-w images and high signal intensity on T2-w images. Marrow conversion from hematopoietic marrow to fatty marrow progresses from the distal appendicular skeleton proximally in the first two decades of life. Marrow conversion in long bones starts in the diaphysis from distal to proximal, proceed to the distal metaphysis, and, finally, the proximal metaphysis. The epiphyses demonstrate fatty marrow within 6 months of formation of the ossification center (37). Under stress, marrow can reconvert from fatty to red marrow; the reconversion progresses in the reverse order. Thus, the epiphyses are the last site to reconvert to red marrow.

Congenital and Developmental Abnormalities.
MRI is useful in imaging patients with failed reduction or with complicated DDH (38, 39). MRI can be used for identifying the cause of failed reduction, such as infolding of the labrum, thickened ligamentum teres, or hypertrophy of the pulvinar (40). Perfusion imaging with contrast-enhanced MRI has been used to identify hips at risk for avascular necrosis after hip reduction. MRI can also be performed to confirm adequate reduction after a spica cast has been applied.

MRI of congenital anomalies of the extremities is helpful in evaluating the nonosseous components for treatment planning (41, 42). In patients with PFFD, MRI is used for

assessing the acetabulum, the cartilaginous femoral head, its connection to the shaft, and the status of the musculature. Congenital lymphatic and vascular malformations can be exquisitely evaluated using MRI to confirm diagnosis, determine the extent of lesion, and assess vascular anatomy using MR angiography and venography (Fig. 3-26). Mesenchymal

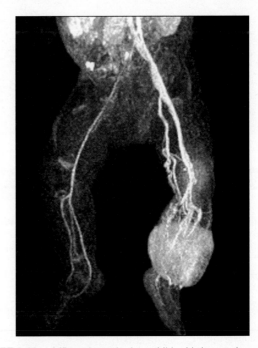

FIGURE 3-26. MR angiography in a child with hemangioma of the lower extremity. Maximum intensity projection image from angiography shows enlarged arterial feeders with prominent early venous drainage secondary to the hemangioma, as compared to the normal right side.

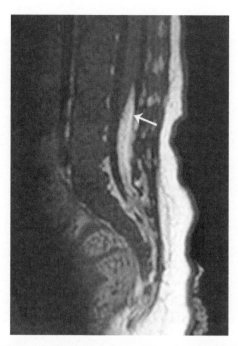

FIGURE 3-27. Tethered cord. Sagittal T1-w image of a child born with a sacral hairy patch demonstrates a tethered cord, ending at the L3 level, with an associated lipoma of the filum (*arrow*).

abnormalities, such as neurofibromatosis, macrodystrophia lipomatosa, congenital fibromatosis, and proteus syndrome, are also well evaluated with MRI.

Spinal dysraphism is the most common congenital anomaly of the central nervous system (CNS). MRI is the definitive modality for diagnosis, treatment planning, and follow-up of patients with tethered cord. If a tethered cord is suspected, clinically or by ultrasonography, MRI evaluation of the conus helps in identifying the cause of tethering, such as a thickened filum or filar lipoma (Fig. 3-27). In patients with atypical scoliosis, MRI evaluation of the craniospinal axis is performed to evaluate for Chiari I malformation, tethered cord, and hydrosyringomyelia. If a syrinx is detected, postcontrast images are imperative in order to exclude an underlying cord tumor.

In patients with suspected or known Legg Calve Perthes disease, MRI is useful in confirming the diagnosis, determining the extent of disease in the femoral head, and defining the severity of the resulting deformity (43). Both diffusion-weighted and perfusion imaging have been used for early diagnosis of avascular necrosis of the femoral head. Pre- and post-Gd images reveal decreased perfusion. In patients with a known diagnosis of Legg Calve Perthes disease, sagittal images are essential to determine the amount of femoral head involvement (44). In patients with suspected slipped capital femoral epiphysis (SCFE), MRI has been used for early detection of the slippage. Physeal widening, periphyseal edema, synovitis, and joint effusion are seen with SCFE. Perfusion MRI can also be used to identify cases of SCFE at risk for avascular necrosis (45).

Infection.   MRI has become the primary imaging modality for the diagnosis of osteomyelitis and soft-tissue infections. Radiography has low sensitivity in the early diagnosis of acute osteomyelitis, especially in the first 10 to 14 days. MRI has been shown to be 88% to 100% sensitive in the diagnosis of osteomyelitis and 75% to 100% specific (46, 47). The extent of the bone marrow, cortical, and soft-tissue changes, as well as joint involvement, can be precisely delineated by MRI. Acute inflammation shows hypointensity on T1-w images and hyperintensity on T2-w images as early as 24 to 48 hours after the onset of symptoms. As the infection spreads up and down the marrow space, it can penetrate the cortex, elevate the periosteum, and then break into the soft tissues. MRI can demonstrate accompanying cellulitis, myositis, sinus tracts, phlegmon, and abscess formation. T1-w fat-suppressed post-contrast images are key for the evaluation of devitalized tissues and abscess formation (48–50). An abscess appears as a peripherally enhancing lesion with a central hypointense fluid collection (Fig. 3-28).

Rheumatic Diseases.   MRI is the most sensitive imaging modality for assessing arthritis in children (51, 52). It can detect early synovial inflammation and subtle cartilage destruction, whereas radiography is able to show only late manifestations of inflammatory arthritis, such as osteoporosis, epiphyseal enlargement, bony erosions, subchondral cysts, and deformity of the joint surface (53). Imaging of arthritis requires sequences that depict the synovium (T2-w and Gd-enhanced T1-w sequences) and articular cartilage (proton density and fat-suppressed spoiled-gradient echo sequences). Inflamed synovium demonstrates low to intermediate signal intensity on T1-w images, high signal intensity on T2-w images, and intense enhancement on postcontrast images. The post-Gd images should be obtained within 5 minutes of intravenous contrast administration, otherwise the contrast can diffuse into the joint space, leading to overestimation of synovial thickness (54). Multiple small filling defects or rice bodies can be seen in the joint, which are synovial cells encased in a fibrinous exudate. Children with inflammatory arthropathy can also develop inflammatory tenosynovitis, which manifests as fluid within the tendon sheath which enhances on the postcontrast images. Cartilage demonstrates high signal intensity on proton density, T2-w, and gradient-echo images. MRI can also be used for assessing thinning, erosions, and traumatic cartilage defects (54).

In diseases producing hemosiderin deposits, such as hemophiliac arthropathy and pigmented villonodular synovitis, GRE images are the most sensitive in detecting hemosiderin due to magnetic susceptibility (Fig. 3-22).

Tumors

Bone Marrow Tumors.   Leukemia, lymphoma, and neuroblastoma are common malignancies in children that can cause marrow replacement. Marrow replacement with neoplasm can be diffuse or focal. When the involvement is focal, metastatic deposits have well-circumscribed margins, and differentiation

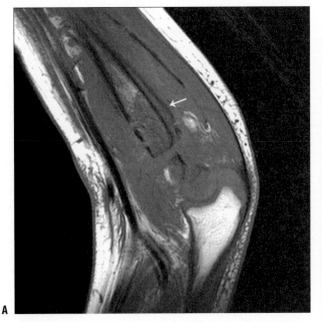

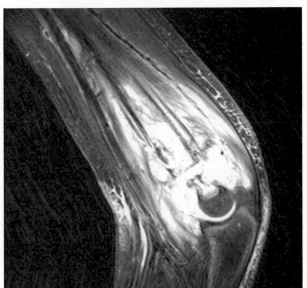

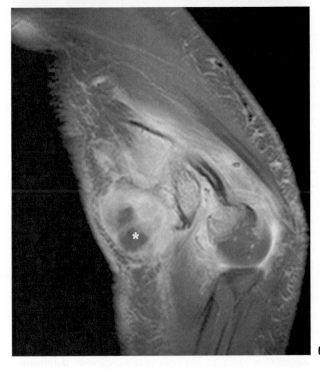

FIGURE 3-28. Osteomyelitis demonstrated by MRI. Sagittal **(A)** T1- and **(B)** T2-w images demonstrate loss of normal marrow signal in the distal humeral shaft, with associated infiltration of the surrounding soft tissues and periosteal elevation (*arrow*), secondary to osteomyelitis. **C:** Post-Gd fat-suppressed T1-w image demonstrates a peripherally enhancing fluid pocket in the ventral aspect, consistent with an abscess (*).

from the surrounding normal marrow is easier than when marrow infiltration is diffuse (Fig. 3-29). The metastatic foci will be hyperintense, compared with muscle on STIR or fat-suppressed T2-w images and will demonstrate enhancement on the T1-w post-Gd images. In diffuse metastatic replacement, the abnormal signal intensity is more extensive and may be more difficult to separate from normal hematopoietic marrow (Fig. 3-25). Loss of fatty marrow signal from the epiphysis gives a good indication of marrow replacement by tumor. Hematopoietic marrow is usually isointense to muscle on T2-w images. However, this may not be true if the patient is receiving granulocyte colony-stimulating factor (GCSF). Out-of-phase

gradient-echo images have been used to differentiate between metastases and hematopoietic marrow; the latter loses signal on out-of-phase sequence, whereas metastases remain bright (56).

Soft-Tissue Tumors. MRI is the imaging modality of choice in the evaluation of soft-tissue tumors (55-58). In cases of suspected soft-tissue masses, MRI has a 100% negative predictive value. Its ability to histologically characterize the mass remains limited. Features that favor benignity include lesion diameters of <3 cm, well-delineated margins, homogeneous signal, lack of peritumoral edema, and absence of neurovascular encasement (59). There are, however,

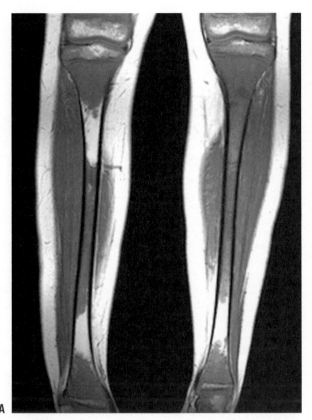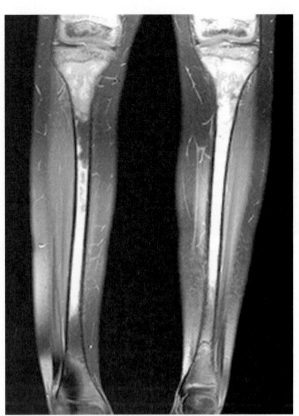

A   B

FIGURE 3-29.   MRI for detection of metastatic disease. **A:** Coronal T1-w image of both tibias demonstrates extensive areas of loss of normal fat signal of the marrow. **B:** The corresponding fat-suppressed T2-w FSE image demonstrates abnormal hyperintensity in the areas of marrow replacement in this child with metastatic neuroblastomas.

considerable overlaps in the MRI appearances of benign and malignant soft-tissue masses, and a correct histologic diagnosis can be reached in only 25% to 35% of cases. Soft-tissue lesions, such as lipomas, hemangiomas, lymphangiomas, and cysts, produce characteristic MRI images, thereby obviating the need for a biopsy (Fig. 3-30).

Bone Tumors.   Although plain radiographs still remain the most reliable method for predicting the histologic nature of bone lesions, MRI plays an essential role in diagnosis, staging, treatment planning, and posttherapy follow-up of bone tumors. MRI is the imaging modality of choice for local staging. Precontrast T1-w images have been shown to have the highest accuracy in determining the intraosseous extent of marrow replacement (60-62). Although MRI has high sensitivity in detection of transphyseal disease, its specificity has been estimated at 60% for T1-w images and 40% on STIR images, due to the presence of peritumoral edema. Evaluation for intra-articular extension, muscle compartment involvement, and neurovascular encasement is best performed with postcontrast imaging. Postcontrast T1-w images have been reported to have a sensitivity of 100% and a specificity of 69% for detection of intra-articular extension of tumor (63). The absence of a joint effusion has a high negative predictive value for intra-articular extension, but the presence of a joint effusion is a nonspecific finding (63). Extraosseous

tumor growth causing displacement of the joint capsule may result in a false-positive diagnosis of joint invasion (64). The sensitivity of MRI for detection of skip metastasis has been reported at 83%, compared to 46% for technetium-99m bone scans (65). Intravenous administration of Gd–diethylene-triamine pentaacetic acid (DTPA) can differentiate between viable and necrotic portions of a tumor (Fig. 3-31) (66, 67). Viable components show enhancement on the postcontrast images, whereas necrotic parts fail to enhance on MRI, thereby identifying viable tumors for biopsy. MRI also plays a crucial role in monitoring bone tumors after preoperative chemotherapy and radiation. There is moderate evidence that change in tumor volume as estimated at MRI correlates with chemotherapy-induced tumor necrosis in patients with Ewing sarcoma (68, 69). However, in patients with osteosarcoma, while an increase in tumor volume has been shown to correlate with poor histologic response, a decrease or no change in volume of tumor has been shown to be an unreliable predictor of response based on histologic evaluation (70, 71). Hence, several investigators have evaluated the role of functional MRI using perfusion imaging with dynamic contrast-enhanced MRI (DEMRI) for determining the response of sarcoma patient's to therapy (70). While the initial results of DEMRI are promising, the routine use of these techniques is currently limited due to lack of standardization and sophistication of postprocessing mathematical models. Tumor response can be assessed

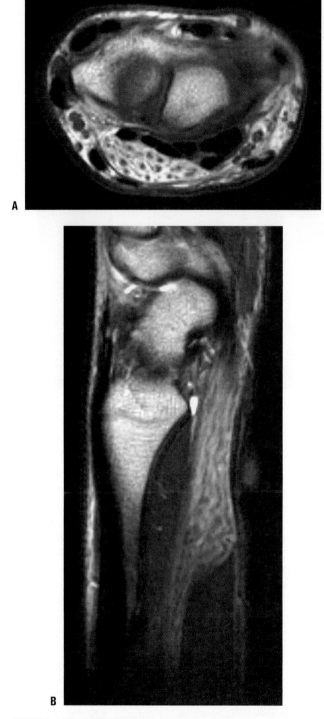

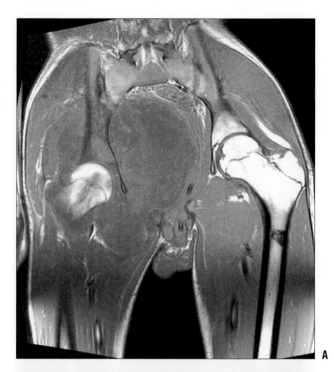

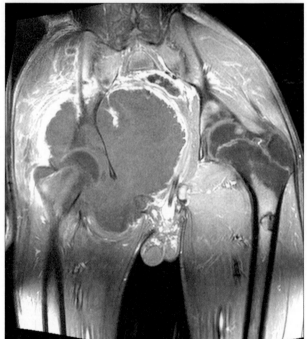

FIGURE 3-30. MRI for characterization of soft-tissue masses. A 10-year-old boy presented with a long-standing mass over the ventral aspect of his wrist. Axial **(A)** and sagittal **(B)** T1-w images show a mass in the region of the median nerve which contains multiple fascicles surrounded by fat. The imaging findings are characteristic of a fibrolipomatous hamartoma of the median nerve.

FIGURE 3-31. MRI for evaluation of primary bone tumors. **A:** Coronal T1-w image demonstrates a T1 hypointense mass in the right hemipelvis. There is loss of normal marrow signal in the right acetabulum and iliac bone. **B:** Postcontrast fat-suppressed T1-w image demonstrates peripheral enhancement, suggesting that central parts of the tumor are mostly necrotic. Biopsy revealed a chondroblastic osteosarcoma.

through estimation of changes in volume, signal intensity, and enhancement pattern (71).

Trauma. Trauma in children often involves radiolucent structures, such as growth plates, unossified epiphyses, muscles, and ligaments (Fig. 3-30). By demonstrating the type, severity, and extent of injury, as well as displacement of bone and soft-tissue structures, MRI provides useful information about traumatic abnormalities of bones, cartilage, menisci joint capsule, tendons, and ligaments (72, 73).

MRI has high diagnostic accuracy in detecting both stress fractures and nondisplaced traumatic fractures (Fig. 3-21) (74). Stress fractures are characterized by focal areas of edema in the bone marrow and periosteum with associated cortical thickening. Fracture lines are best depicted on T1-w images as linear areas of low signal intensity involving the cancellous bone with extension into the cortex. Physeal injury (both acute and chronic) can be well delineated on MRI. MRI can also be used to determine the presence and size of physeal bars (Fig. 3-32) (74).

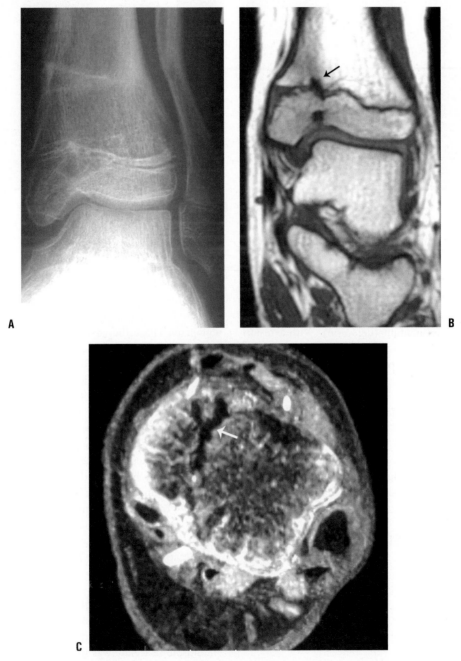

FIGURE 3-32. Mapping of an epiphyseal bar using MRI. **A:** Plain radiograph demonstrates healing fractures of the distal tibia and fibula, with angular deformity and evidence of bony bridging in the medial aspect of the tibial physis. Coronal T1-w **(B)** and **(C)** axial gradient-echo images demonstrate the bony bridge (*arrows*), extending across the medial aspect of the tibial physis.

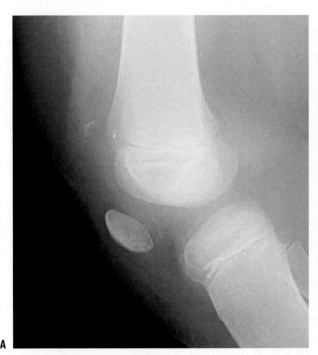
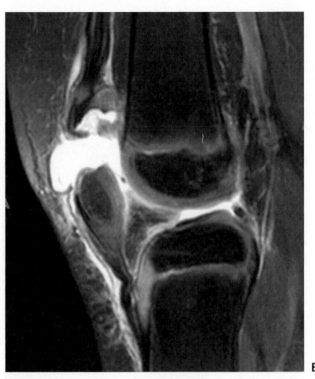

A   B

FIGURE 3-33.   Sleeve fracture of superior pole of patella. **A:** Plain radiograph shows marked suprapatellar soft-tissue swelling with a small ossific fragment in the region of the quadriceps muscle. **B:** Sagittal T2-w MRI shows a sleeve fracture of the superior pole of the patella with a large cartilaginous fragment and extension of fracture into the articular surface of the patella.

Avulsion injuries are much more common in the pediatric age group, as compared to the disruption of the myotendinous junction seen in adults (Fig. 3-33). With avulsion injuries, MRI shows soft-tissue and marrow edema, ligamentous or tendon injury, and the avulsed fragment—which may be difficult to detect by radiography when predominantly cartilaginous (75).

Due to its high-contrast resolution and superb visualization of soft tissues, MRI has become the imaging modality of choice in the evaluation of internal derangements of joints. This can be supplemented with intra-articular Gd for evaluation of the shoulder or hip labrum, the postoperative knee, and stability of osteochondral lesions.

INTERVENTIONAL MUSCULOSKELETAL PROCEDURES

Interventional MSK procedures can be performed for diagnostic and therapeutic reasons. In spite of the tremendous advances in imaging techniques, biopsy remains the ultimate test for tissue characterization of MSK neoplasms and, sometimes, infections.

Needle Biopsy.   Percutaneous needle biopsy (PNB) has been utilized extensively for more than 70 years and is a well-established radiologic procedure. For accurate sampling

of the tumor, guidance with CT, ultrasonography, or fluoroscopy is almost always required. Whereas fluoroscopy and sonography have the advantage of providing real-time guidance, CT can better delineate small and deep skeletal lesions and associated soft-tissue masses (76). In a prospective study of 74 patients, sonographic guidance resulted in a successful biopsy with a diagnostic accuracy of 97% (77). In comparison with open biopsy, the advantages of percutaneous image-guided biopsies include relative ease, safety, low morbidity, and low cost (78). Although percutaneous biopsies can be performed under local anesthesia, either sedation or general anesthesia may be required in small children. Complications such as bleeding, infection, and contamination of the tract are rare (79). Murphy et al. estimated the risk of serious complications to be <0.2% (80). The main drawback of a needle biopsy is the possibility of a false-negative result because the accuracy of a negative result can be established only with follow-up or open biopsy.

Unicameral Cyst Injection.   Percutaneous injection of unicameral bone cysts (UBCs) is simple, safe, and less invasive than open surgery. Treatment of UBCs with methylprednisolone acetate was first proposed by Scaglietti et al. in 1979 (81). Campanacci et al. demonstrated comparable end results in UBCs that were treated with curettage and bone grafting to those treated with cortisone injection (82). A more recent study, however, found that 84% of cysts treated with steroids experienced treatment failure, as compared to 64% treated with curettage and 50% treated with a combination of steroids, demineralized bone matrix, and bone marrow aspirate (83).

The procedure is performed under fluoroscopic guidance, using an 18- or 20-gauge spinal needle. Once the needle is inserted, clear yellow or slightly bloody fluid is aspirated. Radiographic contrast is then injected into the cyst to evaluate for internal loculations (Fig. 3-34). Methylprednisolone acetate (Depo-Medrol) is the most commonly used steroid. Repeated injections are often necessary to achieve complete healing of the cyst. Factors influencing the rate of healing include age of the patient and the location, size, and degree of loculation of the cyst (84). Radiographic changes associated with healing, in the form of cortical thickening and increased opacity of the cyst cavity, are usually seen within 2 to 3 months after the injection (85).

Percutaneous Ablation of Osteoid Osteoma.

Over the last decade, radiofrequency ablation (RFA) has become the treatment of choice for osteoid osteomas (Fig. 3-35).

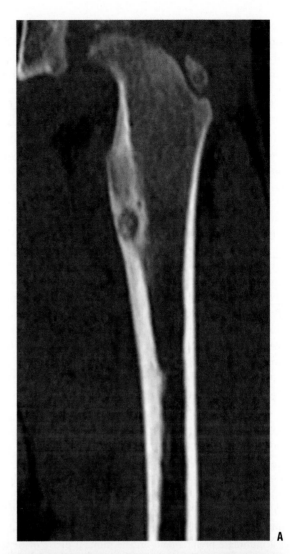

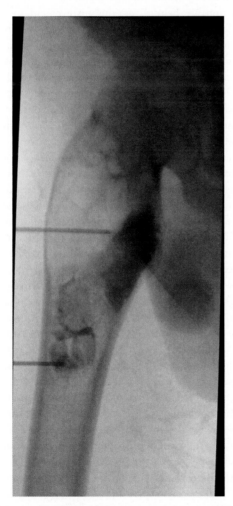

FIGURE 3-34. Treating a UBC with intracavitary steroid injection. After aspiration of the cyst, contrast is injected to confirm its unicameral nature, followed by the injection of steroid.

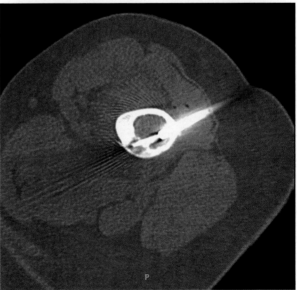

FIGURE 3-35. RFA of osteoid osteoma. **A:** Coronal reconstructed image shows an osteoid osteoma nidus in the medial femoral cortex. **B:** CT guidance is used to ablate the nidus.

The technique of RFA involves the use of electrodes to heat abnormal tissue to a high enough temperature that it results in cell death. As the imaging and clinical findings of osteoid osteoma are fairly specific, it is adequate to perform ablation in the absence of a histopathologic diagnosis. The success rate of RFA of osteoid osteomas has been reported to be as high as 97% (primary success rate) and 100% (secondary success rate) (86). In most studies, there have been few complications with patient's resuming normal activity within 24 hours. Because RFA/laser photocoagulation can cause local thermal injury, there is a risk of injury to vital structures within 1 cm of the lesion. This is why some investigators have advised against ablation of osteoid osteomas located in the posterior elements of the spine. However, other investigators have found that ablation in this location is safe and hypothesize that the surrounding sclerosis and cortical bone acts as an effective insulator.

The advantages of percutaneous treatment include the possibility of performing this procedure on an outpatient and the fact that patients can resume all activities of daily living immediately after the procedure. The cost with percutaneous RFA is estimated at only 25% of the cost of open surgery (86, 87).

Nuclear Imaging in Pediatric Orthopaedics

Bone Scans. Bone scans are obtained using gamma cameras after injection of technetium-99m–labeled phosphonates (Tc-99m MDP, Tc-99m HEDP). At 2 to 4 hours after the injection, approximately one-third of the injected dose of Tc-99m MDP localizes in the bone. When Tc-99m decays (half-life 6 hours), γ rays are emitted, which are detected by a gamma camera which produces an image reflecting the distribution of the radiopharmaceutical. Tc-99m–labeled phosphonates accumulate preferentially in the mineral phase of newly forming bone. Therefore, areas of increased bone remodeling, as a result of infection, trauma, or tumor, will appear "hot" on bone scans. Whole-body and/or regional bone scans of the area of concern are generally obtained 2 to 4 hours after the injection of Tc-99m–labeled phosphonates. To evaluate the blood flow and hyperemia of an area, images may be obtained immediately after the administration of the radiopharmaceutical (three-phase bone scan). Technically, adequate images are usually obtained with moderate restraint, or sedation.

Positron Emission Tomography. Positron emission tomography (PET) imaging utilizes radiopharmaceuticals that are labeled with positron emitters (in contrast to Tc-99m which is a gamma emitter). The most commonly used radiopharmaceutical in clinical PET imaging is a glucose analog, floruine-18 fluorodeoxyglucose (FDG). FDG PET is used for staging, assessment of treatment response, and follow-up of malignant diseases. FDG uptake localizes in cancer cells because of the enhanced transport of glucose and increased rate of glycolysis in tumors. After injection of FDG, the emitted radiation from the body is registered by external detectors and images of tracer distribution are reconstructed to obtain tomographic images. The amount of FDG uptake, that is the glucose metabolism

in the tumor, can be accurately quantified with PET. The most commonly used method for quantification of the radiopharmaceutical uptake is the standardized uptake value (SUV), which is the ratio of concentration of the radiopharmaceutical in the tumor to the product of injected activity and the body weight (SUV = activity concentration in the tumor/injected activity × body weight). Currently, most of the PET imaging is done on integrated PET-CT scanners. The CT portion of PET-CT is used for attenuation correction and localization of metabolically active lesions but may be also utilized to obtain a diagnostic quality CT scan in the same imaging session if a CT scan is also indicated as part of the work-up of the patient. FDG PET scans are performed 60 to 90 minutes after injecting the radiopharmaceutical and take approximately 25 to 45 minutes. Sedation should be considered to avoid motion artifacts.

Clinical Indications

Osteomyelitis. Acute osteomyelitis is most common in young children with half of the cases occurring by 5 years of age. Although clinical examination and laboratory markers of inflammation are helpful, osseous involvement of infection requires radiologic diagnosis. Routine x-rays are insensitive for diagnosis of osteomyelitis in the early phase, and bone scintigraphy becomes positive approximately 2 weeks before routine radiographs for diagnosis of osteomyelitis. The most commonly used imaging modalities for the diagnosis of osteomyelitis in the pediatric group is bone scintigraphy and MRI. Bone scintigraphy may be supplemented with labeled white blood cell scan and gallium scan to improve its accuracy.

Three-phase bone scintigraphy is routinely performed for the evaluation of osteomyelitis. The typical findings of acute osteomyelitis on bone scan are focal area of increased uptake on all three phases reflecting increased blood flow, hyperemia, and increased bone remodeling in the area of osteomyelitis (Fig. 3-36). Whole-body imaging is important, particularly in neonatal osteomyelitis, as osteomyelitis may be multifocal. In neonatal osteomyelitis, the bone scan may demonstrate decreased uptake (cold lesions) because of the highly destructive nature of the disease. Bone scans become positive within 24 to 72 hours after the initial clinical presentation of osteomyelitis and have a sensitivity and specificity of approximately 90%, which is similar to MRI (88). The modality of choice also depends on the local expertise and the clinical presentation. Radionuclide bone scan is ideal for screening if symptoms are poorly localized or multifocal osteomyelitis is suspected. Bone scan is also highly effective in the diagnosis of osteomyelitis in long bones, which rarely develop abscesses that need drainage (89). MRI is the preferred modality for vertebral and pelvic osteomyelitis because of the presence of soft-tissue abscesses with these infections that require drainage for treatment.

The specificity of bone scans is reduced in patients with underlying bone disease, particularly with recent fractures and orthopaedic hardware placement, as these conditions show hyperemia and increased bone remodeling similar to osteomyelitis. The accuracy for diagnosis of osteomyelitis in these patients can be improved

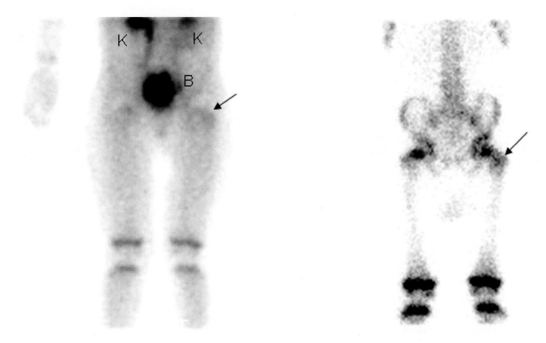

FIGURE 3-36.   Osteomyelitis. Abnormal uptake of the radiotracer (*arrows*) in the left femoral, greater trochanter on blood pool **(left)**, and delayed bone scan images **(right)**. Also note the activity in the kidneys and bladder and the excretion route of the radiopharmaceutical.

with *labeled white blood cell scan (labeled with Tc-99m or In-111)*. Labeled white blood cells accumulate at sites of inflammation. Labeled white blood cells do not usually accumulate at fracture sites after 2 months, whereas bone scan can remain positive in fractures up to 24 months (90, 91). In patients with prosthesis or orthopaedic hardware, labeled white blood cell scan may need to be complemented by a *bone marrow scan* using Tc-99m sulfur colloid. This is because labeled white blood cells localize in normal bone marrow, which may change in distribution with hardware placement. To differentiate between asymmetric marrow uptake from hardware versus infection, bone marrow scan is used to delineate the distribution of bone marrow. With osteomyelitis, there is increased accumulation of labeled white blood cells, which is incongruent with the bone marrow scan (92). In leukopenic patients or in children where blood volume required for labeling leukocytes cannot be withdrawn safely or if white blood cell labeling facilities are not available, *Gallium-67 scans* may be used as an alternative. Gallium-67 is taken up in areas of both bone remodeling and inflammation. Gallium-67 uptake greater than uptake on the bone scan with Tc-99m MDP is considered positive for osteomyelitis; however, Gallium-67 scans are equivocal in a substantial number of patients (93).

Trauma

Occult Traumatic Fractures and Stress Fractures.   Bone scans are almost always positive within 24 hours of fractures in children. In children with unexplained leg pain and refusal to walk and negative plain x-rays, bone scintigraphy is recommended to rule out occult fractures. Bone scans are also highly sensitive in diagnosis of *stress fractures*. The bone scan is positive

at the time of presentation of stress fractures, when x-rays are negative. The typical finding of stress fracture on bone scan is a fusiform pattern of increased uptake (Fig. 3-37). Bone scintigraphy is also very helpful to differentiate stress fractures from *shin splint*, which requires a shorter recovery than stress fractures (94). The typical presentation of shin splints on the bone scan is a linear uptake along the posteromedial aspect of the middle one-third of the involved tibia.

Spondylolysis.   Spondylolysis refers to a bone defect in the pars interarticularis of a vertebra, most commonly at L4 or L5, believed to occur as a result of a stress fracture. Spondylolysis may be asymptomatic and diagnosed as an incidental finding in some patients; however it may cause severe low back pain in others. A positive bone scan with focal uptake in the pars region indicates spondylolysis as the cause of low back pain and correlates with good outcome after fusion surgery (95, 96). Tomographic images of bone scintigraphy (SPECT) of the lumbar spine should always be obtained as more than 50% of active spondylolysis may not be detected with routine planar bone scans (97) (Fig. 3-38). Bone scans should be interpreted in correlation with plain radiographs and/or CT, as other conditions such as osteoid osteoma, infections, and tumors may be also positive on bone scintigraphy.

Child Abuse.   Skeletal injuries are the strongest imaging indicators of child abuse (98). There are usually multiple fractures, involving the long bones, ribs, skull, vertebrae, and facial bones, which usually show different stages of healing. Bone scans are highly sensitive in detecting osseous injury and

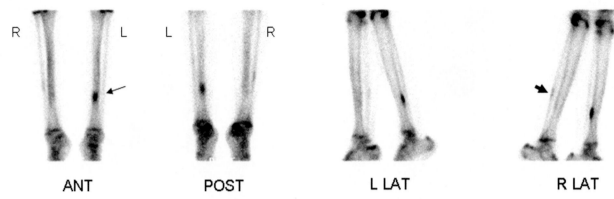

FIGURE 3-37. Acute stress fracture of the left tibia with markedly increased uptake of the radiopharmaceutical (*arrow*). Also note mild uptake in the right fibula (*small arrow*), likely representing a healing old stress fracture.

may be more sensitive than routine radiographs in this clinical setting (99). Bone scintigraphy however does not replace radiographs in the evaluation of child abuse patients because of its relatively limited sensitivity for skull fractures and for metaphyseal fractures, which are in close proximity to normal epiphyseal uptake (100). Bone scans may also be falsely negative in healed fractures. Mandelstam et al. reported that 70% of osseous injuries from child abuse were detected both by bone scans and x-rays, 20% only by scintigraphy, and 10%

only by x-ray (100). Therefore, a combination of x-ray and bone scan is suggested for optimal diagnosis of osseous injury in child abuse.

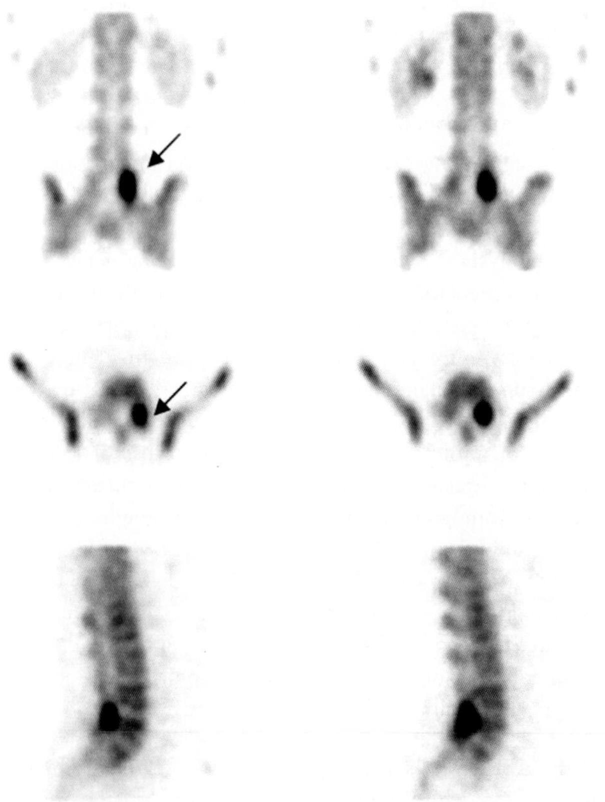

Tumor

Bone Scan. Bone scans are routinely used in pediatric malignancies to evaluate for bone metastases in a number of pediatric neoplasms including osteosarcoma, Ewing sarcoma, rhabdomyosarcoma, lymphoma, and neuroblastoma. Bone scans are obtained as a baseline for staging and during follow-up after treatment. On bone scan, osseous metastases appear as multiple foci of increased uptake throughout the skeleton (Fig. 3-39). Primary lesions of *osteosarcoma and Ewing sarcoma* usually demonstrate intense uptake on bone scans with the area of increased uptake usually larger than the extent of the tumor because of the peritumoral reactive changes particularly in osteosarcomas. In neuroblastoma, bone scintigraphy is used as complementary to MIBG (meta-iodobenzylguanidine) scans for detection of cortical osseous metastases (101). Occasionally highly destructive metastases may appear cold on bone scans (102).

Bone scans are also positive in a number of benign bone tumors and tumor-like lesions. Osteoid osteoma demonstrates intense uptake on bone scan and may show intense accumulation of the bone tracer in the nidus surrounded by a halo of less intense uptake. A negative bone scan essentially rules out osteoid osteoma. Lesions of Langerhans cell *histiocytosis* may show decreased, normal, or increased uptake on bone scans. In one study, whole-body bone scans were found to be complementary to x-ray skeletal surveys, with many rib lesions detected only on bone scan (103).

FDG PET Scan. FDG PET is being increasingly used in management of patients with sarcoma. The role of FDG PET in staging of pediatric sarcoma patients was evaluated in a multicenter prospective study, which included 46 patients with osteosarcoma, Ewing sarcoma, and rhabdomyosarcoma. This study found FDG PET to be more sensitive than conventional imaging for detection of nodal and osseous metastases for nodal metastasis and inferior to CT for pulmonary metastases (25% versus 100%) (104). Inclusion of PET changed the treatment decisions in a substantial group of patients, with

FIGURE 3-38. Spondylolysis. SPECT of the lumbar spine with coronal, transaxial, and sagittal images demonstrate focal increased uptake in the left pars region of L5 (*arrows*).

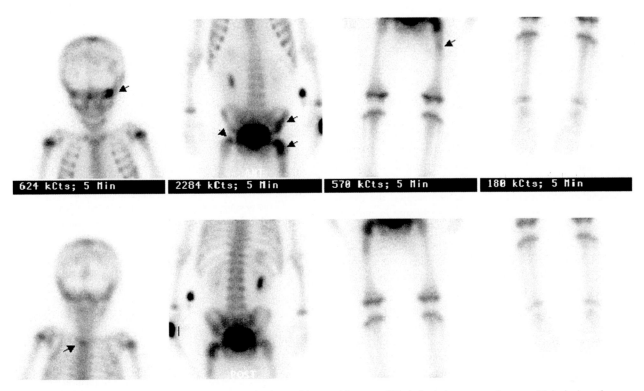

FIGURE 3-39. Metastatic bone disease in a patient with neuroblastoma. Whole-body bone scan shows multiple lesion of increased uptake (*arrows*) in the left orbit, upper thoracic spine, left ileum, and bilateral proximal femurs.

correct treatment decisions made in 91% of patients with combined PET and conventional imaging versus 59% for conventional imaging only (104). In a similar study, Tateishi et al. found a sensitivity of 88% for PET-CT in nodal staging of 117 patients with sarcoma compared to 53% for conventional imaging (105). PET-CT was also more sensitive for detection of distant metastasis, with a sensitivity of 92% compared to 65% for conventional imaging (105). The sensitivity of PET is limited for lung metastases, particularly if it is <1 cm (106); however, these can be diagnosed on the CT component of the PET-CT scan. FDG PET-CT was also found to be useful in detection of recurrent and metastatic disease after therapy (107, 108) (Fig. 3-40).

Although higher grade sarcomas are generally more FDG avid, FDG PET is not sufficiently accurate for grading

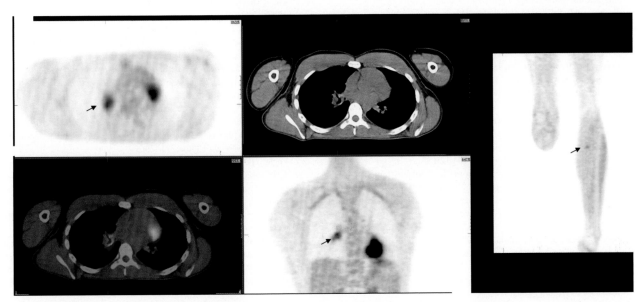

FIGURE 3-40. Recurrent metastatic soft-tissue sarcoma. FDG PET-CT scan shows hypermetabolic lesions in the right hilum and left leg (*arrows*). Normal FDG uptake in the myocardium, liver, and spleen.

of sarcomas because of significant overlap of FDG uptake between low-grade and high-grade tumors. In a meta-analysis that included 15 studies with 441 lesions, SUV was above 2.0 in 89.4% of intermediate/high-grade lesions, in 33.3% of low-grade lesions, and in 19.1% of benign lesions, with no significant difference in FDG uptake between low-grade malignancies and benign lesions (109). False-positive PET is seen in a number of benign bone lesions including giant cell tumors, fibrous dysplasia, eosinophilic granuloma, chondroblastoma, aneurysmal bone cysts, nonossifying fibroma, and osteomyelitis (110).

Several single-center studies have reported on the use of FDG PET to evaluate response to chemotherapy in patients with sarcomas. In 33 pediatric patients with osteosarcoma and Ewing sarcoma, Hawkins et al. found a postchemotherapy SUV of 2.0 to be a good predictor for histopathologic response to neoadjuvant chemotherapy (111). In another study with soft-tissue sarcomas, 40% or greater reduction in tumor SUV between baseline and postchemotherapy scan correlated with good histologic response and predicted significant improvement of recurrence-free and overall survival (112). Change in FDG uptake was found to be a significantly better predictor than change in size for evaluation of response to neoadjuvant therapy (113). Larger multicenter trials are needed to further define the role and criteria for PET in assessment of response to chemotherapy in pediatric patients with sarcoma.

REFERENCES

1. Frush DP, Applegate K. Computed tomography and radiation: understanding the issues. *J Am Coll Radiol* 2004;1:113–119.
2. McCollough CH. The AAPM/RSNA physics tutorial for residents. X-ray production. *Radiographics* 1997;17:967–984.
3. Zink FE. X-ray tubes. *Radiographics* 1997;17:1259–1268.
4. Bushberg JT. The AAPM/RSNA physics tutorial for residents. X-ray interactions. *Radiographics* 1998;18:457–468.
5. Bushberg JT, Seibert JA, Leidholdt EM Jr, et al. *The essential physics of medical imaging*, 2nd ed. Philadelphia, PA: Lippincott Williams & Wilkins, 2002.
6. Schueler BA. The AAPM/RSNA physics tutorial for residents: general overview of fluoroscopic imaging. *Radiographics* 2000;20:1115–1126.
7. Samei E, Seibert A, Andriole K, et al. General guidelines for purchasing and acceptance testing of PACS equipment. *Radiographics* 2004;24: 313–334.
8. Liu BJ, Hwang HK, Cao F, et al. A complete continuous-availability PACS archive server. *Radiographics* 2004;24:1203–1209.
9. El-Khoury GY, Bennett DL, Ondr GJ. Multidetector-row computed tomography. *J Am Acad Orthop Surg* 2004;12:1–5.
10. Cody DD. AAPM/RSNA physics tutorial for residents: topics in CT. Image processing in CT. *Radiographics* 2002;22:1255–1268.
11. Brown GA, Firoozbakhsh K, DeCoster TA, et al. Rapid prototyping: the future of trauma surgery? *J Bone Joint Surg Am* 2003;85-A(Suppl 4): 49–55.
12. Broder J, Fordham LA, Warshauer DM. Increasing utilization of computed tomography in the pediatric emergency department, 2000–2006. *Emerg Radiol* 2007;14:227–232.
13. Erickson SJ. High-resolution imaging of the musculoskeletal system. *Radiology* 1997;205:593–618.
14. Bellah R. Ultrasound in pediatric musculoskeletal disease: techniques and applications. *Radiol Clin North Am* 2001;39:597–618, ix.
15. Rosendahl K, Markestad T, Lie RT. Ultrasound screening for developmental dysplasia of the hip in the neonate: the effect on treatment rate and prevalence of late cases. *Pediatrics* 1994;94:47–52.
16. Screening for developmental dysplasia of the hip: recommendation statement. *Am Fam Physician* 2006;73:1992–1996.
17. Clarke NM, Harcke HT, McHugh P, et al. Real-time ultrasound in the diagnosis of congenital dislocation and dysplasia of the hip. *J Bone Joint Surg Br* 1985;67:406–412.
18. Keller MS, Nijs EL. The role of radiographs and US in developmental dysplasia of the hip: how good are they? *Pediatr Radiol* 2009;39(Suppl 2):S211–S215.
19. Graf R. The diagnosis of congenital hip-joint dislocation by the ultrasonic Combound treatment. *Arch Orthop Trauma Surg* 1980;97:117–133.
20. Harcke HT. Screening newborns for developmental dysplasia of the hip: the role of sonography. *Am J Roentgenol* 1994;162:395–397.
21. Elbourne D, Dezateux C, Arthur R, et al. Ultrasonography in the diagnosis and management of developmental hip dysplasia (UK Hip Trial): clinical and economic results of a multicentre randomised controlled trial. *Lancet* 2002;360:2009–2017.
22. Bearcroft PW, Berman LH, Robinson AH, et al. Vascularity of the neonatal femoral head: in vivo demonstration with power Doppler US. *Radiology* 1996;200:209–211.
23. Shiels WE II, Coley BD, Kean J, et al. Focused dynamic sonographic examination of the congenital clubfoot. *Pediatr Radiol* 2007;37: 1118–1124.
24. Jeanty P, Kleinman G. Proximal femoral focal deficiency. *J Ultrasound Med* 1989;8:639–642.
25. Marchal GJ, Van Holsbeeck MT, Raes M, et al. Transient synovitis of the hip in children: role of US. *Radiology* 1987;162:825–828.
26. Miralles M, Gonzalez G, Pulpeiro JR, et al. Sonography of the painful hip in children: 500 consecutive cases. *Am J Roentgenol* 1989;152:579–582.
27. Zawin JK, Hoffer FA, Rand FF, et al. Joint effusion in children with an irritable hip: US diagnosis and aspiration. *Radiology* 1993;187:459–463.
28. Mizel MS, Steinmetz ND, Trepman E. Detection of wooden foreign bodies in muscle tissue: experimental comparison of computed tomography, magnetic resonance imaging, and ultrasonography. *Foot Ankle Int* 1994;15:437–443.
29. Cellerini M, Salti S, Trapani S, et al. Correlation between clinical and ultrasound assessment of the knee in children with monoarticular or pauci-articular juvenile rheumatoid arthritis. *Pediatr Radiol* 1999;29:117–123.
30. Glasier CM, Seibert JJ, Williamson SL, et al. High resolution ultrasound characterization of soft tissue masses in children. *Pediatr Radiol* 1987;17:233–237.
31. Barnewolt CE, Chung T. Techniques, coils, pulse sequences, and contrast enhancement in pediatric musculoskeletal MR imaging. *Magn Reson Imaging Clin N Am* 1998;6:441–453.
32. Hendrick RE. The AAPM/RSNA physics tutorial for residents. Basic physics of MR imaging: an introduction. *Radiographics* 1994;14:829–846; quiz 847–848.
33. Sadowski EA, Bennett LK, Chan MR, et al. Nephrogenic systemic fibrosis: risk factors and incidence estimation. *Radiology* 2007;243:148–157.
34. Siegel MJ, Luker GG. Bone marrow imaging in children. *Magn Reson Imaging Clin N Am* 1996;4:771–796.
35. Vogler JB III, Murphy WA. Bone marrow imaging. *Radiology* 1988;168:679–693.
36. Laor T, Jaramillo D. MR imaging insights into skeletal maturation: what is normal? *Radiology* 2009;250:28–38.
37. Jaramillo D, Laor T, Hoffer FA, et al. Epiphyseal marrow in infancy: MR imaging. *Radiology* 1991;180:809–812.
38. Bos CF, Bloem JL, Obermann WR, et al. Magnetic resonance imaging in congenital dislocation of the hip. *J Bone Joint Surg Br* 1988;70:174–178.
39. Johnson ND, Wood BP, Jackman KV. Complex infantile and congenital hip dislocation: assessment with MR imaging. *Radiology* 1988;168: 151–156.
40. Jaramillo D, Villegas-Medina O, Laor T, et al. Gadolinium-enhanced MR imaging of pediatric patients after reduction of dysplastic hips:

assessment of femoral head position, factors impeding reduction, and femoral head ischemia. *Am J Roentgenol* 1998;170:1633–1637.

41. Laor T, Jaramillo D, Hoffer FA, et al. MR imaging in congenital lower limb deformities. *Pediatr Radiol* 1996;26:381–387.

42. Mazur JM, Ross G, Cummings J, et al. Usefulness of magnetic resonance imaging for the diagnosis of acute musculoskeletal infections in children. *J Pediatr Orthop* 1995;15:144–147.

43. Jaramillo D. What is the optimal imaging of osteonecrosis, Perthes, and bone infarcts? *Pediatr Radiol* 2009;39(Suppl 2):S216–S219.

44. Ha AS, Wells L, Jaramillo D. Importance of sagittal MR imaging in nontraumatic femoral head osteonecrosis in children. *Pediatr Radiol* 2008;38:1195–1200.

45. Restrepo R, Reed MH. Impact of obesity in the diagnosis of SCFE and knee problems in obese children. *Pediatr Radiol* 2009;39 (Suppl 2): S220–S225.

46. Morrison WB, Schweitzer ME, Bock GW, et al. Diagnosis of osteomyelitis: utility of fat-suppressed contrast-enhanced MR imaging. *Radiology* 1993;189:251–257.

47. Stover B, Sigmund G, Langer M, et al. MRI in diagnostic evaluation of osteomyelitis in children. *Eur Radiol* 1994;4:347–352.

48. Gold RH, Hawkins RA, Katz RD. Bacterial osteomyelitis: findings on plain radiography, CT, MR, and scintigraphy. *Am J Roentgenol* 1991;157:365–370.

49. Towers JD. The use of intravenous contrast in MRI of extremity infection. *Semin Ultrasound CT MR* 1997;18:269–275.

50. Gylys-Morin VM. MR imaging of pediatric musculoskeletal inflammatory and infectious disorders. *Magn Reson Imaging Clin N Am* 1998;6:537–559.

51. Argyropoulou MI, Fanis SL, Xenakis T, et al. The role of MRI in the evaluation of hip joint disease in clinical subtypes of juvenile idiopathic arthritis. *Br J Radiol* 2002;75:229–233.

52. Winalski CS, Aliabadi P, Wright RJ, et al. Enhancement of joint fluid with intravenously administered gadopentetate dimeglumine: technique, rationale, and implications. *Radiology* 1993;187:179–185.

53. Azouz EM. Juvenile idiopathic arthritis: how can the radiologist help the clinician? *Pediatr Radiol* 2008;38(Suppl 3):S403–S408.

54. Peterfy CG, Genant HK. Emerging applications of magnetic resonance imaging in the evaluation of articular cartilage. *Radiol Clin North Am* 1996;34:195–213, ix.

55. Sundaram M, McGuire MH, Herbold DR. Magnetic resonance imaging of soft tissue masses: an evaluation of fifty-three histologically proven tumors. *Magn Reson Imaging* 1988;6:237–248.

56. Totty WG, Murphy WA, Lee JK. Soft-tissue tumors: MR imaging. *Radiology* 1986;160:135–141.

57. Berquist TH, Ehman RL, King BF, et al. Value of MR imaging in differentiating benign from malignant soft-tissue masses: study of 95 lesions. *Am J Roentgenol* 1990;155:1251–1255.

58. Kransdorf MJ, Jelinek JS, Moser RP Jr, et al. Soft-tissue masses: diagnosis using MR imaging. *Am J Roentgenol* 1989;153:541–547.

59. Crim JR, Seeger LL, Yao L, et al. Diagnosis of soft-tissue masses with MR imaging: can benign masses be differentiated from malignant ones? *Radiology* 1992;185:581–586.

60. Gillespy T III, Manfrini M, Ruggieri P, et al. Staging of intraosseous extent of osteosarcoma: correlation of preoperative CT and MR imaging with pathologic macroslides. *Radiology* 1988;167:765–767.

61. Onikul E, Fletcher BD, Parham DM, et al. Accuracy of MR imaging for estimating intraosseous extent of osteosarcoma. *Am J Roentgenol* 1996;167:1211–1215.

62. Hoffer FA, Nikanorov AY, Reddick WE, et al. Accuracy of MR imaging for detecting epiphyseal extension of osteosarcoma. *Pediatr Radiol* 2000;30:289–298.

63. Schima W, Amann G, Stiglbauer R, et al. Preoperative staging of osteosarcoma: efficacy of MR imaging in detecting joint involvement. *Am J Roentgenol* 1994;163:1171–1175.

64. Kager L, Zoubek A, Kastner U, et al. Skip metastases in osteosarcoma: experience of the Cooperative Osteosarcoma Study Group. *J Clin Oncol* 2006;24:1535–1541.

65. Disler DG, McCauley TR, Ratner LM, et al. In-phase and out-of-phase MR imaging of bone marrow: prediction of neoplasia based on the detection of coexistent fat and water. *Am J Roentgenol* 1997;169:1439–1447.

66. Abudu A, Davies AM, Pynsent PB, et al. Tumour volume as a predictor of necrosis after chemotherapy in Ewing's sarcoma. *J Bone Joint Surg Br* 1999;81:317–322.

67. van der Woude HJ, Bloem JL, Holscher HC, et al. Monitoring the effect of chemotherapy in Ewing's sarcoma of bone with MR imaging. *Skeletal Radiol* 1994;23:493–500.

68. Holscher HC, Bloem JL, Nooy MA, et al. The value of MR imaging in monitoring the effect of chemotherapy on bone sarcomas. *Am J Roentgenol* 1990;154:763–769.

69. Holscher HC, Bloem JL, Vanel D, et al. Osteosarcoma: chemotherapy-induced changes at MR imaging. *Radiology* 1992;182:839–844.

70. Dyke JP, Panicek DM, Healey JH, et al. Osteogenic and Ewing sarcomas: estimation of necrotic fraction during induction chemotherapy with dynamic contrast-enhanced MR imaging. *Radiology* 2003;228:271–278.

71. Erlemann R, Sciuk J, Bosse A, et al. Response of osteosarcoma and Ewing sarcoma to preoperative chemotherapy: assessment with dynamic and static MR imaging and skeletal scintigraphy. *Radiology* 1990;175:791–796.

72. Naranja RJ Jr, Gregg JR, Dormans JP, et al. Pediatric fracture without radiographic abnormality. Description and significance. *Clin Orthop Relat Res* 1997;342:141–146.

73. Ahn JM, El-Khoury GY. Occult fractures of extremities. *Radiol Clin North Am* 2007;45:561–579, ix.

74. Laor T, Wall EJ, Vu LP. Physeal widening in the knee due to stress injury in child athletes. *Am J Roentgenol* 2006;186:1260–1264.

75. Bates DG, Hresko MT, Jaramillo D. Patellar sleeve fracture: demonstration with MR imaging. *Radiology* 1994;193:825–827.

76. Puri A, Shingade VU, Agarwal MG, et al. CT-guided percutaneous core needle biopsy in deep seated musculoskeletal lesions: a prospective study of 128 cases. *Skeletal Radiol* 2006;35:138–143.

77. Torriani M, Etchebehere M, Amstalden E. Sonographically guided core needle biopsy of bone and soft tissue tumors. *J Ultrasound Med* 2002;21:275–281.

78. Fraser-Hill MA, Renfrew DL, Hilsenrath PE. Percutaneous needle biopsy of musculoskeletal lesions. 2. Cost-effectiveness. *Am J Roentgenol* 1992;158:813–818.

79. Mankin HJ, Mankin CJ, Simon MA. The hazards of the biopsy, revisited. Members of the Musculoskeletal Tumor Society. *J Bone Joint Surg Am* 1996;78:656–663.

80. Murphy WA, Destouet JM, Gilula LA. Percutaneous skeletal biopsy 1981: a procedure for radiologists—results, review, and recommendations. *Radiology* 1981;139:545–549.

81. Scaglietti O, Marchetti PG, Bartolozzi P. The effects of methylprednisolone acetate in the treatment of bone cysts. Results of three years follow-up. *J Bone Joint Surg Br* 1979;61-B:200–61-B:204.

82. Campanacci M, Capanna R, Picci P. Unicameral and aneurysmal bone cysts. *Clin Orthop Relat Res* 1986;204:25–36.

83. Sung AD, Anderson ME, Zurakowski D, et al. Unicameral bone cyst: a retrospective study of three surgical treatments. *Clin Orthop Relat Res* 2008;466:2519–2526.

84. Capanna R, Albisinni U, Caroli GC, et al. Contrast examination as a prognostic factor in the treatment of solitary bone cyst by cortisone injection. *Skeletal Radiol* 1984;12:97–102.

85. Fernbach SK, Blumenthal DH, Poznanski AK, et al. Radiographic changes in unicameral bone cysts following direct injection of steroids: a report on 14 cases. *Radiology* 1981;140:689–695.

86. Torriani M, Rosenthal DI. Percutaneous radiofrequency treatment of osteoid osteoma. *Pediatr Radiol* 2002;32:615–618.

87. Hoffmann RT, Jakobs TF, Kubisch CH, et al. Radiofrequency ablation in the treatment of osteoid osteoma-5-year experience. *Eur J Radiol* 2010;73(2)374–379.

88. Connolly LP, Connolly SA. Skeletal scintigraphy in the multimodality assessment of young children with acute skeletal symptoms. *Clin Nucl Med* 2003;28:746–754.

89. Connolly LP, Connolly SA, Drubach LA, et al. Acute hematogenous osteomyelitis of children: assessment of skeletal scintigraphy-based diagnosis in the era of MRI. *J Nucl Med* 2002;43:1310–1316.

90. Matin P. The appearance of bone scans following fractures, including immediate and long-term studies. *J Nucl Med* 1979;20:1227–1231.

91. Seabold JE, Forstrom LA, Schauwecker DS, et al. Procedure guideline for indium-111-leukocyte scintigraphy for suspected infection/inflammation. Society of Nuclear Medicine. *J Nucl Med* 1997;38:997–1001.

92. Palestro CJ, Love C, Tronco GG, et al. Combined labeled leukocyte and technetium 99m sulfur colloid bone marrow imaging for diagnosing musculoskeletal infection. *Radiographics* 2006;26:859–870.

93. Schauwecker DS, Park HM, Mock BH, et al. Evaluation of complicating osteomyelitis with Tc-99m MDP, In-111 granulocytes, and Ga-67 citrate. *J Nucl Med* 1984;25:849–853.

94. Minoves M. Bone and joint sports injuries: the role of bone scintigraphy. *Nucl Med Commun* 2003;24:3–10.

95. Raby N, Mathews S. Symptomatic spondylolysis: correlation of CT and SPECT with clinical outcome. *Clin Radiol* 1993;48:97–99.

96. Collier BD, Johnson RP, Carrera GF, et al. Painful spondylolysis or spondylolisthesis studied by radiography and single-photon emission computed tomography. *Radiology* 1985;154:207–211.

97. Bellah RD, Summerville DA, Treves ST, et al. Low-back pain in adolescent athletes: detection of stress injury to the pars interarticularis with SPECT. *Radiology* 1991;180:509–512.

98. Diagnostic imaging of child abuse. *Pediatrics* 2000;105:1345–1348.

99. Jaudes PK. Comparison of radiography and radionuclide bone scanning in the detection of child abuse. *Pediatrics* 1984;73:166–168.

100. Mandelstam SA, Cook D, Fitzgerald M, et al. Complementary use of radiological skeletal survey and bone scintigraphy in detection of bony injuries in suspected child abuse. *Arch Dis Child* 2003;88:387–390; discussion 387–390.

101. Turba E, Fagioli G, Mancini AF, et al. Evaluation of stage 4 neuroblastoma patients by means of MIBG and 99m Tc-MDP scintigraphy. *J Nucl Biol Med* 1993;37:107–114.

102. Cook AM, Waller S, Loken MK. Multiple "cold" areas demonstrated on bone scintigraphy in a patient with neuroblastoma. *Clin Nucl Med* 1982;7:21–24.

103. Dogan AS, Conway JJ, Miller JH, et al. Detection of bone lesions in Langerhans cell histiocytosis: complementary roles of scintigraphy and conventional radiography. *J Pediatr Hematol Oncol* 1996;18:51–58.

104. Volker T, Denecke T, Steffen I, et al. Positron emission tomography for staging of pediatric sarcoma patients: results of a prospective multicenter trial. *J Clin Oncol* 2007;25:5435–5441.

105. Tateishi U, Yamaguchi U, Seki K, et al. Bone and soft-tissue sarcoma: preoperative staging with fluorine 18 fluorodeoxyglucose PET/CT and conventional imaging. *Radiology* 2007;245:839–847.

106. Franzius C, Daldrup-Link HE, Sciuk J, et al. FDG-PET for detection of pulmonary metastases from malignant primary bone tumors: comparison with spiral CT. *Ann Oncol* 2001;12:479–486.

107. Johnson GR, Zhuang H, Khan J, et al. Roles of positron emission tomography with fluorine-18-deoxyglucose in the detection of local recurrent and distant metastatic sarcoma. *Clin Nucl Med* 2003;28:815–820.

108. Arush MW, Israel O, Postovsky S, et al. Positron emission tomography/computed tomography with 18fluoro-deoxyglucose in the detection of local recurrence and distant metastases of pediatric sarcoma. *Pediatr Blood Cancer* 2007;49:901–905.

109. Ioannidis JP, Lau J. 18F-FDG PET for the diagnosis and grading of soft-tissue sarcoma: a meta-analysis. *J Nucl Med* 2003;44:717–724.

110. Schulte M, Brecht-Krauss D, Heymer B, et al. Grading of tumors and tumor-like lesions of bone: evaluation by FDG PET. *J Nucl Med* 2000;41:1695–1701.

111. Hawkins DS, Rajendran JG, Conrad EU, 3rd, et al. Evaluation of chemotherapy response in pediatric bone sarcomas by [F-18]-fluorodeoxy-D-glucose positron emission tomography. *Cancer* 2002;94:3277–3284.

112. Schuetze SM, Rubin BP, Vernon C, et al. Use of positron emission tomography in localized extremity soft tissue sarcoma treated with neoadjuvant chemotherapy. *Cancer* 2005;103:339–348.

113. Evilevitch V, Weber WA, Tap WD, et al. Reduction of glucose metabolic activity is more accurate than change in size at predicting histopathologic response to neoadjuvant therapy in high-grade soft-tissue sarcomas. *Clin Cancer Res* 2008;14:715–720.

CHAPTER 4

David D. Aronsson
Jennifer W. Lisle

The Pediatric Orthopaedic Examination

INTRODUCTION

The pediatric orthopaedic examination can vary considerably depending on the age of the child, chief complaint, magnitude of the problem, and the level of concern of the patient and family. In all situations, the clinician should respect the dignity of the child, family, and other health care professionals that accompany the patient. It is important for the child to feel comfortable in the office environment, so having a bright child-friendly waiting room with toys and age-appropriate books can be very beneficial. It is helpful to have the family or caregivers fill out a patient intake form (Fig. 4-1) prior to the visit to expedite the history so the clinician can focus on engaging the child and gaining the child's trust. In some cases, this may be the most important aspect of the pediatric orthopaedic examination, as it is almost impossible to perform an adequate examination on an uncooperative child. Currently, the paper chart is gradually being replaced by the electronic medical record (EMR). In cases where the EMR is utilized, patients and their families can fill out the patient intake form electronically at home through a security enable portal, or through special computer kiosks, set up in the waiting room. Many hospitals, including ours, are mandating that patients or families fill out a pain assessment form such as the Wong-Baker FACES pain rating scale.

Recent studies have shown that clinician–patient communication underlies successful medical care, yet medical training has paid little attention to the importance of developing communication skills. Research has shown that improved communication improves diagnostic accuracy, fosters shared decision making, and increases the likelihood that the patient will follow the treatment recommendations. In addition, patient and clinician satisfaction increases and the risks of malpractice litigation decrease. The American Academy of Orthopaedic Surgeons (AAOS) has developed the "Clinician-Patient Communication to Enhance Health Outcomes Workshop" to address communication skills.

The AAOS approach identifies the different goals of the clinician and patient and emphasizes how they can all be addressed with improved communication. While the clinician wants to solve the problem with the "find it" and "fix it" approach, the patient has already made a self-diagnosis and wants the clinician to address an agenda of concerns including the self-diagnosis. To achieve the medical goals, the clinician needs to use the "4 Es" of communication skills: engage, empathize, educate, and enlist. To "find it," the clinician must engage and empathize with the patient and not interrupt them while they are explaining their agenda. If this person-to-person or professional–partner engagement is attained, the accuracy of the diagnosis is improved and the "fix it" is achieved by improved patient education and enlisting the patient in shared decision making in the treatment. Improved communication results in improved patient outcomes. In today's world, parents and young people expect to be heard, and their input often helps the clinician work with them.

The clinician begins by introducing himself or herself to the patient and family. If a resident physician or medical student accompanies the clinician into the exam room, it is important to introduce them and explain that they are learning. The clinician sits down to make direct eye contact with the child and listens attentively while taking an accurate history from the patient, family, and caregivers. Although a brief history and limited physical examination may be appropriate for a 5-year-old boy with a torus fracture, a complete history and physical examination are necessary to evaluate a 2-year-old boy who is still not walking.

HISTORY

The history always should begin with the *chief complaint*, a sentence or short statement in the exact words of the patient. If the patient is nonverbal or not yet talking, the chief complaint can be recorded in the exact words of the family or caregivers.

The *history of present illness* includes the details of how and when the chief complaint started and whether the symptoms are constant or intermittent. The clinician asks how the symptoms have evolved and if there are certain circumstances that aggravate the symptoms, such as exercise, or certain circumstances that relieve the symptoms, such as rest. It is important to document if any prior treatment has been recommended or rendered.

Age: Years _____ Months _____   Grade in School _____
Brothers _____   Sisters _____
Height of Mother: _____   Height of Father: _____
Referring Physician: _____   Family Physician: _____
_____   _____

What is the reason for today's visit? _____
When did this problem first start? _____
Is it better, worse or the same from when you first noted it? _____
Have you had any treatment? _____
If yes, please list the treating physician(s) and treatment _____

Past History:

Medical Problems?	Yes _____	No _____	If yes, please list	_____
Operations?	Yes _____	No _____	If yes, please list	_____
Medications?	Yes _____	No _____	If yes, please list	_____
Drug Allergies?	Yes _____	No _____	If yes, please list	_____
Latex Allergies?	Yes _____	No _____		
Other Allergies?	Yes _____	No _____	If yes, please list	_____

Birth History of Patient:

Premature?	Yes _____	No _____	Reason?	_____
Problems?	Yes _____	No _____	Reason?	_____
Breech?	Yes _____	No _____	Reason?	_____
Caesarian?	Yes _____	No _____	Reason?	_____

Birth Place: _____ Hospital: _____ Birth weight: _____ lbs. _____ oz.

Developmental Milestone of the Patient:
At what age did the child:
Roll over? _____ months   Sit up? _____ months   Walk? _____ months

Family History of Patient:
Please describe any family history of medical problems related to patient's condition:

_____

_____

Social History of Patient:
Please describe any sports or extracurricular activities:

_____

General Conditions/Treatments

Yes	No		Yes	No	
_____	_____	frequent or severe headaches	_____	_____	dizziness
_____	_____	blurring or other problems with vision	_____	_____	bladder problems or infection
_____	_____	hearing difficulty	_____	_____	cancer
_____	_____	shortness of breath or wheezing	_____	_____	diabetes
_____	_____	chest pain or palpitations	_____	_____	blood clots or phlebitis
_____	_____	abdominal pain, nausea or vomiting	_____	_____	high blood pressure
_____	_____	abdominal bleeding	_____	_____	stroke
_____	_____	depression	_____	_____	thyroid gland disorder
_____	_____	persistent or repeated rashes	_____	_____	epilepsy or seizures
_____	_____	repeated fevers	_____	_____	weight loss or gain
_____	_____	arthritis			
_____		Other: _____			If yes, please explain briefly: _____

FIGURE 4-1. Patient intake form. This form, when filled out by the patient or family, prior to the office visit can save valuable time while conducting the history and physical examination.

The *past medical history* includes any prior major illnesses, hospitalizations, operations, and if the patient is taking any medications. The patient's medications are reconciled and the patient's allergies are recorded, particularly any allergies to medications.

The *developmental history* includes the details concerning the pregnancy, delivery, and perinatal course. Any complications associated with this pregnancy or any prior pregnancies are documented. Any problems associated with the delivery, such as an emergency cesarean section, or the newborn period, such as transfer to the Neonatal Intensive Care Unit (NICU), are noted. The clinician asks the family if anyone has raised concerns about developmental delay and records the developmental milestones, including when the child first sat, pulled to standing, cruised around furniture, walked independently, and developed handedness.

The *family history* focuses mainly on the immediate family including siblings, parents, grandparents, and any other close relatives. The clinician asks if any family members had a similar problem or a major illness.

The *review of systems* includes a general medical overview with questions about each system, such as the respiratory, cardiovascular, or genitourinary systems, to detect any other medical problems. Detecting a medical problem that may be associated with the chief complaint may lead directly to diagnose the problem (e.g., a patient with scoliosis that has a genitourinary problem).

The *personal and social history* reviews the living situation of the patient and may be extremely valuable in diagnosing the problem. The clinician asks about school and sports activities that interest the patient. Hobbies are important as they may reveal more about strengths, relationships, and other issues. Personal questions may be of value since smoking or secondary smoke in the home has been associated with several orthopaedic conditions such as Legg-Calvé-Perthes disease.

PHYSICAL EXAMINATION

The physical examination begins with the height and weight of the patient that is typically performed by the staff prior to placing the patient and family in the exam room. The clinician begins with a thorough examination of the skin, spine, upper and lower extremities, and a brief neurologic examination. The pediatric orthopaedic physical examination does not typically include the vital signs or a detailed examination of the head, eyes, ears, nose, throat, chest, heart, abdomen, or genitals, but any of these areas may require a detailed examination depending on the chief complaint. If there are concerns about certain aspects of the physical examination, these areas are examined in detail.

The history and physical examination varies considerably depending on the age of the patient. Infants and young children are unable to give a history, whereas an older child will often give a more accurate history than the family or caregivers. A teenage boy with a round back may have no concerns, but the family may be concerned that he will develop a severe

hunchback deformity like his grandmother. Many pediatric orthopaedic conditions develop only in certain age groups, such as Legg-Calvé-Perthes disease, which typically develops in boys between 4 and 10 years of age. To highlight these important conditions that often develop only in certain age groups, this chapter is divided into three sections, according to the age of the patient. In all cases, once the history and physical examination is completed the clinician should communicate the findings with the referring primary care pediatrician or family physician.

The first section includes newborns, infants, and young children from birth to 4 years of age. These patients are usually unable to give an accurate history, so most of the history is obtained from the family or caregivers. The child may be apprehensive about going to the doctor and afraid of being examined. A toy or sticker may be helpful to divert the child's focus away from the situation and allow the clinician to do a physical examination. The majority of the physical examination of a young child can be done in the mother's lap. Once relaxed, the pertinent aspects of the examination can be performed on the examination table. If the infant is afraid and upset, a pause to allow bottle or breast feeding can be helpful. Once the clinician gains the respect and trust of the child and family, the physical examination can easily be performed.

The second section includes children from 4 to 10 years of age. These patients are not usually afraid and are interested in being a part of the examination. They will often correct their parents or caregivers about certain aspects of the history. They are typically calm and eager to participate and cooperate with the physical examination. In the age group, many children do not like removing their clothes or wearing a hospital gown. This situation can be avoided if the patient wears a T-shirt and a pair of shorts for the office visit. It is helpful to have extra pairs of gym shorts in the office to address this issue. Some children with special health needs are particularly resistant to anyone attempting to conduct a physical examination. In this situation, it is often helpful to tell the family exactly what you would like to accomplish. For example, the clinician can explain to the family that he or she would like to examine the child for scoliosis by having the child bend forward at the waist. The family can then place the child on a relative's lap in the seated position while another family member bends the child forward at the waist to allow the clinician to examine the spine.

The third section includes children and adolescents from 10 to 18 years of age. These patients are usually very motivated to get better and will give an accurate history. Teenagers are also concerned about removing their clothes, so it is reassuring to know that they do not need to remove their T-shirt or shorts. Having extra pairs of gym shorts in the office is again helpful if they come to the office in jeans. If conducted appropriately and in a manner that respects their privacy, teenagers will allow the clinician to perform a complete physical examination. In all age groups, it saves time and avoids repetition to begin by reviewing the patient intake form that was filled out by the family, caregivers, or the patient prior to entering the examination room (Fig. 4-1).

THE ORTHOPAEDIC EXAMINATION FROM BIRTH TO 4 YEARS OF AGE

A 1-Month-Old Girl Is Referred for Evaluation of a Hip Click.
A hip click was detected by the pediatrician shortly after birth and was still present at the 2-week appointment. The pediatrician was concerned that the baby might have developmental dysplasia of the hip (DDH) and referred her for evaluation. The history reveals that this is the mother's first child and the pregnancy was normal, but the baby was in the breech presentation and they had to do a cesarean section. The birth weight was 3500 g (7 lb 11 oz) and the baby is otherwise healthy. There is no family history of DDH or hip problems.

A hip click may be a benign click that occurs when the ligamentum teres gets trapped between the femoral head and the acetabulum, or it may indicate a subluxatable or dislocatable hip as is seen in DDH. To distinguish between these two different entities, the clinician focuses on certain aspects of the history and physical examination that are associated with DDH. The birth history may be helpful as DDH is associated with primigravida mothers, oligohydramnios, breech presentations, and congenital muscular torticollis. Of these, the breech presentation is the most important because, even if born by cesarean section, if the infant was in the frank (single) breech presentation, the frequency of DDH is 20% to 30%. The developmental history may reveal that the infant has a neuromuscular disorder, such as arthrogryposis multiplex congenita. The family history is helpful because the frequency of DDH is higher when other family members have the disorder.

The physical examination can be started with the infant in the mother's lap. In this position, the infant is comfortable, and the clinician can examine the range of motion of the hands, wrists, elbows, and shoulders. The neck range of motion is evaluated to rule out a contracture of the sternocleidomastoid muscle that may be secondary to a congenital muscular torticollis. The knees, ankles, and feet are examined to look for any anomalies that might be associated with DDH. The baby can then be placed prone over the mother's shoulder, similar to the position for burping, while the clinician examines the spine. A sacral dimple or hairy patch above the natal cleft may be a sign of an underlying tethered spinal cord or lipomeningocele (Fig. 4-2). These disorders can cause partial paralysis of the lower extremities resulting in a paralytic hip dislocation. Finally, after the rest of the physical examination has been completed, the infant is placed on the examining table to examine the hips.

The key to the early diagnosis of DDH is the physical examination. The examination should be performed on a firm surface with the infant relaxed. If the infant is crying or upset with tensing of the muscles, the DDH may not be detected. In this situation, allow the family to feed or soothe the infant and begin the examination when the infant is calm and relaxed. Barlow recommends the examination be performed in two parts (1).

Part one is termed the "Ortolani maneuver." To perform the Ortolani maneuver, each hip is examined individually

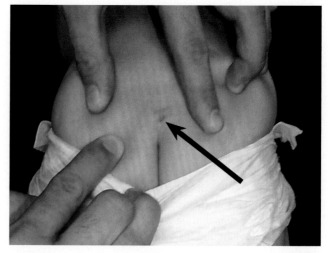

FIGURE 4-2. A sacral dimple (*arrow*) or hairy patch above the natal cleft may indicate an underlying tethered spinal cord or lipomeningocele.

while holding the pelvis steady with the other hand grasping the sacrum and pubic rami, or by using the other hand to hold and stabilize the opposite lower extremity and pelvis. The hips and knees are flexed to 90 degrees and the examiner places the long finger of each hand laterally, along the axis of the femur over the greater trochanter, and the thumb of each hand is placed on the inner side of the thigh opposite the lesser trochanter (Fig. 4-3). With the opposite hip and pelvis stabilized, the thigh of the hip to be examined is carried into abduction with forward pressure applied behind the greater trochanter by the long finger simultaneously. If the femoral head "clunks"

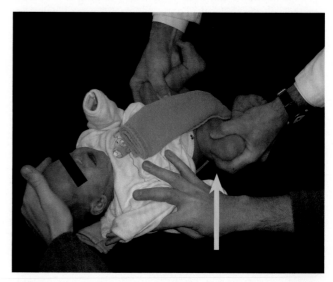

FIGURE 4-3. The first part of the Barlow provocative test is the Ortolani maneuver. This test is performed by gently abducting the hip and pushing forward with the long finger over the greater trochanter (*arrow*). A clunk is palpated as the femoral head slides over the posterior lip into the acetabulum.

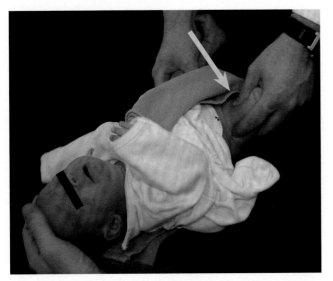

FIGURE 4-4. The second part of the Barlow provocative test involves applying pressure backward and outward with the thumb on the inner side of the thigh (*arrow*) while adducting the hip. If the femoral head clunks or slips out over the posterior lip of the acetabulum and back again after the pressure is released, the hip is unstable.

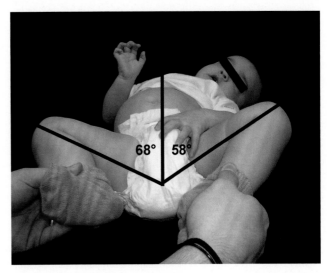

FIGURE 4-5. After 3 months of age, the most common physical finding in a patient with DDH is limited abduction of the hip. The asymmetry may be subtle as in this 15-month-old girl with a dislocated left hip. She has decreased abduction of the left hip (58 degrees) compared with the right (68 degrees).

forward into the acetabulum as the hip is abducted, the hip was dislocated. This maneuver, originally described by Ortolani, represents a "sign of entry" as the femoral head reduces into the acetabulum (Fig. 4-3). The Ortolani maneuver completes the first part of the Barlow test.

Part two of the Barlow test is termed the "provocative test." To perform the Barlow provocative test, each hip is again examined individually. With the hips and knees flexed to 90 degrees, the examiner places the long finger of each hand laterally, along the axis of the femur over the greater trochanter, and the thumb of each hand is placed on the inner side of the thigh opposite the lesser trochanter. With the opposite hip and pelvis stabilized, the examiner applies pressure laterally and posteriorly with the thumb on the inner side of the thigh as the hip is adducted. The hip is unstable if the femoral head "clunks" or slides over the posterior lip of the acetabulum and relocates when the pressure is released. This maneuver represents a "sign of exit," as the femoral head subluxates or dislocates from the acetabulum (Fig. 4-4). In a subluxating hip, the examiner may only detect a sliding sensation as the femoral head slides posteriorly in the acetabulum.

Although some investigators prefer to examine both hips simultaneously and others prefer to examine each hip separately, the most important aspect of the hip examination is to focus closely on each hip during the examination. The Barlow and Ortolani tests detect hip instability with ligamentous laxity, and although they are valuable during the neonatal period, they usually become negative by 3 months of age (2).

Once the infant is 3 months of age, if the femoral head is subluxated or dislocated the adductor and flexor muscles gradually develop contractures. The most common physical finding in older infants with DDH is limited abduction of the hip (Fig. 4-5). The limited abduction may be subtle, so it is important that the infant is positioned supine on a firm table. An infant with bilateral DDH may have symmetrically limited abduction that can only be detected by a careful examination. If the DDH is unilateral, the superolateral subluxation or dislocation of the femoral head causes a limb-length discrepancy that may be detected by the family or primary care physician. The subluxation or dislocation shortens the thigh causing an increased number of thigh folds (telescoping) compared with the uninvolved side. Although asymmetric thigh folds may be a normal finding, it alerts the clinician to the possibility of DDH. If the hips are flexed to 90 degrees, the subtle limb-length discrepancy can be detected, as the knee on the side with DDH will be lower than the opposite side. This finding is termed a positive Galeazzi sign (Fig. 4-6). In this patient, the Ortolani maneuver is positive, so treatment with a Pavlik harness is recommended.

A 2-Year-Old Boy Is Referred for Evaluation of Bowed Legs, Intoeing, and Tripping Over His Feet.

The family first noted that his legs were bowed at 3 months of age. When he began walking at 16 months of age, the bowing was worse and his feet turned in. His feet now turn in so much that he trips over them falling frequently. The birth history reveals that he was born after a 40-week gestation via normal vaginal delivery with a birth weight of 4000 g (8 lb 13 oz). His developmental milestones reveal that he first sat at 7 months of age and began walking at 16 months of age. The family history reveals that the father wore a brace until he was 2 years old because his feet turned in.

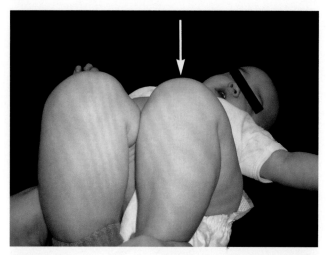

FIGURE 4-6. The subtle femoral-length discrepancy that is seen with the hips flexed to 90 degrees is termed a positive Galeazzi sign. The Galeazzi sign is seen in DDH when the knee on the side with DDH is lower than the opposite side (*arrow*).

TABLE 4-1	Average Developmental Achievement by Age
Age	**Achievement**
1 mo	Partial head control in prone position
2 mo	Good head control in prone position; partial head control in supine position
4 mo	Good head control in supine position; rolls over prone to supine
5 mo	Rolls over supine to prone
6 mo	When prone, lifts head and chest with weight on hands; sits with support
8 mo	Sits independently; reaches for toys
10 mo	Crawls; stands holding onto furniture
12 mo	Walks independently or with hand support
18 mo	Developing handedness
2 yr	Jumps; knows full name
3 yr	Goes upstairs alternating feet; stands momentarily on one foot; knows age and gender
4 yr	Hops on one foot; throws ball overhand
5 yr	Skips; dresses independently

Since most 2-year-old children fall frequently, the clinician focuses on certain aspects of the history and physical examination to determine if the child has developmental delay. If so, he may have problems with coordination or retention of primitive reflexes that should have already disappeared. If the bowed legs represent physiologic bowing, one would expect the deformity to be improving by 2 years of age. If the intoeing is physiologic and represents a normal rotational variation, it will usually be symmetric and is often not noticed until the child begins walking. A unilateral problem, involving the foot, may indicate a mild clubfoot or a neurologic problem such as a tethered spinal cord. The clinician reviews the developmental history as most children will sit independently by 6 to 9 months of age, cruise (walk around furniture) by 10 to 14 months of age, and walk independently by 8 to 18 months of age (Table 4-1).

If the child has developmental delay, it is important to verify the details surrounding the birth to determine if the child was born premature, or if there were any perinatal complications. Premature infants born after 25 to 30 weeks of gestation, with a birth weight of 750 g (1 lb 10 oz) to 1500 g (3 lb 5 oz), have an increased incidence of cerebral palsy with spastic diplegia. The first sign of this disorder may occur when the family notes that their child is delayed in walking, limping, or tripping over his feet. When evaluating for developmental delay, it is valuable to ask if the infant is ambidextrous. Most children will remain ambidextrous until 18 months to 3 years of age (Table 4-1). If a child who is tripping over his left foot is also strongly right-handed, the birth history may reveal an intrauterine cerebral vascular accident causing cerebral palsy with spastic left hemiplegia.

A 2-year-old boy may be apprehensive and uncomfortable in the exam room, so it may be helpful to begin the physical examination by opening the door and asking the family if they would like to take their son for a walk down the

hall. Most 2-year-olds will enjoy walking away from the clinician and the exam room, but they often need to be carried back. While the family and child are walking down the hall, the clinician observes the child's gait pattern including the foot-progression angle (3). The foot-progression angle is the angle between the axis of the foot and an imaginary straight line on the floor (Fig. 4-7). The axis of the foot is derived from a line connecting a bisector of the heel with the center of the second metatarsal head. The foot-progression angle in children 1 to 4 years of age can vary from 15 degrees of inward to 25 degrees of outward rotation. The gait pattern can also vary considerably in this age group, but usually it will be relatively symmetric, with a similar amount of time being spent in stance phase (60% of the gait cycle) and swing phase (40% of the gait cycle). Rotational values within two standard deviations of the mean are termed "rotational variations," and values outside two standard deviations are termed "torsional deformities" (4).

The degree and location of any rotational variations can be documented by creating a rotational profile (Table 4-2). The rotational profile includes the foot-progression angle, internal and external rotation of the hips, the thigh-foot angle, and any foot deformities. The foot-progression angle measures the degree of intoeing or outtoeing compared with an imaginary straight line on the floor (normal range 15 degrees inward to 25 degrees outward rotation) (Fig. 4-7). The internal and external rotation of the hips measures the femoral rotational variation or torsion. Measuring internal rotation of the hips in the prone position is a very important test in pediatric orthopaedics because many hip disorders can be detected by this examination including toxic synovitis, Legg-Calvé-Perthes disease, slipped capital femoral epiphysis (SCFE), and septic

TABLE 4-2	Rotational Profile	
Parameter	Right	Left
Foot-progression angle[a]	15 degrees	15 degrees
Hip internal rotation	70 degrees	70 degrees
Hip external rotation	30 degrees	30 degrees
Thigh-foot angle[a]	20 degrees	20 degrees
Sole of foot	Straight	Straight

The rotational profile includes the foot-progression angles, internal rotation of the hips, external rotation of the hips, the thigh-foot angles, and any foot deformities. The angles should be recorded in degrees, and the foot deformities should be described. The example shows that this child has internal femoral and internal tibial variations.

[a]For foot-progression angle and thigh-foot angle, a positive number indicates inward rotation and a negative number indicates lateral rotation.

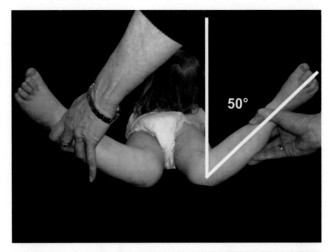

FIGURE 4-8. The internal rotation of the hips can be measured in the supine or prone position. Standing at the foot of the bed, with the patient prone, gravity allows the hips to fall into internal rotation. The angle between the leg and a line perpendicular to the tabletop measures the internal rotation (50 degrees in this patient).

arthritis (Fig. 4-8). The normal range of internal rotation is 20 to 80 degrees (Fig. 4-8), and the normal range of external rotation is 25 to 80 degrees (Fig. 4-9). The thigh-foot angle is the angle between the axis of the thigh and the axis of the foot, with the patient prone and the knee flexed 90 degrees (Fig. 4-10). The thigh-foot angle measures tibial rotational variation or torsion, and the normal ranges are 25 degrees of inward to 25 degrees of outward rotation (4). The foot examination documents any foot deformities that may be contributing to the intoeing. Once the profile is filled out, it gives an

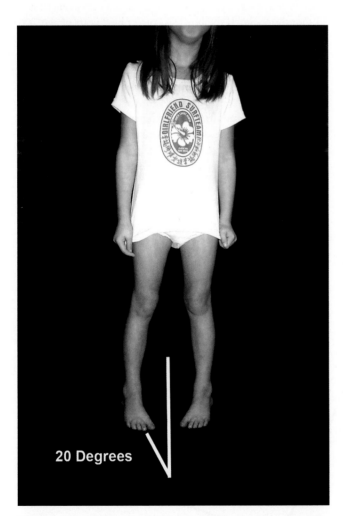

FIGURE 4-7. While the patient is walking, the foot-progression angle is the angle between the axis of the foot and an imaginary straight line on the floor representing the direction of movement. The axis of the foot is derived from a line connecting a bisector of the heel with the center of the second metatarsal head. This patient has a foot-progression angle of 20 degrees of internal rotation.

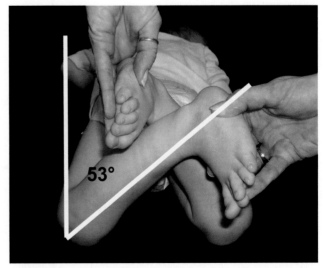

FIGURE 4-9. Standing at the foot of the bed, with the patient prone, gravity allows the hips to fall into external rotation. The angle between the leg and a line perpendicular to the tabletop measures the external rotation (53 degrees in this patient).

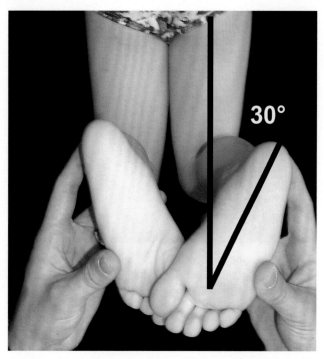

FIGURE 4-10. Standing at the foot of the bed, with the patient prone, the thigh-foot angle is the angle between the axis of the thigh and the axis of the foot, with the foot held in neutral position. The axis of the foot is derived from a line connecting a bisector of the heel with the center of the second metatarsal head. The thigh-foot angle measures the amount of tibial torsion (30 degrees in this patient).

objective view of the location and magnitude of any rotational variations or torsional deformities. This 2-year-old boy has internal rotational variations of both femurs and tibias. The rotational profile can be used as a baseline while following the child to document that rotational variations are indeed changing with growth.

In describing bowlegs and knock knees, the terms "varus" and "valgus" refer to the orientation of the distal fragment (leg) compared with the midline or proximal fragment (thigh). In a child with bowlegs, the distal fragment (tibia) is angulated toward the midline compared with the proximal fragment (femur) and is termed "genu varum." In a child with knock knees, the tibia is angulated away from the midline compared with the femur and is termed "genu valgum." In a child with bowlegs, when the ankles are touching, there is a gap between the knees, whereas in a child with knock knees, when the knees are touching there is a gap between the ankles. Most infants are born with bowlegs that spontaneously correct between 12 and 24 months of age. If the bowlegs correct by 2 years of age, it is termed physiologic bowing. The lower extremities then gradually develop genu valgum, which peaks between 3 and 4 years of age, then decreases to reach the normal adult tibiofemoral alignment of 7 degrees of genu valgum by 7 to 8 years of age (Fig. 4-11) (5).

On physical examination, the lower extremities are closely inspected to determine exactly where the deformity is located. If the deformity is mainly located in the proximal tibia, it may indicate tibia vara or Blount disease. If the deformity

FIGURE 4-11. Graph demonstrating the development of the tibiofemoral angle. Infants have genu varum that typically corrects by 18 to 24 months of age. The lower extremities then gradually develop genu valgum, which peaks between 3 and 4 years of age. The genu valgum then decreases to reach the normal adult tibiofemoral alignment of 7 degrees of valgus by 7 to 8 years of age.

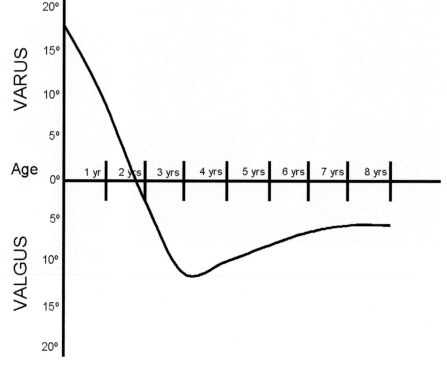

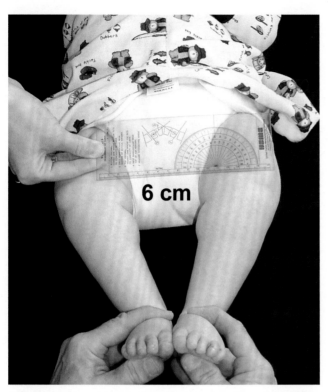

FIGURE 4-12. To measure the intercondylar distance, the child is supine with the lower extremities in extension. The feet are brought together until the medial malleoli just touch; the intercondylar distance is the distance between the femoral condyles (6 cm in this patient).

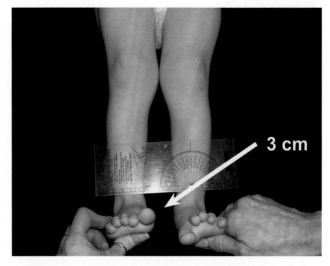

FIGURE 4-13. To measure the intermalleolar distance, the child is supine with the lower extremities in extension. The feet are brought together until the femoral condyles just touch; the intermalleolar distance is the distance between the medial malleoli (3 cm in this patient).

is symmetric, involving both the distal femur and proximal tibia, it may indicate physiologic bowing (6). The genu varum deformity is documented by measuring the "intercondylar distance." The intercondylar distance is measured in the supine position with the hips and knee in extension. The feet are brought together until the medial malleoli are just touching, and the intercondylar distance is the distance between the femoral condyles (Fig. 4-12).

A genu valgum deformity is documented in a similar fashion by measuring the "intermalleolar distance." With the child in the same position, the feet are brought together until the femoral condyles are just touching, and the intermalleolar distance is the distance between the medial malleoli (Fig. 4-13). This 2-year-old boy likely has physiologic bowing with internal tibial torsion, so the clinician anticipates that the intercondylar distance and thigh-foot angles will decrease over the next 6 months.

A Newborn Boy Is Referred for Evaluation of a Right Foot Deformity.
A newborn boy was noted in the neonatal nursery to have a right foot deformity. The birth history reveals that he was the mother's first child. Routine ultrasound screening at 28 weeks of gestation revealed concern for a possible right clubfoot deformity. The pregnancy was otherwise uncomplicated, and the baby was born by spontaneous vaginal delivery at full term weighing 3500 g (7 lb and

11 oz). The family history reveals that a maternal uncle had multiple foot surgeries performed at a young age.

Foot deformities are commonly seen in newborn infants, with an incidence of approximately 4% (7). The most common foot deformity is metatarsus adductus with talipes equinovarus and vertical talus much less frequently seen. The physical examination of the foot can easily be performed with the baby lying supine of the examination table or on the parents lap if the child is fussy. The upper extremities, neck, spine, hips, and knees are all examined first and determined to be within normal limits. The foot is then visually inspected and found to have multiple deformities as well as abnormal creases. There is only a single heel crease as well as the presence of a deep medial plantar crease.

Palpation and physical examination of the foot reveals the forefoot is adducted (indicating metatarsus adductus), the arch is high (indicating pes cavus), and the hindfoot is rolled into varus and equinus (Fig. 4-14). The tibiotalar, subtalar, and calcaneocuboid joints are gently taken through a full range of motion and reveal decreased movement compared to the other side.

Metatarsus adductus is the most common foot deformity and may be a result of intrauterine positional deformity (Fig. 4-15). Metatarsus adductus has forefoot adductus, but unlike a clubfoot there is no hindfoot equinovarus deformity. It is associated with DDH and torticollis, highlighting the importance of a careful examination of face, neck, and hips (8). The forefoot alignment in relation to the hindfoot can be evaluated by the "heel bisector line" (9). This line is generated by drawing a line down the foot that is center over the calcaneus and parallel to its axis (Fig. 4-16). A normal heel bisector should intersect between the second and the third ray. The metatarsus adductus is mild if the line bisects the third ray, moderate if

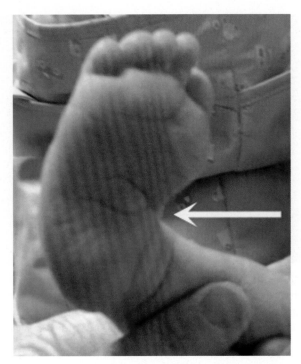

FIGURE 4-14. A clubfoot has forefoot adduction (metatarsus adductus), a high arch (pes cavus), and hindfoot varus and equinus. Depending on the severity of the deformity, a clubfoot may have a posterior and medial skin crease (*arrow*).

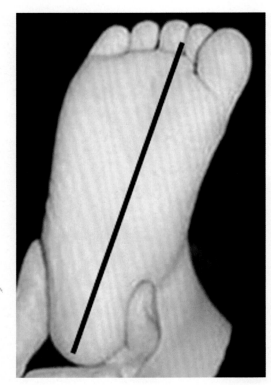

FIGURE 4-16. The normal heel bisector line intersects between the first and second rays.

it bisects the third and fourth rays, or severe if it bisects the fourth or the fifth ray. The lateral border of the foot is inspected and unlike a normal foot that has a straight lateral border, the lateral border is convex or bean shaped indicating metatarsus adductus. A foot that only has metatarsus adductus will have a neutral hindfoot, whereas a clubfoot will have an equinovarus

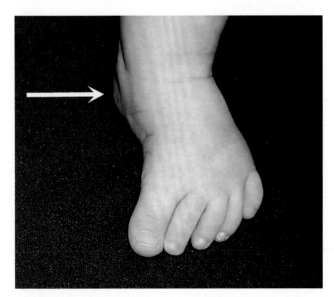

FIGURE 4-15. Metatarsus has forefoot adduction, but unlike a clubfoot the hindfoot is in neutral alignment (*arrow*).

hindfoot deformity. The flexibility of the metatarsus adductus can be assessed by placing the thumb of one hand on the calcaneocuboid joint laterally and grasping the medial forefoot with the other and passively abducting the forefoot (Fig. 4-17). If the metatarsus adductus can be corrected beyond the neutral axis, it is considered flexible. If the metatarsus adductus does not correct beyond the neutral axis, it is considered rigid.

Talipes equinovarus or a clubfoot presents as a spectrum of deformity characterized by midfoot cavus, forefoot adductus, and hindfoot varus and equinus (CAVE). Inspection of the skin of a clubfoot reveals varying degrees of posterior and medial skin creases depending on the severity of the deformity (Fig. 4-14). The hindfoot is palpated to evaluate the position of the calcaneus. When the calcaneus is markedly plantarflexed (equinus), the heel pad is displaced and appears absent. This phenomenon is termed an "empty heel pad sign." In a congenital clubfoot deformity, both the foot and calf are typically smaller than the normal side. In addition, the thigh-foot angles (Fig. 4-10) typically reveal internal tibial torsion and a shortened tibia on the side with the clubfoot (10).

The foot is then examined to assess the rigidity of the deformity by gently attempting to correct the midfoot cavus, forefoot adductus, and hindfoot varus and equinus. The most frequently used classification system to objectively quantify clubfoot rigidity is the Dimeglio clubfoot score (11). A clubfoot can also be classified as typical or atypical. A typical clubfoot is the classic clubfoot that is found most often in otherwise normal infants. An atypical clubfoot is often seen in association

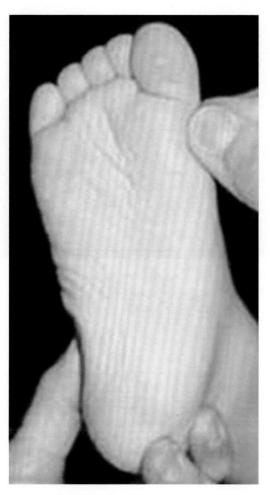

FIGURE 4-17. The flexibility of the metatarsus adductus can be assessed by placing the thumb of one hand on the calcaneocuboid joint laterally and abducting the forefoot with the other hand. If the metatarsus adductus corrects beyond the neutral axis, it is classified as flexible; if the metatarsus adductus does not correct beyond the neutral axis, it is classified as rigid.

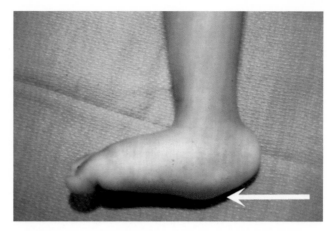

FIGURE 4-18. CVT has forefoot abduction and hindfoot equinovalgus, often described as a "rocker bottom foot." The talar head is palpable on the plantar surface of the foot (*arrow*).

with other neuromuscular disorders, such as arthrogryposis and myelomeningocele, and is usually less responsive to nonoperative management. The atypical clubfoot can be thin or fat and are frequently stiff, short, and chubby and with a deep crease on the plantar surface of the foot and behind the ankle. They may have shortening of the first metatarsal with hyperextension of the metatarsophalangeal joint reflecting a plantarflexed first ray.

A congenital clubfoot deformity is easily differentiated from congenital vertical talus (CVT) even though hindfoot equinus is prominent in both disorders. As opposed to the clubfoot that is typically seen in otherwise normal children, CVT is often associated with neuromuscular disorders including myelomeningocele, arthrogryposis multiplex congenital, spinal muscular atrophy, and prune-belly syndrome. On examination, in contrast to the clubfoot that has forefoot adductus and hindfoot varus, the CVT foot has forefoot abduction and hindfoot valgus, often described as a "rocker

bottom foot." The talar head is palpable on the plantar surface of the foot and creates the apex of the convex plantar surface (Fig. 4-18). In a CVT, the medial border of the foot is convex or bean shaped, whereas in a clubfoot the lateral border of the foot is convex or bean shaped.

This boy has a typical right congenital idiopathic clubfoot deformity. The clinician discusses the natural history of the congenital clubfoot deformity as well as the current treatment and recommends that stretching and treatment should begin preferably within the next few weeks.

An 18-Month-Old Boy Is Referred for Developmental Delay and Inability to Walk. The family first suspected a problem when he was 4 months old and was still having difficulty holding his head up. They became more concerned when he was not sitting at 10 months of age. He finally began sitting independently at 14 months of age and he just recently began pulling to standing, but is not yet cruising are the furniture. He was born after a 28-week gestation, with a birth weight of 1100 g (2 lb 7 oz). He had perinatal respiratory difficulties and was hospitalized in the NICU for 2 months. He developed a seizure disorder at 1 year of age, and his seizures are now under good control with medication.

This patient has developmental delay so the standard physical examination will also include a detailed neurologic examination and developmental assessment. An 18-month-old boy with developmental delay will usually not be apprehensive, and it is convenient to begin the physical examination with the boy in the supine position. The clinician grasps his hands, gradually pulling him into the sitting position, while looking for head and trunk control. A child will usually have head control by 2 to 4 months of age and trunk control by 6 to 8 months of age (Table 4-1). In children, there are a series of primitive reflexes, including the Moro, grasp, neck-righting, symmetric tonic neck, and asymmetric tonic neck reflexes, which are present at birth and then gradually disappear with

TABLE 4-3	Primitive and Postural Reflexes
Reflex	**Age When It Disappears**
Primitive reflex	
Moro	6 mo
Grasp	3 mo
Neck righting	10 mo
Symmetric tonic neck	6 mo
Asymmetric tonic neck	6 mo
Postural reflex	
Foot placement	Early infancy
Parachute	12 mo

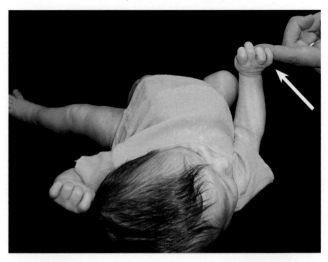

FIGURE 4-20. The grasp reflex is elicited by placing a finger in the infant's palm from the ulnar side (*arrow*). The infant's fingers will firmly grasp the finger and if traction is applied to the hand, the grasp reflex is stronger.

normal development by 3 to 10 months of age (Table 4-3). If these reflexes persist beyond 10 months of age, it may be a sign of a neuromuscular disorder.

The Moro reflex is elicited by introducing a sudden extension of the neck. The sudden neck extension causes the reflex where the shoulders abduct and the upper limbs extend, with spreading of the fingers, followed by an embrace (Fig. 4-19). The Moro reflex usually disappears by 6 months of age (12). The grasp reflex is elicited by placing a finger in the infant's palm from the ulnar side. The infant's fingers will firmly grasp the clinician's finger. If traction is applied to the hand, the grasp reflex is so strong that the clinician can lift the infant's shoulder off the table (Fig. 4-20). The grasp reflex usually disappears by 3 months of age. The neck-righting reflex is elicited by turning the head to one side; it is positive if the trunk and limbs spontaneously turn toward the same side. This reflex usually disappears by 10 months of age. The symmetric tonic neck reflex is elicited

by flexion of the neck, which causes flexion of the upper limbs and extension of the lower limbs. Similarly, extension of the neck causes extension of the upper limbs and flexion of the lower limbs. The asymmetric tonic neck reflex is elicited by turning the head to the side, which causes extension of the upper and lower extremities on the side toward which the head is turned, and flexion of the upper and lower extremities on the opposite side. This position is termed the "fencing position." The symmetric and asymmetric tonic neck reflexes usually disappear by 6 months of age.

The extensor thrust, an abnormal reflex, is elicited by holding the infant under the arms and touching the feet to the floor, which causes a rapid extension of all of the joints of the lower limb, progressing from the feet to the trunk. A normal infant will flex rather than extend the joints of the lower extremities when placed in this position. These primitive reflexes need to resolve with growth and development before the child will be able to walk independently.

There are other primitive reflexes that gradually disappear in normal children at different stages of development, including the rooting, startle, Gallant, and Landau reflexes. The rooting reflex is elicited by touching the corner of the mouth, which causes the mouth and tongue to turn toward the side that was stimulated. The startle reflex is elicited by making a loud noise, which causes a mass myoclonic response resembling a Moro reflex, except that the elbows remain flexed. The startle reflex may persist into adulthood. The Gallant reflex is elicited by stroking the side of the trunk, which causes the infant to bend the spine toward the side that was stimulated, creating a scoliosis convex to the opposite side that was stimulated. The Landau reflex is elicited by supporting the infant by the trunk in the horizontal prone position; the typical response is extension of the neck, spine, and extremities. If the infant collapses into an upside-down U, it may indicate hypotonia.

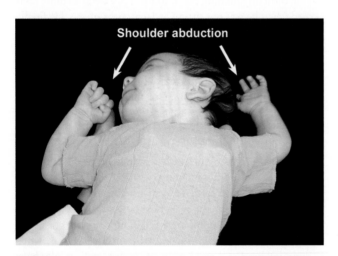

FIGURE 4-19. The Moro reflex is elicited by gently lifting the infant with the right hand under the upper thoracic spine and the left hand under the head. The left hand is dropped to allow sudden neck extension. The infant abducts the upper limbs, with spreading of the fingers, followed by an embrace.

There is another group of reflexes (postural reflexes) that gradually appear with normal development of the nervous system, including the parachute reflex and the foot-placement reaction (Table 4-3). The parachute reflex is elicited by holding the infant in the air in the prone position, then suddenly lowering the infant headfirst toward the table, simulating a fall (Fig. 4-21). The reflex is positive if the infant extends the upper extremities to break the fall. This reflex usually appears by 12 months of age and remains into adulthood. The foot-placement reaction is elicited by holding the infant under the arms, then gently lifting the infant so that the dorsum of the foot or the anterior surface of the tibia touches the side of the table. It is positive if the infant picks up the extremity and steps up onto the table (Figs. 4-22). The foot-placement reaction usually develops early in infancy and may persist until the age of 3 or 4 years.

Bleck (12) evaluated 73 children who were 12 months of age or older and were still not yet walking to determine their prognosis for walking. He used seven tests to predict if an infant would subsequently walk. One point was assigned for each primitive reflex that was still present, and one point was assigned for each postural reflex that was still absent (Table 4-4). A score of two points or more indicated a poor prognosis for walking, a one-point score indicated a guarded prognosis, and a zero-point score indicated a good prognosis.

The physical examination continues by evaluating the spine for any scoliosis or kyphosis. The upper and lower extremities are examined to assess range of motion and to document any contractures. If a contracture is identified, the clinician attempts to passively correct it to determine if it is flexible or rigid. An 18-month-old boy with cerebral palsy and spastic diplegia will typically have contractures that can be passively corrected, whereas a similar child with cerebral

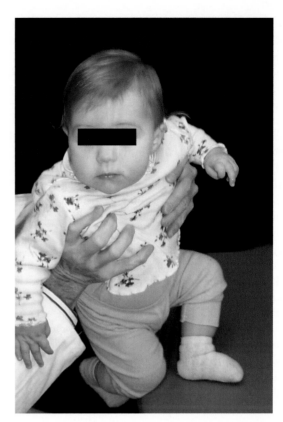

FIGURE 4-22. The foot-placement reaction is elicited by gently lifting the infant so that the dorsum of the foot or the anterior surface of the tibia touches the side of the table. It is positive if the infant picks up the extremity and steps up onto the table.

palsy and spastic quadriplegia may have already developed rigid contractures. When the clinician gradually attempts to passively correct a rigid contracture, if the contracture has continuous resistance to passive correction, it is termed "lead-pipe rigidity." If the contracture has discontinuous resistance to passive correction, it is termed "cog-wheel rigidity" (12). A patient with cerebral palsy and athetosis may have purposeless

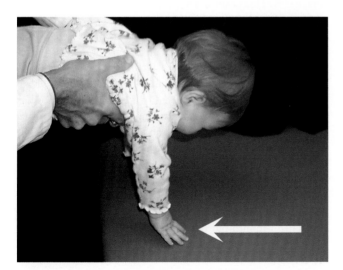

FIGURE 4-21. The parachute reflex is elicited by holding the infant in the air in the prone position, then suddenly lowering the infant headfirst toward the table, simulating a fall. The reflex is positive if the infant extends the upper extremities as if to break the fall (*arrow*).

TABLE 4-4	Prognosis for Walking
Reflex	**Points**
Primitive reflex	
Asymmetric tonic neck	1
Neck righting	1
Moro	1
Symmetric tonic neck	1
Extensor thrust	1
Postural reflex	
Parachute	1 if absent
Foot placement	1 if absent

Prognosis for walking: 2 points, poor; 1 point, guarded (might walk); 0 points, good.

type movement patterns, particularly involving the hands and upper extremities. If the athetosis is of the tension type, it can often be "shaken out" of the limb by the clinician. The reflexes are also tested to determine if the patient has hyperreflexia, clonus, and a positive Babinski reflex. This boy has cerebral palsy with spastic diplegia.

A 3-Month-Old Boy Is Referred for Evaluation Because He Is Not Moving His Right Arm.
Shortly after delivering a healthy 5250 g (11 lb 9 oz) baby boy, the mother was told that the baby was not moving his right arm. The pregnancy was normal, but the delivery was difficult because of right shoulder dystocia. The delivery team had to apply considerable traction on the head to deliver the baby. They noted some swelling and tenderness on the right side of the baby's neck shortly after birth, but this resolved in the first week. At the 2-month appointment with the pediatrician, he was moving his hand but always kept the upper extremity at his side.

After a pediatric orthopaedic history and physical examination, the clinician focuses on a detailed examination of the upper extremities, comparing the paralyzed right side with the uninvolved side. It is important to distinguish between a brachial plexus palsy (a traumatic paralysis involving the upper extremity) and a pseudoparalysis secondary to osteomyelitis of the proximal humerus, septic arthritis of the shoulder, or a birth fracture. The treatment for each of these conditions is different, and a delay in treatment of osteomyelitis or septic arthritis can be devastating. An infant with osteomyelitis, septic arthritis, or a birth fracture will usually have swelling at the site, whereas an infant with traumatic brachial plexus palsy will have no swelling in the extremity, but may have swelling in the neck. An infant with a brachial plexus birth palsy or birth fracture of the humerus will usually have paralysis at birth, whereas an infant with osteomyelitis or septic arthritis may be normal after birth, and then suddenly develop the pseudoparalysis.

Traumatic brachial plexus palsy is a common birth injury, typically seen in primigravida mothers with large babies after difficult deliveries. It occurs because of traction and lateral tilting of the head to deliver the shoulder. If the baby is in the breech presentation, it occurs because of traction and lateral tilting of the trunk and shoulders to deliver the head. Traumatic brachial plexus palsy may have an associated fracture of the clavicle or humerus. There are three types of brachial plexus palsies, depending on which part of the brachial plexus is affected.

The Erb palsy affects the upper roots (C5–C6), the Klumpke palsy affects the lower roots (C8 and T1), and total plexus palsy affects all of the roots in the brachial plexus. The Erb type is the most common and the Klumpke type is rare in newborns. The prognosis for recovery depends on the level and magnitude of the injury and the time at which certain key muscles recover function. If the biceps recovers function before 3 months of age, the prognosis is excellent for a full recovery. The presence of a Horner syndrome usually indicates a poor prognosis (13).

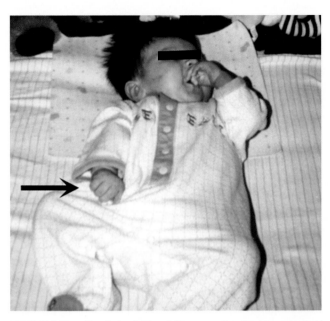

FIGURE 4-23. Paralysis of C5 and C6 causes the shoulder to be held in adduction and internal rotation, with the elbow in extension, the forearm in pronation, and the wrist and fingers in flexion. This posture is termed the waiter's tip, as if the infant is cleverly asking for a tip (*arrow*).

On physical examination, an infant with upper brachial plexus palsy is easily recognized by the absence of active motion of the involved extremity in the Moro reflex (Fig. 4-19), or the asymmetric tonic neck reflex. The paralysis of C5 and C6 causes the shoulder to be held in adduction and internal rotation, with the elbow in extension, the forearm in pronation, and the wrist and fingers in flexion. This posture is termed the "waiter's tip" as if the infant is cleverly asking for a tip (Fig. 4-23). This posture is not seen in an infant with osteomyelitis, septic arthritis, or birth fracture.

An infant with a lower brachial plexus palsy or total brachial plexus palsy is recognized by an absence of the grasp reflex in the involved extremity (Fig. 4-20). The hand is flaccid, with little or no voluntary control. When there is total plexus involvement and the entire extremity is flaccid, the Moro (Fig. 4-19) and grasp (Fig. 4-20) reflexes are both absent. A Horner syndrome refers to the constellation of signs resulting from the interruption of sympathetic innervations to the eye and ocular adnexae. The clinical findings include a triad of ipsilateral blepharoptosis, pupillary miosis, and facial anhidrosis. If the infant has a Horner syndrome, the prognosis for spontaneously recovery is decreased.

This 3-month-old boy is already starting to show biceps motor function at 3 months of age, so the prognosis for recovery is good.

An 18-Month-Old Boy Is Referred Because He Refuses to Walk After His Mother Fell While Carrying Him.
The mother states that she was carrying her son on her hip when she twisted her foot and fell going

down the stairs. She was fine but her son immediately began crying and refused to walk. When she tried to stand him up, he would not put any weight on his right lower extremity. She believes that when she fell, she may have landed on his right leg. She has not noticed any swelling and he stopped crying after she gave him some anti-inflammatory medication. He is in good health and he has not had any chills or fever. She is a single mother with four other children. She called the pediatrician who evaluated him and recommended a radiograph. The radiograph showed a fractured tibia so he referred them for evaluation and treatment.

A minimally displaced spiral fracture involving the distal tibia in a toddler between 9 months and 3 years of age is termed a "toddler's fracture." Although toddler's fractures are relatively common, it is important to review the details concerning the history, physical examination, and radiographs to rule out nonaccidental trauma or "battered-child syndrome." Although children have been harmed by their caregivers for centuries, the medical profession did not officially acknowledge the battered-child syndrome until 1962 (14). The age of the boy is important because most child abuse involves children younger than 3 years of age. It has been estimated that 10% of cases of trauma seen in emergency departments in children under 3 years old are nonaccidental (15). Although a number of risk factors have been identified, it is important to remember that children of all socioeconomic statuses, backgrounds, and ages can be victims of abuse.

The clinician spends time in a quiet environment talking with the mother about the details surrounding the injury to determine if the history is consistent with the child's physical findings. If the history is not consistent with the physical findings, it may cause the clinician to suspect child abuse. While going over the details of the injury, the clinician closely observes the mother's demeanor to determine if she is being forthright with her answers. If the mother seems nervous or uneasy in describing the circumstances surrounding the accident, it should raise a red flag alerting the clinician that someone may have deliberately harmed the child. After reviewing the details of the mechanism of injury, the clinician reviews the past medical history to determine if this is her son's first fracture. A history of multiple previous fractures may be consistent with battered-child syndrome or osteogenesis imperfecta. The birth and developmental history are reviewed to determine if there is any underlying disorder that may make this child more susceptible to fracture. The clinician reviews the family history, review of systems, and personal and social history to evaluate for any family issues and to get a better feel for the home environment.

To check that the history is accurate and further evaluate the home environment, the clinician interviews other family members about the injury. It is important to rule out battered-child syndrome because if missed, there is possibility that the child will be injured again, and the next injury could be life threatening. Each year, more than 1 million children in the United States sustain injuries that are inflicted by their caregivers.

In this case, the physical examination includes the whole child, as the clinician is looking for other injuries that may indicate a battered-child syndrome. The height and weight are recorded to determine if there is any evidence of growth retardation or failure to thrive (16). The skin is closely inspected for any contusions, echymoses, abrasions, welts, or burn scars. Skin lesions are the most common presentation of physical abuse and may be the only physical finding. Bruises are common over the shins and knees in 18-month-old boys, but bruises over the buttocks or genitalia should raise a red flag. The head, eyes, ears, nose, and throat are closely examined for bruises or contusions. Head trauma is the most frequent cause of morbidity and mortality in abused children.

After the skin is inspected, the soft tissues and bones of the upper and lower extremities are palpated to evaluate for injuries. An 18-month-old boy should not have any discomfort when the clinician gently squeezes his arms, forearms, thighs, and legs, but will have considerable discomfort if there is a contusion or fracture. After skin lesions, fractures are the second most common presentation of physical abuse. If the clinician believes there is any question about the possibility of battered-child syndrome, it may be beneficial to contact the referring pediatrician to determine if any question of neglect has ever previously been considered. If the story is straightforward and the mother is forthcoming, treatment of the tibia fracture can proceed without any further studies.

A 4-Year-Old Boy Is Referred Because He Began Limping Yesterday and When He Awoke This Morning, He Refused to Walk on His Right Lower Extremity.

He was apparently in good health until yesterday afternoon, when his mother noticed that he seemed to be limping on the right side at the grocery store. Later that evening, his limp became more obvious and he complained of pain in his right knee. This morning he awoke complaining of right knee pain and refused to walk. They called their pediatrician who evaluated him and referred him for a possible infection in the right knee. The past history reveals that 2 weeks ago he had a fever and cough that lasted for 5 days.

The clinician understands that although the history is typical for a patient with transient synovitis of the hip, it may also be consistent with septic arthritis, osteomyelitis, or Legg-Calvé-Perthes disease. A 4-year-old boy will often describe exactly where it hurts and may point to the groin, thigh, or the knee. It is important to remember that pain can be referred, and a hip problem presenting as knee pain is a classic example of referred pain. The clinician asks if the pain is constant or intermittent as children with infections tend to have constant pain. The fever and cough 2 weeks ago is an important part of the history, as an upper respiratory infection is often a precursor of transient synovitis of the hip.

Kocher et al. (17) compared a group of patients with transient synovitis with a group of patients with septic arthritis. They reported that the patients with septic arthritis appeared to be sicker with fever, chills, inability to bear weight, elevated erythrocyte sedimentation rate, leukocytosis, lower hematocrit, and an altered peripheral blood differential. A patient with acute septic arthritis involving the hip would typically have a history of 1 to 2 days of severe pain, whereas a patient with juvenile arthritis may have had intermittent low-grade pain for several weeks to months. The pain associated with juvenile arthritis is typically worse in the morning, and this is not usually seen in other disorders. If the history revealed he had chicken pox 2 weeks ago, the clinician may be concerned the he is immunocompromised and may have an infection.

The physical examination can start by asking if the patient will stand and take a few steps. If he will walk, the gait pattern is observed to determine if it is symmetric. If the child has an antalgic (painful) gait on the right side, the stance phase of gait would typically be shortened and he would lean over the painful hip. Although it may be difficult to convince a 4-year-old boy to stand, particularly if he has pain, if he will corporate, he is asked to stand on one leg and then on the opposite leg. When a child stands on one leg, the hip abductor muscles contract to hold the pelvis up on the opposite side and avoid falling. The combination of weight-bearing and contracted abductor muscles markedly increases the joint reactive forces in the hip. If the patient has hip pain, the increased joint reactive forces caused by standing on one leg are so painful that he will not contract the hip abductor muscles. This causes the pelvis to drop on the opposite side and is termed a positive Trendelenburg test (Fig. 4-24).

Since the child is having pain, the uninvolved side is examined first before proceeding to the symptomatic side. The lower extremities are observed for any swelling or asymmetry. The clinician palpates the spine, pelvis, and lower extremities for tenderness. The hips are examined with the child in the supine position, and the clinician looks for any asymmetry as the hips are attempted to be taken through a full range of motion. The range of motion of both hips, especially internal rotation, should be symmetric. If the patient has an irritable hip, he will guard and contract his muscles, not allowing the clinician to take the hip through a full range of motion. This is particularly noted in attempting to internally and externally rotate the hip, with the hip and knee in 90 degrees of flexion. If the hip is painful, the clinician can gently "log roll" the extremity with the hip and knee in full extension (Fig. 4-25). This is more comfortable for the patient, and if he has severe pain with log rolling, the pain will be unbearable with the hip and knee in flexion. If there is any question about the possibility of a septic hip, urgent hip aspiration under fluoroscopic guidance is recommended.

After examining the hip, the limb can then be placed in the figure-4 position, with the hip in flexion, abduction, and external rotation (FABER test) (Fig. 4-26). In this position, if the knee is pushed toward the examining table, it transmits a tensile force to the sacroiliac joint. If the patient has pyogenic arthritis involving the sacroiliac joint, he will experience discomfort with this test. This boy has transient synovitis of the right hip, so activity modification and close follow-up are recommended to be certain that the symptoms are resolving.

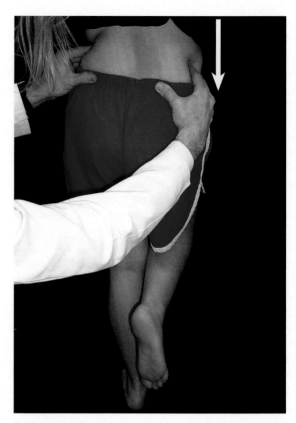

FIGURE 4-24. The clinician palpates the iliac crests while the patient stands on the left lower extremity. In single limb support on the left lower extremity, the right iliac crest should rise as the left hip abductor muscles contract to support the pelvis. If the right iliac crest drops (*arrow*), it is termed a positive Trendelenburg test, indicating weakness of the left hip abductor muscles. The Trendelenburg test can also be positive if the patient has an irritable left hip. In this case, the increased joint reactive forces are painful, so the patient will not contract the left hip abductor muscles.

A 3-Year-Old Girl Is Referred for Evaluation of Flat Feet.

The family states that her feet roll in when she walks. The problem was first noted by the maternal grandmother when she began walking at 13 months of age. The family is concerned that the problem is getting worse and they want to know if she should have arch supports or special shoes. The past medical history as well as the birth and developmental history are within normal limits. The family history reveals that her father had flat feet and wore special shoes until he was 2 years old.

The clinician reviews the details of the history to determine when the flat feet were first noted. This information may be helpful because a rigid pes planus deformity, such as that seen in a child with a CVT, is typically noted at birth. In contrast, a rigid pes planus deformity, such as that seen in a child with a tarsal coalition, is typically not noted until the child is 10 years of age, when the cartilaginous bar begins to ossify causing pain and decreased motion of the foot. A flexible

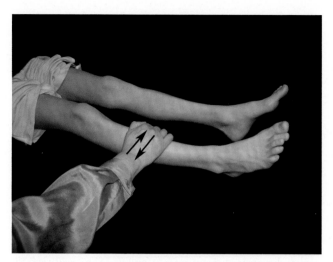

FIGURE 4-25. The clinician can gently "log roll" the extremity with the hip and knee in full extension to determine the severity of the pain. This is more comfortable for the patient and if he has severe pain with log rolling, the pain will be unbearable with the hip and knee in flexion.

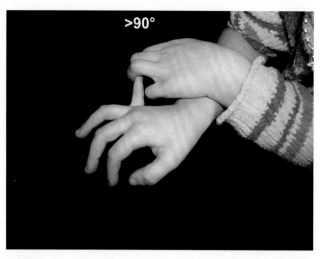

FIGURE 4-27. Ligamentous laxity can be detected by asking the patient to try and hyperextend the little finger metacarpophalangeal joint (>90 degrees indicates laxity).

pes planus deformity collapses with weight bearing, so it is not unusual that the flat feet were first noted when she first began walking. A 3-year-old girl with flexible flat feet will not usually have any pain.

The physical examination begins by opening the door and asking the family if they would take her for a walk in the hall. The clinician notes that she walks with a symmetric heel-toe gait pattern, with a foot-progression angle of 25 degrees

of external rotation (Fig. 4-7). A patient with a planovalgus deformity will often toe-out, whereas a patient with a cavovarus deformity will often toe-in. Before focusing on the feet, a general physical examination of the back, upper, and lower extremities is performed. A patient with flexible pes planovalgus will often have generalized ligamentous laxity. Ligamentous laxity can be detected by asking the patient to hyperextend the little finger metacarpophalangeal joint (>90 degrees indicates ligamentous laxity, Fig. 4-27), hyperextend the elbows, hyperextend the knees, and touch the thumb to the volar surface of the forearm (Fig. 4-28). Flexible pes planus is common and is most likely caused by excessive laxity of the ligaments and joint capsules, allowing the tarsal arch to collapse with weight bearing. It is important to differentiate this benign condition

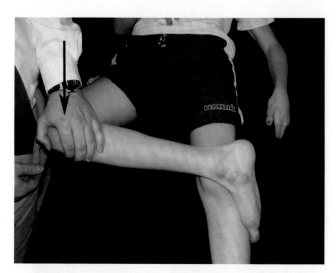

FIGURE 4-26. With the patient supine, the right lower extremity is placed in the figure-4 position with the hip in flexion, abduction, and external rotation (FABER test). The knee is gently pushed toward the examination table (*arrow*) transmitting a tensile force to the sacroiliac joint that may cause pain if the sacroiliac joint is inflamed.

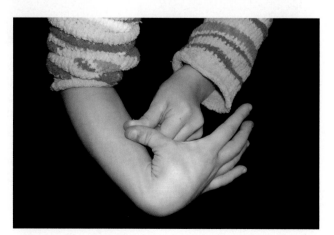

FIGURE 4-28. Ligamentous laxity can be detected by asking the patient to try and touch the thumb to the volar surface of the forearm.

from the more serious types of flat feet, such as CVT or tarsal coalition.

The clinician examines the range of motion of the ankle, subtalar, and tarsal joints to determine if there is any loss of motion. A contracture of the Achilles tendon may accompany a symptomatic flat foot (18). To determine if she has a contracture of the Achilles tendon, it is crucial to supinate the forefoot and lock the subtalar and tarsal joints before attempting to passively dorsiflex the foot and ankle to test for a contracture of the Achilles tendon. If the foot is not first supinated, passive dorsiflexion may occur at the subtalar and tarsal joints rather than the ankle, masking the contracture of the Achilles tendon. In standing, a child with flexible pes planus has a collapsed medial longitudinal arch, a valgus hindfoot, and a supinated externally rotated forefoot (Fig. 4-29A). The arch returns when the child is sitting, because the weight-bearing force that caused the collapsed arch is relieved. The arch also returns when she stands on her tip toes (Fig. 4-29B), or with passive extension of the metatarsophalangeal joint of the great toe, the "toe-raise test," because of the windlass effect of the plantar fascia (Fig. 4-29C). The clinician uses these tests to document that this patient has ligamentous laxity with flexible pes planus, a benign condition that usually does not benefit from treatment.

THE ORTHOPAEDIC EXAMINATION FROM 4 TO 10 YEARS OF AGE

A 7-Year-Old Boy Is Referred for Evaluation of Right Groin Pain and a Limp.
The family first noted that he was limping on the right side after a soccer game 2 months ago. The limp went away, but 3 days later he complained of right groin pain and they noticed that he was limping again. They went to their pediatrician, who questioned whether he may have pulled a muscle while playing soccer. The pediatrician documented that he was in the 5th percentile for height and the 95th percentile for weight. The pain and limp are worse with activity and relieved by rest. He is otherwise in excellent health.

It is unusual to sustain a groin muscle injury at this age, and symptoms from a groin muscle injury will typically improve in 2 to 3 weeks. If the child was black, the clinician may consider that he may have sickle cell disease with a bone infarct involving the proximal femur. A bone infarct in a patient with sickle cell disease will typically present with the sudden onset of pain in the groin, rather than having pain and limping for 2 months. A child with Legg-Calvé-Perthes disease will often complain of pain in the groin and may have short stature and a delayed bone age. It is important to remember that a child with Legg-Calvé-Perthes disease may

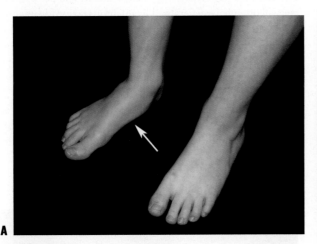

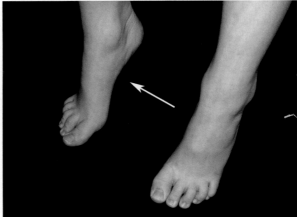

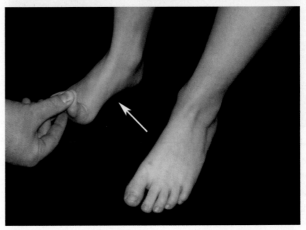

FIGURE 4-29. **A:** In standing, a patient with a flexible pes planus has a collapsed medial longitudinal arch (*arrow*), a valgus hindfoot, a supinated forefoot, and an externally rotated forefoot. **B:** If the pes planus is flexible, the arch will correct when she stands on her tip toes (*arrow*). **C:** If the pes planus is flexible, the "toe-raise test" is positive. When the great toe is dorsiflexed at the metatarsophalangeal, the arch is restored (*arrow*) because of the windlass effect of the plantar fascia.

develop symptoms well after the actual onset of the disease. Children with Legg-Calvé-Perthes disease go through several stages that can be summarized as destructive and reparative phases (19). The majority of symptoms develop early during the destructive phases.

A child with multiple epiphyseal dysplasia may have short stature and may have pain and a limp. Multiple epiphyseal dysplasia is inherited as an autosomal dominant trait, so there may be a family history of the disorder. The insidious onset of pain and a limp may develop in a child with a bone cyst or tumor involving the proximal femur. A child with an osteoid osteoma involving the proximal femur will often complain of night pain that is relieved by aspirin. This boy is 7 years old and osteoid osteomas typically develop in older children.

The physical examination begins by asking the child to walk in the hall. A child with pain and a limp may have an antalgic (painful) limp during gait. This is characterized by a decreased time in the stance phase on the involved side. The clinician also notes swaying or bending of the trunk over the painful hip, to decrease the joint reactive forces. This is termed a Trendelenburg gait pattern and is an important clinical observation, because it leads the clinician to suspect a hip problem. A patient with a Trendelenburg gait pattern will usually have a positive Trendelenburg test (Fig. 4-24). After observing the child's gait pattern, the clinician examines the back and upper and lower extremities, looking for any asymmetry between the symptomatic side and the uninvolved side. A child with Legg-Calvé-Perthes disease and synovitis involving the hip will typically have a loss of internal rotation, abduction, and extension. The loss of internal rotation is usually the most pronounced and is best demonstrated by examining the child in the prone position with the hips in extension (Fig. 4-8).

In the supine position, each hip is flexed to 90 degrees, and gently internally and externally rotated through a range of motion. The clinician notes the amount of internal and external rotation of each hip and feels for any involuntary muscle guarding. Guarding usually indicates that the child has synovitis in the hip with an associated hip joint effusion. In a child with Legg-Calvé-Perthes disease, the finding of persistent synovitis is associated with a guarded prognosis (20). If there is decreased internal rotation without guarding, it may indicate a retroversion deformity of the femoral neck which is often seen in children with developmental coxa vara. This boy likely has Legg-Calvé-Perthes disease, so anteroposterior and frog pelvis radiographs are recommended.

A 6-Year-Old Boy in the Emergency Room Has Severe Pain and Swelling of the Left Elbow After Falling from the Monkey Bars at School.
This boy was apparently in satisfactory health until earlier today, when he fell from the monkey bars at school and complained of severe pain in his left elbow. The school nurse called the family, and they picked him up at school and took him immediately to the emergency room. He was evaluated by the emergency room physician who believes that he may have a fracture of the distal left humerus.

In this situation, the boy and his family are anxious about the accident and apprehensive about being in the emergency room. The patient is usually found on a gurney, with the elbow in a temporary splint. The history of present illness is important because the mechanism of injury reflects the magnitude of the injury and the likelihood of an associated neurovascular injury. The child recalls falling about 6 ft landing on his outstretched arms. A fall on an outstretched arm is a mechanism that can cause a distal humerus fracture, an elbow dislocation, a forearm fracture, a distal radius fracture, or a combination of these injuries. The frequency of associated neurovascular injuries correlates with the magnitude of injury. The past history may be helpful to detect an underlying disorder such as osteogenesis imperfecta. If the patient had osteogenesis imperfecta, he may have a pathologic fracture. A pathologic fracture is a fracture through weakened bone. Pathologic fractures typically are minimally displaced with minimal swelling, and it is unusual to have a neurovascular injury in association with a pathologic fracture. Pathologic fractures in children heal normally in most cases.

The child is reassured that his family can stay with him during the physical examination. After a general examination of the spine and lower extremities to evaluate for other injuries, the splint is removed. The uninjured upper extremity is examined first, so the patient is more at ease with the examination. The injured arm is then observed and compared with the uninjured side. Observation demonstrates marked swelling and ecchymosis over the distal humerus and elbow, findings consistent with a supracondylar fracture of the distal humerus. The clinician gently palpates the distal humerus to locate the point of maximum tenderness. The point of maximum tenderness will be on the tension side of the fracture, because there is more soft-tissue injury on the tension side than the compression side.

In a patient with a supracondylar fracture, the immediate concern is whether there are associated neurovascular injuries. Prior to treatment, a complete neurocirculatory examination of the forearms and hands is performed to document pulses, capillary fill, pain, light touch, strength, and range of motion of the fingers. A detailed motor and sensory examination of the median, anterior interosseus, ulnar, and radial nerves is conducted. A supracondylar fracture can interfere with the circulation to the hand by directly injuring the brachial artery, kinking the artery, or by causing too much swelling in the volar compartment of the forearm (21, 22).

A "compartment syndrome" may develop before or after treatment. A compartment syndrome develops when there is too much swelling within a closed space. After a supracondylar fracture, the compartment that most often develops excessive swelling is the volar compartment of the forearm. When the pressure in the compartment surpasses the systolic blood pressure, it will obliterate the radial and ulnar pulses at the wrist. A compartment syndrome may be first detected by noticing that the patient is experiencing pain that seems out of proportion to the physical findings. Another early sign is pain to passive stretching of the ischemic muscles. In a volar compartment syndrome, the flexor muscles are ischemic, so the patient may complain of pain with passive extension of the fingers. Early detection is crucial because once the pulses are absent, the muscles in the forearm may already be necrotic. When the necrotic muscles develop fibrosis and scarring, a "Volkmann ischemic contracture" develops causing a flexion deformity of the wrist and fingers that can markedly interfere with hand function. If there is any question about a possible compartment syndrome, urgent measuring of compartmental pressures is crucial, and early fasciotomy of the compartments is recommended.

To evaluate the sensory component of a nerve in a 6-year-old boy, it is accurate and painless to test two-point discrimination using a paper clip, comparing the injured side with the uninjured side (Fig. 4-30). The index (median nerve sensory distribution) and little finger (ulnar nerve sensory distribution) are tested; most patients can distinguish between one point and two points if they are separated by more than 2 to 4 mm. The radial nerve is tested checking the sensation in the dorsal web space between the thumb and the index finger (sensory), and by asking the patient to extend his fingers (motor). The median nerve is tested by checking the sensation on the volar aspect of the index finger (sensory), and asking the patient to flex the long and ring fingers (motor). The anterior interosseous nerve has no sensory component, but the motor component can easily be evaluated by having him form a ring between the thumb and index finger. If he is unable to form a ring because of weakness of the flexor pollicis longus and the flexor digitorum profundus of the index finger, it indicates an anterior interosseous nerve palsy (Fig. 4-31). Another way to test the motor function of the anterior interosseous nerve is to hold the index finger in extension at the metacarpophalangeal and proximal interphalangeal joints and ask the patient to flex

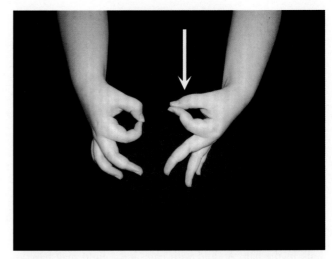

FIGURE 4-31. If the patient is unable to form a ring between the thumb and index finger because of weakness of the flexor pollicis longus and the flexor digitorum profundus of the index finger (*arrow*), it indicates an anterior interosseous nerve palsy.

the tip of the finger (Fig. 4-32). The ulnar nerve is tested by checking the sensation on the volar aspect of the little finger (sensory), and asking the patient to spread his fingers apart (motor). The last muscle innervated by the ulnar nerve is the first dorsal interosseous muscle. This muscle can be tested by placing a finger on the radial side of the distal phalanx and another finger on the muscle belly of the first dorsal interosseous muscle. The patient is asked to push against the finger on the distal phalanx, and the clinician palpates a contracture of the first dorsal interosseous muscle if motor function is intact (Fig. 4-33).

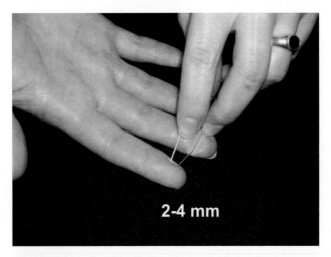

FIGURE 4-30. To evaluate the sensory component of a nerve in a child, it is accurate and painless to test two-point discrimination using a paper clip, comparing the injured side with the uninjured side. Most people have two-point discrimination of 2 to 4 mm in the index (median nerve sensation) and little fingers (ulnar nerve sensation).

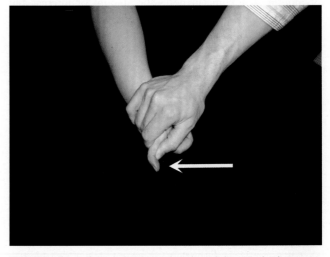

FIGURE 4-32. To test the motor function of the anterior interosseous nerve, the clinician holds the index finger with the metacarpophalangeal and proximal interphalangeal joints in extension, and asks the patient to flex the tip of the finger (*arrow*). Inability to flex the tip of the index finger indicates an anterior interosseous nerve palsy.

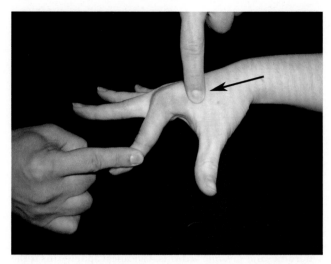

FIGURE 4-33. The first dorsal interosseous muscle is tested by flexing the metacarpophalangeal of the index finger to 60 degrees and placing a finger on the radial side of the distal phalanx and another finger on the muscle belly of the first dorsal interosseous muscle. The patient is asked to push the index finger in a radial direction, and a contraction of the first dorsal interosseous muscle is palpable (*arrow*) if motor function is intact.

If the patient is apprehensive and experiencing severe pain, the physical examination may be compromised. If this occurs, it is important to document the problem in the medical record. In this case, a supracondylar fracture of the distal humerus is suspected, so anteroposterior and lateral radiographs of the elbow are recommended.

A 9-Year-Old Boy Is Referred for Painless Swelling in the Back of His Knees.

The patient's grandmother first noticed a swelling in the back of both of her grandson's knees during the summer while playing at the beach. The patient never noticed the masses until they were pointed out to him. He cannot recall any history of trauma to his knees. Since the masses have been pointed out to him, he has noticed that they get bigger and smaller most notably with exercise. He also notes a dull ache in the area behind the knees that is aggravated by increased activity. He denies any weakness, numbness, or loss of function in the low extremities. He has not had any problems with fatigue, weight loss, or fevers and has otherwise been doing well.

The clinician understands that although soft-tissue masses in children are common and almost always benign (23), it is extremely important and sometimes difficult to differentiate between benign and malignant soft-tissue lesions. The most common benign and malignant soft-tissue masses seen in children are listed in Table 4-5. Unlike bone tumors where the physical examination and radiographs are equally important in developing a differential diagnosis, with soft-tissue tumors the differential diagnosis is almost entirely reliant on the history and physical examination.

TABLE 4-5	Common Benign and Malignant Soft-Tissue Masses in Children
Benign	**Malignant**
Lipoma	Rhabdomyosarcoma
Hemangioma	Synovial sarcoma
Baker cyst	Well-differentiated liposarcoma
Ganglion cyst	Extraskeletal chondrosarcoma
Fibrous tumors	Extraskeletal osteosarcoma
Myositis ossificans	

The majority of soft-tissue sarcomas are painless masses until they become large enough to impinge upon the neurovascular structures. Conversely, many benign pediatric soft-tissue masses present with symptoms. Intramuscular hemangiomas and synovial cysts can present with a waxing and waning dull ache due to changes in blood flow and size during activity and rest. Benign fibrous tumors, such as nodular fasciitis, myositis ossificans, and glomus tumors can be very painful. Some soft-tissue tumors can mimic soft-tissue neoplasms. Epitrochlear lymph nodes secondary to Bartonella hensela (cat scratch disease), foreign-body granuloma, and intramuscular inflammatory reactions to immunizations are well known for generating a confusing clinical and radiologic scenarios. Soft-tissue sarcomas metastasize to the lungs primarily; however, a small subset of sarcomas, specifically rhabdomyosarcoma, alveolar soft parts sarcoma, clear cell sarcoma, epithelial sarcoma, and synovial sarcoma (RACES), will locally metastasize to regional lymph nodes. Therefore, palpation of regional lymph nodes for increases in size is an important part of the physical examination in this patient.

On physical examination, the size, location, consistency, and mobility of the mass or tumor are key parameters to evaluate. Masses that are >5 cm in diameter, firm, fixed, and deep to the fascia should be considered sarcomas until proven otherwise (24). Benign soft-tissue masses are typically soft and mobile. These findings are important because mobility of the tumor reflects the fact the tumor has not invaded the fascia and points to a benign lesion. Benign nerve sheath tumors, such as Schwannomas, arise from the epineurium and will be extensively mobile in a medial to lateral direction, but firmly fixed in a cephalad to caudad direction in line with the nerve. Lipomas and hemangiomas are described as doughy in texture and cysts are easily compressible. Ganglion cysts will occur adjacent to or attached to a joint capsule or tendon sheath. Fluid-filled lesions such as a popliteal cyst (Baker cyst) will transilluminate with a penlight or flashlight. To perform this test on a patient with a Baker cyst, the clinician has the patient lie prone on the exam table in a darkened room and extend the knee while the clinician places a penlight against the skin. If the patient has a Baker cyst, the entire cavity should be illuminated by the penlight. Absence of any dark nonilluminated areas within the lesion helps confirm the diagnosis of a pediatric Baker cyst. If the patient has a hemangioma, the clinician may occasionally palpate a thrill or audible bruit over the lesion.

Masses that increase in size over time should raise a red flag and warrant consideration for biopsy, whereas masses that have been present for a long time are most likely benign. Two exceptions to this rule include synovial cell and clear cell sarcomas as these malignant tumors are known to frequently grow slowly. Two other exceptions to this rule include nodular fasciitis and desmoid tumors as these benign tumors are rapidly growing and locally invasive.

Large, firm, deep masses should raise a red flag requiring further workup and often warrant a biopsy. Plain radiographs can identify soft-tissue mineralization, but this does not differentiate between benign and malignant lesions. Magnetic resonance imaging with gadolinium contrast is the imaging study of choice for the differential diagnosis and treatment of soft-tissue tumors.

After careful examination of this patient, both tumors are located on the posteromedial aspect of the knees and are best seen with the patient standing and looking at him from behind (Fig. 4-34). They are relatively large, and both tumors are somewhat mobile and transilluminate with a penlight. These finding are consistent with bilateral Baker cysts that originate from the joint capsule of the knee and protrude between the medial head of the gastrocnemius and the semimembranosus tendons. Since Baker cysts have a high probability of spontaneous resolution in children, close observation is recommended. If there is any doubt about the diagnosis or

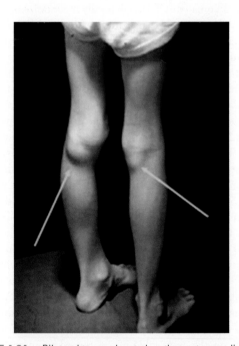

FIGURE 4-34. Bilateral tumors located on the posteromedial aspect of the knees best seen from behind with the patient standing (*arrows*). They are relatively large, somewhat mobile, and transilluminate with a penlight. These findings are consistent with bilateral Baker cysts.

the family has concerns, the diagnosis can be confirmed by ultrasonography.

A 10-Year-Old Boy Is Referred for Evaluation of Right Heel Pain That Is Aggravated by Playing Soccer.
The family noticed that he began complaining of right heel pain 1 month ago after playing soccer. The pain is worse in the evenings, particularly if he played soccer earlier in the day. He does not have any pain in the left foot or ankle. The pain seems to be aggravated by running and relieved by rest. The family has noted mild swelling over the right heel. He is otherwise in excellent health.

The history is consistent with calcaneal apophysitis, also termed "Sever disease," but the differential diagnosis includes tumor, infection, bone cyst, tarsal coalition, leukemia, Reiter syndrome, and juvenile arthritis. Calcaneal apophysitis is the most common cause of heel pain in the immature athlete and is more common in boys (25). Symptoms develop bilaterally in approximately 60% of cases. In 1912, Sever described the condition as an inflammatory injury to the apophysis associated with muscle strain, but recent investigators attribute the symptoms to overuse and repetitive microtrauma. This patient denies any morning pain or stiffness, as one might see in patients with juvenile arthritis. He denies any pain at night, as might be seen in a patient with a tumor or bone cyst. Heel pain that is persistent may be a sign of childhood leukemia, so it is important to ask about any associated symptoms.

On physical examination, the spine, upper extremities, hips, and knees are within normal limits. The feet appear symmetric with no swelling, erythema, or skin changes. The pain is located right over the calcaneal apophysis and is aggravated by medial and lateral compression of the apophysis; this is termed the "heel-squeeze test" (Fig. 4-35). There is no pain at the insertion of the Achilles tendon, as would be seen in a patient with Achilles tendonitis, and there is no pain at the origin of the plantar fascia, as would be seen in a patient with plantar fasciitis. Achilles tendonitis and plantar fasciitis, although common in adults, are not frequently seen in children. Ankle dorsiflexion is tested with the forefoot fully supinated, locking the subtalar and tarsal joints, to avoid masking an Achilles tendon contracture secondary to hypermobility at the subtalar and tarsal joints. Ankle dorsiflexion on the left is to 30 degrees and on the right is only to 20 degrees. It is common to have associated heel cord tightness in a patient with calcaneal apophysitis. In the standing position, he has mild pes planovalgus and forefoot pronation; conditions also seen in association with calcaneal apophysitis. Calcaneal apophysitis is an overuse syndrome and the symptoms should subside with activity modification. Close follow-up is recommended to document symptom resolution.

A 5-Year-Old Boy Is Referred for Evaluation Because He Is Walking on His Toes.
The family first noted that he walked on his toes when he began walking

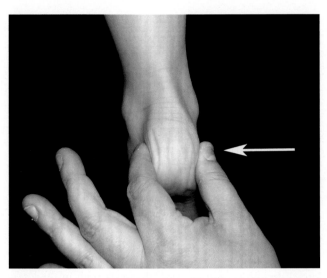

FIGURE 4-35.   A patient with calcaneal apophysitis (Sever disease) has pain over the calcaneal apophysis. The pain is reproduced by medial and lateral compression of the apophysis; this is termed the "heel-squeeze test" (*arrow*).

at 2 years of age. Although able to walk with his feet flat on the floor, he walks on his toes 95% of the time. The birth history reveals that he was born after a 28-week gestation, when his mother spontaneously went into labor. The birth was via normal vaginal delivery with a birth weight of 1400 g (3 lb 1 oz). The perinatal course was complicated, and the patient was hospitalized in the NICU for 6 weeks because of respiratory problems. The developmental history reveals that he sat at 11 months and walked at 2 years of age. The family first noted that he was right-handed at 12 months of age when he preferred playing with toys using the right hand. He has been receiving physical, occupational, and speech therapy through an early intervention program.

The boy wore shorts and T-shirt for the office visit so he would not have to change clothes. The exam begins by asking him to walk in the hall with his mother. He walks on his toes, but will occasionally bring the heel to the floor. Sutherland et al. reported that a mature gait pattern is well established at the age of 3 years (26). Normal gait has a heel-toe pattern in stance phase, beginning with heel strike, followed by foot flat, and ending with toe-off. This patient has a toe-toe gait pattern and occasionally has a toe-heel gait pattern. In normal gait during early stance, the foot plantarflexes between heel strike and foot flat. This early ankle plantarflexion is termed the "first rocker." In midstance, there is forward rotation of the leg over the foot, and the ankle dorsiflexes to accommodate this forward motion. This ankle dorsiflexion is termed the "second rocker." In terminal stance, the ankle plantarflexes at push off and this plantarflexion is termed the "third rocker." When this patient ambulates with a toe-toe gait pattern, there is a loss of the first rocker and a decrease of the second and third rockers. When he ambulates with a

toe-heel gait pattern, the first rocker is reversed as the ankle dorsiflexes to get to foot flat, and there is a decrease of the second and third rockers.

His gait pattern is not symmetrical, as he spends more time in the stance phase on his right side, compared with the left. This is an important observation, because a patient with muscular dystrophy or idiopathic toe walking will typically have a symmetric gait pattern. In this patient, the knees do not extend completely at the end of the swing phase, and the hips do not extend completely at the end of the stance phase. When walking at a faster pace, he lacks the symmetric fluid reciprocating swinging motion of the upper extremities. Instead, he postures both upper extremities, left more than right, with the elbows in flexion, the forearms in pronation, and the wrists in flexion. This is an important observation, as posturing of the upper extremities during gait is commonly seen in patients with spastic cerebral palsy. During gait, he is noted to have a foot-progression angle of 10 degrees of inward rotation on the left and 5 degrees of inward rotation on the right (Fig. 4-7).

After observing the patient's gait, the physical examination includes the spine, upper, and lower extremities. The spine is examined from the back with the patient standing looking for any asymmetry. The clinician's hands are placed on the patient's iliac crests; the right iliac crest is 5 mm higher than the left, indicating a slight limb-length discrepancy, with the right longer than the left. Patients with cerebral palsy and spastic diplegia will often have some asymmetry, and the lower extremity will often be slightly shorter on the more involved side. The patient is then asked to bend forward at the waist, as if he is touching his toes, and the examiner observes for a rib or lumbar prominence that may be associated with a spinal deformity.

The patient is then asked to sit for the upper extremity examination. He is asked to pick up an object, to determine if there is hand preference, and to see if he can do it with both hands. Grip strength is tested by having the patient squeeze the clinician's index and long fingers of both hands at the same time. Pinch strength is tested by having the patient pick up a pen between the index finger and the thumb. Stereognosis is tested by placing a known object, such as a coin, into the hand, and asking the patient to identify the object without looking at it. The shoulders, elbows, forearms, and wrists are taken through a full range of motion, to determine if there are any contractures. A patient with spastic cerebral palsy may have an adduction contracture of the shoulder, a flexion contracture of the elbow, a pronation contracture of the forearm, a flexion contracture of the wrist, and a thumb-in-palm deformity in the hand.

The patient is placed supine for examination of the lower extremities. The hips are passively taken through a full range of motion. Patients with spastic cerebral palsy will often have flexion and adduction contractures of the hips. The Thomas test or the prone hip extension test (Staheli test) can be used to examine for a hip flexion contracture. The Thomas test is performed by flexing one hip completely, to flatten the lumbar spine, and observing the amount of residual flexion of the other hip. The residual flexion represents the hip flexion contracture (Fig. 4-36A). The prone hip extension test is performed by placing the patient prone with the lower extremities flexed over the end of the table. This position flattens the lumbar spine leveling the pelvis. One hip remains flexed at 90 degrees; the clinician gradually extends the other hip while palpating the pelvis (27). As soon as pelvic motion is detected, the amount of residual hip flexion represents the flexion contracture (Fig. 4-36B). A flexion contracture in a patient with spastic cerebral palsy is often secondary to an iliopsoas contracture, but may be secondary to a rectus femoris contracture. The Duncan-Ely test, sometimes referred to as the "prone rectus test," is used to test the rectus femoris muscle. Since the rectus femoris muscle spans both the hip and the knee, this test is performed in the prone position. With the hip extended, the knee is flexed quickly while the clinician looks for arise of the buttocks and feels for increased tone in the limb. If the hip spontaneously flexes, causing the buttocks to rise off the table, it indicates a contracture of the rectus femoris muscle. A positive Duncan-Ely test is an accurate predictor for rectus femoris dysfunction during gait (Fig. 4-37) (28).

Internal and external rotation of the hips can be tested in the supine or prone position, but we prefer the prone position (Figs. 4-8 and 4-9). Patients with spastic cerebral palsy often have increased anteversion of the proximal femur, which causes an increase in internal rotation and a decrease in external rotation of the hips. In contrast, patients with developmental

coxa vara often have a retroversion deformity proximal femur, which causes an increase in external rotation and a decrease in internal rotation of the hips.

In the supine position with the hips flexed to 90 degrees, the hips should abduct symmetrically to at least 75 degrees. Limited abduction, particularly if associated with flexion contracture, may indicate hip subluxation or dislocation (Fig. 4-5). The Phelps-Baker test is used to determine the hamstring contribution to the hip adduction contracture. This test is performed with the patient in the prone position, and the amount of hip abduction with the knees flexed is compared to that with the knees extended. The amount of decreased abduction with the knees extended represents the contribution of the medial hamstrings to the adduction contracture. The Ober test is used to examine for a hip abduction contracture. The Ober test is performed in the lateral decubitus position, with the lower limb in the knee-chest position. The hip on the upper limb is extended and adducted with the knee extended and with the knee flexed (29). The upper limb should easily adduct to the table, and any loss of adduction represents the hip abduction contracture (Fig. 4-38). The amount of increased abduction with the knee extended compared with the knee flexed represents the contribution of the tensor fascia lata to the abduction contracture. A patient with spastic cerebral palsy will usually develop an adduction contracture of the hip, whereas a patient with poliomyelitis will often develop an abduction contracture.

Knee range of motion is examined with the patient supine on the exam table. The range should be from 0 to 130 degrees.

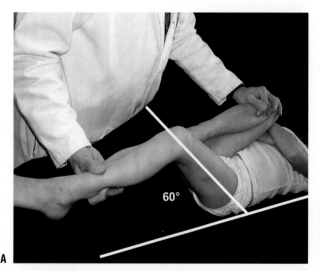
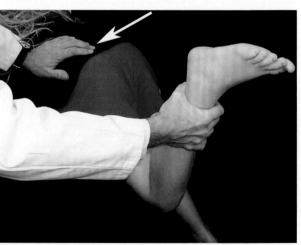

FIGURE 4-36. **A:** The Thomas test is performed by flexing one hip to the knee-chest position, flattening the lumbar spine and leveling the pelvis, while allowing gravity to extend the hip that is being examined. Any residual flexion represents the hip flexion contracture (60 degrees in this patient). **B:** The prone hip extension test is performed in the prone position with the lower extremities flexed over the end of the table flattening the lumbar spine leveling the pelvis. One hip remains flexed at 90 degrees, while the clinician simultaneously extends the other hip while palpating the pelvis (*arrow*). As soon as pelvic motion is detected, the amount of residual hip flexion represents the flexion contracture.

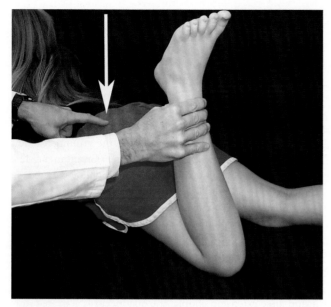

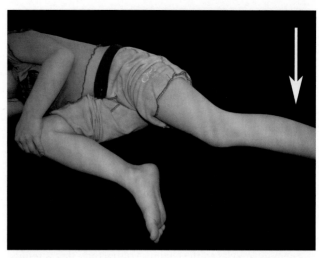

FIGURE 4-37. The Duncan-Ely test is performed in the prone position because the rectus femoris muscle spans both the hip and the knee. With the hip extended, the knee is flexed quickly while the clinician looks for a rise of the buttocks (*arrow*) and feels for increased tone in the limb. If the hip spontaneously flexes, causing the buttocks to rise off the table, it indicates a contracture of the rectus femoris muscle.

FIGURE 4-38. The Ober test is performed in the lateral decubitus position with the lower limb in the knee-chest position. The hip on the upper limb is extended and adducted with the knee extended and with the knee flexed (*arrow*). The upper limb should easily adduct to the table, and any loss of adduction represents the hip abduction contracture.

A flexion contracture may be caused by a hamstring contracture. A hamstring contracture is detected by performing a straight-leg-raising test (Fig. 4-39A). Straight-leg raising should range from 60 to 90 degrees. Limited straight-leg raising often indicates a contracture of the hamstring muscles, but it may be associated with a neurologic problem such as a tethered spinal cord. A hamstring contracture can also be detected by measuring the popliteal angle. To measure the popliteal angle, the hip is flexed to 90 degrees and the knee is gradually extended to the first sign of resistance. The angle between the thigh and the calf is the popliteal angle (Fig. 4-39B). This popliteal angle

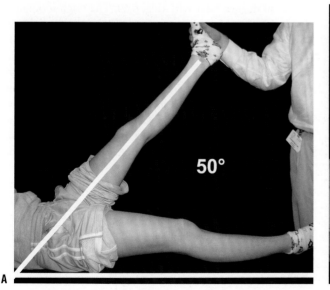

A

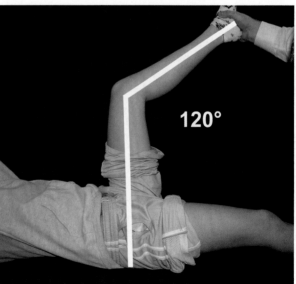

B

FIGURE 4-39. **A:** With the patient supine, the clinician gradually raises one lower extremity by flexing the hip with the knee in extension. The straight-leg-raising test measures the angle between the lower limb and the tabletop (50 degrees in this patient). **B:** With the patient supine, the clinician gradually flexes the hip and knee to 90 degrees. The knee is gradually extended to the first sign of resistance. The angle between the thigh and the calf is the popliteal angle (120 degrees in this patient). This popliteal angle should be distinguished from its complement, which is also called the popliteal angle by some investigators.

should be distinguished from its complement, which is also called the popliteal angle by some investigators (12). Elmer et al. (30) chose to call the angle between the calf and the thigh the popliteal angle, as originally described by Amiel-Tison, because they believed it was a more appropriate description of the angle subtended by the popliteal fossa.

The feet are examined to determine if there is an equinus or equinovarus contracture. The ankles should easily dorsiflex to 30 degrees, plantarflex to 40 degrees, and the hindfoot should be supple. When testing dorsiflexion of the ankle, it is important to supinate the hindfoot, locking the subtalar joint, because hypermobility in the subtalar and tarsal joints can mask an equinus contracture. The decrease in the amount of ankle dorsiflexion with the knee extended, compared to that with the knee flexed, represents the contribution of the gastrocnemius muscles to the equinus contracture; this is termed the Silverskiold test (31). This patient has cerebral palsy with asymmetric spastic diplegia and may have a neuromuscular hip subluxation or dislocation, so an anteroposterior pelvis radiograph is recommended.

A 9-Year-Old Boy with Cerebral Palsy and Spastic Diplegia Is Referred Because His Feet Turn Out and He Fatigues Easily.

His mother first noticed that his feet turned out shortly after he began walking at 3 years of age. According to his mother, his feet have gradually deteriorated over the last 4 years to the point where he now "walks like a duck." She has also noticed that over the last 2 years his endurance has decreased to the point where he actually needs to rest several times when she takes him shopping. She states that 2 years ago he walked upright, but now he walks bent over at the knees. His birth history reveals that he was born after a 26-week gestation with a birth weight of 1300 g (2 lb 14 oz). Immediately after birth, he had difficulty breathing. He was intubated and transferred to the NICU for care. He remained in the NICU for 3 months prior to going home. His subsequent development was delayed as he first sat at 14 months and did not walk independently until he was 3 years old. He has been receiving physical therapy services and his therapist has noted tight hamstrings and questions whether the hamstring spasticity may be contributing to his crouch gait pattern.

On physical examination, he ambulates with a crouched gait pattern with pes planus and a foot-progression angle of 45-degree external rotation on the right and 50-degree external rotation on the left (Fig. 4-7). Stance phase is longer on the right compared with the left, and he seems more stable when he stands on the right lower extremity. During gait, he crouches with bilateral hip flexion of 30 degrees and bilateral knee flexion of 40 degrees in midstance. He swings his arms during gait to control his balance during single-limb stance. There is an absent first rocker with his flat-foot gait pattern, an excessive second rocker as the tibia rolls freely over the foot with minimal resistance from the soleus, and a markedly weakened third rocker or lack of push off secondary to weak ankle plantarflexors.

The lack of push off is an important clinical finding as the ankle plantarflexors play a key role in preventing a crouch gait pattern by a mechanism termed the "plantar flexion knee extension couple." In normal gait, during midstance as the tibia rolls freely over the foot, it creates a large external dorsiflexion moment at the ankle that is balanced by an internal ankle plantarflexion moment created primarily by the soleus. This ankle plantarflexion moment drives the tibia and knee posteriorly in the sagittal plane keeping the ground reaction force anterior to the knee creating an extension moment. The resulting plantar flexion knee extension couple generated by the soleus muscle results in an efficient gait pattern with the knee flexed no more than 15 degrees in midstance (32). In this patient, the soleus muscle is not generating enough power to balance the dorsiflexion moment at the ankle. The resulting weakened plantar flexion knee extension couple causes the ground reaction force to fall anterior to the knee causing the crouch gait pattern. To compensate for the decreased plantar flexion knee extension couple, the quadriceps is activated during midstance resulting in increased patellofemoral pressure and considerable energy consumption.

In the supine position, the Thomas test reveals bilateral hip flexion contractures of 25 degrees (Fig. 4-36A). The straight-leg-raising test only reaches 50 degrees bilaterally indicating hamstring contractures (Fig. 4-39A). The hamstring contractures are further evaluated by measuring the popliteal angles, which reveals a popliteal angle of 130 degrees on the right and 120 degrees on the left (Fig. 4-39B). The foot examination reveals dorsiflexion to 35 degrees and plantarflexion to 40 degrees bilaterally.

In the prone position, maximum internal rotation of the hips is 60 degrees bilaterally (Fig. 4-8), and external rotation is 50 degrees bilaterally (Fig. 4-9). The thigh-foot angles (Fig. 4-10) reveal 50 degrees external rotation on the right and 55 degrees on the left (Fig. 4-40). The marked external tibial torsion in this patient decreases the power of the plantarflexor muscles by shortening their joint moments. Although the plantarflexors may be strong, their decreased joint moments result in decreased function, and this loss of function is termed "lever arm dysfunction." Schwartz and Lakin (32) used an induced acceleration analysis model to analyze the vertical support function of the soleus muscle and reported that external tibial torsion of 50 degrees caused a 40% loss of support.

This patient's external tibial torsion is causing considerable lever arm dysfunction of the ankle plantarflexors causing him to crouch and use the quadriceps muscles to compensate for the loss of support. This gait pattern is very inefficient, causing a loss of endurance and early fatigue. He may benefit from bilateral distal tibial osteotomies to correct the external tibial torsion to restore plantarflexion power and improve the function of the plantar flexion knee extension couple.

A 5-Year-Old Boy Is Referred Because He Has Been Limping.

The mother first noticed that he seemed to walk funny last year, but he definitely began limping on the

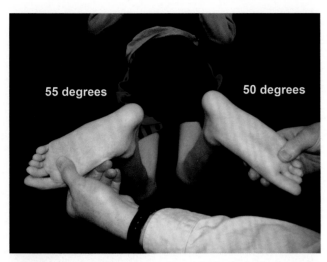

FIGURE 4-40.   The thigh-foot angles in this patient are 55 degrees on the left and 50 degrees on the right. This amount of external tibial torsion decreases the power of the plantarflexor muscles by shortening their joint moments. Although the plantarflexors may be strong, their decreased joint moments results in decreased function termed "lever arm dysfunction."

right side shortly after his fifth birthday. He has been limping for 3 months, and the limp is worse at the end of the day when he is tired. He never complains of pain and she has not previously noticed any swelling.

The physical examination begins by observing his gait pattern in the hall. He walks with an obvious limp on the right, but he spends an equal amount of time in stance phase on both limbs, indicating a painless limp. The differential diagnosis of a painless limp is different than that of a painful (antalgic) limp. A painless limp could be caused by DDH or a limb-length discrepancy, whereas a painful limp could be caused by Legg-Calvé-Perthes disease or transient synovitis. If the patient had bilateral DDH, the limp may be subtle with a waddling gait pattern associated with increased lumbar lordosis.

With the boy standing, the clinician places both hands on the iliac crests and notes that the left iliac crest is 2 cm higher than the right, indicating a limb-length discrepancy with the left lower extremity longer than the right. When he is asked to stand on the left leg, the right iliac crest elevates 5 mm. When he is asked to stand on the right leg, the left iliac crest drops 15 mm. The inability of the hip abductor muscles to hold the pelvis is single-limb support is termed a positive Trendelenburg test (Fig. 4-24). Since the patient has no pain, the positive Trendelenburg test indicates weakness of the hip abductor muscles. In a patient with developmental coxa vara, the decrease in the neck-shaft angle decreases the articulotrochanteric distance between the femoral head and the greater trochanter. This disrupts the normal length–tension relationship of the abductor muscles causing weakness.

The hip exam reveals flexion to 130 degrees on the left and 120 degrees on the right. The Thomas test (Fig. 4-36A) reveals extension to 0 degrees on the left and a flexion contracture of 25 degrees on the right. Abduction is to 80 degrees on the left and 50 degrees on the right, and adduction is to 30 degrees bilaterally. Internal rotation is to 60 degrees on the left and only 0 degrees on the right, and external rotation is to 60 degrees on the left and to 70 degrees on the right (Figs. 4-8 and 4-9). These changes in range of motion may be secondary to a retroversion deformity of the proximal femur, often seen in a patient with developmental coxa vara or SCFE. Since SCFE typically occurs during puberty, it would be unlikely in a 5-year-old boy unless he had an underlying endocrine disorder.

A simple method to assess femoral and tibial lengths and foot heights in a patient with a limb-length discrepancy is to first place him in the supine position with the hips flexed to 90 degrees to measure the femoral lengths. The Galeazzi sign (Fig. 4-6) reveals the difference in height of the knees, indicating the difference in the femoral lengths. To measure tibial lengths, including the heights of the feet, he is placed in the prone position with the hips extended and the knees flexed to 90 degrees. The difference in the heights of the heels represents the discrepancy in the length of the tibias plus the heights of the feet (Fig. 4-41). This method, although an estimate of the total limb-length discrepancy, may be more accurate than a CT scan because, unlike the CT scan, it takes into account the heights of the feet.

This patient has a limb-length discrepancy with abductor weakness and a loss of internal rotation of the right hip. These findings are consistent with the diagnosis of developmental coxa vara so an anteroposterior pelvis radiograph is recommended.

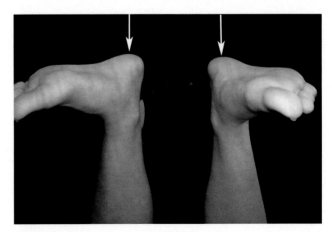

FIGURE 4-41.   To measure tibial lengths and foot heights, the patient is placed in the prone position with the hips extended and the knees are flexed to 90 degrees. The difference in the heights of the heels (arrows) represents the discrepancy in the length of the tibias plus the heights of the feet.

THE ORTHOPAEDIC EXAMINATION FROM 10 TO 18 YEARS OF AGE

A 13-Year-Old Girl Is Referred for Evaluation of Scoliosis.
After a scoliosis screening examination at school, the patient was given a note from the nurse recommending an evaluation for possible scoliosis. The girl's pediatrician detected shoulder asymmetry and a rib prominence and referred her for evaluation. The patient has never noticed any spinal deformity and is active in sports. She occasionally gets pain in the lower back, but this does not interfere with her activities. She denies any problems with bowel or bladder function, and she first began menses 1 month ago, indicating that she is now past her peak growth velocity. The family history reveals that she has two maternal cousins with scoliosis, and one of them required surgery for the spinal deformity. The mother states that she has grown 5 cm (2 in.) in the last 6 months. She is 178 cm (5 ft 10 in.) tall, and her mother is 175 cm (5 ft 9 in.) and her father is 188 cm (6 ft 2 in.) tall.

A history of mild back pain that does not interfere with activities is common in patients with scoliosis. Ramirez et al. (33) evaluated 2442 patients with idiopathic scoliosis and reported that 560 (23%) had back pain at the time of presentation, and an additional 210 (9%) had back pain during the period of observation. In contrast, a history of severe back pain associated with rapid progression of the scoliosis, weakness or sensory changes, bowel or bladder complaints, or balance problems is not typical in a patient with idiopathic scoliosis and suggests a possible intraspinal problem.

The physical examination begins with the patient standing. The trunk shape and balance are observed from the back. The clinician looks for any asymmetry in the neck, level of the shoulders, level of the scapular spines, prominence of the scapulae, surface shape of the rib cage, or the contour of the waist. A patient with lumbar scoliosis convex to the left will have asymmetry of the waist, with the left side being straight and the right side contouring inward, giving the appearance of a limb-length discrepancy. The iliac crest is more accentuated on the concave side, and the patient often interprets this as the right hip sticking out. The skin is observed for any café-au-lait marks or freckling in the axilla that may indicate neurofibromatosis. If the patient is tall and has long prominent fingers (arachnodactyly), it may indicate Marfan syndrome.

If the patient is standing erect and the spine is compensated, the head should be centered directly over the pelvis and a plumb bob suspended from the spinous process of the seventh cervical vertebra should fall directly over the gluteal cleft (Fig. 4-42). If the spine is decompensated to either side, the distance from the plumb bob to the gluteal cleft is recorded in centimeters. The posterior iliac dimples in stance are observed to determine if they are symmetric and level, indicating equal limb lengths. The clinician's hands are placed on the iliac crests to determine if the pelvis is level, or if there is a limb-length discrepancy (Fig. 4-43). If there is a limb-length discrepancy, the difference in the level of the iliac

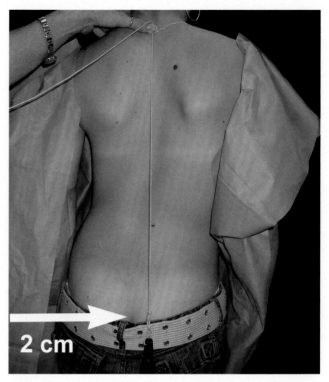

FIGURE 4-42. If the spine is compensated, the head should be centered over the pelvis, and a plumb bob suspended from the spinous process of the seventh cervical vertebra should fall directly over the gluteal cleft. If the spine is decompensated, the distance from the plumb bob to the gluteal cleft is recorded in centimeters (2 cm to the right in this patient).

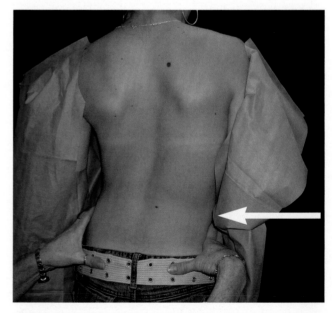

FIGURE 4-43. The patient is observed from the back looking for any asymmetry in the neck, level of the shoulders, level of the scapular spines, prominence of the scapulae, surface shape of the rib cage, contour of the waist, and the level of the iliac crests (*arrow*).

crests is recorded in centimeters. A limb-length discrepancy causes a compensatory postural scoliosis deformity, convex toward the shorter limb, to balance the head over the pelvis. This postural scoliosis will correct when the limb-length discrepancy is corrected by placing an appropriate sized wooden block under the foot of the short leg to equalize the limb lengths. The spinous processes are palpated to determine if there is any focal tenderness, and the patient is asked to arch her back, to see if it causes discomfort (Fig. 4-44). Patients who have a spondylolysis will often have discomfort when the spinous process of the involved vertebra is palpated, or when they attempt to extend the spine.

The patient places the hands together in front of her and bends forward as if she were touching her toes. This is the "Adams forward-bending test" and is one of the most sensitive clinical tests to detect scoliosis (Fig. 4-45). As the patient bends forward, the clinician observes the spine to determine if it is supple and flexes symmetrically. If the patient bends to one side instead of straight ahead, it may indicate a hamstring contracture associated with a spondylolisthesis, disk herniation, or neoplasm. As the patient bends forward, if the spine flexes excessively in the thoracic area, it may indicate Scheuermann disease or kyphosis (Fig. 4.46). When the patient is in the forward-bending position, the clinician looks for any asymmetry of the trunk and measures the angle of trunk rotation, or rib prominence, using a scoliometer (Fig. 4-45) (34). In

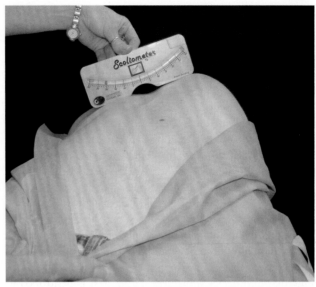

FIGURE 4-45. The Adams forward-bending test is performed by asking the patient to place the hands together in front of her and bend forward at the waist, as if she were touching her toes. As the patient bends forward, the clinician observes the spine to determine if it is supple and flexes symmetrically. Once the patient has bent forward so that the spine is parallel to the floor, the clinician looks for asymmetry of the trunk and measures the angle of trunk rotation using a scoliometer (Fig. 4-45). In this patient, the angle of trunk rotation is 21 degrees at T8.

this patient, the angle of trunk rotation measures 21 degrees at T8 with the right side higher than the left. The angle of trunk rotation or rib prominence reflects the rotational component of the scoliosis deformity that occurs in the axial plane. The most common type of scoliosis is a convex right thoracic curve, in which the vertebrae rotate into the convexity of the curve, causing the ribs to be more prominent posteriorly on

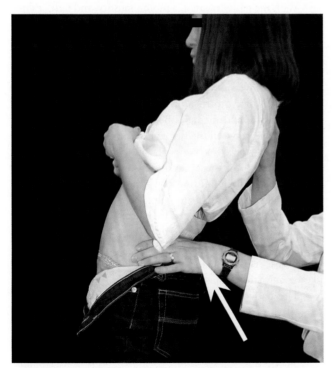

FIGURE 4-44. The patient is asked to arch her back, to determine if it causes discomfort. Pain or discomfort to palpation in to lower back (*arrow*) or pain that is aggravated by arching the back are important findings often seen in patients with a spondylolysis.

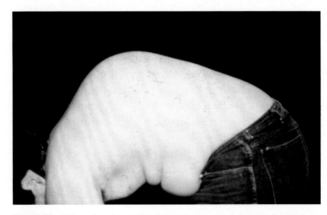

FIGURE 4-46. As the patient bends forward during the Adams forward-bending test, the clinician observes closely to determine if the spine flexes symmetrically. Any excessive flexion in the thoracic area, as seen in this patient, may indicate Scheuermann disease.

the patient's right side. The ribs are also more prominent anteriorly on the patient's left side, which may cause breast asymmetry. While the patient is in the forward-bending position, she is asked to bend to the right and left to assess the flexibility of the scoliosis.

Scoliosis is seen in association with neuromuscular disorders, such as muscular dystrophy, and is also seen in association with spinal cord anomalies, such as a tethered spinal cord. A thorough neurologic examination is essential to rule out a neuromuscular disorder. In standing, the Romberg sign is elicited by asking the patient to place the feet closely together. She then closes her eyes and the clinician looks for any sway or instability. A patient with cerebellar ataxia will sway or move her feet to maintain balance. This test may be helpful because scoliosis is frequently seen in patients with Friedreich ataxia. An evaluation of the upper and lower extremity strength, sensation, and reflexes is essential to rule out an occult neuromuscular disorder. A straight-leg-raising test is performed to look for hamstring tightness or a radiculopathy (Fig. 4-39A). Straight-leg raising to <40 degrees may indicate tight hamstrings associated with a spondylolisthesis, disc herniation, or neoplasm. The abdominal reflexes are tested by gently stroking the side of the abdomen, and the umbilicus should deviate toward the stimulus. Any asymmetry of the abdominal reflexes is important because it may indicate an intraspinal problem.

In a patient with adolescent idiopathic scoliosis, it is important to assess their maturity, because the risk of curve progression is higher in young patients and in patients with larger curves (35). The risk of progression is highest when the patient is at their peak growth velocity. The peak growth velocity typically occurs about 12 months before the onset of menses and 12 months after closure of the triradiate cartilage. Most investigators recommend radiographs if the angle of trunk rotation is >7 degrees, so scoliosis posteroanterior and lateral radiographs are recommended, to be taken with a tube-to-film distance of 183 cm (72 in.) on a 91 cm (36 in.) cassette.

A 14-Year-Old Girl Is Referred for Evaluation of Low Back Pain Aggravated by Playing Soccer.

The patient was apparently in satisfactory health until 4 months ago when she developed low back pain after a soccer game. Over the last 3 months, the pain has increased to the point that she is unable to play for more than 5 minutes without resting. She describes the pain as being in the lower back in the L5–S1 area and it is worse on the right side. The pain does not radiate into the buttocks or lower extremities, and it is aggravated by exercise and relieved by rest. Her past medical history reveals no major illnesses or prior hospitalizations.

The physical examination begins by observing her gait and she has a normal heel-toe gait pattern. A patient with low back pain may have subtle changes in gait that can be detected by an astute observer. A patient with spondylolisthesis may have a hamstring contracture that prevents full extension of the knee in terminal swing, causing a decrease in step length and stride length. Step length is the distance from the foot strike of one foot to the foot strike of the other foot. Stride length is the distance from one foot strike to the next foot strike by the same foot. Thus, each stride length includes one right and one left step length (36). In a patient with a severe spondylolisthesis, the hamstring contractures may be so severe that the patient actually walks on their toes with a toe-toe gait pattern.

In standing, the trunk shape and balance are observed from the back. The clinician looks for any asymmetry in the neck, scapulae, shoulders, rib cage, waist, or hips (Fig. 4-43). Low back pain can cause muscle spasms on the side with the pain, causing a scoliosis convex to the opposite side. The paraspinal muscles are palpated to determine if they are in spasm. An osteoid osteoma involving the posterior elements of the spine may be associated with a painful scoliosis. This patient describes increased pain when she attempts to arch her back (Fig. 4-44). Hyperextension of the lumbar spine increases the pressure on the posterior elements, causing a patient with spondylolysis to experience increased pain with this maneuver. This test is important because most patients with back pain will not have increased in pain with this maneuver. The spinous processes of the lumbar vertebrae are palpated to determine if palpation causes discomfort. A patient with a spondylolysis at L5 will often experience pain with palpation of the L5 spinous process because the palpation increases the pressure on the pars interarticularis (Fig. 4-44).

With the patient seated, a motor, sensory, and reflex examination of the upper and lower extremities is performed. A disc protrusion affecting the L5 nerve root may compromise function of the extensor hallucis longus and posterior tibial muscles and is detected by weakness in dorsiflexion of the great toe, weakness in inversion, and a decreased posterior tibial tendon reflex. A L5 disc protrusion may also cause sensory changes over the dorsal and medial aspect of the foot, particularly in the web space between the first and second toes. A disc protrusion affecting the S1 nerve root could compromise function of the gastrocsoleus muscle and is detected by weakness in the gastrocsoleus muscle and a decreased Achilles tendon reflex. Occasionally it is difficult to elicit the Achilles tendon reflex. This problem can be resolved by having the patient kneel on a chair with the feet dangling over the edge. In this position, the reflex hammer typically elicits a good ankle jerk. A patient with an S1 disc protrusion may have sensory changes over the plantar and lateral aspect of the foot.

The patient is placed supine, and a straight-leg-raising test is performed (Fig. 4-39A). Limited straight-leg raising may indicate hamstring tightness associated with spondylolisthesis or nerve root irritation from disc herniation or neoplasm. Young athletes with spondylolysis will often experience increased pain while playing soccer. Debnath et al. (37) evaluated 22 young athletes who had surgery for low back pain associated with a spondylolysis and 13 (59%) were soccer players. This patient's pain may be secondary to a spondylolysis, so radiographs of the lumbar spine are recommended.

A 14-Year-Old Boy Is Referred for Evaluation of Left Knee Pain and Limping.

The patient was in satisfactory health until 4 months ago when he developed pain in his left knee. Several weeks later, his mother noticed he was limping on his left leg. The pain and limping has increased and are aggravated by activities. There is no history of injury, and he has not had any swelling in the knee. The past medical history and family history are unremarkable. The personal and social history reveals that he has always been overweight.

A 14-year-old boy who is obese and complaining of left knee pain and a limp should cause the clinician to immediately consider the diagnosis of SCFE. The majority of children with SCFE are obese. Obesity is also associated with femoral retroversion, with anteversion averaging 10.6 degrees in adolescents of average weight, but only 0.4 degrees in obese adolescents (38). Obesity and femoral retroversion increase the mechanical shear stresses across the physis, increasing the risk of slip progression in a patient with SCFE.

On physical examination, he weighs 95 kg (208 lb) (greater than the 95th percentile for weight). In observing his gait pattern, he ambulates with an antalgic (painful) limp on the left lower extremity. He leans his head and trunk to his left during the stance phase. The shifting of weight over the left lower extremity in stance phase decreases the joint reactive forces in the hip and is termed a Trendelenburg gait pattern. A patient with a Trendelenburg gait will usually have a positive Trendelenburg test (Fig. 4-24). He has a shortened stance phase on the left, and his foot-progression angle is 10 degrees of external rotation on the right and 35 degrees of external rotation on the left (Fig. 4-7). In standing, the shoulders, scapular spines, and spine are observed from the back, and no asymmetry is noted. The clinician's hands are placed on the iliac crests, and the left iliac crest is noted to be 1 cm lower than the right, indicating a limb-length discrepancy (Fig. 4-43). In single-limb stance, he is noted to have a negative Trendelenburg test when he stands on his right lower extremity and a positive Trendelenburg test when he stands on his left lower extremity (Fig. 4-24).

In describing his pain, he points to the anterior aspect of the left knee. A patient with SCFE may complain of knee pain, rather than hip, thigh, or groin pain. This phenomenon occurs because the obturator and femoral nerves that supply the hip also supply the knee. A patient with hip pathology complaining of knee pain is a classic example of referred pain. The range of motion of his hips reveals flexion to 130 degrees on the right and 120 degrees on the left. When the right hip is flexed to the knee-chest position, it remains in neutral rotation, but when the left hip is flexed it spontaneously goes into abduction and external rotation. This abduction and external rotation occurs because a patient with SCFE has a retroversion deformity of the proximal femur. The femoral neck displaces anteriorly, through the physis, creating apex-anterior angulation of the proximal femur (39). Abduction is to 70 degrees on the right and 50 degrees on the left. Internal rotation is to 20 degrees on the right and minus 20 degrees on the left (Fig. 4-8). External rotation is to 70 degrees on the right and

85 degrees on the left (Fig. 4-9). These physical findings indicate a retroversion deformity of the left femoral neck, with an increase in external and a decrease in internal rotation of the left hip. An obese adolescent boy with these physical findings has a high probability of having SCFE, so anteroposterior and frog-lateral pelvis radiographs are recommended.

A 14-Year-Old Girl Is Referred for Evaluation of Left Knee Pain and giving Way.

The patient states that she was fine until 6 months ago, when she collided with another player in a soccer game and landed directly on her left knee. She had moderate swelling that resolved in 7 days and she gradually resumed playing soccer. The knee felt better after the soccer season, but recurred when she began playing basketball. She describes the pain as being located circumferentially around the kneecap. The pain is aggravated by sitting in the back seat of the car with the knee flexed. The pain is also worse going up and down the stairs.

A patient with anterior knee pain or patellofemoral pain syndrome will often experience pain when sitting with the knee flexed for a prolonged period of time. This finding has been termed a positive "movie sign" from sitting for several hours in the movie theater. In a similar fashion, the pain occurs after sitting in the back seat of a car for several hours. Patients with anterior knee pain will often have increased pain going upstairs and downstairs. The patient may note catching, subpatellar crepitus, and giving way, but true locking is unusual.

On physical examination, the clinician compares the injured knee with the uninjured knee looking for loss of the "dimples" on either side of the patella, indicating an effusion (Fig. 4-47). If the patient does not have an observable effusion, the suprapatellar pouch is milked from medial to lateral moving any fluid into the lateral compartment of the knee. The lateral side is then milked while observing for a fluid wave on the medial side (Fig. 4-48). Visualizing the fluid wave is

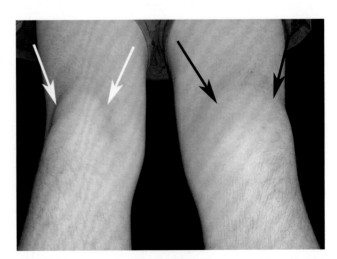

FIGURE 4-47. In this patient, the uninjured right knee has "dimples" (*white arrows*) on either side of the patella. The injured left knee has a large effusion that stretches out the dimples (*black arrows*).

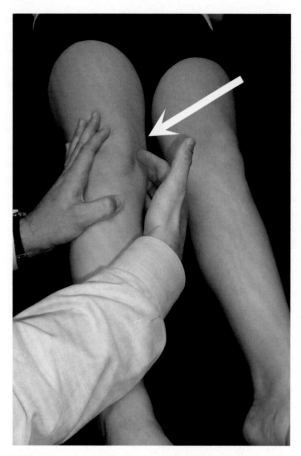

FIGURE 4-48. If a mild knee effusion is suspected, the suprapatellar pouch is milked from lateral to medial moving any fluid into the medial compartment of the knee. As the lateral side is milked, the clinician observes for a fluid wave on the medial side (*arrow*).

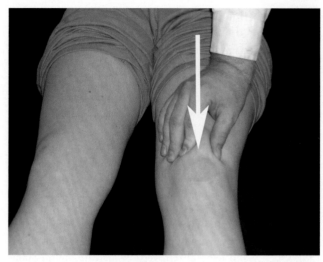

FIGURE 4-49. The patellar inhibition test is performed with the patient supine and the knee in extension. The clinician holds the patella (*arrow*), inhibiting it from ascending along the femur, while the patient performs a straight-leg raise. This maneuver increases the forces in the patellofemoral joint causing discomfort in a patient with patellofemoral pain.

If the patient immediately contracts her quadriceps to prevent the patella from subluxating, the test is positive and often occurs in patients who have previously had a subluxation or dislocation of the patella.

A patient with "miserable malalignment syndrome" may be more susceptible to lateral subluxation of the patella. This syndrome includes a combination of internal femoral torsion and external tibial torsion which causes patellae to face in

the most sensitive test to detect a trace effusion. In describing the pain, she points to the medial and lateral sides of the patella. She has tenderness on the undersurface of the medial and lateral facets of the patella, which is elicited by gently palpating the facets while pushing the patella laterally and medially with the knee in extension. A patient with anterior knee pain may have a contracture of the lateral retinaculum. This is detected by the inability to elevate the lateral margin of the patella when tilting the patella medially and laterally during the tilt test. If the pain is caused by patellofemoral joint reaction forces, it can be reproduced by the "patellar inhibition test." This test is performed in the supine position with the knee in extension. The patient is asked to do a straight-leg raise while the clinician holds the patella distally, preventing it from ascending along the anterior femur (Fig. 4-49). This maneuver increases the pressure between the patella and femur, reproducing the pain in a patient with patellofemoral pain syndrome. If the pain is caused by patellofemoral instability, it can be reproduced by the "patellar apprehension test." This test is performed with the knee flexed to 30 degrees, and the clinician gently pushes the patella laterally (Fig. 4-50).

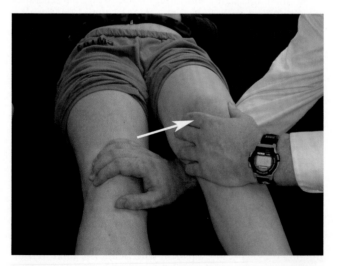

FIGURE 4-50. The patellar apprehension test is performed with the patient supine and the knee flexed to 30 degrees. The clinician gently pushes the patella laterally (*arrow*). If the patient immediately contracts her quadriceps to prevent the patella from subluxating, the test is positive.

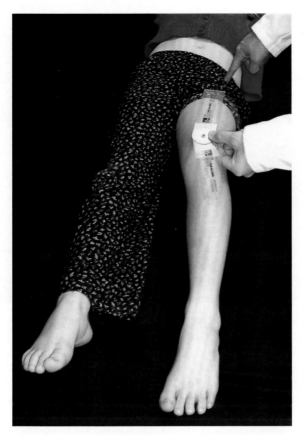

FIGURE 4-51. The Q angle is the angle formed by a line connecting the anterior superior iliac spine with the center of the patella and a second line connecting the center of the patella with the tibial tubercle. The Q angle is measured with the knee in 30 degrees of flexion, so that the patella is in contact with the femoral sulcus.

(squinting patellae) when the feet are pointing straight ahead. Patients with miserable malalignment syndrome may have knee pain and often have an increased Q angle. The Q angle is the angle formed by a line connecting the anterior superior iliac spine with the center of the patella and a second line connecting the center of the patella with the tibial tubercle (Fig. 4-51). The Q angle is measured with the knee in 30 degrees of flexion so that the patella is in contact with the femoral sulcus. Patients with an increased Q angle (>15 degrees) may have knee pain because of lateral tracking of the patella in the femoral sulcus resulting in a small contact area between the patella and femur. The maltracking can be detected by observing the patella as the patient actively extends the knee. Sitting over the side of the table with the knees flexed to 90 degrees, the patient is asked to gradually extend the knee. The patella is observed to remain in the femoral sulcus as it ascends along the axis of the femur, but as the knee reaches full extension, the patella deviates laterally like an upside-down J. This is termed a positive "J sign," and if the patient has patellofemoral instability, the patella may subluxate with this maneuver. It is important to note that a normal knee has a "J sign," but in an unstable

knee it is exaggerated or occurs earlier or more dramatically compared to the normal side as the knee extends.

A patient with anterior knee pain will typically have a full range of motion from 0 to 135 degrees. The pain is often described as being circumferential around the patella, and there is usually no evidence of an effusion. A patient with Osgood-Schlatter disease will have pain over the tibial tubercle, and a patient with Sinding-Larsen-Johansson disease (jumper's knee) will have pain at the inferior pole of the patella (40). A patient with osteochondritis dissecans (OCD) will have pain elicited by direct palpation over the femoral articular surface at the site of the lesion. OCD most frequently occurs on the lateral aspect of the medial femoral condyle, but can also occur over the lateral femoral condyle, femoral sulcus, or the patella. If the lesion is in the lateral aspect of the medial femoral condyle, the pain can be reproduced by flexing the knee to 90 degrees, internally rotating the tibia, then gradually extending the knee. As the knee approaches 30 degrees of flexion, a patient with an OCD involving the medial femoral condyle will experience pain that is relieved by externally rotating the tibia. This phenomenon is termed a positive Wilson test (41).

A patient with a torn meniscus will typically have pain at the joint line. A torn meniscus can be evaluated by maximally flexing the knee and circumducting the tibia on the femur. If the clinician palpates a clunk with this maneuver, a meniscus tear is likely and this is termed a positive "McMurray test." The Apley's grinding test is another method to identify a torn meniscus. With the patient in the prone position, this test is performed by applying pressure directly to the heel, loading the knee in compression, while the tibia is internally and externally rotated. A patient with a torn meniscus will experience pain with this maneuver when the meniscus gets trapped between the tibia and the femur. A painful test is termed a positive "Apley test." The bounce test is another method to identify a torn meniscus. With the patient supine and the knee extended, the clinician elevates the foot, then drops it several inches causing the knee to hyperextend, flex, then hyperextend again. Most patients will not have discomfort with this maneuver, but if there is a torn meniscus the maneuver causes pain at the medial joint line and a reflex contraction of the hamstrings preventing the knee from hyperextending. This inability to hyperextend the knee associated with medial joint line pain is termed a positive "bounce test."

Although the patient with anterior knee pain would not typically have any abnormal ligamentous laxity, these important knee stabilizers are examined. With the patient in the supine position and the knees flexed to 90 degrees and the foot flat on the exam table, the clinician looks for a posterior sag of the tibia, which is often seen in a patient with a posterior cruciate ligament (PCL)-deficient knee. A torn PCL can be detected by the "quadriceps active test" (42). This test is performed with the patient in the supine position and the knee flexed to 90 degrees with the foot flat on the exam table. The patient is asked to slide her foot directly down the table by contracting the quadriceps muscles, while the clinician prevents the foot from moving. The force of the quadriceps muscle will

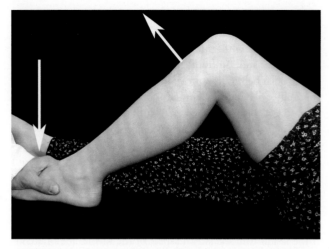

FIGURE 4-52. The quadriceps active test is performed with the patient supine and the knee flexed to 90 degrees. In this position, the tibia is subluxated posteriorly in a patient with a ruptured PCL. The patient is asked to slide her foot down the table, while the clinician prevents the foot from moving (*down arrow*). The force of the quadriceps muscle pulls the tibia anteriorly (*up arrow*), reducing the posterior subluxation.

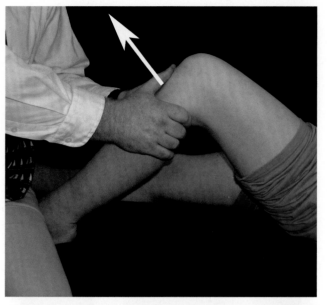

FIGURE 4-53. The anterior drawer test is performed with the patient supine and the knee flexed to 90 degrees. The foot is stabilized by the clinician's thigh, while the tibia is pulled forward at the knee (*arrow*). The clinician should feel a solid stop after 3 to 4 mm of translation, indicating an intact ACL. It is important to palpate the hamstring tendons to be sure the hamstring muscles are relaxed, because contracting hamstrings can mask an ACL-deficient knee.

pull the tibia anteriorly, reducing the posterior subluxation in a patient with a PCL-deficient knee (Fig. 4-52).

An anterior cruciate ligament (ACL)-deficient knee is evaluated by performing the anterior drawer test. This test is performed with the patient supine and the knee flexed to 90 degrees with the foot flat on the exam table. The foot is stabilized under the clinician's thigh, while the proximal tibia is pulled forward. The clinician should feel a solid stop after 3 to 5 mm of anterior translation of the proximal tibia on the femur, indicating an intact ACL (Fig. 4-53). It is important to palpate the hamstring tendons while performing this test, because a torn ACL may not be detected if the patient contracts the hamstring muscles during the test. A negative anterior drawer test does not always guarantee that the ACL is normal. A more sensitive test to detect a ruptured ACL is the Lachman test. This test is performed with the patient supine and the knee flexed to 30 degrees. The lateral femoral condyle is held motionless in one hand, while the tibia is pulled anteriorly with the other hand (Fig. 4-54). If anterior subluxation greater than the normal knee is detected, without a solid end point, it indicates a ruptured ACL. An ACL-deficient knee that is not painful can be detected by the pivot-shift test. This test is performed with the patient supine and the knee in extension. A valgus and internal rotation force is applied to the lateral tibia while the calcaneus is grasped with the other hand. This maneuver causes the tibia to translate anteriorly in an ACL-deficient knee. As the knee is flexed, when the iliotibial band crosses the axis of the knee joint, the tibia rapidly shifts to its normal position, and a pivot shift or jerk is felt by the clinician and the patient. This test can only be reliably performed when the patient is completely relaxed, so it is usually not helpful in an acutely injured patient.

The medial and lateral collateral ligaments are located just under the skin, so an injury to these ligaments is associated with pain to palpation over the ligament. By gently palpating the uninjured side and comparing it with the injured side, the

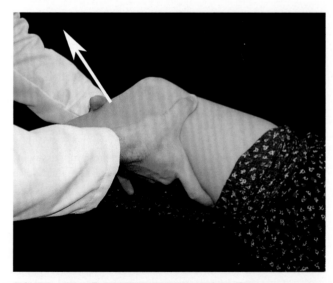

FIGURE 4-54. The Lachman test is performed with the patient supine and the knee flexed to 30 degrees. To test the left knee, the femoral condyles are held with the right hand, while the tibia is pulled anteriorly with the left hand (*arrow*). Anterior subluxation >5 mm, without a solid end point, indicates an ACL-deficient knee.

clinician can often pinpoint the location of the injury. The medial and lateral collateral ligaments are tested with the knee in 30 degrees of flexion, because varus or valgus instability can be masked by intact cruciate ligaments with the knee in extension. The medial joint line is palpated with a finger, while the examiner applies a valgus stress to the knee, and the lateral joint line is similarly palpated while the examiner applies a varus stress to the knee. The amount of joint line opening is recorded in millimeters, and 0 to 5 mm of opening with a solid end point is considered a normal amount of ligamentous laxity. Medial and lateral collateral ligament sprains are classified according to the amount of opening of the joint space on physical examination. A grade I sprain has pain over the ligament and opens 0 to 5 mm, a grade II sprain opens 6 to 10 mm, and a grade III sprain opens more than 10 mm.

This patient has anterior knee pain or patellofemoral pain secondary to a direct blow to the patella when she fell on the knee. Activity modification and physical therapy is recommended in anticipation of gradual improvement.

A 15-Year-Old Boy Is Referred for Evaluation of Bilateral Foot Pain.

The patient first noted pain under the arch of his left foot 2 years ago. Six months later, he developed similar symptoms in the right foot. He describes several episodes where the left ankle gave out while walking. The last episode occurred 1 month ago, when he was walking downstairs and the left ankle gave out, causing swelling over the lateral aspect of the ankle. The swelling resolved over the next few days. The pain under both arches has worsened over the last year and is aggravated by exercise. His mother states that he has always had high arches. There is a family history of high arches in his father and paternal grandfather.

The clinician understands that pes cavus is associated with a neuromuscular disorder until proven otherwise. The most common neurologic disorder associated with pes cavus is Charcot-Marie-tooth disease. The inheritance pattern for Charcot-Marie-tooth disease is autosomal dominant, so the clinician suspects that this boy may have Charcot-Marie-tooth disease, since his father and grandfather both have high arches.

On physical examination, he ambulates with a heel-toe-gait pattern, but walks on the lateral side of the foot with the heel in varus. In standing, he has high-arched feet and points to the medial arch of both feet when describing the pain. He has painful callosities on both feet under the heels, the first and fifth metatarsals, over the dorsal surfaces of the proximal interphalangeal joints of the lateral toes. The lateral toes have moderate claw-toe deformities. A detailed motor, sensory, and reflex examination of the upper and lower extremities is within normal limits.

The longitudinal arch of each foot is elevated, shortening the medial border of the foot, creating a concave appearance. The lateral side of each foot is convex, with lengthening of the lateral border of the foot, creating a bean-shaped deformity. On both feet, the first metatarsal is plantarflexed, forcing the hindfoot to rotate into a varus position. The normal foot has a "tripod" structure with weight bearing balanced between the heel, the first metatarsal head, and the fifth metatarsal

head. If the forefoot develops a pronation deformity, with plantarflexion of the first metatarsal, weight bearing will force the hindfoot into varus. The flexible hindfoot varus deformity will eventually become a structural deformity as the soft tissues of the subtalar joint contract over time. The flexibility of the hindfoot deformity is important when contemplating surgical reconstruction of a cavus foot. The forefoot contribution to the hindfoot varus deformity is determined by the Coleman block test (43). This test is performed with the patient standing with his back facing the clinician, and the amount of hindfoot varus is noted (Fig. 4-55A). A 2- to 3-cm block is placed under the lateral aspect of the foot and heel, allowing the first metatarsal to hang freely, negating any effect it may have upon the hindfoot by eliminating the tripod mechanism (Fig. 4-55B). The amount of correction of the hindfoot deformity, when standing on the block with the first metatarsal off the medial side of the block, represents the forefoot contribution to the hindfoot varus deformity. A similar test can be performed with the patient prone and the knee flexed to 90 degrees. The foot is dorsiflexed by applying pressure over the fifth metatarsal head, allowing the first metatarsal to remain plantarflexed, and the amount of correction of the hindfoot varus is observed.

These tests are crucial in preoperative planning because a flexible hindfoot will correct when the forefoot deformity is corrected, whereas a rigid hindfoot will not. This patient has pes cavus that may be associated with Charcot-Marie-tooth disease, so a referral to a geneticist is recommended. In addition, standing anteroposterior, lateral, oblique, and Harris axial radiographs of the calcaneus are recommended.

A 17-Year-Old Girl Is Referred Because She Has Pain in the Left Hip That Is Aggravated by Playing Soccer and Prolonged Sitting.

She states that she first noted some discomfort in the left hip area when playing soccer on the high school team 9 months ago. Recently she has noted pain over the lateral aspect of the left hip that is aggravated by prolonged sitting and getting in and out of a car. She believes that the pain has gradually increased over the last 6 months, and she currently has a dull ache when leaning forward and often gets a sharp pain or catching sensation when turning or pivoting, especially toward the affected side. She is referred for evaluation because the pain has increased to the point where she is considering not playing soccer this year.

The differential diagnosis of hip pain in an adolescent includes avascular necrosis of the femoral head, SCFE, bursitis, tumor, hernia, infection, intra-articular loose body, lumbar spine pathology, pelvic pathology, muscle strain, early osteoarthritis, and femoroacetabular impingement (FAI). The clinician asks the patient to point to the exact location of the pain and she makes a cup with the thumb and index finger of the left hand in the shape of the letter "C," and then places her cupped hand around the anterolateral aspect of the left hip just above the greater trochanter (Fig. 4-56). This method of describing the pain is termed a positive "C sign" and is often seen in patients with FAI (44). The clinician asks if other

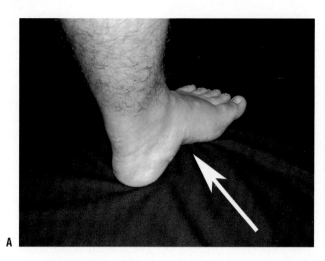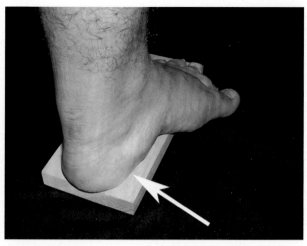

FIGURE 4-55. **A:** This foot has a pes cavus deformity with a high longitudinal arch (*arrow*), hindfoot varus, and a plantarflexed first metatarsal. **B:** The "Coleman block test" evaluates the forefoot contribution to the hindfoot varus deformity. The patient stands with the lateral aspect of the foot and heel on a 2- to 3-cm block, allowing the first metatarsal to hang freely, negating any effect it may have upon the hindfoot by eliminating the tripod mechanism. The amount of correction of the hindfoot varus deformity (*arrow*) represents the forefoot contribution to the hindfoot varus deformity.

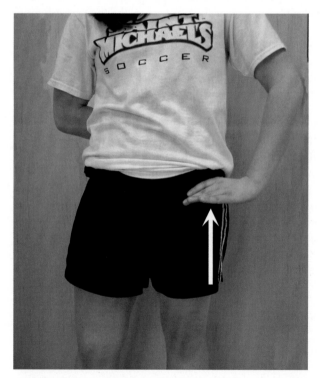

FIGURE 4-56. In describing the pain associated with left FAI, the patient makes a cup with the thumb and index finger of the left hand in the shape of the letter "C," and then places her cupped hand over the anterolateral aspect of the hip just above the greater trochanter. This method of describing the pain is termed a positive "C sign" and is often seen in patients with FAI.

activities aggravate the pain, and the patient states that she has been noting discomfort when getting out of the car.

The physical examination often begins by asking the patient to walk in the hallway to determine if there is a limp or any asymmetry to the gait pattern, and this patient walks without a limp and a symmetric gait pattern. The examination of the hip includes inspection, palpation, and an assessment of range of motion. Inspection evaluates for asymmetry as might be seen with a limb-length discrepancy or a joint contracture secondary to pain and muscle spasm. Palpation of bony landmarks may illicit pain over the anterior inferior iliac spine indicating an avulsion injury of the rectus femoris, pain over the greater trochanter indicating a greater trochanteric bursitis, or a mass indicating a tumor. Range of motion is performed to determine if there is pain associated with any particular movement. Pain in a muscle under tension indicates a muscle strain and severe pain with any motion may indicate an infection. The patient is placed in the figure-4 position, and the FABER test is performed to determine if the patient has pain with this maneuver (Fig. 4-26). Groin pain may indicate a muscle strain involving the iliopsoas muscles, whereas pain over the sacroiliac joint may indicate sacroilitis. The flexion, adduction, and internal rotation test (FADIR test) is performed to determine if placing the hip in this position causes pain (Fig. 4-57). This test is performed with the patient supine; the clinician positions the hip in 90 degrees of flexion and maximum adduction while internally and externally rotating the hip. If pain similar to the pain the patient has been experiencing occurs with internal rotation, it may indicate FAI. In a patient with hip pain caused by

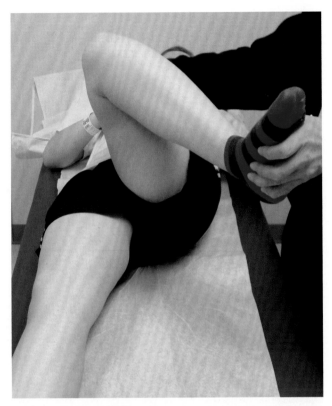

FIGURE 4-57. The flexion, adduction, and internal rotation (FADIR) test is the most sensitive test to detect FAI in a patient with groin pain. The hip is flexed to 90 degrees and adducted, while the clinician internally and externally rotates the hip. Groin pain with internal rotation, similar to the pain the patient has been experiencing, often indicates FAI.

A 15-Year-Old Boy Is Referred for a Painful Enlarging Mass on the Back of His Left Knee.

The patient is an active skateboarder who first noticed some pain and swelling on the back of the left knee several weeks ago. He cannot recall any history of trauma to the area and has recently been treated with physical therapy for patellar tendonitis. He has had no difficulty with walking or going to school, but had to quit skateboarding recently due to increasing pain. He now has pain all the time and has been taking nonsteroidal anti-inflammatory drugs (NSAIDs) to help him sleep at night. He maintains a good appetite and denies fevers, night sweats, or fatigue. His mother states that he recently had a growth spurt and grew 5 cm (2 in.) over the last 6 months. She is concerned that the mass seems to be increasing in size. His past history and family history are unremarkable.

A detailed history and physical examination is important to formulate an accurate differential diagnosis in a patient with a suspected bone lesion. The clinician understands that infections (osteomyelitis) are the most common cause of bone lesions in children. Primary bone tumors do not typically present with fever, loss of appetite, or weight loss, but they can mimic an infection with a serendipitous onset of pain, swelling, or limp with increasing lethargy. The presence of pain at the time of diagnosis is important because a painful bone lesion, or a painful lesion that subsequently develops a pathologic fracture, is often a sign of malignancy. In general, asymptomatic bone lesions that are detected as incidental findings on radiographs are usually benign lesions. Nonossifying fibromas, osteochondromas, and unicameral bone cysts are common benign lesions that are often identified incidentally on radiographs taken for other purposes.

Pain is a very important symptom when evaluating a patient with a possible tumor. It is crucial to accurately characterize the type of pain when it first occurred, how the pain has progressed, and the level of severity. Activity-related pain that is associated with benign conditions must be differentiated from more worrisome night pain and pain at rest. Although night pain can occur with a benign bone tumor, such as an osteoid osteoma, night pain is more commonly associated with malignant tumors that cause pain that insidiously progresses over time ultimately leading to severe pain that even occurs at rest.

Although the patient can frequently remember exactly when the pain first started, it is often difficult to determine how long a mass has been present. A slow-growing osteochondroma may not be noticed until just prior to the consultation, giving the patient and family a false impression that the tumor is growing quickly. Masses in the proximal femur, humerus, and pelvis may be present for several months prior to detection because of abundant soft-tissue covering.

The age of the patient is also helpful in the differential diagnosis because the most common bone lesions in children <5 years of age are eosinophilic granulomas and simple bone cysts, whereas in older children and adolescents the most

FAI, the FADIR test is the most sensitive test to detect the FAI (44). The patient is asked to hop on the involved lower extremity to determine if hopping causes pain. Pain with hopping is of concern and may indicate a muscle strain, FAI, or stress fracture. In a patient with hip pain, it is extremely important to examine the spine, abdomen, and pelvis to evaluate for conditions that may cause referred pain to the hip such as discitis, hernia, or pelvic inflammatory disease. Finally, since some of these maneuvers can cause pain or discomfort, it is important to test the other side for comparison.

This patient has FAI, an abutment between the proximal femur and the rim of the acetabulum. The impingement typically occurs with flexion, adduction, and internal rotation of the femur. The impingement may cause labral tears and early cartilage damage that tend to gradually progress and limit her ability to exercise and play soccer. FAI is now a well-recognized cause of early osteoarthritis of the hip. Since FAI may not be detected by standard radiographs (45), a referral to an orthopaedic surgeon that specializes in hip disorders is recommended.

TABLE 4-6	Locations of Common Bone Tumors in Children	
	Benign	**Malignant**
Spine		
Anterior elements	Langerhan cell histiocytosis	Ewing sarcoma Lymphoma
Posterior elements	Osteoid osteoma	Metastatic neuroblastoma
	Osteoblastoma	
	Osteochondroma	
	Aneurysmal bone cyst	
Extremity		
Epiphyseal	Chondroblastoma	
	Aneurysmal bone cyst	
	Giant cell (adolescent)	
Metaphyseal	Osteochondroma	Osteosarcoma
	Nonossifying fibroma	
Diaphyseal	Fibrous dysplasia	Ewing sarcoma
	Osteofibrous dysplasia	Lymphoma
	Langerhan cell histiocytosis	

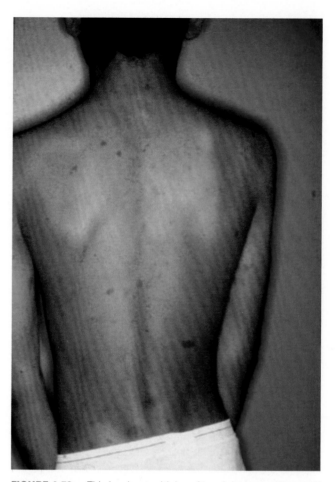

FIGURE 4-58. This boy has multiple café-au-lait spots with smooth borders like the coast of California. He has type 1 neurofibromatosis and also has numerous cutaneous neurofibromas. Most patients with type 1 neurofibromatosis will have five or more café-au-lait spots that are >1.5 cm in diameter.

common bone lesions are osteoblastomas, osteoid osteomas, and chondroblastomas.

Finally, the location of the tumor is extremely important as several tumors appear only in certain locations (Table 4-6). Bone tumors that occur in the posterior elements of the spine are most commonly osteoid osteomas, osteoblastomas, and aneurysmal bone cysts, whereas bone tumors that occur in the anterior elements are most commonly eosinophilic granulomas. In the appendicular skeleton, the most common epiphyseal tumors are chondroblastomas and aneurysmal bone cysts, whereas the most common diaphyseal tumors are fibrous dysplasias and eosinophilic granulomas. The most common metaphyseal tumors are nonossifying fibromas and unicameral bone cysts.

Some bone tumors, including fibrous dysplasia, enchondromas, nonossifying fibromas, and osteochondromas, may present with multiple lesions. A patient presenting with a single bony osteochondroma or exostosis should have a careful review of the family history to determine if other family members had similar bumps, suggesting the diagnosis of multiple hereditary exostosis, an autosomal dominant condition. If the physical examination detects other osteochondromas, a careful examination may detect angular deformity at wrists (ulnar deviation) and valgus deformity at the ankles secondary to tethering by the osteochondromas. In addition, these patients may have short stature and a limb-length discrepancy.

The clinician must be careful to perform a complete physical examination including inspection and palpation of the skin and soft tissues of the upper and lower extremities. Pigmented skin lesions termed café-au-lait spots can be very helpful in the differential diagnosis. Café-au-lait spots with smooth borders (coast of California) are often seen in patients with type 1 neurofibromatosis or Jaffe-Campanacci syndrome (Fig. 4-58) (46). These patients may also have axillary freckling, and patients with type 1 neurofibromatosis will often have cutaneous neurofibromas. Most patients with type 1 neurofibromatosis will have five or more café-au-lait spots that are greater than 1.5 cm in diameter. Café-au-lait spots with rugged borders (coast of Maine) are often seen in patients with McCune-Albright syndrome (Fig. 4-59). Multiple cutaneous hemangiomas are often seen in patients with Maffuci disease. The skin is also inspected for any overlying changes such as erythema or vascular engorgement from hyperemia. These findings are often seen in association with primary bone sarcomas such as an osteosarcoma.

The bone tumor is palpated to identify a point of maximal tenderness and determine if there is an associated soft-tissue mass. Benign inactive tumors do not usually have an associated soft-tissue mass, whereas benign aggressive tumors such as

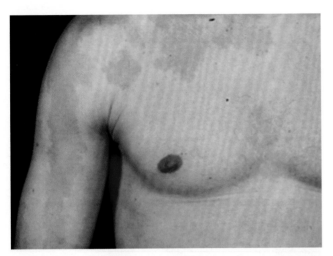

FIGURE 4-59. This boy has multiple café-au-lait spots with rugged borders like the coast of Maine. These skin lesions are often seen in patients with McCune-Albright syndrome.

TABLE 4-7		Grading of Muscle Strength Using the Medical Research Council Rating System	
Grade	Rating	Muscle Strength	Assessment
0	Zero	No palpable contraction	Nothing
1	Trace	Muscle contracts, but no movement of bone	Trace
2	Poor	Muscle moves the bone, but not against gravity	With gravity eliminated
3	Fair	Muscle moves the bone through a full range of motion against gravity	Against gravity
4	Good	Muscle moves the bone against resistance	Near normal
5	Excellent	Normal strength against full resistance	Normal

chondroblastomas and eosinophilic granuloma, and malignant bone sarcomas, especially Ewing sarcoma, will often have a large soft-tissue mass. The adjacent joint is thoroughly examined to check for swelling, range of motion, and muscle atrophy to differentiate between pain secondary to the tumor and pain secondary to an intra-articular derangement.

This patient has a painful proximal tibial lesion with a large associated soft-tissue mass measuring 4 by 8 cm protruding posteromedially. These findings suggest an aggressive tumor such as an osteosarcoma, so anteroposterior and lateral radiographs of the knee are recommended.

A 13-Year-Old Boy Is Referred for Left Shoulder Pain That Is Aggravated by Swimming.
He first developed pain in the left shoulder after swim practice 3 months ago. The pain is aggravated by swimming freestyle (crawl) and relieved by rest. He describes the pain as an ache in front of the left shoulder. He has never noted any swelling and he cannot recall any injury. He has been a competitive swimmer since he was 6 years old and currently practices 6 days a week. He has taken anti-inflammatory medication with some relief of his symptoms.

The clinician understands that a competitive swimmer who is having difficulty with shoulder pain will often have an overuse injury caused by extensive or improper training. If that were the case, activity modification, such as cross-training, or correction of a simple training error may resolve his symptoms. It is important to follow a patient with an overuse injury, because if the symptoms are not resolving with activity modification, it may indicate a more serious problem.

On physical examination, inspection of the shoulder reveals no muscle wasting, swelling, or deformity. Palpation reveals that he is tender over the supraspinatus tendon and the anterior aspect of the acromion. A patient with imbalance of the rotator cuff muscles may have impingement with tendonitis involving the supraspinatus tendon. Range of motion of the

shoulders reveals elevation to 180 degrees bilaterally, external rotation with the arm at the side to 70 degrees bilaterally, and internal rotation to the point where the thumbs touch the spinous process of T4 on the right and T9 on the left. The limited internal rotation on the left side indicates tight posterior structures, a common finding in patients who do overhead athletics. Muscle strength testing of shoulder flexion, abduction, internal, and external rotation are graded from 0 to 5, according to the scale of the Medical Research Council (Table 4-7) (47). Rotator cuff imbalance is often seen in patients with weakness of the periscapular muscles, including the rhomboids, serratus anterior, subscapularis, and trapezius muscles.

A swimmer with shoulder pain may have ligamentous laxity with multidirectional instability, or rotator cuff tendonitis with impingement. There are several tests to detect instability and impingement. Ligamentous laxity with instability can be evaluated by palpating glenohumeral translation. With the patient seated, the clinician evaluates the amount of glenohumeral translation by stabilizing the scapula and clavicle with one hand while pushing and pulling the proximal humerus in an anterior and posterior direction with the other hand. The amount of glenohumeral translation is measured in millimeters and compared with the uninjured shoulder (Fig. 4-60). Another test for ligamentous laxity is the "sulcus sign." With the patient standing, the clinician applies a longitudinal inferior traction force on the upper extremity while palpating the distance between the humeral head and the acromion (Fig. 4-61). Excessive laxity of the superior glenohumeral ligament will allow the humeral head to subluxate inferiorly.

The apprehension test is used to evaluate for anterior shoulder instability. This test can be performed with the

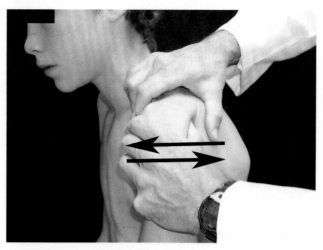

FIGURE 4-60. Ligamentous laxity of the left shoulder is evaluated with the patient seated, by holding the scapula and clavicle with the right hand while pushing the humeral head anteriorly and pulling it posteriorly with the left hand (*arrows*). The amount of glenohumeral translation is measured in millimeters and compared with the uninjured shoulder. This test is a shoulder drawer sign.

patient sitting or in the supine position. If the left shoulder is being examined, the clinician abducts the shoulder to 90 degrees and gradually increases the amount of external rotation using the left hand. The clinician's right hand is placed over the humeral head, and the clinician gently pushes the humeral head forward with the right thumb with the fingers strategically placed anteriorly to control any instability. A patient with anterior instability will experience discomfort or apprehension with this test when the humeral head subluxates anteriorly (Fig. 4-62).

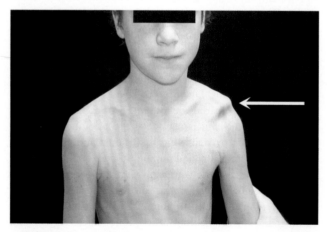

FIGURE 4-61. Ligamentous laxity of the shoulder can also be evaluated by applying a longitudinal inferior traction force to the upper extremity while observing the distance between the humeral head and the acromion (*arrow*). Excessive laxity of the superior glenohumeral ligament will allow the humeral head to subluxate inferiorly; this phenomenon is termed a "sulcus sign."

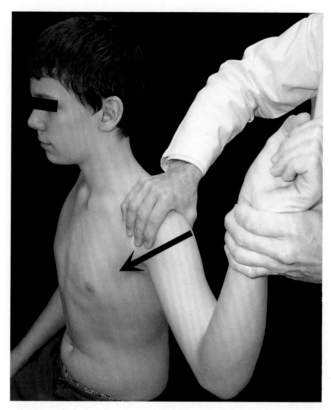

FIGURE 4-62. The apprehension test of the left shoulder is performed with the shoulder abducted to 90 degrees and externally rotated by the clinician's left hand. The clinician gently pushes the humeral head forward with the right thumb (*arrow*), while the fingers are strategically placed anteriorly in front of the humeral head, to prevent any sudden instability. Apprehension with this maneuver indicates anterior instability of the shoulder.

The relocation test can be performed with the patient sitting or supine. In the supine position, the apprehension test is performed first, and the clinician notes the amount of shoulder external rotation when the patient first experiences apprehension (Fig. 4-63A). The apprehension is relieved when the clinician pushes posteriorly on the humeral head, reducing it in the glenoid, and allowing increased external rotation of the shoulder (Fig. 4-63B). If the apprehension is relieved with this maneuver, it is termed a positive relocation test.

A swimmer with shoulder pain may have tendonitis involving the rotator cuff muscles, particularly the supraspinatus tendon. To determine if the patient has tendonitis, the clinician performs impingement tests. If the patient has tendonitis involving the supraspinatus tendon, elevation of the arm to 180 degrees, with the shoulder internally rotated, will cause discomfort as the inflamed tendon impinges against the anterior inferior acromion and coracoacromial ligament. This discomfort is termed a positive Neer impingement sign (Fig. 4-64) (48). Another method to detect impingement is to flex the shoulder forward to 90 degrees in neutral rotation, with the elbow flexed to 90 degrees. In this position, internal rotation of the shoulder by pushing down on the forearm will

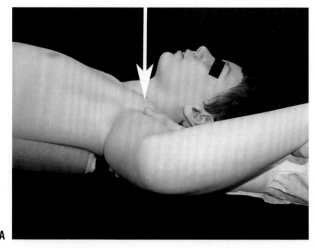 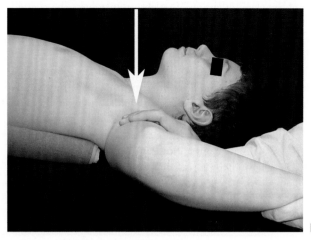

FIGURE 4-63.   A: The relocation test is a two-part test performed with the shoulder abducted to 90 degrees. The clinician first performs an apprehension test and notes the amount of shoulder external rotation when the patient first experiences apprehension (*arrow*). **B:** The clinician then stabilizes the humeral head by pushing it posteriorly (*downward arrow*). If the patient has increased external rotation and loss of apprehension, it is a positive relocation test.

cause discomfort as the supraspinatus tendon impinges against the coracoacromial ligament. This maneuver is termed a positive Hawkins sign (Fig. 4-65) (48).

A patient with shoulder pain that is aggravated by swimming may have multidirectional instability, with an associated

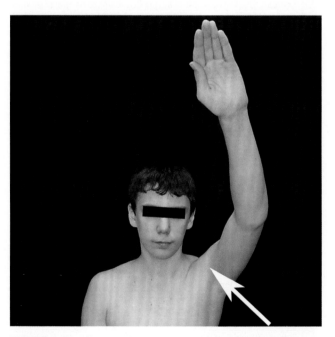 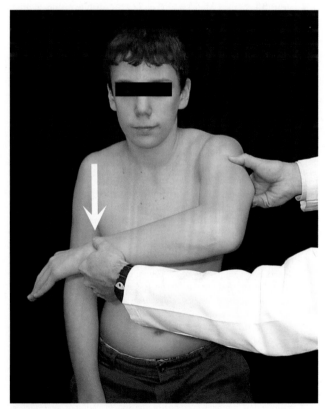

FIGURE 4-64.   If the patient has tendonitis involving the supraspinatus tendon, elevation of the arm to 180 degrees with internal rotation of the shoulder will cause discomfort when the inflamed tendon impinges against the anterior inferior acromion and coracoacromial ligament (*arrow*). This is termed a positive "Neer impingement sign."

FIGURE 4-65.   The Hawkins test is performed with the shoulder flexed forward to 90 degrees. While supporting the arm with one hand, the clinician then pushes down on the forearm with the other hand (*arrow*), internally rotating the shoulder. Discomfort with this maneuver indicates impingement between the inflamed supraspinatus tendon and the anterior inferior acromion and the coracoacromial ligament.

tear of the glenoid labrum. The labrum surrounds the glenoid cavity, deepening the glenohumeral joint, and the humeral head rests against the labrum. If there is a tear of the superior labrum, it is termed an SLAP (superior labrum anterior and posterior) lesion. If the labral tear involves the anteroinferior labrum, it is termed a Bankart lesion. If the attachment of the labrum to the glenoid is torn, it causes increased shoulder instability because the capsular attachment to the glenoid has been disrupted.

This patient has an overuse injury involving the rotator cuff muscles. Activity modification, in consultation with the swim coach to alter the training program, is recommended. As in any overuse injury, close follow-up is important to document that the symptoms are indeed resolving.

REFERENCES

1. Barlow TG. Early diagnosis and treatment of congenital dislocation of the hip. *J Bone Joint Surg Br* 1962;44B(2):292–301.
2. Aronsson DD, Goldberg MJ, Kling TF Jr, et al. Developmental dysplasia of the hip. *Pediatrics* 1994;94:201–208.
3. Yngve DA. Foot-progression angle in clubfeet. *J Pediatr Orthop* 1990; 10(4):467–472.
4. Staheli LT, Corbett M, Wyss C, et al. Lower-extremity rotational problems in children. Normal values to guide management. *J Bone Joint Surg Am* 1985;67(1):39–47.
5. Salenius P, Vankka E. The development of the tibiofemoral angle in children. *J Bone Joint Surg Am* 1975;57(2):259–261.
6. Illingworth R. *The development of the infant and young child: normal and abnormal*, 9th ed. New York, NY: Churchill Livingstone, 1987.
7. Sankar WN, Weiss J, Skaggs DL. Orthopaedic conditions in the newborn. *J Am Acad Orthop Surg* 2009;17(2):112–122.
8. Paton RW, Choudry Q. Neonatal foot deformities and their relationship to developmental dysplasia of the hip: an 11-year prospective, longitudinal observational study. *J Bone Joint Surg Br* 2009;91(5):655–658.
9. Bleck EE. Metatarsus adductus: classification and relationship to outcomes of treatment. *J Pediatr Orthop* 1983;3(1):2–9.
10. Spiegel DA, Loder RT. Leg-length discrepancy and bone age in unilateral idiopathic talipes equinovarus. *J Pediatr Orthop* 2003;23(2):246–250.
11. Dimeglio A, Bensahel H, Souchet P, et al. Classification of clubfoot. *J Pediatr Orthop B* 1995;4(2):129–136.
12. Bleck D. *Orthopaedic management in cerebral palsy*. Philadelphia, PA: JB Lippincott Co, 1987.
13. Waters PM. Comparison of the natural history, the outcome of microsurgical repair, and the outcome of operative reconstruction in brachial plexus birth palsy. *J Bone Joint Surg Am* 1999;81(5):649–659.
14. Kempe CH, Silverman FN, Steele BF, et al. The battered-child syndrome. *JAMA* 1962;181:17–24.
15. Kocher MS, Kasser JR. Orthopaedic aspects of child abuse. *J Am Acad Orthop Surg* 2000;8(1):10–20.
16. Akbarnia B, Torg JS, Kirkpatrick J, et al. Manifestations of the battered-child syndrome. *J Bone Joint Surg Am* 1974;56(6):1159–1166.
17. Kocher MS, Zurakowski D, Kasser JR. Differentiating between septic arthritis and transient synovitis of the hip in children: an evidence-based clinical prediction algorithm. *J Bone Joint Surg Am* 1999;81(12): 1662–1670.
18. Mosca VS. Calcaneal lengthening for valgus deformity of the hindfoot. Results in children who had severe, symptomatic flatfoot and skewfoot. *J Bone Joint Surg Am* 1995;77(4):500–512.
19. Joseph B, Varghese G, Mulpuri K, et al. Natural evolution of Perthes disease: a study of 610 children under 12 years of age at disease onset. *J Pediatr Orthop* 2003;23(5):590–600.
20. Wingstrand H. Significance of synovitis in Legg–Calve–Perthes disease. *J Pediatr Orthop B* 1999;8(3):156–160.
21. Boyd DW, Aronson DD. Supracondylar fractures of the humerus: a prospective study of percutaneous pinning. *J Pediatr Orthop* 1992;12(6): 789–794.
22. Garbuz DS, Leitch K, Wright JG. The treatment of supracondylar fractures in children with an absent radial pulse. *J Pediatr Orthop* 1996; 16(5):594–596.
23. Aflatoon K, Aboulafia AJ, McCarthy EF Jr, et al. Pediatric soft-tissue tumors. *J Am Acad Orthop Surg* 2003;11(5):332–343.
24. Damron TA, Beauchamp CP, Rougraff BT, et al. Soft-tissue lumps and bumps. *Instr Course Lect* 2004;53:625–637.
25. Micheli LJ, Ireland ML. Prevention and management of calcaneal apophysitis in children: an overuse syndrome. *J Pediatr Orthop* 1987;7(1): 34–38.
26. Sutherland DH, Olshen R, Cooper L, et al. The development of mature gait. *J Bone Joint Surg Am* 1980;62(3):336–353.
27. Staheli LT. The prone hip extension test: a method of measuring hip flexion deformity. *Clin Orthop Relat Res* 1977(123):12–15.
28. Marks MC, Alexander J, Sutherland DH, et al. Clinical utility of the Duncan-Ely test for rectus femoris dysfunction during the swing phase of gait. *Dev Med Child Neurol* 2003;45(11):763–768.
29. Ober FR. The role of the iliotibial band and fascia: a factor in the causation of low back disorders and sciatica. *J Bone Joint Surg Am* 1936; 18(1):105–110.
30. Elmer EB, Wenger DR, Mubarak SJ, et al. Proximal hamstring lengthening in the sitting cerebral palsy patient. *J Pediatr Orthop* 1992; 12(3):329–336.
31. Silverskiold N. Reduction of the uncrossed two joint muscles of the one-to-one muscle in spastic conditions. *Acta Chir Scand* 1923;56:315.
32. Schwartz M, Lakin G. The effect of tibial torsion on the dynamic function of the soleus during gait. *Gait Posture* 2003;17(2):113–118.
33. Ramirez N, Johnston CE, Browne RH. The prevalence of back pain in children who have idiopathic scoliosis. *J Bone Joint Surg Am* 1997;79(3):364–368.
34. Bunnell WP. An objective criterion for scoliosis screening. *J Bone Joint Surg Am* 1984;66(9):1381–1387.
35. Lonstein JE, Carlson JM. The prediction of curve progression in untreated idiopathic scoliosis during growth. *J Bone Joint Surg Am* 1984; 66(7):1061–1071.
36. Chambers HG, Sutherland DH. A practical guide to gait analysis. *J Am Acad Orthop Surg* 2002;10(3):222–231.
37. Debnath UK, Freeman BJ, Gregory P, et al. Clinical outcome and return to sport after the surgical treatment of spondylolysis in young athletes. *J Bone Joint Surg Br* 2003;85(2):244–249.
38. Loder RT, Aronson DD, Dobbs MB, et al. Slipped capital femoral epiphysis. *Instr Course Lect* 2001;50:555–570.
39. Aronson DD, Loder RT, Breur GJ, et al. Slipped capital femoral epiphysis: current concepts. *J Am Acad Orthop Surg* 2006;14(12):666–679.
40. Medlar RC, Lyne ED. Sinding–Larsen–Johansson disease. Its etiology and natural history. *J Bone Joint Surg Am* 1978;60(8):1113–1116.
41. Wilson JN. A new diagnostic sign in osteochondritis dissecans of the knee. *J Bone Joint Surg Am* 1967;49:477–480.
42. Daniel DM, Stone ML, Barnett P, et al. Use of the quadriceps active test to diagnose posterior cruciate-ligament disruption and measure posterior laxity of the knee. *J Bone Joint Surg Am* 1988;70(3):386–391.
43. Coleman SS, Chesnut WJ. A simple test for hindfoot flexibility in the cavovarus foot. *Clin Orthop Relat Res* 1977;123:60–62.
44. Kuhlman GS, Domb BG. Hip impingement: identifying and treating a common cause of hip pain. *Am Fam Physician* 2009;80(12):1429–1434.
45. Dudda M, Albers C, Mamisch TC, et al. Do normal radiographs exclude asphericity of the femoral head-neck junction? *Clin Orthop Relat Res* 2009;467(3):651–659.
46. Mankin HJ, Trahan CA, Fondren G, et al. Non-ossifying fibroma, fibrous cortical defect and Jaffe–Campanacci syndrome: a biologic and clinical review. *Chir Organi Mov* 2009;93(1):1–7.
47. Council MR. *Aids to the examination of the peripheral nervous system.* Memorandum 45 ed. London, UK: Her Majesty's Stationery Office, 1943.
48. Yamamoto N, Muraki T, Sperling JW, et al. Impingement mechanisms of the Neer and Hawkins signs. *J Shoulder Elbow Surg* 2009;18(6):942–947.

Evaluation of the Medical Literature

INTRODUCTION

Evaluation of the medical literature is an essential task of the pediatric orthopaedic surgeon in order to evaluate the efficacy of treatments, to stay abreast of new technology, and to provide optimal patient care. However, this task can be daunting as the clinician is inundated with medical information from scientific journals, scientific meetings, the lay press, industry, and even the Internet. Critical evaluation of the medical literature is vital to assess which studies are scientifically sound and sufficiently compelling to change practice from those that are methodologically flawed or biased. A working understanding of clinical epidemiology and biostatistics is necessary for critical evaluation of the medical literature.

This chapter provides an overview of the concepts of study design, hypothesis testing, measures of effect, diagnostic performance, evidence-based medicine (EBM), outcomes assessment, and biostatistics. Examples from the orthopaedic literature and a glossary of terminology (terms italicized throughout the text) are provided.

STUDY DESIGN

Clinical research study design has evolved from cataloguing vital statistics from birth and death records in the 1600s, to correlational studies associating cholera with water contamination, to case-control studies linking smoking with lung cancer, to prospective cohort studies such as the Framingham Heart Study, and to the randomized clinical trial (RCT) for the polio vaccine (1).

The EBM and patient-derived outcomes assessment movements burst onto the scene of clinical medicine in the 1980s and 1990s as a result of contemporaneous medical, societal, and economic influences. Pioneers, such as Sackett

and Feinstein, emphasized levels of evidence and patient-centered outcomes assessment (2–10). Work by Wennberg and colleagues revealed large small-area variations in clinical practice, with some patients 30 times more likely to undergo an operative procedure than other patients with identical symptoms merely because of their geographic location (11–16). Further critical research suggested that up to 40% of some surgical procedures might be inappropriate and that up to 85% of common medical treatments were not rigorously validated (17–19). Meanwhile, the costs of health care were rapidly rising to over 2 billion dollars per day, increasing from 5.2% of the gross domestic product in 1960 to 16.6% in 2008 (20). Health maintenance organizations and managed care emerged. In addition, increasing federal, state, and consumer oversight were brought to bear on the practice of clinical medicine. These forces have led to an increased focus on the effectiveness of clinical care and the design of clinical research studies.

In *observational studies*, researchers observe patient groups without allocation of the intervention, whereas in *experimental studies*, researchers allocate the treatment. Experimental studies involving humans are called *trials*. Research studies may be *retrospective*, meaning that the direction of inquiry is backward from the cases and that the events of interest transpired before the onset of the study, or they may be *prospective*, meaning that the direction of inquiry is forward from the cohort inception and that the events of interest transpire after the onset of the study (Fig. 5-1). *Cross-sectional* studies are used to survey one point in time. *Longitudinal* studies follow the same patients over multiple points in time.

All research studies are susceptible to invalid conclusions due to bias, confounding, and chance. *Bias* is the nonrandom systematic error in the design or conduct of a study. Bias usually is not intentional; however, it is pervasive and insidious. Forms of bias can corrupt a study at any phase, including patient selection (selection and membership bias), study

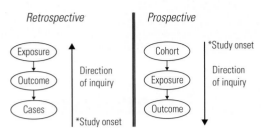

FIGURE 5-1. Prospective versus retrospective study design defined based on the direction of inquiry and the onset of the study.

performance (performance and information bias), patient follow-up (nonresponder and transfer bias), and outcome determination (detection, recall, acceptability, and interviewer bias). Frequent biases in the orthopaedic literature include selection bias when unlike groups are being compared, nonresponder bias in studies with low follow-up rates, and interviewer bias when the investigator is determining outcome. A *confounder* is a variable having independent associations with both the *independent* (predictor) and *dependent* (outcome) variables, thus potentially distorting their relationship. For example, an association between knee laxity and anterior cruciate ligament injury may be confounded by female sex since females may have greater knee laxity and a higher risk of anterior cruciate ligament injury. Frequent confounders in clinical research include gender, age, socioeconomic status, and comorbidities. As discussed below in the section on hypothesis testing, chance may lead to invalid conclusions based on the probability of *type I* and *type II errors*, which are related to *P values* and *power*.

The adverse effects of bias, confounding, and chance can be minimized by study design and statistical analysis. Prospective studies minimize bias associated with patient selection, quality of information, trying to recall preoperative status, and nonresponders. *Randomization* minimizes selection bias and equally distributes confounders. *Blinding* can further decrease bias, and *matching* can decrease confounding. Confounders can sometimes be controlled *post hoc* with use of stratified analysis or multivariable methods. The effects of chance can be minimized by an adequate sample size based on *power* calculations and use of appropriate levels of significance in hypothesis testing. The ability of study design to optimize validity while minimizing bias, confounding, and chance is recognized by the adoption of hierarchical levels of evidence on the basis of study design (Table 5-1).

Observational study designs include case series, case-control studies, cross-sectional surveys, and cohort studies. A *case series* is a retrospective, descriptive account of a group of patients with interesting characteristics or a series of patients who have undergone an intervention. A case series of one patient is a *case report*. Case series are easy to construct and can provide a forum for the presentation of interesting or unusual observations. However, case series are often anecdotal, are subject

to many possible biases, lack a hypothesis, and are difficult to compare with other series. Thus, case series are usually viewed as a means of generating hypotheses for further studies but are not viewed as conclusive. A *case-control study* is one in which the investigator identifies patients with an outcome of interest (cases) and patients without the outcome (controls) and then compares the two groups in terms of possible risk factors. The effects in a case-control study are frequently reported with use of the *odds ratio*. Case-control studies are efficient (particularly for the evaluation of unusual conditions or outcomes) and are relatively easy to perform. However, an appropriate control group may be difficult to identify, and preexisting high-quality medical records are essential. Moreover, case-control studies are susceptible to multiple biases, particularly selection and detection bias based on the identification of cases and controls. *Cross-sectional surveys* are often used to determine the prevalence of disease or to identify coexisting associations in patients with a particular condition at one particular point in time. *Prevalence* of a condition is the number of individuals with the condition divided by the total number of individuals at one point in time. *Incidence*, in contradistinction, refers to the number of individuals with the condition divided by the total number of individuals over a defined time period. Thus, prevalence data are usually obtained from a cross-sectional survey and are a proportion, whereas incidence data are usually obtained from a prospective cohort study and contain a time value in the denominator. Surveys are also frequently performed to determine preferences and treatment patterns. Because cross-sectional studies represent a snapshot in time, they may be misleading if the research question involves the disease process over time. Surveys also present unique challenges in terms of adequate response rate, representative samples, and acceptability bias. A traditional *cohort study* is one in which a population of interest is identified and followed prospectively in order to determine outcomes and associations with risk factors. Retrospective cohort studies, or historical cohort studies, can also be performed in which cohort members are identified based on records and the follow-up period occurs entirely or partly in the past. Cohort studies are optimal for studying the incidence, course, and risk factors of a disease because they are longitudinal, meaning that a group of subjects is followed over time. The effects in a cohort study are frequently reported in terms of *relative risk*. Because traditional cohort studies are prospective, they can optimize follow-up and data quality and can minimize bias associated with selection, information, and measurement. In addition, they have the correct time sequence to provide strong evidence regarding associations. However, these studies are costly, are logistically demanding, often require long time periods for completion, and are inefficient for the assessment of unusual outcomes or diseases.

Experimental study designs may involve the use of concurrent controls, sequential controls *(cross-over trials)*, or historical controls. The *randomized clinical trial (RCT)* with concurrent controls is the so-called gold standard of clinical evidence as it provides the most valid conclusions (internal

TABLE 5-1	Levels of Evidence for Primary Research Question Used by the *Journal of Bone and Joint Surgery*

Levels of Evidence for Primary Research Question

	Types of Studies			
	Therapeutic Studies—Investigating the Results of Treatment	Prognostic Studies—Investigating the Outcome of Disease	Diagnostic Studies—Investigating a Diagnostic Test	Economic and Decision Analyses—Developing an Economic or Decision Model

Level I	1. Randomized controlled trial
	  a. Significant difference
	  b. No significant difference but narrow confidence intervals
	2. Systematic review[2] of Level I randomized controlled trials (studies were homogeneous)
		1. Prospective study[1]
		2. Systematic review[2] of Level I studies
			1. Testing of previously developed diagnostic criteria in series of consecutive patients (with universally applied reference "gold" standard)
			2. Systematic review[2] of Level I studies
				1. Clinically sensible costs and alternatives; values obtained from many studies; multiway sensitivity analyses
				2. Systematic review[2] of Level I studies

Level II	1. Prospective cohort study[3]
	2. Poor-quality randomized controlled trial (e.g., <80% follow-up)
	3. Systematic review[2]
	  a. Level II studies
	  b. Nonhomogeneous Level I studies
		1. Retrospective study[4]
		2. Study of untreated controls from a previous randomized controlled trial
		3. Systematic review[2] of Level II studies
			1. Development of diagnostic criteria on basis of consecutive patients (with universally applied reference "gold" standard)
			2. Systematic review[2] of Level II studies
				1. Clinically sensible costs and alternatives; values obtained from limited studies; multiway sensitivity analyses
				2. Systematic review[2] of Level II studies

Level III	1. Case-control study[5] 2. Retrospective cohort study[4] 3. Systematic review[2] of Level III studies		1. Study of nonconsecutive patients (no consistently applied reference "gold" standard) 2. Systematic review[2] of Level III studies	1. Limited alternatives and costs; poor estimates 2. Systematic review[2] of Level III studies
Level IV	Case series (no, or historical, control group)	Case series	1. Case-control study 2. Poor reference standard	No sensitivity analyses
Level V	Expert opinion	Expert opinion	Expert opinion	Expert opinion

1. All patients were enrolled at the same point in their disease course (inception cohort) with greater than or equal to 80% follow-up of enrolled patients.
2. A study of results from two or more previous studies.
3. Patients were compared with a control group of patients treated at the same time and institution.
4. The study was initiated after treatment was performed.
5. Patients with a particular outcome ("cases" with, e.g., a failed total arthroplasty) were compared with those who did not have the outcome ("controls" with, e.g., a total hip arthroplasty that did not fail).

validity) by minimizing the effects of bias and confounding. A rigorous randomization with enough patients is the best means of avoiding confounding. The performance of an RCT involves the construction of a protocol document that explicitly establishes eligibility criteria, sample size, informed consent, randomization, stopping rules, blinding, measurement, monitoring of compliance, assessment of safety, and data analysis. Because allocation is random, selection bias is minimized and confounders (known and unknown) are theoretically equally distributed between groups. *Blinding* minimizes performance, detection, interviewer, and acceptability bias.

Blinding may be practiced at four levels: participants, investigators applying the intervention, outcome assessors, and analysts. *Intention-to-treat analysis* minimizes nonresponder and transfer bias, while sample-size determination ensures adequate power. The intention-to-treat principle states that all patients should be analyzed within the treatment group to which they were randomized in order to preserve the goals of randomization. Although the RCT is the epitome of clinical research designs, the disadvantages of RCTs include their expense, logistics, and time to completion. Accrual of patients and acceptance by clinicians may be problematic. With rapidly evolving technology, a new technique may become rapidly well accepted, making an existing RCT obsolete or a potential RCT difficult to accept. Ethically, RCTs require clinical equipoise (equality of treatment options in the clinician's judgment) for enrollment, interim stopping rules to avoid harm and evaluate adverse events, and truly informed consent. Finally, while RCTs have excellent internal validity, some have questioned their generalizability (external validity) because the practice pattern and the population of patients enrolled in an RCT may be overly constrained and nonrepresentative.

Ethical considerations are intrinsic to the design and conduct of clinical research studies. Informed consent is of paramount importance, and it is the focus of much of the activity of Institutional Review Boards. Investigators should be familiar with the Nuremberg Code and the Declaration of Helsinki as they pertain to ethical issues of risks and benefits, protection of privacy, and respect for autonomy (21, 22).

HYPOTHESIS TESTING

The purpose of hypothesis testing is to permit generalizations from a sample to the population from which it came. Hypothesis testing confirms or refutes the assertion that the observed findings did not occur by chance alone but rather occurred because of a true association between variables. By default, the *null hypothesis* of a study asserts that there is no significant association between variables, whereas the *alternative hypothesis* asserts that there is a significant association. If the findings of a study are not significant, we cannot reject the null hypothesis, whereas if the findings are significant, we can reject the null hypothesis and accept the alternative hypothesis.

Thus, all research studies that are based on a sample make an inference about the truth in the overall population. By constructing a 2 × 2 table of the possible outcomes of a study (Table 5-2), we can see that the inference of a study is correct if a significant association is not found when there is no true association or if a significant association is found when there is a true association. However, a study can have two types of errors. A *type I* or *alpha (α) error* occurs when a significant association is found when there is no true association (resulting in a "false-positive" study that rejects a true null hypothesis). A *type II* or *beta (β) error* wrongly concludes that there is no

significant association (resulting in a "false-negative" study that rejects a true alternative hypothesis).

The alpha level refers to the probability of the type I (α) error. By convention, the alpha level of significance is set at 0.05, which means we accept the finding of a significant association if there is less than a one in twenty chance that the observed association was due to chance alone. Thus, the *P* value, which is calculated from a statistical test, is a measure of the strength of evidence from the data in favor of the null hypothesis. If the *P* value is less than the alpha level, then the evidence against the null hypothesis is strong enough to reject it and conclude that the result is statistically significant. *P* values frequently are used in clinical research and are given great importance by journals and readers; however, there is a strong movement in biostatistics to de-emphasize *P* values because a significance level of *P* < 0.05 is arbitrary, a strict cutoff point can be misleading (there is little difference between *P* = 0.049 and *P* = 0.051, yet only the former is considered "significant"), the *P* value gives no information about the strength of the association, and the *P* value may be statistically significant without the results being clinically important. Alternatives to the traditional reliance on *P* values include the use of variable alpha levels of significance based on the consequences of the type I error and the reporting of *P* values without using the term "significant." Use of *95% confidence intervals* in lieu of *P* values has gained acceptance as these intervals convey information regarding the significance of findings (95% confidence intervals do not overlap if they are significantly different), the magnitude of differences, and the precision of measurement (indicated by the range of the 95% confidence interval).

Power is the probability of finding a significant association if one truly exists and is defined as 1—the probability of type II (β) error. By convention, acceptable power is set at ≥80%, which means there is ≤20% chance that the study will demonstrate no significant association when there is a true association. In practice, when a study demonstrates a significant association, the potential error of concern is the type I (α) error as expressed by the *P* value. However, when a study demonstrates no significant association, the potential error of concern is the type II (β) error as expressed by power. That is, in a study that demonstrates no significant effect, there may truly be no significant effect, or there may actually be a significant effect, but the study was underpowered because the sample size may have been too small or the measurements may have been too imprecise. Thus, in a study that demonstrates no significant effect, the power of the study should be reported. The calculations for power analyses differ depending on the statistical methods utilized for analysis; however, four elements are involved in a power analysis: α, β, effect size, and sample size (*n*). Effect size is the difference that you want to be able to detect with the given α and β. It is based on a clinical sense about how large a difference would be clinically meaningful. Effect sizes are often defined in dimensionless terms, based on a difference in mean values divided by the pooled standard deviation for a comparison

TABLE 5-2	Hypothesis Testing	
	Truth	
Experiment	No association	Association
No association	Correct	Type II (β) error
Association	Type I (α) error	Correct

P value: probability of type I (α) error
Power: 1 – probability of type II (β) error

of two groups. Low sample sizes, small effect sizes, and large variance decrease the power of a study. An understanding of power issues is important in clinical research to minimize resources when planning a study and to ensure the validity of a study. Sample size calculations are performed when planning a study. Typically, power is set at 80%, alpha is set at 0.05, the effect size and variance are estimated from pilot data or the literature, and the equation is solved for the necessary sample size. The calculation of power after the study has been completed, post-hoc power analysis, is controversial and is not recommended.

DIAGNOSTIC PERFORMANCE

A diagnostic test can result in four possible scenarios: (a) *true positive* if the test is positive and the disease is present, (b) *false positive* if the test is positive and the disease is absent, (c) *true negative* if the test is negative and the disease is absent, and (d) *false negative* if the test is negative and the disease is present (Table 5-3). The *sensitivity* of a test is the percentage (or proportion) of patients who have the disease that are classified positive (true-positive rate). A test with 97% sensitivity implies that of 100 patients with disease, 97 will have a positive test. Sensitive tests have a low false-negative rate. A negative result on a highly sensitive test rules disease out (SNout). The *specificity* of a test is the percentage (or proportion) of patients without the disease who are classified negative (true-negative rate). A test with 91% specificity implies that of 100 patients without the disease, 91 will have a negative test. Specific tests have a low false-positive rate. A positive result on a highly specific test rules disease in (SPin). Sensitivity and specificity can be combined into a single parameter, the *likelihood ratio (LR)*, which is the probability of a true positive

divided by the probability of a false positive. Sensitivity and specificity can be established in studies in which the results of a diagnostic test are compared with the gold standard of diagnosis in the same patients—for example, by comparing the results of magnetic resonance imaging with arthroscopic findings (24).

Sensitivity and specificity are technical parameters of diagnostic testing performance and have important implications for screening and clinical practice guidelines (25, 26); however, they are less relevant in the typical clinical setting because the clinician does not know whether or not the patient has the disease. The clinically relevant questions are the probability that a patient has the disease given a positive result *(positive predictive value)* and the probability that a patient does not have the disease given a negative result *(negative predictive value)*. The positive and negative predictive values are probabilities that require an estimate of the prevalence of the disease in the population and can be calculated using equations that utilize Bayes theorem (27).

There is an inherent trade-off between sensitivity and specificity. Because there is typically some overlap between the diseased and nondiseased groups with respect to a test distribution, the investigator can select a positivity criterion with a low false-negative rate (to optimize sensitivity) or one with a low false-positive rate (to optimize specificity) (Fig. 5-2). In practice, positivity criteria are selected on the basis of the consequences of a false-positive or a false-negative diagnosis. If the consequences of a false-negative diagnosis outweigh the consequences of a false-positive diagnosis of a condition (such as septic arthritis of the hip in children (28)), a more sensitive

TABLE 5-3	Diagnostic Test Performance	
	Disease Positive	**Disease Negative**
Test positive	a (true positive)	b (false positive)
Test negative	c (false negative)	d (true negative)
Sensitivity:	a/(a + c)	
Specificity:	d/(b + d)	
Accuracy:	(a + c)/(a + b + c + d)	
False-negative rate:	1 − sensitivity	
False-positive rate:	1 − specificity	
Likelihood ratio (+):	sensitivity/false-positive rate	
Likelihood ratio (−):	false-negative rate/specificity	
Positive predictive value:	[(prevalence)(sensitivity)] /[(prevalence)(sensitivity) + (1 − prevalence)(1 − specificity)]	
Negative predictive value:	[(1 − prevalence)(specificity)] /[(1 − prevalence)(specificity) + (prevalence)(1 − sensitivity)]	

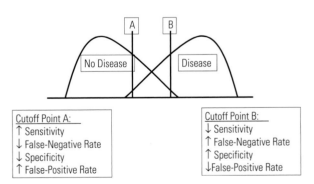

FIGURE 5-2. Selecting positivity criterion. Because there is typically overlap between the diseased population and the nondiseased population over a range of diagnostic values (*x*-axis), there is an intrinsic trade-off between sensitivity and specificity. Identifying positive test results to the right of cutoff point A, there is high sensitivity because most diseased patients are correctly identified as positive; however, there is lower specificity because some nondiseased patients are incorrectly identified as positive (false positives). Identifying positive test results to the right of cutoff point B, there is lower sensitivity because some diseased patients are incorrectly identified as negative (false negatives); however, there is high specificity because most nondiseased patients are correctly identified as negative.

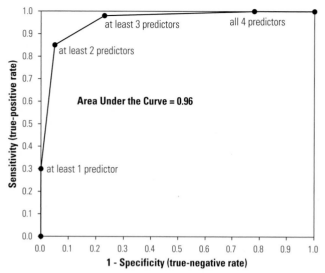

FIGURE 5-3. Receiver-operating characteristic (ROC) curve for a clinical prediction rule for differentiating septic arthritis and transient synovitis of the hip in children (28). The false-positive rate (1 – specificity) is plotted on the x-axis and sensitivity is plotted on the y-axis. The area under the curve represents the overall diagnostic performance of a prediction rule or a diagnostic test. For a perfect test, the area under the curve is 1.0. For random guessing, the area under the curve is 0.5.

TABLE 5-4	Treatment Effects	
	Adverse Events	**No Adverse Events**
Experimental group	a	b
Control group	c	d
Control event rate (CER):	c/(c + d)	
Experimental event rate (EER):	a/(a + b)	
Control event odds (CEO):	c/d	
Experimental event odds (EEO):	a/b	
Relative risk (RR):	EER/CER	
Odds ratio (OR:	EEO/CEO	
Relative risk reduction (RRR):	(EER – CER)/CER	
Absolute risk reduction (ARR):	EER – CER	
Number needed to treat (NNT):	1/ARR	

criterion is chosen. This relationship between the sensitivity and specificity of a diagnostic test can be portrayed with use of a *receiver operating characteristic (ROC) curve*. An ROC graph shows the relationship between the true-positive rate (sensitivity) on the y-axis and the false-positive rate (100-specificity) on the x-axis plotted at each possible cutoff (Fig. 5-3). Overall diagnostic performance can be evaluated by the area under the ROC curve (29).

MEASURES OF EFFECT

Measures of likelihood include probability and odds. *Probability* is a number, between 0 and 1, that indicates how likely an event is to occur based on the number of events per the number of trials. The probability of heads on a coin toss is 0.5. *Odds* are the ratio of the probability of an event occurring to the probability of the event not occurring. The odds of flipping a heads on a coin toss is 1 (0.5/0.5). Because probability and odds are related, they can be converted where odds = probability/(1 – probability).

Relative risk (RR) can be determined in a prospective cohort study, where RR equals the incidence of disease in the exposed cohort divided by the incidence of disease in the nonexposed cohort (Table 5-4). A similar measurement in a retrospective case-control study (where incidence cannot be determined) is the *odds ratio (OR)*, which is the ratio of the odds of having the disease in the study group compared with the odds of having the disease in the control group (Table 5-4). For example, a prospective cohort study of anterior cruciate

ligament–deficient skiers that finds a significantly higher proportion of subsequent knee injuries in nonbraced (12.7%) versus braced (2.0%) skiers may report a risk ratio of 6.4 (12.7%/2.0%) (30). This can be interpreted as a nonbraced anterior cruciate ligament–deficient skier has a 6.4 times higher risk of subsequent knee injury than a braced skier.

Factors that are likely to increase the incidence, prevalence, morbidity, or mortality of a disease are called risk factors. The effect of a factor that reduces the probability of an adverse outcome can be quantified by the *relative risk reduction (RRR), the absolute risk reduction (ARR)*, and the *number needed to treat (NNT)* (Table 5-4). The effect of a factor that increases the probability of an adverse outcome can be quantified by the *relative risk increase (RRI)*, the *absolute risk increase (ARI)*, and the *number needed to harm (NNH)* (Table 5-4).

OUTCOMES ASSESSMENT

Process refers to the medical care that a patient receives, whereas *outcome* refers to the result of that medical care. The emphasis of the outcomes assessment movement has been patient-derived outcomes assessment. Outcome measures include generic measures, condition-specific measures, and measures of patient satisfaction (31). *Generic measures*, such as the Short Form-36 (SF-36), are used to assess health status or health-related quality of life, as based on the World Heath Organization's multiple-domain definition of health (32, 33). *Condition-specific* measures, such as the International Knee Documentation Committee knee score or the Constant shoulder score, are used to assess aspects of a specific condition or body system. Measures of *patient satisfaction* are used to assess various components of care and have diverse applications, including quality of care, health care delivery, patient-centered models of care, and continuous quality improvement (34–37).

The process of developing an outcomes instrument involves identifying the construct, devising items, scaling responses, selecting items, forming factors, and creating scales.

A large number of outcome instruments have been developed and used without formal psychometric assessment of their reliability, validity, and responsiveness to change. *Reliability* refers to the repeatability of an instrument. *Interobserver* and *intraobserver reliability* refer to the repeatability of the instrument when used by different observers or by the same observer at different time points, respectively. *Test–retest reliability* can be assessed by using the instrument to evaluate the same patient on two different occasions without an interval change in medical status. These results are usually reported using the *kappa statistic* or intraclass correlation coefficient. *Validity* refers to whether the instrument measures what it purports to measure. *Content validity* assesses whether an instrument is representative of the characteristic being measured using expert consensus opinion (face validity). *Criterion validity* assesses an instrument's relationship to an accepted, gold-standard instrument. *Construct validity* assesses whether an instrument follows accepted hypotheses (constructs) and produces results consistent with theoretical expectations. *Responsiveness to change* assesses how an instrument's values change over the disease course and treatment.

EVIDENCE-BASED MEDICINE

Evidence-based medicine (EBM) involves the conscientious, explicit, and judicious use of current best evidence in making decisions about the care of individual patients (38). EBM integrates best research evidence with clinical expertise and patient values. The steps of EBM involve converting the need for information into an answerable question; tracking down the best evidence to answer that question; critically appraising the evidence with regard to its validity, impact, and applicability; and integrating the critical appraisal with clinical expertise and the patient's unique values and circumstances (39, 40). The types of questions asked in EBM are foreground questions pertaining to specific knowledge about managing patients who have a particular disorder. Evidence is graded on the basis of

study design (Table 5-1), with an emphasis on RCTs, and can be found on evidence-based databases (Evidence-Based Medicine Reviews from Ovid Technologies, the Cochrane Database of Systematic Reviews, Best Evidence, Clinical Evidence, National Guidelines Clearinghouse, CancerNet, and Medline) and evidence-based journals *(Evidence-Based Medicine, ACP Journal Club).*

A *systematic review (SR)* is a summary of the medical literature in which explicit methods are used to perform a thorough literature search and critical appraisal of studies. A more specialized type of SR is *meta-analysis*, in which quantitative methods are used to combine the results of several independent studies (usually RCTs) to produce summary statistics. For example, a study that systematically reviews the literature (with inclusion and exclusion criteria for studies) regarding internal fixation versus arthroplasty for femoral neck fractures and then summarizes the subsequent outcomes and complications would be considered a systematic review. On the other hand, a study that systematically reviews the literature (with inclusion and exclusion criteria for studies) and then combines the patients to perform new statistical analyses would be considered a meta-analysis (41). *Clinical pathways* or *clinical practice guidelines (CPG)* are algorithms that are developed, on the basis of the best available evidence, to standardize processes and optimize outcomes. They may also potentially reduce errors of omission and commission, reduce variations in practice patterns, and decrease costs.

Decision analysis is a methodological tool that allows for the quantitative analysis of decision making under conditions of uncertainty (42–44). The rationale underlying explicit decision analysis is that a decision must be made, often under circumstances of uncertainty, and that rational decision theory optimizes expected value. The process of expected-value decision analysis involves the creation of a decision tree to structure the decision problem, determination of outcome probabilities and utilities (patient values), fold-back analysis to calculate the expected value of each decision path to determine the optimal decision-making strategy (Fig. 5-4), and sensitivity analysis

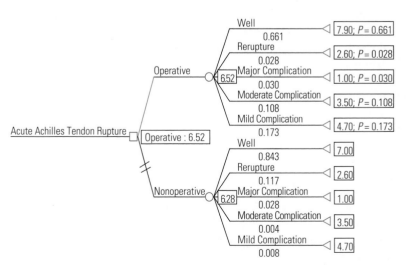

FIGURE 5-4. Expected-value decision analysis tree for operative versus nonoperative management of acute Achilles tendon rupture (50). Decision nodes are represented by □, chance nodes are represented by O, and terminal nodes are represented by Δ. Mean outcome utility scores are listed to the right of the terminal node [0–10]. Outcome probabilities are listed under the terminal node title [0–1]. Operative treatment is favored because it has a higher expected value (6.52 versus 6.28).

FIGURE 5-5. Sensitivity analysis for operative versus nonoperative management of acute Achilles tendon rupture (50). The probability of wound complication from operative treatment is varied on the *x*-axis. The lines represent the expected value for the operative and nonoperative decisions. Above the threshold value (probability of wound complication from operative treatment = 21%), nonoperative treatment is favored.

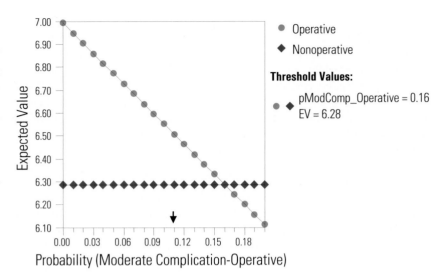

to determine the effect of varying outcome probabilities and utilities on decision making (Fig. 5-5). Decision analysis can identify the optimal decision strategy and how this strategy changes with variations in outcome probabilities or patient values. This process, whether used explicitly or implicitly, integrates well with the newer doctor–patient model of shared decision making.

Economic evaluative study designs in medicine include cost-identification studies, cost-effectiveness analysis, cost–benefit analysis, and cost–utility analysis (45, 46). In *cost-identification studies*, the costs of providing the treatment are identified. In *cost-effectiveness analysis*, the costs and clinical outcome are assessed and reported as cost per clinical outcome. In *cost–benefit analysis*, both costs and benefits are assessed in monetary units. In *cost–utility analysis*, cost and utility are measured and reported as cost per *quality-adjusted life-year (QALY)*.

BIOSTATISTICS

The scale on which a characteristic is measured has implications for the way in which information is summarized and analyzed. Data can be categorical, ordinal, or continuous. *Categorical data* indicate types or categories and can be thought of as counts. The categories do not represent an underlying order. Examples include gender and a dichotomous (yes/no, successful/failure) outcome. Categorical data are also called nominal data. Categorical data generally are described in terms of proportions or percentages and are reported in tables or bar charts. If there is an inherent order among categories, then the data are *ordinal*. The numbers that are used represent an order but are not necessarily to scale. Examples include cancer stages and injury grades. Ordinal data generally are also described in terms of proportions or percentages and are reported in tables or bar charts. *Continuous data* are observations on a continuum for which the differences between numbers have meaning on a numerical scale. Examples include age, weight, and distance. When a numerical observation can take on only integer values,

the scale of measurement is called *discrete*. Continuous data are generally described in terms of mean and standard deviation and can be reported in tables or graphs.

Data can be summarized in terms of measures of central tendency, such as *mean, median*, and *mode*, and in terms of measures of dispersion, such as *range, standard deviation*, and *percentiles*. Data can be characterized by different distributions, such as the normal (Gaussian) distribution, skewed distributions, and bimodal distributions (Fig. 5-6).

Survivorship analysis is used to analyze data when the outcome of interest is time until an event occurs. A group of patients is followed to see if they experience the event of interest. The endpoint in survivorship analysis can be mortality or a clinical end point such as revision of a total joint replacement. Survivorship data are typically analyzed using the Kaplan-Meier (KM) product-limit method and depicted graphically by KM curves (47–49) (Fig. 5-7).

Univariate, or *bivariate*, analysis assesses the relationship of an independent variable to a dependent variable. Commonly used statistical tests and their indications are listed in Table 5-5. *Multivariate analysis* explores relationships between multiple variables. Regression is a method of obtaining a mathematical relationship between an outcome variable (Y) and an explanatory variable (X) or set of independent variables (X_is). Linear regression is used when the outcome variable

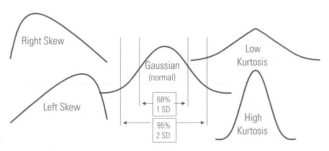

FIGURE 5-6. Data distributions.

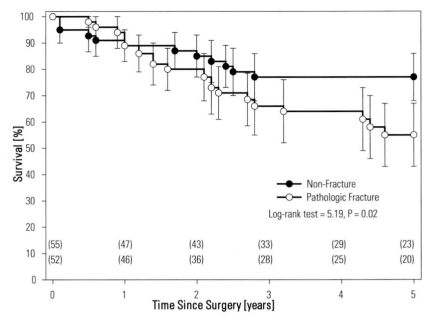

FIGURE 5-7. Kaplan-Meier estimated survivorship curves comparing survival rates between patients who had osteosarcoma with a pathologic fracture and those without a fracture (51). The estimated rates were significantly lower for patients with a pathologic fracture (log-rank test = 5.19, *P* = 0.02). The error bars around the survivorship curves represent 95% confidence intervals derived by Greenwood's formula. The numbers of patients on whom the estimates were based are shown in parentheses.

is continuous with the goal of finding the line that best predicts *Y* from *X*. Logistic regression is used when the outcome variable is binary or dichotomous and has become the most common form of multivariable analysis for non–time-related outcomes. Other regression methods include time-to-event data (Cox proportional-hazards regression) or count data (Poisson regression). Regression modeling is commonly used to predict outcomes (Table 5-6) or to establish independent associations (controlling for confounding and collinearity) among predictor or explanatory variables. For example, logistic regression can be used to determine predictors of septic arthritis versus transient synovitis of the hip in children from an array of presenting demographic, laboratory, and imaging variables (23, 28). Similarly, linear regression can be used to determine independent determinants of patient outcome measured using a continuous outcome instrument (37). Because many variables usually influence a particular outcome, it is often necessary to use multivariable analysis.

CASE EXAMPLE: SCOLIOSIS

The management of adolescent idiopathic scoliosis is illustrative of the impact of the medical literature in the understanding of a pediatric orthopaedic condition and the importance of well-designed clinical research studies.

In the medical literature, Hippocrates ascribed scoliosis to chronic poor posture: "lateral curvatures also occur, the proximate cause of which is the attitudes in which these patients lie" (52). This concept of a postural etiology persisted for the next 2000 years and was supported by the writings of Nicolas Andry in the 1700s, James Paget in the 1800s, and Robert Lovett in the 1900s (53). Various forms of historical treatment were subsequently developed and described in the medical literature, including various braces and appliances, traction devices, gymnastic exercises, subcutaneous tenotomy, and plaster of Paris casts (53). Modern surgical management of scoliosis is based on the results of case series of in situ

TABLE 5-5	Statistical Tests for Comparing Independent Groups and Paired Samples		
Type of Data	**Number of Groups**	**Independent Groups**	**Paired Samples**
Continuous			
Normal	2	Student *t*-test	Paired *t*-test
Non-normal	2	Mann-Whitney U-test	Wilcoxon signed-rank test
Normal	3 or more	ANOVA	Repeated-measures ANOVA
Non-normal	3 or more	Kruskal-Wallis test	Friedman test
Ordinal	2	Mann-Whitney U-test	Wilcoxon signed-rank test
	3 or more	Kruskal-Wallis test	Friedman test
Nominal	2	Fisher exact test	McNemar test
	3 or more	Pearson chi-square test	Cochran's *Q* test
Survival	2 or more	Log-rank test	Conditional logistic regression

TABLE 5-6	Multivariable Methods: Logistic Regression for Prediction of Septic Arthritis of the Hip in Children			
History of Fever	Non–Weight-Bearing	Erythrocyte Sedimentation Rate ≥40 mm/h	Serum White Blood Cell Count > 12,000 (×1000/mm^3)	Predicted Probability of Septic Arthritis
Yes	Yes	Yes	Yes	99.8%
Yes	Yes	Yes	No	97.3%
Yes	Yes	No	Yes	95.2%
Yes	Yes	No	No	57.8%
Yes	No	Yes	Yes	95.5%
Yes	No	Yes	No	62.2%
Yes	No	No	Yes	44.8%
Yes	No	No	No	5.3%
No	Yes	Yes	Yes	93.0%
No	Yes	Yes	No	48.0%
No	Yes	No	Yes	33.8%
No	Yes	No	No	3.4%
No	No	Yes	Yes	35.3%
No	No	Yes	No	3.7%
No	No	No	Yes	2.1%
No	No	No	No	1 in 700

Kocher MS, Zurakowski D, Kasser JR. Differentiating between septic arthritis and transient synovitis of the hip in children: an evidence-based clinical prediction algorithm. *J Bone Joint Surg Am* 1999;81:1662–1670.

fusion in 360 patients by Russell Hibbs in 1931 and fusion with instrumentation in 129 patients by Paul Harrington in 1962 (54, 55).

An evidence-based approach to the management of scoliosis was advocated. In 1941, a committee of the American Orthopaedic Association, headed by Alfred Shands, investigated the treatment of scoliosis in the United States and reviewed the records of 425 patients (56). This committee concluded that bracing and exercise programs were effective only in some patients and that those with progressive deformity were best treated with correction followed by fusion. John Moe established the Scoliosis Research Society in 1966. Classical epidemiologic methods were utilized to establish the incidence of scoliosis and to study the value of screening programs (57, 58). A nomogram was developed for the prediction of curve progression to aid in planning treatment and advising families (59).Case series purported the efficacy of the Milwaukee brace and the Boston brace (60, 61). The long-term results of natural history, bracing, and surgery were reported (62–65). The health, function, and psychosocial characteristics of patients with idiopathic scoliosis were investigated (66, 67).

Future clinical research in scoliosis aims to utilize highly rigorous epidemiologic methods to improve the effectiveness of scoliosis treatment. RCTs of different spinal instrumentation systems are under way. A large, multicenter trial regarding the effectiveness of bracing for adolescent idiopathic scoliosis is also under way. Further inquiry into the effect of scoliosis on health-related quality of life has been advocated.

REFERENCES

1. Hennekens CH, Buring JE. *Epidemiology in medicine*. Boston, MA: Little Brown, 1987.
2. Oxman AD, Sackett DL, Guyatt GH. Users' guides to the medical literature. I. How to get started. The Evidence-Based Medicine Working Group. *JAMA* 1993;270(17):2093–2095.
3. Davidoff F, Haynes B, Sackett D, et al. Evidence based medicine. *BMJ* 1995;310:1085–1086.
4. Sackett DL, Rosenberg WM. On the need for evidence-based medicine. *J Public Health Med* 1995;17:330–334.
5. Sackett DL, Rosenberg WM, Gray JA, et al. Evidence based medicine: what it is and what it isn't. *BMJ* 1996;312:71–72.
6. Straus SE, Sackett DL. Using research findings in clinical practice. *BMJ* 1998;317:339–342.
7. Feinstein AR, Spitz H. The epidemiology of cancer therapy. I. Clinical problems of statistical surveys. *Arch Intern Med* 1969;123:171–186.
8. Feinstein AR, Pritchett JA, Schimpff CR. The epidemiology of cancer therapy. II. The clinical course: data, decisions, and temporal demarcations. *Arch Intern Med* 1969;123:323–344.
9. Feinstein AR, Pritchett JA, Schimpff CR. The epidemiology of cancer therapy. 3. The management of imperfect data. *Arch Intern Med* 1969; 123:448–461.
10. Wright JG, Feinstein AR. A comparative contrast of clinimetric and psychometric methods for constructing indexes and rating scales. *J Clin Epidemiol* 1992;45:1201–1218.
11. Wennberg J, Gittelsohn A. Small area variations in health care delivery. *Science* 1973;182(117):1102–1108.
12. Wennberg J, Gittelsohn A. Variations in medical care among small areas. *Sci Am* 1982;246(4):120–134.
13. Wennberg JE. Dealing with medical practice variations: a proposal for action. *Health Aff (Millwood)* 1984;3(2):6–32.
14. Wennberg JE. Outcomes research: the art of making the right decision. *Internist* 1990;31(7):26, 28.

15. Wennberg JE. Practice variations: why all the fuss? *Internist* 1985; 26(4):6–8.

16. Wennberg JE, Bunker JP, Barnes B. The need for assessing the outcome of common medical practices. *Annu Rev Public Health* 1980;1:277–295.

17. Chassin MR. Does inappropriate use explain geographic variations in the use of health care services? A study of three procedures [see comments]. *JAMA* 1987;258(18):2533–2537.

18. Kahn KL, Kosecoff J, Chassin MR, et al. Measuring the clinical appropriateness of the use of a procedure. Can we do it? *Med Care* 1988;26(4): 415–422.

19. Park RE, Fink A, Brook RH, et al. Physician ratings of appropriate indications for three procedures: theoretical indications vs indications used in practice. *Am J Public Health* 1989;79(4):445–447.

20. Millenson ML. *Demanding medical excellence.* Chicago, IL: University of Chicago Press, 1997.

21. Katz J. The Nuremberg Code and the Nuremberg Trial. *JAMA* 1996; 276:1662–1666.

22. World Medical Organization. Declaration of Helsinki: recommendations guiding physicians in biomedical research involving human subjects. *JAMA* 1997;277:925–926.

23. Kocher MS, Mandiga R, Murphy J, et al. A clinical practice guideline for septic arthritis in children: efficacy on process and outcome for septic arthritis of the hip. *J Bone Joint Surg Am* 2003;85:994–999.

24. Kocher MS, DiCanzio J, Zurakowski D, et al. Diagnostic performance of clinical examination and selective magnetic resonance imaging in the evaluation of intra-articular knee disorders in children and adolescents. *Am J Sports Med* 2001;29:292–296.

25. Kocher MS. Ultrasonographic screening for developmental dysplasia of the hip: an epidemiologic analysis. Part I. *Am J Orthop* 2000;29: 929–933.

26. Kocher MS. Ultrasonographic screening for developmental dysplasia of the hip: an epidemiologic analysis. Part II. *Am J Orthop* 2001;30:19–24.

27. Baron JA. Uncertainty in Bayes. *Med Dec Making* 1994;14:46–51.

28. Kocher MS, Zurakowski D, Kasser JR. Differentiating between septic arthritis and transient synovitis of the hip in children: an evidence-based clinical prediction algorithm. *J Bone Joint Surg Am* 1999;81: 1662–1670.

29. Hanley JA, McNeil BJ. The meaning and use of the area under a receiver operating characteristic (ROC) curve. *Radiology* 1982;143:29–36.

30. Kocher MS, Sterett WI, Briggs KK, et al. Effect of functional bracing on subsequent knee injury in ACL-deficient professional skiers. *J Knee Surg* 2003;16:87–92.

31. Kane RL. Outcome measures. In: Kane R, ed. *Understanding health care outcomes research.* Gaithersberg, MD: Aspen Publishers, 1997:17–18.

32. Patrick DL, Deyo RA. Generic and disease-specific measures is assessing health status and quality of life. *Med Care* 1989;27:217–232.

33. Stewart AL, Ware JE, eds. *Measuring functioning and well-being.* Durham, UK: Duke University Press, 1992.

34. Carr-Hill RA. The measurement of patient satisfaction. *J Public Health Med* 1992;14(3):236–249.

35. Strasser S, Aharony L, Greenberger D. The patient satisfaction process: moving toward a comprehensive model. *Med Care Rev* 1993;50(2):219–248.

36. Ware JE Jr, Davies-Avery A, Stewart AL. The measurement and meaning of patient satisfaction. *Health Med Care Serv Rev* 1978;1(1):1, 3–15.

37. Kocher MS, Steadman JR, Zurakowski D, et al. Determinants of patient satisfaction after anterior cruciate ligament reconstruction. *J Bone Joint Surg Am* 2002;84:1560–1572.

38. Sackett DL, Rosenberg WMC, Gray JAM, et al. Evidence-based medicine: what it is and what it isn't. *BMJ* 1996;312:71–72.

39. Evidence-Based Medicine Working Group. Evidence-based medicine. A new approach to teaching the practice of medicine. *JAMA* 1992;268: 2420–2425.

40. Sackett DL, Strauss SE, Richardson WS, et al. *Evidence-based medicine: how to practice and teach EBM.* Edinburgh, UK: Churchill-Livingstone, 2000.

41. Bhandari M, Devereaux PJ, Swiontkowski MF, et al. Internal fixation compared with arthroplasty for displaced fractures of the femoral neck. A meta-analysis. *J Bone Joint Surg Am* 2003;85:1673–1681.

42. Birkmeyer JD, Welch HG. A reader's guide to surgical decision analysis. *J Am Coll Surg* 1997;184(6):589–595.

43. Krahn MD, Naglie G, Naimark D, et al. Primer on medical decision analysis: part 4—Analyzing the model and interpreting the results [see comments]. *Med Decis Making* 1997;17(2):142–151.

44. Pauker SG, Kassirer JP. Decision analysis. *N Engl J Med* 1987;316(5): 250–258.

45. Detsky AS, Naglie IG: A clinician's guide to cost-effectiveness analysis. *Ann Intern Med* 1990;113:147–154.

46. Weinstein MC, Stason WB. Foundations of cost-effectiveness analysis for health and medical practices. *N Engl J Med* 1977;13:716–721.

47. Kaplan EL, Meier P. Nonparametric estimation from incomplete observations. *J Am Stat Assoc* 1958;53:457–481.

48. Kalbfleisch JD, Prentice RL. *The statistical analysis of failure time data.* New York, NY: John Wiley & Sons, 1980:10–14.

49. Mantel N. Evaluation of survival data and two new rank order statistics arising in its consideration. *Cancer Chemother Rep* 1996;50:163–170.

50. Kocher MS, Bishop J, Luke A, et al. Operative vs nonoperative management of acute Achilles tendon ruptures: expected-value decision analysis. *Am J Sports Med* 2002;30:783–90.

51. Scully SP, Ghert MA, Zurakowski D, et al. Pathologic fracture in osteosarcoma: prognostic importance and treatment implications. *J Bone Joint Surg Am* 2002;84:49–57.

52. Adams F. *The genuine works of Hippocrates.* Baltimore, MD: William & Wilkins, 1939:237.

53. Peltier LF. *Orthopedics: a history and iconography.* San Francisco, CA: Norman Publishing, 1993:195–222.

54. Hibbs RA, Risser JC, Ferguson AB. Scoliosis treated by the fusion operation: An end-result study of three hundred and sixty cases. *J Bone Joint Surg Am* 1931;13:91–104.

55. Harrington PR. Treatment of scoliosis: correction and internal fixation by spine instrumentation. *J Bone Joint Surg Am* 1962;44:591–610.

56. Research Committee of the American Orthopaedic Association. End-result study of the treatment of idiopathic scoliosis. *J Bone Joint Surg Am* 1941;23:962–977.

57. Rogala EJ, Drummond DS, Gurr J. Scoliosis: incidence and natural history. *J Bone Joint Surg Am* 1978;60:173–176.

58. Lonstein JE. Screening for spinal deformities in Minnesota schools. *Clin Orthop* 1977;126:33–42.

59. Lonstein JE, Carlson JM. The prediction of curve progression in untreated idiopathic scoliosis during growth. *J Bone Joint Surg Am* 1984;66: 1061–1071.

60. Blount WP, Schmidt AC, Keever ED, et al. The Milwaukee brace in the operative treatment of scoliosis. *J Bone Joint Surg Am* 1958;40:511–525.

61. Emans JB, Kaelin A, Bancel P, et al. The Boston bracing system for idiopathic scoliosis. Follow-up results in 295 patients. *Spine* 1986;11: 792–801.

62. Ponsetti IV, Friedman B. Prognosis in idiopathic scoliosis. *J Bone Joint Surg Am* 1950;32:381–395.

63. Ponsetti IV, Friedman B. Changes in scoliotic spines after fusion. *J Bone Joint Surg Am* 1950;32:751–766.

64. Weinstein SL, Zavala DC, Ponseti IV. Idiopathic scoliosis: long-term follow-up and prognosis in untreated patients. *J Bone Joint Surg Am* 1981; 63:702–712.

65. Weinstein SL, Ponseti IV. Curve progression in idiopathic scoliosis. *J Bone Joint Surg Am* 1983;65:447–455.

66. Weinstein SL, Dolan LA, Spratt KF, et al. Health and function of patients with untreated idiopathic scoliosis: a 50-year natural history study. *JAMA* 2003;289:559–567.

67. Noonan KJ, Dolan LA, Jacobson WC, et al. Long-term psychosocial characteristics of patients treated for idiopathic scoliosis. *J Pediatr Orthop* 1997;17:712–717.

CHAPTER 6

Andrew W. Howard
Benjamin A. Alman

Metabolic and Endocrine Abnormalities

INTRODUCTION

Biologic Functions of Bone. Although orthopaedists tend to focus on the role of bone as the structural support for the body, bone also plays a crucial role in maintaining serum mineral homeostasis. The serum levels of calcium and phosphorus need to be maintained under tight control, to allow for normal function of a variety of cells. The cancellous bone has a tremendously large surface area that allows for the rapid transfer of minerals stored in the bone, such as calcium, to the serum. This process occurs at over a million sites in the human skeleton, mediated by osteoblast and osteoclast cells. A variety of endocrine, metabolic, and cellular factors are crucial to maintain this tight homeostatic balance. Not only do these various factors maintain serum minerals at their proper level, but they also act to regulate the amount of bone present. The interrelationship between these metabolic and endocrine factors with the distribution of minerals between the bone and serum results in metabolic and endocrine disorders altering the quantity and quality of bone. This same interrelationship occasionally results in disorders altering bone structure dysregulating serum mineral balance (1).

Growing Bone. The effect of metabolic and endocrine disorders on the skeleton is very different in children than in adults. This is because many endocrine and metabolic factors have an effect on the growth plate. Chondrocytes in the growth plate go through a coordinated process of differentiation, beginning with a proliferative phase at the epiphyseal side of the growth plate and progressing to terminal differentiation and apoptotic cell death at the metaphyseal side of the physis. Terminal differentiation is associated with the expression of Type X collagen and the formation of scaffolding for bone formation. Blood vessels located adjacent to the physis in the metaphyseal bone bring pluripotential mesenchymal cells to the region, which differentiate into osteoblasts, producing new bone on the scaffolding left behind by the growth plate chondrocytes. This coordinated differentiation process results in longitudinal growth of long bones. The process of growth plate chondrocyte differentiation needs to be tightly regulated, since if chondrocytes on one side of the body go though this process at a different rate than growth plate chondrocytes on the other side of the body, a limb length inequality would result. The process of growth plate chondrocyte maturation is regulated by both local and systemic factors (2). Conditions in which these systemic factors are dysregulated, as is the case in several endocrinopathies, there is an associated growth plate abnormality (3). In addition, some endocrine factors that regulate bone mineral homeostasis, such as thyroid hormone, also regulate the growth plate chondrocytes. Thus, while thyroid hormone dysregulation has implications in bone density in adults, in growing children, thyroid hormone dysregulation also can cause an abnormality in the growth plate.

FACTORS THAT REGULATE BONE DENSITY

Cells. Bone density is regulated by osteoblast, osteocyte, and osteoclast cells that add to or break down bone. These cells are regulated by local and systemic factors, some of which can be modulated by the mechanical environment. All of these factors are interrelated, in a complex way that is still not completely elucidated.

Osteoblasts. Osteoblasts are the main cells responsible for lying down of new bone in the form of osteoid. These cells are derived from pluripotential stromal precursor cells (sometimes called mesenchymal stem cells) and are the active cells that lay down new bone during skeletal growth and remodeling. Mesenchymal stem cells are very similar too and likely arise from the pericytes or perivascular cells present just deep to the endothelium of blood vessels. A very active area of basic science and translational research is harnessing the regenerative potential of mesenchymal stem cells to treat a variety of diseases (4–6). As the bone matures, osteoblasts become encased in the new bone. They produce alkaline phosphatase, an enzyme that is often used to identify osteoblasts and osteoblastic activity. Once they become encased in osteoid, they become relatively quiescent and are termed osteocytes. In mature bone, osteocytes are located extremely far away from neighboring cells, and communicate with other cells through long cytoplasmic processes. The osteocytes remain quiescent until stimulated by hormonal or mechanical factors to begin to reabsorb or lay down bone. Although osteoblasts and osteocytes are thought of as cells responsible for building new bone, they also are able to rapidly reabsorb small quantities of bone. They are able to do this in a relatively rapid manner, in contrast to osteoclasts, which require cellular differentiation and recruitment to reabsorb bone. Thus, they are the first cells that the body activates when bone reabsorption is required (7).

Osteoclasts.

Osteoclasts are derived from circulating monocytes. After differentiation and recruitment to the site of bone where required, osteoclasts are able to reabsorb bone in a very robust manner. They form a ruffled boarder that attaches to the osteoid, in which proteins that degrade the bone matrix are secreted. As such, osteolasts form active reabsorption cavities called Howship lacunae. There is an intimate relationship between osteocyte and osteoclast activities, and many of the signals to activate osteoclasts are mediated by osteocytes. For instance, PTH does not directly regulate osteoclast activity but conveys information via osteocytes, which produce secondary factors that regulate the differentiation of monocytes to osteoclasts. The major signaling pathway that is used by osteocytes to regulate osteoclasts involves a member of the tumor necrosis factor superfamily called RANKL, its receptor, RANK, and a circulating inhibitor, osteoprotegerin (OPG). The receptor, RANK, is present on osteoclast precursor cells, and when stimulated, it causes these precursors to differentiate into active osteoclasts. RANKL is produced by osteocytes that are stimulated to reabsorb bone. OPG also binds to RANKL, but inhibits its ability to activate RANK, and thus inactivates osteoclasts. The balance between OPG and RANKL regulates the number of osteoclasts available (Fig. 6-1) (7, 8). Since OPG inhibits osteoclast production, its use is a promising approach to inhibiting osteoclastic activity, and as such, it has the potential to be developed into useful therapy for osteoporosis, neoplastic bone loss, and even loosening surrounding total joint implants (9, 10). Denosumab, another RANKL inhibitor, has been used in clinical trials to decrease bone turnover and increase bone mineral density (BMD) in postmenopausal females but has not yet been described for clinical use in children (11).

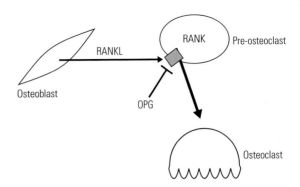

FIGURE 6-1. Expression of RANKL by osteoblasts and osteocytes activates RANK receptor on preosteoclasts to cause differentiation into active osteoclasts. OPG is a circulating factor that can also bind to RANK, but inhibits its ability to cause differentiation to osteoclasts.

Genetic Mechanisms Controlling Bone Density.

In recent years, there have been tremendous advances made into understanding genes that regulate how these cells develop. Much of this information is covered in several review articles (1, 2) and is beyond the scope of this textbook. For the purpose of this chapter, we consider three modulators of bone density: physical forces, hormone factors, and calcium homeostasis.

Hierarchy in the Regulation of Bone Mass.

There is a hierarchy among the various factors regulating bone mass. Calcium mobilization overrides the other functions of the skeleton. Calcium deficiency due to renal disease, malabsorption, or poor calcium diet invariably causes bone loss, which cannot be overcome by modulating any of the other factors that regulate bone mass. Hormone effects, such as that of estrogen, seem to be more potent than the effect of physical forces. This is suggested by the fact that exercise is limited in its ability to maintain or restore bone mass in postmenopausal women and amenorrhoeic marathon runners lose bone. Of the three modulators of bone mass—calcium availability, hormonal, and physical forces—the last has the least pronounced effects, although this is the one that orthopaedic surgery concentrates most of its efforts on (7).

Calcium Homeostasis

Biologic Functions of Calcium.

Calcium plays a crucial role in the irritability, conductivity, and contractility of smooth and skeletal muscle, and the irritability and conductivity of nerves. Small changes in extracellular and intracellular calcium levels lead to dysfunction of these cells. For the case of neurons, the cellular activity is inversely proportional to the calcium ion concentration, while for cardiac myocytes there is a direct proportionality. Thus, decreases in ionic calcium concentration can lead to tetany, convulsions, or diastolic death. Conversely, increases in the concentration of calcium can lead to muscle weakness, somnolence, and ventricular fibrillation. It is obviously important for the body to guard the concentration of ionized calcium, thus providing a rationale for the overriding importance of calcium homeostasis in modulating bone density (12, 13).

Normal Calcium Balance. Calcium is absorbed from the gut, stored in bone, and excreted primarily by the kidney. Thus, diseases that effect gut absorption or renal function have the potential to deregulate normal calcium homeostasis, and bone mass. In addition, some conditions that cause massive loss of bone mass, such as widespread metastatic disease or prolonged bed rest, also can alter serum calcium levels. Almost all of the body's calcium is stored in the bones and is held in the form of hydroxyapatite, a salt that is composed of calcium, phosphorus, hydrogen, and oxygen $Ca_{10}(PO_4)_6(OH)_2$ in very tiny crystals embedded in the collagen fibers of the cortical and cancellous bone (14–17). The small size of the crystals provides an enormous surface area, and this factor, combined with the reactivity of the crystal surface and the hydration shell that surrounds it, allows a rapid exchange process with the extracellular fluid (ECF). This process converts the mechanically solid structure of bone to a highly interactive reservoir for calcium, phosphorus, and a number of other ions (16, 18).

Serum Calcium and Phosphate Naturally Crystallizes. Hydroxyapatite is not freely soluble in water. At the pH of body fluids, calcium and phosphate concentrations in the serum exceed the critical solubility product, and are predicted to precipitate into a solid form. It is thought that various plasma proteins act to inhibit the precipitation, and keep these ions in solution. This metastable state is important for bone structure, as it allows the deposition of hydroxyapatite during bone formation with a minimal expenditure of energy. Unfortunately, it also makes ectopic calcification and ossification easy to occur as a result of increments in levels of either or both of these ions.

Active Transport of Calcium Regulators. Calcium cannot passively diffuse across mammalian cell membranes, and as such, requires an active transport machinery to move into or out of cells (12, 16, 18–20). Although the mechanism to control this transport is regulated in a large part by the action of the active form of vitamin D, parathyroid hormone (PTH), and the concentration of phosphate (18, 21, 22), a variety of other cell signaling pathways also play a role in calcium transport across cell membranes. These other cell signaling pathways, however, seem to act in specialized cell types under specific physiologic states, and as such, likely play only a small role regulating the total serum calcium level. As such, PTH, vitamin D, and phosphate are the three factors that play the most crucial roles in the calcium transport process, and thus in maintaining the normal extracellular soluble calcium level.

Parathyroid Hormone. PTH is produced by cells of the parathyroid glands, and the expression level of PTH is regulated by the serum level of ionized calcium. When serum calcium levels are low, there is an increase in PTH expression, protein production, and ultimately increased PTH levels in the serum. There are four parathyroid glands, and any one gland has the potential to produce enough PTH to maintain calcium homeostasis. This is of importance in the surgical management of thyroid neoplasia, in which it is preferable to maintain the viability of at least one parathyroid gland. PTH binds to a family of cell membrane receptors (parathyroid hormone receptors, PTHR), which activate a number of cell signaling pathways. The pathway studied most in the control of calcium is one that regulates adenyl cyclase activity, resulting in an increased cellular level of cyclic adenosine monophosphate (cAMP). cAMP renders the cell membrane more permeable to ionic calcium, and it induces the mitochondria, which are intracellular storehouses for calcium, to release their calcium. These actions increase the intracellular concentration of calcium, but do not promote transport to the extracellular space, a function that also requires vitamin D. PTH acts with 1,25-dihydroxyvitamin D to facilitate cellular calcium transport in the gut, the renal tubule, and in the lysis of hydroxyapatite crystal (20, 21, 23). PTH directly stimulates osteoblasts to begin to degrade the surrounding calcium-rich osteoid. Osteoclasts do not contain receptors for PTH, but are stimulated by PTH activation in osteoblasts through induction of the expression of RANKL, which activates osteoclasts (23, 24). Another action of PTH is to diminish the tubular reabsorption of phosphate, which causes the renal excretion of phosphate (23, 25, 26).

Vitamin D. Active vitamin D is produced from provitamins through conversion steps in the skin, liver, and kidney (Fig. 6-2). The provitamins are ingested in animal fats (ergosterol) or synthesized by the liver (7-dehydrocholesterol) (14, 20, 27) and are converted to calciferol and cholecalciferol by ultraviolet light, a process that occurs in the skin. In the absence of ultraviolet light, this conversion cannot occur, explaining the vitamin D deficiency associated with prolonged periods indoors away from ultraviolet light sources, such as in chronically ill individuals, or in people living in extremely cold climates (14, 28). The compounds are then transported to the liver, where they are converted to 25-hydroxyvitamin D by a specific hydrolase (29–33). Severe liver disease or drugs that block hydrolase activity will inhibit the production of 25-hydroxyvitamin D, also potentially leading to vitamin D deficiency. The final conversion occurs in the kidney. In the presence of specific hydrolases and a number of biochemical cofactors, 25-hydroxyvitamin D is converted to either 24,25-dihydroxyvitamin D or 1,25-dihydroxyvitamin D. The latter serves as the potent calcium transport promoter (34–36). A low serum calcium level and a high PTH level cause conversion to the 1,25 analog, while a high serum calcium level, a higher serum phosphate level, and a low PTH level favor formation of 24,25-dihydroxyvitamin D, which is less potent in activating calcium transport (Fig. 6-3) (34, 37–40). Serum phosphate also plays an important role here, as a high concentration of phosphate shunts the 25-hydroxyvitamin D into the 24,25-dihydroxy form. Although the 24,25-dihydroxy form is less active in its effects regulating calcium, it has an important role in growth plate chondrocytes. This crucial role for conversion of vitamin D in the kidney, as well as the kidney's important role excreting excess calcium and phosphorus, explains the particularly deleterious effect of renal failure on bone homeostasis, causing

Factors that Regulate Bone Density

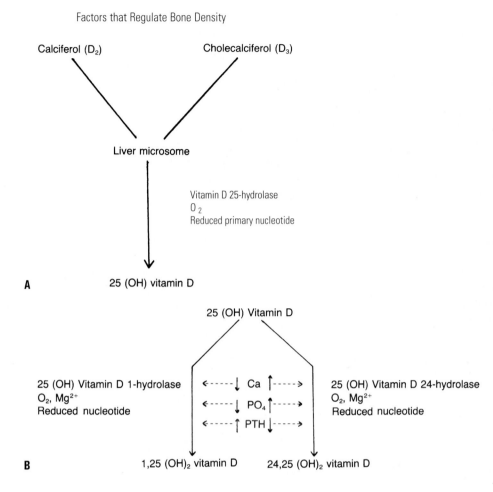

FIGURE 6-2. The conversion of vitamin D from the skin or from dietary sources takes place in the liver and kidney. **A:** In the liver, the enzyme vitamin D 25-hydrolase acts to form 25-hydroxy vitamin D. **B:** The second conversion of vitamin D takes place in the kidney, where at least two pathways have been described. The *maintenance* pathway (when the need is minimal, as defined by a normal calcium and phosphorus and low PTH level) occurs in the presence of a specific enzyme (25-hydroxyvitamin D 24-hydrolase) and results in the less active 24,25-dihydroxyvitamin D. If calcium transport is required, as signaled by the presence of low serum calcium and phosphorus levels and a high PTH level, the body converts the 25-hydroxyvitamine D to the much more active form, 1,25-dihydroxyvitamin D.

vitamin D deficiency as well as directly deregulating normal calcium excretion. Because of the crucial role of vitamin D in calcium metabolism, the National Academy of Sciences and the American Academy of Pediatrics recommend 200 IU per day of vitamin D (41). This dose will prevent physical signs of vitamin D deficiency and maintain serum 25-hydroxyvitamin D at or above 27.5 nmol/L (11 ng/mL). Many professional bodies and experts are currently advocating for increased intake of vitamin D for healthy children, with credible recommendations ranging from 400 to 1000 IU (42, 43). The generic name of 1,25-dihydroxyvitamin D is calcitriol. Recent studies found that vitamin D also has a variety of extraskeletal effects, including modulating the immune response, and as a chemoprotective agent against certain cancers (42–44).

Dietary Calcium Intake. Dietary calcium is crucial to the maintenance of bone mass. Daily requirements vary with the need of calcium during periods of rapid bone growth. Recommendations from the American Academy of Pediatrics are summarized in Table 6-1 (12, 28, 45, 46). Adequate calcium in the diet during adolescent years is important in the maintenance of bone mass over the long-term, and the orthopaedist should counsel their patients about the importance of appropriate amounts of calcium, as well as vitamin D, in their diet. Several dietary factors alter calcium absorption. Calcium

salts are more soluble in acid media, and loss of the normal contribution of acid from the stomach reduces the solubility of the calcium salts and decreases the absorption of the ionized cation. A diet rich in phosphate may decrease the absorption of calcium by binding the cation to HPO_4^{2-} and precipitating most of the ingested calcium as insoluble material (16, 47). Ionic calcium can be chelated by some organic materials with a high affinity for the element, such as phytate, oxalate, and citrate. Although these materials may remain soluble, they cannot be absorbed (16, 47–49). Calcium, in the presence of a free fatty acid, forms an insoluble soap that cannot be absorbed (47, 50). Disorders of the biliary or enteric tracts, associated with steatorrhea, are likely to reduce the absorption of calcium, because it forms an insoluble compound, and because ingested fat-soluble vitamin D is less likely to be absorbed under these circumstances (51).

Dietary Phosphate Intake. Phosphate (PO_4) is absorbed lower in the gastrointestinal tract than calcium and is freely transported across the gut cell to enter the extracellular space, in which it represents a major buffer system. Transport into and out of the bone is passive and related to the kinetics of the formation and breakdown of hydroxyapatite crystals. Tubular reabsorption of phosphate, however, is highly variable, with reabsorption ranging from almost 100% to <50%. The principal factor in decreasing tubular reabsorption of phosphate is *PTH*.

FIGURE 6-3. The roles of the bone, kidneys, gastrointestinal tract, parathyroid gland, and thyroid gland in calcium kinetics. These organs act to maintain calcium in the ECF at the appropriate levels for normal cellular function. **A:** Vitamin D and PTH act to transport calcium ions across the gut wall and regulate renal excretion and, thereby, bone calcium content. Depending on the need for increased transport, 25-hydroxy vitamin D is converted to 24,25- or 1,25-dihydroxyvitamin D. **B:** In the normocalcemic state, a reduced concentration of calcium signals the parathyroid glands to release more PTH, which acts at the levels of the gut cell, renal tubule, and bone to increase transport of calcium and rapidly replenish body fluids with it. An increase in PTH also favors the synthesis of 1,25-dihydroxvitamin D in the kidney and acts to promote renal phosphate excretion by markedly diminishing the tubular reabsorption of phosphate. **C:** In the hypercalcemic state, low concentrations of calcium and PTH act independently to diminish the synthesis of 1,25-dihydroxyvitamin D and decrease transport of calcium in the gut cell, tubule, and bone. Increased concentrations of calcium also cause the release of CT from the C cells of the thyroid gland, thereby diminishing calcium concentration. This mechanism principally involves stabilizing the osteoclast and decreasing its action on the bone, but it is not very effective in humans.

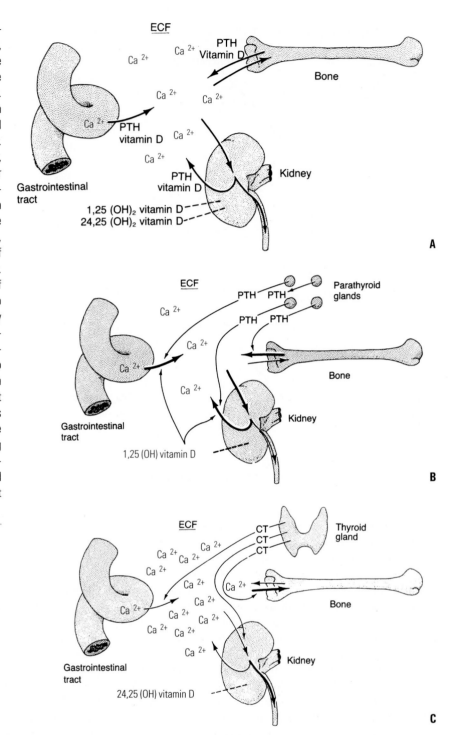

Endocrine Factors

Sex Steroids. The most potent endocrine regulator of bone density is estrogen. Much of the clinical and experimental data on the role of estrogen in bone have been generated from data on postmenopausal women. However, clinical data from children with deficiencies in sex hormones, such as in Turner syndrome, show that a lack of estrogen in growing girls also is responsible for profound loss of bone density. The exact mechanism by which estrogen regulates bone formation and loss is unknown. Estrogen receptors are present on both osteoblasts and osteoclasts, yet the cellular mechanism by which estrogen alters these cells' behavior is not clear. Studies in animals suggest that estrogen exhibits at least some of its effects through the regulation of pluripotential stromal cells in the bone marrow, a process which may be mediated by interleukin-6. Estrogen also suppresses the activation of osteoclasts by inhibiting the activation of RANK in the precursor cells (52, 53).

Androgens also seem to regulate bone mass, although the mechanism is less well understood than for estrogen. Idiopathic hypogonadotropic hypogonadism is associated

TABLE 6-1	Dietary Calcium Requirements
Age	**Calcium Requirement (mg/d)**
0 to 6 mo	210
6 mo to 1 y	270
1 through 3 y	500
4 through 8 y	800
9 through 18 y	1300

with decreased bone mass, and there is an association between delayed puberty and low bone mass in boys, suggesting a positive role for androgens regulating bone mass (54).

Thyroid Hormones. Thyroid hormones act in the cell nucleus, interacting with nuclear proteins and DNA to increase the expression of a variety of genes, ultimately positively regulating cell activity. As such, thyroid hormone activates both osteoblasts and osteoclasts. The actual effect on bone mass depends on the body's balance between these two cell types and how well the normal control of calcium level is able to counteract the heightened activity of these cell types. In general, the balance is in favor of the osteoclast, and most often increased thyroid hormone levels result in bone loss (55, 56).

Corticosteroids. Corticosteroids have a variety of effects on cells. They inhibit cellular activity in general, potentially decreasing the ability of osteoblasts to lay down new bone. They also have profound effects on the skeleton based on their effect on calcium regulation in the kidney, where they increase calcium excretion. This leads secondarily to elevated PTH levels, with its negative effects on bone density (57, 58).

Calcitonin. Calcitonin (CT) is produced by parafollicular thyroid cells. Although CT causes inhibition of bone resorption by osteoclasts and osteoblasts and decreases reabsorption of calcium and phosphate in the kidneys in animal models and cell cultures, it seems to play little role in humans (59, 60).

Mechanical Factors. Excessive reductions in bone strain produced by weightlessness (microgravity in outer space) or immobilization (paralysis, prolonged bed rest, or application of casts) can cause significant bone loss, while strenuous athletic activity can augment certain bones (60, 61). This effect is important in the pediatric orthopaedic population, in which many of the neuromuscular disorders are associated with decreased weight bearing and associated osteoporosis. Bone remodels according to the mechanical stresses applied, a phenomenon termed Wolff law. It is well known that mechanical environment alters cell behavior and gene expression, and it is thought that such a mechanism, most likely acting through osteocytes, is responsible for the effect of weight bearing on bone density as well as for the changes attributable to Wolff's law (62, 63).

FACTORS THAT REGULATE GROWTH PLATE CHONDROCYTES

In recent years, a number of signaling pathways that regulate the function of growth plate chondrocytes have been elucidated (2). General information about growth plate development and its local regulation is covered in the chapter on developmental biology. However, it is apparent that the growth plate chondrocytes are affected either primarily or secondarily by a variety of endocrine regulatory factors, and as such, a short review here is warranted. Growth plate chondrocytes at the epiphyseal side of the growth plate reside in the resting zone. They begin to proliferate and as such advance toward the metaphyseal side of the growth plate in the proliferative zone. Following this, they enter a prehypertrophic zone, where they shift from proliferation to differentiation. It is also in this prehypertrophic zone that important signals that regulate the differentiation process such as PTH-related protein and Indian hedgehog are present. Following this, the cells hypertrophy form columns in the hypertrophic zone, and then undergo terminal differentiation and cell death. Blood vessels from the metaphysis are present adjacent to the terminally differentiated chondrocytes, bringing in new pluripotential mesenchymal cells, which will differentiate into osteoblasts, forming the new bone on the scaffolding left behind by the chondrocytes. This last region is sometimes called the zone of provisional calcification.

It is easy to imagine how hormones can tip the balance in favor of or against the differentiation process in these cells. In addition, agents that alter normal bone formation by osteoblasts can also alter the growth plate, by preventing the normal replacement of the terminally differentiating chondrocytes with new bone. This inhibition of normal ossification results in the characteristic growth plate changes in rickets, in which there is an increased zone of terminal differentiation. Endocrinopathies can also alter the size and matrix components in the various zones of the growth plate. Such disorders effect terminal differentiation and may make the growth plate mechanically weaker in this region, predisposing to conditions such as slipped capital femoral epiphysis. In a similar manner, it may make the growth plate chondrocytes easier to deform with compressive pressure, causing deformities such as genu varum. This explains the high frequency of these growth plate deformities in children with endocrine disorders. Like in bone, mechanical factors can also play a role in growth pate function. The Hueter-Volkmann principle states that growth plates exhibit increased growth in response to tension and decreased growth in response to compression (64). Thus, an endocrinopathy can cause growth plate deformities, which can then be exacerbated by the effect of the changing mechanical axis in the effected limb.

Similar to the situation in bone, there is also a hierarchal regulation of the growth plate, with endocrine factors playing a dominant role over mechanical factors (3, 65). This is readily apparent in conditions such as rickets, where surgery will not result in correction of genu varum in the absence of correction of the underlying endocrinopathy in the growing child. Thus, it is important to avoid the temptation for surgical correction of a deformity in a growing child with an endocrine disorder until the endocrinopathy is also treated.

There are a large number of endocrine factors that play a role regulating growth plate function. In many cases, not much is known about the intracellular signaling mechanisms utilized by these factors. Growth hormone plays an important role regulating growth plate chondrocytes proliferation, mediated by somatomedins. In an absence of growth hormone, there is a slowing of growth plate maturation, as well as a slowing of the rate of long bone growth. Thyroid hormone also plays a role regulating chondrocyte activity, by increasing the metabolic and proliferative rate of the growth plate chondrocytes. PTH may alter growth pate chondrocyte maturation, as the PTH receptor, PTHR1 is expressed in prehypertrophic chondrocytes, and its stimulation results in an inhibition of terminal differentiation. Nutrition and insulin also regulate growth plate chondrocytes, in a similar manner to growth hormone, by regulating growth plate chondrocyte proliferation. A lack of dietary protein exerts a negative control over the somatomedins. Excess glucocorticoids also inhibit growth, partly by an inhibitory effect on protein synthesis in cartilage, but also by interference with somatomedin production and action (3). Although these factors all play roles regulating growth plate chondrocytes, in the coming years we will likely learn more about the role of such factors in a variety of growth plate pathologies, including disorders such as slipped capital femoral epiphysis, where it is well known that a variety of endocrinopathies are predisposing conditions.

DISEASES OF BONE

Rickets

Context/Common Features. Rickets describes the clinical condition of inadequate mineralization of growing bone. Severe nutritional rickets was endemic in early industrialized societies particularly where sunlight was scarce. Accordingly, severe rachitic deformities were commonly seen in the early days of orthopaedics (66, 67). In developed countries, nutritional rickets is now a rarity, although it may present *de novo* to pediatric orthopaedists for diagnosis. Inherited form of rickets remain commonly seen in the United States (68). The surgeon should also be familiar with renal tubular abnormalities, which can result in rickets, as well as with the clinical entity of renal osteodystrophy, which describes the bone disease associated with end-stage renal disease and includes features of rickets as well as secondary hyperparathyroidism.

The clinical manifestations of all forms of rickets are similar and, therefore, clinical presentation will be covered separately prior to breaking down the various etiologies.

Clinical Presentation. Rickets is failure or delay of calcification of newly formed bone at long bone physes. The manifestations include changes in the growth plate morphology with decreased longitudinal growth and angular deformities of the long bones. Osteomalacia, which is failure of mineralization of osteoid formed at cortical and trabecular surfaces, often accompanies

rickets in childhood. Osteomalacia is the only result in the adult of the mechanisms, which cause rickets in childhood.

The skeletal abnormalities of severe rickets present in early childhood and often before the age of 2 years. The child may have a history consistent with hypocalcemia in infancy including apneic spells, convulsions, tetany, and stridor prior to age of 6 months (69). The child is often hypotonic with delayed motor milestones for sitting, crawling, and walking. There is proximal muscle weakness and sometimes perfuse sweating. Cardiomyopathy and respiratory and gastrointestinal infections can accompany the clinical presentation (70–75).

Skeletal deformities can be evident at every physis. The wrists, elbows, and knees are thickened, and the long bones are short. Genu varum or valgum may be present. Coxa vara may be present. Costochondral enlargement leads to the characteristic rachitic rosary appearance of the chest. Harrison sulcus is an indentation of the lower ribs caused by indrawing against the soft bone. Kyphoscoliosis can be present. Closure of the anterior fontanelle is delayed. Frontal and parietal bossing of the skull is evident. Plagiocephaly may be related to positioning on a soft skull. Delayed primary dentition is common (68, 76).

Radiographic Changes. The radiographic hallmark of rickets is widened and indistinct growth plates (Fig. 6-4). In a normal child, the distance between the metaphysis and epiphysis of the distal radius should never be >1 mm (77).

Lateral expansion of the growth plates also occurs, particularly with weight bearing. Crawling children weight bear on their wrists, explaining the thickened wrists as well as knees. The metaphysis typically takes on a cupped and splayed appearance. The long bones are short for age. The long bones show evidence of the coxa vara, genu varum, or valgum described above in the clinical deformities. Further evidence of osteomalacia radiographically may also be present. The hallmark is Looser zones. These are transverse bands of unmineralised osteoid, which typically appear in the medial aspect of the proximal femur and at the posterior aspect of the ribs. These are described as pseudofractures and often have an osteosclerotic reaction around them. In an adult, they can progress to true fractures. Acetabular protrusion and pathologic fractures complete the radiographic signs of rickets (70, 76–78).

Overview of Classification of Rickets. Bone is mineralized by the crystallization of calcium and phosphate in the presence of alkaline phosphatase enzyme. Calcium and phosphate are maintained in the body very close to their solubility coefficient by complex series of inhibitors. The control mechanisms in the physiologic state are discussed in sections above.

A useful way of thinking about rickets is to consider those conditions that reduce the availability of calcium, those conditions that reduce the availability of phosphate, and the rare condition that reduces the availability of alkaline phosphatase at the osteoblast–bone junction (Table 6-2). Nutritional rickets and end-organ insensitivity to calcitriol are problems on the calcium side. X-linked hypophosphatemia is the most common form of rickets seen today in the United States and

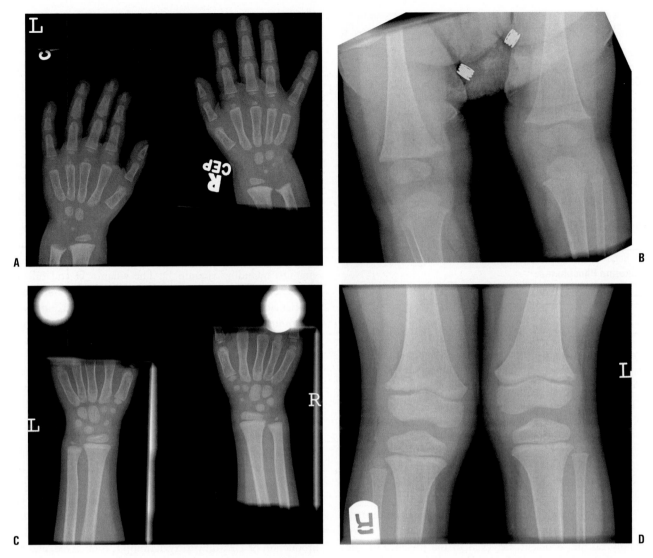

FIGURE 6-4. Rickets. Changes caused by rickets can be seen **(A)** at the wrist and **(B)** at the knees of this 1-year-old child with X-linked hypophosphatemia. The growth plates are widened and the metaphyses are cupped, particularly at the ulna and femur. At 4 years of age **(C,D)**, the changes have resolved with medical treatment.

is caused by renal tubular phosphate wasting in isolation (79). Renal tubular abnormalities including Fanconi syndrome feature renal wasting of phosphate, calcium, magnesium, and bicarbonate. Alkaline phosphatase is deficient only in one rare recessive condition, appropriately called hypophosphatasia.

Finally, renal osteodystrophy is often discussed with rickets and appropriately so since many children with renal osteodystrophy manifest findings of rickets. However, renal osteodystrophy classically includes changes of secondary hyperparathyroidism as well as those of rickets.

Nutritional Rickets. Nutritional rickets had near universal prevalence in Northern industrialized societies in the 19th century. It has now largely disappeared in developed countries. It remains a significant clinical problem in the developing world with, for example, a 66% prevalence of clinical rickets in preschool children in Tibet in 2001 (80).

The main cause of nutritional rickets is vitamin D deficiency. Vitamin D_3 (Cholecalciferol) can be produced in the skin by a process that requires ultraviolet B (UVB) radiation, or it can be ingested in the diet. Peak age of presentation of nutritional rickets is between 3 and 18 months in children who have inadequate exposure to sunlight and no vitamin D supplementation in the diet (81–83). Breast milk is poor in vitamin D and prolonged breast-feeding is a risk factor (84, 85). Vitamin D is supplemented in dairy foods in North America and diets deficient in dairy foods are therefore a risk factor (85–87). Two hundred international units of vitamin D per day is the recommended dietary amount for preventing rickets (41, 68, 68). Increasing amounts are now being recommended for optimization of bone health, with the Canadian Paediatric Society recommending 800 IU per day for northern children and the AAP recommending 400 IU per day (42). Some experts advocate 1000 IU of vitamin D per

TABLE 6-2	Classification of Rickets According to What Is Lacking at the Osteoblast-Bone Interface

Calcium
 Nutritional rickets
  Vitamin D deficiency (common)
  Isolated calcium deficiency (rare)
  Combined calcium deficiency and marginal vitamin D intake (common)
 Gastrointestinal rickets
 1α hydroxylase deficiency
 End organ insensitivity to vitamin D
 Rickets of end-stage renal disease (renal osteodystrophy)
Phosphorus
 X-linked hypophosphatemia (common)
 Renal tubular abnormalities
Alkaline Phosphatase
 Hypophosphatasia

day for all healthy children and adults (43). Sunlight exposure also prevents rickets. Two hours per week of summer sunshine at the latitude of Cincinnati (39 degrees North) is sufficient to produce adequate vitamin D in the skin. However, during the winter months in Edmonton (52 degrees North), there is insufficient UVB exposure to allow for adequate intrinsic production of vitamin D (68). A recent national survey in Canada estimated a prevalence of vitamin D deficiency rickets of at least 3 per 100,000 children, with a higher risk among breast-fed children and those dwelling in the north (88).

Although vitamin D deficiency is the principal cause of nutritional rickets, it is possible to have rickets from a profoundly calcium-deficient diet even in the presence of adequate vitamin D intake (89). Probably much more common is a subtle combination of calcium deficiency and vitamin D deficiency interacting to produce dietary rickets (90). This has been described among the modern Asian population in the United Kingdom (91, 92) and black populations in the United States (68). A diet that is low in calcium and high in phytate, oxalate, or citrate (substances found in almost all fresh and cooked vegetables and that bind calcium) means that calcium intake is poor. Vegetarians, especially those who avoid dairy products, are particularly at risk. This produces an increase in PTH that in turn increases vitamin D catabolism. Vitamin D status may have been marginal due to low sun exposure and poor dietary intake. The increased catabolism of vitamin D with marginal intake results in a vitamin D deficiency and a clinical presentation of rickets. This combination or relative deficiencies of both calcium and vitamin D together has a high prevalence among adolescents presenting with rickets in the United Kingdom and the United States.

Treatment of nutritional rickets involves adequate provision of vitamin D. The treatment dose of 5000 to 10,000 international units per day for 4 to 8 weeks should be provided along with calcium to 500 to 1000 mg per day in the diet (93). Where

daily dosing and compliance were a problem, much larger doses of vitamin D (200,000 to 600,000 IU orally or intramuscularly) have given as single doses with good results (94).

Laboratory abnormalities in established nutritional rickets can include a low normal or decreased calcium ion concentration, a low serum phosphate, a low serum 25-hydroxyvitamin D_3, and a high alkaline phosphate. Alkaline phosphate drops to normal in response to successful therapy.

Gastrointestinal Rickets. Even if adequate calcium and vitamin D are present in the diet, some gastrointestinal diseases prevent its appropriate absorption (95). Gluten-sensitive enteropathy, Crohn disease, ulcerative colitis, sarcoidosis, short-gut syndromes have been implicated. If liver disease interferes with the production of bile salts, then fat accumulates in the GI tract and prevents the absorption of fat-soluble vitamins including vitamin D. The vitamin D and calcium deficiency cause bone disease in the same way as nutritional deficiencies, but the treatments are aimed at the underlying gastrointestinal problem as well as at supplementing the missing vitamin and mineral.

X-Linked Hypophosphatemia. X-linked hypophosphatemia is the most common inherited etiology for rickets with a prevalence of 1 in 20, 000 persons (96). It is an x-linked dominant disorder. This means a female-to-male patient ratio is approximately 2:1, and no male-to-male transmission. Approximately one-third of cases are sporadic (96). People with sporadic occurrence do transmit the defect to their offspring. The defect is in a gene called PHEX (79). This gene product indirectly regulates renal phosphate's transport. The defect at the kidney is isolated renal phosphate wasting leading to hypophosphatemia. In addition, a low or normal kidney production of 1,25-dihydroxyvitamin D_3 is observed, and this would be inappropriate in the hypophosphatemic state.

The clinical presentation includes rickets and mild short stature (97, 98). Dental abscesses occur in childhood, even prior to the development of dental carries (99). Adults with the condition have osteomalacia accompanied by degenerative joint disease, enthesopathies, dental abscesses, and short stature (100–102). Specific treatment for the condition is oral administration of phosphate as well as the active form of vitamin D_3 calcitriol, which is 1 alpha-hydroxylated. Treatment requires careful metabolic monitoring. Hyperparathyroidism, soft-tissue calcification, and death due to vitamin D intoxication have been problems with medical therapy in the past. Calcitriol can be used in much lower doses than the less active vitamin D metabolites previously used and are thought to be a safer therapy (79, 103, 104). Angular deformities, particularly genu valgum, may persist after medical treatment and require osteotomy (105–107). Although good initial corrections are obtained with standard techniques including external fixators, Petje reported a 90% recurrence of deformity after the first surgery and a 60% recurrence of deformity after the second surgery due to ongoing disease activity (108).

A small number of those patients with McCune-Albright syndrome also develop hypophosphatemic rickets. This syndrome includes patients with café au lait spots, precocious puberty, and fibrous dysplasia of multiple long bones. This syndrome is caused by constitutional activation of the cyclic AMP-PKA signaling pathway related to genetic defects in G signaling proteins (109).

1 Alpha-Hydroxylase Deficiency.

In 1961, Prader described what was initially called vitamin D–dependent rickets (110). This was because the initial patients were treated with very large doses of vitamin D. It turns out that these patients have 1 alpha-hydroxylase deficiency and they can be treated with much smaller quantities of the biologically active 1 alpha-hydroxylated calcitriol (111). Typically, the patients present <24 weeks of age with weakness, pneumonia, seizures, bone pain, and the skeletal bone changes of rickets. Serum findings include low calcium and phosphorus, high alkaline phosphatase, and PTH with a normal level of 25-hydroxyvitamin D_3, but a markedly decreased level of 1,25-dihydroxyvitamin D_3. The patients are not able to convert the accumulated 25-hydroxyvitamin D_3 to its biologically active form of 1,25-dihydroxyvitamin D_3 and, therefore, develop clinical rickets. The autosomal recessive genetic pattern has been described (112), and the specific mutations were initially described in 1997 (113) since which time at least 31 distinct mutations in the 1 alpha-hydroxylase gene have been identified (111).

Current treatment is oral provision of activated vitamin D_3, which is curative.

End-Organ Insensitivity.

In 1978, Marx (114) described two sisters with clinical rickets. The unusual clinical feature was an exceedingly high circulating level of 1,25-dihydroxyvitamin D_3. Levels can be 3 to 30 fold higher than normal (115). A striking clinical finding is alopecia or near total loss of hair from the head and the body. These patients have an end-organ insensitivity to vitamin D_3 (115). Treatment with very high doses of vitamin D produces a variable but incomplete clinical response. Intravenous high doses of calcium followed by oral calcium supplementation in large quantities have also been tried, but as yet, this rare form of rickets cannot be completely treated medically (111).

Renal Tubular Abnormalities.

There is a large group of causes of the Fanconi syndrome. This syndrome implies failure of tubular reabsorption of many small molecules <50 Da. The kidneys lose phosphate, calcium, magnesium, bicarbonate, sodium, potassium, glucose, uric acid, and small amino acids. With this renal tubular abnormality, there are multiple mechanisms by which bone mineral homeostasis is disrupted (95, 116). As a result, these patients are short with rickets and delayed bone age. The predominant cause of bone disease is hypophosphatemia from renal phosphate wasting, very similar to that seen in x-linked hypophosphatemic rickets. Other mechanisms include calcium and magnesium loss, the meta-

bolic acidosis caused by bicarbonate loss, renal osteodystrophy if renal disease is sufficient that less 1,25-dihydroxyvitamin D_3 is produced, and finally decreased calcium and phosphate reabsorption.

Treatment is similar to that of x-linked hypophosphatemia with provision of oral phosphate and vitamin D. Electrolyte imbalances from other causes need monitoring and treatment, and the underlying renal disease can also be treated if possible.

Hypophosphatasia.

This is another disease with clinical overlap with rickets. Hypophosphatasia is caused by alkaline phosphatase deficiency. Like most enzyme deficiencies, this is a recessive condition with over 112 mutations described in the alkaline phosphatase gene in chromosome 1 (117–119). Clinically, alkaline phosphatase deficiency produces abnormal mineralization of bone with a presentation of rickets in the child or osteomalacia in the adult (120). Pathologic fractures can occur in children and in adults (121, 122). This is accompanied by abnormal formation of dental cementum that causes loss of teeth. The primary teeth are lost early and with minimal root resorption (123). Additional clinical manifestation can include failure to thrive, increased intercranial pressure, and craniosynostosis.

Hypophosphatasia has an estimated prevalence of 1 per 100,000 people (124). There is a perinatal lethal form. A childhood form presents with rickets at 2 or 3 years of age and remission of the disease in adolescence. An adult form presents with mild osteomalacia with pathologic fractures (117).

There is no satisfactory medical treatment of the underlying defect. Bone marrow transplantation has been used experimentally in severe cases, with the aim of repopulating the bone marrow with osteoblasts capable of producing alkaline phosphatase (117). Surgical treatment of femoral fractures and pseudofractures in the adult has been reported, with rodding techniques superior to plating techniques in the abnormal bone (121).

Renal Osteodystrophy.

Renal osteodystrophy describes the bony changes accompanying end stage renal disease and is commonly seen in patients on dialysis. The clinical presentation includes hyperparathyroidism as well as rickets/osteomalacia in varying combinations (125–128).

Renal failure means inadequate clearance of phosphate from the blood once the renal function drops below 25% to 30% of normal. The hyperphosphatemia drives the solubility equilibrium to produce hypocalcemia. This hypocalcemia signals the parathyroid glands to produce PTH, causing secondary hyperparathyroidism. The bony changes of hyperparathyroidism then become evident. These include subperiosteal erosions and brown tumors (Fig. 6-5). The subperiosteal erosions are described as classically appearing on the radial margins of the middle phalanges of digit 2 and digit 3 in adults. In children, they can also be seen at the lateral aspects of the distal radius and ulna and at the medial aspect of the proximal tibia (Fig. 6-6) (129). Prolonged stimulation of the parathyroid glands can produce sufficient hyperplasia that the glands

FIGURE 6-5. Radiograph of the pelvis of a patient with renal osteodystrophy shows the marked changes of secondary hyperparathyroidism. Several brown tumors are seen in the femoral shafts and ischial rami. These appear as expanded destructive lesions, resembling primary or metastatic bone tumors.

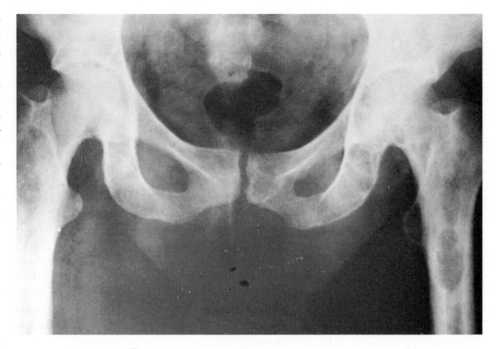

remain autonomous and maintain a hyperparathyroid state even if the end stage renal disease is treated by transplantation. In this case, the ongoing hyperparathyroidism is described as tertiary rather than secondary.

The other aspect of renal osteodystrophy is rickets. If there is inadequate renal mass to produce sufficient 1,25-dihydroxyvitamin D_3, rickets (clinical and radiographic) will accompany renal osteodystrophy. The clinical manifestations can include varus or valgus deformities at the knees or ankles, with widened and deformed growth plates radiographically, and other radiographic signs of rickets/osteomalacia such as Looser zones (Fig. 6-7).

Treatment of renal osteodystrophy includes

- Dietary phosphate restriction
- Phosphate binding agents, especially those that contain calcium

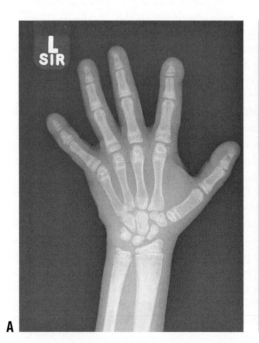
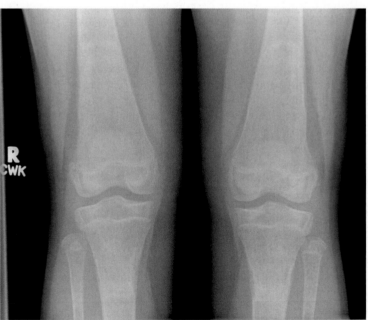

FIGURE 6-6. Renal osteodystrophy in an 8-year-old boy. **A:** Radiographs of the hand show sclerosis, acroosteolysis, and soft-tissue calcification around the metacarpal phalangeal and proximal interphalangeal joints. **B:** Radiographs of the knees show subperiosteal resorption at the medial border of the proximal tibia.

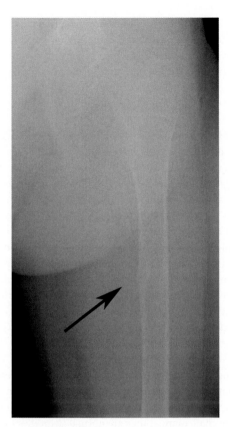

FIGURE 6-7. Renal osteodystrophy. A Looser zone is evident (*arrow*) in the medial femoral diaphysis.

- Vitamin D particularly calcitriol to decrease the secondary hyperparathyroidism as well as to treat clinical rickets or osteomalacia
- Restoration of renal function by transplantation often improves the musculoskeletal manifestations.

Slipped capital femoral epiphysis occurs frequently in patients with renal osteodystrophy and is not common in other presentations of rickets (Fig. 6-8) (130–132). The slip occurs through the metaphyseal side of the physis (126, 133, 134) and occurs at a younger age, in children who are typically small because of their chronic disease. Therefore, stabilization of the slip should permit ongoing growth of the proximal femur if possible. Unstable slips and avascular necrosis are rare in patients with renal osteodystrophy, but avascular necrosis possibly associated with steroid use post transplant has been reported (134). If the child is young and the slip is severe and the bone disease is not yet treated medically, then traction plus medical treatment have shown very good results. When considering the surgical treatment of the slipped epiphysis associated with renal osteodystrophy, the high incidence of bilaterality suggests stabilizing both epiphyses. In young patients, a pinning technique, which allows for growth (smooth pins across the physis), can be considered (133). Hardware cutout, including pin protrusion into the joint, is more likely with the soft bone of renal osteodystrophy but has generally been associated with inadequate medical control of the hyperparathyroidism (133, 134).

Osteoporosis in Children

Implications to General and Lifelong Health. The National Institutes of Health (NIH) Consensus Panel (2000) has defined osteoporosis as "a skeletal disorder characterized by compromised bone strength predisposing to an increasing risk of fracture." They note that bone strength includes both bone density and bone quality. Childhood osteoporosis can come from numerous primary and secondary etiologies, summarized in Table 6-3.

There are 10 million people in the United States with osteoporosis, and 18 million more with low bone mass at risk for osteoporosis (135). We associate osteoporosis with senescence, and certainly most of the individuals currently

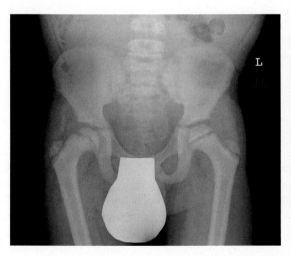
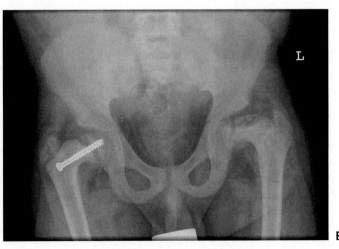

FIGURE 6-8. Renal osteodystrophy in a 12-year-old boy. **A:** An anteroposterior pelvis x-ray reveals an early capital femoral epiphysis on the right. Slipped capital femoral epiphysis is common in renal osteodystrophy and rare in rickets. **B:** Three years after fixation the right proximal femoral epiphysis remains open and stable; the left hip now shows signs of epiphyseal avascular necrosis and fragmentation.

TABLE 6-3	Classification of Childhood Osteoporosis

Primary
  Structural gene abnormalities
    Osteogenesis imperfecta
    Marfan syndrome
    Ehlers-Danlos syndrome
    Bruck syndrome
  Genes important in bone development
  Homocystinuria
  Osteoporosis pseudoglioma syndrome
  Idiopathic juvenile osteoporosis

Secondary
  Neuromuscular
    Duchenne muscular dystrophy
    Cerebral palsy
    Myelomeningocele
  Endocrine
    Growth hormone deficiency
    Hyperthyroidism
    Disorders of puberty
  Drug-related
    Glucocorticoids
    Anticonvulsants
  Miscellaneous (methotrexate, heparin, cyclosporine)

affected are old, and not likely seeing paediatric orthopaedists. However, the NIH emphasizes that "sub-optimal bone growth in childhood and adolescence is as important as bone loss to the development of osteoporosis." An epidemiologic study compared rickets mortality in 1942 to 1948 with hip fracture rates in 1986 to 1993 across birth regions in the United States, and found a very high correlation, suggesting that early deficiency of vitamin D could have important effects on the skeleton decades later (136). The recommended intake of calcium for children aged 9 to 17 is 1300 mg per day, and it is estimated that only 10% of girls and 25% of boys meet this minimum requirement (135). While consumption of dairy-based beverages supplying calcium has declined, consumption of carbonated beverages has increased (137). Phosphoric acid is used in cola soft drinks, and teenage girls who drink soft drinks are three to four times more likely to report fractures than those who do not, the association being strongest among active girls drinking cola (138). A meta-analysis of calcium supplementation including 19 randomized trials and 2859 children showed no effect of calcium supplementation alone on BMD at the femoral neck or the lumbar spine (139). Self-reported physical activity in adolescence (but not during adulthood), on the other hand, was a strong determinant of BMD after menopause (140). A meta-analysis of 22 randomized controlled trials of physical activity in childhood showed 1% to 5% increases in bone mineral accrual among the exercising groups, with a greater effect before puberty was complete (141). Vitamin D supplementation has not been so well studied but is receiving increasing attention, with advocates pointing to

epidemiologic studies linking vitamin D intake or latitude to lower incidences of cancer and cardiovascular disease as well as to improved bone health (43). A challenge is determining the appropriate level for supplementation of vitamin D, although recent opinion suggests increasing the amount of oral vitamin D_3 to 1000 units per day for both children and adults (43).

Collagen Mutations—Osteogenesis Imperfecta. Osteogenesis imperfecta (OI) or brittle bone disease describes a spectrum of clinical disorders that have in common abnormal bone fragility. The vast majority of patients with OI have disorders of collagen production, which affects either the quantity or quality of collagen produced. Many of these disorders can be traced to specific mutations in collagen genes, but there are myriad such mutations. The phenotype of OI is quite variable and can include mildly affected individuals who are of normal stature without any skeletal deformities, and can extend to include people with extensive bony fragility who suffer dozens of fractures during childhood and are short with deformed bowed extremities and abnormal facial appearance. The most severe form of OI is fatal in the perinatal period.

The orthopaedic surgeon may be involved in operative management of the fractures and deformities that result from OI. Diagnosis of milder forms of OI among children with frequent fractures is easy if the sclerae are abnormal (blue or grey) but can be challenging if they are normal (white). It can be particularly difficult to distinguish mild OI from inflicted injury.

Clinical Presentation. OI is a rare condition with an estimated prevalence of 1 in 15,000 to 1 in 20,000 children (142). The hallmark of OI is brittle bones and the tendency to fracture with recurrent fractures occurring in childhood, in particular during the preschool years. Bone pain is a feature in many patients. It is described as chronic and unremitting and usually relates to old fractures. Muscle weakness may be variously present. Ligamentous laxity and joint hypermobility may be present. Wormian bones are present in the skull in approximately 60% of patients. Abnormal collagen in the eye leads to the blue or gray–blue sclerae classically associated with OI. Abnormal collagen in the teeth leads to dentinogenesis imperfecta (clinically small, deformed teeth which are "opalescent" due to a higher ratio of transparent enamel to opaque dentin), which is present in some, but not all, patients with OI (143–148).

The clinical presentation of OI is heterogeneous across a very wide spectrum. The most utilized clinical classification scheme is based on that first proposed by Sillence in 1979 (148). The Sillence classification has stood the test of time and is a useful way of dividing the phenotype. This classification has recently been modified (146, 149) to incorporate the genetic and biochemical abnormalities (Table 6-4). Greater genetic understanding has led to the addition of extra types to the four OI types initially described by Sillence.

Type I Osteogenesis Imperfecta—Mild. Type I OI is nondeforming. Patients are of normal or low normal height and

TABLE 6-4	Classification of Osteogenesis Imperfecta			
Type	Skeletal Manifestation	Sclerae	Teeth	Collagen Defect
I	Mild	Blue	Normal (IA) or dentinogenesis imperfecta (IB)	Quantitative deficiency, but normal collagen
II	Lethal			Abnormal collagen or severe quantitative deficiency
III	Severe	White	Dentinogenesis imperfecta	Abnormal collagen
IV	Moderate	White	Normal (IVA) or dentinogenesis imperfecta (IVB)	Abnormal collagen

do not have limb deformities. They share the hallmark of bony fragility and often have multiple fractures during childhood. Fractures become less common after puberty. Blue sclerae are present in Type I OI. Fifty percent of patients also have pre-senile deafness (150, 151). This presents typically in the third decade of life and therefore is not helpful for diagnosing children (152). The deafness itself has a conductive component and a sensorineural component and sometimes of a sufficient severity to require surgery for the ossicles of the ears, or cochlear implantation in severe cases (153, 154). Fractures that occur in Type I OI include spiral and transverse fractures of long bones, particularly lower extremity bones. In addition, avulsion type fractures such as olecranon fractures (155) and patellar fractures are common and are related to the decreased tensile strength of the bone because of its underlying low collagen content.

Type II Osteogenesis Imperfecta—Lethal Perinatal. This is the most severe form of OI, and patients die at or shortly after birth. They are born with crumpled femora and crumpled ribs accompanied by pulmonary hypoplasia, which usually leads to death. Central nervous system malformations and hemorrhages are common due to markedly abnormal collagen being produced. Lethal OI can be diagnosed by prenatal utlrasonography. Short broad limbs are identified with low echogenicity and low shadowing, and it is easier to see soft-tissue features such as orbits or arterial pulsations within the fetus. At present, it is not possible to reliably distinguish on prenatal ultrasound between lethal Type II OI and severe but survivable OI Type III described below. Most patients with the lethal form of OI have blue sclerae, though some are born with white sclerae (147, 148, 156, 157).

Type III Osteogenesis Imperfecta—Severe. This is the most severe survivable OI group. These patients have a relatively large skull but undeveloped facial bones leading to a characteristic triangular appearance of the face. The sclerae of patients with Type III OI are described as pale blue at birth, but they become normal in color by puberty. Patients are short with severe limb deformities including bowing and coxa vara (Fig. 6-9). Multiple vertebral compression fractures lead to severe scoliosis and kyphosis and rib cage deformity. Many patients use a wheelchair for mobility or require a walking aid if they walk. Radiographic characteristics include very osteopenic

bones with deformity related to previous fracturing. A characteristic popcorn appearance of the epiphysis and metaphysis occurs in early childhood. Up to 25% of these patients will have a coxa vara deformity (158). Pedicles of the vertebrae are elongated. The vertebrae are wedged and may assume a codfish biconcave morphology. Posterior rib fractures are seen. Additional clinical features can include basilar invagination of the skull. This can present with headache, lower cranial nerve palsy, dysphagia, limb hyperreflexia, nystagmus, hearing loss, or quadriparesis. These patients often have multiple fractures when they are born, but they do not have the severe thoracic deformities seen in Type II OI. Fractures heal at the normal rate but recur frequently during childhood particularly in the pre-school years, and some patients have over 100 fractures with this form of OI (156, 157).

Type IV Osteogenesis Imperfecta—Moderate. Type IV OI describes patients with a moderate clinical presentation. Most have short stature and many have bowing and vertebral fractures; although they are not as severely involved as those with Type III OI. Most of them are ambulatory, though some use walking aids. There is a wide range of age at the first fracture and number of fractures in people with Type IV OI. Dentinogenesis imperfecta may be present or absent in these patients. The sclerae are typically white (147, 148).

Additional Types. The four main presentations described by Sillence cover the vast majority of people presenting with OI. There is some overlap in the phenotypes that can be difficult to distinguish—for instance, Type III from Type IV OI. As the genetic defects are understood, there has been the addition of at least three more types of OI, which do not fit into the scheme above. Type V OI is described as hypercallus variety of OI (159). These patients develop profuse amounts of extraosseous callus following their fractures (Fig. 6-10), and the presentation can be confused clinically and radiographically with an osteosarcoma, although Type V OI usually occurs in a much younger child. An additional clinical feature is the ossification of interosseous membranes in between the tibia and fibula, and between the radius and ulna. This leads to the clinical sign of diminished or absent pronation and supination of the forearm, which can help suggest the diagnosis. Over 80% of patients with Type V OI have subluxation or dislocation

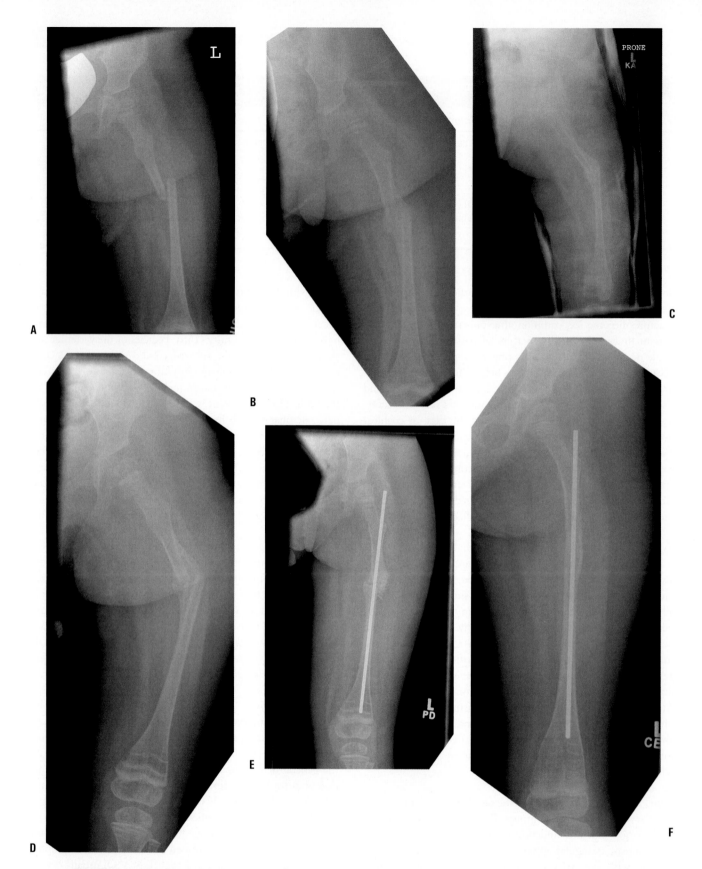

FIGURE 6-9. This female infant with severe OI presented at 19 months of age with a left femoral fracture **(A)** which was treated in a spica cast and healed **(B)**. A refracture was treated in a spica **(C)** with progressive varus. At age 2, a second refracture occurred through the varus malunion **(D)** and was treated with open IM Williams rodding **(E)**. Three years later the femur is intact and has grown distally, as evidenced by the position of the rod and by the transverse metaphyseal lines that occur with each pamidronate treatment cycle **(F)**.

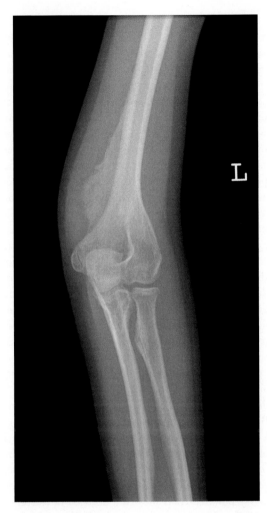

FIGURE 6-10. Osteogenesis imperfecta. The excess callus formation around the distal humerus following injury (no displaced fracture was seen) is typical of type V OI.

of the radial head, which is related to the ossification of the interosseous membrane and may be difficult to treat (160). Type VI OI includes people who phenotypically appear to have moderate or severe OI similar to a Type IV presentation (161). However, they are known to have normal collagen, and they have a defect in new bone mineralization without having any of the biochemical abnormalities or growth plate deformities associated with rickets. The exact etiology of this condition remains uncertain. Type VII OI was initially described in a cohort of First Nations individuals from Quebec, Canada (162). These patients are rhizomelic with deformities characteristically coxa vara of the long bones. The bone is histologically similar to that as seen in Type I OI. Linkage analysis shows that the defect is on chromosome 3 and, therefore, is not in a collagen gene.

Etiology of Osteogenesis Imperfecta.   Most presentations of OI are caused by mutations within the collagen 1A1 gene found on chromosome 7q, or mutations in the collagen 1A2

gene found on chromosome 17q. The complete list of mutations found is kept up-to-date at the Osteogenesis Imperfecta Mutation Database at www.le.ac.uk/genetics/collagen.

Two different types of mutations produce OI. OI Type I, which is the mild form, is a *quantitative* defect in collagen production resulting from a silenced allele of the collagen 1A1 gene (146, 163, 164). This is usually the result of a premature stop code on within the gene. This results in the production of nonsense messenger RNA instead of proper messenger RNA coding for the preprocollagen molecule. The nonsense messenger RNA is detected and destroyed, and the result is production of a diminished number of alpha 1 chains, and consequently a decreased quantity of normal collagen being produced. With the decreased quantity of collagen, the bone is weakened and more susceptible to microfractures. Bone can sense its mechanical environment, and microfractures cause a new round of bone removal and reformation. This leads to constant activation of bone remodeling in OI. This demands an increased transcriptional activity of Type I collagen and induces an increased number of osteoclasts and an increase in the excretion of collagen degradation of products. Bone turns over rapidly but remains of poor quality. When growth ceases at puberty, and the transcriptional activity demand is reduced and bone turnover can slow down, then the bone strength and architecture becomes closer to normal and the fracture rate drops.

OI Types II, III, and IV are usually caused by production of *abnormal types of collagen* (146, 165). The collagen molecule is a triple helix formed by spontaneous self-assembly of three long linear procollagen molecules. These procollagen molecules have a typical repeating amino acid pattern of glycine XY-glycine XY-glycine XY. Glycine appears every third position because it is the smallest amino acid and can be folded into the interior of the triple helix. Glycine substitutions place a larger amino acid where the glycine residue belongs, so the collagen triple helix cannot assemble appropriately. The collagen molecule begins assembling at the C-terminal end and assembles toward the N-terminal end. If the mutation substitutes for a glycine close to the C-terminus at the beginning of the molecule, then a very short strand of abnormal gene product is produced and the corresponding clinical diseases are severe. If the glycine substitution mutation is toward the distal N-terminus end, then a longer partial collagen molecule can be formed, and the clinical phenotype is less severe.

The primary defect in OI is the osteoporosis produced by abnormal quantity or quality of collagen. Mechanically the bone is more ductile, rather than being more brittle (166). To this is added secondary osteoporosis caused by immobilization following fractures or surgery, or because of decreased physical activity and weight bearing with severe deformity. Prevention of the secondary osteoporosis is an important concept when treating fractures, planning surgery, or recommending general care.

Diagnosis.   The clinical diagnosis of OI is the mainstay. There is no single laboratory test that distinguishes people with OI from those with normal bone. The clinical features of severe OI Type II and Type III are distinct enough that physical findings and plain radiography are usually sufficient to arrive at a diagnosis. Patients with Type I OI have blue or blue–grey sclerae and are readily identified clinically. Normal babies may have blue sclerae until 1 year of age, so this finding is only diagnostic in the older child. Patients with mild presentations of Type IV OI are easy to diagnose if they have dentinogenesis imperfecta, but those with normal teeth may benefit from additional investigation depending on the purpose of making the diagnosis. Dual energy x-ray absorptiometry (DEXA) scanning shows low lumbar and femoral BMD in mild OI patients (167, 168). Published values for BMD in healthy normal children are available for comparison (169). Caution must be exercised in interpreting DEXA scans in children, and overdiagnosis of osteoporosis is reported to be frequent (170). This is because DEXA scanning reports BMD per square centimeter surface area of bone, ignoring the third dimension (thickness of the bone in the path of the photon) which is larger in adults leading to greater area density even if true volumetric density were the same.

Dozens of individual mutations have been found within collagen 1A1 and collagen 1A2 genes producing the main phenotypes of Type I, Type II, Type III, and Type IV OI (146, 156, 157, 164, 171). As such, many new patients often have new mutations specific to themselves. Accordingly, a DNA-based genetic test for OI is usually performed only at reference laboratories at present. An intermediate level of testing involves culturing dermal fibroblasts and studying the amount and quality of collagen that they produce. Quantitatively, abnormal collagen production can be detected in 87% of individuals with known OI. Conversely, 13% of individuals with known OI would be missed by a cultured dermal fibroblast test. One common question is whether a person has OI or inflicted trauma. OI is very rare and inflicted injury remains significantly more prevalent. Clinical diagnosis remains a gold standard to distinguish these two entities and cultured dermal fibroblast testing is not considered useful as a routine part of such investigation (172). In cases with legal implications, positive findings in the history, past history, family history, clinical examination, or properly interpreted DEXA scan may assist in the diagnosis of osteoporosis or OI. OI cannot be entirely ruled out in patients with negative findings, but is a highly unlikely diagnosis in the presence of positive findings suggesting child abuse (discussed elsewhere). Finally, a diagnosis of OI does not exclude the possibility of child abuse.

Osteogenesis Imperfecta—Medical Treatment. Cyclical administration of intravenous bisphosphonates has recently become popular in the pharmacologic management of *severe* OI, but cannot currently be recommended for mild OI. Bisphosphonates are widely used drugs based on the pyrophosphate molecule, which is the only natural inhibitor to bone resorption. The drugs all bind strongly to bone, with the primary action at the level of the osteoclast. Osteoclast toxicity from ATP analogues is thought to be important to the mechanism of action.

Clinical reports of the use of bisphosphonate in OI began with case series, and much of the published evidence remains case series. Glorieux reported the effects of bisphosphonate treatment in uncontrolled observational study of 30 patients with severe OI (173). The intravenous dosing given was 3 mg/kg of pamidronate per cycle by slow intravenous infusion at 4-month intervals. All patients were given 800 to 1000 mg calcium per day and 400 international units of vitamin D per day. Marked improvement in patient's clinical status was noted. There was an average of 42% per year increase of BMD. There was an increase in the cortical width of the metacarpals and in the size of the vertebral bodies. Average number of fractures dropped from 2.3 per year to 0.6 per year. No nonunions or delayed unions of any fractures were noted. Patients reported a marked reduction of bone pain 1 to 6 weeks following initiation of treatment. The only adverse effect noted was the acute phase reaction comprising fever, back pain, and limb pain on day 2 of the first cycle. This was treated with acetaminophen and did not recur with subsequent infusion cycles. Patient's mobility improved in 16 of the 30 patients treated with no change in 14. Growth rates increased. Patients under 3 years of age showed a faster and more pronounced effect of the bisphosphonate. The direct effect of the bisphosphonate is decreasing bone resorption and turnover. The resulting decreasing bone pain and fractures resulted in increased weight bearing and mobility. It is likely that the increased weight bearing and mobility resulted in further strengthening of bone and muscle.

Bisphosphonate treatment has become a standard for severe OI, and the clinical literature supporting it now includes randomized clinical trials. A Cochrane review found eight randomized clinical trials supporting the use of bisphosphonates in severe OI (174). All trials showed an increase in BMD, and adequately powered trials showed a decrease in fracture rates. Oral or IV bisphosphonates were both effective. A high-quality placebo-controlled trial showed oral olpadronate effective at increasing BMD and decreasing fractures (175). Improvements in functional outcomes and quality of life have not been shown in randomized trials to date, although case series suggest they are present (176, 177). It should be noted that this drug does not address the basic abnormality underlying OI, but it does alter the natural course of the disease. Radiographs of patients with OI treated with cyclic intravenous bisphosphonates show characteristic dense sclerotic lines which form at the growth plate, one per treatment cycle (178).

Duration and continuity of bisphosphonate therapy has not been optimized in children. Stopping bisphosphonate treatment while rapid growth remains may result in a marked reduction in metaphyseal bone mineral content (179), and prolonged use has not been shown to adversely affect the mechanical properties of bone in children with OI (180), so there is a tendency to continue treatment, perhaps at a lower dose, while growth remains. Fracture healing in children is not impaired by bisphosphonates, and the evidence regarding osteotomy treatment is contradictory (181, 182) with one series reporting no delay and another reporting delay—in the latter case, the osteotomies were done open and with powered saws. Lower extremity nonunions in the presence of rods are often asymptomatic and clinically unimportant, but distal humeral malunions can be disabling and challenging to treat (183). Some surgeons recommend discontinuing bisphosphonate treatment for 6 weeks before and after planned osteotomy surgery, but this recommendation may change as evidence accumulates.

Concerns about the potential negative consequences of using bisphosphonates over the long term still exist. Pamidronate binds strongly to bone and is released only slowly, so demonstrable amounts have been reported in the urine of patients many years after the cessation of therapy (184). Animal studies show bisphosphonate crosses from the placenta to the fetus, although no adverse fetal outcomes have yet been reported in series of mothers who were taking bisphosphonates prior to or during pregnancy (185, 186). Similarly, despite the concern about osteonecrosis of the jaw in adult patients taking bisphosphonates, there is no clinical evidence of this complication among 64 pediatric patients with 38 dental procedures (187) nor is the author aware of case reports of this complication in children.

Caution must be exercised in extending the indications for bisphosphonate treatment to patients with milder forms of OI. Reported clinical results apply only to patients with severe OI. Osteopetrosis is a reported complication of bisphosphonates in humans (188). Animal studies suggest reduced longitudinal bone growth with these drugs (189–191). Randomized controlled clinical trials are needed before routine clinical use of bisphosphonates in milder forms of OI is considered.

Other medical treatments for OI include anabolic agents, specifically human growth hormone. Human growth hormone is an anabolic agent, therefore, stimulates increased bone turnover—causing a higher demand for collagen transcription and perhaps exacerbating the underlying abnormality while attempting to ameliorate the decreased stature. Because growth hormone may have both beneficial and negative effects in OI, clinical research results are required before indications can be stated. We suggest at present that growth hormone be used in OI patients only in the context of clinical research studies.

Osteogenesis Imperfecta—Surgical Treatment.
Patients with mild (nondeforming) OI require little modification of standard surgical treatments, whereas those with severe (deforming) OI require multiple specialized surgical techniques and implants.

A newer elongating rod design, the Fassier-Duval rod (Figs. 6-11 to 6-18) has cancellous screw threads at either end to provide stable anchorage in the epiphysis or metaphysis (192). The need for revision due to bone growth and rod migration was reported as higher for nonelongating rods in one series (193), but approximately equal to that seen with elongating rods in another (194). Methods of rod exchange via percutaneous techniques have been described (195, 196), and a stereotactic device to assist this has been developed (196) but is not in wide clinical use.

Tiley reported on 129 roddings among 13 children, of whom 11 maintained or gained the ability to ambulate (197). Most reports suggest that ambulation is improved by rodding (198–201), but one emphasizes the possibility of ambulatory status worsening in a large number of patients (202). The ultimate walking prognosis in OI is much more strongly influenced by subtype than by treatment (203–205), but modern combinations of medical and surgical treatment combined with rapid advances in the understanding of the biology of the disease may one day change this. Current trends are toward percutaneous or minimal open osteotomies, multiple bones rodded simultaneously, elongating rods, and postoperative splinting instead of casting with early supervised ambulation (206).

The Spine in Osteogenesis Imperfecta.
Scoliosis (Fig. 6-19) can be very challenging to treat in patients with OI (207–216). Progressive curves beyond 25 degrees are more common in Type III OI, and are associated with lower BMD (217). There is no evidence yet that bisphosphonate treatment prevents scoliosis. Bracing appears to be ineffective at preventing curve progression even when curves are small (213, 216). Patients with large progressive curves may suffer from pulmonary compromise, and bracing can cause rib deformities which worsen this. It is unknown whether operative management of the scoliosis leads to improved pulmonary function, quality of life, and survival. Accordingly, operative decision making must be individualized for each patient. Spinal fusions have a higher complication rate in OI, with 20 patients of 60 experiencing a total of 33 major complications (213). The most common complications were blood loss >2.5L (9 cases), intraoperative hook pullout (5 cases), postoperative hook pullout (5 cases), and pseudarthrosis (5 cases). Strategies to prevent hook pullout include load sharing via segmental instrumentation, supplementation of hook site bone with methylmethacrylate, and consideration of fusion without instrumentation. Preoperative medical treatment (bisphosphonate) to strengthen the bone is logical but results are not yet reported. Progression of the curve postoperatively, with or without pseudarthrosis, may occur (213). The natural history, expectations, likelihood of complications, and likelihood of success must be carefully assessed for each patient, and decisions not to embark on surgical reconstruction are sometimes correct.

Spondylolysis of the lumbar spine was found in only 5.3% of patients with OI at a national referral program clinic, a rate similar to that in the normal population (218).

Cervical Spinal Conditions in Osteogenesis Imperfecta.
Anterior decompression and posterior stabilization of the cervical spine for basilar invagination was reported in 20 patients with a median follow-up of 10 years. Twenty-five percent of patients had recurrence of deformity or death, 15% had no improvement, and 60% improved or stabilized (219). In addition to surgery for basilar invagination, some OI patients have required anterior corpectomy for upper cervical kyphosis with spinal cord compression (220) and some have required shunting for obstructive hydrocephalus, or craniotomy for subdural and epidural bleeding following no or minor trauma (221).

Text continued on page 161

Fassier-Duval Technique for Growing Rods of Femur in Osteogenesis Imperfecta (Figs. 6-11 to 6-18)

FIGURE 6-11. Fassier-Duval Technique for Growing Rods of Femur in Osteogenesis Imperfecta: Step 1. Perform the first osteotomy through a lateral incision where the proximal apex of deformity will permit a straight rod to reach the trochanter. Image intensifier control is recommended. Pay extra attention to the lateral view when planning this osteotomy as there is often marked apex anterior angulation in addition to a varus deformity.

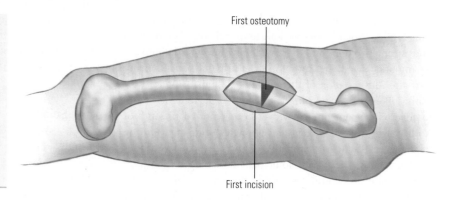

FIGURE 6-12. Step 2. Ream the proximal fragment up to the tip of the greater trochanter over a flexible guide wire.

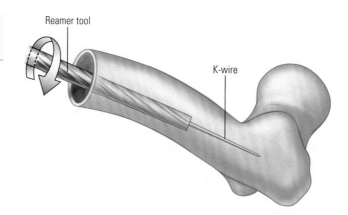

FIGURE 6-13. Step 3. Perform a second more distal osteotomy if needed to place a straight rod. Insert a male size K-wire retrograde from the more distal osteotomy and make an incision in the buttock to allow the K-wire to exit proximally.

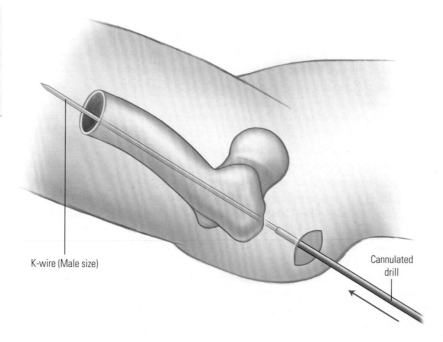

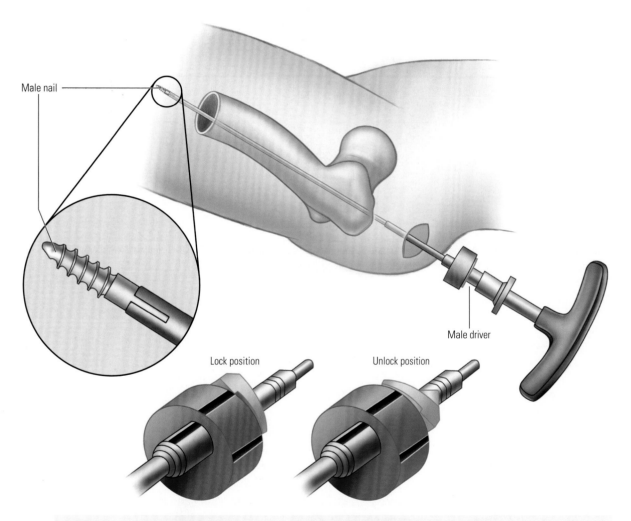

Male nail

Male driver

Lock position

Unlock position

FIGURE 6-14. **Step 4.** Introduce the male driver over the K-wire. Remove the K-wire and introduce the male nail into the driver working retrograde through the more distal osteotomy.

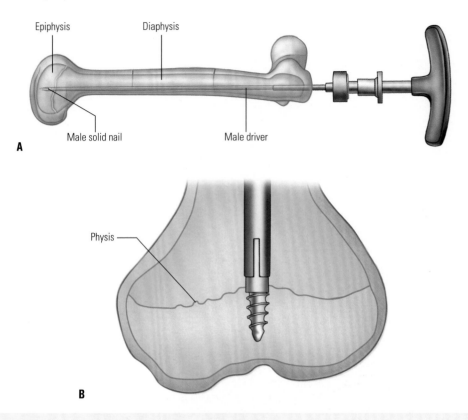

FIGURE 6-15. **Step 5. A:** Reduce the femur and push the male nail and driver into the distal fragment. Avoid bending the nail. **B:** Screw the threaded portion into the centre of the epiphysis.

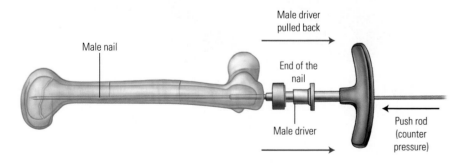

FIGURE 6-16. **Step 6.** Stabilize the male nail with a pushrod while removing the male driver.

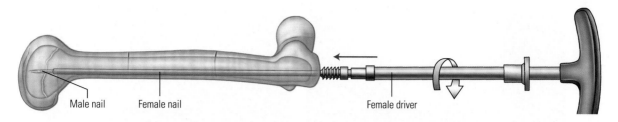

Male nail   Female nail   Female driver

FIGURE 6-17. **Step 7.** Introduce the precut hollow female nail over the male nail and screw it in to the trochanter.

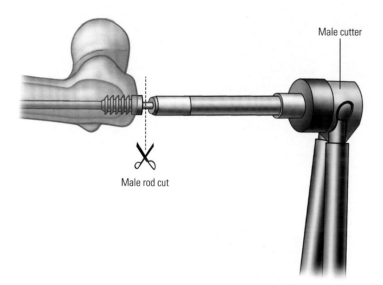

Male cutter

Male rod cut

FIGURE 6-18. **Step 8.** Cut the male nail leaving 10 to 15 mm prominent and confirm a smooth end for gliding with growth.

Juvenile Idiopathic Osteoporosis. Idiopathic juvenile osteoporosis is a rare condition (222). Onset is typically 2 to 3 years prior to puberty, and patients present with vertebral (Fig. 6-20) or long bone fractures and bone pain. Fractures are typically metaphyseal in location. Kyphosis, scoliosis, and pectus carinatum deformities can be present. BMD is decreased 2.5 standard deviations below age-appropriate norms. Idiopathic juvenile osteoporosis is a diagnosis of exclusion, other primary and secondary causes of osteoporosis must be excluded (Table 6-3). There are no lab abnormalities specific to the diagnosis and the genetic cause is as yet unknown. Treatment includes optimizing calcium and vitamin D intake and promoting physical activity including weight bearing and strength training but avoiding trauma. Bracing can be used to treat vertebral pain and to prevent progression of kyphotic deformities (223). Judicious use of bisphosphonate therapy may be considered in severe cases. A remarkable remission of the condition at puberty is common.

Other Forms of Primary Osteoporosis in Children. As well as OI and idiopathic juvenile osteoporosis, there are several other primary causes of reduced BMD in children. Children with Ehlers-Danlos syndrome, Marfan syndrome, and homocystinuria have reduced bone mass. Those who suffer fractures or bone pain as well can be considered to have a form of primary osteoporosis, but fractures are not as typical a feature of these conditions as they are of OI. Like OI, these conditions are based on known deficiencies in the production of structural proteins. They are discussed in other chapters.

Bruck syndrome is a rare primary form of osteoporosis. The phenotype is similar to OI with thin bones, fractures, bone pain, and blue or white sclerae. Joint contractures are a distinctive clinical characteristic of Bruck syndrome (224). The condition is a result of failure to crosslink collagen fibrils, which is specific to bone tissue (225).

Osteoporosis pseudoglioma syndrome is an autosomal recessive disorder phenotypically similar to OI but accompanied

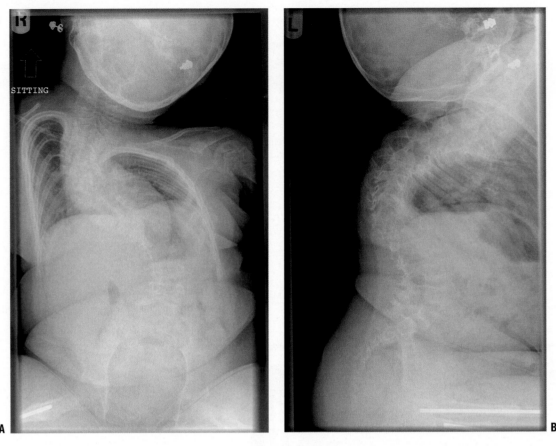

FIGURE 6-19. **A,B:** Osteogenesis imperfecta. Marked spinal deformity in a 5-year-old girl with severe OI.

FIGURE 6-20. Juvenile idiopathic osteoporosis. This 14-year-old boy has marked osteoporosis evident on plain radiographs (DEXA scans indicated bone mineral densities 2.8 standard deviations below mean) and a healed compression fracture at T7.

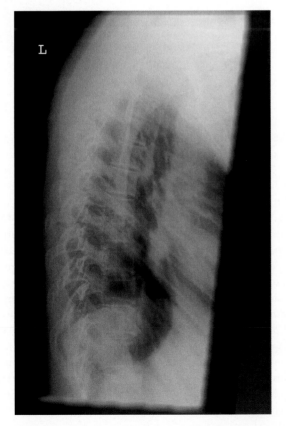

by congenital blindness due to hyperplasia of the vitreous (226, 227). The mutation is in the low-density lipoprotein receptor related protein 5 gene (228). Treatment with bisphosphonates has been successful (229). Operative management of fractures with IM rodding techniques has encountered complications related to severe fragility of bone (230).

Secondary Osteoporosis in Children.

Bone mass responds to biochemical, hormonal, and mechanical signals as described in the first part of the chapter. Interference with normal homeostatic mechanisms leads to a reduced bone mass—for example, many children have disuse osteopenia following fracture treatment. Resumption of load bearing after healing allows this to normalize. In conditions where weight bearing is reduced, persistent low bone mass can lead to low energy fractures and a fracture cascade of repeated fractures in the same extremity.

Neuromuscular Disorders.

The central nervous system exerts direct control over BMD. The fat-derived hormone leptin acts on hypothalamic neurons, which mediate bone mass via the sympathetic nerves (231–234). Clinical significance of this recent finding has not been elucidated, but it may become important in managing osteoporosis and related regional conditions such as reflex sympathetic dystrophy. At present, the management of neuromuscular osteoporosis focuses on the downstream effects of the neuromuscular abnormalities on load bearing and nutrition.

Low bone mass is observed in cerebral palsy (CP) patients (235–239). Typically, it is nonambulatory patients with the lowest bone masses who are at risk for pathologic and low energy fractures, but the reduced bone mass has been observed in the affected limb of ambulatory hemiplegics (240, 241), suggesting that both weight bearing and muscle forces play a role in establishment and maintenance of bone mass. Undernutrition is the second most important predictor of low bone mass in CP patients, after ambulation (239, 242). Fractures and a "fracture cascade" of increasing disuse osteoporosis from treatment-related immobilization can cause significant problems for many patients (243, 244). Fracture prevalence among children and adolescents with moderate to severe CP was 26% in one study (239). The orthopaedic surgeon should focus as much on the prevention as on the treatment of osteoporosis in the CP population. Increasing weight bearing, optimizing nutrition, and minimizing the extent and duration of immobilization following surgery are important. A controlled trial of weight bearing in CP patients showed significant increases in femoral neck bone mineral content (245). Medical treatments including vitamin D and calcium (246) or bisphosphonates (236, 247, 248) have also been reported to increase BMD in CP patients, although the precise indications for their prescription are unclear. More recent evidence shows that BMD returns toward pretreatment baseline in nonambulatory CP patients after discontinuation of bisphosphonate therapy (249). Approximately one-third of children without CP sustain a fracture during childhood, so the 26% fracture prevalence among children with CP does not seem out of line. Accordingly, if weight bearing is easy to achieve and

enjoyable for the child, it can be recommended; but if extensive surgery, elaborate standers, and many hours of professional care are required, then perhaps it is not of benefit to the child.

Patients with Duchenne muscular dystrophy (DMD) lose bone mass as lower extremities weaken, with bone densities 1.6 standard deviations below the mean while still walking and 4 standard deviations below the mean once nonambulatory. Of 41 boys followed, 18 sustained a fracture, 12 of which were lower extremity fractures, and 4 of which caused loss of ambulation (250). BMD has been reported as lower among boys treated with steroids (prednisone) than among untreated boys with DMD (251). Deflazacort is a steroid medication which preserves muscle strength, ambulation, and respiratory function as well as prevents the onset of scoliosis. Despite being a glucocorticoid analogue, it is reported as having bone sparing effects (252) and randomized trial evidence (in juvenile arthritis) shows less bone loss among deflazacort treated patients compared with prednisone treated patients (253). Vertebral fractures have been reported in patients treated with deflazacort (254) while they are rare among untreated boys (250). A single clinical case series reported positive effects on BMD following daily oral alendronate for 2 years, with better response seen in younger boys (255).

Endocrine/Metabolic Disorders

Growth Hormone Deficiency. Growth hormone deficiency results in extreme short stature and low muscle mass. BMD is low in both adults and children, and adults have a 2.7 times increased fracture rate compared with normal controls (256). Treating the deficiency with growth hormone improves longitudinal growth and muscle mass as well as improving calcium absorption, so exerts beneficial effects on the osteoporosis both mechanically and biologically. Improved BMD with growth hormone treatment has been documented in adults but requires further study in children (257, 258).

It is noteworthy that growth hormone deficiency is the second most common endocrinologic cause of slipped capital femoral epiphysis (after hypothyroidism). Ninety-two percent of children with growth hormone deficiency and SCFE present with the slip *after* growth hormone treatment has been initiated perhaps because the growth plate becomes more active, and potentially mechanically weaker relative to the larger size of the body. The prevalence of bilaterality in slips with endocrinopathies has been reported to be as high as 61%, so prophylactic pinning of the contralateral side is suggested by some (259). Among 2922 children followed prospectively while receiving growth hormone in Australia and New Zealand, only 10 slipped epiphyses were reported by clinicians performing active surveillance for complications (260).

Hyperthyroidism. Hyperthyroidism leads to bone loss through increased bone turnover. T3 directly stimulates osteoblasts, which results in linked osteoclast activation and bone resorption. The increase in serum calcium and phosphate suppresses PTH and 1,25-dihydroxyvitamin D production, which decreases calcium and phosphate absorption and increases calcium excretion. The net result is bone resorption in a high turnover state (222). Treatment of the underlying disease to achieve a euthyroid state is the appropriate management for the osteoporosis.

Disorders of Puberty. One-third to one-half of adult bone mass is accrued during the pubertal years, and sex steroids are necessary for this accelerated bone mineral accrual. Mineral accrual lags behind the longitudinal growth spurt by a year or two, perhaps partially explaining the increased fracture rate documented during and just after the growth spurt (261). Over the past 30 years, there has been a statistically significant increase in the incidence of distal forearm fractures in adolescents, but it is unclear whether this relates to changes in diet or in physical activity (262).

Precocious puberty results in accelerated growth and bone mineral accrual. It can be treated with GnRH analogues to preserve epiphyseal function and allow attainment of greater final height. Such treatment does not adversely affect peak bone mass. Constitutionally, delayed puberty in boys is associated with lower BMD, but it is unclear whether testosterone treatment improves overall mineral acquisition (222).

Athletic amenorrhea is common among young women training for endurance sports, particularly distance running. Thirty-one percent of college-level athletes not using oral contraceptives reported athletic amenorrhea or oligomenorrhea (263). Athletic amenorrhea plus disordered eating plus osteoporosis has been dubbed the "female athlete triad" (264, 265). The full triad is rare among athletes (266) and was found to be nonexistent among female army recruits (267). Not all sports are equal in propensity to bone loss. Gymnasts exhibit higher bone mass than do runners despite similar prevalence of amenorrhea, (268), gymnasts have both higher muscle strength (269) and higher serum insulin like growth factor 1 (IGF-I) (270) than do runners and these are both protective of bone mass. It must be remembered that for the general population, more exercise means more bone, as has been demonstrated in randomized trials of physical activity in prepubescent and pubescent children (271, 272).

Untreated anorexia nervosa is associated with 4% to 10% trabecular and cortical bone loss per year (273). The long-term prevalence of fractures among people with anorexia nervosa is 57% at 40-year follow-up, 2.9 times higher than that in the general population (274). Estrogen alone is insufficient to restore BMD, particularly if nutrition is compromised (275, 276). Restoration of body mass, provision of adequate calcium and vitamin D, and correction of the hormonal environment should all occur.

Primary amenorrhea from pure dysfunction of the hypothalamic–pituitary axis was associated with osteoporosis in three and osteopenia in 10 of 19 girls (ages 16 to 18), compared with 0 of 20 controls with regular cycles (277).

Drug Related

Glucocorticoids. Steroids are commonly used to treat a variety of acute and chronic medical conditions. Frequent short courses of oral glucocorticoids (for asthma exacerbations) have been shown not to adversely affect BMD in children (278), but chronic glucocorticoid use is a well-established cause of osteoporosis and is common among patients with juvenile arthritis, leukemia, and organ transplantation. The underlying mechanism includes osteoblast apoptosis and decreased intestinal calcium absorption and renal reabsorption (222). Deflazacort is a bone sparing glucocorticoid (252) and randomized trial evidence (in juvenile arthritis) shows less bone loss among deflazacort treated patients compared with prednisone treated patients (253). In adults using glucocorticoids, there are now multiple trials demonstrating that bisphosphonates and teriparatide (a synthetic analogue of PTH) are useful for prevention and treatment of bone loss, and for prevention of fractures (279–284). Case series of bisphosphonate use in children on chronic glucocorticoid treatment have shown similar promising results; however, teriparatide is not used in children because of the potential for malignancy in growing bone (255, 285, 286).

Anticonvulsants. An association between altered bone mineral metabolism and anticonvulsant drugs has long been discussed (287–293), although the exact mechanism by which anticonvulsants interfere with bone metabolism remains unknown. Induction of liver enzymes with increased vitamin D catabolism has been proposed (294, 295), but vitamin D metabolism has been conflictingly reported as normal (296, 297). There is laboratory evidence that phenytoin and carbamazepine exert a direct effect on bone cells (298). Quantitative CT studies of the distal radius in patients using carbamazepine or valproic acid (for isolated epilepsy, without CP) showed decreased trabecular BMD but a compensatory increase in cortical BMD in a high bone turnover state (299). A controlled trial has shown that treatment with vitamin D and calcium increases BMD in children with severe CP, who are receiving anticonvulsants (246).

Miscellaneous. Other drugs reported to cause osteopenia and osteoporosis in children include methotrexate, cyclosporine, and heparin. Little information on prevention and treatment of the iatrogenic osteoporosis in children is available (222).

SCLEROSING BONE CONDITIONS IN CHILDREN

Osteopetrosis. Osteopetrosis is the most common and the most well-known of the sclerosing bony dysplasias. All of these conditions are characterized by an imbalance between the formation and the resorption of bone favoring formation. In osteopetrosis, it is decreased or completely failed resorption of bone due to an osteoclast defect which tips the balance to favor formation.

Three clinical presentations of osteopetrosis are traditionally described (300). The infantile or autosomal recessive form is the most severe and can be fatal in the first decade. Patients present with pathologic fractures or with an exceedingly dense radiographic appearance of the bones (Fig. 6-21). They can have cranial nerve problems including optic nerve compression and blindness, facial nerve dysfunction, and sensorineural deafness due to narrowing of the skull foramina. They can have bone pain related to fractures or stress fractures.

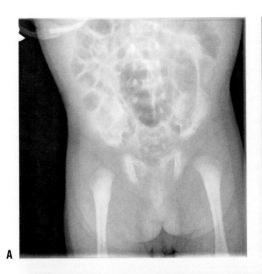

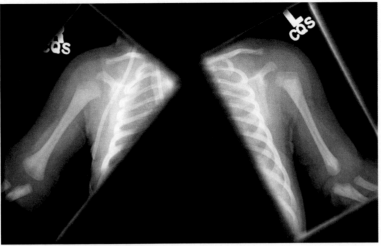

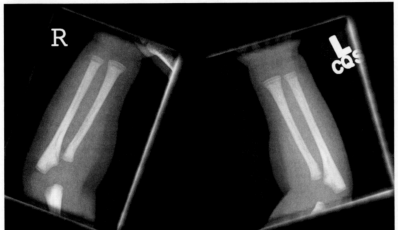

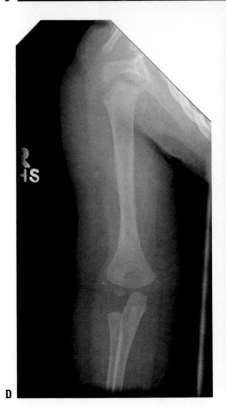

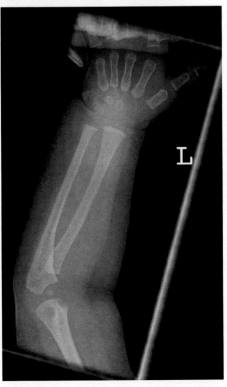

FIGURE 6-21. Six-month-old male infant with severe osteopetrosis and pancytopenia. **A–E:** Dense sclerotic bones at the pelvis **(A)**, humerus **(B)**, and forearm **(C)**, without evident medullary cavities. **D, E:** After successful bone marrow transplant the bony architecture in the humerus **(D)** and forearm **(E)** were normalized.

They frequently have infections of the bones or mandibles. Searching nystagmus is described. Patients are pale due to anemia and hepatosplenomegaly due to extramedullary hematopoiesis. A prominent forehead and broad upper skull with hypertelorism are common features.

The milder autosomal dominant adult form of osteopetrosis can present with pathologic fractures and dull pain in people with mild degrees of short stature and prominent forehead. Other people with the autosomal dominant form are so mildly affected that the diagnosis is made incidentally based on the very curious appearance of the bones.

An intermediate clinical type of osteopetrosis is described and includes patients with more severe phenotypes who survive into adulthood. Classifications, which are based on identification of genetic defect, have begun to expand, so that there are at least six types of osteopetrosis based on the genetic aspects, but the genetic classification is not currently comprehensive enough to replace the clinical classification of the disease (301).

The striking radiographic characteristic is that the bones are dense white without medullary cavities and appear marble-like. A bone within bone or endobone appearance can be seen within the pelvis. Marked sclerosis of the end plates of the vertebral bodies can give a rugger–jersey spine appearance (Fig. 6-22). They can be significant sclerosis of the base of the skull. Failure of metaphyseal cutback by osteoclast leads to an Erlenmeyer flask shape of the epiphysis. Secondary deformities including progressive coxa vara or apex lateral bowing of the femur may be present (300, 302, 303).

Etiology. Osteopetrosis is caused by specific osteoclast defects, which prevent the osteoclast from carrying out its normal function in resorbing bone. Many specific defects have been identified. These include carbonic and hydrase deficiency which prevents the osteoclasts from acidifying the extracellular space at the ruffled border. This is associated with the milder clinical forms and can be associated with distal renal tubular

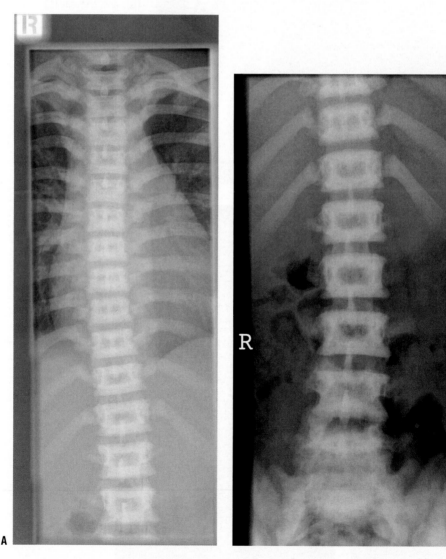

FIGURE 6-22.   A,B: The classic rugger jersey appearance of the spine is seen in this 15-year-old girl with osteopetrosis.

acidosis and with intercranial calcifications which are unique to this form (304–306). Fatal infantile forms of osteopetrosis have been associated with defects in the genes coding for proton pump or chloride channel protein production (307). More recent case reports describe iatrogenic osteopetrosis as a result of bisphosphonate treatment (188, 308).

All causes of osteopetrosis decrease the function of the osteoclast resorbing of bone. The histologic hallmark is remnants of primary spongiosa within the bone. These are areas of calcified cartilage that are precursor to enchondral bone formation and are normally removed during the first pass remodeling in the fetal life. The ongoing failure to resolve and remodel bone leads to the skeletal manifestations of the diseases, limits the narrow space available and contributes to the pancytopenia and hepatosplenomegaly, and is also responsible for the cranial nerve compression at the skull base. The predisposition toward musculoskeletal infections is thought to be a combination of the abnormal bony architecture and the absence of sufficient white blood cells.

Medical Treatment.

Bone marrow transplantation for the severe forms of infantile osteopetrosis was first described in 1977 (309) and this has since been widely reported (310–312). Successful bone marrow transplant corrects both the skeletal and hematologic abnormalities associated with osteopetrosis. However, not all bone marrow transplantations are successful and not all patients have survived. Additional medical treatment can include very high doses of calcitriol to stimulate osteoclastic activity, and the administration of interferon gamma to stimulate superoxide production by osteoclasts. Long-term therapy with interferon gamma in patients with osteopetrosis increases bone resorption and hematopoiesis and improves leukocyte function (313).

Orthopaedic Treatment.

Most patients presenting to pediatric orthopaedists do so because of fractures (314). The majority of fractures in children with osteopetrosis will heal well if treated with closed means, although healing can be delayed (Fig. 6-23). The principle exception to this are fractures of the femoral neck and intratrochanteric region, which can be extremely difficult to manage (Fig. 6-24). In Armstrong's survey of the experience of the Pediatric Orthopaedic Society of North America, there was a high incidence of nonunion and varus deformity of the femur if femoral neck intertrochanteric fractures were treated by closed means. The results of early operative treatment of femoral neck and intertrochanteric fractures were good, but technical difficulties of obtaining fixation in the dense bone were noted. Worn out or broken drills and even drivers were reported. Subtrochanteric and femoral shaft fractures did well with both closed and open management. Most tibial fractures were managed closed. Multiple fractures of the tibia were reported in some patients but could be well managed with cast management.

Cervical spine fractures are rare and involve the posterior elements and were treated with immobilization. Lumbar spondylolysis and listhesis have also been described (314, 315) and have responded well to nonoperative treatment in children and adolescents, but occasionally required spinal fusion in adults.

Acquired coxa vara can be treated with proximal femoral valgus osteotomies fix by conventional plates or screws with similar technical difficulties noted to those encountered treating femoral fractures.

Some patients with osteopetrosis get osteoarthritis of the hip and knee during midlife. These can be treated with total knee arthroplasty and total hip arthroplasty, although difficulty with reaming the canal and cutting the bone surfaces has been noted.

Caffey Disease.

Caffey disease, or infantile cortical hyperostosis, characteristically presents between the ages of 6 weeks and 6 months. The clinical features are of an irritable child, sometimes with fever and with tender soft-tissue swelling over the affected bone. Radiographically, there is abundant subperiosteal new bone and eventually thickening of the cortex (Fig. 6-25). Episodes are usually self-limiting and may recur episodically, but typically resolves by the age of 2 years and most cases do not require any active orthopaedic treatment. Laboratory investigation can show an increased erythrocyte sedimentation rate (ESR), an increased white blood cell count, an increased alkaline phosphatase and an iron deficiency anemia. Differential diagnosis includes child abuse, infection, and metastatic neoplasms. Caffey was a radiologist who initially described the condition while working on the radiographic presentation of child abuse. A recent linkage analysis has demonstrated a mutation in the COL1A1 gene in patients with Caffey disease (316). This mutation is believed to make the periosteum easily separate from the bone in early infancy, accounting for the typical clinical findings. In addition, older patients in the kindred had voluntary subluxation and hyperextension of joints, suggesting ongoing problems related to the abnormal collagen. Table 6-5 presents a listing of other causes of periosteal reaction and cortical thickening in infancy and early childhood.

Pyknodysostosis.

This is similar to osteopetrosis in that it is a manifestation of a failure of bone resorption (Fig.6-26). These patients do not produce cathepsin K which normally degrades bone proteins during bone resorption (317–320). It is inherited as autosomal recessive condition. Patients are mildly short with deformities including pectus excavatum, kyphoscoliosis, an oblique angle of the mandible, failure fusion of the sutures of the skull in adulthood, proptosis, oblique nose, and frontal bossing (321–323). Growth hormone therapy has been used for stature (323). Orthopaedic management is similar to that of osteopetrosis.

Over Production of Bone by Osteoblasts.

There are several rare conditions in which osteoblasts overproduce bone because of abnormalities in normal regulation. These conditions are caused by defects in the transforming growth factor beta (TGF β) super family of proteins which are known to regulate bone growth. The three clinical conditions include melorheostosis, Camurati-Engelmann disease, and sclerostenosis.

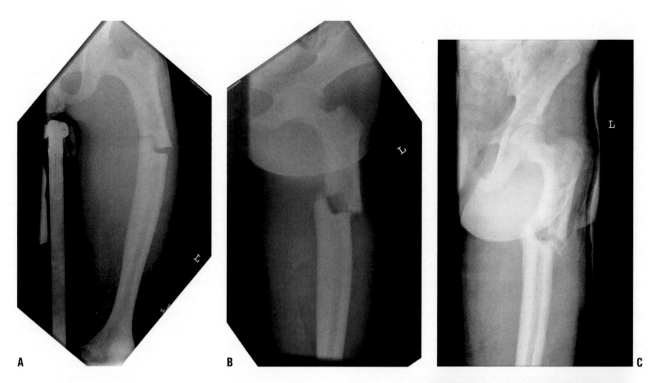

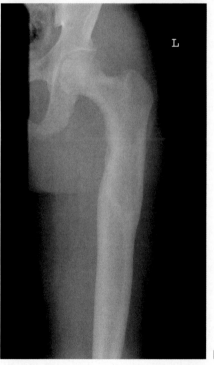

FIGURE 6-23.   A–C: This 15-year-old boy with osteopetrosis sustained a fractured femoral shaft from a fall while running **(A)**. He was successfully treated by traction **(B)** followed by spica casting **(C)**. **D:** One-year follow-up exam.

Melorheostosis is best remembered by its Greek name which describes flowing wax on a burning candle. The condition is characterized by new periosteal and endosteal bone, which resembles dripping wax radiographically. It typically affects one limb or one side and produces irregularities of cortical bone with a lesion or rash overlying on the skin. The etiology is believed to be downregulation of beta IG-H$_3$ (324). Somatic mosaicism is thought to explain the usual single limb manifestation (325). There may be stiffness in the soft tissues and shortening or contracture of the affected extremity and the lesion may present with pain (326). Sarcomas arising in melorheostotic lesions have been reported (327–329). Ilizarov treatment has been useful in treating limb shortening and deformity (330, 331), but abnormal bone and soft-tissue–related complications are recorded (332). Soft-tissue contractures are often more problematic for the patient than the bony deformity, but they are difficult to treat operatively with an over 50% recurrence rate, and complications including distal ischemia (326).

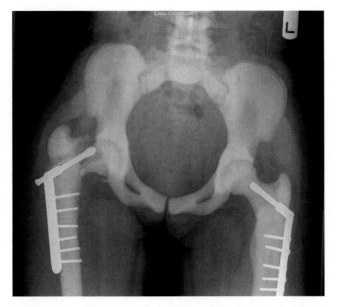

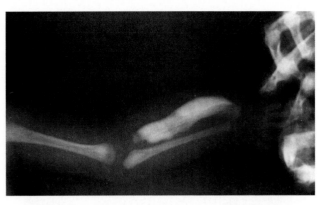

FIGURE 6-25. The ulna is the most frequently affected bone in the extremities of patients with Caffey disease.

FIGURE 6-24. This 12-year-old girl with osteopetrosis has had bilateral femoral neck fractures treated with open reduction and internal fixation. The left has united but the right has had nonunion and cutout despite revisions of hardware. The bone has been likened to chalk—dense but brittle—leading to a high rate of complications associated with internal fixation.

TABLE 6-5	Causes of Conditions Associated with Periosteal Reaction and cortical Thickening in Infancy and Early Childhood	
Cause	**Time of Presentation**	**Characteristics**
Physiologic periosteal reaction of newborn	Age 1–6 mo	Thin, even periosteal reaction symmetric along femora, tibiae, humeri
Congenital or Genetic Condition		
Menkes kinky-hair syndrome	Newborn	Failure to thrive; X-linked defective copper absorption; boys; sparse, kinky hair; central nervous system degeneration, metaphyseal fractures, and periosteal reaction; can be mistaken for abuse or rickets
Camurati-Engelmann (diaphyseal dysplasia)	Age 4–6 yr	Autosomal dominant; progressive midshaft thickening of long bones; waddling gait; normal laboratory findings, except slight elevation of alkaline phosphatase
Infection		
Osteomyelitis	Any age	Classic bacterial osteomyelitis with lytic or blastic changes at metaphysis and periosteal reaction as disease progresses; elevated ESR; viral and fungal types exist; *Salmonella* osteomyelitis in sickle cell disease may begin at diaphysis; ESR not elevated
Congenital syphilis	Age >3 mo (severe spirochetal infection can cause fetal loss)	Many manifestations possible; osteochondritis with metaphyseal lytic lesions; diaphyseal osteitis; periostitis; positive serology for syphilis
Inflammatory Disease		
Juvenile chronic arthritis	Age 5–10 yr	Periarticular reaction at phalanges, metacarpals, and metatarsals
Trauma		
Accidental or nonaccidental injury	Any age	Accidental injury should result in local reaction consistent with age-appropriate activities (i.e., single tibial reaction 7–10 d after injury in a child who is walking); nonaccidental injury can result in multiple areas of periosteal reaction inconsistent with age-appropriate activities

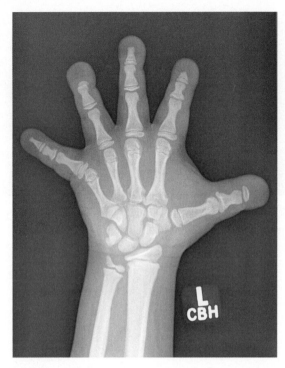

FIGURE 6-26. Pykodysostosis. This 12-year-old boy has the dense bones and acroosteolysis characteristic of pyknodysostosis.

Camurati-Engelmann disease is an autosomal dominant condition that includes hyperostosis, typically with accumulation of the bone within the medullary canal and the diaphyseal region and in the skull. Clinical features include an enlarged head, proptosis, and thin limbs, with weak proximal muscle leading sometimes to a waddling gait and musculoskeletal pain (322, 333). Spontaneous improvement at puberty has been described. Cranial nerve abnormalities and increased intracranial pressure are possible sequelae. The disorder is called by an excess of active TGF beta1 which leads to continuous stimulation of osteoblastic bone deposition (301, 334, 335).

Sclerostenosis is a rare condition inherited in an autosomal recessive pattern (336). It is characterized by skeletal overgrowth particularly of the skull and of the mandible. In addition, patients have sclerotic long bones and gigantism. Bony syndactyly is a characteristic clinical tip off (337–342). Increased intracranial pressure in this condition may lead to sudden death, so recognition of this condition is important (343). The underlying defect is loss of function and mutation in the SOST gene (344, 345). No specific medical treatment is currently available.

REFERENCES

1. Karsenty G. The complexities of skeletal biology. *Nature* 2003;423(6937):316–318.
2. Kronenberg HM. Developmental regulation of the growth plate. *Nature* 2003;423(6937):332–336.
3. Siebler T, Robson H, Shalet SM, et al. Glucocorticoids, thyroid hormone and growth hormone interactions: implications for the growth plate. *Horm Res* 2001;56(1):7–12.
4. Caplan AI. New era of cell-based orthopaedic therapies. *Tissue Eng Part B Rev* 2009;15(2):195–200.
5. Caplan AI. All MSCs are pericytes? *Cell Stem Cell* 2008;3(3):229–230.
6. Crisan M, Yap S, Casteilla L, et al. A perivascular origin for mesenchymal stem cells in multiple human organs. *Cell Stem Cell* 2008;3(3):301–313.
7. Harada S, Rodan GA. Control of osteoblast function and regulation of bone mass. *Nature* 2003;423(6937):349–355.
8. Troen BR. Molecular mechanisms underlying osteoclast formation and activation. *Exp Gerontol* 2003;38(6):605–614.
9. Khosla S. Minireview: the OPG/RANKL/RANK system. *Endocrinology* 2001;142(12):5050–5055.
10. Doggrell SA. Present and future pharmacotherapy for osteoporosis. *Drugs Today* 2003;39(8):633–657.
11. McClung MR, Lewiecki EM, Cohen SB, et al. Denosumab in postmenopausal women with low bone mineral density. *N Engl J Med* 2006;354(8):821–831.
12. Fourman P, Royer P. *Calcium metabolism and bone*, 2nd ed. Philadelphia, PA: 1968.
13. Rasmussen H. The calcium messenger system. *N Engl J Med* 1986;314:1094.
14. Avioli LV, Haddad JG. Progress in endocrinology and metabolism. Vitamin D: current concepts. *Metab Clin Exp* 1973;22:507.
15. Hoffman WS. *The biochemistry of clinical medicine*, 4th ed. Chicago, IL: Year Book, 1970.
16. Morgan B. *Osteomalacia, renal osteodystrophy, and osteoporosis*. Springfield, IL: Charles C. Thomas, 1973.
17. Widdowson EM, McCance RA. The metabolism of calcium, phosphorus, magnesium and strontium. *Pediatr Clin North Am* 1965;12:595.
18. Raisz LG. Bone metabolism and calcium regulation. In: Avioli LV, Krane SM, eds. *Metabolic bone disease*. New York, NY: Academic Press, 1978.
19. Borle AB. Membrane transfer of calcium. *Clin Orthop* 1967;52:267.
20. DeLuca HF. Vitamin D: new horizons. *Clin Orthop* 1971;78:423.
21. Arnaud C, Fischer J, Rasmussen H. The role of the parathyroids in the phosphaturia of vitamin D deficiency. *J Clin Invest* 1964;43.
22. Arnaud C, Tsao HS, Littledike T. Calcium homeostasis, parathyroid hormone and calcitonin: preliminary report. *Mayo Clin Proc* 1970;45:125.
23. Arnaud CD, Tenenhouse AM, Rasmussen H. Parathyroid hormone. *Annu Rev Physiol* 1967;29:349.
24. Harrison HE, Harrison HC. The interaction of vitamin D and parathyroid hormone on calcium, phosphorus and magnesium homeostasis in the rat. *Metab Clin Exp* 1964;13:952.
25. Rasmussen H. Ionic and hormonal control of calcium homeostasis. *Am J Med* 1971;50:567.
26. Bijovet OLM. Kidney function in calcium and phosphate metabolism. In: Avioli LV, Krane SM, eds. *Metabolic bone disease*. New York, NY: Academic Press, 1977:49.
27. Harmeyer J, DeLuca HF. Calcium-binding protein and calcium absorption after vitamin D administration. *Arch Biochem Biophys* 1969;133:247.
28. Beal VA. Calcium and phosphorus in infancy. *J Am Diet Assoc* 1968;53:450.
29. Blunt JW, DeLuca HF. The synthesis of 25-hydroxycholecalciferol: a biologically active metabolite of vitamin D3. *Biochemistry* 1969;8:671.
30. Blunt JW, DeLuca HF, Schnoes HK. 25-Hydroxycholecalciferol: a biologically active metabolite of vitamin D3. *Biochemistry* 1968;7:3317.
31. Blunt JW, Tanaka Y, DeLuca HF. The biological activity of 25-hydroxycholecalciferol: a metabolite of vitamin D3. *Proc Natl Acad Sci USA* 1968;61:1503.
32. Jones G, Schnoes HK, DeLuca HF. Isolation and identification of 1,25 dihydroxy vitamin D_2. 1975;14:1250.
33. Lund J, DeLuca HF. Biologically active metabolite of vitamin D from bone, liver and blood serum. *J Lipid Res* 1966;7:739.
34. Cheeney RW. Current clinical applications of vitamin D metabolite research. *Clin Orthop* 1981;161:285.
35. Holick MF, Schnoes HK, DeLuca HF. Isolation and identification of 24,25-hydroxycholecalciferol, a metabolite of D3 made in the kidney. *Biochemistry* 1972;11:4251.
36. Holick MF, Schnoes HK, DeLuca HF, et al. Isolation and identification of 1,24-dihydroxycholecalciferol: a metabolite of vitamin D active in intestine. *Biochemistry* 1971;10:2799.

37. DeLuca HF. Parathyroid hormone as a trophic hormone for 1,25-dihydroxy vitamin D3, the metabolically active form of vitamin D. *N Engl J Med* 1972;287:250.

38. Boyle IT, Gray RW, DeLuca HF. Regulation by calcium of in vivo synthesis of 1,25-dihydroxycholecalciferol and 21,25-dihydroxycholecalciferol. *Proc Natl Acad Sci USA* 1971;68:2131.

39. Fraser DR, Kodicek E. Regulation of 25-hydroxycholecalciferol-1-hydrolase activity in kidney by parathyroid hormone. *Nature* 1973; 241:163.

40. Rasmussen H, Wong M, Bikle D, et al. Hormonal control of 25-hydroxycholecalciferol to 1,25-dihydroxycholecalciferol. *J Clin Invest* 1972;51:2502.

41. Gartner LM, Greer FR, Section on Breastfeeding and Committee on Nutrition. American Academy of Pediatrics. Prevention of rickets and vitamin D deficiency: new guidelines for vitamin D intake. *Pediatrics* 2003;111(4 Pt 1):908–910.

42. Misra M, Pacaud D, Petryk A, et al. Drug and Therapeutics Committee of the Lawson Wilkins Pediatric Endocrine Society. Vitamin D deficiency in children and its management: review of current knowledge and recommendations. *Pediatrics* 2008;122(2):398–417.

43. Holick MF. Vitamin D deficiency. *N Engl J Med* 2007;357(3):266–281.

44. Lin R, White JH. The pleiotropic actions of vitamin D. *Bioessays* 2004;26(1):21–28.

45. *Food and Nutrition Board recommended dietary allowances*, 10th ed. Washington, DC: 1989.

46. Committee on Nutrition (AAP). Calcium requirements of infants, children, and adolescents. *Pediatrics* 1999;104(5):1152–1157.

47. Avioli LV. Intestinal absorption of calcium. *Arch Intern Med* 1972;129:345.

48. Bruce HM, Callow RK. Cereals and rickets: the role of inositalhexaphosphoric acid. *Biochem J* 1934;28:517.

49. Wills MR, Phillips JB, Day RC, et al. Phytic acid and nutritional rickets in immigrants. *Lancet* 1972;1:771.

50. DeToni G. Renal rickets with phospho-gluco-amino renal diabetes. *Ann Paediatr* 1956;187:42.

51. Tryfus H. Hepatic rickets. *Ann Paediatr* 1959;192:81.

52. Raisz LG, Rodan GA. Pathogenesis of osteoporosis. *Endocrinol Metab Clin North Am* 2003;32(1):15–24.

53. Manolagas SC, Kousteni S, Jilka RL. Sex steroids and bone. *Recent Prog Horm Res* 2002;57:385–409.

54. Vanderschueren D, Bouillon R. Androgens and bone. *Calcif Tissue Int* 1995;56(5):341–346.

55. Burman KD. Thyroid disease and osteoporosis. *Hosp Pract* 1997;32(12):71–73, 78–85.

56. Ramos-Remus C, Sahagun RM, Perla-Navarro AV. Endocrine disorders and musculoskeletal diseases. *Curr Opin Rheumatol* 1996;8(1):77–84.

57. Sambrook PN. Corticosteroid induced osteoporosis. *J Rheumatol Suppl* 1996;45:19–22.

58. Adachi JD. Corticosteroid-induced osteoporosis. *Int J Fertil Womens Med* 2001;46(4):190–205.

59. Wallach S, Farley JR, Baylink DJ, et al. Effects of calcitonin on bone quality and osteoblastic function. *Calcif Tissue Int* 1993;52(5):335–339.

60. Ferretti JL, Cointry GR, Capozza RF, et al. Bone mass, bone strength, muscle-bone interactions, osteopenias and osteoporoses. *Mech Ageing Dev* 2003;124(3):269–279.

61. Berard A, Bravo G, Gauthier P. Meta-analysis of the effectiveness of physical activity for the prevention of bone loss in postmenopausal women. *Osteoporos Int* 1997;7(4):331–337.

62. Brighton CT, Strafford B, Gross SB, et al. The proliferative and synthetic response of isolated calvarial bone cells of rats to cyclic biaxial mechanical strain. *J Bone Joint Surg Am* 1991;73:320.

63. Greco F, DePalma L, Speddia N, et al. Growth plate cartilage metabolic response to mechanical stress. *J Pediatr Orthop* 1989;9:520.

64. Hueter C. Anatomische Studien an den Extremitatengelenken Neugeborner und Erwachsener. *Virchows Arch* 1862;25:572.

65. Ohlsson C, Isgaard J, Tornell J, et al. Endocrine regulation of longitudinal bone growth. *Acta Paediatr Suppl* 1993;82(Suppl 391):33–40; discussion 41.

66. Whistler D. *Disputatio Medica Inauguralis de Morbo puerili Anglorum quem patrio idiomate indigenae vocant the rickets*. London, UK: Wilhemi, Christiani, Boxii, 1645.

67. Glisson R. *De rachitide sive marbo puerili qui vulgo The Rickets Dicitur Tracttatus. Adscitis in operis societatem Georgio Bate et Ahasuero Regemortero*. London, UK: G Du-Gardi, 1650.

68. Pettifor JM. Nutritional rickets. In: Glorieux F, Pettifor JM, Juppner H, eds. *Pediatric bone: biology & diseases*. California: Academic Press, 2003:541.

69. Buchanan N, Pettifor JM, Cane RD, et al. Infantile apnoea due to profound hypocalcaemia associated with vitamin D deficiency. A case report. *S Afr Med J* 1978;53(19):766–767.

70. Fraser DR, Salter RB. The diagnosis and management of the various types of rickets. *Pediatr Clin North Am* 1958;26:417.

71. Arnstein AR, Frame B, Frost HM. Recent progress in osteomalacia and rickets. *Ann Intern Med* 1967;67:1296.

72. Smith R. The pathophysiology and management of rickets. *Orthop Clin North Am* 1972;3:601.

73. Laditan AA, Adeniyi A. Rickets in Nigerian children: response to vitamin D. *J Trop Med Hyg* 1975;78:206.

74. Harrison HE, Harrison HC. Rickets then and now. *J Pediatr* 1975;87:1144.

75. Goel KM, Sweet EM, Logan RW, et al. Florid and subclinical rickets among immigrant children in Glasgow. *Lancet* 1976;1(7970): 1141–1145.

76. Mughal Z. Rickets in childhood. *Semin Musculoskelet Radiol* 2002;6(3): 183–190.

77. Steinbach HG, Noetzli M. Roentgen appearance of the skeleton in osteomalacia and rickets. *AJR Am J Roentgenol* 1964;91:955.

78. Opie WH, Muller CJ, Kamfer H. The diagnosis of vitamin D deficiency rickets. *Pediatr Radiol* 1975;3(2):105–110.

79. Holm IA, Econs MJ, Carpenter TO. Familial hypophosphatemia and related disorders. In: Glorieux F, Pettifor JM, Juppner H, eds. *Pediatric bone: biology & diseases*. California: Academic Press, 2003:603.

80. Harris NS, Crawford PB, Yangzom Y, et al. Nutritional and health status of Tibetan children living at high altitudes. *N Engl J Med* 2001;344(5):341–347.

81. Salimpour R. Rickets in Tehran: study of 200 cases. *Arch Dis Child* 1975;50:63.

82. Majid Molla A, Badawi MH, al-Yaish S, et al. Risk factors for nutritional rickets among children in Kuwait. *Pediatr Int* 2000;42(3):280–284.

83. el Hag AI, Karrar ZA. Nutritional vitamin D deficiency rickets in Sudanese children. *Ann Trop Paediatr* 1995;15(1):69–76.

84. Biser-Rohrbaugh A, Hadley-Miller N. Vitamin D deficiency in breast-fed toddlers. *J Pediatr Orthop* 2001;21(4):508–511.

85. Feldman KW, Marcuse EK, Springer DA. Nutritional rickets. *Am Fam Physician* 1990;42(5):1311–1318.

86. Carvalho NF, Kenney RD, Carrington PH, et al. Severe nutritional deficiencies in toddlers resulting from health food milk alternatives. *Pediatrics* 2001;107(4):E46.

87. Rudolf M, Arulanantham K, Greenstein RM. Unsuspected nutritional rickets. *Pediatrics* 1980;66(1):72–76.

88. Ward LM, Gaboury I, Ladhani M, et al. Vitamin D-deficiency rickets among children in Canada. *CMAJ* 2007;177(2):161–166.

89. Marie PJ, Pettifor JM, Ross FP, et al. Histological osteomalacia due to dietary calcium deficiency in children. *N Engl J Med* 1982;307(10): 584–588.

90. Clements MR, Johnson L, Fraser DR. A new mechanism for induced vitamin D deficiency in calcium deprivation. *Nature* 1987;325(6099): 62–65.

91. Henderson JB, Dunnigan MG, McIntosh WB, et al. Asian osteomalacia is determined by dietary factors when exposure to ultraviolet radiation is restricted: a risk factor model. *Q J Med* 1990;76(281):923–933.

92. Henderson JB, Dunnigan MG, McIntosh WB, et al. The importance of limited exposure to ultraviolet radiation and dietary factors in the aetiology of Asian rickets: a risk-factor model. *Q J Med* 1987;63(241): 413–425.

93. Kruse K. Pathophysiology of calcium metabolism in children with vitamin D-deficiency rickets. *J Pediatr* 1995;126(5 Pt 1):736–741.

94. Shah BR, Finberg L. Single-day therapy for nutritional vitamin D-deficiency rickets: a preferred method. *J Pediatr* 1994;125(3):487–490.

95. Mankin HJ. Metabolic bone disease. *J Bone Joint Surg Am* 1994;76:760.

96. Burnett CH, Dent CE, Harper C, et al. Vitamin D-resistant rickets: analysis of twenty-four pedigrees with hereditary and sporadic cases. *Am J Med* 1964;36:222.

97. Albright F, Butler AM, Bloomberg E. Rickets resistant to vitamin D therapy. *Am J Dis Child* 1937;54:529.

98. Harrison HE. The varieties of rickets and osteomalacia associated with hypophosphatemia. *Clin Orthop* 1957;9:61.

99. McWhorter AG, Seale NS. Prevalence of dental abscess in a population of children with vitamin D-resistant rickets. *Pediatr Dent* 1991;13(2):91–96.

100. Berndt M, Ehrich JH, Lazovic D, et al. Clinical course of hypophosphatemic rickets in 23 adults. *Clin Nephrol* 1996;45(1):33–41.

101. Chung WT, Niu DM, Lin CY. Clinical aspects of X-linked hypophosphatemic rickets. *Acta Paediatr Taiwan* 2002;43(1):26–34.

102. Stickler GB, Morgenstern BZ. Hypophosphataemic rickets: final height and clinical symptoms in adults. *Lancet* 1989;2(8668):902–905.

103. Carpenter TO. New perspectives on the biology and treatment of X-linked hypophosphatemic rickets. *Pediatr Clin North Am* 1997;44(2): 443–466.

104. Carpenter TO, Keller M, Schwartz D, et al. 24,25-dihydroxyvitamin D supplementation corrects hyperparathyroidism and improves skeletal abnormalities in X-linked hypophosphatemic rickets—a clinical research center study. *J Clin Endocrinol Metab* 1996;81(6):2381–2388.

105. Ferris B, Walker C, Jackson A, et al. The orthopaedic management of hypophosphataemic rickets. *J Pediatr Orthop* 1991;11:367.

106. Rohmiller MT, Tylkowski C, Kriss VM, et al. The effect of osteotomy on bowing and height in children with X-linked hypophosphatemia. *J Pediatr Orthop* 1999;19(1):114–118.

107. Loeffler RD Jr, Sherman FC. The effect of treatment on growth and deformity in hypophosphatemic vitamin D-resistant rickets. *Clin Orthop* 1982;162:4–10.

108. Petje G, Meizer R, Radler C, et al. Deformity correction in children with hereditary hypophosphatemic rickets. *Clin Orthop Relat Res* 2008;466(12):3078–3085.

109. Ringel MD, Schwindinger WF, Levine MA. Clinical implications of genetic defects in G proteins: the molecular basis of McCune-Albright syndrome and Albright hereditary osteodystrophy. *Medicine* 1996;75:171.

110. Prader A, Illig R, Heierli E. Eine besondere form des primare vitamin D resistenten rachitis mit hypocalcemie und autosomal-dominanten erbgang: Die hereditare pseudomangelrachitis. *Helv Paediatr Acta* 1961;16:452–468.

111. Portale AA, Miller WL. Rickets due to hereditary abnormalities of vitamin D synthesis or action. In: Glorieux F, Pettifor JM, Juppner H, eds. *Pediatric bone: biology & diseases*. California: Academic Press, 2003:583.

112. De Braekeleer M, Larochelle J. Population genetics of vitamin D-dependent rickets in northeastern Quebec. *Ann Hum Genet* 1991;55(Pt 4):283–290.

113. Fu GK, Lin D, Zhang MY, et al. Cloning of human 25-hydroxyvitamin D-1 alpha-hydroxylase and mutations causing vitamin D-dependent rickets type 1. *Mol Endocrinol* 1997;11(13):1961–1970.

114. Marx SJ, Spiegel AM, Brown EM, et al. A familial syndrome of decrease in sensitivity to 1,25-dihydroxyvitamin D. *J Clin Endocrinol Metab* 1978;47(6):1303–1310.

115. Brooks MH, Bell NH, Love L, et al. Vitamin D-dependent rickets, type II: resistance of target organs to 1,25-dihydroxy-vitamin D. *N Engl J Med* 1978;298:996.

116. Chesney RW. Rickets: an old form for a new century. *Pediatr Int* 2003;45(5):509–511.

117. Cole DEC. Hypophosphatasia. In: Glorieux F, Pettifor JM, Juppner H, eds. *Pediatric bone: biology & diseases*. California: Academic Press, 2003:651.

118. Zurutuza L, Muller F, Gibrat JF, et al. Correlations of genotype and phenotype in hypophosphatasia. *Hum Mol Genet* 1999;8(6):1039–1046.

119. Sato S, Matsuo N. Genetic analysis of hypophosphatasia. *Acta Paediatr Jpn* 1997;39(4):528–532.

120. McCane RA, Fairweathr DVI, Barrett AM, et al. Genetic, clinical, biochemical, and pathological features of hypophosphatasia. *Q J Med* 1956;25:523.

121. Coe JD, Murphy WA, Whyte MP. Management of femoral fractures and pseudofractures in adult hypophosphatasia. *J Bone Joint Surg Am* 1986;68:981.

122. Anderton JM. Orthopaedic problems in adult hypophosphatasia: a report of two cases. *J Bone Joint Surg Br* 1979;61:82.

123. Hu CC, King DL, Thomas HF, et al. A clinical and research protocol for characterizing patients with hypophosphatasia. *Pediatr Dent* 1996;18(1):17–23.

124. Fraser D. Hypophosphatasia. *Am J Med* 1957;22:730.

125. Kuizon BD, Salusky IB. Renal osteodystrophy: pathogenesis, diagnosis, and treatment. In: Glorieux F, Pettifor JM, Juppner H, eds. *Pediatric bone: biology & diseases*. California: Academic Press, 2003:679.

126. Oppenheim WL, Salusky IB, Kaplan D, et al. Renal osteodystrophy in children. In: Castells S, Finberg L, eds. *Metabolic bone disease in children*. New York, NY: Marcel Dekker, 1990:197.

127. Weller M, Edeiken J, Hodes PJ. Renal osteodystrophy. *AJR Am J Roentgenol* 1968;104:354.

128. Parfitt AM. Renal osteodystrophy. *Orthop Clin North Am* 1972;3:681.

129. States LJ. Imaging of metabolic bone disease and marrow disorders in children. *Radiol Clin North Am* 2001;39(4):749–772.

130. Mehls O, Ritz E, Krempien B, et al. Slipped epiphyses in renal osteodystrophy. *Arch Dis Child* 1975;50:545.

131. Floman Y, Yosipovitch Z, Licht A, et al. Bilateral slipped upper femoral epiphysis: a rare manifestation of renal osteodystrophy. Case report with discussion of its pathogenesis. *Isr J Med Sci* 1975;11:15.

132. Goldman AB, Lane JM, Salvati E. Slipped capital femoral epiphyses complicating renal osteodystrophy: a report of three cases. *Radiology* 1978;126:33.

133. Oppenheim WL, Bowen RE, McDonough PW, et al. Outcome of slipped capital femoral epiphysis in renal osteodystrophy. *J Pediatr Orthop* 2003;23(2):169–174.

134. Loder RT, Hensinger RN. Slipped capital femoral epiphysis associated with renal failure osteodystrophy. *J Pediatr Orthop* 1997;17(2):205–211.

135. Osteoporosis prevention, diagnosis, and therapy. NIH Consensus Statement. 2000;17(1):1–45.

136. Paulozzi LJ. Does inadequate diet during childhood explain the higher high fracture rates in the Southern United States? *Osteoporos Int* 2009.

137. Calvo MS. Dietary considerations to prevent loss of bone and renal function. *Nutrition* 2000;16(7–8):564–566.

138. Wyshak G. Teenaged girls, carbonated beverage consumption, and bone fractures. *Arch Pediatr Adolesc Med* 2000;154(6):610–613.

139. Winzenberg TM, Shaw K, Fryer J, et al. Calcium supplementation for improving bone mineral density in children. *Cochrane Database Syst Rev* 2006;(2):CD005119.

140. Rideout CA, McKay HA, Barr SI. Self-reported lifetime physical activity and areal bone mineral density in healthy postmenopausal women: the importance of teenage activity. *Calcif Tissue Int* 2006;79(4): 214–222.

141. Hind K, Burrows M. Weight-bearing exercise and bone mineral accrual in children and adolescents: a review of controlled trials. *Bone* 2007;40(1):14–27.

142. Orioli IM, Castilla EE, Barbosa-Neto JG. The birth prevalence rates for the skeletal dysplasias. *J Med Genet* 1986;23(4):328–332.

143. Seedorff KS. *Osteogenesis imperfecta: a study of clinical features and heredity based on 55 Danish families comprising 180 affected persons*. Copenhagen, Denmark: Ejnar Munksgaard, 1949.

144. Smith R, Francis MJO, Bauze RJ. Osteogenesis imperfecta: a clinical and biochemical study of a generalized connective tissue disorder. *Q J Med* 1975;44:555.

145. Wynne-Davis R, Gormley J. Clinical and genetic patterns in osteogenesis imperfecta. *Clin Orthop* 1981;159:26.

146. Cole WG. The Nicholas Andry Award-1996. The molecular pathology of osteogenesis imperfecta. *Clin Orthop* 1997;343:235–248.

147. Sillence DO. Osteogenesis imperfecta: an expanding panorama of variance. *Clin Orthop* 1981;159:11.

148. Sillence DO, Senn A, Danks DM. Genetic heterogeneity in osteogenesis imperfecta. *J Med Genet* 1979;16:101.

149. Cole WG. Etiology and pathogenesis of heritable connective tissue diseases. *J Pediatr Orthop* 1993;13:392.

150. Kuurila K, Grenman R, Johansson R, et al. Hearing loss in children with osteogenesis imperfecta. *Eur J Pediatr* 2000;159(7):515–519.

151. Imani P, Vijayasekaran S, Lannigan F. Is it necessary to screen for hearing loss in the paediatric population with osteogenesis imperfecta? *Clin Otolaryngol* 2003;28(3):199–202.

152. Kuurila K, Kaitila I, Johansson R, et al. Hearing loss in Finnish adults with osteogenesis imperfecta: a nationwide survey. *Ann Otol Rhinol Laryngol* 2002;111(10):939–946.

153. van der Rijt AJ, Cremers CW. Stapes surgery in osteogenesis imperfecta: results of a new series. *Otol Neurotol* 2003;24(5):717–722.

154. Szilvassy J, Jori J, Czigner J, et al. Cochlear implantation in osteogenesis imperfecta. *Acta Otorhinolaryngol Belg* 1998;52(3):253–256.

155. Stott NS, Zionts LE. Displaced fractures of the apophysis of the olecranon in children who have osteogenesis imperfecta. *J Bone Joint Surg Am* 1993;75(7):1026–1033.

156. Zeitlin L, Fassier F, Glorieux FH. Modern approach to children with osteogenesis imperfecta. *J Pediatr Orthop B* 2003;12(2):77–87.

157. Plotkin H, Primorac D, Rowe D. Osteogenesis Imperfecta. In: Glorieux F, Pettifor JM, Juppner H, eds. *Pediatric bone: biology & diseases.* California: Academic Press, 2003:443.

158. Aarabi M, Rauch F, Hamdy RC, et al. High prevalence of coxa vara in patients with severe osteogenesis imperfecta. *J Pediatr Orthop* 2006;26(1):24–28.

159. Glorieux FH, Rauch F, Plotkin H, et al. Type V osteogenesis imperfecta: a new form of brittle bone disease. *J Bone Miner Res* 2000;15(9):1650–1658.

160. Fassier AM, Rauch F, Aarabi M, et al. Radial head dislocation and subluxation in osteogenesis imperfecta. *J Bone Joint Surg Am* 2007;89(12):2694–2704.

161. Glorieux FH, Ward LM, Rauch F, et al. Osteogenesis imperfecta type VI: a form of brittle bone disease with a mineralization defect. *J Bone Miner Res* 2002;17(1):30–38.

162. Ward LM, Rauch F, Travers R, et al. Osteogenesis imperfecta type VII: an autosomal recessive form of brittle bone disease. *Bone* 2002;31(1):12–18.

163. Pettinen RP, Lichtenstein JR, Martin GR, et al. Abnormal collagen metabolism in cultured cells in osteogenesis imperfecta. *Proc Natl Acad Sci USA* 1975;72:586.

164. Barsh GS, David KE, Byers PH. Type I osteogenesis imperfecta: a nonfunctional allele for pro alpha (I) chains for type I procollagen. *Proc Natl Acad Sci USA* 1982;79:3838.

165. Peltonen L, Palotie A, Prockop DJ. A defect in the structure of type I procollagen in a patient who had osteogenesis imperfecta: excessive mannose in the COOH-terminal peptide. *Proc Natl Acad Sci USA* 1980;77:6179.

166. Alman B, Frasca P. Fracture failure mechanisms in patients with osteogenesis imperfecta. *J Orthop Res* 1987;5(1):139–143.

167. Moore MS, Minch CM, Kruse RW, et al. The role of dual energy x-ray absorptiometry in aiding the diagnosis of pediatric osteogenesis imperfecta. *Am J Orthop* 1998;27(12):797–801.

168. Zionts LE, Nash JP, Rude R, et al. Bone mineral density in children with mild osteogenesis imperfecta. *J Bone Joint Surg Br* 1995;77(1):143–147.

169. Faulkner RA, Bailey DA, Drinkwater DT, et al. Bone densitometry in Canadian children 8–17 years of Age. *Calcif Tissue Int* 1996;59(5):344–351.

170. Gafni RI, Baron J. Overdiagnosis of osteoporosis in children due to misinterpretation of dual-energy x-ray absorptiometry (DEXA). *J Pediatr Orthop* 2004;144(2):253–257.

171. Minch CM, Kruse RW. Osteogenesis imperfecta: a review of basic science and diagnosis. *Orthopedics* 1998;21:558.

172. Marlowe A, Pepin MG, Byers PH. Testing for osteogenesis imperfecta in cases of suspected non-accidental injury. *J Med Genet* 2002;39(6):382–386.

173. Glorieux FH, Bishop NJ, Plotkin H, et al. Cyclic administration of pamidronate in children with severe osteogenesis imperfecta. *N Engl J Med* 1998;339(14):947–952.

174. Phillipi CA, Remmington T, Steiner RD. Bisphosphonate therapy for osteogenesis imperfecta. *Cochrane Database Syst Rev* 2008;(4):CD005088.

175. Sakkers R, Kok D, Engelbert R, et al. Skeletal effects and functional outcome with olpadronate in children with osteogenesis imperfecta: a 2-year randomised placebo-controlled study. *Lancet* 2004;363(9419):1427–1431.

176. Land C, Rauch F, Munns CF, et al. Vertebral morphometry in children and adolescents with osteogenesis imperfecta: effect of intravenous pamidronate treatment. *Bone* 2006;39(4):901–906.

177. Lowing K, Astrom E, Oscarsson KA, et al. Effect of intravenous pamidronate therapy on everyday activities in children with osteogenesis imperfecta. *Acta Paediatr* 2007;96(8):1180–1183.

178. Grissom LE, Harcke HT. Radiographic features of bisphosphonate therapy in pediatric patients. *Pediatr Radiol* 2003;33(4):226–229.

179. Rauch F, Cornibert S, Cheung M, et al. Long-bone changes after pamidronate discontinuation in children and adolescents with osteogenesis imperfecta. *Bone* 2007;40(4):821–827.

180. Weber M, Roschger P, Fratzl-Zelman N, et al. Pamidronate does not adversely affect bone intrinsic material properties in children with osteogenesis imperfecta. *Bone* 2006;39(3):616–622.

181. Pizones J, Plotkin H, Parra-Garcia JI, et al. Bone healing in children with osteogenesis imperfecta treated with bisphosphonates. *J Pediatr Orthop* 2005;25(3):332–335.

182. Munns CF, Rauch F, Zeitlin L, et al. Delayed osteotomy but not fracture healing in pediatric osteogenesis imperfecta patients receiving pamidronate. *J Bone Miner Res* 2004;19(11):1779–1786.

183. Agarwal V, Joseph B. Non-union in osteogenesis imperfecta. *J Pediatr Orthop B* 2005;14(6):451–455.

184. Papapoulos SE, Cremers SC. Prolonged bisphosphonate release after treatment in children. *N Engl J Med* 2007;356(10):1075–1076.

185. Levy S, Fayez I, Taguchi N, et al. Pregnancy outcome following in utero exposure to bisphosphonates. *Bone* 2009;44(3):428–430.

186. Ornoy A, Wajnberg R, Diav-Citrin O. The outcome of pregnancy following pre-pregnancy or early pregnancy alendronate treatment. *Reprod Toxicol* 2006;22(4):578–579.

187. Malmgren B, Astrom E, Soderhall S. No osteonecrosis in jaws of young patients with osteogenesis imperfecta treated with bisphosphonates. *J Oral Pathol Med* 2008;37(4):196–200.

188. Whyte MP, Wenkert D, Clements KL, et al. Bisphosphonate-induced osteopetrosis. *N Engl J Med* 2003;349(5):457–463.

189. Evans KD, Lau ST, Oberbauer AM, et al. Alendronate affects long bone length and growth plate morphology in the oim mouse model for osteogenesis imperfecta. *Bone* 2003;32(3):268–274.

190. Lepola VT, Hannuniemi R, Kippo K, et al. Long-term effects of clodronate on growing rat bone. *Bone* 1996;18(2):191–196.

191. Miller SC, Jee WS, Woodbury DM, et al. Effects of N,N,N′,N′-ethylenediaminetetramethylene phosphonic acid and 1-hydroxyethylidene-1,1-bisphosphonic acid on calcium absorption, plasma calcium, longitudinal bone growth, and bone histology in the growing rat. *Toxicol Appl Pharmacol* 1985;77(2):230–239.

192. Fassier F, Glorieux FH. Surgical management of osteogenesis imperfecta. Surgical Techniques in Orthopaedics and Traumatology Elsevier SAS, Paris, France: 2003.

193. Gamble JG, Strudwick WJ, Rinsky LA, et al. Complications of intramedullary rods in osteogenesis imperfecta: Bailey-Dubow rods versus nonelongating rods. *J Pediatr Orthop* 1988;8:645.

194. Porat S, Heller E, Seidman DS, et al. Functional results of operation in osteogenesis imperfecta: elongating and nonelongating rods. *J Pediatr Orthop* 1991;11:200.

195. Ryoppy S, Alberty A, Kaitila I. Early semiclosed intramedullary stabilization in osteogenesis imperfecta. *J Pediatr Orthop* 1987;7:139.

196. Middleton RWD, Frost RB. Percutaneous intramedullary rod interchange in osteogenesis imperfecta. *J Bone Joint Surg Br* 1987;69:429.

197. Tiley F, Albright JA. Osteogenesis imperfecta: treatment by multiple osteotomy and intramedullary rod insertion. *J Bone Joint Surg Am* 1973;55:701.

198. Luhmann SJ, Sheridan JJ, Capelli AM, et al. Management of lower-extremity deformities in osteogenesis imperfecta with extensible intramedullary rod technique: a 20-year experience. *J Pediatr Orthop* 1998;18(1):88–94.

199. Engelbert RH, Pruijs HE, Beemer FA, et al. Osteogenesis imperfecta in childhood: treatment strategies. *Arch Phys Med Rehabil* 1998;79(12):1590–1594.

200. Antoniazzi F, Mottes M, Fraschini P, et al. Osteogenesis imperfecta: practical treatment guidelines. *Paediatr Drugs* 2000;2(6):465–488.

201. Mulpuri K, Joseph B. Intramedullary rodding in osteogenesis imperfecta. *J Pediatr Orthop* 2000;20(2):267–273.

202. Khoshhal KI, Ellis RD. Effect of lower limb Sofield procedure on ambulation in osteogenesis imperfecta. *J Pediatr Orthop* 2001;21(2):233–235.

203. Engelbert RH, Uiterwaal CS, Gulmans VA, et al. Osteogenesis imperfecta in childhood: prognosis for walking. *J Pediatr* 2000;137(3):397–402.

204. Engelbert RH, Uiterwaal CS, Gulmans VA, et al. Osteogenesis imperfecta: profiles of motor development as assessed by a postal questionnaire. *Eur J Pediatr* 2000;159(8):615–620.

205. Engelbert RH, Beemer FA, van der Graaf Y, et al. Osteogenesis imperfecta in childhood: impairment and disability—a follow-up study. *Arch Phys Med Rehabil* 1999;80(8):896–903.

206. Esposito P, Plotkin H. Surgical treatment of osteogenesis imperfecta: current concepts. *Curr Opin Pediatr* 2008;20(1):52–57.

207. Engelbert RH, Uiterwaal CS, van der Hulst A, et al. Scoliosis in children with osteogenesis imperfecta: influence of severity of disease and age of reaching motor milestones. *Eur Spine J* 2003;12(2):130–134.

208. Janus GJ, Finidori G, Engelbert RH, et al. Operative treatment of severe scoliosis in osteogenesis imperfecta: results of 20 patients after halo traction and posterior spondylodesis with instrumentation. *Eur Spine J* 2000;9(6):486–491.

209. Widmann RF, Bitan FD, Laplaza FJ, et al. Spinal deformity, pulmonary compromise, and quality of life in osteogenesis imperfecta. *Spine* 1999;24(16):1673–1678.

210. Engelbert RH, Gerver WJ, Breslau-Siderius LJ, et al. Spinal complications in osteogenesis imperfecta: 47 patients 1–16 years of age. *Acta Orthop Scand* 1998;69(3):283–286.

211. Hanscom DA, Winter RB, Lutter L, et al. Osteogenesis imperfecta. Radiographic classification, natural history, and treatment of spinal deformities. *J Bone Joint Surg Am* 1992;74(4):598–616.

212. Hanscom DA, Bloom BA. The spine in osteogenesis imperfecta. *Orthop Clin North Am* 1988;19(2):449–458.

213. Yong-Hing K, MacEwen GD. Scoliosis associated with osteogenesis imperfecta. *J Bone Joint Surg Br* 1982;64(1):36–43.

214. Benson DR, Newman DC. The spine and surgical treatment in osteogenesis imperfecta. *Clin Orthop* 1981;159:147–153.

215. Cristofaro RL, Hoek KJ, Bonnett CA, et al. Operative treatment of spine deformity in osteogenesis imperfecta. *Clin Orthop* 1979;139:40–48.

216. Benson DR, Donaldson DH, Millar EA. The spine in osteogenesis imperfecta. *J Bone Joint Surg Am* 1978;60(7):925–929.

217. Watanabe G, Kawaguchi S, Matsuyama T, et al. Correlation of scoliotic curvature with Z-score bone mineral density and body mass index in patients with osteogenesis imperfecta. *Spine (Phila Pa.1976)* 2007;32(17):E488–E494.

218. Verra WC, Pruijs HJ, Beek EJ, et al. Prevalence of vertebral pars defects (spondylolysis) in a population with osteogenesis imperfecta. *Spine (Phila Pa.1976)* 2009;34(13):1399–1401.

219. Ibrahim AG, Crockard HA. Basilar impression and osteogenesis imperfecta: a 21-year retrospective review of outcomes in 20 patients. *J Neurosurg Spine* 2007;7(6):594–600.

220. Daivajna S, Jones A, Hossein Mehdian SM. Surgical management of severe cervical kyphosis with myelopathy in osteogenesis imperfecta: a case report. *Spine (Phila Pa.1976)* 2005;30(7):E191–E194.

221. Sasaki-Adams D, Kulkarni A, Rutka J, et al. Neurosurgical implications of osteogenesis imperfecta in children. Report of 4 cases. *J Neurosurg Pediatr* 2008;1(3):229–236.

222. Ward LM, Glorieux HF. The spectrum of pediatric osteoporosis. In: Glorieux F, Pettifor JM, Juppner H, eds. *Pediatric bone: biology & diseases.* California: Academic Press, 2003:401.

223. Jones ET, Hensinger RN. Spinal deformity in idiopathic juvenile osteoporosis. *Spine* 1981;6:1.

224. Breslau-Siderius EJ, Engelbert RH, Pals G, et al. Bruck syndrome: a rare combination of bone fragility and multiple congenital joint contractures. *J Pediatr Orthop B* 1998;7(1):35–38.

225. Bank RA, Robins SP, Wijmenga C, et al. Defective collagen crosslinking in bone, but not in ligament or cartilage, in Bruck syndrome: indications for a bone-specific telopeptide lysyl hydroxylase on chromosome 17. *Proc Natl Acad Sci USA* 1999;96(3):1054–1058.

226. Frontali M, Stomeo C, Dallapiccola B. Osteoporosis-pseudoglioma syndrome: report of three affected sibs and an overview. *Am J Med Genet* 1985;22(1):35–47.

227. McDowell CL, Moore JD. Multiple fractures in a child: the osteoporosis pseudoglioma syndrome. A case report. *J Bone Joint Surg Am* 1992;74(8):1247–1249.

228. Gong Y, Slee RB, Fukai N, et al. LDL receptor-related protein 5 (LRP5) affects bone accrual and eye development. *Cell* 2001;107(4):513–523.

229. Zacharin M, Cundy T. Osteoporosis pseudoglioma syndrome: treatment of spinal osteoporosis with intravenous bisphosphonates. *J Pediatr* 2000;137(3):410–415.

230. Kasten P, Bastian L, Schmid H, et al. Failure of operative treatment in a child with osteoporosis-pseudoglioma syndrome. *Clin Orthop* 2003;410:262–266.

231. Ducy P, Schinke T, Karsenty G. The osteoblast: a sophisticated fibroblast under central surveillance. *Science* 2000;289(5484):1501–1504.

232. Ducy P, Amling M, Takeda S, et al. Leptin inhibits bone formation through a hypothalamic relay: a central control of bone mass. *Cell* 2000;100(2):197–207.

233. Takeda S, Elefteriou F, Levasseur R, et al. Leptin regulates bone formation via the sympathetic nervous system. *Cell* 2002;111(3):305–317.

234. Flier JS. Physiology: is brain sympathetic to bone? *Nature* 2002;420(6916):619, 621–622.

235. King W, Levin R, Schmidt R, et al. Prevalence of reduced bone mass in children and adults with spastic quadriplegia. *Dev Med Child Neurol* 2003;45(1):12–16.

236. Henderson RC, Lark RK, Gurka MJ, et al. Bone density and metabolism in children and adolescents with moderate to severe cerebral palsy. *Pediatrics* 2002;110(1 Pt 1):e5.

237. Ihkkan DY, Yalcin E. Changes in skeletal maturation and mineralization in children with cerebral palsy and evaluation of related factors. *J Child Neurol* 2001;16(6):425–430.

238. Tasdemir HA, Buyukavci M, Akcay F, et al. Bone mineral density in children with cerebral palsy. *Pediatr Int* 2001;43(2):157–160.

239. Henderson RC, Lin PP, Greene WB. Bone-mineral density in children and adolescents who have spastic cerebral palsy. *J Bone Joint Surg Am* 1995;77(11):1671–1681.

240. Lin PP, Henderson RC. Bone mineralization in the affected extremities of children with spastic hemiplegia. *Dev Med Child Neurol* 1996;38(9):782–786.

241. Naftchi NE, Viau AT, Marshall CH, et al. Bone mineralization in the distal forearm of hemiplegic patients. *Arch Phys Med Rehabil* 1975;56(11):487–492.

242. Duncan B, Barton LL, Lloyd J, et al. Dietary considerations in osteopenia in tube-fed nonambulatory children with cerebral palsy. *Clin Pediatr (Phila)* 1999;38(3):133–137.

243. Brunner R, Doderlein L. Pathological fractures in patients with cerebral palsy. *J Pediatr Orthop B* 1996 Fall;5(4):232–238.

244. Bischof F, Basu D, Pettifor JM. Pathological long-bone fractures in residents with cerebral palsy in a long-term care facility in South Africa. *Dev Med Child Neurol* 2002;44(2):119–122.

245. Chad KE, Bailey DA, McKay HA, et al. The effect of a weight-bearing physical activity program on bone mineral content and estimated volumetric density in children with spastic cerebral palsy. *J Pediatr* 1999;135(1):115–117.

246. Jekovec-Vrhovsek M, Kocijancic A, Prezelj J. Effect of vitamin D and calcium on bone mineral density in children with CP and epilepsy in full-time care. *Dev Med Child Neurol* 2000;42(6):403–405.

247. Allington N, Vivegnis D, Gerard P. Cyclic administration of pamidronate to treat osteoporosis in children with cerebral palsy or a neuromuscular disorder: a clinical study. *Acta Orthop Belg* 2005;71(1):91–97.

248. Plotkin H, Coughlin S, Kreikemeier R, et al. Low doses of pamidronate to treat osteopenia in children with severe cerebral palsy: a pilot study. *Dev Med Child Neurol* 2006;48(9):709–712.

249. Bachrach SJ, Kecskemethy HH, Harcke HT, et al. Pamidronate treatment and posttreatment bone density in children with spastic quadriplegic cerebral palsy. *J Clin Densitom* 2006;9(2):167–174.

250. Larson CM, Henderson RC. Bone mineral density and fractures in boys with Duchenne muscular dystrophy. *J Pediatr Orthop* 2000;20(1):71–74.

251. Bianchi ML, Mazzanti A, Galbiati E, et al. Bone mineral density and bone metabolism in Duchenne muscular dystrophy. *Osteoporos Int* 2003;14(9):761–767.

252. Markham A, Bryson HM. Deflazacort. A review of its pharmacological properties and therapeutic efficacy. *Drugs* 1995;50(2):317–333.

253. Loftus J, Allen R, Hesp R, et al. Randomized, double-blind trial of deflazacort versus prednisone in juvenile chronic (or rheumatoid) arthritis: a relatively bone-sparing effect of deflazacort. *Pediatrics* 1991;88(3):428–436.

254. Talim B, Malaguti C, Gnudi S, et al. Vertebral compression in Duchenne muscular dystrophy following deflazacort. *Neuromuscul Disord* 2002;12(3):294–295.

255. Hawker GA, Ridout R, Harris VA, et al. Alendronate in the treatment of low bone mass in steroid-treated boys with Duchennes muscular dystrophy. *Arch Phys Med Rehabil* 2005;86(2):284–288.

256. Wuster C. Fracture rates in patients with growth hormone deficiency. *Horm Res* 2000;54(Suppl 1):31–35.

257. Cowell CT, Wuster C. The effects of growth hormone deficiency and growth hormone replacement therapy on bone. A meeting report. *Horm Res* 2000;54(Suppl 1):68–74.

258. Clanget C, Seck T, Hinke V, et al. Effects of 6 years of growth hormone (GH) treatment on bone mineral density in GH-deficient adults. *Clin Endocrinol (Oxf)* 2001;55(1):93–99.

259. Loder RT, Wittenberg B, DeSilva G. Slipped capital femoral epiphysis associated with endocrine disorders. *J Pediatr Orthop* 1995;15(3):349–356.

260. Cowell CT, Dietsch S. Adverse events during growth hormone therapy. *J Pediatr Endocrinol Metab* 1995;8(4):243–252.

261. Bailey DA, Wedge JH, McCulloch RG, et al. Epidemiology of fractures of the distal end of the radius in children as associated with growth. *J Bone Joint Surg Am* 1989;71(8):1225–1231.

262. Khosla S, Melton LJ III, Dekutoski MB, et al. Incidence of childhood distal forearm fractures over 30 years: a population-based study. *JAMA* 2003;290(11):1479–1485.

263. Beals KA, Manore MM. Disorders of the female athlete triad among collegiate athletes. *Int J Sport Nutr Exerc Metab* 2002;12(3):281–293.

264. Kazis K, Iglesias E. The female athlete triad. *Adolesc Med* 2003;14(1):87–95.

265. Skolnick AA. 'Female athlete triad' risk for women. *JAMA* 1993;270(8):921–923.

266. Khan KM, Liu-Ambrose T, Sran MM, et al. New criteria for female athlete triad syndrome? As osteoporosis is rare, should osteopenia be among the criteria for defining the female athlete triad syndrome? *Br J Sports Med* 2002;36(1):10–13.

267. Lauder TD, Williams MV, Campbell CS, et al. The female athlete triad: prevalence in military women. *Mil Med* 1999;164(9):630–635.

268. Robinson TL, Snow-Harter C, Taaffe DR, et al. Gymnasts exhibit higher bone mass than runners despite similar prevalence of amenorrhea and oligomenorrhea. *J Bone Miner Res* 1995;10(1):26–35.

269. Bale P, Doust J, Dawson D. Gymnasts, distance runners, anorexics body composition and menstrual status. *J Sports Med Phys Fitness* 1996;36(1):49–53.

270. Snow CM, Rosen CJ, Robinson TL. Serum IGF-I is higher in gymnasts than runners and predicts bone and lean mass. *Med Sci Sports Exerc* 2000;32(11):1902–1907.

271. Fuchs RK, Bauer JJ, Snow CM. Jumping improves hip and lumbar spine bone mass in prepubescent children: a randomized controlled trial. *J Bone Miner Res* 2001;16(1):148–156.

272. McKay HA, Petit MA, Schutz RW, et al. Augmented trochanteric bone mineral density after modified physical education classes: a randomized school-based exercise intervention study in prepubescent and early pubescent children. *J Pediatr* 2000;136(2):156–162.

273. Maugars YM, Berthelot JM, Forestier R, et al. Follow-up of bone mineral density in 27 cases of anorexia nervosa. *Eur J Endocrinol* 1996;135(5):591–597.

274. Lucas AR, Melton LJ III, Crowson CS, et al. Long-term fracture risk among women with anorexia nervosa: a population-based cohort study. *Mayo Clin Proc* 1999;74(10):972–977.

275. Seeman E, Szmukler GI, Formica C, et al. Osteoporosis in anorexia nervosa: the influence of peak bone density, bone loss, oral contraceptive use, and exercise. *J Bone Miner Res* 1992;7(12):1467–1474.

276. Golden NH, Lanzkowsky L, Schebendach J, et al The effect of estrogen-progestin treatment on bone mineral density in anorexia nervosa. *J Pediatr Adolesc Gynecol* 2002;15(3):135–143.

277. Csermely T, Halvax L, Schmidt E, et al. Occurrence of osteopenia among adolescent girls with oligo/amenorrhea. *Gynecol Endocrinol* 2002;16(2):99–105.

278. Ducharme FM, Chabot G, Polychronakos C, et al. Safety profile of frequent short courses of oral glucocorticoids in acute pediatric asthma: impact on bone metabolism, bone density, and adrenal function. *Pediatrics* 2003;111(2):376–383.

279. Adachi JD, Roux C, Pitt PI, et al. A pooled data analysis on the use of intermittent cyclical etidronate therapy for the prevention and treatment of corticosteroid induced bone loss. *J Rheumatol* 2000;27(10):2424–2431.

280. Adachi JD, Bensen WG, Brown J, et al. Intermittent etidronate therapy to prevent corticosteroid-induced osteoporosis. *N Engl J Med* 1997;337(6):382–387.

281. Reid DM, Hughes RA, Laan RF, et al. Efficacy and safety of daily risedronate in the treatment of corticosteroid-induced osteoporosis in men and women: a randomized trial. European Corticosteroid-Induced Osteoporosis Treatment Study. *J Bone Miner Res* 2000;15(6):1006–1013.

282. Wallach S, Cohen S, Reid DM, et al. Effects of risedronate treatment on bone density and vertebral fracture in patients on corticosteroid therapy. *Calcif Tissue Int* 2000;67(4):277–285.

283. Reid DM, Devogelaer JP, Saag K, et al. Zoledronic acid and risedronate in the prevention and treatment of glucocorticoid-induced osteoporosis (HORIZON): a multicentre, double-blind, double-dummy, randomised controlled trial. *Lancet* 2009;373(9671):1253–1263.

284. Saag KG, Shane E, Boonen S, et al. Teriparatide or alendronate in glucocorticoid-induced osteoporosis. *N Engl J Med* 2007;357(20):2028–2039.

285. Noguera A, Ros JB, Pavia C, et al. Bisphosphonates, a new treatment for glucocorticoid-induced osteoporosis in children. *J Pediatr Endocrinol Metab* 2003;16(4):529–536.

286. Rudge S, Hailwood S, Horne A, et al. Effects of once-weekly oral alendronate on bone in children on glucocorticoid treatment. *Rheumatology (Oxford)* 2005;44(6):813–818.

287. Dent CE, Richens A, Rowe DJF, et al. Osteomalacia with long-term anticonvulsant therapy in epilepsy. *Br Med J* 1970;4:69.

288. Frame B. Hypocalcemia and osteomalacia associated with anticonvulsant therapy. *Ann Intern Med* 1971;74:294.

289. Aponte CJ, Petrelli MP. Anticonvulsants and vitamin D metabolism. *JAMA* 1973;225:1248.

290. Crosley CJ, Chee C, Berman PH. Rickets associated with long-term anticonvulsant therapy in a pediatric outpatient population. *Pediatrics* 1975;56:52.

291. Winnacker JL, Yeager H, Saunders RB, et al. Rickets in children receiving anticonvulsant drugs: biochemical and hormonal markers. *Am J Dis Child* 1977;131:286.

292. Morijiri Y, Sato T. Factors causing rickets in institutionalised handicapped children on anticonvulsant therapy. *Arch Dis Child* 1981;56(6):446–449.

293. Timperlake RW, Cook SD, Thomas KA, et al. Effects of anticonvulsant drug therapy on bone mineral density in a pediatric population. *J Pediatr Orthop* 1988;8:467.

294. Hahn TJ, Halstead LR. Anticonvulsant drug-induced osteomalacia: alterations in mineral metabolism and response to vitamin D₃ administration. *Calcif Tissue Int* 1979;27(1):13–18.

295. Hahn TJ. Bone complications of anticonvulsants. *Drugs* 1976;12(3): 201–211.

296. Henderson RC. Vitamin D levels in noninstitutionalized children with cerebral palsy. *J Child Neurol* 1997;12(7):443–447.

297. Camfield CS, Delvin EE, Camfield PR, et al. Normal serum 25-hydroxyvitamin D levels in phenobarbital-treated toddlers. *Dev Pharmacol Ther* 1983;6(3):157–161.

298. Feldkamp J, Becker A, Witte OW, et al. Long-term anticonvulsant therapy leads to low bone mineral density—evidence for direct drug effects of phenytoin and carbamazepine on human osteoblast-like cells. *Exp Clin Endocrinol Diabetes* 2000;108(1):37–43.

299. Rieger-Wettengl G, Tutlewski B, Stabrey A, et al. Analysis of the musculoskeletal system in children and adolescents receiving anticonvulsant monotherapy with valproic acid or carbamazepine. *Pediatrics* 2001;108(6):E107.

300. Shapiro F. Osteopetrosis. Current clinical considerations. *Clin Orthop* 1993;294:34–44.

301. Key LLJ, Ries WL. Sclerosing bony dysplasia. In: Glorieux F, Pettifor JM, Juppner H, eds. *Pediatric bone: biology & diseases*. California: Academic Press, 2003:473.

302. Milgram JW, Jasty M. Osteopetrosis. *J Bone Joint Surg Am* 1982;64:912.

303. Hinkel CL, Beiler DD. Osteopetrosis in adults. *AJR Am J Roentgenol* 1955;74:46.

304. Whyte MP. Carbonic anhydrase II deficiency. *Clin Orthop* 1993;294:52–63.

305. Sly WS, Whyte MP, Sundaram V, et al. Carbonic anhydrase II deficiency in 12 families with the autosomal recessive syndrome of osteopetrosis with renal tubular acidosis and cerebral calcification. *N Engl J Med* 1985;313(3):139–145.

306. Sly WS, Hewett-Emmett D, Whyte MP, et al. Carbonic anhydrase II deficiency identified as the primary defect in the autosomal recessive syndrome of osteopetrosis with renal tubular acidosis and cerebral calcification. *Proc Natl Acad Sci USA* 1983;80(9):2752–2756.

307. Cleiren E, Benichou O, Van Hul E, et al. Albers-Schonberg disease (autosomal dominant osteopetrosis, type II) results from mutations in the ClCN7 chloride channel gene. *Hum Mol Genet* 2001;10(25):2861–2867.

308. Whyte MP, McAlister WH, Novack DV, et al. Bisphosphonate-induced osteopetrosis: novel bone modeling defects, metaphyseal osteopenia, and osteosclerosis fractures after drug exposure ceases. *J Bone Miner Res* 2008;23(10):1698–1707.

309. Ballet JJ, Griscelli C, Coutris C, et al. Bone marrow transplantation in osteopetrosis. *Lancet* 1977;2:1137.

310. Coccia BF, Krivit W, Cervenka J. Successful bone marrow transplantation for infantile osteopetrosis. *N Engl J Med* 1980;302:701.

311. Sieff CA, Levinsky RJ, Rogers DW, et al. Allogeneic bone-marrow transplantation in infantile malignant osteopetrosis. *Lancet* 1983;1:437.

312. Kaplan FS, August CS, Fallon MD, et al. Successful treatment of infantile malignant osteopetrosis by bone-marrow transplantation. *J Bone Joint Surg Am* 1988;70:617.

313. Key LLJ, Rodgriguiz RM, Willi SM, et al. Long-term treatment of osteopetrosis with recombinant human interferon gamma. *N Engl J Med* 1995;332:1594.

314. Armstrong DG, Newfield JT, Gillespie R. Orthopedic management of osteopetrosis: results of a survey and review of the literature. *J Pediatr Orthop* 1999;19(1):122–132.

315. Szappanos L, Szepesi K, Thomazy V. Spondylolysis in osteopetrosis. *J Bone Joint Surg Br* 1988;70(3):428–430.

316. Glorieux FH. Caffey disease: an unlikely collagenopathy. *J Clin Invest* 2005; 115(5):1142–1144.

317. Everts V, Hou WS, Rialland X, et al. Cathepsin K deficiency in pycnodysostosis results in accumulation of non-digested phagocytosed collagen in fibroblasts. *Calcif Tissue Int* 2003;73(4):380–386.

318. Goto T, Yamaza T, Tanaka T. Cathepsins in the osteoclast. *J Electron Microsc (Tokyo)* 2003;52(6):551–558.

319. Motyckova G, Fisher DE. Pycnodysostosis: role and regulation of cathepsin K in osteoclast function and human disease. *Curr Mol Med* 2002;2(5):407–421.

320. Fujita Y, Nakata K, Yasui N, et al. Novel mutations of the cathepsin K gene in patients with pycnodysostosis and their characterization. *J Clin Endocrinol Metab* 2000;85(1):425–431.

321. Edelson JG, Obad S, Geiger R, et al. Pycnodysostosis. Orthopedic aspects with a description of 14 new cases. *Clin Orthop* 1992;280:263–276.

322. Vanhoenacker FM, De Beuckeleer LH, Van Hul W, et al. Sclerosing bone dysplasias: genetic and radioclinical features. *Eur Radiol* 2000;10(9):1423–1433.

323. Soliman AT, Ramadan MA, Sherif A, et al. Pycnodysostosis: clinical, radiologic, and endocrine evaluation and linear growth after growth hormone therapy. *Metabolism* 2001;50(8):905–911.

324. Kim JE, Kim EH, Han EH, et al. A TGF-beta-inducible cell adhesion molecule, betaig-h3, is downregulated in melorheostosis and involved in osteogenesis. *J Cell Biochem* 2000;77(2):169–178.

325. Fryns JP. Melorheostosis and somatic mosaicism. *Am J Med Genet* 1995;58(2):199.

326. Younge D, Drummond D, Herring J, et al. Melorheostosis in children. Clinical features and natural history. *J Bone Joint Surg Br* 1979; 61-B(4):415–418.

327. Murphy M, Kearns S, Cavanagh M, et al. Occurrence of osteosarcoma in a melorheostotic femur. *Ir Med J* 2003;96(2):55–56.

328. Brennan DD, Bruzzi JF, Thakore H, et al. Osteosarcoma arising in a femur with melorheostosis and osteopathia striata. *Skeletal Radiol* 2002;31(8):471–474.

329. Bostman OM, Holmstrom T, Riska EB. Osteosarcoma arising in a melorheostotic femur. A case report. *J Bone Joint Surg Am* 1987;69(8):1232–1237.

330. Choi IH, Kim JI, Yoo WJ, et al. Ilizarov treatment for equinoplanovalgus foot deformity caused by melorheostosis. *Clin Orthop* 2003;414: 238–241.

331. Atar D, Lehman WB, Grant AD, et al. The Ilizarov apparatus for treatment of melorheostosis. Case report and review of the literature. *Clin Orthop* 1992;281:163–167.

332. Griffet J, el Hayek T, Giboin P. Melorheostosis: complications of a tibial lengthening with the Ilizarov apparatus. *Eur J Pediatr Surg* 1998;8(3):186–189.

333. Vanhoenacker FM, Janssens K, Van Hul W, et al. Camurati-Engelmann disease. Review of radioclinical features. *Acta Radiol* 2003;44(4):430–434.

334. Janssens K, ten Dijke P, Ralston SH, et al. Transforming growth factor-beta 1 mutations in Camurati-Engelmann disease lead to increased signaling by altering either activation or secretion of the mutant protein. *J Biol Chem* 2003;278(9):7718–7724.

335. Campos-Xavier B, Saraiva JM, Savarirayan R, et al. Phenotypic variability at the TGF-beta1 locus in Camurati-Engelmann disease. *Hum Genet* 2001;109(6):653–658.

336. Beighton P, Davidson J, Durr L, et al. Sclerosteosis—an autosomal recessive disorder. *Clin Genet* 1977;11(1):1–7.

337. Hamersma H, Gardner J, Beighton P. The natural history of sclerosteosis. *Clin Genet* 2003;63(3):192–197.

338. Itin PH, Keseru B, Hauser V. Syndactyly/brachyphalangy and nail dysplasias as marker lesions for sclerosteosis. *Dermatology* 2001;202(3): 259–262.

339. Stephen LX, Hamersma H, Gardner J, et al. Dental and oral manifestations of sclerosteosis. *Int Dent J* 2001;51(4):287–290.

340. Cremin BJ. Sclerosteosis in children. *Pediatr Radiol* 1979;8(3): 173–177.

341. Beighton P, Cremin BJ, Hamersma H. The radiology of sclerosteosis. *Br J Radiol* 1976;49(587):934–939.

342. Beighton P, Durr L, Hamersma H. The clinical features of sclerosteosis. A review of the manifestations in twenty-five affected individuals. *Ann Intern Med* 1976;84(4):393–397.

343. du Plessis JJ. Sclerosteosis: neurosurgical experience with 14 cases. *J Neurosurg* 1993;78(3):388–392.

344. Balemans W, Ebeling M, Patel N, et al. Increased bone density in sclerosteosis is due to the deficiency of a novel secreted protein (SOST). *Hum Mol Genet* 2001;10(5):537–543.

345. Brunkow ME, Gardner JC, Van Ness J, et al. Bone dysplasia sclerosteosis results from loss of the SOST gene product, a novel cystine knot-containing protein. *Am J Hum Genet* 2001;68(3):577–589.

Paul D. Sponseller
Michael C. Ain

CHAPTER 7

The Skeletal Dysplasias

GENERAL PRINCIPLES

Osteochondral dysplasias are rare disorders of growth and development that affect cartilage and bone. Knowledge about these dysplasias is important to orthopaedic surgeons as an aid to understanding skeletal development. In the preface to the classic text, *McKusick's Heritable Disorders of Connective Tissue* (1), the late Victor McKusick stated, "Nature is nowhere more openly to display her secret mysteries than in cases where she shows traces of her workings apart from the beaten path...." It may be true that there is a mutation and a disorder representing nearly each step of skeletal development. Although there is substantial overlap between conditions that primarily affect cartilage and those that primarily affect bone because of shared matrix elements, metabolic pathways, hormonal influences, and other processes (2), this chapter focuses on those that affect cartilage (for a summary, see Appendix 1).

A useful tool for diagnosis and additional research is the Online Mendelian Inheritance in Man. This web-based compendium is publicly available and readily accessible on the PubMed Web site of the National Library of Medicine (http://www.ncbi.nlm.nih.gov/omim). It allows a user to search by physical features or diagnosis and provides a compilation of applicable knowledge on each (3).

Terminology. Most skeletal dysplasias result in short stature, defined as height more than 2 standard deviations below the mean for the population at a given age. The term "dwarfing condition" is used to refer to disproportionate short stature. The disproportion is commonly referred to as "short trunk" or "short limb." The short-limb types are further subdivided into categories based on which segment of the limb is short. "Rhizomelic" refers to shortening of the root (proximal) portion of the limb; "mesomelic," to the middle segment; and "acromelic," to the distal segment. Achondroplasia is a classic example of rhizomelic involvement, with the femora and especially the humeri being most affected by shortening. Some of these disorders are named after the appearance of the skeleton (diastrophic means "to grow twisted," camptomelic means "bent limbs," and chondrodysplasia punctata refers to stippled cartilage). Eponyms such as Kneist, Morquio, and McKusick are used to name others.

Pathogenesis. Although their pathogenesis is only slowly being investigated, a number of mechanisms have been discovered to lead to skeletal dysplasia. Some result from an alteration in transcription or in the intracellular or extracellular processing of structural molecules of the skeleton (Fig. 7-1). Others are caused by a defect in a receptor or signal transduction in pathways of skeletal differentiation and proliferation. These abnormalities tend to occur in the pathway of cartilage differentiation, growth, and development.

Abnormalities in the form of a structural macromolecule may occur, as in type-II collagen causing spondyloepiphyseal dysplasia (SED). In some cases, the effect may be magnified—a phenomenon termed a "dominant negative" effect. This phenomenon occurs as the defective gene product binds to normal copies of the product, leading to early destruction of normal and defective copies, as seen in osteogenesis imperfecta type II. Pseudoachondroplasia provides another example, with the abnormal cartilage oligomeric matrix protein (COMP) accumulating in the rough endoplasmic reticulum and causing secondary retention of type-IX collagen and other proteins. By contrast, models in which COMP is completely knocked out and not expressed display no disease.

Another pathway through which mutations may act is the alteration of the transport of structural molecules. One example of this mechanism is the group of conditions that includes diastrophic dysplasia (DD) and achondrogenesis type 1, the result of a defect in sulfate transport. This alteration disturbs proteoglycan assembly, leading to diffuse changes in the articular surface cartilage, growth plate, and other areas. An example of receptors gone awry is the family of disorders that includes achondroplasia, hypochondroplasia, and thanatophoric dysplasia. These disorders occur as a result of varying defects in fibroblast growth factor receptor protein. These mutations result in a constitutively active receptor (gain of function). Because this receptor down-regulates endochondral growth, mutations result in decreased endochondral growth. Another example is Jansson metaphyseal dysplasia, which is the result of a constitutively active mutation in parathyroid hormone receptor protein. This protein inhibits the expression of the signaling factor Indian hedgehog, which is needed to stimulate terminal differentiation to hypertrophic chondrocytes and produce normal metaphyseal growth. Disorders of transcription may also cause skeletal dysplasia, as seen in cleidocranial dysplasia, a defect in core-binding factor 1. Because this transcription factor stimulates osteoblast differentiation, a defect in this factor leads to a cartilage model that is well formed but not normally ossified.

Classification. The classification of skeletal dysplasias has traditionally been structured according to the pattern of bone involvement, as in the International Classification of Osteochondrodysplasias (4) (Table 7-1). Another approach, however, is to group them according to the specific causative gene defect for cases in which the defect is known (Table 7-2). A schematic representation of the effects of the known mutations on cartilage development is shown in Figure 7-1. It is also useful for the orthopaedic surgeon to classify the dysplasias into those that are free from spinal deformity [for instance, hypochondroplasia and multiple epiphyseal dysplasia (MED) rarely have significant spinal abnormalities] versus those for which spinal deformity is a frequent problem (such as SED, DD, and metatropic dysplasia). Which disorders are free from epiphyseal involvement and therefore from risk of subsequent degenerative joint disease (DJD)? Achondroplasia and hypochondroplasia, cleidocranial dysplasia, and diaphyseal aclasia

TABLE 7-2	Classification of Skeletal Dysplasias Based on Pathogenesis (Partial List)

Defects in extracellular structural proteins
  COL1 (OI)
  COL2 (achondrogenesis, hypochondrogenesis, SEDC, SEDC, Stickler, Kneist)
  COL9 (MED)
  COL10 (Schmidt)
  COL11 (Stickler variant)
  COMP (pseudoachondroplasia, MED)
  MATN3 (MED)
Defects in metabolic pathways
  AP (hypophosphatasia)
  DTDST (achondrogenesis B, DD, rMED)
Defects in processing and degradation of macromolecules
  Sedlin (SED-X-linked type)
  Lysosomal enzymes (mucopolysaccharidoses, mucolipidoses)
  EXT1, EXT2 (*MHE*1,2)
Defects in hormones, growth factors, receptors, and signal transduction
  *FCGR*s 1–3 (craniosynostoses, achondroplasia, thanatophoric)
  PTH/PTHrP (Jansen metaphyseal dysplasia)
  *GNAS*1 (McCune Albright, pseudohypoparathyroidism)
Defects in nuclear proteins and transcription factors
  SOX1 (camptomelic dysplasia)
  *CBFA*1 (cleidocranial dysplasia)
  SHOX (Leri-Weill)
Defects in RNA processing and metabolism
  RMRP (cartilage-hair hypoplasia)
Defects in cytoskeletal proteins
  Filamins (Larsen syndrome, Melnick-Needles)

TABLE 7-1	International Nosology and Classification of Genetic Skeletal Disorders 2006 (Partial List)

FGFR3 group
Type-II collagen group
Sulfation disorder group
Perlecan group
Filman group
MED/pseudoachondroplasia group
Metaphyseal dysplasias
Spondylometaphyseal dysplasias
Spondyloepimetaphyseal dysplasias
Acromesomelic dysplasias
Mesomelic and rhizomelic dysplasias
Bent bone dysplasias
Slender bone dysplasias
Dysplasias with multiple joint dislocations
Chondrodysplasia punctata group
Increased bone density group
Decreased bone density group
Lysosomal storage diseases
Cleidocranial dysplasia group

rarely present these problems in adulthood, but SED, MED, DD, and others commonly do.

Prenatal Diagnosis With the increasing availability of prenatal screening, many individuals with skeletal dysplasia are being diagnosed before birth. When ultrasound shows a fetus with shortening of the skeleton, femur length is the best biometric parameter to distinguish among the five most common possible conditions. In one study, fetuses with femur length <40% of the mean for gestational age most commonly had achondrogenesis, those with femur length between 40% and 60% most commonly had thanatophoric dysplasia or osteogenesis imperfecta type II, and those with femur length >80% most commonly had achondroplasia or osteogenesis imperfecta type III (5). Additional testing may be performed, if indicated, by chorionic villous sampling and mutation analysis.

Evaluation. In evaluating for skeletal dysplasia in a patient with short stature or abnormal bone development, there are several aspects of the medical history that should be investigated as an aid to diagnosis and coordination of care. Birth length

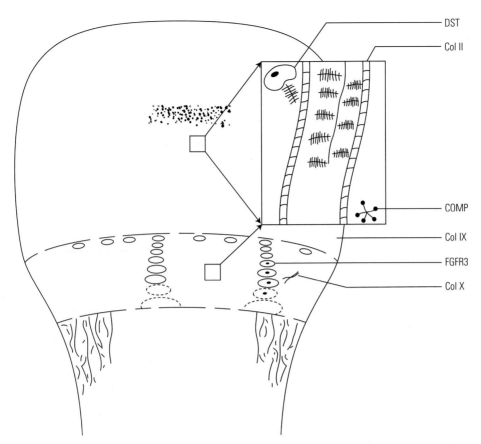

FIGURE 7-1. Schematic illustration of the sites and effects of the known cartilage defects in the skeletal dysplasias. Section of cartilage matrix of physis and epiphysis is simplified and enlarged; genetic abnormalities often affect both regions. *DST,* diastrophic sulfate transporter, deficiency of which leads to undersulfation of proteoglycans in epiphysis and physis of DD and achondrogenesis types 1B and 2; *Col II,* type-II collagen, which is defective in Kneist dysplasia and SED; *COMP,* cartilage oligomeric matrix protein, abnormal pseudoachondroplasia, and some forms of MED; *Col IX,* type-IX collagen, which is closely linked to type-II collagen and is abnormal in some forms of MED; *FGFR3,* fibroblast growth factor receptor 3, which inhibits chondrocyte proliferation in achondroplasia, hypochondroplasia, and thanatophoric dysplasia; *Col X,* type-X collagen, which is synthesized only by the hypertrophic cells of the growth plate and is abnormal in Schmidt-type metaphyseal chondrodysplasia.

is usually shorter than normal in patients with achondroplasia, SED, and most dysplasias but not in those with pseudoachondroplasia or storage disorders. Head circumference is usually larger than normal in patients with achondroplasia. Respiratory difficulty in infancy may occur as a result of restrictive problems in the syndromes with a small thorax, neurologic problems such as foramen magnum stenosis in achondroplasia, or upper airway obstruction in various conditions. A history of heart disease suggests the possibilities of chondroectodermal dysplasia, which may be associated with congenital heart malformations, or storage disorders, such as Hurler or Morquio syndromes, in which cardiac dysfunction may be acquired. A history of immune deficiency or malabsorption is common in cartilage-hair hypoplasia. Retinal detachment may occur with Kneist syndrome or SED. The clinician should elicit information about a family history of short stature or dysmorphism any previous skeletal surgery the patient may have had.

The presence of unusual facial characteristics, a cleft palate, or extremity malformations should be noted. Height percentile

for age should be determined using standard charts. Most skeletal dysplasias result in adult height of <60 in. Measurement of the upper:lower segment ratio may be helpful in distinguishing disproportion early. This value can be obtained by measuring the distance from the top of the pubic symphysis to the sole of the plantigrade foot and subtracting it from the overall length. The normal ratio is 1.6 at birth (given that extremities develop later than the trunk) and diminishes to 0.93 in adults and teens. If shortening of the extremities is noted, it is helpful to classify it as rhizomelic (shortest in the humerus and femur), as in achondroplasia, mesomelia (shortest in the forearms and the legs), or acromelia (shortest distally). The extremities should be examined for ligamentous laxity or contracture (6, 7).

A thorough neurologic examination is needed because of the frequent incidence of spinal compromise at the upper cervical level in SED, DD, Larsen syndrome, and metatropic dysplasia, or at any level in achondroplasia.

A skeletal survey should be ordered, including lateral radiographs of skull and neck and anteroposterior views of the entire spine, pelvis, arms, hands, and legs. Much of this information can be gleaned from reviewing previous radiographs of the child's chest and abdomen that may have been obtained. Sometimes, pathognomonic features will be revealed, such as the caudal narrowing of the interpediculate distances in achondroplasia, double-layered patella in MED, and the iliac horns in nail–patella syndrome. Flexion–extension radiographs of the cervical spine should be ordered if instability is suspected to be causing delay in reaching milestones, loss of strength, or loss of endurance. In many syndromes in which cervical instability is common, such as SED, such radiographs should be ordered as a matter of course. Magnetic resonance imaging (MRI) in flexion and extension may be helpful in some cases to determine if the instability is causing critical risk. However, the limitation of this test is that it often must be done under anesthesia or sedation and the degree of cervical movement is less. If conventional radiographs show substantial motion and a static MRI shows signal changes at the same location, then flexion and extension images are usually not needed.

Laboratory tests may include calcium, phosphate, alkaline phosphatase, and protein to rule out metabolic disorders such as hypophosphatemia or hypophosphatasia. If a progressive disorder is found, the patient's urine should be screened for storage products (under the guidance of a geneticist). To rule out hypothyroidism, serum thyroxine should be measured if the fontanels in an infant are bulging and bone development is delayed. After the differential diagnosis is clinically focused, DNA testing for mutation analysis is increasingly being done in the clinical setting for patients with skeletal dysplasias. A geneticist should be consulted to help establish a diagnosis and a prognosis and to address medical problems. The geneticist sometimes functions as a primary physician for a patient with a genetic disorder because a geneticist has the best overview of the medical issues facing the patient.

Treatment. An orthopaedic surgeon caring for a person with skeletal dysplasia should focus on three aspects: prevention of future limitations, treatment of current deformity, and treatment of pain. The patient's parents should be counseled about the mode of inheritance and the risk of recurrence so that they can make future family plans appropriately. In most cases, it is advisable to see such patients on a routine basis for surveillance so that skeletal problems can be detected at the optimum time for treatment. Weight management is a continuing challenge for many and requires attention. One study of the quality of life in patients with achondroplasia has shown that, although many individuals are able to function at a high level, as a group there are significantly lower scores in all domains (8). Physical difficulties in an environment that is not scaled for such individuals were some of the most commonly cited factors, indicating that treatments to increase stature may have functional benefit.

If surgery becomes necessary for a person with skeletal dysplasia, special considerations apply. Anesthetic management is more difficult if the dysplasia involves oropharyngeal malformations, limited neck mobility, cervical instability, or stenosis (9). Cervical instability is so common in the skeletal dysplasias that the surgeon should make a point of ruling it out by knowledge of the patient or by knowledge of the condition and whether cervical instability is associated with it, or by obtaining special radiographs in flexion and extension (10–12). Restrictive airway problems accompany some dysplasias, and laryngotracheomalacia affects many young diastrophic children. Skeletal distortion may make deep venous access challenging and, in some cases, a general surgeon should be consulted in advance. Intraoperative positioning must accommodate small stature and any contractures that are present. Limb lengthening is an option for many patients who do not have a high risk of DJD. In the tibia, for instance, concomitant stabilization of the tibiofibular joints during lengthening and Achilles lengthening can decrease complications (13). However, the achievement of substantial lengthening in multiple extremities requires a major commitment of a patient's time. Total joint arthroplasty is more difficult in individuals with skeletal dysplasia because of patients' contractures and abnormal skeletal shape and size and because extensive soft-tissue releases may be necessary. However, pain and function scores have been shown to improve substantially after arthroplasty (13).

Postoperative planning must be done in advance because most of these patients have a decreased ability to accommodate postoperative immobilization, stiffness, or functional restrictions. In some situations, postoperative placement in a rehabilitative setting may be most helpful to the patient and family. The Little People of America organization (www.lpaonline.org) may be an important resource for information and support.

ACHONDROPLASIA

Overview. Achondroplasia, an abnormality of endochondral ossification, is the most common form of skeletal dysplasia and occurs in approximately 1 of 25,000 live births (14, 15).

Achondroplasia is caused by a gain of function in the mutation of a gene that encodes for fibroblast growth factor receptor 3 (FGFR3) (16–19). Achondroplasia arises from a point mutation on the short arm of chromosome 4 at nucleotide 1138 of the FGFR3 gene. The mutation is located on the distal short arm of chromosome 4. The result of this mutation is endochondral-ossification-engendered underdevelopment and shortening of the long bones that does not involve intramembranous or periosteal components.

Achondroplasia is inherited as a fully penetrant autosomal dominant trait, but more than 80% of such cases are sporadic, meaning both parents are unaffected (20). If one of the parents is affected, there is a 50/50 chance that the child will develop achondroplasia (14, 15, 20). However, because there is also an increased incidence when the parents are more than 33 years old at the time of conception, a *de novo* mutation is implied (21).

Etiology. The cause of achondroplasia is a single-point mutation in the gene that encodes for *FGFR3*. *FGFR3* mutations have also been found in individuals with thanatophoric dysplasia and hypochondroplasia. Almost all people with achondroplasia have the same recurrent *G-380Rlocus* mutation, which causes a change in a single amino acid. This mutation substitutes an arginine for a glycine residue in the transmembrane domain of the tyrosine-coupled transmembrane receptor in the physis (1, 22). *FGFR3* is expressed in the cartilaginous precursors of bone, where it is believed to decrease chondrocyte proliferation in the proliferative zone of the physis and to regulate growth by limiting endochondral ossification (23). However, in persons with achondroplasia, articular cartilage formation, articular cartilage development, and the intramembranous and periosteal ossification processes are unaffected (24).

It is not known why the proximal portions of the long bones (rhizomelic) are affected more than the distal aspects.

Clinical Features. In the achondroplastic population, the extremities are most affected, that is, they are shorter than those in an unaffected individual. The most commonly affected bones are the humerus and femur, which present a rhizomelic appearance (25). The trunk length is within normal limits or at the lower end of normal limits. This combination typically results in the fingertips reaching only to the tops of the greater trochanter (26), a condition that can lead to possible difficulties in personal hygiene and care and that can worsen as decreasing amount of flexibility occurs in the normal aging process (Fig. 7-2).

The hands are described as trident in nature, that is, the individual is unable to oppose the third and the fourth ray, leaving a space that cannot be closed. There are flexion contractures at the elbow and decreased ability to supinate, most often secondary to the fact that the radial head can be subluxed, as evidenced on radiographs. None of the above features are clinically important, but a nonknowledgeable physician might misdiagnose such a presentation as a "nursemaid's elbow" and incorrectly attempt a reduction.

The facial appearance of patients with achondroplasia is characterized by an enlarged head, mandibular protrusion, frontal bossing (flattened or depressed nasal bridge), and midface hypoplasia. The bones in the midface are more affected than the other facial bones because of their endochondral origin (16).

Although the lower extremities are typically in varus secondary to knee and ankle morphology, the lower extremities can be straight or occasionally in valgus, and internal tibial torsion may also be seen. Typically, the knee and ankle joints have excessive laxity, although usually such patients do not develop premature arthritis. The femoral necks are often shortened, giving an appearance of coxa breva.

In terms of the spine, kyphosis at the thoracolumbar junction is very common and is typically seen in the first 1 to 2 years of life (Fig. 7-3). In most children, this condition will correct spontaneously within a few months of ambulation, although ambulation is often delayed in patients with

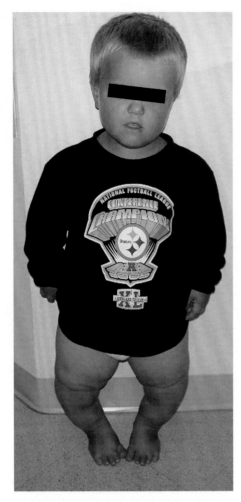

FIGURE 7-2. Photograph of a 5-year-old male with achondroplasia. Note the typical bowing and fingertips reaching to the top of the hips.

achondroplasia (27). As kyphosis improves, lumbosacral lordosis may seem to progress.

One study found that life expectancy is not substantially diminished in individuals with achondroplasia (28), but a more recent report has indicated a higher mortality rate in 30- to 50-year-old people with achondroplasia compared with age-matched controls (29). This reported increased mortality is typically secondary to heart disease. One indicator for heart disease is abnormal blood pressure, but it is possible that standard blood pressure cuffs may underestimate the pressures in the achondroplastic population, leading to the nonidentification and nontreatment of a large number of patients with high blood pressure. New cuffs have been developed and their use for this population is being reviewed.

Growth and Development. In most children with achondroplasia, growth and development fall behind those of unaffected children.

Widely available growth charts (25) indicate that the infant with achondroplasia is shorter than an unaffected infant, a

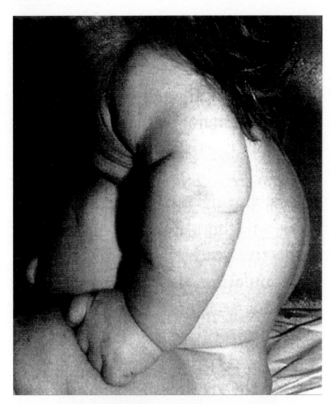

FIGURE 7-3. Photograph of an 18-month-old female with achondroplasia sitting with typical postural kyphosis.

height deficit that increases markedly during the first few years of life and becomes even more marked during the growth spurt at puberty (30). The average height for an adult with achondroplasia is 132 cm for men and 125 cm for women (20).

Children with achondroplasia also have delayed motor milestones (head control, 4 months; sitting up independently, 10 months; ambulation, 18 to 20 months) (31, 32), and three-quarters of them have ventriculomegaly (33).

Historically, hydrocephalus was thought to be the cause, leading also to macrocephaly, but only a very small subset has been shown to have clinically significant hydrocephalus (34); standardized head circumference charts can help track such children (35). Ventricular peroneal shunting is indicated only for rapid progression of head circumference, or for signs and symptoms of increased intracranial pressure.

Mental development is typically normal in children with achondroplasia, but physical manifestations are often delayed, especially in the first 2 to 3 years of life (36). Typically, motor development normalizes by 3 years of age. There are standardized developmental charts that are available for monitoring such children.

Foramen magnum stenosis is one of the earliest serious health consequences faced by some children with achondroplasia. Its symptoms, which most commonly occur in the first 2 years of life but which may present later (37), include chronic brain stem compression, sleep apnea, lower cranial nerve dysfunction, difficulty in swallowing, hyperreflexia,

hypotonia, weakness, paresis or clonus, and severe developmental delay, and are quantified in sleep studies (34, 38–42). The most common presenting symptom of foramen magnum stenosis is respiratory difficulty with excessive snoring or apnea (43). Apnea can be central in nature (because of brainstem compression) or just obstructive because of the individual's small midface. The American Academy of Pediatrics recommends screening for foramen magnum stenosis with polysonography and computed tomography (CT) or MRI in all infants with achondroplasia. Because CT and MRI in the first year of life require sedation, the child who is developing well, has no abnormal reflexes, and is alert, oriented, and meeting all milestones can typically just be followed clinically. If head circumference changes or if a patient is not reaching milestones, a sleep study should be ordered. If the sleep study is abnormal, then a CT or an MRI scan should be obtained. We prefer MRI because, in our opinion, it produces a better image of the brain stem and the upper cervical spinal cord.

Some studies have shown a high mortality rate (2% to 5%) in infants with achondroplasia and have indicated foramen magnum stenosis as the responsible factor (33).

Radiographic Characteristics. There are several features typically seen on the radiographs of individuals with achondroplasia, but caution should be exercised in interpreting the absence of such findings: not all affected individuals exhibit such radiographic characteristics.

The key feature is the typical narrowing intrapedicular distance from L1 to L5 seen on the anteroposterior radiographs of affected individuals (44, 45); in the unaffected population, the intrapedicular distance from L1 to L5 increases. The presence of such narrowing is an absolute indicator of achondroplasia, but the lack of such narrowing does not rule out the presence of achondroplasia. In addition, pedicles in those with achondroplasia are approximately 30% to 40% thicker than those in unaffected individuals (46). In this patient population, the vertebral bodies have a scalloped appearance (20), lumbar lordosis increases to the sacrum segment and may even become horizontal, and severe scoliosis is rare but can be seen; however, the incidence of cervical instability is not higher than that in the unaffected population (20, 46).

Other radiographic abnormalities include underdeveloped facial bones, skull base, and foramen magnum; square iliac rings; rhizomelic shortening; and flared metaphysis of the long bones. Affected individuals also have a pronounced, inverted "v" shape of the distal femoral physis with normal distal femoral epiphysis, and the metacarpals and metatarsals are almost all equal in length. The iliac wings have a squared appearance. The metaphysis of all long bones is flared in appearance. Despite being short, the diaphyses of all long bones are thick. The sites of major muscle insertions, such as the tibial tubercle, greater trochanter, and insertion of the deltoid, are more prominent than usual. The epiphysis throughout the skeleton is normal in appearance and development; consequently, degenerative joint arthritis or changes are rarely seen.

General Medical Treatment. Although children with achondroplasia are typically healthier than those with other dysplasias, infants and young children with achondroplasia should be closely monitored and evaluated, especially during the first few years of life, for signs and symptoms of foramen magnum stenosis (see earlier). If the diagnosis is made clinically, an MRI should be ordered to show the stenosis. At this point, neurosurgery can enlarge the foramen magnum. Sometimes, surgeons may need to perform a durotomy or an expansion of the dura and a C1 laminectomy. Many of these children also have dilatation of the veins of their cranium secondary to venous distension, which can also be relieved by such surgery. As indicated earlier, children with achondroplasia have delayed motor milestones; for example, most unaffected children walk by 12 months, whereas most of those with achondroplasia do not walk until 18 months. Postsurgery, patients typically are able to start achieving milestones much more quickly and progress rapidly (38, 40). In addition, children with achondroplasia have a higher risk of respiratory complications than do unaffected children, not only because of midface hypoplasia and upper airway obstruction, but also because of a decreased respiratory drive that can be secondary to foramen magnum stenosis. Early brain stem decompression can decrease the risk (37).

Otolaryngeal problems are also prevalent: 90% of the patients with achondroplasia can experience otitis media before they are 2 years old (47), and many require ear tube placements. Adenoid and tonsil hypertrophy in the presence of midface hypoplasia can cause obstructive sleep apnea. The otitis media and adenotonsil hypertrophy may result in conductive hearing loss that can impair speech development and delay.

Achieving and maintaining an ideal body weight is also difficult and a lifelong struggle. Currently, because there are no standardized charts for size and weight, observing skin-fold thickness and noting general appearance may be the best clinical option (48, 49).

Children with achondroplasia are typically not deficient in growth hormone levels, but there is a substantial amount of research with regard to the administration of growth hormone to supplement height (18, 50, 51). Typically, in the first year of receiving growth hormone treatment, there is an increase in the growth height velocity, but it diminishes over the next 2 to 3 years, with a net result of no real increase. There has been speculation that too much growth hormone can hasten the development of spinal stenosis, which is one of the worst complications of achondroplasia (18, 50, 51).

There are several other otolaryngologic problems that are usually secondary to the underdevelopment of midface skeletal structures. Maxillary hypoplasia can lead to dental overcrowding and malocclusion (52). Many children with this condition require orthodontic attention. In such children, Eustachian tubes often do not function properly because the children are smaller than the unaffected population and more horizontally than vertically positioned, decreasing the ability to drain middle ear fluid (53).

Orthopaedic problems include angular deformities of the lower extremities, genu varum at the knees, thoracolumbar kyphosis, and spinal stenosis (which can occur at any level of the spinal canal). Malalignment of the lower extremities is typically secondary to genu varum or ankle varus (24, 54). A very small percentage of patients have genu valgum, which rarely becomes severe enough to require treatment, but genu varum may progress to cause substantial pain and difficulty in ambulation (24, 55). Some clinicians have postulated that the longer fibula is the cause of this pain, but others have shown that the length of the fibula has no direct relationship on the amount of bowing on the knee (56–58) (Fig. 7-4). Leg malalignment has been shown to be the result of ankle, distal femur, or proximal tibia deformity, or from a combination thereof. Incomplete ossification epiphysis often makes it quite challenging to elicit the source of this malalignment. Arthrograms are typically used at our institution to help identify the exact location of the deformity and are especially helpful in patients <8 years old (12). Although bracing has been used elsewhere to help control ligamentous laxity and to try to correct bowing, we have found that the short and often pendulous nature of the legs of patients with achondroplasia makes it difficult to provide a brace with proper fit and enough of a mechanical advantage to correct the malalignment. During the past 10 years of our practice, no brace has been used to control malalignment, and surgical decisions are not made until the child is at least 3 years old. The indication for surgery is persistent pain that is secondary to malalignment (not to spinal stenosis) deformity severe enough to cause a fibular thrust, resulting in a gap between the proximal tibia and the femur on ambulation (40, 57, 59). Again, in our practice, if the decision has been made for surgical intervention, an arthrogram is obtained to evaluate the optimal location of the osteotomy. Such arthrography also often identifies internal tibial torsion, which can then be corrected concurrently. Although fibular shortening has been advocated in the past (55), we and others (60, 61) do not think it is ever indicated. Treatment indications are difficult to define clearly because there are no natural history studies showing which degree of deformity causes early degeneration.

Short Stature and Limb Lengthening. Infants with achondroplasia are shorter than other individuals and the deficit progresses until skeletal maturity.

Everyday difficulties as the result of short stature include using public restrooms, face washing in public restrooms, hair combing, engaging in hobbies involving physical activity, playing sports with average-statured individuals, conducting routine business transactions (often at countertop level), and driving a car. Nevertheless, the decision to augment stature is difficult and controversial because the procedure is time consuming, complicated (40, 62), and fraught with complications (38, 40).

First, surgical lengthening can achieve quite a bit of height if done safely and correctly (13, 63, 64), but because it is a time-consuming process, it removes these children from their normal activities of school and socialization. The psychologic impact can be tremendous, especially if the lengthening goals

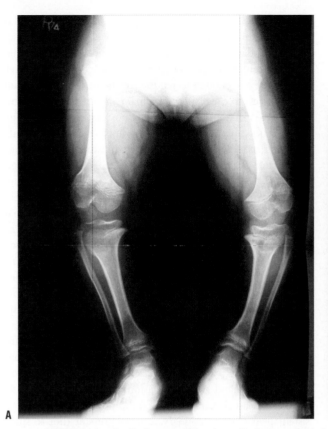
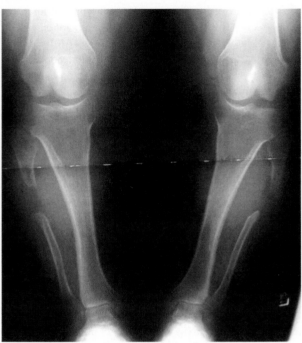

FIGURE 7-4. Prefibulectomy **(A)** and postfibulectomy **(B)** (without change of alignment) radiographs of a 14-year-old male with achondroplasia and tibia vara.

are not achieved. At some centers, lengthening is performed at two separate time intervals, the first typically at the age of 7 years old and the second at preadolescence. The overall time frame for surgery and postoperative therapy may be up to 3 years. Some centers prefer to delay lengthening until early adolescence to increase the patient's participation for the rehabilitation process and also the decision making as to whether or not the lengthening should be done. We know of only one child with achondroplasia who has had limb lengthening and whose parents were also affected.

Second, surgical limb lengthening is a very complicated endeavor (40, 62), and one that is fraught with complications (38, 40). In one study by Aldegheri and Dall'Oca (65), 43% of the patients who underwent limb lengthening had complications, including fracture, failure of premature consolidation, malunion, malalignment, joint stiffness, and infection. One report in the literature indicates increased symptoms of lumbar spinal stenosis (66). The effect of limb lengthening on spinal stenosis needs additional investigation. Humeral lengthening, often is combined with lower extremity limb lengthening, may be the most functionally appreciated because it makes it is easier to perform personal care, put on shoes and socks, and perform extended reaching. The procedure also has lower risks than lower limb lengthening.

Despite the fact that limb lengthening has been a procedure in frequent use for several decades, to our knowledge, the

functional benefits after elective limb lengthening have never been studied.

Spinal Aspects Thoracolumbar kyphosis develops in most infants with achondroplasia. A newborn with achondroplasia typically has a thoracolumbar kyphosis centered at approximately T12–L1. When sitting begins, the infant slumps forward because of trunk hypotonia, in combination with a relatively large head, flat chest, and protuberant abdomen. The apex of the vertebral deformity becomes wedge-shaped anteriorly, although it usually is a reversible phenomenon. This condition should not be confused with a diagnosis of congenital kyphosis. Most of these patients improve by the 2nd or the 3rd year of life, after walking begins and muscle strength increases (15, 27, 67, 68). However, persistent kyphosis can increase the risk of symptomatic stenosis, putting pressure on the conus (Fig. 7-5). To prevent persistent kyphosis, Pauli et al. (27) recommended early parental counseling (before the infant is 1 year old) for prohibition of unsupported sitting or sitting up at more than a 45-degree angle and for the use of the following measures: firm, back-seating devices; curling the infant into a "C" position; hand counterpressure when holding the infant; and bracing as needed. In the study by Pauli et al. (27), bracing is initiated for patients who develop kyphosis that does not correct to <30 degrees on prone lateral radiographs. Those authors initially used bracing but found it cumbersome

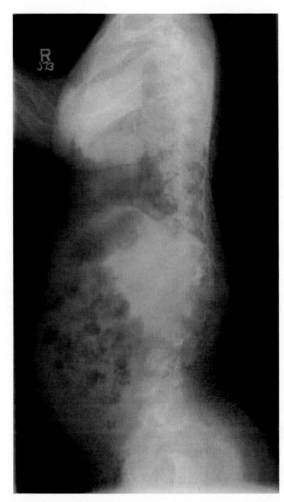

FIGURE 7-5. Radiograph of a 4-year-old patient with achondroplasia and thoracolumbar wedging and kyphosis.

has decreased with increased rigidity instrumentation by the placement of pedicle screws at every level (70–76).

For the child with achondroplasia, thoracolumbar kyphosis, and concurrent spinal stenosis symptoms, MRI will be obtained; if it shows anterior cord impingement, a corpectomy via an anterior approach will be performed. In this situation, we would not perform a vertebral body resection posteriorly because we think the achondroplastic spinal cord is not mobile enough to tolerate such a procedure. Currently, any child >3 years old who can accommodate pedicle screws, including cervical spine screws, is not placed in a cast or brace postoperatively. However, for a child <3 years old with pedicle screws, a bracing protocol is instituted for 3 months.

Lumbar stenosis typically can present during the second or third decade of life of an individual with achondroplasia, but it can be seen as early as 18 months (Fig. 7-6). Patients typically present with complaints of lower back pain, leg pain, progressive weakness of the extremities, numbness, and tingling, symptoms that often are decreased or alleviated completely by squatting or bending over—maneuvers that reduce the lumbar lordosis, increase the size of the canal, and relieve the pressure. Surgical indications include myelopathy, progressive signs and symptoms, inability to ambulate more than one or two city

and not very helpful. In addition, the braced patient may be at an increased risk for falls because of the brace's large size and the patient's small body, poor trunk control, and developmental delay. Bracing may also have a detrimental effect on pulmonary function in children with small thoracic cages. In our practice, we have found that bracing has delayed the onset of walking. If wedging of the vertebrae persists beyond the ages of 4 or 5 years, and surgical intervention is not sought, we recommend a trial of using hyperextension casts to see if it will help with the wedging. Although some surgeons have used this technique with some benefit (69), we have seen several instances of such use that have resulted in numerous complications, including skin breakdowns, the inability to tolerate the casts, decreased ability to ambulate, and others. Currently, the indication for safe surgical intervention in our practice is kyphosis ≥50 degrees at 5 years of age with no sign of improvement (70). The key is twofold: (a) no hooks, wires, or any other hardware in the canal and (b) no overcorrection. Correction should limited to what is obtainable preoperatively with the awake child hyperextended laterally over a bolster. The threshold for performing an anterior arthrodesis

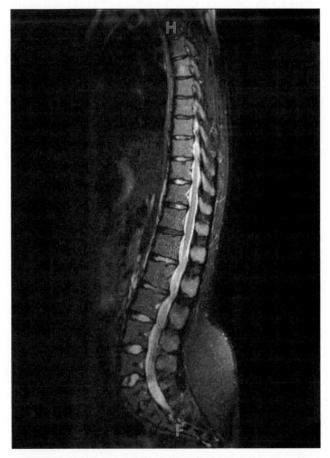

FIGURE 7-6. T2-weighted MRI of a 12-year-old patient with achondroplasia and lumbar stenosis.

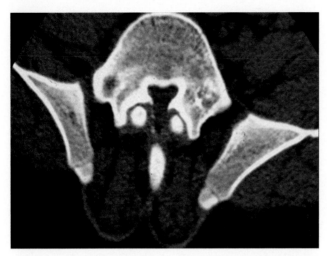

FIGURE 7-7. CT myelogram in a patient with achondroplasia and severe lumbar/sacral stenosis.

blocks without having to stop or squat to relieve the pressure. Preoperative workup includes MRI and possibly a CT scan (Fig. 7-7). By correlating the physical examination and the MRI study, the clinician can identify the approximate level of the most severe stenosis. Usually, treatment is a wide decompression that extends at least two levels above the point of the most severe stenosis and down to the sacrum. In skeletally immature patients, a posterior spinal fusion with pedicle screw instrumentation needs to be done concurrently to prevent progressive kyphosis. If the patient is skeletally mature and has no underlying kyphosis, posterior decompression can be done alone, without a concurrent fusion (40, 46, 71–74, 77).

HYPOCHONDROPLASIA

Etiology and Pathogenesis. Hypochondroplasia is an autosomal dominant disorder, and the chance of passing it on to offspring is approximately 50% (1). Although hypochondroplasia and achondroplasia have similar names and are similar phenotypically (individuals with mild achondroplasia can appear similar to individuals with severe hypochondroplasia), they are two distinct disorders. The mutation that causes hypochondroplasia is located on the short arm of chromosome 4, in gene *FGFR3,* as it is in achondroplasia and thanatophoric dysplasia. However, the nucleotide change is in a different region, the tyrosine kinase domain. In hypochondroplasia, the mutation results in increased activation of factors that slow cell growth (16, 78–81).

Clinical Features. Hypochondroplasia can usually be identified at birth, but it can also be unrecognized until early puberty if the individual is only mildly affected. The presentation is more varied than that of achondroplasia; foramen magnum stenosis and thoracolumbar stenosis are extremely rare in patients with hypochondroplasia.

Compared with the achondroplastic population, individuals with hypochondroplasia have less of a height discrepancy

(118 to 160 cm) (20, 82); similar, but less pronounced, facial characteristics; limbs shorter than the trunk, but to a lesser extent; milder other features such as thoracolumbar kyphosis, spinal stenosis, and genu varum; and mesomelic rather than rhizomelic long-bone shortening. In addition, the need for surgical intervention for patients with hypochondroplasia is much lower than that for those with achondroplasia. In our practice, we have surgically treated several hundred patients who had achondroplasia with spinal stenosis and/or kyphosis, but only a few patients with hypochondroplasia have required surgical intervention. Unlike individuals with achondroplasia, in whom intelligence is normal, a small portion (<10%) of those with hypochondroplasia have been associated with mental retardation (83).

Radiographic Features. Hall and Spranger (84) have proposed primary and secondary criteria for making this diagnosis. Primary criteria are narrowing of the pedicles in the lumbar spine, squaring of the iliac crest, broad femoral necks, mild metaphyseal flaring, and brachydactyly. Secondary criteria are shortening lumbar pedicles, mild posterior scalloping of the vertebral bodies, elongation of the distal fibula, and ulnar styloid. In patients with achondroplasia, the sciatic notches are narrow in nature; in patients with hypochondroplasia, the notches are unaffected and normal in appearance.

Differential Diagnosis. Compared with achondroplasia, hypochondroplasia is a much milder form of skeletal dysplasia and has a much more variable presentation; it can also go unrecognized until early puberty. However, severe cases of hypochondroplasia can overlap mild forms of achondroplasia. Occasionally, hypochondroplasia can be confused with Schmidt metaphyseal dysplasia because both disorders have mild short stature, typically normal faces, and mild genu varum.

Treatment. Surgery is rarely indicated. The administration of growth hormone therapy can have a positive initial impact (51, 85, 86), but to our knowledge, no long-term studies have been done. If limb lengthening is chosen, the risks and complications are the same as those for individuals with achondroplasia, but the benefits may be greater because the patients are taller initially and successful lengthening may enable them to achieve low-to-normal adult height and stature. However, patients should still be advised of all of the risks and complications and that there are no long-term studies.

METATROPIC DYSPLASIA

Overview. The term "metatropic dwarfism" comes from the Greek word metatropos, or "changing form," because patients with this condition appear to have short-limb dwarfism early in life, but later develop a short-trunk pattern as spinal length is lost with the development of kyphosis and scoliosis. The condition has been likened to Morquio syndrome because of the enlarged appearance of the metaphyses and the contractures (87).

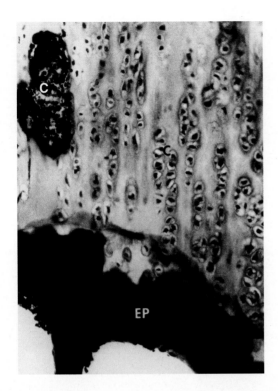

FIGURE 7-8. Histology of the growth plate in metatropic dysplasia, showing relatively normal columns of proliferating chondrocytes (*C*), but absence of the hypertrophic or the degenerating zones, as well as a "seal," or bony end plate (*EP*), over the metaphysis. (From Boden SD, Kaplan FS, Fallon MD, et al. Metatropic dwarfism: uncoupling of endochondral and perichondral growth. *J Bone Joint Surg Am* 1987;69:174, with permission.)

It is a rare condition that may be inherited in an autosomal dominant or recessive manner (88). The cause of this dysplasia has not been elucidated. However, histologic abnormalities of the growth plate have been studied and appear to be characteristic, as shown in the study by Boden et al. (89). The physis shows relatively normal columns of proliferating chondrocytes. However, there is an abrupt arrest of further development, with absence of a zone of hypertrophic or degenerating chondrocytes. Instead, there is a mineralized seal of bone over the metaphyseal end of the growth plate (Fig. 7-8). The perichondral ring remains intact, and circumferential growth is preserved. This uncoupling of endochondral and perichondral growth appears to account for the characteristic "knobby" metaphyses and the platyspondyly. Additional understanding of the defect in this disorder will shed light on the normal maturation of the physis.

Clinical Features.   One of the most characteristic features of this condition is the presence of the "coccygeal tail," a cartilaginous prolongation of the coccyx that is not present in other dysplasias (Fig. 7-9A,B). It is usually a few centimeters long and arises from the gluteal fold. The facial appearance includes a high forehead, and there may be a high arched palate. The sternum may display a pectus carinatum, the limbs have flexion contractures of up to 30 to 40 degrees from infancy, and other joints may have ligamentous laxity. The limbs appear relatively short with respect to the trunk. The metaphyses are enlarged, which, when combined with underdeveloped musculature, gives a "bulky" appearance to the limbs. Some patients have been reported to have ventriculomegaly or hydrocephalus (90) or to develop upper cervical spine instability and/or stenosis (90, 91). Scoliosis develops in early childhood and is progressive (92, 93). Some restrictive lung disease is usually present,

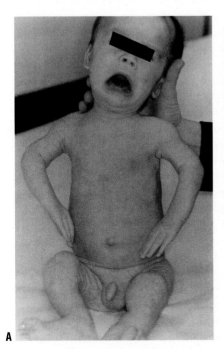
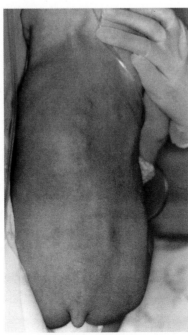

FIGURE 7-9. A 1-year-old infant with metatropic dysplasia, illustrating knee-flexion contractures, "bulky" metaphyses **(A)**, and a coccygeal tail **(B)**.

A

B

and it may cause death in infancy for the one-third of patients who are afflicted by the autosomal recessive form of the disease (88, 93). However, for those who survive into adulthood, height varies from 110 to 120 cm.

Radiographic Features.

Prenatal sonographic diagnosis may be possible in the first or second trimester, with the finding of substantial dwarfism, narrow thorax, and enlarged metaphyses (94, 95). Odontoid hypoplasia frequently exists in patients with this condition, as in many patients with skeletal dysplasia. In infancy, the vertebrae are markedly flattened throughout the spine, but normal in width. Kyphosis and scoliosis develop in most patients. The ribs are short and flared, with cupping at the costochondral junctions (Fig. 7-10).

The epiphyses and metaphyses are enlarged, giving the long bones an appearance that has been likened to that of a barbell (Fig. 7-11). The epiphyses have delayed and irregular ossification. Protrusio acetabuli has been reported (93). Genu varum of mild-to-moderate degree usually develops. Degenerative changes of major joints often occur in adulthood.

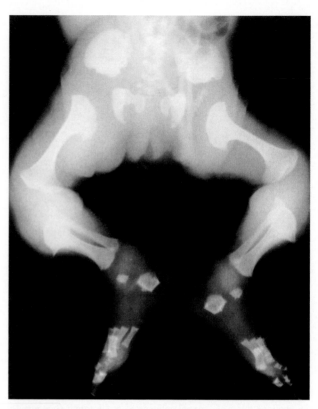

FIGURE 7-11. Newborn with metatropic dysplasia. The diaphyses are short and the metaphyses are broad and flared; their appearance has been likened to dumbbells. The iliac wings are flared, and the acetabulae are deep. (Courtesy of George S. Bassett, MD.)

Treatment/Orthopaedic Considerations.

Respiratory problems often dominate infancy and may be fatal. They result from the small thorax and may also result, in part, from cervical instability. Such children need to be observed on a follow-up basis at a center with clinicians who have pediatric pulmonary expertise. The neck should be imaged early with MRI and possibly flexion–extension radiographs. Because cervical quadriplegia has been reported (91), fusion is recommended if atlantooccipital translation is more than approximately 8 mm, or neurologic compromise is present. If a patient has atlantoaxial instability of 5 to 8 mm but is neurologically intact, MRI should be obtained in flexion and extension. Fusion should be recommended if cord compromise is seen. Severe stenosis should be decompressed (91).

The patients should be examined early for spinal curvature. There is no documentation of efficacy of brace treatment for this condition. It may be tried in small curves (<45 degrees) in young patients or those who need support to sit, but it has no proven value for large curves, even if the patients are young and still actively growing. Spinal fusion for scoliosis may be advisable in patients with more severe curves. Deciding exactly when to intervene is more of an informed judgment call than a science. To document medical health and to have a chance of bone size adequate for instrumentation, we recommend observation and accepting a larger curve

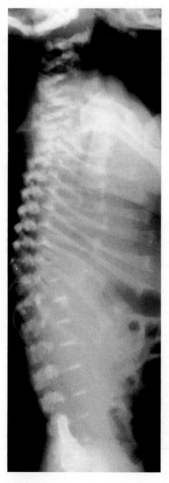

FIGURE 7-10. Newborn with metatropic dysplasia. Note platyspondyly with delayed vertebral ossification and flared ribs. (Courtesy of Judy Hall, Vancouver, BC.)

threshold for surgery in patients <10 years old. However, progressive, sharp, angular kyphosis with paraparesis may occur in metatropic dysplasia and should be treated early with growth-sparing procedures or fusion if, in the surgeon's estimation, neurologic compromise is a risk. When surgery is undertaken, anterior as well as posterior fusion should be considered if the patient is able to tolerate it, because rigid fixation is difficult and there is a high rate of pseudarthrosis in this condition (10). Given that the curves are often rigid, only the amount of correction that can be achieved safely should be attempted. Halo-cast immobilization is an option if patient size, stenosis, or poor bone density make instrumentation inadvisable.

CHONDROECTODERMAL DYSPLASIA

Overview.   Chondroectodermal dysplasia is an uncommon disorder. It is also known as Ellis-Van-Creveld syndrome and is prevalent among the Amish (96). It results in disproportional short stature and abnormalities in the teeth, limbs, and cardiac areas. The pathognomonic characteristic of this condition is severe flattening or wedging of the lateral proximal tibial physis, which leads to the severe genu valgum (Fig. 7-12).

It is a defect in *EVC* gene, or in the short arm of chromosome 4 (97–99). It results in the defect of maturation of endochondral ossification. It is transmitted as an autosomal recessive condition.

Orthopaedic Treatment.   The first priority for patients with chondroectodermal dysplasia is stabilization of the heart.

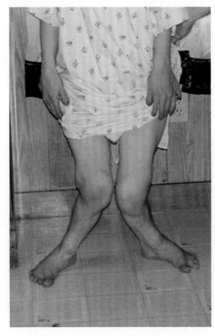

FIGURE 7-12.   Photograph of a 16-year-old Amish male with Ellis-Van-Creveld syndrome and severe genu valgum.

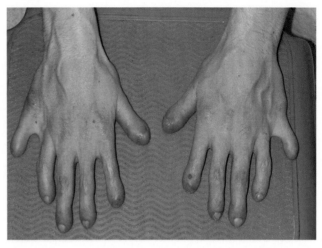

FIGURE 7-13.   Photograph of a 21-year-old male with Ellis-Van-Creveld syndrome who did not undergo polydactyly correction.

Approximately one-third of these infants die in the first few weeks of life (100). In the first year, most patients with this condition have polydactyly, which can be reconstructed (Fig. 7-13). Genu valgum frequently occurs and can be quite severe. If seen early, genu valgum can be treated with guided growth, such as a hemiepiphysiodesis with an 8-plate. In our practice, bracing has had no effect on this condition and does not help control the severe ligamentous laxity. If surgical intervention (i.e., osteotomies) is warranted because of severe valgus angulation, rotational malalignment should be considered along with any genu valgum. The distal femur is typically externally rotated, and the tibia is internally rotated. It appears as though there is a flexion contracture in the lower extremities, but after correcting the malrotation, the flexion contracture typically disappears and then the malalignment needs to be corrected (62, 101). Clinicians can correct the malalignment with external or internal fixation. In these children and young adults, there is an increased risk of patellar subluxation and dislocation. Many times, lateral release, medial reefing, and even tibial tubercle osteotomies are required. In the presence of genu valgum, after correcting the malrotation, lateral proximal tibial elevation can also be entertained. Before the plateau elevation, an external fixator across the knee can be placed to open the lateral joint line. Osteotomy is necessary in severe cases because there is a high rate of recurrence.

Clinical Features.   Approximately half of the children with chondroectodermal dysplasia have cardiac defects, most commonly atrial septal defects. One-third of children with this condition die during the neonatal period, most from cardiac abnormalities.

Patients with this disorder develop hypospadious and epispadious. They have narrow chests, abnormal dentition (with crooked, sparse, and sometimes lost teeth), abnormal nails, and postaxial polydactyly. This condition presents as acromesomelic shortening of the middle and distal segments of the upper and lower extremities (102–105). The spine is typically uninvolved. The lower extremities have significant genu valgum secondary to a hypoplastic proximal laterotibial plateau and lax ligaments, and rotational abnormalities (such as external rotation of the femur or internal rotation of the tibia) are often present, as though there were a flexion contracture.

Radiographic Features.

The ribs are short, the chest is narrow, and there is uneven growth of the proximal tibial epiphysis laterally. Exostosis can develop from the proximal tibial epiphysis medially and acetabular spike of the medial and lateral edges. The greater trochanteric epiphyses are quite pronounced, and the wrists can display fusion of the capitates, hamate, and (sometimes) other carpal bones. Carpal bones typically have delayed maturation, in contrast to the accelerated maturation of the phalanges.

DIASTROPHIC DYSPLASIA

Overview.

DD is perhaps the dysplasia with the most numerous, disparate, and severe skeletal abnormalities. The term "diastrophic" comes from a Greek root meaning "distorted," which aptly describes the ears, spine, long bones, and feet. Before the current level of understanding of the skeletal dysplasias was developed, early authorities referred to this condition as "achondroplasia with clubbed feet" (106, 107). Certainly, the skeletal abnormalities are much more extensive than that.

The disorder is autosomal recessive and is extremely rare, except in Finland, where between 1% and 2% of the population are carriers, and there are more than 160 people known to be affected because of an apparent founder effect (108). The defect is on chromosome 5 in the gene that codes for a sulfate transporter protein (aptly named "diastrophic dysplasia sulfate transporter" or *DTDST*) (109, 110). This protein is expressed in virtually all cell types. Decreased content of sulfate in cartilage from patients with DD has been shown (111). A defect in this gene leads to undersulfation of proteoglycan in the cartilage matrix. If one considers proteoglycans to be the "hydraulic jacks" of cartilage at the ultrastructural level, it is understandable that there should be such impairment of performance of physeal, epiphyseal, and articular cartilage throughout the body. Achondrogenesis types 1B and 2 are more serious disorders causing mutations on the same gene.

Histopathology reveals that chondrocytes appear to degenerate prematurely, and collagen is present in excess (112, 113). Tracheal cartilage has some of the same abnormalities seen in other cartilage types, but it still does not explain some of the specific focal malformations seen in DD, such as proximal interphalangeal joint fusion in the hands, short first metacarpal causing hitchhiker thumbs, or cervical spina bifida. Additional work on the role of this sulfate transporter on skeletal growth and development must be done to explain these curious findings.

Clinical Features.

Prominent cheeks gave rise to the previously used name "cherub dwarf" (Fig. 7-14). The nasal bridge is flattened. Up to one-half of patients have a cleft palate, which may contribute to aspiration pneumonia (112). The cartilage of the trachea is abnormally soft, and its diameter may be narrowed. The ear is normal at birth but develops a peculiar acute swelling of the pinna at 3 to 6 weeks in 80% to 85% of cases (114). The reasons for this event and this timing are not known. The cartilage hardens in a deformed shape—the "cauliflower ear," which is one of the pathognomonic features of this dysplasia.

Patients with diastrophism have a slightly increased [approximately 5% (106, 107)] perinatal mortality as a result of respiratory problems, especially aspiration pneumonia and tracheomalacia. Motor milestones are delayed: sitting occurs at a mean age of 8 months, pulling up to a stand at 13 months, and walking at 24 months (115).

The skeleton displays abnormalities from the cervical spine down to the feet (6). The posterior arches of the lower cervical spine are often bifid. There are no external clues to this occult underlying abnormality. Cervical kyphosis is seen in one-third to one-half of patients (11, 116); it may be present in infancy, and its course is variable. Spontaneous resolution has been reported in a number of patients, even with curves of up to

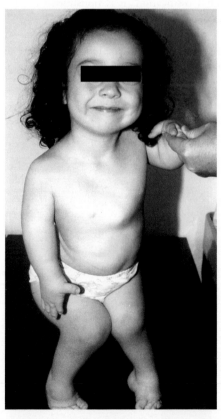

FIGURE 7-14. A 5-year-old girl with DD. Note prominent cheeks, circumoral fullness, equinovarus feet, valgus knees with flexion contracture, and abducted or "hitchhiker" thumbs.

80 degrees (117, 118) (Fig. 7-15A–C). However, others progress, and several reports of quadriparesis from this deformity exist (11, 119). Scoliosis develops in at least one-third of patients (116), but many curves do not exceed 50 degrees. Tolo (120) has stated that the scoliosis may be one of two types: idiopathic-like or sharply angular. The sharply angular type is usually characterized by kyphosis at the same level as the scoliosis. Spinal stenosis is not common, in contrast to achondroplasia. Most patients have substantial lumbar lordosis, likely to compensate for the hip flexion contractures in diastrophism.

The extremities display rhizomelic shortening. The shoulders may be subluxated, as may the radial heads (possibly because of ulnar shortening). The hands are short, broad, and ulnarly deviated. The hitchhiker thumb is the result of a short, proximally placed, often triangular, first metacarpal that may be hypermobile. This finding is seen in up to 95% of persons with DD (106). The proximal interphalangeal joints of the fingers are often fused (symphalangism).

The hips maintain a persistent flexion contracture. The proximal femoral epiphyses progressively deform, and even subluxate, in some patients. Epiphyseal flattening and hinge abduction develop in many patients (121). Arthritic changes develop by early to middle adulthood. The knees usually have flexion contractures, which result from a combination of ligamentous contracture and epiphyseal deformation (Fig. 7-16A,B). Excessive valgus is also common. Up to one-fourth of patients

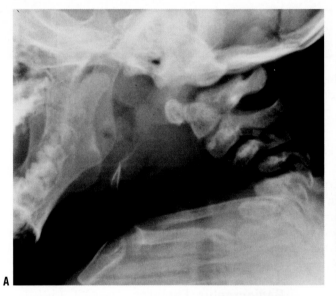

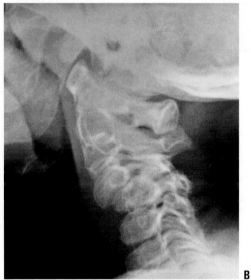

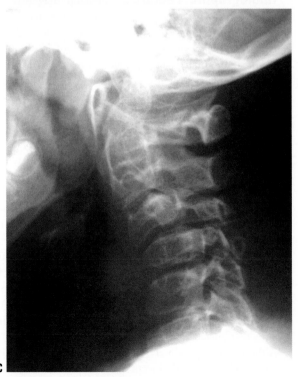

FIGURE 7-15. Cervical kyphosis in a 1-year-old child **(A)** with DD is pronounced with marked deformity of C4. Results of findings on neurologic examination are normal. Four years later, it is markedly improved without any intervention **(B)**, and 7 years later, the vertebral bodies have restored to nearly normal shape, although the canal remains narrow **(C)**.

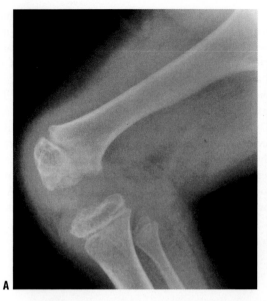
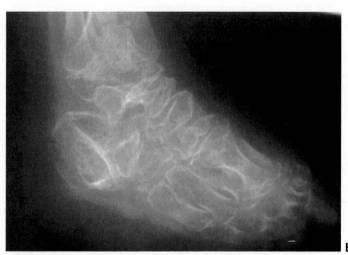

FIGURE 7-16. The extremities and the feet are involved in DD. Joint contracture is accompanied by epiphyseal deformity, as this knee radiograph illustrates (**A**). A rigid, severe equinovarus foot is common (**B**).

have a dislocated patella (106). DJD of the hips and knees develops in early to midadulthood.

The feet of diastrophic persons are commonly described as being clubfeet, but many different variations exist. In the large Finnish series by Ryoppy et al. (107), the most common finding was adduction and valgus (seen in 43%), followed in prevalence by equinovarus in 37%, and then by pure equinus. Diastrophic feet have significantly marked differences from idiopathic clubfeet (122). In the former, the equinus is more extreme, and the talocalcaneal joint is usually in valgus. Cavus often occurs with wedging of the calcaneocuboid joint. Adduction of the foot occurs mostly through the cuneiforms and metatarsals. The great toe may be in varus beyond the degree commonly seen in idiopathic clubfoot, analogous to the hitchhiker thumb. The foot deformities are very stiff and involve bony malformations, contracture, and malalignment. These feet are as difficult to correct as any type of clubfoot, and rarely have substantial or lasting improvement from serial cast treatment (122).

There is great variation in the severity of DD. Height is related to overall severity of involvement, with taller people being less severely affected (123, 124). The variation in stature is an example of the same spectrum of disorder. Growth curves for persons with DD are available (125). The median adult height is 136 cm for males and 129 cm for females (126). Therefore, people with achondroplasia are shorter in stature, and are approximately equal to those with pseudoachondroplasia and SED congenita. The pubertal growth spurt is diminished or absent, so the overall growth failure is progressive, suggesting that the physes are unable to respond to normal hormonal influences.

The life expectancy of persons with DD is not substantially less than that of the unaffected population, except for a small number of patients [approximately 8% (106)] who die in infancy from respiratory causes or during childhood from cervical myelopathy. Patients with severe spinal deformities are more prone to develop respiratory problems. Many patients are able to lead productive work and family lives, but walking ability is progressively limited and 10% do not walk at all, mostly because of the limitation of joint movement (127).

Radiographic Features. Prenatal diagnosis may be made by sonography in the second trimester with demonstration of long-bone measurements at least 3 standard deviations below normal, as well as clubfeet and adducted thumbs. In infancy, calcification develops in the pinna of the ear, and later in the cranium and the costal cartilages. The vertebrae are poorly ossified. The lower cervical spine may show kyphosis in infancy and early childhood, usually having an apex at approximately C4; this finding tends to decrease with time (118). MRI may be necessary to judge the severity of this condition in relation to the spinal cord. To our knowledge, only one case (116) of atlantoaxial instability has been reported in this condition. The vertebral "wedging" decreases with time in most patients (128). Spina bifida occulta is seen in more than three-fourths of patients (128). Unlike the spine in achondroplasia, the interpediculate distances in individuals with DD narrow only slightly at descending levels of the lumbar spine. Scoliosis may occur in the form of either a sharp, angular curve or a gradual, idiopathic-like one (Fig. 7-17A,B).

Images of the hand are characterized by several findings. The first metacarpal is small, oval, and proximally placed. Although the proximal interphalangeal joints of the digits are ankylosed, a radiolucent space is present early and later

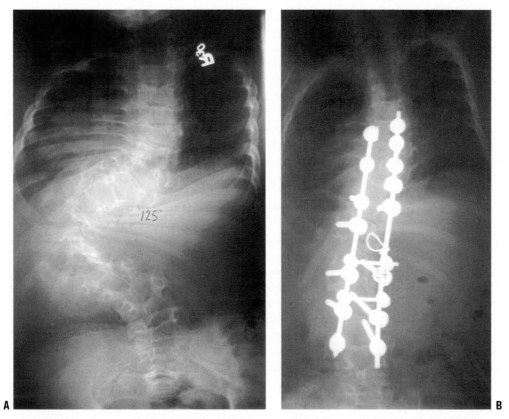

FIGURE 7-17. Severe scoliosis may occur early in DD, as in this 125-degree curve in an 8-year-old child **(A)**. After correction **(B)**.

fuses. The ulna and the fibula are shortened, contributing to the valgus of the knees and the radial head subluxation, which is sometimes seen. The diaphyses of the long bones are short and broad. The epiphyses of the proximal and the distal femur are delayed in appearance. The capital femoral epiphyses may show signs of osteonecrosis well into childhood. Arthrograms show flattening of the proximal and the distal femur, accounting for the stiffness observed clinically. The proximal femur is usually in varus, but, even so, hip dysplasia or subluxation may develop progressively with time.

Treatment

Cervical Spine. A neurologic examination should be performed periodically on all children, and a lateral cervical radiograph should also be obtained during the first 2 years of life. If cervical kyphosis is noted, the patient should be followed with clinical and radiographic examinations every 6 months. The behavior of the kyphosis appears to be related to the severity of the DD (121). If the kyphosis is nonprogressive, and there is no neurologic deficit, the only treatment should be observation because most kyphosis in this disorder will improve with time and growth, probably as a result of strengthening of the extensor muscles (121, 123). However, if the kyphosis progresses, but there is no neurologic deficit, bracing may be used. Successful control of cervical kyphosis by full-time use of the Milwaukee brace was reported by Bethem et al. (10, 11). If the curve continues to progress despite the brace, or a neurologic deficit

occurs, posterior fusion should be performed. The surgeon should be cognizant of the bifid lamina during the exposure. Instrumentation may not be technically possible. If adequate bone graft is not available from the iliac crests, it may be taken from the proximal tibia(s) or other sources. Immobilization by a halo and vest is needed for 2 to 4 months postoperatively. For children, the pins should be inserted at a lower torque than in adults (4 inch-pounds), and the surgeon may elect to use a slight distractive moment and a slight posterior translation of the head. A pad may be used behind the apex of the kyphosis to help keep it from increasing. If neurologic deficit is present along with the curve, MRI in a neutral position and in extension will help to determine the degree of anterior compression and the type of procedure required. If there is severe anterior cord compression, corpectomy and strut graft may be indicated. Posterior fusion is also indicated.

Thoracolumbar Spine. Scoliosis affects more than one-half of diastrophic patients (116), follows one of three patterns (early progressive, idiopathic-like, or mild nonprogressive) (129), and has been shown to be unrelated to the type of mutation in *DTST* (108, 128). To our knowledge, the success of bracing in preventing or slowing curve progression has not been documented. It seems reasonable to offer it to patients, if the curve is <45 degrees, but to discontinue it for those in whom there would be no apparent benefit. Large curves often continue to progress in adulthood (116), and surgery has a role in preventing progression for curves >~50 degrees. Posterior fusion is the mainstay of treatment (120). For younger patients, or those whose associated kyphosis is >50 degrees, anterior fusion may also be added. Instrumentation should be used carefully, bearing in mind the short stature, the stiffness of the spine, and the slightly diminished bone density. Small hooks may be used if needed (120). Spinal stenosis is seen in this condition much less often than it is in achondroplasia, but it may occur if degenerative changes are superimposed on the baseline canal size. Mild stenosis may be masked in some cases by the patients' relative inactivity.

Hips. Hip flexion contractures and knee flexion contractures should be assessed together. If they are severe (>40 degrees), release may be considered if an arthrogram shows no epiphyseal flattening and good potential for gaining range of motion. If there is epiphyseal flattening, it is probably better to avoid releases, given that recurrence is likely. Hip dysplasia is often progressive because of deformation of the abnormal cartilage under muscle forces and body weight. No long-term series has been done to show the ability of surgery to arrest this process. Therefore, the surgeon should use individual judgment as to whether an acetabular augmentation or a femoral osteotomy will help provide good coverage without restricting range of motion or function. Nonoperative treatment cannot be faulted in this condition.

Degenerative changes in the hip are one of the main reasons for decreasing walking ability in those with diastrophism. Hip joint arthroplasty is an option, when the pain becomes severe enough. Small or custom components are needed (130). The femur often has an increased anterior bow, probably in compensation for the hip flexion contracture. The isthmus of the femur is only 13 mm on average. Femoral shortening osteotomy is often needed. Contracture release (adductor, rectus, and sartorius) may be needed along with the arthroplasty, but femoral nerve palsy may follow if it is done extensively. Autograft augmentation of the acetabulum is often necessary. The largest series of hip arthroplasty in this condition is by Helenius et al. (131), with 41 hips in 10 patients (mean age, 41 years). Trochanteric transfer was performed in nearly one-half of the hips. Two patients had femoral palsies, but recovered. Hip range of motion was increased slightly, and Harris hip score nearly doubled. At a mean follow-up of 8 years, revision rate was 24%; all involved the acetabular side.

Knees. The knees in diastrophism usually lack flexion and extension. Complete correction of knee flexion contractures is prohibited by the shape of the condyles, which may be triangular, creating a bony block to flexion, extension, or both. Residual contracture at maturity may be diminished by distal femoral osteotomy. Patellar subluxation is present in one-fourth of those with DD (106); correcting it may help improve extensor power.

Knee arthroplasty often becomes necessary because of pain. Unique features of the procedure for patients with DD include extensive lateral release with patellar relocation, use of constrained prostheses whose stems must be shortened or bent,

and femoral osteotomy (132). Mean age at surgery is similar to that for total hip arthroplasty (mid-40s). Pain and function are improved, although many patients lose a slight amount of knee motion (132).

Feet. Although the classic foot deformity in this condition is equinovarus, other types may be seen, including isolated equinus, forefoot adduction, or valgus. The feet are rigid, and cast treatment is usually futile. A plantigrade foot is the goal of treatment. Surgical treatment should be deferred until the feet are large enough to work on (usually after 1 year), and the neck is free of marked kyphosis. If soft-tissue release is performed, it should be as extensive as needed to correct the deformity. Sometimes, it requires release of the posteroinferior tibiofibular ligament to bring the dome of the talus into the mortise. Partial recurrence of deformity is common (107), and salvage procedures include talectomy, talocalcaneal decancellation, and arthrodesis (in the older child).

KNEIST SYNDROME

Overview. This syndrome results from a type-II collagen defect. Most mutations occur between exons 12 and 24 of the *COL2A1* gene. There have been numerous mutations described in literature, but all are phenotypically similar. It behaves as an autosomal dominant condition. Pathologically, the cartilage has been termed "soft" and "crumbly," with a "Swiss cheese" appearance (133).

The syndrome is characterized by large, stiff and knobby joints, with substantial contractures (134, 135). Patients with Kneist syndrome have unique facial features. This type of dysplasia results in severe disability. The spine and the epiphysis are also involved.

Clinical Features. The characteristic facial features of patients with Kneist syndrome are prominent eyes and forehead and a depressed midface. The joints appear enlarged, are very pronounced (secondary to the broad metaphysis of the long bones), and very stiff. The stiffness, which affects the large joints (e.g., the knees and hips) and the small joints of the fingers, progresses as the patients age and delays ambulation and fine motor skills. There is an increased incidence of inguinal and abdominal hernias. Many patients have a cleft palate, which can result in aspiration, a broad trunk, and a depressed sternum. Intellectual development is normal.

Compared with unaffected individuals, patients with Kneist syndrome have a higher incidence of aspiration secondary to the cleft palate or tracheal malacia and of otitis media (which can result in chronic hearing loss and myopia). Other eye problems include glaucoma and retinal detachment, which can lead to blindness early in life (135).

Radiographic Features. There is a generalized osteopenia of the spine and extremities, most probably secondary to disuse from increasing pain on ambulation, myelopathy, and difficulty in ambulation from joint stiffness and premature arthritis.

Atlantoaxial instability is seen and can be secondary to odontoid hypoplasia. The vertebrae are flattened, and the vertebral bodies have clefts. As patients age, they can develop a severe kyphoscoliosis that needs to be corrected.

The femoral necks are short and broad with a substantial loss of joint space seen early into adolescence. There are regular calcifications in the epiphyseal and the metaphyseal regions. The epiphyses are flattened and irregular. Valgus can develop in the distal femur and the proximal tibia, leading to severe genu valgum.

Orthopaedic Treatment.
Cervical instability must be checked routinely every 3 years with flexion and extension radiographs (136). If the space available for the cord is <13 mm or if the atlantodens internal is >8 mm, prophylactic cervical fusion is indicated. For many patients, halo-cast immobilization is used.

Kyphosis or scoliosis can present early and be progressive. We have found brace treatment to be ineffective in these patients. Early on, when the spine is still growing, growing rods can be used, followed by a definitive fusion at maturity.

For many of these patients with dysplasia, joint stiffness, and early arthritis, aqua therapy is recommended to keep the muscles strong and help preserve some joint motion (130).

Osteotomies around the hip for containment of the femoral head can be done. Arthrograms are recommended, especially for lower extremity malalignment, when surgical correction is performed. Many of these patients also have substantial flexion contractures, and using some extension in the osteotomies can help or diminish the arc of motion rather than increase it.

Clubfoot is seen fairly commonly. In our experience, the Ponseti method (137) has been less than satisfying in such patients. Aggressive posterior releases are recommended but a painful hallux can develop. Fusion of this joint can also be beneficial for hallux rigidus.

SPONDYLOEPIPHYSEAL DYSPLASIA CONGENITA

Overview.
SED congenita is a rare disorder with an estimated prevalence of approximately 3 to 4 per 1 million people (1, 2). Its key features include substantial spinal and epiphyseal involvement, without metaphyseal enlargement or contractures of other joints (138). It is heritable in an autosomal dominant form, but most patients acquire the disease because of a new mutation. The etiology of this disorder has been characterized as a defect type-II collagen, the gene for which is located on chromosome 1293. This gene is the predominant protein of the cartilage matrix, and mutations have been observed in the α1 chain, resulting in alteration in length (139). As for many skeletal dysplasias, electron microscopy has shown intracellular inclusions in SED, which are probably a result of intracellular retention of procollagen (140).

Clinical Features.
In general, the face is taut, and the mouth is small. Cleft palate is common. The trunk and extremities are shortened, although the extremities are more shortened proximally because of the coxa vara (Fig. 7-18A,B). Pectus carinatum develops, possibly because the rib growth outpaces the increase in trunk height. There are similarities to Morquio syndrome but a lack of visceral involvement. Scoliosis and kyphosis usually develop before the teen years. Back pain is also common by this time.

The hips are most commonly in varus, but this finding varies. The degree of varus has been thought to be the best marker for the severity of the disease (141), which varies. If the varus is severe, it is often accompanied by a substantial hip flexion contracture. Patients often walk with the trunk and head held back to compensate for this contracture. The knees are often in mild varus, and a combination of external rotation of the femora and internal rotation of the tibiae often coexists.

The most common foot deformity is equinovarus, but this it is not nearly as stiff as it is when associated with DD. Growth curves are available for this condition (141). Adult height varies from 90 to 125 cm.

Radiographic Features.
One of the traits of this condition is that ossification is delayed in almost all regions (142, 143). There is often odontoid hypoplasia or os odontoideum. Flattened vertebral ossification centers with posterior wedging give the vertebral appearance, on lateral view, a pear shape. If scoliosis is present, it is often sharply angulated over a few vertebrae (Fig. 7-19). Disc spaces become narrow and irregular by maturity. Ossification of the pubis is delayed. The proximal femora are in varus with short necks, but the degree of this involvement varies. The proximal femur may not ossify for up to 9 years (141). Often, the varus is progressive (Fig. 7-20), and there may be progressive extrusion of the femoral head, which requires an arthrogram to show it clearly. The distal femoral metaphyses are flared. Genu valgum is more common than genu varum. Early osteoarthritis is likely in the hips, more so than in the knee. The carpal bones are delayed in ossification, but the tubular bones of the hands are near normal.

Medical Problems.
Respiratory problems occur in infants, often because of a small thorax. The most common disabling problem in this syndrome involves the eyes: retinal detachment is frequent. It is reported to occur especially during the adolescent growth spurt (144). Regular ophthalmologic examinations are recommended. Hearing impairment is noted in a minority of patients.

Orthopaedic Problems and Treatment.
Orthopaedically, the most potentially serious sequelae can involve neck instability. Os odontoideum, odontoid hypoplasia, or aplasia may all cause instability and, potentially, myelopathy (Fig. 7-21A–C). Numerous cases have been reported (10). Careful neurologic examination should be done at each clinic visit. Flexion-extension radiographs should be performed

FIGURE 7-18. SED congenita produces the most extreme short stature. This 12-year-old boy is with his 14-year-old brother **(A)**. Note extreme spinal shortening, increased lumbar lordosis, and hip flexion contracture **(B)**.

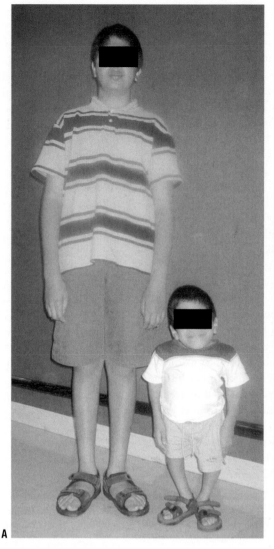

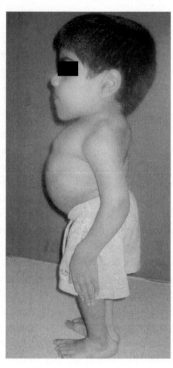

A   B

approximately every 3 years if an upper cervical anomaly is identified. If the odontoid is difficult to see, one can use CT or MRI. Stenosis often coexists and makes subluxation more critical. It is recommended to fuse the atlantoaxial interval if instability exceeds 8 mm, or if symptoms develop. If severe stenosis exists, or if a fixed subluxation cannot be reduced, it may be necessary to perform a decompression of the atlas and, consequently, fusion to the occiput (145). Transarticular screw fixation is often possible after children are 6 to 8 years old. However, in younger children, bone strength or size of the neural arches may make rigid internal fixation impractical; in such patients, bone graft and halo-cast immobilization are usually successful. Scoliosis is present in more than one-half of patients with SED (138, 139, 142), and it may become severe. Curve control with a brace may be attempted if the curve is <40 degrees. However, long-term efficacy has not been shown. Fusion may be necessary if the curve is progressive. Thoracolumbar stenosis is not as severe as in achondroplasia. Instrumentation is not contraindicated but should be used judiciously. If internal stabilization is not judged

to be strong, the use of halo-brace immobilization postoperatively should be considered. Correction is usually modest [17% in one series (10)]. Anterior surgery should be used if the patient is young (<11 years old) or the curve is rigid (correcting to <45 degrees). Kyphosis is also common; use of a Milwaukee brace has been shown to be effective if it can be worn until maturity (10).

Hip osteotomies are indicated if the neck-shaft angle is <100 degrees. Insufficient correction makes recurrence more likely. It is helpful to correct any flexion contracture at the same time, leaving adequate flexion for function. Malrotation should be also corrected. If a patient is experiencing painful hinge abduction, a valgus osteotomy may improve symptoms (146). An arthrogram may help in operative planning.

Hip subluxation may be reconstructed using a combination of femoral and iliac osteotomies. When doing any procedure on the hip, knee alignment should be assessed at the same time and corrected if necessary. The clinician should also consider the effect that knee angular correction will have on the hip. For instance, correction of severe knee valgus deformity

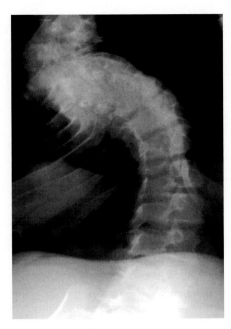

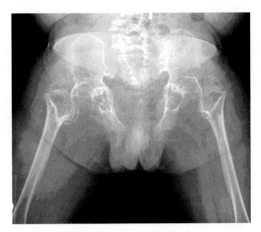

FIGURE 7-20. The hips in this 15-year-old with SED congenita show severe coxa vara, with delayed ossification of the capital femoral epiphyses and metaphyses.

FIGURE 7-19. Scoliosis, with a sharp apex concentrated over a limited number of vertebrae, is characteristic of SED congenita.

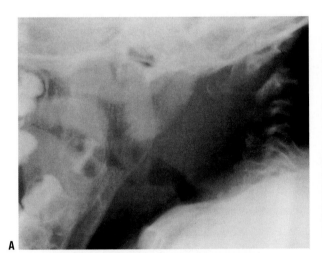

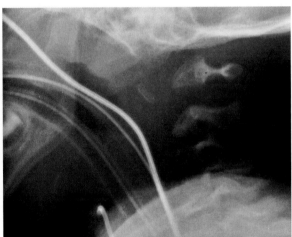

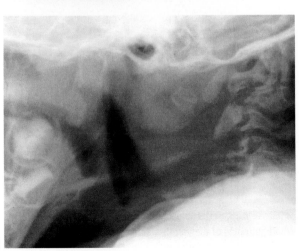

FIGURE 7-21. Atlantoaxial instability is common in SED congenita. This 2-year-old patient had delayed motor milestones. The upright lateral radiograph (A) of the cervical spine shows odontoid hypoplasia with marked atlantoaxial subluxation. Less evident is the stenosis of the ring of the atlas. When supine in a neutral position (B), the alignment improved. After decompression of the atlas and fusion of occiput to C2 (C), he gained the ability to walk.

has the same effect on hip congruity as does a varus osteotomy of the proximal femur.

Total joint replacement is a very difficult procedure: the hip is stiff, custom components are often needed, and concomitant osteotomy is sometimes necessary (130).

Foot deformities can usually be treated according to standard clubfoot principles. If the foot is stiff, an osteotomy or a decancellation of the talus, calcaneus, and/or cuboid may be needed.

SPONDYLOEPIPHYSEAL DYSPLASIA TARDA

Overview. SED tarda is distinguished from the congenita form by later age at diagnosis and milder features. Manifestations first appear in later childhood, or even in adulthood. The spine and only the larger joints are affected. Several genetic patterns of transmission have been reported (105, 147, 148). The most common is X-linked, in which male patients are more commonly or more severely affected and female patients may show milder (or no) manifestations. It is the result of a defect in the gene *SEDL* (149), whose function is not yet known. A recessive form has also been reported. SED tarda is one of several conditions (termed the *COL2A1* group or the SED family), which may result from a mutation in type-II collagen (14, 78). The mechanism by which the particular mutation for this condition produces the mildest phenotype in this family has yet to be elucidated.

Clinical Features. In the earliest cases, manifestations are first called to clinical attention when the child is approximately 4 years old. Stature is mildly shortened. Arm span is substantially longer than height. The condition may be first diagnosed as bilateral Perthes syndrome (150). Back pain and hip or knee pain may be present in childhood. Joint range of motion is minimally limited, if at all. Varus or valgus deformities are rare. Degenerative changes may occur in the hip or the knee by young adulthood. Adult height may be 60 in. or more (105).

Radiographic Features. Involvement of shoulders, hips, and knees predominates. The hips manifest varying degrees of coxa magna, epiphyseal flattening (Fig. 7-22), or epiphyseal extrusion, differing markedly even within the same family. A minority of patients present with bilateral coxa vara. Odontoid hypoplasia or os odontoideum may cause atlantoaxial instability. Spinal involvement ranges from mild platyspondyly (Fig. 7-23), with axe-like configuration of the vertebral bodies on the lateral view, to isolated disc-space narrowing. Mild-to-moderate scoliosis develops in a minority of patients.

Orthopaedic Problems and Treatment. The severity of orthopaedic conditions varies widely, even within a family. There are undoubtedly many affected individuals whose problems are so mild that no diagnosis is ever made. In one large family, only 4 of the 31 affected members requested

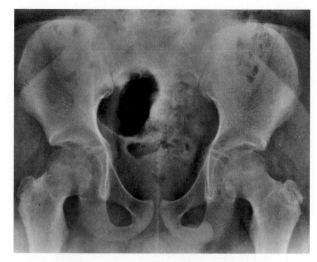

FIGURE 7-22. The pelvis in this patient with SED tarda shows small, flattened epiphyses.

any orthopaedic treatment (151). This condition should be considered whenever spine, hip, and/or knee pains run in a family, and the radiographs seem to be just a little atypical. Bracing may be recommended if scoliosis exceeds 30 degrees in the skeletally immature patient. Surgery should be offered for the rare patient in whom it exceeds 50 degrees. All patients should be screened for atlantoaxial instability. Fusion should be recommended if the spine is unstable in either flexion or extension, according to criteria given earlier for the congenita form. The role for procedures to increase coverage of the dysplastic, extruded femoral head by the acetabulum during the childhood years is not well documented. However, it may

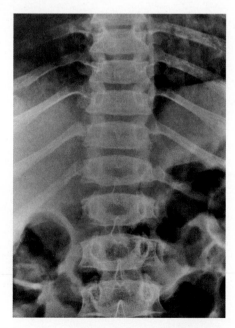

FIGURE 7-23. The spine in this patient with SED tarda shows typical mild flattening of the vertebral bodies, but no scoliosis.

be helpful in the rare young patient with increasing extrusion and persistent pain, in whom the hip contact surface is markedly compromised. If hip pain becomes a problem after the femoral heads are mature or nearly mature, osteotomy may help to increase congruity or decrease hinge abduction. Usually, a valgus or valgus-extension osteotomy is most appropriate, as long as there is reasonable joint space and adequate contact remaining. A preoperative arthrogram is helpful in the young patient to see the full outline of the articular surface. Osteotomies of knees or ankles are rarely needed. Total joint arthroplasty is often needed for the hips or knees, at an age much younger than that for the general population.

PSEUDOACHONDROPLASIA

Overview.   Pseudoachondroplasia is one of the more common forms of skeletal dysplasia, occurring in approximately 4 per 1 million live births in the United States (152). Although the name is similar to achondroplasia, it is a phenotypically and genotypically distinct condition. It was originally described by Maroteaux and Lamy (153) in 1959, at which time they identified it as a subset of SED. Later on, it became its own distinct dysplasia. Clinical features are not recognized during the first few years of life, and there is less involvement of the spine than is seen in SED.

Pseudoachondroplasia results from a mutation in the COMP protein (154, 155). This protein is the same as that seen in MED. Chondrocytes of people affected with pseudoachondroplasia have lamellae inclusion bodies located within the endoplasmic reticulum.

MED and pseudoachondroplasia have been described as a family of dysplasias, with MED being the milder and pseudoachondroplasia being the more severe form. COMP is a large extracellular matrix glycol-protein that is found surrounding chondrocytes and also in the extracellular matrix of ligaments and tendons. Multiple mutations in the COMP gene have been found to result in pseudoachondroplasia. In this case, it is an overproduction of COMP gene, not a deletion, that results in pseudoachondroplasia. Abnormal COMP deposits in the rough endoplasmic reticulum of chondrocytes and into the extracellular matrix (92, 156) leads to an abnormal, flatter cell shape (157, 158). Somatic and germinal line mosaicism is present, which allows this condition to act as a recessive disorder in terms of inheritance, even though it is a dominant gene.

Clinical Features.   This is one of the skeletal dysplasias that are not recognized until later on in life because it is essentially a storage disorder. It is typically recognized between 2 and 4 years old. As patients age, more COMP is deposited and the condition progresses. The height of children with pseudoachondroplasia is within the normal parameters at birth, but trails down to less than the 5th percentile at 2 years old (125). In addition, the atypical normal faces prevent the diagnosis of this condition until later on in life (159, 160).

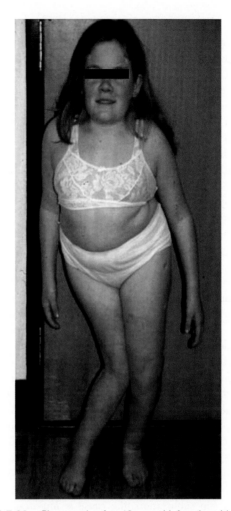

FIGURE 7-24.   Photograph of a 16-year-old female with pseudoachondroplasia and windswept deformity.

Patients with pseudoachondroplasia have a rhizomelic appearance of shortening of the extremities, the same as that seen in achondroplasia. However, the trident hand, typically seen in achondroplasia, is not seen in pseudoachondroplasia. These children typically develop substantial malalignment of the lower extremities, with genu varum on one side and genu valgum on the other side (i.e., the windswept deformity) (Fig. 7-24). Femoral heads typically get misshapen with time and are flattened. The hips, knees, and ankles develop premature arthritis in early adulthood. Spinal involvement is to a lesser degree. Cervical instability that will need stabilization may occur with this disorder (12); therefore, it needs to be checked on a routine basis. There is an increased kyphosis and lumbar lordosis (157). Scoliosis can also affect these patients.

Typically, these people have normal life expectancies and intelligence. They do not develop changes outside of the skeleton.

Radiographic Features.   The vertebral bodies are very flat with anterior indentation, which is seen early on in life. It would be very helpful to identify these patients early on and make a diagnosis.

Cervical instability is common, secondary to odontoid hypoplasia. These patients need to be monitored in a routine fashion, with radiographs every 2 to 3 years in flexion and extension.

The epiphyses are regularly shaped and ossify later in life. In the long bones, the metaphyses are broad, irregular at the ends, and flared. The pubic rami and the greater trochanteric apophyses are delayed in closing (161).

As the femoral head enlarges, it takes on a flattened appearance and can sublux from the acetabulum. An arthrogram can be helpful in eliciting the cause and identifying the surgical options. Much of the ossification between the carpals is delayed, which can make it challenging to decide how to correct the malalignment of lower extremities, which is why we think arthrograms are critical.

Orthopaedic Problems and Treatment. The cervical spine should be evaluated early on and often. If the atlanto-dens interval is >8 mm, or if the space available for the cord is <14 mm, prophylactic posterior fusion (Fig. 7-25) is indicated with a halo brace. If myelopathy develops, it is another indication for surgical treatment. Even with internal fixation, a halo brace has been found to be helpful (162), and using it may increase the rate of union. Kyphosis and scoliosis are seen, and we use the same indications for surgical treatment as those for patients of average stature. However, in our experience, brace treatment is not helpful. Although stenosis is not usually seen, we prefer to use pedicle screws during operative treatment. If a large curve is seen early on in life, growing rods can be an effective interim treatment before a definitive fusion.

With hip subluxation, the cause is important. If it is secondary to valgus at the knees, it needs to be addressed first. If it is primary to hip abnormality, then this also needs to be addressed. Arthrograms are obtained to see if surgical varus of the hip, which can be combined with an iliac osteotomy, would be appropriate. Typically, an acetabular shelf

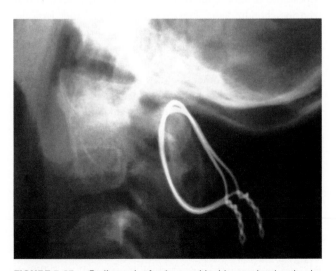

FIGURE 7-25. Radiograph of a 4-year-old with pseudoachondroplasia after cervical fusion and sublaminar wiring for cervical instability.

augmentation can also be done to increase the volume in the acetabulum. However, despite a clinician's best efforts, many of these hips will develop premature arthritis (22, 130, 157). Total hip arthroplasty for patients with pseudoachondroplasia can be done safely and effectively at facilities that have experience with this procedure and patient population (130).

In such patients, lower extremity malalignment usually consists of the "windswept deformity," that is, varus of one limb and valgus of the other. Arthrograms followed by lower extremity osteotomies can be helpful, but overcorrection must be avoided, or the same problems will rapidly develop in the opposite direction. As with the hips, these knees can develop premature arthritis, requiring total knee arthroplasty, which requires a constrained prosthesis because the arthritis is secondary to ligamentous laxity. We have seen nonconstrained prosthesis in total knee arthroplasties dislocating immediately after surgery.

MULTIPLE EPIPHYSEAL DYSPLASIA

Overview. MED is one of the most widely known, variable, and commonly occurring skeletal dysplasias. It is usually dominantly inherited, although recessive cases have recently been described as a result of mutations in transport protein (152). It affects many epiphyses, produces symptoms mainly in those with substantial load bearing, and has few changes in the physes or metaphyses. Historically, it was described as occurring in two separate forms, with eponyms that are still used today: Ribbing dysplasia, having mild involvement, or Fairbank dysplasia, a more severe type (163–165). However, with the current understanding of the genetic basis, this distinction may not be scientific, and a wide variability is recognized (166).

Histologically, intracytoplasmic inclusions are seen that are similar to, but not as severe as, those seen in pseudoachondroplasia. Growth plate organization is still noticeably abnormal, despite the minimal changes seen in the metaphyses. The genetic basis for this disorder is now reasonably well understood. It is a heterogeneous disorder. Mutations in many patients have been found in the gene for the matrix glycoprotein COMP on chromosome 19, as in pseudoachondroplasia. This product accumulates in cartilage cells and causes premature apoptosis. It also weakens the integrity of the matrix, allowing deformation and wear under normal loads. However, in other cases of MED, abnormalities have been found in the α_2 fibers of collagen type IX (COL9A2). Collagen type IX is normally a trimer that is found on the surface of type-II collagen in cartilage. It may form a macromolecular bridge between type-II collagen fibrils and other matrix components—it therefore may be important for the adhesive properties of cartilage. A COL9A2 mutation has been described in one large family, with peripheral joint involvement only (167). In addition, dominant MED in some cases is caused by defects in matrilin-3, another oligomeric extracellular matrix protein (152, 168). Rarer, recessive forms of MED are caused by mutations in transporters (152). Therefore, it appears that MED is a very heterogeneous disorder, which may help clinicians to understand some of the more common epiphyseal cartilage disorders such as Perthes disease, osteochondritis dissecans, and osteoarthritis (152).

Clinical Features.
Patients typically present later in childhood for one of several reasons. They may be referred for joint pain in the lower extremities, decreased range of motion, gait disturbance, or angular deformities of the knees (169). There may be flexion contractures of knees or elbows. Symptoms may develop as late as adulthood. These patients have minimal short stature, ranging in height from 145 to 170 cm (164). The face and the spine are normal. There is no visceral involvement.

Radiographic Features.
Most changes in MED involve the epiphyses; any of the ossification centers may be delayed in appearance. There are occasional irregularities of streaking in the metaphyses, but they are minor. The appearances of the epiphyses in the immature and in the mature patients are characteristic (170). In the growing patient, the epiphyses are fragmented and small in size (Fig. 7-26). The epiphyseal ossification centers eventually coalesce, but the overall shape of the epiphysis is smaller. An arthrogram may be helpful for assessing the shape of the joint surface. The more fragmentation there is in the capital femoral epiphysis, the earlier is the onset of osteoarthritis (171). Coxa vara occurs in some patients. By maturity, there is some degree of flattening of the major load-bearing epiphyses: flattening of the femoral condyles, an

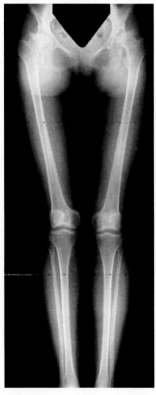

FIGURE 7-26. Multiple epiphyseal dysplasia.

ovoid femoral head, decreased sphericity of the humeral head, and squaring of the talus. In adulthood, major joints develop premature osteoarthritis. This condition is most common and most severe in the hips.

Avascular necrosis may be superimposed on MED, a combination that occurs in approximately one-half of the femoral heads (172). It can be recognized by the appearance of a crescent sign, resorption of bone that had already been formed, and, sometimes, by the presence of metaphyseal cysts (172). MRI at this time may show loss of signal in a portion of the femoral head. A "sagging rope sign" may develop later (173).

An orthopaedic surgeon must be able to differentiate MED from Perthes disease (150). Several radiographic clues may be helpful. In MED, abnormalities in the acetabulum are primary and are more pronounced. The radiographic changes are symmetric and fairly synchronous. It is also helpful to obtain radiographs of the knees, ankles, shoulders, and wrists.

Radiographs of the knees show that the femoral condyles are flattened and may be in valgus. There may be irregular ossification, just as in the hip. The condyles are somewhat squared on lateral view. Osteochondritis dissecans may be superimposed. MED patients with a *DTDST* mutation also show a double-layered patella on the lateral view (174, 175). This is a complete or partial double radiodensity, which is rarely seen in other conditions.

The ankles in MED are also in valgus; changes occur in the talus and in the distal tibia. Upper extremity involvement is less severe; there may be irregularities in the proximal and distal humerus and radius. The humeral head involvement in adulthood has been termed a "hatchet-head" appearance, and results from undergrowth of the head and neck. It occurs in children more severely affected with MED. Radial ray hypoplasia may occur sporadically (176). The carpal ossification centers are delayed in appearing. The hand and wrist involvement may predict stature, that is more severely disordered epiphyses (177). The spine may be normal, or it may have slight endplate irregularities or ossification defects on the anterior margins of the vertebrae (178).

Orthopaedic Implications.
The orthopaedic surgeon may become involved in the care of the patient with MED in one of two periods. There is a small role for realignment procedures in the early, deforming period of the hip if there is progressive subluxation or pain. However, with substantial delay in epiphyseal ossification, recurrent deformity has been reported (179). Pain is more likely to occur in cases in which avascular necrosis has supervened (172). Although the principle of coverage is the same as that used in Perthes disease, there is often a degree of coxa vara pre-existing in hips with MED, which may contraindicate the use of a femoral osteotomy. Acetabular shelf augmentation is a worthwhile procedure in these instances (180, 181).

Not all patients need surgical treatment; however, it can help some. Hemiepiphysiodesis may guide growth to help correct knee and ankle deformities. Even though the physes may not be normal, correction of 15 to 20 degrees has been reported in 18 months (182). Severe deformities may be corrected by osteotomy at maturity in the femur or tibia, depending on the site of abnormality. Patients having a double-layered patella may have symptoms because of the relative movement of one over the other. This situation may be treated by excision of one or fusion of the two segments, as appropriate (183). DJD is the biggest problem, and it occurs in the second or third decade. It results not so much from malalignment of the joints, but from intrinsic defect in cartilage. It produces stiffness, from an early age, and pain leading to a total joint arthroplasty. Differences from standard osteotomy include a shallow or an anteverted acetabulum or narrow femoral canal (184). Even the shoulder is commonly affected by degeneration, and shoulder arthroplasty may be necessary (185).

CHONDRODYSPLASIA PUNCTATA

Overview. This skeletal dysplasia is named for a radiographic finding of calcification in skeletal cartilage, which can arise through several different pathways (186). It is also known by the synonym "congenital stippled epiphysis." Key features include depressed nasal bridge and multiple punctate calcifications in infancy, which are best visualized on the newborn's radiographs (187). There are many different types, the most common being an X-linked dominant type (Conradi-Hünermann syndrome), followed by an autosomal recessive rhizomelic type (which is usually fatal in infancy) and a rare X-linked recessive type. Four other types have been described that are even more rare (188). Although the appearance of neonatal epiphyseal calcification is striking, it is not very specific. There are various conditions that may present with the same phenomenon: Zellweger (cerebrohepatorenal) syndrome, gangliosidosis, rubella, trisomy 18 or 21, vitamin K deficiency, hypothyroidism, or fetal alcohol or hydantoin syndromes (188–193). Rhizomelic chondrodysplasia punctata is a peroxisomal deficiency of dihydroxyacetone-phosphate acyltransferase that is often (but not always) fatal in the first year of life (194, 195). The genetic defect and pathogenesis of the Conradi-Hünermann syndrome is related to a defect in sterol metabolism (186). The final common pathway of the various types is a defect in cholesterol synthesis (196) or peroxisomal enzymes. Histologic examination shows perilacunar calcifications throughout the cartilage matrix (197).

Clinical Features. Patients with Conradi-Hünermann syndrome are characterized by hypertelorism, a depressed nasal bridge, and a bifid nasal tip (198–201). In addition, many have alopecia, congenital heart and/or renal malformations, and mental retardation. In rhizomelic chondrodysplasia punctata, findings include microcephaly, a high incidence of congenital cataracts, growth retardation, and a well-formed nasal bridge (202–205). Some have feeding difficulties, and many succumb to death from respiratory issues or seizures in the first year. Diagnosis may be made by amniocentesis, with measurement of plasmalogen biosynthesis and phytanic acid oxidation.

Skeletal findings in the extremities include limb-length inequality, coxa vara, and clubfoot or other foot deformities (206). Spinal findings include atlantoaxial instability, congenital scoliosis, spinal stenosis or kyphosis (196, 207, 208).

Radiographic Features. Skeletal calcifications are visible at birth, but most disappear by 1 year. These calcifications involve the epiphyses, carpal bones, ribs, and pelvis (209) (Fig. 7-27A,B). Extraskeletal sites include the trachea and larynx. The appearance is of small flecks of calcium, "which appear as if paint had been flecked on by a brush" (210). The

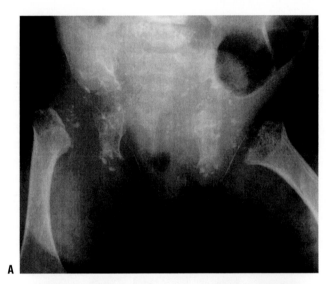

A

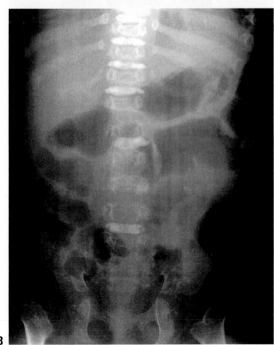

B

FIGURE 7-27. **A:** Diffuse punctate epiphyseal calcifications in infancy are a hallmark for which chondrodysplasia punctata was named. **B:** At 2.5 years old, the epiphyseal calcifications are mostly resolved, but calcification of the intervertebral discs persists.

ossification centers themselves may be delayed in appearance. Coxa vara may affect one or both hips, or it may be absent (211). The fibula often substantially overgrows the tibia. Spine radiographs may have the appearance of a hemivertebra or a congenital bar. Calcification of the intervertebral discs may develop (Fig. 7-27B). Odontoid hypoplasia and os odontoideum have been described (208).

Orthopaedic Implications. Because of the risk of cervical instability or stenosis, each patient should have a lateral cervical radiograph and, if instability appears possible, a flexion-extension view. Scoliosis may occur early because of secondary congenital anomalies. It may require early fusion if progression is documented and the patient, medically, is a candidate. Anterior structural grafting, followed by posterior fusion and cast immobilization, has the highest rate of success (196). Coxa vara should be treated if it is symptomatic and the neck-shaft angle is <100 degrees. Lower limb-length inequality should be monitored and treated appropriately.

METAPHYSEAL CHONDRODYSPLASIAS

Overview. Metaphyseal chondrodysplasias are a family of disorders resulting in metaphyseal irregularities and limb deformity (211–214); however, the epiphyses are uninvolved. There are four named disorders in this family: McKusick type, Schmidt type, Jansen metaphyseal dysplasia, and Kozlowski type.

McKusick Type. Also known as *cartilage-hair dysplasia*, the McKusick type is most commonly found among the Amish population in Lancaster, Pennsylvania, but it can also be found outside this community. The condition is autosomal recessive and maps to chromosome 9 (215). The defect is in the *RMRP* gene, which encodes a mitochondrial RNA process (216).

Clinical Features. Individuals with McKusick-type dysplasia have light, fine, and sparse hair (Fig. 7-28). They might have a change in T-cell immunity, which causes an increased risk of infection, especially varicella zoster (217, 218).

Anemia occurs frequently in young children, but the incidence lessens as they become adolescents (219). A high risk of malignancies, such as lymphoma, sarcoma, and skin cancers, can be seen in this patient population (217, 220), and life expectancy is decreased, warranting medical treatment into adulthood more than with most of the other dysplasias.

In addition, individuals with McKusick-type dysplasia have generalized ligamentous laxity of the elbows and can develop substantial instability even though they might have flexion contractures. Pectus deformities can also develop. These individuals also have genu varum that might require operative intervention. Bracing is ineffective in controlling the genu varum in these patients, so if it is progressive and painful, operative intervention is warranted.

Radiographic Features. Compared with individuals who have Schmidt-type dysplasia, those with McKusick-type

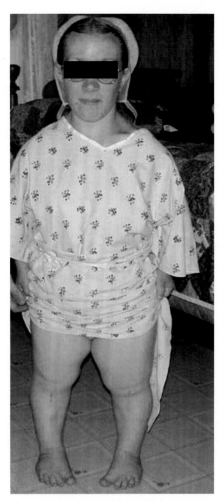

FIGURE 7-28. Photograph of a 24-year-old Amish female with McKusick-type dysplasia and mild genu varum.

dysplasia have more shortening and less varus of the long bones. The metaphyseal involvement is seen uniformly throughout and there is a distal fibula overgrowth. Atlantoaxial instability has been reported secondary to odontoid hypoplasia, but it is not common in this population (220).

Orthopaedic Implications. Routine radiographs with flexion/extension every 3 years are warranted. If there is more than 8 mm of movement, prophylactic fusion is indicated. Early observation of scoliosis is warranted; if the scoliosis is progressive or reaches more than 45 degrees, posterior spinal fusion is indicated. If the individual is still skeletally immature, growing rods can be used. Bracing in this population has not been helpful.

Hip dislocation occurs in approximately 3% of the population (220). Traditional treatment can be used with good success, but it must be implemented early and aggressively (217). Lower extremity malalignment can be corrected if it is progressive or causing pain. Later on in life, if premature arthritis develops, total hip and total knee arthroplasty can be done safely with good results.

Schmidt Type.   This type is more common than the McKusick type; it is autosomal dominant. The defect is seen in the α-1 chain of type-X collagen (221–223). Histologically, cartilage islands that extend into the metaphyses are visible. Sometimes, it is necessary to differentiate this type of dysplasia from rickets or hypophosphatasia.

Clinical Features.   The adult height is minimally shortened. Minimal features with typical normal faces are seen. Patients can develop leg pain later in life, with mild varus at the knees and ankles accompanied by a mild form of short stature, and it may be at this late presentation that it is first diagnosed.

Radiographic Features.   Radiographically, the metaphysis of the long bones are wedged and flared and can contain cysts. The physes are slightly widened, there may be mild varus at the knees, and atlantoaxial instability can be seen, although the latter is not very common.

Orthopaedic Implications.   These patients do not develop premature arthritis. Occasionally, clinicians may see varus needing operative correction, secondary to progressive pain.

Jansen Metaphyseal Dysplasia.   This type of dysplasia is less common than the other two and is an autosomal dominant disorder that is linked to a defect in the receptor for parathyroid hormone and parathyroid hormone–related proteins (224).

Patients with this disorder can develop hypercalcemia and have more pronounced metaphyseal changes than those seen in the Schmidt and McKusick types.

Kozlowski Type.   This autosomal dominant disorder is fairly rare. It is characterized by spinal metaphyseal involvement seen in the first few years of life, secondary to short stature, and a progressive kyphosis. Patients with this disorder can have limitation of movement, a Trendelenburg gait, and an early onset of arthritic changes.

Mild platyspondyly is seen, which is in direct contrast to the other three metaphyseal chondrodysplasias previously described. The most visible area to detect metaphyseal dysplasia in the Kozlowski type is in the proximal femur. The bone age of the carpals and tarsals is delayed.

DIAPHYSEAL ACLASIA (HEREDITARY MULTIPLE EXOSTOSES)

Overview.   Although solitary exostoses do not qualify as skeletal dysplasias, it is clear that patients with hereditary multiple exostoses (HME) have a generalized disturbance of skeletal growth. The condition has been localized to mutations on chromosomes 8 and 11. The genes involved are referred to as *EXT1* and *EXT2*. The differing locations of mutation account for the phenotypic variability of the condition. Patients affected because of a mutation in *EXT1* have a more

severe phenotype (225). These genes produce transmembrane glycoproteins that affect cell signaling, interact with fibroblast growth factor, and affect endochondral development and maturation (226). Most cases of HME are transmitted in an autosomal dominant fashion, but a large number of patients acquire it as a spontaneous mutation. The metaphysis of a person with HME is characterized by thinning of the cortex, innumerable small bumps, and cartilage rests extending into the trabecular bone.

Clinical Features.   The condition is not usually diagnosed until the child is 3 to 4 years old, at which time the first exostoses are noted and other features develop. The features become progressively more pronounced until maturity, at which point exostoses should cease to grow. Affected persons are at the low end of normal for stature. The metaphyses are circumferentially enlarged throughout the body, not only in the regions in which there are obvious exostoses. This enlargement gives the child a rather "stocky" appearance, which is then further exaggerated by the appearance of the exostoses. The exostoses may cause soreness when they arise under tendons or in an area vulnerable to contusion, such as the knee or shoulder. The exostoses tend to steal from the longitudinal growth of the long bones. The categories of problems caused by HME are fourfold:

1. Localized pressure on tendons, vessels and nerves, among other places. Peroneal palsy may arise from a lateral exostosis, and it may occur in such a way as to cause brachial plexus compression. Intraspinal lesions have been reported in a substantial minority of patients (227). Pseudoaneurysms may occur.
2. Angular growth of two-bone segments—the arms and forearms. Usually, the thinner of these two bones is more inhibited in its growth than the wider one, so it tethers the growth of the latter. Valgus may develop at the wrist, knee, and ankle. The radial head may subluxate or dislocate.
3. Limb-length inequality. Often, one limb is more involved than the other with exostoses, and it may undergrow as much as 4 cm.
4. Malignant degeneration. Transformation to chondrosarcoma occurs in approximately 5% of patients after maturity (226). It is more likely in *EXT1* than *EXT2* mutations (228). Such change may be signaled by increased growth of an exostosis, or pain over an exostosis. Bone scans every 2 years in adulthood have been advocated as one way to detect this change. Self-examination and periodic orthopaedic examination, with MRI in the case of an apparent change, is another way to follow these patients in adulthood (226).

Radiographic Features.   The metaphyses are very wide, and internal irregularities can be seen. The exostoses may be sessile or pedunculated, and have continuity with the main cortex, as do solitary exostoses. Exostoses on the undersurface of the scapula may be identified on conventional radiographs, but they are best evaluated by CT. The femoral necks are usually wide and in valgus (Fig. 7-29). Valgus is much more common than varus at the knee (Fig. 7-30), and the distal

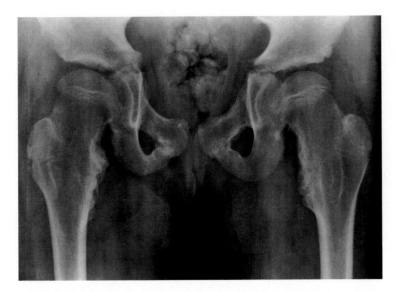

FIGURE 7-29.   The hips in diaphyseal aclasia are characterized by broad, irregular femoral necks that are usually in valgus. There are osteochondromas and irregularities in formation of the pelvis also, which can be difficult to monitor over time.

tibial epiphysis may be triangular if the fibula is pulling the ankle into valgus. Radial head subluxation may occur with ulnar shortening, and the resultant carpal subluxation can readily be identified by wrist radiographs.

Orthopaedic Implications.   Monitoring in childhood should mostly be done by clinical examination because all bones are affected and the lesions are too numerous to image routinely. Clinicians should perform a brief neurologic exami-

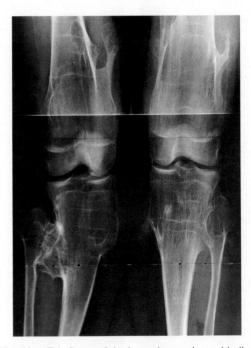

FIGURE 7-30.   This figure of the knees in a patient with diaphyseal aclasia best illustrates that this defect is a systemic abnormality of bone formation, rather than a series of discrete tumors. The metaphyses are broad and irregular in the region where the exostoses are located. The knees are developing a valgus alignment because of the short fibulae, as are the ankles (not shown).

nation; check joint range of motion; measure knee, ankle, elbow, and wrist angulation and limb lengths; and remove any exostoses that are causing severe symptoms, but warn the patients that the metaphyseal widening will persist, so the effect on appearance may not match expectations. Removal of lesions impairing radioulnar motion may result in slight increase in range of motion, especially if an exostosis is located on only the ulna but not on the radius (229). Ulnar lengthening may help avert radial head subluxation. However, studies of the function after osteotomies of the forearm show that there is not often functional benefit (229, 230). Hemiepiphysiodesis is a minimally invasive way to correct angulation at the wrist, knee, and ankle (231). Valgus angulation at the distal tibia is correlated with degenerative changes in the long term (232). If the patient is near maturity and needs correction, osteotomy may be indicated. Limb-length inequality can be corrected by the standard methods. Patients with HME are more likely than others to form keloids (233). Some experts recommend screening patients with HME by MRI for intraspinal lesions at least once during growing years (227) (Fig. 7-31).

Patients should be taught to examine themselves for signs of growth after maturity because it may signal malignant degeneration. A bone scan may be a helpful adjunct if a problem is suspected.

DYSCHONDROSTEOSIS (LERI-WEILL SYNDROME)

Overview.   Dyschondrosteosis, which was described by Leri and Weill (234) in 1929, is characterized by mild mesomelic short stature (middle segments of the limbs are shortest) (235, 236). This growth disturbance of the middle segments is most notable in the distal radius, which usually develops a Madelung deformity (234, 237, 238). It is inherited in an autosomal dominant fashion, with approximately 50% penetrance (237, 239). The expression is more severe in female patients than in males. It has

FIGURE 7-31. Two patients with multiple hereditary osteochondromas had severe lesions in the spinal canal that were not visible on conventional radiographs. **A:** MRI scan showing osteochondroma arising from the undersurface of the C5 lamina in one patient. **B:** CT scan showing lesion arising from a rib and invading the spinal canal in another patient. (Figures courtesy of Dr. James Roach.)

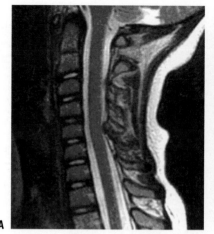
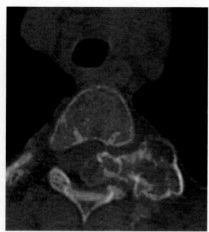

been shown to involve a mutation or deletion in the *S*hort-stature *H*omeobox-containing gene *O*n chromosome *X* [*SHOX* (240)], which also causes the short stature seen in Turner syndrome and other causes of short stature (241, 242).

Clinical Features. Patients usually present in juvenile or adolescent years because of short stature, forearm disproportion or deformity, or wrist pain or deformity (243). The deformity of the distal forearm, or Madelung deformity, is characterized by a deficiency of growth of the volar-ulnar portion of the radius. The differential diagnosis of this phenomenon includes Turner syndrome, trauma, Ollier disease, or multiple hereditary exostoses. Most patients begin to experience pain in the wrist during adolescence, and limitation of pronation and supination. A variation on this theme, seen in some patients with dyschondrosteosis, is shortening of both radius and ulna without angulation. The mesomelic shortening also involves the lower extremities, specifically the tibiofibular segments. There, however, angular deformity is not pronounced—only a mild genu varum or an ankle valgus usually exists. Short stature is usually, but not always, a feature; adult height ranges from 135 to 170 cm. In one series of patients, deficiency in growth hormone was found, and stature was increased by growth hormone supplementation (244).

Radiographic Features. Madelung deformity is a failure of development of the volar-ulnar part of the distal radial epiphysis. The distal radial epiphysis develops a triangular appearance and a tilt of joint surface (243) (Fig. 7-32A,B). A physeal bar may be seen on CT at the lunate facet (239). The ulna is subluxated or dislocated dorsally. In contrast to other causes of Madelung deformity, the ulna is as long as, or longer than, the radius (244). The tibia and fibula are short, with the fibula longer than the tibia at the ankle and/or the knee. There may be some degree of genu varum or ankle valgus. Cubitus valgus, hypoplasia of the humeral head, short fourth metacarpal, and coxa valga have all been noted, but rarely do all occur in the same patient.

Orthopaedic Implications. Human growth hormone treatment may produce a sustained response, and patients concerned about short stature may be referred to an endocrinologist for discussion of this treatment (244, 245).

Patients who experience wrist pain may be treated initially by a wrist splint and anti-inflammatory agents. If still symptomatic, a reconstruction with a double osteotomy of the distal radius and an ulnar recession can provide good results (246). In one study, this procedure provided improvement in symptoms and clinical appearance, but lunate subluxation, grip strength, and range of motion were minimally influenced (238). Although it has been described, it is unclear whether bar resection can allow normal growth to occur. Osteotomy of the tibia is occasionally indicated to correct genu varum (237).

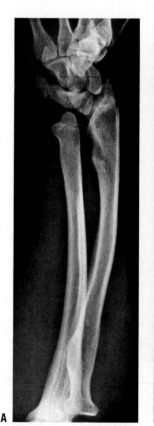
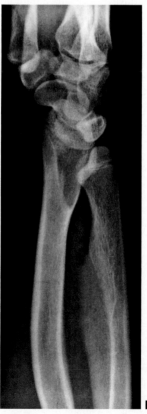

FIGURE 7-32. **A:** Madelung deformity in the forearm of a patient with dyschondrosteosis. **B:** The distal radial epiphysis has a markedly triangular epiphysis, and the ulna is dorsally subluxated.

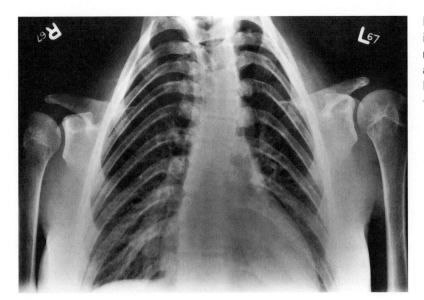

FIGURE 7-33.   The clavicles are completely absent in the patient with cleidocranial dysplasia, although in many patients they are merely hypoplastic. There is also a characteristic mild scoliosis and an occult bifid lamina of T2.

CLEIDOCRANIAL DYSPLASIA

Overview.   Cleidocranial dysplasia is a true skeletal dysplasia because it affects the growth of many bones in all parts of the skeleton, primarily those of membranous origin. Classic features include a widening of the cranium, and dysplasia of the clavicle and the pelvis (247, 248). The incidence is estimated at 1 per 200,000 (249). It is transmitted as an autosomal dominant condition, and the defect is in the *RUNX2/CFBA1* gene on chromosome 6, which encodes an osteoblast-specific transcription factor required for osteoblast differentiation (250–252). *RUNX2* activity is regulated by mechanical stress (253).

Clinical Features.   Although the name suggests that only two bones are affected, there are numerous abnormalities. Patients have mildly to moderately diminished stature, with most male and some female patients below the 5th percentile for age. Mean adult height for males is 64 in. There is bossing in the frontal parietal and occipital regions. The maxillary region is underdeveloped, giving apparent exophthalmos and maxillary micrognathism. Cleft palate and dental abnormalities are common (254–257).

The clavicles are partially or completely absent (256); there is complete absence only 10% of the time (256). This clavicle deficit causes the shoulders to drop and the neck to appear longer. The classic diagnostic feature is that the shoulders can be approximated, which is an ability that helped one college wrestler to escape holds (257). The pelvis is narrow. The hips are occasionally unstable at birth. Coxa vara may occur, causing limitation of abduction and a Trendelenburg gait. There is an increased incidence of scoliosis and, often, a double thoracic curve. Syringomyelia has been reported in several patients with cleidocranial dysplasia and scoliosis (258–260). It has been recommended that MRI be obtained for patients with this dysplasia who have progressive scoliosis.

Radiographic Features.   Prenatal radiographic diagnosis may be made on the basis of small or absent clavicles (Fig. 7-33). Nomograms are available for clavicular size during gestation (261). If there is uncertainty, molecular prenatal diagnosis may be performed. If a portion of the clavicle is present, it is usually the medial end. The skull of a newborn with this disorder has the maturation of a 20-week fetus (254). Wormian bones are present in the skull. The anterior fontanel may be open in adulthood (Fig. 7-34). In the vertebral column, spina bifida occulta and spondylolysis are common (262). The pelvis

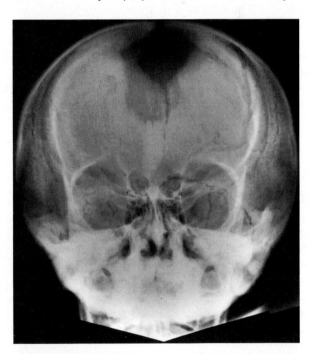

FIGURE 7-34.   The skull in this teenager with cleidocranial dysplasia shows an enlarged cranium, widened sutures, and a persistent anterior fontanel.

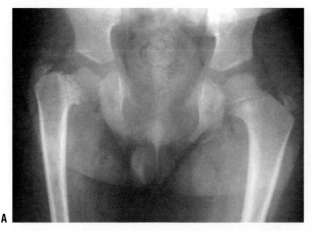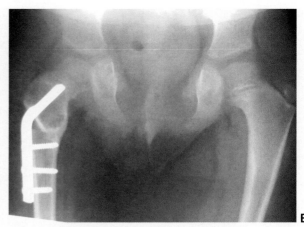

FIGURE 7-35. In cleidocranial dysplasia, the pelvis is narrow, the symphysis pubis is widened, the ischiopubic synchondrosis is unossified, and there may be coxa vara. Preoperative **(A)** and postoperative **(B)** radiographs.

is narrow and shows widening of the triradiate cartilage, delay in pubic ossification, and progressive deformation of the base of the femoral neck into varus (Fig. 7-35A,B), with a triangular metaphyseal fragment typical of coxa vara (263). Skeletal maturation may be delayed.

Orthopaedic Implications. No treatment is indicated for the clavicles. Scapulothoracic arthrodesis has been reported for symptomatic shoulder dysfunction (264). The coxa vara may be treated by valgus-rotational osteotomy if the neck shaft angle is <100 degrees and the patient has a Trendelenburg gait (265). If acetabular dysplasia is present, it should be corrected first. Scoliosis should be treated according to usual guidelines. MRI should be obtained if the curve is progressive because of the increased risk of syringomyelia.

Cesarean section is often necessary. Craniofacial surgery may be helpful in correcting the skull defects, and many dental problems may develop. Affected pregnant women may have cephalopelvic disproportion, especially if the fetus has the same disorder, because of the mother's narrow pelvis and the fetus' enlarged cranium.

LARSEN SYNDROME

Overview. This syndrome was first described in 1950; the six patients were described having the unique combination of hypertelorism, multiple joint dislocations, and focal bone deformities (266). This syndrome has been reported in autosomal dominant and -recessive patterns. The gene is on chromosome 3 near, but distinct from, *COL7A1* locus 4207 (267). The dominant form has been associated with a mutation in filamin B, a cytoskeletal structural protein (268, 269). It remains a rare condition, with an incidence estimated at 1 per 100,000 (270).

Clinical Features. The facial appearance involves widely spaced eyes, a depressed nasal bridge, and a prominent forehead.

Cleft palate is common. The thumb has a wide distal phalanx, and the fingers do not taper distally. Hypotonia has also been reported, but it may result from cervical compression (271). Sudden death has been reported (266, 272); most instances were likely a result of exacerbation of this compression. Dislocations most commonly involve the elbows (or radial heads), hips, and knees (Fig. 7-36), followed by the midfoot and shoulders. Characteristic foot deformities involve equinovarus or equinovalgus. Atrial and ventricular septal defects have been reported (267). Within the range of abnormalities just described, every patient with this syndrome is unique in his or her pattern of associated problems.

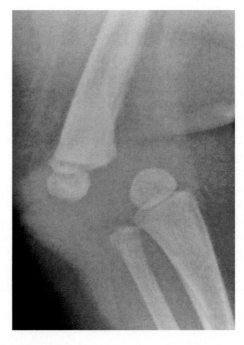

FIGURE 7-36. Congenital anterior knee dislocation is common in Larsen syndrome.

Radiographic Features. There does not appear to be a theme to the radiographic findings in this syndrome. Virtually every patient described, however, has some abnormality in some part of the spine. The cervical spine is the most commonly and severely affected, and spina bifida is very common in that location. Perhaps as a result, the cervical vertebrae may develop progressive kyphosis (Fig. 7-37A–C). The vertebral

bodies in this situation, especially C4 and C5, are very hypoplastic. It is not clear whether this vertebral hypoplasia is a result of pressure from the kyphosis, or a separate, coincidental phenomenon that coexists with the posterior element deficiency. The reported incidence of cervical kyphosis ranges from none to 60% (270, 271, 273). Other cervical problems that may occur include atlantoaxial or subaxial instability (273)

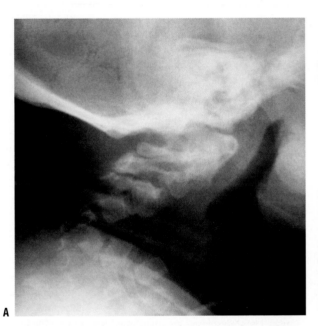
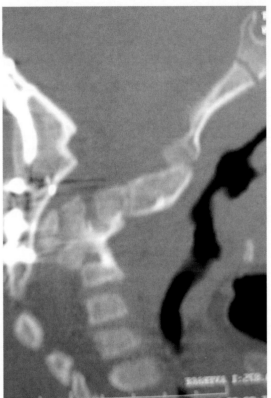
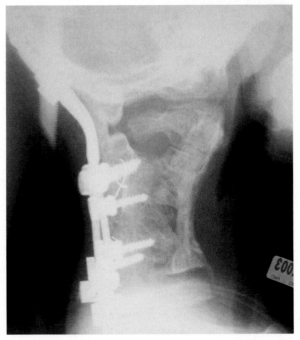

FIGURE 7-37. Cervical kyphosis occurs in many patients with Larsen syndrome, in association with spina bifida occulta of this region **(A)**. The disorder is usually progressive **(B)** and may require decompression and fusion if myelopathy from focal kyphosis occurs **(C)**.

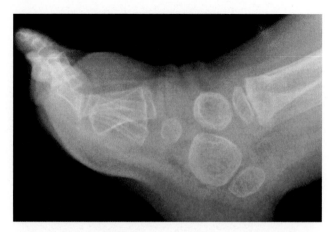

FIGURE 7-38.   The feet in Larsen syndrome are usually in equinovarus and show a characteristic accessory calcaneal ossification center.

and spondylolisthesis of vertebrae. The thoracic spine may also manifest spina bifida; scoliosis is seen in many individuals, but it is usually mild and rarely requires treatment (273). In the lumbar spine, spondylolysis, kyphosis, scoliosis, and back pain may occur (273). Sacral spina bifida is common, but no neurologic compromise is reported.

One of the characteristic (although not universal) findings in Larsen syndrome is the presence of accessory calcaneal or carpal ossification centers (Fig. 7-38). Shortened metacarpals are also noted.

Orthopaedic Implications.   At the beginning of treatment, the orthopaedic surgeon must rule out the cervical kyphosis that may accompany this syndrome because of the catastrophic complications, such as paraparesis, that have been reported. It may be easy to ascribe any developmental delay to the many other skeletal problems these children have, when in fact the cervical kyphosis may cause a neurologic basis for it. Because spontaneous improvement has not been reported with this kyphosis, as it has been with DD, the involved cervical segments should be fused posteriorly if the kyphosis exceeds 35 to 45 degrees. At this level, posterior fusion alone over the involved segments may be successful and may result in spontaneous correction with growth by acting as a posterior tether. Segmental fixation may be helpful in obtaining and maintaining some correction. If the kyphosis progresses to the point of myelopathy, an anterior corpectomy and fusion may be needed, and anterior growth will not occur (274). If enough iliac crest bone is not available for fusion, tibial bone may be used. After surgery, the patient should be in a brace or cast for 4 to 6 months (271). Laryngotracheomalacia may complicate induction of anesthesia.

The lower extremity problems are usually treated in a sequence beginning with the feet and the knees, and then the hips. Treatment for clubfeet may be started early, because some respond to manipulation and cast treatment with tenotomy. Recurrence is common and should be treated with complete subtalar release and shortening osteotomy or decancellation, as necessary. Knees that are hyperextended or subluxatable may

also be treated with casts, but this treatment is unlikely to succeed for patients with complete dislocation who usually require open reduction with V-Y quadricepsplasty, anterior capsulotomy, and release of the anterior portions of the collateral ligaments. A successful result after serial cast treatment and quadriceps tenotomy has been reported (275). If cruciate deficiency leads to persistent anterior instability, reconstruction using parapatellar fascia is usually successful.

Whether to reduce hip dislocations in this condition remains controversial. Some series report that they are resistant to treatment (270, 273), whereas others report some successful results (270, 272). A dislocated hip after failed treatment is less functional than one left untreated. A reasonable approach is to consider treatment of those hips in which the dislocation is not too high and the acetabulum is not too shallow, for patients with otherwise good prospects for activity. The medial approach may be used for infants, but for older children or those with a shallow acetabulum, an anterolateral approach is preferred, with osteotomy or augmentation. If the hip subluxates easily or has a narrow safe zone, the clinician should not hesitate to perform a femoral shortening and derotation. We prefer to begin cast treatment for the feet and knees together, then to operate on the knees if, as usual, they are resistant, then the feet if they are resistant. By that time, the surgeon will have a better idea of the patient's potential and can decide on the most appropriate approach to the hips.

PERINATAL LETHAL SKELETAL DYSPLASIAS

With the increasing use of prenatal diagnostic tests, the orthopaedic surgeon may be questioned about some of the lethal dysplasias that would not otherwise be encountered in practice. These dysplasias are mentioned here to provide some basic information. The combined incidence of lethal dysplasias has been estimated at 15 per 100,000 births in one population. The natural history of these conditions should be considered carefully if one is facing a decision to provide respiratory support.

Thanatophoric dysplasia is characterized by disproportionately small limbs, normal trunk length, a protuberant abdomen, and a large head with frontal bossing. The chest is narrow and the lungs are hypoplastic. The femora are bowed, and their appearance has been likened to old-style telephone receivers. There is phenotypic resemblance to homozygous achondroplasia, and in fact this condition results from a mutation in the same gene, *FGFR3*. Only a few children with this disorder have been reported to survive past 2 years old, even with full respiratory support (1).

Achondrogenesis is characterized by a short trunk, large head, distended abdomen, and severely underdeveloped limbs. It has been subclassified into four types. It may be autosomal dominant or recessive. Achondrogenesis type I results from a mutation in the *DTDST*.

Survival beyond birth is very rare. Currently, there is no treatment available for prolonging the lifespan. Atelosteogenesis, of which there are two types, is characterized by dislocations of large joints and, in some cases, clubfeet. Midface hypoplasia, micrognathism, and a narrow chest are also seen. At least one of the two types results from a mutation in the *DTDST*.

Short-rib-polydactyly syndrome is autosomal recessive and is characterized by polydactyly, which is classically post-axial but may be preaxial, short horizontal ribs, and defects in the kidneys and lungs.

Osteogenesis imperfecta type II is arguably a skeletal dysplasia. Because of the poor prognosis, some of these children have been treated by bone marrow transplants, with reportedly prolonged survival (276).

Conditions that may be, but are not always, fatal in the neonatal period include achondroplasia (homozygous form), rhizomelic chondrodysplasia punctata, camptomelic dysplasia, and a congenital form of hypophosphatasia.

APPENDIX 1: SUMMARIES OF IMPORTANT SKELETAL DYSPLASIAS

Achondroplasia

Genetic Transmission: Autosomal dominant, but most patients have *de novo* mutation

Gene Defect: Highly uniform mutation in *FGFR3* (gain of function)

Key Clinical Features: Stenosis of spine (especially lumbar) or foramen magnum; thoracolumbar kyphosis; genu varum

Key Treatment Points: Brace thoracolumbar kyphosis if more than 2 years old; decompress symptomatic stenosis; cervical spine is stable; osteotomies for genu varum if symptomatic.

Hypochondroplasia

Genetic Transmission: Autosomal dominant

Genetic Defect: Most in *FGFR3* (different domain)

Key Clinical Features: Mild short stature; mild spinal stenosis

Key Treatment Implications: May benefit from growth hormone and/or limb lengthening

Metatropic Dysplasia

Genetic Transmission: Autosomal dominant or recessive

Genetic Defects: Unknown

Key Clinical Features: Infant mortality risk; coccygeal tail, enlarged metaphyses, and contractures; kyphoscoliosis

Key Treatment Points: Rule out cervical instability; possible role for spine fusion.

Chondroectodermal Dysplasia

Genetic Transmission: Autosomal recessive

Genetic Defect: *EVC* with defective maturation or endochondral ossification

Key Clinical Features: Cardiac defects, teeth and nails abnormal, postaxial polydactyly; genu valgus, external femoral rotation

Key Treatment Points: Lateral knee subluxation and depression of tibial plateau are pathognomonic features.

Diastrophic Dysplasia

Genetic Transmission: Autosomal recessive

Genetic Defect: Diastrophic dysplasia sulfate transporter abnormal in all cartilage

Key Clinical Features: "Hitchhiker" thumbs and "cauliflower" ears; joint contractures, cervical kyphosis; scoliosis; DJD, equinovarus feet

Key Treatment Points: Monitor cervical kyphosis, fuse if increasing; correct feet; treat scoliosis, DJD

Kneist Dysplasia

Genetic Transmission: Autosomal dominant

Genetic Defect: Type-II collagen, *COL2A1*, usually exons 12 to 24

Key Clinical Features: Large stiff joints; equinovarus; risk retinal detachment and odontoid hypoplasia

Key Treatment Points: Severe scoliosis and epiphyseal dysplasia occur.

SED Congenita

Genetic Transmission: Autosomal dominant

Genetic Defect: Type-II collagen, *COL2A1*

Key Clinical Features: Severely short stature, C1–C2 instability, scoliosis, hip dysplasia, possible equinovarus foot

Key Treatment Points: Rule out cervical instability. Monitor for scoliosis.

SED Tarda

Genetic Transmission: X-linked most common

Genetic Defect: Type-II collagen (*COL2AI*) or SEDLIN

Key Clinical Features: Hip, back, or knee pain develop in later childhood/adolescence; mild scoliosis

Key Treatment Points: Monitor for scoliosis and kyphosis. Premature DJD may occur.

Pseudoachondroplasia

Genetic Transmission: Autosomal dominant

Genetic Defect: COMP

Key Clinical Features: Ligamentous laxity, windswept knees; size normal at birth, but falls behind

Key Treatment Points: Correct windswept knees; screen for cervical instability. Degenerative changes in hips and knees may occur in adulthood.

Multiple Epiphyseal Dysplasia

Genetic Transmission: Autosomal dominant

Genetic Defect: COMP, other forms from type-IX collagen or Maitrilin 3

Key Clinical Features: Near-normal stature; epiphyseal deformation of large joints with symptoms in late childhood or adulthood

Key Treatment Points: Observation versus acetabular coverage in childhood; joint replacement in adulthood

Chondrodysplasia Punctata

Genetic Transmission: Multiple

Genetic Defect: Rhizomelic form from peroxisomal enzyme deficiency; other forms affect cholesterol synthesis

Key Clinical Features: Neonatal stippling of epiphyses; early mortality (most rhizomelic patients)

Key Treatment Points: Evaluate and treat atlantoaxial instability, congenital scoliosis, coxa vara.

Metaphyseal Chondrodysplasias

Genetic Transmission and Defect: McKusick, autosomal recessive; Schmidt, Jansen, and Kozlowski, autosomal dominant

Key Clinical Features: Metaphyseal irregularities with normal epiphyses; genu varum, mild short stature, fine sparse hair; immune and gastrointestinal disorders in McKusick type

Key Treatment Points: Rule out rare atlantoaxial instability; correct genu varum if severe; monitor medical problems in McKusick type.

Diaphyseal Aclasia (Multiple Osteocartilaginous Exostosis)

Genetic Transmission: Autosomal dominant

Genetic Defect: *EXT1* and *EXT2* gene mutations found on chromosomes 8 and 11, respectively

Key Clinical Features: Short stature, impingement on tendons and nerves, angular deformities, limb-length inequality, malignant degeneration

Key Treatment Points: Monitor for growth disturbances, remove symptomatic exostoses, educate about signs of slight malignant degeneration, monitor spine

Dyschondrosteosis (Leri-Weill Syndrome)

Genetic Transmission: Autosomal dominant

Genetic Mutation: Short stature homeobox gene on chromosome X(*SHOX*)

Key Clinical Features: Mild mesomelic short stature, mild knee angulation, bilateral Madelung deformities

Key Treatment Points: Osteotomies may be indicated to correct forearm deformities.

Cleidocranial Dysplasia

Genetic Transmission: Autosomal dominant

Genetic Defect: Defect in human *RUNX2* (*CBFA1*) gene

Key Clinical Features: Widened cranium, clavicles partially or completely absent, unossified pubic rami; hip abnormalities

Key Treatment Points: Hip surgery for dysplasia or varus; care of dental, cranial, and obstetric problems

Larsen Syndrome

Genetic Transmission: Autosomal dominant or recessive

Genetic Defect: Defect in filamin B, a cytoskeletal protein

Key Clinical Features: Widely spaced eyes, depressed nasal bridge, multiple joint dislocations, cervical kyphosis

Key Treatment Points: Screen for, and aggressively treat, cervical kyphosis. Joint dislocations treated according to standard principles.

REFERENCES

1. Beighton P, ed. *McKusick's Heritable Disorders of Connective Tissue.* St. Louis, MO: Mosby, 1993.
2. Rimoin DL, Cohn D, Krakow D, et al. The skeletal dysplasias: clinical-molecular correlations. *Ann N Y Acad Sci* 2007;1117:302.
3. Boyadjiev SA, Jabs EW. Online Mendelian Inheritance in Man (OMIM) as a knowledge base for human developmental disorders. *Clin Genet* 2000;57:253.
4. Beighton P, Giedion A, Gorlin R, et al. International classification of osteochondrodysplasias. *Am J Med Genet* 1992;44:223.
5. Dreyer SD, Zhou G, Lee B. The long and the short of it: developmental genetics of the skeletal dysplasias. *Clin Genet* 1998;54:464.
6. Walker BA, Scott CI, Hall JG, et al. Diastrophic dwarfism. *Medicine (Baltimore)* 1972;51:41.
7. Unger S. A genetic approach to the diagnosis of skeletal dysplasia. *Clin Orthop Relat Res* 2002;401:32.
8. Gollust SE, Thompson RE, Gooding HC, et al. Living with achondroplasia in an average-sized world: an assessment of quality of life. *Am J Med Genet A* 2003;120:447.
9. Tobias JD. Anesthetic implications of Larsen syndrome. *J Clin Anesth* 1996;8:255.
10. Bethem D, Winter RB, Lutter L, et al. Spinal disorders of dwarfism. Review of the literature and report of eighty cases. *J Bone Joint Surg Am* 1981;63:1412.
11. Bethem D, Winter RB, Lutter L. Disorders of the spine in diastrophic dwarfism. A discussion of nine patients and review of the literature. *J Bone Joint Surg Am* 1980;62:529.
12. Ain MC, Chaichana KL, Schkrohowsky JG. Retrospective study of cervical arthrodesis in patients with various types of skeletal dysplasia. *Spine (Phila Pa 1976)* 2006;31:E169.
13. Aldegheri R. Distraction osteogenesis for lengthening of the tibia in patients who have limb-length discrepancy or short stature. *J Bone Joint Surg Am* 1999;81:624.
14. Dietz FR, Mathews KD. Update on the genetic bases of disorders with orthopaedic manifestations. *J Bone Joint Surg Am* 1996;78:1583.
15. Hall JG. The natural history of achondroplasia. *Basic Life Sci* 1988;48:3.
16. Horton WA. Fibroblast growth factor receptor 3 and the human chondrodysplasias. *Curr Opin Pediatr* 1997;9:437.
17. Muenke M, Schell U. Fibroblast-growth-factor receptor mutations in human skeletal disorders. *Trends Genet* 1995;11:308.
18. Seino Y, Moriwake T, Tanaka H, et al. Molecular defects in achondroplasia and the effects of growth hormone treatment. *Acta Paediatr Suppl* 1999;88:118.
19. Shiang R, Thompson LM, Zhu YZ, et al. Mutations in the transmembrane domain of FGFR3 cause the most common genetic form of dwarfism, achondroplasia. *Cell* 1994;78:335.
20. Wynne-Davies R, Walsh WK, Gormley J. Achondroplasia and hypochondroplasia. Clinical variation and spinal stenosis. *J Bone Joint Surg Br* 1981;63:508.
21. Giudicelli MD, Serazin V, Le Sciellour CR, et al. Increased achondroplasia mutation frequency with advanced age and evidence for G1138A mosaicism in human testis biopsies. *Fertil Steril* 2008;89:1651.
22. McKeand J, Rotta J, Hecht JT. Natural history study of pseudoachondroplasia. *Am J Med Genet* 1996;63:406.
23. Maynard JA, Ippolito EG, Ponseti IV, et al. Histochemistry and ultrastructure of the growth plate in achondroplasia. *J Bone Joint Surg Am* 1981;63:969.
24. Ponseti IV. Skeletal growth in achondroplasia. *J Bone Joint Surg Am* 1970;52:701.
25. Nehme AME, Riseborough EJ, Tredwell SJ. Skeletal growth and development of the achondroplastic dwarf. *Clin Orthop Relat Res* 1976;116:8.
26. Bailey JA II. Orthopaedic aspects of achondroplasia. *J Bone Joint Surg Am* 1970;52:1285.

27. Pauli RM, Breed A, Horton VK, et al. Prevention of fixed, angular kyphosis in achondroplasia. *J Pediatr Orthop* 1997;17:726.
28. Mahomed NN, Spellmann M, Goldberg MJ. Functional health status of adults with achondroplasia. *Am J Med Genet* 1998;78:30.
29. Wynn J, King TM, Gambello MJ, et al. Mortality in achondroplasia study: a 42-year follow-up. *Am J Med Genet A* 2007;143:2502.
30. Scott CI Jr. Achondroplastic and hypochondroplastic dwarfism. *Clin Orthop Relat Res* 1976;114:18.
31. Ireland PJ, Johnson S, Donaghey S, et al. Developmental milestones in infants and young Australasian children with achondroplasia. *J Dev Behav Pediatr* 2010;31:41.
32. Trotter TL, Hall JG. Health supervision for children with achondroplasia. *Pediatrics* 2005;116:771.
33. Keiper GL Jr, Koch B, Crone KR. Achondroplasia and cervicomedullary compression: prospective evaluation and surgical treatment. *Pediatr Neurosurg* 1999;31:78.
34. Pauli RM, Horton VK, Glinski LP, et al. Prospective assessment of risks for cervicomedullary-junction compression in infants with achondroplasia. *Am J Hum Genet* 1995;56:732.
35. Pierre-Kahn A, Hirsch JF, Renier D, et al. Hydrocephalus and achondroplasia. A study of 25 observations. *Childs Brain* 1980;7:205.
36. Todorov AB, Scott CI Jr, Warren AE, et al. Developmental screening tests in achondroplastic children. *Am J Med Genet* 1981;9:19.
37. Bagley CA, Pindrik JA, Bookland MJ, et al. Cervicomedullary decompression for foramen magnum stenosis in achondroplasia. *J Neurosurg* 2006;104:166.
38. Hecht JT, Nelson FW, Butler IJ, et al. Computerized tomography of the foramen magnum: achondroplastic values compared to normal standards. *Am J Med Genet* 1985;20:355.
39. Hecht JT, Horton WA, Reid CS, et al. Growth of the foramen magnum in achondroplasia. *Am J Med Genet* 1989;32:528.
40. Shirley ED, Ain MC. Achondroplasia: manifestations and treatment. *J Am Acad Orthop Surg* 2009;17:231.
41. Waters KA, Everett F, Sillence DO, et al. Treatment of obstructive sleep apnea in achondroplasia: evaluation of sleep, breathing, and somatosensory-evoked potentials. *Am J Med Genet* 1995;59:460.
42. Zucconi M, Weber G, Castronovo V, et al. Sleep and upper airway obstruction in children with achondroplasia. *J Pediatr* 1996;129:743.
43. Reynolds KK, Modaff P, Pauli RM. Absence of correlation between infantile hypotonia and foramen magnum size in achondroplasia. *Am J Med Genet* 2001;101:40.
44. Lutter LD, Longstein JE, Winter RB, et al. Anatomy of the achondroplastic lumbar canal. *Clin Orthop Relat Res* 1977;126:139.
45. Lutter LD, Langer LO. Neurological symptoms in achondroplastic dwarfs—surgical treatment. *J Bone Joint Surg Am* 1977;59:87.
46. Srikumaran U, Woodard EJ, Leet AI, et al. Pedicle and spinal canal parameters of the lower thoracic and lumbar vertebrae in the achondroplast population. *Spine (Phila Pa 1976)* 2007;32:2423.
47. Collins WO, Choi SS. Otolaryngologic manifestations of achondroplasia. *Arch Otolaryngol Head Neck Surg* 2007;133:237.
48. Hoover-Fong JE, Schulze KJ, McGready J, et al. Age-appropriate body mass index in children with achondroplasia: interpretation in relation to indexes of height. *Am J Clin Nutr* 2008;88:364.
49. Hecht JT, Francomano CA, Horton WA, et al. Mortality in achondroplasia. *Am J Hum Genet* 1987;41:454.
50. Horton WA, Hecht JT, Hood OJ, et al. Growth hormone therapy in achondroplasia. *Am J Med Genet* 1992;42:667.
51. Tanaka H, Kubo T, Yamate T, et al. Effect of growth hormone therapy in children with achondroplasia: growth pattern, hypothalamic-pituitary function, and genotype. *Eur J Endocrinol* 1998;138:275.
52. Berkowitz RG, Grundfast KM, Scott C, et al. Middle ear disease in childhood achondroplasia. *Ear Nose Throat J* 1991;70:305.
53. Glass L, Shapiro I, Hodge SE, et al. Audiological findings of patients with achondroplasia. *Int J Pediatr Otorhinolaryngol* 1981;3:129.
54. Stanley G, McLoughlin S, Beals RK. Observations on the cause of bowlegs in achondroplasia. *J Pediatr Orthop* 2002;22:112.
55. Kopits SE. Correction of bowleg deformity in achondroplasia. *Johns Hopkins Med J* 1980;146:206.
56. Lee ST, Song HR, Mahajan R, et al. Development of genu varum in achondroplasia. Relation to fibular overgrowth. *J Bone Joint Surg Br* 2007;89:57.
57. Ain MC, Shirley ED, Pirouzmanesh A, et al. Genu varum in achondroplasia. *J Pediatr Orthop* 2006;26:375.
58. Beals RK, Stanley G. Surgical correction of bowlegs in achondroplasia. *J Pediatr Orthop B* 2005;14:245.
59. Bober M, Johnson C, Nicholson L, et al. Scott sign: a clinical measure of ligamentous laxity in achondroplastic infants. *Am J Med Genet A* 2008;146:2291.
60. Dietz FR, Weinstein SL. Spike osteotomy for angular deformities of the long bones in children. *J Bone Joint Surg Am* 1988;70:848.
61. Rab GT. Oblique tibial osteotomy for Blount's disease (tibia vara). *J Pediatr Orthop* 1988;8:715.
62. Paley D, Tetsworth K. Mechanical axis deviation of the lower limbs. Preoperative planning of multiapical frontal plane angular and bowing deformities of the femur and tibia. *Clin Orthop Relat Res* 1992;280:65.
63. Aldegheri R. Femoral callotasis. *J Pediatr Orthop B* 1997;6:42.
64. Kashiwagi N, Suzuki S, Seto Y, et al. Bilateral humeral lengthening in achondroplasia. *Clin Orthop Relat Res* 2001;391:251.
65. Aldegheri R, Dall'Oca C. Limb lengthening in short stature patients. *J Pediatr Orthop B* 2001;10:238.
66. Park HW, Kim HS, Hahn SB, et al. Correction of lumbosacral hyperlordosis in achondroplasia. *Clin Orthop Relat Res* 2003;414:242.
67. Siebens AA, Hungerford DS, Kirby NA. Curves of the achondroplastic spine: a new hypothesis. *Johns Hopkins Med J* 1978;142:205.
68. Kopits SE. Orthopedic complications of dwarfism. *Clin Orthop Relat Res* 1976;114:153.
69. Tolo VT. Surgical treatment of kyphosis in achondroplasia. In: Nicoletti B, Kopits SE, Ascani E, et al., eds. *Human Achondroplasia: A Multidisciplinary Approach.* New York, NY: Plenum Press, 1988:257.
70. Ain MC, Shirley ED. Spinal fusion for kyphosis in achondroplasia. *J Pediatr Orthop* 2004;24:541.
71. Sciubba DM, Noggle JC, Marupudi NI, et al. Spinal stenosis surgery in pediatric patients with achondroplasia. *J Neurosurg* 2007;106:372.
72. Ain MC, Chang TL, Schkrohowsky JG. Laminectomies and achondroplasia: does body mass index influence surgical outcomes? *Am J Med Genet A* 2007;143A:1032.
73. Schkrohowsky JG, Carlisle ES, Chaichana KL, et al. Intraoperative dural tears secondary to lumbar decompression in adults with achondroplasia. *Neurosurg Q* 2006;16:92.
74. Ain MC, Shirley ED, Pirouzmanesh A, et al. Postlaminectomy kyphosis in the skeletally immature achondroplast. *Spine (Phila Pa 1976)* 2006;31:197.
75. Ain MC, Browne JA. Spinal arthrodesis with instrumentation for thoracolumbar kyphosis in pediatric achondroplasia. *Spine (Phila Pa 1976)* 2004;29:2075.
76. Farmer KW, Brinkley MF, Skolasky RL, et al. Lumbar fusion in achondroplasia. Does fusion to the sacrum affect function? *J Pediatr Orthop* 2009;29:476.
77. Ain MC, Chang TL, Schkrohowsky JG, et al. Rates of perioperative complications associated with laminectomies in patients with achondroplasia. *J Bone Joint Surg Am* 2008;90:295.
78. Horton WA. Evolution of the bone dysplasia family [editorial comment]. *Am J Med Genet* 1996;63:4.
79. Rousseau F, Bonaventure J, Legeai-Mallet L, et al. Clinical and genetic heterogeneity of hypochondroplasia. *J Med Genet* 1996;33:749.
80. Cohen MM Jr. Some chondrodysplasias with short limbs: molecular perspectives. *Am J Med Genet* 2002;112:304.

81. Su WC, Kitagawa M, Xue N, et al. Activation of Stat1 by mutant fibroblast growth-factor receptor in thanatophoric dysplasia type II dwarfism. *Nature* 1997;386:288.

82. Beals RK. Hypochondroplasia. A report of five kindreds. *J Bone Joint Surg Am* 1969;51:728.

83. Wynne-Davies R, Patton MA. The frequency of mental retardation in hypochondroplasia [letter to the editor]. *J Med Genet* 1991;28:644.

84. Hall BD, Spranger J. Hypochondroplasia: clinical and radiological aspects in 39 cases. *Radiology* 1979;133:95.

85. Oberklaid F, Danks DM, Jensen F, et al. Achondroplasia and hypochondroplasia. Comments on frequency, mutation rate, and radiological features in skull and spine. *J Med Genet* 1979;16:140.

86. Ramaswami U, Hindmarsh PC, Brook CG. Growth hormone therapy in hypochondroplasia. *Acta Paediatr Suppl* 1999;88:116.

87. Rimoin DL, Siggers DC, Lachman RS, et al. Metatropic dwarfism, the Kniest syndrome and the pseudoachondroplastic dysplasias. *Clin Orthop Relat Res* 1976;114:70.

88. Genevieve D, Le Merrer M, Feingold J, et al. Revisiting metatropic dysplasia: presentation of a series of 19 novel patients and review of the literature. *Am J Med Genet A* 2008;146:992.

89. Boden SD, Kaplan FS, Fallon MD, et al. Metatropic dwarfism: uncoupling of endochondral and perichondral growth. *J Bone Joint Surg Am* 1987;69:174.

90. Shohat M, Lachman R, Rimoin DL. Odontoid hypoplasia with vertebral cervical subluxation and ventriculomegaly in metatropic dysplasia. *J Pediatr* 1989;114:239.

91. Leet AI, Sampath JS, Scott CI Jr, et al. Cervical spinal stenosis in metatropic dysplasia. *J Pediatr Orthop* 2006;26:347.

92. Beck M, Roubicek M, Rogers JG, et al. Heterogeneity of metatropic dysplasia. *Eur J Pediatr* 1983;140:231.

93. Maroteaux P, Spranger J, Wiedemann HR. Metatrophic dwarfism. *Arch Kinderheilkd* 1966;173:211.

94. Gordienko IY, Grechanina EY, Sopko NI, et al. Prenatal diagnosis of osteochondrodysplasias in high risk pregnancy. *Am J Med Genet* 1996;63:90.

95. Manouvrier-Hanu S, Devisme L, Zelasko MC, et al. Prenatal diagnosis of metatropic dwarfism. *Prenat Diagn* 1995;15:753.

96. Ellis RWB, Van Creveld S. A syndrome characterized by ectodermal dysplasia, polydactyly, chondro-dysplasia and congenital morbus cordis. Report of three cases. *Arch Dis Child* 1940;15:65.

97. Ide SE, Ortiz de Luna RI, Francomano CA, et al. Exclusion of the MSX1 homeobox gene as the gene for the Ellis van Creveld syndrome in the Amish. *Hum Genet* 1996;98:572.

98. Polymeropoulos MH, Ide SE, Wright M, et al. The gene for the Ellis-van Creveld syndrome is located on chromosome 4p16. *Genomics* 1996;35:1.

99. McKusick VA. Ellis-van Creveld syndrome and the Amish. *Nat Genet* 2000;24:203.

100. Baujat G, Le Merrer M. Ellis-Van Creveld syndrome. *Orphanet J Rare Dis* 2007;2:27.

101. Kruse RW, Bowen JR, Heithoff S. Oblique tibial osteotomy in the correction of tibial deformity in children. *J Pediatr Orthop* 1989;9:476.

102. Qureshi F, Jacques SM, Evans MI, et al. Skeletal histopathology in fetuses with chondroectodermal dysplasia (Ellis-van Creveld syndrome). *Am J Med Genet* 1993;45:471.

103. McKusick VA, Egeland JA, Eldridge R, et al. Dwarfism in the Amish I. The Ellis-Van Creveld syndrome. *Bull Johns Hopkins Hosp* 1964;115:306.

104. Kaitila II, Leisti JT, Rimoin DL. Mesomelic skeletal dysplasias. *Clin Orthop Relat Res* 1976;114:94.

105. Pinelli G, Cottafava F, Senes FM, et al. Ellis-Van Creveld syndrome: description of four cases. Orthopaedic aspects. *Ital J Orthop Traumatol* 1990;16:113.

106. Hollister DW, Lachman RS. Diastrophic dwarfism. *Clin Orthop Relat Res* 1976;114:61.

107. Ryoppy S, Poussa M, Merikanto J, et al. Foot deformities in diastrophic dysplasia. An analysis of 102 patients. *J Bone Joint Surg Am* 1992;74:441.

108. Remes VM, Hastbacka JR, Poussa MS, et al. Does genotype predict development of the spinal deformity in patients with diastrophic dysplasia? *Eur Spine J* 2002;11:327.

109. Hastbacka J, de la Chapelle A, Mahtani MM, et al. The diastrophic dysplasia gene encodes a novel sulfate transporter: positional cloning by fine-structure linkage disequilibrium mapping. *Cell* 1994;78:1073.

110. Hastbacka J, Sistonen P, Kaitila I, et al. A linkage map spanning the locus for diastrophic dysplasia (DTD). *Genomics* 1991;11:968.

111. Superti-Furga A, Rossi A, Steinmann B, et al. A chondrodysplasia family produced by mutations in the diastrophic dysplasia sulfate transporter gene: genotype/phenotype correlations. *Am J Med Genet* 1996;63:144.

112. Lamy M, Maroteaux P. Diastrophic nanism. *Presse Med* 1960;68:1977.

113. Qureshi F, Jacques SM, Johnson SF, et al. Histopathology of fetal diastrophic dysplasia. *Am J Med Genet* 1995;56:300.

114. Godbersen GS, Hosenfeld D, Pankau R. Diastrophic dysplasia. A congenital syndrome with remarkable changes of the external ear and stridor. *HNO* 1990;38:256.

115. Crockett MM, Carten MF, Hurko O, et al. Motor milestones in children with diastrophic dysplasia. *J Pediatr Orthop* 2000;20:437.

116. Poussa M, Merikanto J, Ryoppy S, et al. The spine in diastrophic dysplasia. *Spine (Phila Pa 1976)* 1991;16:881.

117. Herring JA. The spinal disorders in diastrophic dwarfism. *J Bone Joint Surg Am* 1978;60:177.

118. Remes V, Marttinen E, Poussa M, et al. Cervical kyphosis in diastrophic dysplasia. *Spine (Phila Pa 1976)* 1999;24:1990.

119. Kash IJ, Sane SM, Samaha FJ, et al. Cervical cord compression in diastrophic dwarfism. *J Pediatr* 1974;84:862.

120. Tolo VT. Spinal deformity in skeletal dysplasias. In: Weinstein SL, ed. *The Pediatric Spine: Principles and Practice.* New York, NY: Raven Press, 1994:369.

121. Vaara P, Peltonen J, Poussa M, et al. Development of the hip in diastrophic dysplasia. *J Bone Joint Surg Br* 1998;80:315.

122. Weiner DS, Jonah D, Kopits S. The 3-dimensional configuration of the typical foot and ankle in diastrophic dysplasia. *J Pediatr Orthop* 2008;28:60.

123. Horton WA, Rimoin DL, Lachman RS, et al. The phenotypic variability of diastrophic dysplasia. *J Pediatr* 1978;93:609.

124. Merrill KD, Schmidt TL. Occipitoatlantal instability in a child with Kniest syndrome. *J Pediatr Orthop* 1989;9:338.

125. Horton WA, Hall JG, Scott CI, et al. Growth curves for height for diastrophic dysplasia, spondyloepiphyseal dysplasia congenita, and pseudoachondroplasia. *Am J Dis Child* 1982;136:316.

126. Makitie O, Kaitila I. Growth in diastrophic dysplasia. *J Pediatr* 1997;130:641.

127. Remes V, Poussa M, Lonnqvist T, et al. Walking ability in patients with diastrophic dysplasia: a clinical, electroneurophysiological, treadmill, and MRI analysis. *J Pediatr Orthop* 2004;24:546.

128. Remes VM, Marttinen EJ, Poussa MS, et al. Cervical spine in patients with diastrophic dysplasia—radiographic findings in 122 patients. *Pediatr Radiol* 2002;32:621.

129. Remes V, Poussa M, Peltonen J. Scoliosis in patients with diastrophic dysplasia: a new classification. *Spine (Phila Pa 1976)* 2001;26:1689.

130. Ain MC, Andres BM, Somel DS, et al. Total hip arthroplasty in skeletal dysplasias: patient selection, preoperative planning, and operative techniques. *J Arthroplasty* 2004;19:1.

131. Helenius I, Remes V, Tallroth K, et al. Total hip arthroplasty in diastrophic dysplasia. *J Bone Joint Surg Am* 2003;85:441.

132. Helenius I, Remes V, Lohman M, et al. Total knee arthroplasty in patients with diastrophic dysplasia. *J Bone Joint Surg Am* 2003;85:2097.

133. Gilbert-Barnes E, Langer LO Jr, Opitz JM, et al. Kniest dysplasia: radiologic, histopathological, and scanning electron microscopic findings. *Am J Med Genet* 1996;63:34.

134. Kneist W. Zur abgrenzung der dysostosis endochondralis von der chondrodystrophie. *Z Kinder* 1952;70:633.

135. Spranger J, Winterpacht A, Zabel B. Kniest dysplasia: Dr. W. Kniest, his patient, the molecular defect. *Am J Med Genet* 1997;69:79.

136. Siggers CD, Rimoin DL, Dorst JP, et al. The Kniest syndrome. *Birth Defects Orig Artic Ser* 1974;10:193.

137. Dobbs MB, Gurnett CA. Update on clubfoot: etiology and treatment. *Clin Orthop Relat Res* 2009;467:1146.

138. Cole WG, Hall RK, Rogers JG. The clinical features of spondyloepiphyseal dysplasia congenita resulting from the substitution of glycine 997 by serine in the alpha 1(II) chain of type II collagen. *J Med Genet* 1993;30:27.

139. Harrod MJE, Friedman JM, Currarino G, et al. Genetic heterogeneity in spondyloepiphyseal dysplasia congenita. *Am J Med Genet* 1984;18:311.

140. Tiller GE, Weis MA, Polumbo PA, et al. An RNA-splicing mutation (G + 5IVS20) in the type II collagen gene (COL2A1) in a family with spondyloepiphyseal dysplasia congenita. *Am J Hum Genet* 1995;56:388.

141. Wynne-Davies R, Hall C. Two clinical variants of spondylo-epiphysial dysplasia congenita. *J Bone Joint Surg Br* 1982;64:435.

142. Spranger JW, Langer LO Jr. Spondyloepiphyseal dysplasia congenita. *Radiology* 1970;94:313.

143. Williams BR, Cranley RE. Morphologic observations on four cases of SED congenita. *Birth Defects Orig Artic Ser* 1974;10:75.

144. Ikegawa S, Iwaya T, Taniguchi K, et al. Retinal detachment in spondyloepiphyseal dysplasia congenita. *J Pediatr Orthop* 1993;13:791.

145. LeDoux MS, Naftalis RC, Aronin PA. Stabilization of the cervical spine in spondyloepiphyseal dysplasia congenita. *Neurosurgery* 1991;28:580.

146. Shetty GM, Song HR, Lee SH, et al. Bilateral valgus-extension osteotomy of hip using hybrid external fixator in spondyloepiphyseal dysplasia: early results of a salvage procedure. *J Pediatr Orthop B* 2008;17:21.

147. Kaibara N, Takagishi K, Katsuki I, et al. Spondyloepiphyseal dysplasia tarda with progressive arthropathy. *Skeletal Radiol* 1983;10:13.

148. Yang SS, Chen H, Williams P, et al. Spondyloepiphyseal dysplasia congenita. A comparative study of chondrocytic inclusions. *Arch Pathol Lab Med* 1980;104:208.

149. Fiedler J, Bergmann C, Brenner RE. X-linked spondyloepiphyseal dysplasia tarda: molecular cause of a heritable disorder associated with early degenerative joint disease. *Acta Orthop Scand* 2003;74:737.

150. Crossan JF, Wynne-Davies R, Fulford GE. Bilateral failure of the capital femoral epiphysis: bilateral Perthes disease, multiple epiphyseal dysplasia, pseudoachondroplasia, and spondyloepiphyseal dysplasia congenita and tarda. *J Pediatr Orthop* 1983;3:297.

151. Diamond LS. A family study of spondyloepiphyseal dysplasia. *J Bone Joint Surg Am* 1970;52:1587.

152. Briggs MD, Chapman KL. Pseudoachondroplasia and multiple epiphyseal dysplasia: mutation review, molecular interactions, and genotype to phenotype correlations. *Hum Mutat* 2002;19:465.

153. Maroteaux P, Lamy M. Pseudo-achondroplastic forms of spondyloepiphyseal dysplasias. *Presse Med* 1959;67:383.

154. Deere M, Sanford T, Francomano CA, et al. Identification of nine novel mutations in cartilage oligomeric matrix protein in patients with pseudoachondroplasia and multiple epiphyseal dysplasia. *Am J Med Genet* 1999;85:486.

155. Ferguson HL, Deere M, Evans R, et al. Mosaicism in pseudoachondroplasia. *Am J Med Genet* 1997;70:287.

156. Cooper RR, Ponseti IV, Maynard JA. Pseudoachondroplastic dwarfism. A rough-surfaced endoplasmic reticulum storage disorder. *J Bone Joint Surg Am* 1973;55:475.

157. Hecht JT, Montufar-Solis D, Decker G, et al. Retention of cartilage oligomeric matrix protein (COMP) and cell death in redifferentiated pseudoachondroplasia chondrocytes. *Matrix Biol* 1998;17:625.

158. Pedrini-Mille A, Maynard JA, Pedrini VA. Pseudoachondroplasia: biochemical and histochemical studies of cartilage. *J Bone Joint Surg Am* 1984;66:1408.

159. Hall JG. Pseudoachondroplasia. *Birth Defects Orig Artic Ser* 1975;11:187.

160. Hall JG, Dorst JP. Pseudoachondroplastic SED, recessive Maroteaux-Lamy type. *Birth Defects Orig Artic Ser* 1969;5:254.

161. Wynne-Davies R, Hall CM, Young ID. Pseudoachondroplasia: clinical diagnosis at different ages and comparison of autosomal dominant and recessive types. A review of 32 patients (26 kindreds). *J Med Genet* 1986;23:425.

162. Leet AI, Pichard CP, Ain MC. Surgical treatment of femoral fractures in obese children: does excessive body weight increase the rate of complications? *J Bone Joint Surg Am* 2005;87:2609.

163. Fairbank T. Dysplasia epiphysealis multiplex. *Br J Surg* 1947;34:225.

164. Ribbing S. Studien uber hereditare, multiple epiphysenstorungen. *Acta Radiol Suppl* 1937;34:1.

165. Stanescu R, Stanescu V, Muriel MP, et al. Multiple epiphyseal dysplasia, Fairbank type: morphologic and biochemical study of cartilage. *Am J Med Genet* 1993;45:501.

166. Posey KL, Hecht JT. The role of cartilage oligomeric matrix protein (COMP) in skeletal disease. *Curr Drug Targets* 2008;9:869.

167. van Mourik JB, Hamel BC, Mariman EC. A large family with multiple epiphyseal dysplasia linked to COL9A2 gene. *Am J Med Genet* 1998;77:234.

168. Makitie O, Mortier GR, Czarny-Ratajczak M, et al. Clinical and radiographic findings in multiple epiphyseal dysplasia caused by MATN3 mutations: description of 12 patients. *Am J Med Genet A* 2004;125:278.

169. Jacobs PA. Dysplasia epiphysialis multiplex. *Clin Orthop Relat Res* 1968;58:117.

170. Schlesinger AE, Poznanski AK, Pudlowski RM, et al. Distal femoral epiphysis: normal standards for thickness and application to bone dysplasias. *Radiology* 1986;159:515.

171. Treble NJ, Jensen FO, Bankier A, et al. Development of the hip in multiple epiphyseal dysplasia. Natural history and susceptibility to premature osteoarthritis. *J Bone Joint Surg Br* 1990;72:1061.

172. Mackenzie WG, Bassett GS, Mandell GA, et al. Avascular necrosis of the hip in multiple epiphyseal dysplasia. *J Pediatr Orthop* 1989;9:666.

173. Apley AG, Wientroub S. The sagging rope sign in Perthes' disease and allied disorders. *J Bone Joint Surg Br* 1981;63:43.

174. Hodkinson HM. Double patellae in multiple epiphyseal dysplasia. *J Bone Joint Surg Br* 1962;44:569.

175. Vatanavicharn N, Lachman RS, Rimoin DL. Multilayered patella: similar radiographic findings in pseudoachondroplasia and recessive multiple epiphyseal dysplasia. *Am J Med Genet A* 2008;146A:1682.

176. Eddy MC, Steiner RD, McAlister WH, et al. Bilateral radial ray hypoplasia with multiple epiphyseal dysplasia. *Am J Med Genet* 1998;77:182.

177. Haga N, Nakamura K, Takikawa K, et al. Stature and severity in multiple epiphyseal dysplasia. *J Pediatr Orthop* 1998;18:394.

178. Spranger J. The epiphyseal dysplasias. *Clin Orthop Relat Res* 1976;114:46.

179. Trigui M, Pannier S, Finidori G, et al. Coxa vara in chondrodysplasia: prognosis study of 35 hips in 19 children. *J Pediatr Orthop* 2008;28:599.

180. Kruse RW, Guille JT, Bowen JR. Shelf arthroplasty in patients who have Legg-Calve-Perthes disease. A study of long-term results. *J Bone Joint Surg Am* 1991;73:1338.

181. Willett K, Hudson I, Catterall A. Lateral shelf acetabuloplasty: an operation for older children with Perthes' disease. *J Pediatr Orthop* 1992;12:563.

182. Cho TJ, Choi IH, Chung CY, et al. Hemiepiphyseal stapling for angular deformity correction around the knee joint in children with multiple epiphyseal dysplasia. *J Pediatr Orthop* 2009;29:52.

183. Ramachandran G, Mason D. Double-layered patella: marker for multiple epiphyseal dysplasia. *Am J Orthop (Belle Mead NJ)* 2004;33:35.

184. Pavone V, Costarella L, Privitera V, et al. Bilateral total hip arthroplasty in subjects with multiple epiphyseal dysplasia. *J Arthroplasty* 2009;24:868.

185. Ingram RR. The shoulder in multiple epiphyseal dysplasia. *J Bone Joint Surg Br* 1991;73:277.

186. Irving MD, Chitty LS, Mansour S, et al. Chondrodysplasia punctata: a clinical diagnostic and radiological review. *Clin Dysmorphol* 2008;17:229.

187. Andersen PE Jr, Justesen P. Chondrodysplasia punctata. Report of two cases. *Skeletal Radiol* 1987;16:223.

188. Wulfsberg EA, Curtis J, Jayne CH. Chondrodysplasia punctata: a boy with X-linked recessive chondrodysplasia punctata due to an inherited X-Y translocation with a current classification of these disorders. *Am J Med Genet* 1992;43:823.

189. Borg SA, Fitzer PM, Young LW. Roentgenologic aspects of adult cretinism. Two case reports and review of the literature. *Am J Roentgenol Radium Ther Nucl Med* 1975;123:820.

190. Hanson JW, Smith DW. The fetal hydantoin syndrome. *J Pediatr* 1975;87:285.

191. Harrod MJE, Sherrod PS. Warfarin embryopathy in siblings. *Obstet Gynecol* 1981;57:673.

192. Pauli RM, Lian JB, Mosher DF, et al. Association of congenital deficiency of multiple vitamin K-dependent coagulation factors and the phenotype of the warfarin embryopathy: clues to the mechanism of teratogenicity of coumarin derivatives. *Am J Hum Genet* 1987;41:566.

193. Pike MG, Applegarth DA, Dunn HG, et al. Congenital rubella syndrome associated with calcific epiphyseal stippling and peroxisomal dysfunction. *J Pediatr* 1990;116:88.

194. Curry CJR, Magenis RE, Brown M, et al. Inherited chondrodysplasia punctata due to a deletion of the terminal short arm of an X chromosome. *N Engl J Med* 1984;311:1010.

195. Wardinsky TD, Pagon RA, Powell BR, et al. Rhizomelic chondrodysplasia punctata and survival beyond one year: a review of the literature and five case reports [see comments]. *Clin Genet* 1990;38:84.

196. Mason DE, Sanders JO, Mackenzie WG, et al. Spinal deformity in chondrodysplasia punctata. *Spine (Phila Pa 1976)* 2002;27:1995.

197. Gilbert EF, Opitz JM, Spranger JW, et al. Chondrodysplasia punctata—rhizomelic form. Pathologic and radiologic studies of three infants. *Eur J Pediatr* 1976;123:89.

198. Happle R. X-linked dominant chondrodysplasia punctata. Review of literature and report of a case. *Hum Genet* 1979;53:65.

199. Manzke H, Christophers E, Wiedemann HR. Dominant sex-linked inherited chondrodysplasia punctata: a distinct type of chondrodysplasia punctata. *Clin Genet* 1980;17:97.

200. Silengo MC, Luzzatti L, Silverman FN. Clinical and genetic aspects of Conradi-Hunermann disease. A report of three familial cases and review of the literature. *J Pediatr* 1980;97:911.

201. Spranger JW, Opitz JM, Bidder U. Heterogeneity of chondrodysplasia punctata. *Humangenetik* 1971;11:190.

202. Heymans HSA, Oorthuys JWE, Nelck G, et al. Rhizomelic chondrodysplasia punctata: another peroxisomal disorder [letter to the editor]. *N Engl J Med* 1985;313:187.

203. Hoefler S, Hoefler G, Moser AB, et al. Prenatal diagnosis of rhizomelic chondrodysplasia punctata. *Prenat Diagn* 1988;8:571.

204. Mueller RF, Crowle PM, Jones RAK, et al. X-linked dominant chondrodysplasia punctata: a case report and family studies. *Am J Med Genet* 1985;20:137.

205. Rittler M, Menger H, Spranger J. Chondrodysplasia punctata, tibia-metacarpal (MT) type. *Am J Med Genet* 1990;37:200.

206. Burck U. Mesomelic dysplasia with punctate epiphyseal calcifications—a new entity of chondrodysplasia punctata? *Eur J Pediatr* 1982;138:67.

207. Khanna AJ, Braverman NE, Valle D, et al. Cervical stenosis secondary to rhizomelic chondrodysplasia punctata. *Am J Med Genet* 2001;99:63.

208. Bethem D. Os odontoideum in chondrodystrophia calcificans congenita. A case report. *J Bone Joint Surg Am* 1982;64:1385.

209. Sheffield LJ, Halliday JL, Danks DM, et al. Clinical, radiological and biochemical classification of chondrodysplasia punctata. *Am J Hum Genet* 1989;45:A64.

210. Fairbank HAT. Dysplasia epiphysialis punctata: synonyms—stippled epiphyses, chondrodystrophia calcificans congenita (Hunermann). *J Bone Joint Surg Br* 1949;31:114.

211. Lawrence JJ, Schlesinger AE, Kozlowski K, et al. Unusual radiographic manifestations of chondrodysplasia punctata. *Skeletal Radiol* 1989;18:15.

212. Cooper RR, Ponseti IV. Metaphyseal dysostosis: description of an ultrastructural defect in the epiphyseal plate chondrocytes. *J Bone Joint Surg Am* 1973;55:485.

213. Evans R, Caffey J. Metaphyseal dysostosis resembling vitamin D-refractory rickets. *AMA J Dis Child* 1958;95:640.

214. Kozlowski K. Metaphyseal and spondylometaphyseal chondrodysplasias. *Clin Orthop Relat Res* 1976;114:83.

215. Sulisalo T, van der Burgt I, Rimoin DL, et al. Genetic homogeneity of cartilage-hair hypoplasia. *Hum Genet* 1995;95:157.

216. Ridanpaa M, Jain P, McKusick VA, et al. The major mutation in the RMRP gene causing CHH among the Amish is the same as that found in most Finnish cases. *Am J Med Genet C Semin Med Genet* 2003;121:81.

217. Makitie O, Kaitila I. Cartilage-hair hypoplasia—clinical manifestations in 108 Finnish patients. *Eur J Pediatr* 1993;152:211.

218. Makitie O, Marttinen E, Kaitila I. Skeletal growth in cartilage-hair hypoplasia. A radiological study of 82 patients. *Pediatr Radiol* 1992;22:434.

219. Juvonen E, Makitie O, Makipernaa A, et al. Defective in-vitro colony formation of haematopoietic progenitors in patients with cartilage-hair hypoplasia and history of anaemia. *Eur J Pediatr* 1995;154:30.

220. van der Burgt I, Haraldsson A, Oosterwijk JC, et al. Cartilage hair hypoplasia, metaphyseal chondrodysplasia type McKusick: description of seven patients and review of the literature. *Am J Med Genet* 1991;41:371.

221. Wasylenko MJ, Wedge JH, Houston CS. Metaphyseal chondrodysplasia, Schmid type. A defect of ultrastructural metabolism: case report. *J Bone Joint Surg Am* 1980;62:660.

222. Paschalis EP, Jacenko O, Olsen B, et al. Fourier transform infrared microspectroscopic analysis identifies alterations in mineral properties in bones from mice transgenic for type X collagen. *Bone* 1996;19:151.

223. Wallis GA, Rash B, Sykes B, et al. Mutations within the gene encoding the alpha 1 (X) chain of type X collagen (COL10A1) cause metaphyseal chondrodysplasia type Schmid but not several other forms of metaphyseal chondrodysplasia. *J Med Genet* 1996;33:450.

224. Schipani E, Jensen GS, Pincus J, et al. Constitutive activation of the cyclic adenosine 3′,5′-monophosphate signaling pathway by parathyroid hormone (PTH)/PTH-related peptide receptors mutated at the two loci for Jansen's metaphyseal chondrodysplasia. *Mol Endocrinol* 1997;11:851.

225. Alvarez C, Tredwell S, De Vera M, et al. The genotype-phenotype correlation of hereditary multiple exostoses. *Clin Genet* 2006;70:122.

226. Jones KB, Morcuende JA. Of hedgehogs and hereditary bone tumors: re-examination of the pathogenesis of osteochondromas. *Iowa Orthop J* 2003;23:87.

227. Roach JW, Klatt JW, Faulkner ND. Involvement of the spine in patients with multiple hereditary exostoses. *J Bone Joint Surg Am* 2009;91:1942.

228. Porter DE, Lonie L, Fraser M, et al. Severity of disease and risk of malignant change in hereditary multiple exostoses. A genotype-phenotype study. *J Bone Joint Surg Br* 2004;86:1041.

229. Ishikawa J, Kato H, Fujioka F, et al. Tumor location affects the results of simple excision for multiple osteochondromas in the forearm. *J Bone Joint Surg Am* 2007;89:1238.

230. Akita S, Murase T, Yonenobu K, et al. Long-term results of surgery for forearm deformities in patients with multiple cartilaginous exostoses. *J Bone Joint Surg Am* 2007;89:1993.

231. Beals RK, Shea M. Correlation of chronological age and bone age with the correction of ankle valgus by surface epiphysiodesis of the distal medial tibial physis. *J Pediatr Orthop B* 2005;14:436.

232. Noonan KJ, Feinberg JR, Levenda A, et al. Natural history of multiple hereditary osteochondromatosis of the lower extremity and ankle. *J Pediatr Orthop* 2002;22:120.

233. Hosalkar H, Greenberg J, Gaugler RL, et al. Abnormal scarring with keloid formation after osteochondroma excision in children with multiple hereditary exostoses. *J Pediatr Orthop* 2007;27:333.

234. Leri A, Weill J. Une affection congenitale et symetrique du developpement osseux: la dyschondrosteose. *Bull Mem Soc Med Hosp (Paris)* 1929;53:1491.

235. Felman AH, Kirkpatrick JA Jr. Dyschondrosteose. Mesomelic dwarfism of Lwei and Weill. *Am J Dis Child* 1970;120:329.

236. Langer LO Jr. Dyschondrosteosis, a hereditable bone dysplasia with characteristic roentgenographic features. *Am J Roentgenol Radium Ther Nucl Med* 1965;95:178.

237. Dawe C, Wynne-Davies R, Fulford GE. Clinical variation in dyschondrosteosis. A report on 13 individuals in 8 families. *J Bone Joint Surg Br* 1982;64:377.

238. Murphy MS, Linscheid RL, Dobyns JH, et al. Radial opening wedge osteotomy in Madelung's deformity. *J Hand Surg Am* 1996;21:1035.

239. Mohan V, Gupta RP, Helmi K, et al. Leri-Weill syndrome (dyschondrosteosis): a family study. *J Hand Surg Br* 1988;13:16.

240. Shears DJ, Vassal HJ, Goodman FR, et al. Mutation and deletion of the pseudoautosomal gene SHOX cause Leri-Weill dyschondrosteosis. *Nat Genet* 1998;19:70.

241. Marchini A, Rappold G, Schneider KU. SHOX at a glance: from gene to protein. *Arch Physiol Biochem* 2007;113:116.

242. Rappold GA, Shanske A, Saenger P. All shook up by SHOX deficiency. *J Pediatr* 2005;147:422.

243. Cook PA, Yu JS, Wiand W, et al. Madelung deformity in skeletally immature patients: morphologic assessment using radiography, CT, and MRI. *J Comput Assist Tomogr* 1996;20:505.

244. Thuestad IJ, Ivarsson SA, Nilsson KO, et al. Growth hormone treatment in Leri-Weill syndrome. *J Pediatr Endocrinol Metab* 1996;9:201.

245. Burren CP, Werther GA. Skeletal dysplasias: response to growth hormone therapy. *J Pediatr Endocrinol Metab* 1996;9:31.

246. Vickers D, Nielsen G. Madelung deformity: surgical prophylaxis (physiolysis) during the late growth period by resection of the dyschondrosteosis lesion. *J Hand Surg Br* 1992;17:401.

247. Marie P, Sainton P. On hereditary cleido-cranial dysostosis. *Clin Orthop Relat Res* 1968;58:5.

248. Marie P, Seinton P. Observation d'hydrocephalie hereditaire (pere et fils) par vice de developpement du crane et du cerveau. *Rev Neurol* 1897;5:394.

249. Martinez-Frias ML, Herranz I, Salvador J, et al. Prevalence of dominant mutations in Spain: effect of changes in maternal age distribution. *Am J Med Genet* 1988;31:845.

250. Geoffroy V, Corral DA, Zhou L, et al. Genomic organization, expression of the human CBFA1 gene, and evidence for an alternative splicing event affecting protein function. *Mamm Genome* 1998;9:54.

251. Lee B, Thirunavukkarasu K, Zhou L, et al. Missense mutations abolishing DNA binding of the osteoblast-specific transcription factor OSF2/CBFA1 in cleidocranial dysplasia. *Nat Genet* 1997;16:307.

252. Otto F, Thornell AP, Crompton T, et al. Cbfa1, a candidate gene for cleidocranial dysplasia syndrome, is essential for osteoblast differentiation and bone development. *Cell* 1997;89:765.

253. Ziros PG, Basdra EK, Papavassiliou AG. Runx2: of bone and stretch. *Int J Biochem Cell Biol* 2008;40:1659.

254. Jensen BL. Somatic development in cleidocranial dysplasia. *Am J Med Genet* 1990;35:69.

255. Jensen BL, Kreiborg S. Development of the skull in infants with cleidocranial dysplasia. *J Craniofac Genet Dev Biol* 1993;13:89.

256. Miles PW. Cleidocranial dysostosis: a survey of six new cases and 126 from the literature. *J Kansas Med Soc* 1940;41:462.

257. Gupta SK, Sharma OP, Malhotra S, et al. Cleido-cranial dysostosis—skeletal abnormalities. *Australas Radiol* 1992;36:238.

258. Dore DD, MacEwen GD, Boulos MI. Cleidocranial dysostosis and syringomyelia. Review of the literature and case report. *Clin Orthop Relat Res* 1987;214:229.

259. Taglialavoro G, Fabris D, Agostini S. A case of progressive scoliosis in a patient with craniocleidopelvic dysostosis. *Ital J Orthop Traumatol* 1983;9:507.

260. Vari R, Puca A, Meglio M. Cleidocranial dysplasia and syringomyelia. Case report. *J Neurosurg Sci* 1996;40:125.

261. Hamner LH III, Fabbri EL, Browne PC. Prenatal diagnosis of cleidocranial dysostosis. *Obstet Gynecol* 1994;83:856.

262. Jarvis JL, Keats TE. Cleidocranial dysostosis. A review of 40 new cases. *Am J Roentgenol Radium Ther Nucl Med* 1974;121:5.

263. Kim HT, Chambers HG, Mubarak SJ, et al. Congenital coxa vara: computed tomographic analysis of femoral retroversion and the triangular metaphyseal fragment. *J Pediatr Orthop* 2000;20:551.

264. Krishnan SG, Hawkins RJ, Michelotti JD, et al. Scapulothoracic arthrodesis: indications, technique, and results. *Clin Orthop Relat Res* 2005;435:126.

265. Richie MF, Johnston CE II. Management of developmental coxa vara in cleidocranial dysplasia. *Orthopedics* 1989;12:1001.

266. Larsen LJ, Schottstaedt ER, Bost FC. Multiple congenital dislocations associated with characteristic facial abnormality. *J Pediatr* 1950;37:574.

267. Vujic M, Hallstensson K, Wahlstrom J, et al. Localization of a gene for autosomal dominant Larsen syndrome to chromosome region 3p21.1–14.1 in the proximity of, but distinct from, the COL7A1 locus. *Am J Hum Genet* 1995;57:1104.

268. Krakow D, Robertson SP, King LM, et al. Mutations in the gene encoding filamin B disrupt vertebral segmentation, joint formation and skeletogenesis. *Nat Genet* 2004;36:405.

269. Zhang D, Herring JA, Swaney SS, et al. Mutations responsible for Larsen syndrome cluster in the FLNB protein. *J Med Genet* 2006;43:e24.

270. Laville JM, Lakermance P, Limouzy F. Larsen's syndrome: review of the literature and analysis of thirty-eight cases. *J Pediatr Orthop* 1994;14:63.

271. Johnston CE II, Birch JG, Daniels JL. Cervical kyphosis in patients who have Larsen syndrome. *J Bone Joint Surg Am* 1996;78:538.

272. Micheli LJ, Hall JE, Watts HG. Spinal instability in Larsen's syndrome: report of three cases. *J Bone Joint Surg Am* 1976;58:562.

273. Bowen JR, Ortega K, Ray S, et al. Spinal deformities in Larsen's syndrome. *Clin Orthop Relat Res* 1985;197:159.

274. Sakaura H, Matsuoka T, Iwasaki M, et al. Surgical treatment of cervical kyphosis in Larsen syndrome: report of 3 cases and review of the literature. *Spine (Phila Pa 1976)* 2007;32:E39.

275. Dobbs MB, Boehm S, Grange DK, et al. Congenital knee dislocation in a patient with Larsen syndrome and a novel filamin B mutation. *Clin Orthop Relat Res* 2008;466:1503.

276. Bodian DL, Chan TF, Poon A, et al. Mutation and polymorphism spectrum in osteogenesis imperfecta type II: implications for genotype-phenotype relationships. *Hum Mol Genet* 2009;18:463.

Benjamin A. Alman
Michael J. Goldberg

Syndromes of Orthopaedic Importance

The word *syndrome* is derived from a Greek word that means *to run together*. When several relatively uncommon anomalies occur in the same individual, it may be nothing more than coincidence. However, if all the anomalies result from the same cause, or occur in the same pattern in other children, that particular combination of birth defects is called a *syndrome*. A syndrome should be suspected if a characteristic orthopaedic malformation (e.g., radial clubhand) is encountered, if all four extremities are affected, if limb deformities are symmetric, if there are several associated nonorthopaedic anomalies, or if the patient has a familiarly dysmorphic face. Children who have syndromes look more like one another than like their parents (1–4).

It is not unusual for an orthopaedist to be the first physician to recognize that a child has characteristics of a syndrome. In such cases, appropriate referrals should be made to a geneticist to assist in syndrome identification, order appropriate confirmatory tests, and arrange for management of the nonorthopaedic manifestations of the syndrome. The evaluation of a child for a syndrome includes a family history, a systems review, and a search for minor dysmorphic features, such as abnormal palm creases or abnormal shape of digits or toes. These evaluation processes may not be of immediate orthopaedic importance, but they are the clues to look further.

During fetal development, cell signaling pathways are activated in a coordinated manner to allow cells to divide, differentiate, move, and die off, ultimately resulting in a normally formed individual. These cell signaling pathways play roles in the development of multiple organs. It is not surprising that dysregulation of such developmentally important pathways can cause the malformation of a number of organs, resulting in several otherwise uncommon abnormalities occurring together, producing a syndrome. Such pathways can be dysregulated by a mutation in a key pathway member, by fetal environmental factors (e.g., a teratogen, such as in fetal alcohol syndrome), or both.

The relation between the clinical (phenotypic) features and the cause of a syndrome is not always as simple as one would wish. Even within a family in which all the members carry the identical causative gene mutation, some individuals are minimally affected, whereas others have all of the findings of the syndrome. This may be due to the presence of modifying genes, which may not be inherited in the same way as the gene mutation that causes the syndrome, or due to fetal environmental factors that modify the manner in which the pathways are activated. In addition, different mutations in the same gene can cause different syndromes, because the products of different mutations have different cellular functions. Such is the case with the dystrophin gene, which causes both Duchenne and Becker muscular dystrophies.

Information about the etiology of a syndrome is important, because it has implications for the parents as to the risk of recurrence in subsequent pregnancies, and may hold the key to the development of novel treatments. The rapid pace of basic research in developmental biology and genetics makes it difficult for a traditional textbook to provide the most up-to-date information about syndrome etiology. The Internet is becoming an excellent source for such information. One useful site is the On-line Mendelian Inheritance in Man (OMIM), administered by the National Institutes of Health. This site can be accessed at http://www.ncbi.nlm.nih.gov/Omim/ and can be searched by syndrome name, causative gene, or clinical findings (5).

The care of children with syndromes involves multiple specialists (6). Discussions about the risk of subsequent pregnancies are in the realm of the genetic counselor. While parents often assume that if the condition has a name, it is treatable or curable, this sadly, is not the case. The importance of understanding syndromes is in recognizing associated medical abnormalities that may be life threatening, adversely influence orthopaedic outcomes, or may influence surgical timing and management. Importantly, patients can come to significant harm if an orthopaedist misses recognizing a syndrome. For instance, in the case of Marfan syndrome, starting a child on beta-blockers can prevent a catastrophic cardiovascular event.

Even if parents are not planning subsequent pregnancies, and if there are no plans for their child to undergo surgery in the near future, genetic evaluation is still important for proper syndrome diagnosis. Correct diagnoses are essential for research into syndrome etiology and treatment. Patients should be given the opportunity to participate in such research, especially in cases of relatively rare syndromes.

Nomenclature can confuse syndrome identification, because a single syndrome may have several names. Eponyms are not descriptive of the syndrome, nor do they give information about etiology. Many syndromes are caused by a mutation in a gene, and the causative gene has been identified in most such syndromes. Classifying syndromes by the causative gene alone can be problematic because some genes cause more than one syndrome, some syndromes are caused by more than one gene, and some syndromes are not caused by a gene mutation. Furthermore, gene names are frequently unrelated to clinical findings associated with a given syndrome. A numbering system is used by computer databases; the most widely used is that of the OMIM (5), but this is helpful only for database searches. An ideal nomenclature, which would give information about clinical findings and etiology, has yet to be developed.

Knowledge of the genetic cause of syndromes does not supplant the need for the clinician to know the phenotypic features of individual syndromes (7). For many syndromes, molecular genetic tests are not available or are available only at a very high cost. As such, it is impractical to test a given patient for every known genetic condition (8). A thorough study of the patient's history and a physical examination gives clues as to which supportive tests to order, such as radiographs. This information is used for narrowing down the diagnosis to only a handful of syndromes. In many cases, the ultimate diagnosis can be made on the clinical and radiographic findings alone [e.g., neurofibromatosis (NF) type I]. For syndromes in which molecular genetic tests are available, these are usually performed to confirm a diagnosis rather than to make a diagnosis and should only rarely be ordered by an orthopaedist before consultation with a clinical geneticist or genetic counselor.

It is clinically useful to classify syndromes caused by gene mutations into groups broadly categorized by the function of the causative gene (9, 10). Such syndromes can be broadly classified into those caused by mutation in genes encoding one of the following types of proteins: structural proteins, proteins that regulate developmentally important signaling pathways, proteins implicated in neoplasia, proteins such as enzymes that play a role in processing molecules, and proteins that play a role in nerve or muscle function (7). Syndromes within each broad group share similarities in the mode of inheritance and clinical behavior. For instance, syndromes caused by mutations in genes encoding structural proteins tend to be inherited in an autosomal dominant manner and result in skeletal structures that wear out with time, for which corrective surgery has a high recurrence or failure rate. Most of the disorders in this chapter are grouped using this functional genetic scheme. The one exception is contracture syndromes, which are considered

as a separate group. Although the genetic etiology of many of the contracture syndromes has been identified, it is easiest, from a practical standpoint, to consider them as a few subgroups based on clinical and treatment similarities.

STRUCTURAL GENES

A variety of proteins play important roles in the connective tissues, including the bones, articular cartilage, ligaments, and skin. Mutations in such genes disrupt the structural integrity of the connective tissues in which they are expressed. In most cases, the phenotype is absent or there are only minor manifestations present at birth; the phenotype evolves with time, because the abnormal structural components slowly fail or wear out with time as the individual grows. Deformity often recurs after surgery, because the structural components are abnormal and will wear out again. In cases where the structural abnormality involves cartilage, there may be growth abnormality caused by physeal mechanical failure or early degenerative disease of the joints caused by articular cartilage failure. When a protein that is important for ligament or tendon strength is affected, joints often subluxate. There can be substantial heterogeneity in the severity of the phenotype, depending upon the exact way in which the mutation alters the protein function. In patients with mild disease, life expectancy is normal; however, in patients with more severe disease, life expectancy may be shortened because of secondary effects of the structural defects on vital organs. These disorders tend to be inherited in an autosomal dominant manner (9, 10). Many of the disorders caused by mutations in genes that encode structural proteins, including osteogenesis imperfecta and spondyloepiphyseal dysplasia, are covered in other sections of this textbook.

Marfan Syndrome. Anton Marfan, a French pediatrician, first described this syndrome in 1896, as a condition associated with long limbs and involvement of the cardiovascular, ocular, and skeletal systems (11). Although some authorities believe that Abraham Lincoln had Marfan syndrome, there remains considerable controversy surrounding this, and a decision was made against using DNA from his remains to test for this diagnosis (12). This is one of the few syndromes caused by a mutation in a gene encoding a structural protein that is associated with tall stature. Patients can be recognized by the characteristic tall stature, arachnodactyly (abnormally long and slender digits), dolichostenomelia (long, narrow limbs), pectus deformities, and scoliosis. Stria can be seen in the skin (Fig. 8-1). There are a number of cardiovascular anomalies associated with this condition, including aortic regurgitation, aortic dilatation, aneurysms, and mitral valve prolapse. Ocular findings are myopia and superior displacement of the lens. The lens moves in the opposite direction in homocystinuria, a condition that sometimes is misdiagnosed as Marfan syndrome. Undiagnosed patients with Marfan syndrome not infrequently present to an orthopaedist with a diagnosis of scoliosis. It is

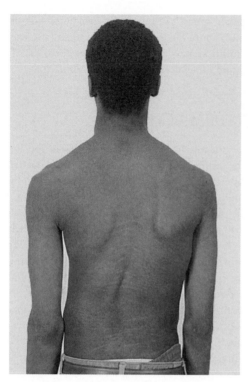

FIGURE 8-1. Stria in a boy with Marfan syndrome, who initially presented for evaluation of scoliosis.

important for an orthopaedist to recognize this condition, since its identification allows for referral for management of the cardiovascular abnormalities, early treatment of which can prevent premature mortality.

Diagnosis and Physical Findings.   The diagnosis is made on the basis of family history and clinical findings, including abnormalities in the ocular, cardiac, and musculoskeletal systems (13). Despite several meetings to develop a consensus about diagnostic criteria, controversy remains as to the best set of diagnostic criteria to employ. If one uses more stringent criteria, this will exclude many individuals who are currently managed as Marfan syndrome patients. The less stringent Berlin criteria and the more stringent Ghent criteria are outlined in Table 8-1 (14–16). To further confound issues of clinical diagnosis, there is controversy about the definition of dural ectasia. The initial definition included a number of morphologic characteristics, as well as a dural volume >7 cm³ below the inferior L5 endplate, as measured using a magnetic resonance image (MRI) study (14, 15). The normal dural volume in younger, growing children is not known, and the reliability and reproducibility of volume measures when used outside of clinical investigative groups is also unclear. A recent retrospective analysis suggests that a sagittal dural sac width at S1 greater than that at L4 is a better criterion for dural ectasia in children, adolescents, and young adults (16).

There are a variety of additional physical findings that are suggestive of Marfan syndrome and while not part of the

diagnostic criteria, should alert one to consider this diagnosis. It was thought that the physical finding of an arm span longer than height would be diagnostic of Marfan syndrome; however, population studies have shown that this is not the case. The ratio of upper segment (head to pubic symphysis) to lower segment (pubic symphysis to plantar surface), which is normally 0.93 in a mature individual, is often decreased in Marfan syndrome to 0.85 or less (17). Two clinical findings associated with arachnodactyly are a thumb that protrudes past the ulnar border of the hand when it is held in a clenched fist (Steinberg sign) and overlap in the thumb and index finger when they are wrapped around the opposite wrist (18).

Radiographic Findings.   Although there are a variety of radiographic findings that are frequently present in patients with Marfan syndrome, none are pathopneumonic. Spinal morphology suggestive of dural ectasia and pedicle dysplasia are suggestive of this disorder. The use of measurements from spine radiographs in making this diagnosis (an interpedicular distance at L5 ≥ 36.0 mm; a sagittal diameter at L5 ≥ 13.5 mm; a transverse process-to-vertebral width ratio at L3 ≥ 2.25 mm) yields a high sensitivity but a relatively poor specificity (16). A arachnodactyly is defined on radiographs as an increase in the ratio of length to width of the second to the fifth metacarpals (Fig. 8-2). The average ratio of the lengths of the second to the fifth metacarpals, divided by the widths of the respective diaphyses, is >8.8 in male patients and >9.4 in female patients with Marfan syndrome (19). There are no studies, however, that determine the sensitivity and specificity of the use of these measures to make a diagnosis of Marfan syndrome.

Etiology.   Marfan syndrome is inherited in an autosomal dominant manner and is caused by mutations in the fibrillin gene (20). Like many inherited genetic disorders, almost a third of cases are sporadic due to a new mutation at embryogenesis. The expression of the mutant gene product inactivates the function of the normal gene product, an effect that is termed *dominant negative*. As such, this condition could potentially be treated by the use of therapies that decrease the expression of the mutant gene (21). The fibrillin protein plays a role in maintaining the normal mechanical properties of the soft tissues, especially in resistance to cyclic stress (22). The clinical findings of laxity and subluxation of the joints, and weakening of arterial walls with resultant aortic dilatation, are easy to understand on the basis of the function of fibrillin. The tall stature and arachnodactyly associated with the syndrome are seemingly difficult to attribute to the fibrillin mutation. However, the extracellular matrix also contains growth factors, which are bound to extracellular matrix proteins. Fibrillin mutations cause some of these extracellular growth factors, such as transforming growth factor β, to become more readily accessible to cell receptors (23). The increased growth factor availability likely causes increased cellular growth and rapid longitudinal bone growth; resulting in long, thin fingers and toes and tall stature. This raises the possibility that growth factor activity modulation could be used to treat some of the sequelae of Marfan syndrome (23).

TABLE 8-1   Diagnostic Criteria for Marfan Syndrome: A Comparison of the Berlin and Ghent Diagnostic Criteria

Berlin

If the patient has an affected first-degree relative, at least two systems of any class must be involved. In the absence of an affected first-degree relative, involvement of the skeleton as well as one major system and two minor systems are required.

Major Involvement

Ocular system
Cardiovascular system
Dural ectasia

Minor Involvement

Skeletal system
Ocular system
Cardiovascular system
Pulmonary system
Skin
Central nervous system

Ghent

Diagnosis requires two major involvements and one minor involvement

Major Involvement

Family history or molecular data
Cardiovascular system
Dural ectasia
Skeletal system
Ocular system

Minor Involvement

Skeletal system
Ocular system
Cardiovascular system
Pulmonary system
Skin

Skeletal system

Presence of at least four of the following manifestations

Major Involvement

Pectus carinatum
Pectus excavatum requiring surgery
Reduced upper to lower segment ratio or arm span to height ratio >1.05
Wrist and thumb signs
Scoliosis of >20 degrees or spondylolisthesis
Reduced extension at the elbows (<170 degrees)
Medial displacement of the medial malleolus causing pes planus
Protrusio acetabula of any degree (ascertained on radiographs)

Minor Involvement

Pectus excavatum of moderate severity
Joint hypermobility
Highly arched palate with crowding of teeth
Facial appearance (dolichocephaly, malar hypoplasia, enophthalmos, retrognathia, down-slanting palpebral fissures)

Ocular System

Major Involvement

Ectopia lentis

Minor Involvement

Abnormally flat cornea (as measured by keratometry)
Increased axial length of globe (as measured by ultrasound)
Hypoplastic iris or hypoplastic ciliary muscle causing decreased miosis

Cardiovascular System

Major Involvement

Dilatation of the ascending aorta with or without aortic regurgitation and involving at least the sinuses of Valsalva

Dissection of the ascending aorta

Minor Involvement

Mitral valve prolapse with or without mitral valve regurgitation
Dilatation of the main pulmonary artery, in the absence of valvular or peripheral pulmonic stenosis or any other obvious cause, below the age of 40 yr
Calcification of the mitral annulus below the age of 40 yr
Dilatation or dissection of the descending thoracic abdominal aorta below the age of 50 yr

Pulmonary System

Major Involvement

None

Minor Involvement

Spontaneous pneumothorax
Apical blebs (ascertained by chest radiographs)

TABLE 8-1	*(continued)*		
Skin and Integument			
Major Involvement		*Minor Involvement*	
None		Striae atrophicae (stretch marks) not associated with marked weight changes, pregnancy, or repetitive stress	
		Recurrent or incision hernias	
Dura			
Major Involvement		*Minor Involvement*	
Lumbosacral dural ectasia by CT scan or MRI		None	
Family/Genetic History			
Major Involvement		*Minor Involvement*	
Having a parent, child, or sibling who meets these diagnostic criteria independently		None	
Presence of a mutation in *FBN1* known to cause the Marfan syndrome			
Presence of a haplotype around *FBN1*, inherited by descent, known to be associated with unequivocally diagnosed Marfan syndrome in the family			

CT, computed tomography; MRI, magnetic resonance imaging.

Although molecular diagnosis for a mutation in the fibrillin gene is available, this is usually not required in making the diagnosis, as physical findings and information from radiographic studies are generally sufficient for this purpose.

Orthopaedic Manifestations and Their Management.
Hyperlaxity is responsible for many of the clinical problems in Marfan syndrome, including subluxation of joints, a predisposition to sprains, and scoliosis. Scoliosis is a common reason for which patients are referred to the orthopaedist. Smaller curves can be managed in a manner similar to that for idiopathic scoliosis, with bracing considered for select curves in skeletally immature individuals. Although bracing is often prescribed, it seems to be less effective than in idiopathic scoliosis (24). This has led some to suggest that bracing only delays the need for surgical treatment. There are no well-controlled studies comparing brace treatment with observation or any other type of management in

these patients. Although the efficacy of brace treatment remains controversial, we offer brace treatment using the same principles as for idiopathic scoliosis. Curves will often be relatively short and associated with deformity of vertebrae termed *dysplastic* (Fig. 8-3). The spinal deformity is often associated with kyphosis, especially in the lumbar spine region. Surgery is considered for rapidly progressive curves in skeletally immature individuals, or for large curves in skeletally mature individuals. Patients with Marfan syndrome have higher complication rates when undergoing scoliosis surgery than in idiopathic scoliosis. Infection, instrumentation fixation failure, pseudarthrosis, or coronal and sagittal curve decompensation occur in 10% to 20% of patients. Infection is often associated with a dural tear. Perioperative death from valvular insufficiency has been reported. To avoid such complications, the cardiopulmonary condition of patients with Marfan syndrome should be evaluated preoperatively (25–32). Overcorrection can also cause cardiovascular complications, and

FIGURE 8-2. Hands showing arachnodactyly. Notice the long, thin metacarpals and phalanges.

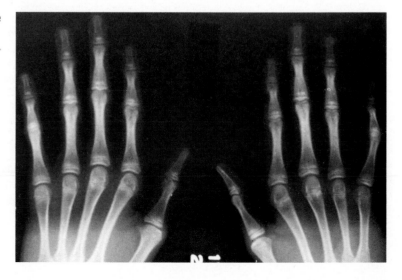

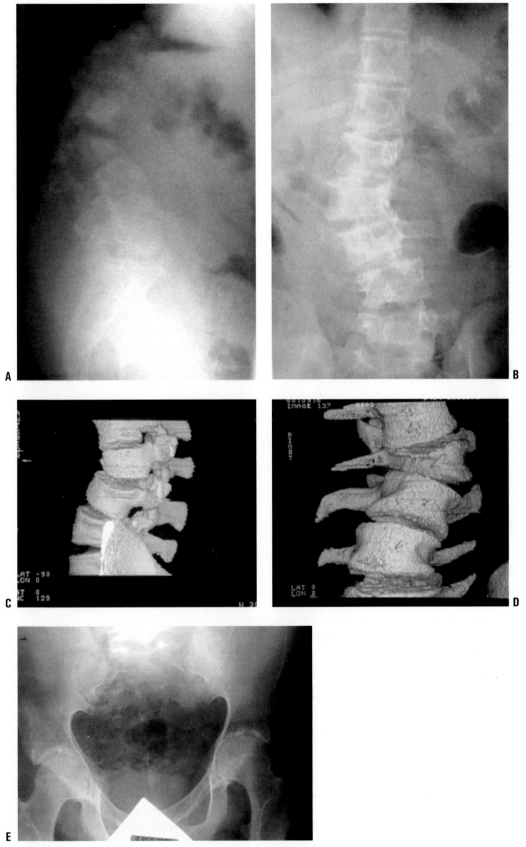

FIGURE 8-3.   Scoliosis **(A,B)** and protrusia of the hips **(E)** in a patient with Marfan syndrome. **C, D:** Deformity of the apical vertebrae is shown in a three-dimensional reconstruction of a computerized tomographic scan image. (Courtesy of Chris Reily, MD, Vancouver, British Columbia, Canada.)

reducing the amount of correction in a patient treated with a growing rod was shown in a case report to reverse cardiac failure (33). Computerized tomography (CT) scan to assess bony anatomy, especially of the pedicles, is quite useful in preoperative planning of hook and screw placement. Other unusual spinal deformities can occur, such as subluxation of vertebrae (25, 34). Traction should be used with caution, especially in cases with underlying kyphosis, as it can worsen and cause subluxation (26).

Dural ectasia is common in individuals with Marfan syndrome and seems to increase in severity with age. Its severity is not related to the severity of other clinical findings; for instance, there is no association between aortic dilatation and dural ectasia (27). Although there is a slightly higher incidence of back pain in patients with dural ectasia than in those without, a 40% incidence of back pain in patients with Marfan syndrome without dural ectasia suggests that dural ectasia itself is not the cause of the pain. One should thus evaluate patients with Marfan syndrome for other causes of back pain even in the presence of dural ectasia.

Mild osteopenia is associated with Marfan syndrome; this may be caused in part by the fibrillin abnormality disrupting the normal extracellular matrix structure of bone, and in some cases it may be related to relative physical inactivity. Susceptibility to fracture does not seem to be a problem, and it is therefore not clear whether intervention for the decreased bone density is warranted (28, 29). Protrusio acetabula is present in about one-third of patients with Marfan syndrome. The radiographic diagnosis can be difficult as there is a deformity of the inner aspect of the pelvis that can distort the normal pelvic landmarks. Protrusion is not related to bone mineral density and is usually asymptomatic (30). Although prophylactic fusion of the triradiate cartilage is reported, for these reasons it is not warranted in the majority of cases.

Nonorthopaedic Manifestations. Cardiovascular failure can lead to premature death in patients with Marfan syndrome. Indeed, many cases of sudden death during athletic activities in the young are in individuals with Marfan syndrome. Despite this, there are no universally accepted criteria for restricting physical activity in individuals with Marfan syndrome. Early intervention using β-blockers can reduce the development of aortic dilatation. New treatments based on reversing the changes associated with the identified mutation are under investigation and will likely change the course for patients with Marfan syndrome. For instance, the antihypertensive agent, Losartan, has also been found to down-regulate the expression of transforming growth factor beta; animal studies as well as small clinical series suggest that its use can slow the progression of the cardiovascular side effects of this condition (23). However, larger scale clinical trials are required before routine use is recommended. Individuals with aortic dilation may also benefit from earlier cardiac surgical intervention. Lens dislocation requires ophthalmologic intervention. In Marfan syndrome the lens is dislocated in a superior direction, whereas in homocystinuria there is an inferior dislocation.

Homocystinuria shares many clinical features with Marfan syndrome but is also associated with a coagulation disorder. As such, it is crucial that an individual suspected of having Marfan syndrome be evaluated for cardiovascular problems, and that the possibility of homocystinuria be excluded before the patient undergoes surgery.

Homocystinuria. It is important for the orthopaedist to be able to distinguish patients with homocystinuria from those with Marfan syndrome, as patients with homocystinuria often present to the orthopaedists with a clinical picture suggesting Marfan syndrome. Unlike Marfan syndrome, homocystinuria is associated with a coagulopathy, which can be fatal if unrecognized, especially during surgery. Although homocystinuria is not caused by a mutation in a gene encoding a structural protein, it shares phenotypic similarities with Marfan syndrome, and it is therefore being discussed here. It is caused by a defect in one of the enzymes that is important in the production of cysteine from methionine, thereby resulting in the accumulation of intermediate metabolites in the blood (homocysteine and homocystine) and in the urine (homocystine) (31, 32). There are several subtypes, and patients with type I have a phenotype similar to that of Marfan syndrome (35). Affected individuals are tall with long limbs and may have arachnodactyly and scoliosis. Dislocation of the lens of the eye is common but in contrast to Marfan syndrome the displacement is inferior. Osteoporosis is often more severe in type I homocystinuria than in Marfan syndrome. Vertebral osteoporosis can produce biconcavity and flattening of vertebral bodies, whereas in Marfan syndrome the vertebral bodies are either normal or excessively long. Widening of the epiphyses and metaphyses of long bones is more typically seen in homocystinuria. Mental retardation is not a feature of Marfan syndrome, but occurs in approximately half of all patients with homocystinuria (36). Patients with type I homocystinuria have an abnormality in clotting, which leads to venous and arterial thromboembolic episodes (37). Such episodes can complicate surgery, and as such a hematology consultation should be considered when planning surgery.

Type I homocystinuria is caused by a deficiency of cystathionine synthetase, which normally catalyzes the chemical union of homocysteine and serine to form cystathionine. The enzyme uses pyridoxine (vitamin B_6) as a cofactor. Blood levels of methionine are increased, and thus screening of patients with Marfan syndrome for homocystine in the urine (with the cyanide nitroprusside test) can differentiate type I homocystinuria from Marfan syndrome. Type II and III homocystinuria are biochemically distinct. Because the errors cause blocks at other points, blood levels of methionine are normal, and other clinical findings such as skeletal changes and thromboses are absent.

The treatment for homocystinuria depends on the type. In type I, the typical course is methionine restriction and pyridoxine supplementation (37). For types II and III, methionine restriction is harmful. Treatment with cofactors also varies for these other types. Vitamin B_{12} is suggested in the management of type II, and folic acid for type III.

Ehlers-Danlos Syndrome. Ehlers-Danlos syndrome (EDS) is a collection of different disorders that are associated with the common phenotypic findings of hyperextensibility of the skin and hypermobility of the joints. Easy bruisability of soft tissue, fragility of bone, calcification of soft tissues, and various degrees of osteopenia are associated with the various subtypes. The hyperlaxity allows affected individuals to have impressively large ranges of motion of the joints. Contortionists are often individuals with this syndrome. Although Tschernogobow first described the syndrome in 1892, the condition derives its name from reports by Edward Ehlers, a Danish dermatologist, in 1901, and Henri-Alexandre Danlos, a French physician, in 1908. These two individuals combined the pertinent features of the condition to provide a detailed description of the phenotype (38).

The main features of classic EDS are loose-jointedness and fragile, bruisable skin that heals with peculiar "cigarette-paper" scars and may show changes resulting from multiple bruises (Fig. 8-4). Children with this condition may be born prematurely because of premature rupture of fetal membranes, because these membranes are derived from the fetus itself. The fragile soft tissues can also cause problems such as "spontaneous" carotid-cavernous fistula, ruptures of large vessels, hiatus hernia, spontaneous rupture of the bowel, diverticula of the bowel, rupture of the colon, aortic dilatation, and retinal detachments (39–43).

Classification and Etiology. The tradition classification of EDS into 11 types (44) has been modified in a way that groups individuals with this disorder into 6 major types (45), based on clinical findings, genetic cause, and inheritance pattern (45) (Table 8-2). There additional subtypes of EDS, but these are very rare, often being reported as a single family. Although an understanding of the genetic cause of the rare types provides important information about how various proteins contribute to the maintenance of the mechanical integrity of the soft tissues, the infrequency of their occurrence makes their incorporation into a general classification scheme less useful to the clinician.

EDS is caused by mutations in either a collagen gene or in a gene that produces a protein that processes collagen. The types of EDS that are caused by a mutation in collagen are inherited in an autosomal dominant manner, whereas those caused by a protein processing defect (kyphoscoliotic and dermatosparaxis types) are inherited in an autosomal recessive pattern. Since collagen is the main structural component of a variety of connective tissues, it is easy to understand how these mutations cause the associated changes in soft-tissue mechanics (38, 46, 47).

There are several characteristics that are unique to the individual subtypes (48–50). The hypermobility type, which is characterized by multiple dislocations of joints, is also associated with a delay in achieving developmental milestones, perhaps because of the dislocations. Individuals with this type have the greatest functional disability. The vascular type is associated with ruptures of vessels or viscera. Such events are rare in childhood, but by the age of 20, one-fourth of those with the condition will have had some vascular or visceral complication. Teenage boys may be at a higher risk for this during their prepubertal growth spurt (51). Early death occurs, most commonly because of vascular rupture, with the median age of survival being <50 years. Individuals with the kyphoscoliosis type often present as "floppy" infants, and this diagnosis should therefore be considered in such children. Although molecular diagnosis is possible for some of the subtypes, these are usually not needed for making the diagnosis, and referral to clinical geneticists is usually sufficient to confirm a diagnosis. There are no universally accepted criteria for restricting participation in physical activity in patients with EDS, so recommendations to limit activity should be made on an individual basis.

Orthopaedic Manifestations and Management. Subluxations and recurrent dislocations of joints are common occurrences in the various subtypes. The chronic pain that such individuals complain of is often attributed to these subluxations. The management of the subluxations is problematic, and a multidisciplinary effort, including pharmacologic and

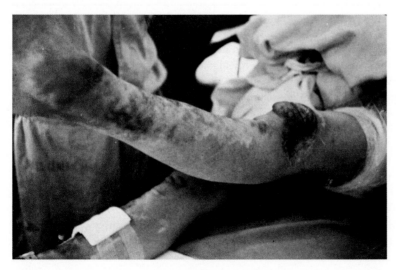

FIGURE 8-4. Patient with Ehlers-Danlos syndrome, type I. The knees and the pretibial regions have been subjected to recurrent injury and have accumulated heme pigmentation. (Courtesy of Michael G. Ehrlich, MD, Providence, Rhode Island.)

TABLE 8-2 **A Modified Classification Scheme for Ehlers-Danlos Syndrome**

New	Former	Major Clinical Findings	Minor Clinical Findings	Genetic Etiology
Classic	Type I	Skin hyperextensibility	Smooth skin (velvety)	*COL5A1* mutations
	Type II	Wide scars	Complications of joint hypermobility	
		Joint hyperlaxity	Easy bruisability	
			Tissue fragility and extensibility resulting in hiatal hernia, anal prolapse, or cervical insufficiency	
			Family history	
Hypermobility	Type III	Skin hyperextensibility	Recurrent joint dislocations	Unknown
		Smooth velvety skin	Chronic joint dislocations	
		Generalized joint hypermobility	Family history	
Vascular	Type IV	Thin, translucent skin	Hypermobility of small joints	*COL3A1* tenascin-XB
		Arterial, intestinal, or uterine rupture or fragility	Tendon or muscle rupture	
			Clubfoot	
			Varicose veins	
		Excessive bleeding	Arteriovenous or carotid-cavernous fistulas	
			Pneumothorax	
			Hemothorax	
			Family history	
			History of sudden death in family	
Kyphoscoliosis	Type VI	Generalized joint laxity	Tissue fragility	Lyslhydroxlyase deficiency
		Hypotonia at birth	Easy bruisability	
		Progressive infantile scoliosis	Arterial rupture	
			Marfanoid habitus	
		Scleral fragility	Microcornea	
		Rupture of the ocular globe	Osteopenia	
			Family history	
Arthrochalasia	Type VIIA	Severe generalized hypermobility	Skin hyperextensibility	*COL1A1* or *COL1A2* mutations
			Tissue fragility	
	Type VIIB	Congenital hip dislocation	Easy bruisability	
			Muscle hypotonia	
			Kyphoscoliosis	
			Osteopenia	
Dermatosparaxis	Type VIIC	Severe skin fragility	Soft doughy skin texture	Procollagen 1
		Sagging, redundant skin	Easy bruising	*N*-terminal peptodase
			Premature fetal membrane rupture	
			Hernias	

physical therapeutic approaches, is often required. As opposed to individuals with normal joint laxity, patients with this condition have patellar instability in multiple planes (39). Since the matrix components that provide the mechanical properties to the soft tissues are defective, surgical approaches focusing on ligaments and tendons (e.g., soft-tissue procedures around the shoulder) have a low success rate. A variety of such operations are reported, such as osteotomies, which change the direction and location of insertion of tendons or osteotomies or that provide a larger joint area (tibial tubercle transfer operations for patellar dislocations, and femoral and pelvic osteotomies for hip subluxation). Procedures that involve surgery to the bones have a higher success rate than operations on ligaments or tendons. In particularly problematic cases, it may be necessary to place a bone graft to limit motion and prevent dislocation (e.g., a posteriorly placed graft at the elbow). Arthrodesis may be required as a last resort in those cases that remain symptomatic despite other managements (52–54).

Scoliosis is common in EDS, and is usually managed using the same principles as those for idiopathic scoliosis, although there is a lack of studies investigating the implications of scoliosis in this population and the efficacy of this management approach. Surgical management can be problematic in the vascular type, as there are a number of complications, and vessel ruptures can occur during surgery (41, 55). It is important not to place undue stretch on vessels during surgery, and it is probably safest to have a vascular surgeon available in case a major disruption is encountered. Spondylolisthesis can occur, and it may be present at multiple levels, including nonadjacent sites (42). Valve problems can occur in EDS, so patients should have a cardiac evaluation before undergoing surgery. Low bone density is identified in EDS; however, when one corrects for the activity level of these patients, the bone density may not be so abnormal (56). Pharmacologic treatment for low bone density should be considered only in rare instances.

OVERGROWTH SYNDROMES AND CONDITIONS CAUSED BY TUMOR-RELATED GENES

There are a variety of cellular proteins and signaling pathways that are important in regulating cell reproduction or proliferation. A mutation that results in dysregulation of such pathways can increase cell proliferation, resulting in overgrowth of a cell type or an organ. Such pathways are frequently dysregulated in neoplasia. In some inherited conditions, when a single copy (one allele) of a gene that is important in regulating cell proliferation is mutated in the germ line, the result is an overgrowth phenotype, but when the second copy becomes mutated in a somatic manner (in a certain cell type), the result is the development of a tumor. Since these disorders are usually caused by one copy of the defective gene, they tend to be inherited in an autosomal dominant manner. The type of tissue or organ involved depends on the cell type in which the gene is expressed. In many syndromes, such as NF, the tissues of the musculoskeletal system are affected, resulting in obvious bone or soft-tissue abnormality. There is a risk of malignant progression, which develops over time as the cells are subjected to genetic damage (second hit), causing the loss of the normal copy of the causative gene. Recurrence of a deformity after surgery is not unusual, because the underlying genetic defect that causes abnormal cell growth cannot be corrected by any surgical procedure. Many children present with limb-length discrepancy, but most of these conditions will not be related to a syndrome and can be managed as described in Chapter 28 on limb-length inequality. It is important to understand the various associated syndromes so that appropriate referrals can be made for nonorthopaedic problems.

Neurofibromatosis. There are several forms of NF, the most common of which are type I and type II (NF1 and NF2). Orthopaedic manifestations are common in NF1, which is also called *von Recklinghausen disease*, whereas they are rare in NF2, which is also called *central neurofibromatosis* or *familial acoustic neuroma*. The clinical findings in NF1 are quite variable, and many of these findings develop over time. Children may exhibit none of the typical findings at birth, but the diagnosis can be made as they grow older and develop the characteristics necessary to confirm a diagnosis of NF1 (48, 57). Although a causative gene for NF1 has been identified, this diagnosis is made by identifying at least two of the clinical findings in Table 8-3.

TABLE 8-3	Neurofibromatosis Type I: Diagnostic Criteria

At least two of the following are necessary for establishing the diagnosis of NF1:

- At least six café-au-lait spots, larger than 5 mm in diameter in children, and larger than 15 mm in adults
- Two neurofibromas, or a single plexiform neurofibroma
- Freckling in the axillae or inguinal region
- An optic glioma
- At least two Lisch nodules (hamartoma of the iris)
- A distinctive osseous lesion, such as vertebral scalloping or cortical thinning
- A first-degree relative with NF1

Cutaneous Markings.   Café-au-lait spots are discrete, tan spots (Fig. 8-5). In patients with NF, these spots often appear after 1 year of age, and then they steadily increase in number and size. The spots have a smooth edge, often described as similar to the coast of California, as opposed to the ragged edge of spots associated with fibrous dysplasia, which are described as

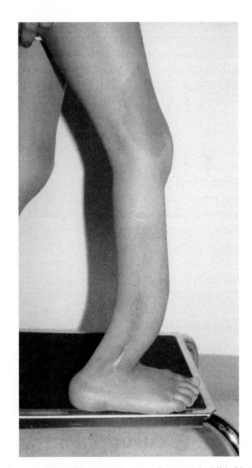

FIGURE 8-5.   Neurofibromatosis in a 6-year-old child. Notice the large café-au-lait spot on the thigh and the anterior bowed tibia typical of pseudarthrosis. (From Goldberg MJ. *The dysmorphic child: an orthopedic perspective.* New York, NY: Raven Press, 1987, with permission.)

FIGURE 8-6. Neurofibromatosis in a 14-year-old patient. Cutaneous neurofibromas make their appearance with the onset of puberty. (From Goldberg MJ. *The dysmorphic child: an orthopedic perspective.* New York, NY: Raven Press, 1987, with permission.)

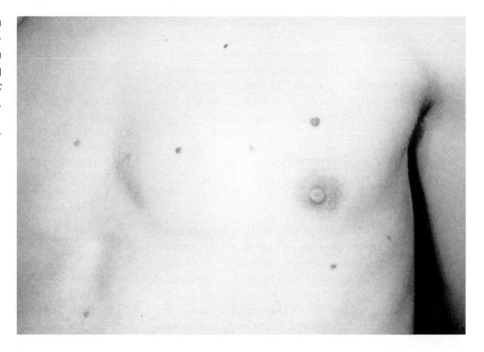

similar to the coast of Maine. The spots vary greatly in number, shape, and size, and six lesions >1 cm in size are required for the diagnostic criteria. Axillary and inguinal freckling are common and serve as good diagnostic markers, because such freckling is exceptionally rare except in people with NF. Hyperpigmented nevi are dark brown areas that are sensitive to the touch; they typically overlie a deeper plexiform neurofibroma.

Neurofibroma. The two types of neurofibroma are different in their anatomic configuration and clinical morbidity. The most common is the cutaneous neurofibroma, composed of benign Schwann cells and fibrous connective tissue (Fig. 8-6). This type of neurofibroma may occur anywhere, but is usually just below the skin. These neurofibromas may not be detectable until 10 years of age, and with puberty there is a rapid increase in their number. When many are grouped together on the skin, it is known as a *fibroma molluscum.* Plexiform neurofibromas are usually present at birth and are highly infiltrative in the surrounding tissues. The overlying skin is often darkly pigmented. They are highly vascular and lead to limb gigantism, facial disfigurement, and invasion of the neuroaxis (Figs. 8-7 and 8-8).

Osseous Lesions. There are many skeletal manifestations, but the presence of an unusual scoliosis, overgrowth of a part, or a congenital pseudarthrosis lesion seen on radiographs should alert the physician to consider a diagnosis of NF (58). There are a variety of anomalies of bone observed in radiographic images, ranging from a scalloping of the cortex, to cystic lesions in long bones that look much like nonossifying fibromas, to permeative bone destruction (Fig. 8-9). These radiographic findings may mimic benign or malignant bone lesions (49, 50, 59). Radiographs of the pelvis usually show various degrees of coxa valga, and in nearly 20% of patients there is radiographic evidence of protrusio acetabuli (52, 60).

Lisch Nodules. Lisch nodules are hamartomas of the iris. These nodules are present in 50% of all 5-year-olds with NF1, and in all adults with NF1. It is unusual for Lisch nodules to be present in individuals who do not have NF1, so the detection of these nodules can aid in making this diagnosis. However, it may be difficult to detect these lesions, and patients should be sent to an experienced ophthalmologist for this diagnosis. The lesions do not cause any visual disturbances. Once the

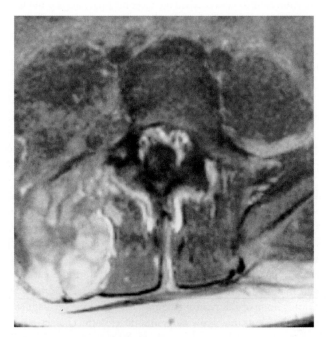

FIGURE 8-7. Neurofibromatosis in a 16-year-old patient. The MRI at the level of L4–L5 demonstrates a large plexiform neurofibroma that invades the neural axis. It extends from the level of L3 to the sacrum.

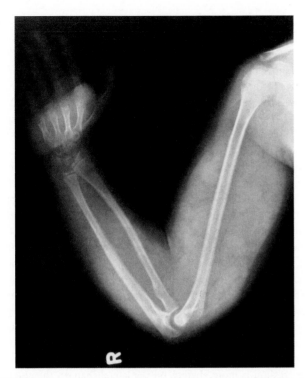

FIGURE 8-8.   Neurofibromatosis in a 10-year-old patient. Hypertrophy affects the arm from the shoulder to the fingertips; the major component is soft tissue. Nodular densities throughout the upper arm are consistent with a plexiform neurofibroma. Notice the lack of skeletal overgrowth and some attenuation of the radius and ulna, caused by external compression by the neurofibroma. (From Goldberg MJ. *The dysmorphic child: an orthopedic perspective.* New York, NY: Raven Press, 1987, with permission.)

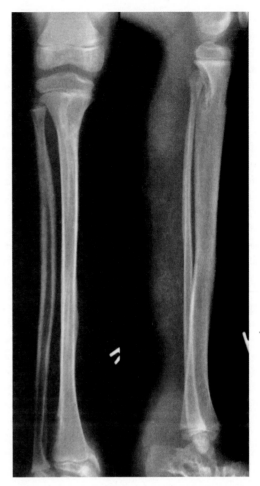

FIGURE 8-9.   Neurofibromatosis in a 10-year-old patient. The radiograph shows an array of cystic and scalloped skeletal lesions in the tibia and os calcis of the right leg. Some of the lesions are characteristic of neurofibromatosis. Other lesions, occurring in isolation, can mimic benign fibrous tumors. Scalloped cortical erosion at the upper end of the femur, permeative bone destruction in the region of the os calcis, and metaphyseal cystic lesions are other features. (From Goldberg MJ. *The dysmorphic child: an orthopedic perspective.* New York, NY: Raven Press, 1987, with permission.)

diagnosis is established, further ophthalmologic evaluation is not necessary (53, 54).

Etiology.   NF is the most common single-gene disorder in humans, affecting 1 in 3000 newborns (61–63). NF1 is an autosomal dominant disorder with 100% penetrance, but one-half of cases are sporadic mutations and are associated with an older-than-average paternal age. The most well-known patient who was presumed to have had NF, Joseph Merrick, also called the *Elephant Man*, probably did not have this condition; his clinical profile better fits Proteus syndrome (64). The *NF1* gene is located on chromosome 17 (65). Its protein product, *neurofibromin*, acts as a tumor suppressor (66). There are also other potential genes located in introns within the *NF1* gene, whose functional significance is unclear.

Neurofibromin plays a role stimulating the conversion of Ras-GTP to Ras-GDP, and as such modulates activation of the Ras signaling system, which is involved in the control of cell growth (67). Mutations in the *NF1* gene cause a disruption in its normal regulatory control of Ras signaling, giving affected cells an abnormal growth pattern. Neurofibromin is expressed at higher levels in the neural crest during development. Cells from the neural crest migrate to become pigmented cells of the skin,

parts of the brain, spinal cord, peripheral nerves, and adrenals, thus explaining the common sites of abnormalities in the disorder. Disruption of the normal Ras signaling cascade is probably responsible for the malignant potential of this disorder. Only one of the two copies of the *NF1* gene is mutated in affected patients; however, tumors from such individuals have been found to have only the mutated gene because of loss of the normal copy (68–71). The gene defect also gives a clue to potential novel therapies, because pharmacologic agents that block Ras signaling could be used to treat the disorder. Farnesyl transferase inhibitors block the downstream effects of Ras signaling activation and thus have the potential to be used in the treatment of some of the neoplastic manifestations of NF (72, 73). Another therapeutic approach is the use of statin inhibitors, such as lovastatin, which is thought to regulate Ras signaling by the membrane binding of Ras (52, 53).

Other Types of Neurofibromatosis. Although patients with other forms of NF rarely present to an orthopaedist, one should be aware of these types because musculoskeletal malformations are occasionally present. Patients with NF2 present with acoustic neuromas, central nervous system tumors, and rare peripheral manifestations. There are usually fewer than six café-au-lait spots, and no peripheral neurofibromata. These patients are very unlikely to present with an orthopaedic deformity. There are two much less common types of NF, type 3 and type 4 (NF3 and NF4), in which patients are more likely to develop a problem requiring orthopaedic intervention. Individuals with NF3 present with some of the characteristics of NF1 but also have acoustic neuromas, which are characteristic of NF2. These individuals often have spinal deformity, especially in the cervical region. NF4 presents with the same clinical findings as NF1, except that one of the cardinal features of NF1, namely, Lisch nodules of the iris, is absent (48, 57).

Orthopaedic Manifestations. The orthopaedic manifestations of NF include scoliosis, overgrowth of the limbs, pseudarthrosis, and specific radiographic appearances of bone lesions. Patients with NF often exhibit overgrowth, ranging from a single digit to an entire limb and from mild anisomelia to massive gigantism. As such, the possibility of NF should be considered in a child with focal gigantism, such as macrodactyly. When NF is compared with the more symmetric idiopathic hemihypertrophy, there is disproportional overgrowth involving the skin and the subcutaneous tissue more than the bone (Fig. 8-8)

Scoliosis is common, and curves fall into two categories: a dystrophic curve and an idiopathic curve. Most curves in NF resemble idiopathic scoliosis curves and can be managed like any other idiopathic curve.

The dystrophic scoliotic curve is a short, sharp, single thoracic curve typically involving four to six segments (Fig. 8-10) (60, 74–81). It is associated with deformity of the ribs and vertebrae. The onset is early in childhood, and it is relentlessly progressive. Curves that initially appear to be idiopathic in children under age 7 have almost a 70% chance of becoming dystrophic over time, although there may be subtle clues, for example, mild rib penciling (thinning of the ribs in a shape similar to a pencil point near the vertebrae), suggesting that the curve is actually dystrophic. The most important risk factors for progression are an early age of onset, a high Cobb angle, and an apical vertebra that is severely rotated, scalloped (concave loss of bone), and located in the middle-to-lower thoracic area (78). The combination of curve progression and vertebral malformation mimics congenital scoliosis in appearance and behavior. Dystrophic curves are refractive to brace treatment. Sagittal plane deformities may occur, including an angular kyphosis (i.e., gibbus) and a scoliosis that has so much rotation that curve progression is more obvious on the lateral than on the anteroposterior radiograph (78). In those with angular kyphosis, there is a risk of paraplegia. Dystrophic curves are difficult to stabilize, and it is best to intervene with early surgery involving both anterior and posterior fusion (78, 82–84). Kyphotic deformities are often the most difficult to manage surgically, and strut grafts across the kyphosis anteriorly may be necessary. In rare

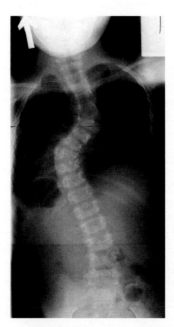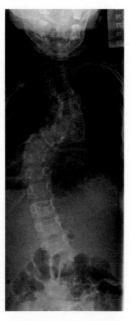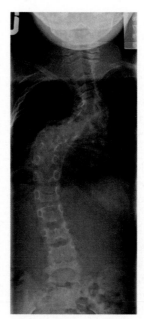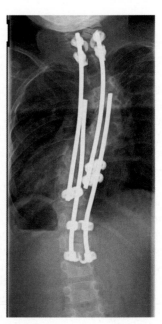

FIGURE 8-10. Neurofibromatosis in a 5-year-old patient. A dystrophic curve is shown in the **left panel**. There is a short-segment scoliosis, with ribboned ribs show cystic irregularities. There was a delay in the recommendation for surgery, and the middle two panels show the rapid progression in the dystrophic curve over the next 12 months. The right panel shows the curve after undergoing surgery including anterior and posterior fusions of the dystrophic segments.

severe cases, the spine can even seem to be "dislocated" because of the kyphosis and scoliosis. In cases with extremely severe deformity, halofemoral or halogravity traction may be necessary to safely straighten the spine to a more acceptable deformity without producing neurologic sequelae. Other reported techniques include inserting a bone graft without instrumentation and then gradually straightening the curve using a cast postoperatively (85). In rare severe cases in which there is a vertebral "dislocation," one can use instrumentation to achieve an overall alignment of the back, while leaving the vertebrae "dislocated" (86). Unusual complications have been reported in the management of such dystrophic curves, such as a rib head migrating into the neural canal resulting in spinal cord compromise (87).

There can be several vertebral abnormalities evident on radiographs. These include scalloping of the posterior body, enlargement of the neural foramina, and defective pedicles, occasionally with a completely dislocated vertebral body (88–92). Such findings may mean that there is a dumbbell-shaped neurofibroma in the spinal canal, extending out through a neural foramina. The dura in NF patients behaves like the dura in patients with a connective tissue disorder, and dural ectasia is common, with pseudomeningoceles protruding through the neural foramina. Unlike neurofibroma, dural ectasia is an outpouching of the dura, without an underlying tumor or overgrowth of spinal elements (Fig. 8-11) (93–96). The incidence of anterolateral meningoceles was underestimated until asymptomatic patients were screened with MRI (58, 97). The erosion of the pedicles may lead to spinal instability, especially in the cervical spine. In rare cases, this can even lead to dislocation of the spine (98, 99). MRI and CT scans are helpful preoperatively in delineating the presence of defective vertebrae or dural abnormalities, and may assist in choosing the levels on which to place instrumentation.

Pseudarthrosis of a long bone is typically associated with NF (76). It usually affects the tibia, with a characteristic antero-

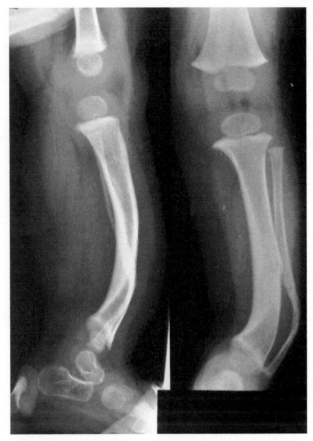

FIGURE 8-12. Neurofibromatosis in a 1-year-old patient. The anterolateral bow of the tibia and the fibula warrant concern about impending fracture and pseudarthrosis. (From Goldberg MJ. *The dysmorphic child: an orthopedic perspective.* New York, NY: Raven Press, 1987, with permission.)

lateral bow that is obvious in infancy (Fig. 8-12) (100, 101). Fracture usually follows, with spontaneous union being rare and surgical union presenting a challenge. An anterolateral bowed tibia is routinely managed with a total-contact orthosis to prevent fracture, although there are no well-designed studies showing that this is indeed effective. Intramedullary rod fixation seems to offer the best results for the initial management of a pseudarthrosis. Recent studies have shown the importance of achieving neutral tibial alignment in the healing of a tibial pseudarthrosis. The presence of an intact fibula is associated with a lower healing rate, perhaps because of associated tibial malalignment (102). There is a hamartoma of undifferentiated mesenchymal cells at the pseudarthrosis site (75), and in some cases, this is associated with loss of the normal allele of the NF1 gene (76). Neurofibromas have not been identified at the pseudarthrosis site. The pseudarthrosis process may affect the ulna, radius, femur, or clavicle (77, 103–109). In each of these locations, there is a course similar to that in the tibia, with bone loss and difficulty in achieving union (Fig. 8-13). Not all pseudarthroses of the forearm require treatment (110), but if they are symptomatic, the available options include proximal

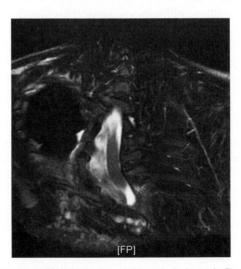

FIGURE 8-11. MRI of the spine of the patient shown in Figure 8-10, showing dural ectasia.

FIGURE 8-13. Neurofibromatosis in a 3-year-old patient. The radiograph shows progressive pseudarthrosis of the radius and ulna after a pathologic fracture. **A:** Fracture through the cystic lesion of the radius and thinning of the midulna. **B:** After 10 months of cast immobilization, pseudarthrosis affects the radius and ulna. (From Goldberg MJ. *The dysmorphic child: an orthopedic perspective.* New York, NY: Raven Press, 1987, with permission.)

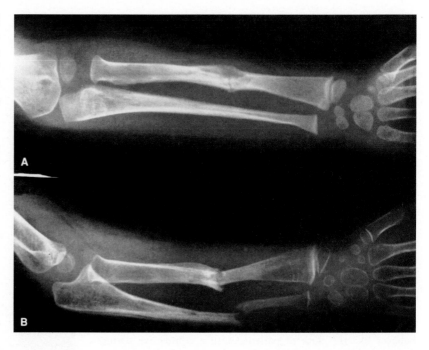

and distal synostosis to produce a single-bone forearm, the use of a vascularized fibula graft, or resection of the pseudarthrosis with shortening of the forearm and internal fixation (111). Pharmacologic approaches to the pseudarthrosis in NF are reported. A mouse model suggests the use of lovastatin, but the mouse does not develop pseudarthroses, only bowing of the bones, and as such human studies of this approach are needed (53). Direct installation of BMP to the pseudarthrosis site may help in the achievement of union, but variable results are reported, and it is not known if the use of BMP in patients with an inherited premalignant condition has long-term harmful consequences (80).

There are a variety of benign and malignant neoplastic lesions that affect individuals with NF1. Most neurofibromas do not require treatment, but symptomatic lesions may require excision. Plexiform neurofibromas that become symptomatic are very difficult to manage. Their vascularity and infiltrative nature make complete excision almost impossible, with a substantial risk of uncontrollable hemorrhage and neurologic deficit. Although speculative, the use of angiogenesis inhibitors, such as interferon, or experimental agents that modulate the effect of the causative gene mutation, such as farnesyl transferase inhibitors or statin inhibitors, may be beneficial (88, 89).

The incidence of malignancy in NF is reported at rates ranging from under 1% to over 20% (90–92, 112, 113). The most common tumor location is in the central nervous system, with lesions such as optic nerve glioma, acoustic neuroma, and astrocytoma (114). There is a risk of malignant degeneration of a neurofibroma to a neurofibrosarcoma. This process can occur in a central or peripheral neurofibroma (115–118). It can be quite difficult to distinguish a malignant lesion from a benign one. CT scans show areas of low-enhancing density in neurofibrosarcomas (119), but

there are no studies confirming the sensitivity and specificity of this finding. Similar patterns can also be visualized using MRI. Routine surveillance for sarcomatous change is impossible because of the large number of neurofibromas. Lesions that increase in size or develop new characteristics should be investigated. There is a propensity for children with neurofibroma to develop other malignancies, such as Wilms tumors or rhabdomyosarcomas.

Hypertension as a result of renal artery stenosis or pheochromocytoma is reported regularly, as is a curious type of metabolic bone disease similar to hypophosphatemic osteomalacia (120, 121). Hypertension is a major risk factor for early death (113). Precocious puberty may occur because of an intracranial lesion (103). Affected children are short, but tend to have large heads. Approximately 50% have an intellectual handicap. Although the mean IQ is low, the range of IQ is quite wide (104). More than the low IQ, it is the difficulty in concentrating (which is common in this condition) that may interfere with the learning process (105). Although it was hoped that lovastatin might help with concentration problems, a recent randomized trial suggests that this is not the case (106).

Beckwith-Wiedemann Syndrome. Beckwith-Wiedemann syndrome is a triad of organomegaly, omphalocele, and a large tongue (107). The incidence is 1 in 14,000, and it is probably an autosomal dominant trait of variable expression. Patients are large, although this feature is not always noticed at birth (108). The child is in the 97th percentile for size by 1 year of age. The tongue is gigantic at birth, and although it tends to regress, hemiglossectomy is sometimes needed. Omphalocele is common, and 15% of the babies born with omphaloceles have Beckwith-Wiedemann syndrome. The abdominal viscera are enlarged, and a single-cell hypertrophy accounts for the large organs: in the adrenals, giant cortical cells; in the gonads, an increased number of interstitial cells; and in the pancreas, islet cell hyperplasia. This underlies the 10% risk of developing benign or malignant tumors. Wilms tumor is the most common.

Beckwith-Wiedemann syndrome is linked to chromosome 11p15, which is near the Wilms tumor gene (11p13) and the insulin-like growth factor gene (11p15.5) (109). There may be some paternal genomic imprinting (122, 123). The closeness of the Beckwith-Wiedemann gene locus and these embryonal tumor gene loci accounts for the dysregulation of the tumor-related genes and the associated overgrowth and higher incidence of tumors seen in this syndrome.

Pancreatic islet cell hyperplasia causes hypoglycemia. It is crucial that the neonatologist diagnose this syndrome early so as to prevent the consequences of hypoglycemia. If it is not managed properly, seizures occur at day 2 or 3. Central nervous system damage from the hypoglycemia leads to a cerebral palsy–like picture. The cerebral palsy–like findings confuse the diagnosis of this syndrome and make the management of these patients more complex. The diagnosis can occasionally be made prenatally by ultrasound (124, 125).

The clinical feature that makes the orthopaedist suspect the presence of this disorder is the unusual combination of two otherwise common problems: spastic cerebral palsy and hemihypertrophy (Fig. 8-14). The spasticity is thought to be a result of the neonatal hypoglycemic episodes, especially if accompanied by neonatal seizures, but spastic hemiplegia is most commonly seen. In general, children with cerebral palsy tend to be small; Beckwith-Wiedemann syndrome should be suspected if a large child has spastic cerebral palsy. Asymmetric growth affects about 20% of the patients. It is usually true hemihypertrophy, but it can be significant if the spastic hemiplegia affects the smaller side.

Children with Beckwith-Wiedemann syndrome are predisposed to a variety of neoplasms, most notably Wilms tumor. Abdominal ultrasounds at regular intervals until the age of 6, to screen for Wilms tumor, are advocated. A series comparing a screened population (ultrasounds every 4 months) with a population that was not screened showed that none of the children in the screened group presented with late-stage Wilms tumor, whereas one-half of the children who developed Wilms tumor in the nonscreened group presented with late-stage disease. This study suggests that screening every 4 months will identify early disease. However, a larger study is needed to determine whether screening improves patient survival (125, 126). Other tumors types, such as alveolar rhabdomyosarcoma, can present in a new born (100).

Scoliosis is common and usually behaves like an idiopathic spinal deformity, but there may be insignificant morphogenic variations, such as 13 ribs. It is managed in the same way as any idiopathic curve. Other orthopaedic findings include cavus feet, dislocated radial heads, and occasional cases of polydactyly (127, 128). All of these can be managed the same as in sporadic deformities.

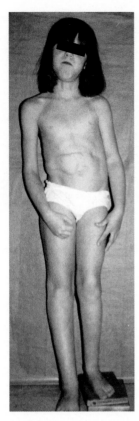

FIGURE 8-14. Beckwith-Wiedemann syndrome in an 8-year-old patient. Hemihypertrophy on the right, a part of this syndrome, is combined with hemiatrophy on the left, caused by acquired encephalopathy secondary to hypoglycemic seizures as a newborn, leading to a significant leg-length discrepancy of 4.6 cm. Abdominal scars are a consequence of omphalocele repair. (From Goldberg MJ. *The dysmorphic child: an orthopedic perspective.* New York, NY: Raven Press, 1987, with permission.)

Russell-Silver Syndrome. The patient with Russell-Silver syndrome is defined clinically as a short child with body asymmetry and a characteristic facial shape (129–131) (Fig. 8-15). The diagnostic characteristics include (i) a birth weight ≤ 2 standard deviations below the mean, (ii) poor postnatal growth ≤ 2 standard deviations from the mean at diagnosis, (iii) preservation of occipitofrontal head circumference, (iv) classic facial features, and (v) asymmetric growth (132). Poor feeding is also a common occurrence. The cause of the disorder is unclear; although some cases are associated with uniparental disomy, there is a suggestion of autosomal dominant inheritance, and there is some evidence implicating an abnormal intrauterine environment (130, 131). The associated genitourinary malformations and the variation in the pattern of sexual maturation chemically (increased gonadotropin secretion) or clinically (precocious sexual development) suggest that hypothalamic or other endocrine disturbances may contribute to the pathogenesis. Affected children are small at birth and remain below the 3rd percentile throughout growth, with a marked delay in skeletal maturation. Body asymmetry with hemihypertrophy affects 80% of them. The asymmetry

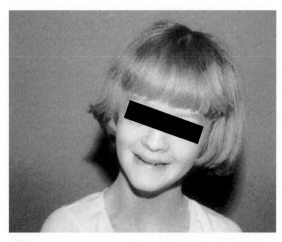

FIGURE 8-15. Russell-Silver syndrome. The triangular face is seemingly small for the size of the skull.

averages approximately 2 cm at maturity, but can be as much as 6 cm. Regardless of the magnitude of the discrepancy, it is clinically more apparent because the child is small. The face is characteristically triangular and seemingly too small for the cranial vault. There have been several reports of variations in sexual maturation pattern and malformations of the genitourinary system.

Radiologic analysis discloses a remarkable array of orthopaedic findings, but it is not clear which form part of the syndrome and which are coincidental (133–137). Scoliosis is usually idiopathic. Hand and foot abnormalities include clinodactyly, polydactyly, and hallux varus. Developmental hip dysplasia, avascular necrosis of the femoral head, and slipped capital femoral epiphysis (SCFE) may be present. Many radiographic changes, such as the minor hand abnormalities, suggest a disturbed morphogenesis.

Treatment consists of managing leg-length equality. This can be difficult because individual growth curves may vary, the skeletal age is very retarded, and puberty may be very abnormal. It is easy to miss the appropriate timing for epiphysiodesis. Growth hormone has been administered in an attempt to improve stature. Although the use of growth hormone will increase growth velocity, it is not yet known whether the ultimate height is increased (138).

Cytogenetic studies found anomalies on chromosomes 1, 7, and 17, but most patients have anomalies involving chromosome 7. However, no single causative gene has yet been identified. It is not known whether screening for Wilms tumor, as is performed in other forms of hemihypertrophy, is necessary. Despite early evidence that the insulinlike growth factor receptor, which plays a causative role in Wilms tumor, is involved in this syndrome, more comprehensive molecular genetic investigations have not found any abnormalities in this gene. However, there is a case report of Wilms tumor developing in an affected patient (139), leading some to recommend screening for Wilms tumor in these patients as one would in any other hemihypertrophy.

Proteus Syndrome. Proteus syndrome is an overgrowth condition in which there is a bizarre array of abnormalities that include hemihypertrophy, macrodactyly, and partial gigantism of the hands or feet, or both. The key to this diagnosis is worsening of existing symptoms and the appearance of new ones over time. There is a characteristic appearance to the plantar surface of the feet, often described as similar to the surface of the brain. Unlike in other overgrowth syndromes, an increased incidence of malignancy has not been reported in Proteus syndrome (140–144).

The cause of this syndrome is not known. Although there are case reports of familial occurrence, the vast majority of cases are sporadic (145–147). It is most likely due to a gene that is mutated in a mosaic manner (mutated in the affected tissues but not in the normal tissues), similar to McCune-Albright syndrome (polyostotic fibrous dysplasia). Such a mutation can occur very early in development in a single cell, which will divide to ultimately form various structures throughout the body.

The Proteus syndrome is named after the ancient Greek demigod who could change appearance and assume different shapes. The progressive nature of the deformities seen in this syndrome can lead to grotesque overgrowth, facial disfigurement, angular malformation, and severe scoliosis (148). Joseph Merrick, called the *Elephant Man*, is now believed to have had this syndrome rather than NF (149).

The signs of Proteus syndrome overlap other hamartomatous overgrowth conditions, such as idiopathic hemihypertrophy, Klippel-Trenaunay syndrome, Maffucci syndrome, and NF. However, unlike these other syndromes, the features here are more grotesque and involve multiple tissue types and sites. Proteus can be differentiated from NF1 by the lack of café-au-lait spots and Lisch nodules (150). A rating scale, which assigns points on the basis of clinical findings (macrodactyly, hemihypertrophy, thickening of the skin, lipomas, subcutaneous tumors, verrucae, epidermal nevus, and macrocephaly), may be used to assist in diagnosis (151). However, the finding of worsening overgrowth features over time is usually sufficient to make this diagnosis.

Most children who present with macrodactyly do not have it as part of Proteus syndrome. In these sporadic cases, an isolated digit is involved or, when multiple digits are involved, these are located adjacent to each other. Macrodactyly affecting nonadjacent toes or fingers or opposite extremities is almost always due to Proteus syndrome. There is a characteristic thickening and deep furrowing of the skin on the palms of the hands and soles of the feet. The array of cutaneous manifestations includes hemangiomas and pigmented nevi of various intensities, and subcutaneous lipomas (Fig. 8-16). Varicosities are present, although true arteriovenous malformations are rare. There are cranial hyperostoses and occasionally exostosis of the hands and feet.

Macrodactyly seems to correspond to overgrowth along the terminal branches of a peripheral sensory nerve. Digital involvement in the hand favors the sensory distribution of the median nerve (1). The index is the most frequently affected

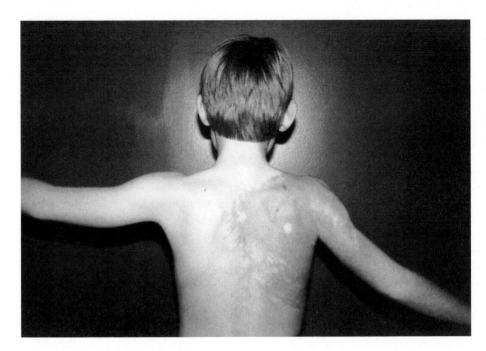

FIGURE 8-16. Proteus syndrome. Notice the cutaneous markings, large hemangioma of the shoulder, and lightly pigmented area on the back. There is some atrophy of the shoulder and arm muscles and a fixed contracture of the elbow.

finger, followed by the long finger and the thumb. It is the second toe that is most commonly macrodactylous. The regional sensory nerve is greatly increased in size, taking a tortuous route through the fatty tissue.

There is a wide range of orthopaedic deformities, including focal and regional gigantism, scoliosis, and kyphosis (152, 153). Rather large vertebral bodies, known as *megaspondylodysplasia*, are present (154). Angular malformations of the lower extremities, especially genu valgum, are common. Because the genu valgum is often associated with restricted range of motion, flexion contractures, and pain in the joints, it is postulated that an intra-articular growth disturbance contributes to the angular malformation. Hip abnormalities that show up in roentgenographic tests, acetabular dysplasia for example, are frequently discovered in asymptomatic patients. Deformities in the hindfoot are frequent and are usually heel valgus, but congenital equinovarus and "Z-foot" deformities have also been described (150, 153, 155).

Recurrences after various surgical intervention are very common. This is probably due to an underlying growth advantage in affected tissues that cannot be corrected operatively. Thus, musculoskeletal deformities caused by Proteus syndrome can be very difficult to manage. When the foot becomes difficult to fit into a shoe because of macrodactyly, it is best managed by ablation rather than debulking (156). Anisomelia is best managed with epiphysiodesis. Osteotomies can correct angular malformations, but the decision to undertake surgical correction must take into account the possibility of a rapid recurrence of the deformity after corrective surgery (152, 153). The use of growth modulation (e.g., 8-plate) to manage limb angular deformity is a rather promising approach (120), but publications on the results of this approach are lacking. In some cases, a sudden overgrowth of the operative limb has been reported. There are anecdotal reports of soft-tissue procedures

to "debulk" overgrown lesions; however, there are no series in the literature reporting results of these procedures, and our experience with them is that the results are only temporary. In rare cases, nerve or spinal cord impingement can occur. Nerve compression can be managed using decompression, but spinal cord compression is difficult, if not impossible, to successfully treat operatively (157, 158). Scoliosis can occur and seems to be caused by overgrowth of one side of the spine (159). Since mixed results are obtained from surgical treatment in this disorder, operative treatment should be reserved for individuals who have exhausted nonsurgical management. Sometimes, the operative procedures can be used as a temporizing measure, and patients may need to have repeat procedures performed throughout life.

Functional ability depends on the severity of the limb deformity and the presence of intracranial abnormalities (143, 160). The life expectancy is unknown, but many adult patients have been reported. Intubations can be difficult because of overgrowth of structures surrounding the trachea.

DEVELOPMENTALLY IMPORTANT SIGNALING PATHWAYS

During embryonic development, cell signaling systems are activated in a coordinated manner to cause cells to proliferate, move, and undergo programmed cell death, so as to allow the organism to pattern normally and develop into an adult. Normal patterning is altered by mutations in the genes that encode proteins that play roles in these pathways. Environmental events such as exposure to a teratogen can also dysregulate these same pathways, resulting in a phenotype similar to that of a gene mutation. Such events occurring in a pathway that is important for skeletal development can result in a musculoskeletal malformation. These disorders can be identified at birth, because the problem is present at the start of development. Despite this, sometimes the abnormalities do not become obvious to parents or physicians until the child is older. Because these are generally patterning problems, surgery to correct malalignment is usually quite successful. There are frequently manifestations in other organ systems, because the same developmental signaling pathways play important roles in the development of multiple organs. These disorders are not associated with an increased rate of neoplasia. Symptoms from the malformations often increase with age because the abnormally shaped structures cannot sustain the stresses of normal activity. This results in the early development of degenerative problems. These disorders are usually inherited in an autosomal dominant manner, although the inheritance pattern is more variable than in disorders caused by genes encoding for structural proteins or for proteins implicated in neoplasia.

Nail-Patella Syndrome.   Children with nail-patella syndrome have a quartet of findings that include nail dysplasia, patellar hypoplasia, elbow dysplasia, and iliac horns (161). The most prominent feature is dystrophic nails (Fig. 8-17A). The nail may be completely absent, hypoplastic, or have grooves and distortions in its surface (162). The thumb is more involved than the small finger, and the ulnar border more involved than the radial. The hands are often very symmetric, and fingernails are more involved than toenails.

The second cardinal feature is hypoplastic patellae (163). They are quite small, or may be entirely absent (Fig. 8-17B). Where present, they are unstable, and may be found in a position of fixed dislocation. The patellar abnormality highlights the total knee dysplasia, with an abnormal femoral condyle and a peculiar septum running from the patella to the intercondylar groove (septum interarticularis), dividing the knee into two compartments. Abnormalities in varus and valgus alignment occur, with valgus more common because of the small, flat lateral femoral condyle (163).

A third feature is a dislocated radial head (163, 164) (Fig. 8-17C). The elbow joint is dysplastic, with abnormalities in the lateral humeral condyle, in many ways mimicking the dysplasia of the knee. The trochlea is large and the capitellum is hypoplastic, creating an asymmetric shape that may predispose the radial head to dislocation.

The fourth and pathognomonic feature is iliac horns: bony exostoses on the posterior surface of the ilium (165) (Fig. 8-17D). They usually cannot be found on physical examination, are asymptomatic, and require no treatment.

Nail-patella syndrome is caused by a mutation in the *LMX1B* gene. This gene is a homeodomain protein, which plays a role regulating transcription in limb patterning during fetal development. Mutation in the gene will disrupt normal limb patterning and alter kidney formation, resulting in deformities in the extremities and an associated nephropathy (166).

Children with the syndrome have short stature, the height being between the 3rd and 10th percentiles. There may be a shoulder girdle dysplasia, and a variety of abnormalities of the

glenoid and the humeral head are possible. These, however, merely represent curious radiographic features and not any significant functional disability (167). There is a foot deformity that is sometimes the chief presenting complaint of children with nail-patella syndrome (163, 168). The foot deformities include variations of stiff calcaneal valgus, metatarsus adductus, and clubfeet.

There is a restricted range of motion, and contractures affect several large joints; these include knee-flexion deformities and external rotation contracture of the hip. When these contractures are severe and accompanied by stiff clubfeet, the condition may be misdiagnosed as arthrogryposis multiplex congenita. Madelung deformity, spondylolysis, and in some adults, inflammatory arthropathy may be present (161, 169, 170).

Knee disability is variable and related to the magnitude of quadriceps dysfunction and the dislocated patella. At long-term follow-up, knee pain is the main musculoskeletal complaint in patients with nail-patella syndrome (171). Small femoral condyles make it difficult to achieve patellar stability. As a rule, limited soft-tissue or capsular releases are ineffective, but combined proximal and distal patella realignments have an overall favorable outcome (163, 172). A contracted and fibrotic quadriceps may result in a knee extension contracture, and in such cases quadricepsplasty is indicated along with the patella realignment. More commonly, an associated knee-flexion deformity may require hamstring release and posterior capsulotomy, although results have been inconsistent (163). Residual deformity, which is usually related to flexion or rotation, is managed by femoral osteotomy toward the end of the first decade of life. Osteochondritis dissecans of the femoral condyle is relatively common (Fig. 8-17B). An intra-articular septum makes arthroscopic management difficult, but the septum can be removed arthroscopically.

The radial head dislocation is asymptomatic in young children, but may become symptomatic with time. In symptomatic individuals, excision of the radial head will improve symptoms arising from the prominent lateral bump, but the range of motion is rarely improved. Although traditional teaching advocates performing radial head excision after skeletal maturity, earlier excision in symptomatic children does not seem to be associated with significant problems (163). Dislocated hips (173) and clubfeet can occur, and can be managed using techniques similar to those in idiopathic cases.

The most important nonorthopaedic condition is kidney failure. The nephropathy of nail-patella syndrome causes significant morbidity, affecting the patient's longevity. There is great variability in the age at onset and severity of the nephropathy (174). All patients should be referred for a nephrology evaluation when this diagnosis is made. Patients may go on to chronic renal failure, requiring long-term nephrology management.

Goldenhar Syndrome.   The association of anomalies in the eye, ear, and vertebrae are termed *ocular–auricular–vertebral dysplasia* or *Goldenhar syndrome* (175). There is variability in the

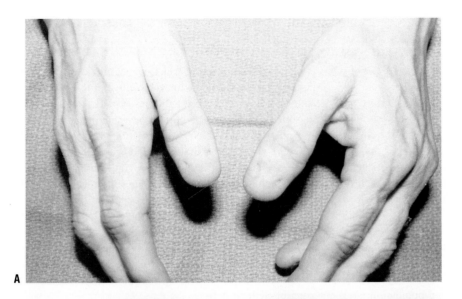

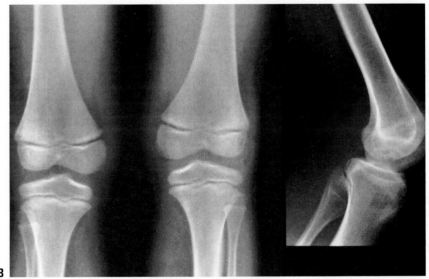

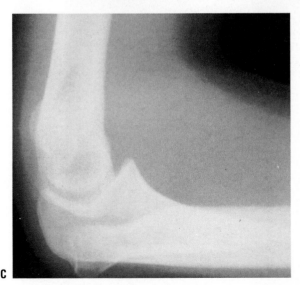

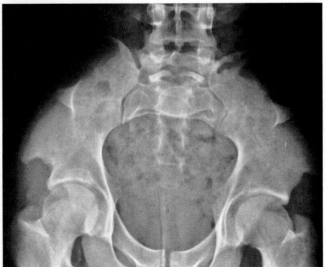

FIGURE 8-17.   Nail-patella syndrome. The classic quartet of features consists of dystrophic nails **(A)**, absent patellae (notice the region of osteochondritis dissecans on the lateral film) **(B)**, posterior dislocation of the radial head **(C)**, and iliac horns **(D)**.

severity of the anomalies and they are frequently associated with other malformations (176, 177). It has an estimated incidence of 1 in 5600 births (178), and roughly 2% of individuals with congenital spinal abnormalities will have another manifestations of ocular–auricular–vertebral dysplasia (138).

The typical eye defect is an epibulbar dermoid on the conjunctiva (Fig. 8-18A). Preauricular fleshy skin tags are found in front of the ear, and pits extend from the tragus to the corner of the mouth (Fig. 8-18B). In some patients, the ear may be hypoplastic or absent. The eye and ear anomalies are unilateral in 85% of these children, and facial asymmetry is the result of a hypoplastic mandibular ramus, invariably on the same side as the ear anomalies (Fig. 8-18C).

Vertebral anomalies may occur anywhere along the spine, although the lower cervical and the upper thoracic locations predominate (Fig. 8-18C). Hemivertebrae are the most common defect, with an occasional block fusion. Neural tube defect occurs more often than in the general population, and it may involve any portion of the spine, or even the skull (an encephalocele). Half of the patients have clinically detectable scoliosis (179).

The congenital curve can cause cosmetic concerns, but these need to be considered in the context of the other abnormalities, which may outweigh the cosmetic implications of the spinal deformity. In addition, Sprengel deformity and rib anomalies may be present in association with the congenital curves in the cervical–thoracic region, and these contribute to the cosmetic implications of the condition. The congenital curves should be managed like congenital scoliosis of other etiologies, although management based on cosmetic concerns needs to be made in the context of the other deformities. Early surgery should be considered when there is progression of the congenital curve. Preoperative CT scan and MRI are recommended to delineate the anatomy of the congenital curve and determine whether there is any intraspinal pathology or occult posterior element defects.

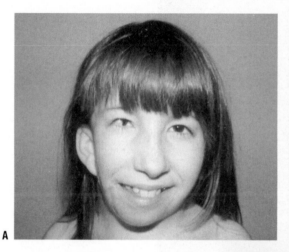

A

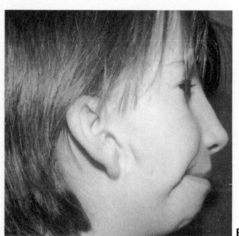

B

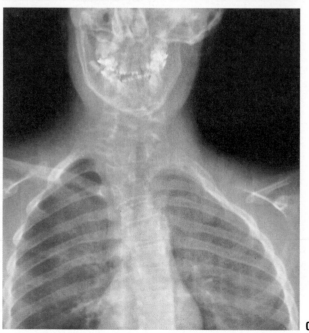

C

FIGURE 8-18. Goldenhar syndrome. **A:** Facial asymmetry and epibulbar dermoid of the right eye. **B:** Malformed ears with preauricular tags and sinuses. **C:** X-ray film demonstrates the congenital anomalies of the lower cervical and the upper thoracic spine. Hypoplasia of the ascending ramus of the mandible accounts for the facial asymmetry. The clavicle is absent on the same side as the deformation of the face. (From Goldberg MJ. *The dysmorphic child: an orthopedic perspective.* New York, NY: Raven Press, 1987, with permission.)

There is frequently a compensatory curve below the congenital curve that can behave like idiopathic scoliosis. The compensatory curve can cause as much, if not more of a problem for the patient as the congenital curve. This curve is managed the same as idiopathic scoliosis. Brace treatment has no effect on the congenital curve, and although orthotic management has been used for the compensatory curve, its success rate seems lower than for idiopathic scoliosis although high-quality comparative studies of its efficacy are lacking.

Intubation for anesthesia may be difficult because of the small jaw, stiff neck, and upper airway dysmorphology (180). Other anomalies include congenital heart disease (e.g., ventricular septal defect) (176), cleft lip, and cleft palate (181). Mental retardation, reported to affect between 10% and 39% of patients, is more common in cases involving microphthalmia or an encephalocele (143, 182).

Cornelia de Lange Syndrome.
Cornelia de Lange syndrome is associated with a characteristic face, and growth retardation, which makes the clinical diagnosis of Cornelia de Lange syndrome reasonably reliable (183). The face has immediately recognizable downturned corners of the mouth, eyebrows meeting in the midline (synophrys), elongated philtrum, and long eyelashes (184, 185) (Fig. 8-19).

Mutations in a number of genes, which all regulate the same signaling pathway, are identified in Cornelia de Lange syndrome. About half of affected individuals have a mutation in the *N1PBL* gene, which encodes a protein that is a component of a multiprotein complex, called the *cohesin complex*. The mutation alters the activity of a developmentally important signaling pathway called *Notch* (186, 187). Notch plays a major role in central nervous system development, hence the associated mental retardation. An X-linked form of the disorder can be caused by mutation in the SMC1L1 gene, which also encodes a component of the cohesin complex.

A mild variant of Cornelia de Lange syndrome is related to mutation in the SMC3 gene, which encodes yet another component of the cohesin complex. Duplication or deletion of the chromosome band 3q25-29 produces a phenotype similar to Cornelia de Lange syndrome (188, 189). In these instances, the mother is always the transmitting parent, suggesting genomic imprinting. The syndrome is relatively common, occurring in 1 in 10,000 live births, and it is possible to make a prenatal diagnosis by ultrasound (135, 136, 190, 191).

Most have mild orthopaedic deformities of the upper extremities (191–197) (Fig. 8-20). They form a curious constellation of a small hand, a proximally placed thumb, clinodactyly of the small finger, and decreased elbow motion, usually caused by a dislocated radial head. This combination rarely causes any disability. Some patients, however, have severe deformities of the upper extremity in the form of an absent ulna and a monodigital hand, a condition that can be unilateral or bilateral (Fig. 8-20).

The lower extremities are less often affected. Tight heel cords and other cerebral palsy–like contractures can be seen. These can be managed similarly to cerebral palsy, but there seems to be a higher rate of recurrence (198). Syndactyly of the toes is fairly constant. Aplasia of the tibia has been reported rarely. There is possibly a higher incidence of Legg-Perthes disease, approaching about 10%. Scoliosis can occur and should be managed similarly to scoliosis in cerebral palsy. Most of the skeletal deformities in Cornelia de Lange syndrome are asymptomatic and probably do not benefit from surgical intervention (198).

The small size begins with intrauterine growth retardation. Children remain small, with a delayed skeletal age. The mortality rate in the first year of life is high because of defective swallowing mechanisms (199), gastroesophageal reflux (200), aspiration, and respiratory infections. If the children survive their first year, they usually do well, but the long-term outcome is unclear.

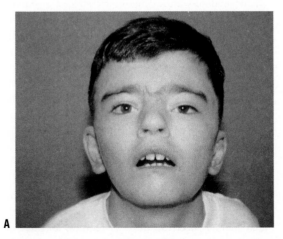 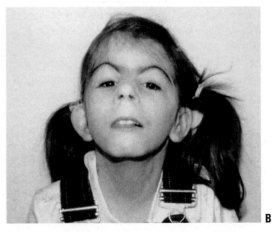

FIGURE 8-19. Cornelia de Lange syndrome. Notice the classic facial features of heavy eyebrows meeting in the midline, upturned nose, downturned corners of the mouth, and long eyelashes in a 13-year-old boy **(A)** and a 7-year-old girl **(B)**. (From Goldberg MJ. *The dysmorphic child: an orthopedic perspective.* New York, NY: Raven Press, 1987, with permission.)

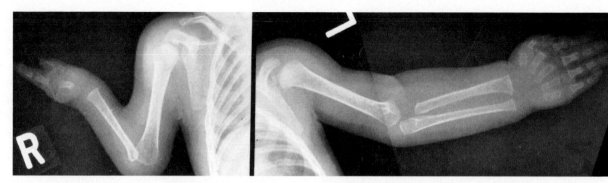

FIGURE 8-20. Cornelia de Lange syndrome: a child with a severely affected upper extremity on her right side (i.e., absent ulna and fingers) and a mildly affected arm on her left (i.e., short thumb and dysplasia of proximal radius). (From Goldberg MJ. *The dysmorphic child: an orthopedic perspective.* New York, NY: Raven Press, 1987, with permission.)

Almost all of them walk, but their milestones are delayed. There is retarded mentation, but the added features of no speech and no interactions cause major disability (201). Self-mutilating behavior can be an obstacle to orthopaedic care (202, 203).

Orthopaedic interventions need to be considered in the overall functional context of the individual. Braces, physical therapy, and surgery for tight heel cords, using similar indications as in cerebral palsy are justifiable. Upper extremity surgery is not indicated unless improved performance capacity is ensured. Patients with Cornelia de Lange syndrome rarely if ever use upper extremity prostheses. Lower extremity prostheses, however, should be prescribed for the rare case with tibial deficiency. Because the gastroesophageal reflux and swallowing disorders may persist well past the first year, there is a higher risk of anesthesia complications (204).

FETAL ENVIRONMENT

Syndromes caused by problems in the fetal environment can share similarities with conditions caused by genes that encode proteins that are important in normal development. Many teratogenic agents modulate the same pathways that are dysregulated by the mutations that cause such syndromes. A good example of this is holoprosencephaly, a midbrain patterning disorder. This can be caused by mutations in a gene called *sonic hedgehog*, and can also be caused by teratogenic agents that block the hedgehog signaling pathway, such as derivatives found in the plant *Veraculum californicum* (205, 206).

Fetal Alcohol Syndrome. Fetal alcohol syndrome is a pattern of malformations found in children of alcoholic mothers. There is a great deal of variability in the findings associated with fetal alcohol exposure and the full-blown syndrome is usually seen only in children of chronic alcoholics who drink throughout pregnancy. Multiple terms are used to describe the effects that result from prenatal exposure to alcohol, including fetal alcohol effects, alcohol-related birth defects, alcohol-related neurodevelopment disorder, and, most recently, fetal alcohol spectrum disorder (207). Although the risk to alcoholic

mothers is known, there is substantial difference of opinion about the effects of moderate alcohol use during pregnancy (208–210). This is in part because fetal exposure to alcohol may be relatively common. Indeed, it is estimated that about 12% of U.S. women who are sexually active, do not use contraception effectively, and drink alcohol frequently or binge drink, thereby putting them at risk for an alcohol-exposed pregnancy. As such, alcohol is the most likely teratogen for a mother to encounter (211). Because no safe threshold of alcohol use during pregnancy has been established, the Centers for Disease Control recommend that women who are pregnant, planning a pregnancy, or at risk for pregnancy should not drink alcohol. The overall incidence of full-blown fetal alcohol syndrome is reported to be between 0.5 and 2.0 per 1000 live births (212, 213), making this condition as common as Down syndrome. For an alcoholic mother, there is a 30% risk for fetal alcohol syndrome in her child.

A cardinal clinical feature is disturbed growth; the children have intrauterine growth retardation, small weight, and small length at birth, and these limitations remain despite good nutrition during childhood (214, 215) (Fig. 8-21). Their smallness and a loss of fat suggest a search for endocrine dysfunction; the patients often look similar to those who are deficient in growth hormone. The second cardinal feature is disturbed central nervous system development. Children with fetal alcohol syndrome present with a diagnosis of cerebral palsy clinics. The typical child has a small head, a small brain, and delayed motor milestones. Accomplishing fine motor skills is also delayed. Hypotonia is present early, but many develop spasticity later. The typical face has three characteristic features: short palpebral fissures (i.e., the eyes appear small), a flat philtrum (i.e., no groove below the nose), and a thin upper lip (216, 217) (Fig. 8-21). Because of the variety of clinical features, a joint consensus conference sponsored by the Centers for Disease Control suggested that a diagnosis of fetal alcohol spectrum disorder requires all three of the characteristic dysmorphic facial features (smooth philtrum, thin vermillion border, and small palpebral fissures), prenatal or postnatal growth deficit in height or weight, and a central nervous system abnormality.

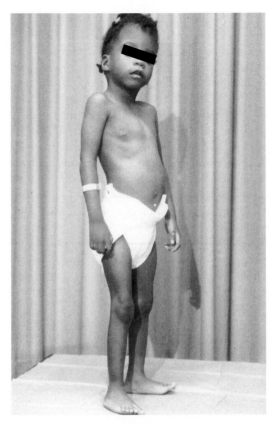

FIGURE 8-21. The 3-year-old patient is small and has the characteristic face of fetal alcohol syndrome. (From Goldberg MJ. *The dysmorphic child: an orthopedic perspective.* New York, NY: Raven Press, 1987, with permission.)

VACTERLS and VATER Association. VATER, as the syndrome was previously known, has been expanded to VACTERLS (229). The letters of VACTERLS in this syndrome's name constitute an acronym for the systems and defects involved: vertebral, anal, cardiac, tracheal, esophageal, renal, limb, and single umbilical artery. One does not need to find examples of all seven categories of anomalies in order to diagnose the syndrome. The syndrome can be diagnosed prenatally by visualizing several of the malformations on ultrasound. The most obvious physical finding at birth is the radial ray defect. Between 5% and 10% of radial clubhands are associated with VACTERLS.

The cause is unknown, but it is a nonrandom association, whose simultaneous occurrence by chance is unlikely (230). Disruption of a developmentally important signaling pathway called *Hedgehog* can give all of the clinical findings associated with VACTERLS, suggesting that an intrauterine event disrupting this signaling pathway is the cause (189). The current thought is that these structures are either all formed at the same time, or are all patterned by the same developmental signaling pathway. An event occurring during fetal development that disrupts either the common signaling pathway or any of a variety of susceptible pathways operating at the same time is probably responsible for the associated malformations.

The vertebral defects include disturbed spinal segmentation, with vertebral bars and blocks (231, 232). Thoracic anomalies are worse in those with tracheoesophageal fistula, and lumbar anomalies are more common in those who have an imperforate anus. Occult intraspinal pathology is common (232, 233), and a screening MR study of the spine is recommended, especially in patients who require operative management of their scoliosis. The curves can be managed like other types of congenital scoliosis.

Congenital heart defects are present in one-half of these patients. A ventricular septal defect is the most common problem. Duodenal atresia may be found in this syndrome. The VACTERLS patient often has a single kidney. Other collecting-system anomalies occur frequently among this group.

The limb anomalies range from a hypoplastic thumb to a radial clubhand. The defect may be unilateral or bilateral; bilateral defects are always asymmetric (231). The legs are spared 80% of the time. When the lower extremities are involved, a duplicated hallux is the most common finding.

The normal umbilical cord has two arteries and one vein. The absence of an artery, detectable only at the time of delivery or in the immediate newborn period, reflects the broad range of morphologic defects dating back to placental formation.

Developmental delay may be observed, and is thought to be the consequence of skeletal anomalies of the arms, scoliosis, and surgery for gastrointestinal or genitourinary malformations. Nevertheless, several central nervous system malformations (e.g., encephalocele hydrocephalus) may be associated with VACTERLS, and must be excluded (233, 234). If the patient survives the gastrointestinal anomalies and correction of the cardiac defects, the prognosis for a normal life is excellent. Each orthopaedic abnormality can be treated as an isolated

Approximately 50% of children with this syndrome have an orthopaedic abnormality, but most of these are not disabling (218–220). At birth, the range of motion is restricted, especially of the hands and feet, and occasionally these contractures are fixed. The contractures typically respond well to physical therapy, although residual stiffness in the proximal interphalangeal joints may remain. Clubfoot is common, and approximately 10% of these patients have developmental dysplasia of the hip. The clubfoot is usually not rigid (221). Cervical spine fusions, usually involving C2 and C3, may be seen on radiographs (220, 222–226). These may resemble the picture seen in Klippel-Feil syndrome, but there are usually none of the other findings associated with that syndrome. Synostoses are also common in the upper extremity, with fusions involving the radial–ulnar articulation and the carpal bones, all without any resultant disability (222, 225, 227). Stippled epiphyses may be seen in the lower extremities, but rarely in the upper extremities (228).

The orthopaedic problems associated with fetal alcohol syndrome can be managed in the same way as in children without this syndrome. The future for children with fetal alcohol syndrome is dim, despite placement away from the alcoholic home. Intellect remains retarded, with little catch up. Social services departments should be involved in these children's care.

problem. The sections in this chapter that deal with congenital scoliosis and radial clubhand contain detailed information. The key point is to recognize this association and to identify other abnormalities that might interfere with treatment.

GENES IMPORTANT FOR NERVE OR MUSCLE FUNCTION

There are a large number of neurologic disorders that can be caused by genes that encode for proteins that are important for nerve or muscle function. The course of these disorders is variable; however, several show progressive weakening effects over time. Various inheritance patterns are possible, but frequently these disorders are linked to the X chromosome. Duchenne muscular dystrophy and Rett syndrome are two such disorders that are inherited in an X-linked recessive manner and X-linked dominant manner, respectively.

Familial Dysautonomia. Familial dysautonomia, also called *Riley-Day syndrome*, is an autosomal recessive disorder occurring primarily in Jews who trace their ancestry to Eastern Europe. Among such individuals, the incidence is estimated to be about 1 in 3700. The clinical manifestations are caused by defective functioning of the autonomic nervous system and sensory system. The autonomic dysfunction causes labile blood pressure, dysphagia, abnormal temperature control, and abnormal gastrointestinal motility. Infants have difficulty swallowing, with misdirected fluids going to the lungs, resulting in pneumonia. There is a poor suck response and a curious absence of tears. During childhood, the autonomic dysfunction becomes more apparent, with wide swings in blood pressure and body temperature. There are cyclic vomiting episodes; these crises often last hours or days. Swallowing remains poor. The skin is blotchy. There is relative insensitivity to pain and poor hot–cold distinction. Intelligence is normal, but the children exhibit emotional liability, and may have unusual personality development, especially in the teenage years. The diagnosis is made on clinical findings and on the basis of the presence of five signs: (i) lack of axon flare after intradermal injection of histamine, (ii) absence of fungiform papillae on the tongue, (iii) miosis of the pupil after conjunctival installation of methacholine chloride, (iv) absence of deep tendon reflexes, and (v) diminished tear flow (235–237).

This disorder is caused by a mutation in the inhibitor of kappa light polypeptide gene enhancer in B cells. The protein product of this gene plays a role in the phosphorylation of other signaling proteins, but the mutant form is expressed only in select tissue types, primarily affecting cells in the autonomic nervous system (238, 239). Since the mutation is expressed only in certain tissue types, one approach to treatment would be to change the tissue-specific expression of the mutant form by using drugs that regulate the expression of only the mutant variant. Such a potential treatment has been proposed using tocotrienols, which are members of the vitamin E family

(240, 241). Pathologic anatomy reveals a paucity of neurons in cervical sympathetic ganglia, dorsal sensory roots, and abdominal parasympathetic nerves (242). A number of small axons are depleted from the sensory nerves and the dorsal columns. Because of a primary failure to develop axons, the symptoms are present at birth, and there is a loss of nerve cells and progression of symptoms as the patient grows older.

Musculoskeletal manifestations include scoliosis, fracture susceptibility, avascular necrosis, and a Charcot joint–like process. Scoliosis affects a majority of patients, and approximately one-fourth will need operative intervention (243–249). It has an early onset, and progression is often rapid. Kyphosis, accentuated by tight anterior pectoralis muscles, appears in approximately one-half of the patients. Bracing does not work well, because of the underlying gastrointestinal and emotional problems. Anesthesia can be challenging in individuals with such autonomic liability, but with proper techniques, operative intervention is successful. Surgery seems to give better results if performed early in the course of the disease (229, 250, 251).

Fractures occur frequently, and often go unrecognized because of the patient's insensitivity to pain (252). The physician should be suspicious of occult fractures in patients who have had trauma and swelling but experience minimal tenderness. Fractures usually heal quite well, but early diagnosis and avoiding displacement is the goal.

Radiographic evidence of avascular necrosis is common, but the pathobiology is entirely unknown (252–254). There are Legg-Perthes changes in the hips. Osteochondritis dissecans of the knees is often extensive, involving both femoral condyles (Fig. 8-22). It may be difficult to determine whether the ossification changes in the knee are because of osteochondritis dissecans or the early stage of Charcot joint (255, 256). Hip dysplasia may be seen in patients with this syndrome.

The natural history of familial dysautonomia is characterized by a relatively high mortality rate in infancy, attributed to aspiration pneumonia (237). Sudden death in childhood and adolescence occurs because the child is unable to respond appropriately to stress or hypoxia. Early recognition of this syndrome and appropriate care lead to a life expectancy of many decades. Management of the gastrointestinal problems and the use of gastrostomy and fundoplications have been extremely successful in such patients. There have been successful pregnancies brought to term in mothers with the syndrome (257, 258).

Rett Syndrome. Rett syndrome is an X-linked dominant disorder that is present almost exclusively in girls and is characterized by normal development for the first 6 to 18 months, followed by rapid deterioration of higher brain functions. This is accompanied by dementia, autism, loss of purposeful use of the hands, and ataxia. After the initial rapid decline, the deterioration slows dramatically, so that affected individuals may have a relatively stable picture for several decades (244). There is variability in the severity of the decline, so that some girls are still walking as teenagers, whereas others stop ambulating in early childhood (245). A hand radiograph may help with

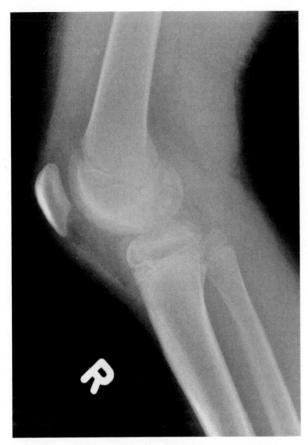

FIGURE 8-22. Familial dysautonomia. Irregular ossifications of the distal femoral epiphysis mimic osteochondritis dissecans.

curves. These can be stabilized surgically when they reach a magnitude that interferes with sitting or balance. Although case series suggest an improvement after surgery (262), as is seen in cerebral palsy, there are no comparative studies showing improved function after spinal surgery. Spinal instrumentation and fusion should include the whole curve and any kyphotic segments. Although, theoretically, walking ability can worsen following extensive fusions, this has not been reported in the small number of cases in which spinal surgery was undertaken in ambulatory girls with Rett syndrome (259, 262, 263). Coxa valga and lower extremity contractures can occur, and these should be managed as in cerebral palsy, with emphasis placed on operative procedures that will improve function or decrease pain (264, 266, 267).

The life span in Rett syndrome is not known, but there are some affected individuals with a normal life span. There are a variety of nonorthopaedic problems, including cardiac conduction abnormalities, epilepsy, and vasomotor instability of the lower limbs. Some of these put the patients at increased risk when undergoing anesthesia (268). Interestingly, there is a high incidence of left handedness (approximately 40%) in girls with Rett syndrome (269).

CHROMOSOMAL (MULTIPLE GENES)

Chromosomal abnormalities involve large portions of DNA, and multiple genes are affected. There can be deletions, duplications, or translocations. Large abnormalities in chromosomes are almost always associated with some degree of mental deficiency. Because there is duplication of multiple genes, there are multiple abnormalities in multiple organ systems. Since multiple genes are abnormal in all cells, normal cell functions (such as the ability to mount an immune response or normal wound healing) also may be abnormal. Except for rare instances, these disorders are not inherited, and occur as sporadic events.

Down Syndrome.   Down syndrome is the most common and perhaps the most readily recognizable malformation in humans (270) (Fig. 8-23). Patients have a characteristic facial appearance including upward-slanting eyes, epicanthal folds, and a flattened profile. Examination of the hands reveals a single flexion crease, often referred to as a *simian crease*. There is also clinodactyly of the small finger. These hand malformations have no clinical significance (271). Milestones are delayed, with most children not walking until 2 to 3 years of age. The classic gait pattern is broad based, toed out, and waddling.

The bones in Down syndrome have subtle malformations. The best-studied changes are in the pelvis, which is characterized by flat acetabula and flared iliac wings (243). These pelvic changes are so characteristic that prior to use of chromosome analysis, pelvic radiographs were used for confirming the diagnosis. Short stature is a cardinal feature; the average for men is 155 cm (61 in.), and the average for women is 145 cm (57 in.) (244). The detection of bone changes can be useful in prenatal

the diagnosis, because 60% will have either a negative ulnar variance or a short fourth metacarpal (246, 247).

Children with this syndrome were initially thought to have cerebral palsy with a movement disorder. Andreas Rett, a pediatrician practicing in Austria, noted that these girls all had normal development in the first month of life, and was thus able to separate them from those with cerebral palsy. It occurs with an incidence of 1 in 40,000. In some patients, it is caused by a mutation in the *MECP2* gene, which encodes X-linked methyl-CpG-binding protein 2. This protein plays an important role in regulating gene expression during development, especially in the central nervous system (259). X-linked dominant diseases are more severe in boys, and Rett is probably fatal in the vast majority of male patients, though few such cases have been reported (260). Genetic testing and prenatal diagnosis (261) are possible, but as in other syndromes, a careful physical examination and history can be used to make the diagnosis in most cases (262).

Children with Rett syndrome present to the orthopaedist with a clinical picture similar to that of a cerebral palsy patient with total body involvement. Scoliosis occurs in over half the girls who are affected with this disorder (260, 263–266). Orthotic management probably does not alter the progression of the curve. There is a typical, usually long "c" pattern to the

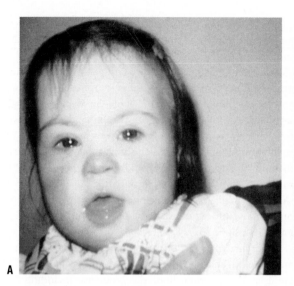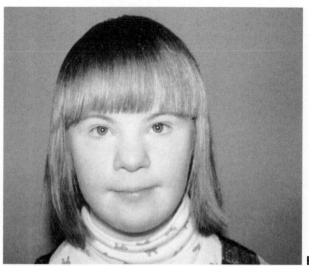

FIGURE 8-23. Down syndrome. The child has the characteristic face, with upward-slanting eyes, epicanthal folds, open mouth of early childhood, and flattened profile. **A:** At 1 year of age. **B:** At 10 years of age. (A, Courtesy of Murray Feingold, MD, Boston, Massachusetts. B, From Goldberg MJ. *The dysmorphic child: an orthopedic perspective.* New York, NY: Raven Press, 1987, with permission.)

diagnosis. A combination of bone length and lab tests on the mother (human chorinoic gonadotropin and alpha-fetoprotein levels) may predict the diagnosis, although the positive and negative predictive values are not as good as had been initially hoped (245). Cytogenetic study, which identifies complete trisomy 21 in 95% of the cases, remains the best confirmative test.

Complete trisomies account for 95% of the cases, with 2% mosaics and 3% translocations. The overall occurrence is 1 per 660 live births, and the incidence is closely related to maternal age. If the mother is younger than 30 years of age, the risk is 1 of 5000 live births, and if the mother is older than 35 years of age, the incidence rises to 1 in 250. The critical region for Down syndrome resides in part of the long arm of chromosome 21. Duplication of a 5-megabase region of chromosome 21 (located at 21q22.2–22.3) causes the classic phenotypic features, such as the characteristic facies, hand anomalies, congenital heart disease, and some aspects of mental retardation (246). This region probably contains a number of genes whose duplication is necessary to produce the syndrome.

The general features of Down syndrome are well known. There is a characteristic flattened face. Mental retardation is typical, but performance is far better than expected from standard IQ testing. Congenital heart disease occurs in about 50% of patients and is usually a septal defect (e.g., arteriovenous communis, ventricular septal defect). Duodenal atresia is found regularly. Leukemia occurs in about 1% of this population (1, 5). There is a high incidence of endocrinopathies, hypothyroidism in particular. Infections are common, and while the precise molecular mechanism is not apparent, it may be due to the same white blood cell abnormality that predisposes to leukemia. The propensity to develop infections may result in a higher than anticipated rate of surgical wound

infections (225). Although problems with fracture repair have not been reported, there is a substantially worse than expected rate of successful arthrodesis in procedures to obtain a surgical fusion, suggesting a defect in osteoblast function (226). The appearance of premature aging is obvious, and there is often an early onset of Alzheimer disease (247).

Approximately 10% of individuals with Down syndrome show an increased atlantodens interval on lateral spine films (248, 249, 272–274) (Fig. 8-24A). In most, the increased interval is not associated with symptoms (249, 275). In addition, there is a broad array of other abnormalities in the upper cervical spine, including instability at occiput and C1 (274, 276–278), odontoid dysplasia (249, 279–281) (Fig. 8-24C), laminal defects at C1 (282) (Fig. 8-24B), spondylolisthesis (Fig. 8-24D), cervical stenosis (235), and precocious arthritis in the midcervical region (283, 284) (Fig. 8-24E). In addition, there is an anomalous course to the vertebral artery at the craniovertebral junction, which can complicate surgical management (238). The cervical spine abnormalities may complicate anesthesia (239).

These other abnormalities often complicate decision making about spinal instability. Although routine screening radiographs often disclose these cervical spine abnormalities, radiographs are not reliable in predicting myelopathy (285–291). Therefore, their efficacy in the management of the cervical spine in patients with Down syndrome is uncertain. The management of cervical instability in Down syndrome is discussed elsewhere in this text.

Approximately 50% of patients with Down syndrome have scoliosis, with an idiopathic pattern in most (292). Scoliosis is five times more likely to be detected in a severely retarded, institutionalized population than in an ambulatory

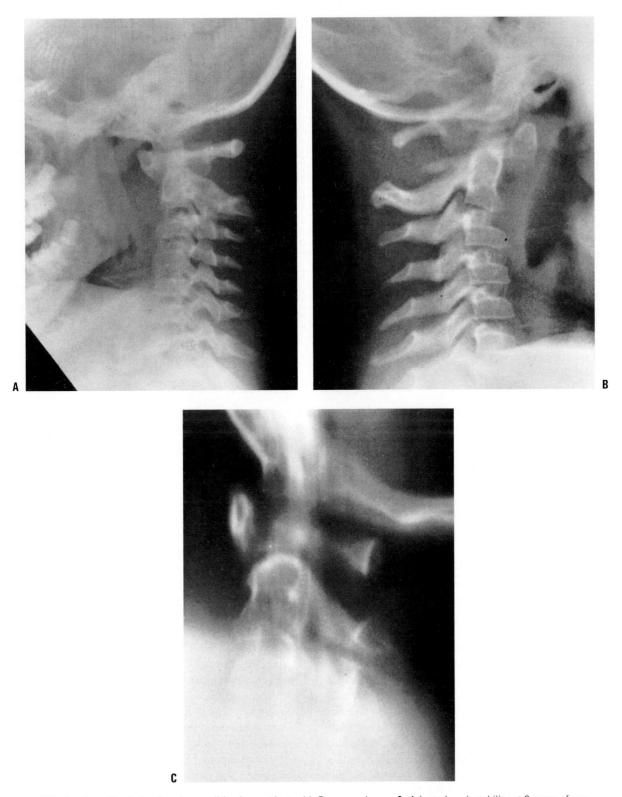

FIGURE 8-24. Cervical spine abnormalities in a patient with Down syndrome. **A:** Atlantodens instability at 8 years of age. **B:** Hypoplastic posterior elements of C1 at 3 years of age. **C:** Os odontoideum and increased atlantodens interval at 14 years of age.

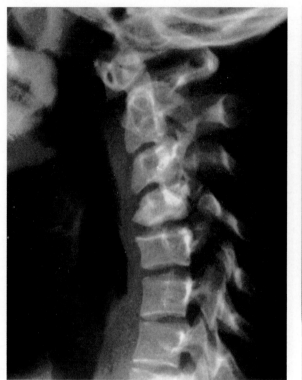
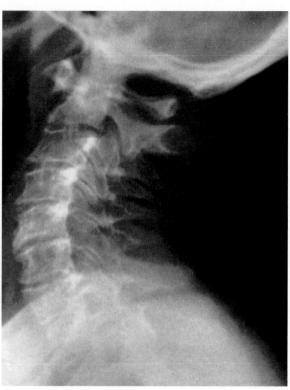

D

E

FIGURE 8-24. (*continued*) **D:** Midcervical spondylolysis at 16 years of age. **E:** Precocious osteoarthritis of the midcervical spine at 40 years of age. (From Goldberg MJ. *The dysmorphic child: an orthopedic perspective.* New York, NY: Raven Press, 1987, with permission.)

setting. This finding raises the possibility that factors such as severity of the phenotype, or other neuromuscular factors contribute to scoliosis. Management is the same as in idiopathic scoliosis. Similar to the case of the cervical spine, there is a higher rate of complications from scoliosis surgery than in the general population (293). Spondylolisthesis occurs in about 6%, with the lower lumbar spine being most commonly involved. Spondylolisthesis can also occur in the cervical spine.

Congenital dislocated hips are rare, but progressive dysplasia may begin during later childhood. This loss of acetabular containment may lead to an acute or a gradual complete dislocation (Fig. 8-25A,B). The onset of acetabular dysplasia can be progressive even after maturity, leading to dislocations in adulthood (294–296) (Fig. 8-25C,D). Although hip instability and developmental dysplasia are thought to lead to functional disability (interfering with walking and reducing independent mobility), there are no studies showing this to be the case. The etiology of the hip instability is probably multifactorial, with ligamentous laxity, subtle changes in the shape of the pelvis and acetabular alignment, and behavior (some children become habitual dislocators) all contributing. Treatment of the unstable hip is difficult, and the multiple causative factors also contribute to higher treatment failure rates. Both operative and nonoperative treatment are reported. Prolonged bracing after reduction for the hip that dislocates acutely has shown success in children younger than 6 years (297). In cases in which there are repeated

dislocations, surgical reconstruction is warranted, especially in children older than 6 years. Operative treatment requires correction of all the deforming factors. Reconstruction must take into account the abnormal bone alignment, and should include femoral and acetabular osteotomies, as well as imbrication of the redundant capsule. Posterior acetabular deficiency has been reported, and was not improved following a traditional Salter-style innominate osteotomy (298); therefore, three-dimensional imaging (such as a CT scan) should be considered before embarking on surgery. The recurrence rate following hip surgery is high, suggesting that other factors related to the underlying disease, but not necessarily related to the hip anatomy itself, are contributory (299–301).

Slipped capital femoral epiphyses are reported in all Down syndrome series, although the precise incidence is unknown (292, 302) (Fig. 8-26). There appears to be a higher-than-expected risk for avascular necrosis. The reasons are not clear, but factors include more acute slips and delayed diagnoses. It is tempting to speculate about an association with the hypothyroid state, which is common in Down syndrome. All children with Down syndrome should have thyroid function tests.

The configuration of the knee is that of genu valgum, with a subluxed and a dislocated patella (Fig. 8-27). Many individuals will have asymptomatic patellar dislocations that do not require treatment (303). Symptomatic cases should be

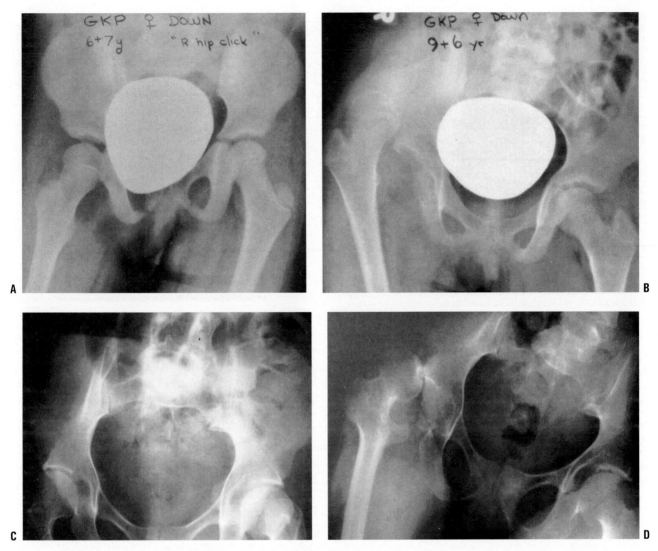

FIGURE 8-25.   Down syndrome patient with late-onset developmental dysplasia of the hip and dislocation. **A:** Pelvic radiograph taken in standing position, at 6.5 years of age. **B:** At 9.5 years of age, the patient suddenly refused to walk because of hip dislocation. **C:** Pelvic radiograph of a 31-year-old man with Down syndrome. **D:** Three years later, dislocation of right hip occurred. (A and B, from Goldberg MJ. *The dysmorphic child: an orthopedic perspective.* New York, NY: Raven Press, 1987; C and D, from Pueschel SM. Should children with Down syndrome be screened for atlantoaxial instability? *Arch Pediatr Adolesc Med* 1998;152:123, with permission.)

initially managed with orthoses and a physiotherapy program. Individuals who continue to be symptomatic can be considered for operative treatment. As in hip dysplasia, operative interventions that correct all of the deformities (bone and soft tissue) have the best success.

The characteristic appearance of the feet in childhood is one of an asymptomatic flexible planovalgus shape, with an increased space between the great and the second toes. Because it is important to maintain mobility in adults with Down syndrome, symptomatic foot problems should be treated. The treatment involves footwear modification in many cases, but may require surgery in cases that are symptomatic despite appropriate footwear. Valgus feet with toe deformities are most likely to become symptomatic. In many, hallux valgus develops in adolescence, and in adulthood the bunions become

symptomatic. Orthotics will improve foot position, but may actually slow the walking speed of children with Down syndrome (304). For that reason, orthotics should be used only in symptomatic cases. Repair of a hallux valgus and bunion may be needed in late adolescence or young adulthood. Because of the hindfoot valgus, pronation, and external tibial torsion, the forces that produce bunions are obvious, and fusion of the first metatarsophalangeal joint should be considered, along with osteotomy, to correct hindfoot valgus.

A polyarticular arthropathy occurs in approximately 10% of those with Down syndrome (305–307). Whether this is true juvenile rheumatoid arthritis or a unique inflammatory arthritis due to genetic or immune defects is unknown; the natural history is not documented. Delayed diagnosis is common. Nonsteroidal anti-inflammatory drugs have been the mainstay

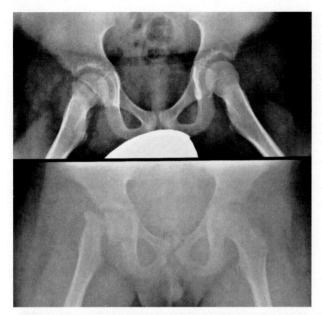

FIGURE 8-26. Effects of Down syndrome in a 12-year-old boy with 4 months of knee pain. The grade I slipped capital femoral epiphysis progressed to a total slip while the patient was undergoing preoperative evaluation and bed rest. (From Goldberg MJ. *The dysmorphic child: an orthopedic perspective.* New York, NY: Raven Press, 1987, with permission.)

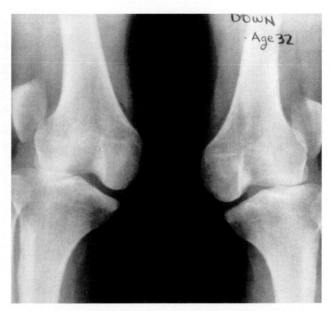

FIGURE 8-27. Effects of Down syndrome in a 32-year-old patient. The radiograph shows bilateral dislocated patellae and an oblique orientation of the joint line. The patient is fully ambulatory, but before standing must manually reduce the patellae to the midline. (From Goldberg MJ. *The dysmorphic child: an orthopedic perspective.* New York, NY: Raven Press, 1987, with permission.)

of treatment. Foot symptoms are exceptionally frequent with the onset of polyarthropathy (Fig. 8-28). Patients with Down syndrome have low bone mineral density, but it is in part a consequence of reduced body size, relative physical inactivity, and low vitamin D levels from a lack of sunlight exposure. As such, it is recommended that patients with Down syndrome engage in regular physical activity and have sufficient levels of vitamin D (256).

Marked joint hypermobility is evident; the children are able to assume the most intriguing sitting postures. Ligamentous laxity was traditionally thought to be the cause of joint hypermobility, and it was assumed that it predisposes patients with Down syndrome to orthopaedic pathology. However, ligamentous laxity correlates poorly with joint hypermobility. This suggests that other factors, such as subtle malformations in the shapes of bones and insertion sites of ligaments, play a role in hypermobility (308, 309).

The natural history of those with Down syndrome has changed in the last few decades. Longevity has increased because of the aggressive surgical approach to congenital heart disease, chemotherapy for leukemia, and antibiotics for infection. Survival into the sixties is common. Approximately one of five persons with Down syndrome has musculoskeletal abnormalities. Many of these, however, are merely radiographic abnormalities or curious physical findings. These patients often have excellent functional performance despite the abnormalities. There is a paucity of well-documented, long-term orthopaedic studies of patients with Down syndrome. Treatment

programs should focus on functional performance rather than on radiographic findings.

Turner Syndrome. Turner syndrome is present only in girls, and consists of short stature, sexual infantilism, a webbed neck, and cubitus valgus. It is a relatively common chromosome disorder affecting 1 in 2500 live births, but the rate of intrauterine lethality is 95%. The syndrome is caused by a single X chromosome. In two-thirds of cases, all cells are XO,

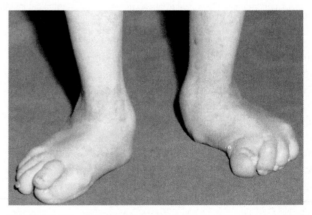

FIGURE 8-28. Polyarthritis of Down syndrome and valgus feet led to significant deformity in a 16-year-old patient. (From Goldberg MJ. *The dysmorphic child: an orthopedic perspective.* New York, NY: Raven Press, 1987, with permission.)

and parental origin of the single X chromosome is the mother in 70% of the cases (310). XO mosaicism occurs in about one-third of patients, and in 1% there is deletion of only a part of an X chromosome (310, 311). Cytogenetic studies will confirm this diagnosis.

The effect of the single X chromosome may be different, depending on whether it is derived from the father or from the mother, and this is probably the result of imprinting (285). Recent studies based on individuals with partial loss of the X chromosome suggest that a critical region at Xp11.2–p22.1 is responsible for the disease (312).

The identification of particular features at a particular age raises suspicion of the presence of this syndrome. At birth, the child has a webbed neck, widely spaced nipples, and edema of the hands and feet. The foot edema may persist for several months. During childhood, the low hairline, webbed neck, cubitus valgus, and short stature become more apparent. The adolescent has short stature and sexual infantilism. The most important features that call for chromosome analysis are edema of the hands and feet at birth, short stature in childhood, and sexual infantilism as an adolescent.

Growth retardation is a cardinal feature, with an ultimate height of approximately 140 cm (56 in.) (286). Bone maturation is normal until 8 to 9 years of age; then, because sex hormone stimulation is absent, there is neither skeletal maturation nor pubertal growth spurt. There is no puberty at all, and the girls remain without secondary sexual characteristics unless exogenous estrogen is administered.

The web neck looks like a feature of Klippel-Feil syndrome, but the cervical spine radiographs are normal. It is a cutaneous web only, and the cause may be related to an intrauterine cystic hygroma (313). It is cosmetically unsightly, and plastic surgery is effective (314).

Scoliosis is common, present in over 10% of affected individuals (315), and the curve usually develops in juveniles. The delayed skeletal maturation allows a long period for curve progression. Growth hormone, which is almost always administered to girls with this syndrome, accelerates curve progression. Although the scoliosis can be managed in the same way as idiopathic scoliosis, patients must be observed more frequently during growth hormone administration. Kyphosis is present in a large proportion of individuals with this condition, but its functional significance is unclear (287).

Cubitus valgus is present in 80%, but there is a normal range of elbow motion and no disability (316). Genu valgum is also apparent, but the vast majority of cases are asymptomatic. Osteotomy is performed for the rare symptomatic case. There is a medial bony protuberance not unlike an osteochondroma, arising off the proximal tibia in some patients (317).

Osteoporosis is a significant problem because of the low estrogen and an altered renal vitamin D metabolism, which may correctable with the administration of adequate calcium, vitamin D, growth hormone, and sex steroid supplementation (270, 288, 289, 318). These measures work best to maintain bone density, rather than to increase it from pathologic levels, and as

such should be instituted early in the course (243, 271). While a high incidence of wrist fractures has been reported in childhood (290), in women who are treated with treated with standard estrogen therapy there is not a higher fracture rate (245).

Intelligence is normal, but there is a high frequency of learning disabilities (291, 319). The life expectancy is normal, overall medical status is excellent, and social acceptance is good (320). There are some heart and kidney abnormalities reported at a somewhat higher incidence than for the normal population (321). Having only one X chromosome enables the patient to have X-linked recessive disorders, such as Duchenne muscular dystrophy.

Children with Turner syndrome are treated with growth hormone through adolescence, which results in a modest increase in growth velocity and final height from an average of 140 cm (55 in.) to just under 149 cm (58.5 in.) (322, 323). Limb lengthening is associated with a very high rate of complications, and is therefore not recommended (324). Cyclic sex hormones are administered during adolescence and throughout adulthood. Estrogen is necessary for the development of secondary sexual characteristics, and the estrogens, and possibly the previously administered growth hormone, help prevent osteoporosis. Many with Turner syndrome marry, and obstetric techniques of hormone supplementation and ovum transplantation can result in pregnancy.

Noonan Syndrome. Although Noonan syndrome is not caused by a chromosomal abnormality, its phenotype is reminiscent of Turner syndrome, with short stature, webbed neck, cubitus valgus, and sexual immaturity (325, 326), which is why it is discussed here. Noonan syndrome is an autosomal dominant disorder, in which approximately half of all cases are caused by a mutation in the *PTPN11* gene, which encodes for a protein—tyrosine phosphatase (327–329). How tyrosine phosphatase causes the observed phenotype has yet to be elucidated. The incidence is between 1 in 1000 and 1 in 2500 (330). Many clinical features are shared with the Turner phenotype, but what distinguishes this syndrome are the normal gonads, a high incidence of mental retardation, and right-sided congenital heart defects, often with hypertrophic cardiomyopathy (331, 332). Scoliosis is more common (40%) than in patients with Turner syndrome, and more severe (333, 334). Minor to major vertebral abnormalities may be seen on radiographs. Skeletal maturation is delayed despite normal puberty and menarche. There is short stature, and the use of growth hormone may be associated with a modest increase in ultimate height (305); however, there are no well-controlled comparative series on the basis of which to evaluate the use of growth hormone in these children. Noonan syndrome is often misdiagnosed, and most frequently confused with King-Denborough syndrome, a myopathic arthrogryposis syndrome characterized by short stature, web neck, spinal deformity, and contractures. Recognizing the difference is important, because a malignant hyperthermia-like picture is part of the King-Denborough syndrome. The use of genetic testing for *PTPN11* mutations may aid in this differentiation.

Trichorhinophalangeal Syndrome. The name *trichorhinophalangeal* (TRP) *syndrome* causes confusion, because textbooks describe trichorhinophalangeal syndrome, trichorhinophalangeal syndrome with exostosis, and Langer-Giedion syndrome. It is best to think of two relatively distinct TRP syndromes: types I and II. Despite the clinical overlaps between the two, there are enough features to separate them into distinct syndromes.

Patients with TRP-I have a pear-shaped, bulbous nose, prominent ears, sparse hair, and cone epiphyses. They have mild growth retardation. The thumbs are broad, and the fingers are often angled at the distal interphalangeal and proximal interphalangeal joints. The hips mimic a Perthes-like disease in radiographs and symptoms (306). There may be lax ligaments.

The key feature distinguishing TRP-II from TRP-I is the presence of multiple exostoses, especially involving the lower extremities. Those with TRP-II have facial features and cone epiphyses similar to patients with TRP-I. There is a higher chance of mental retardation in TRP-II. Langer-Giedion syndrome and TRP-II are identical (307). Patients with TRP-II also have microcephaly, large and protruding ears, a bulbous nose, and sparse scalp hair. In infancy, their skin is redundant and loose, and this condition may be severe enough to mimic EDS. Marked ligamentous laxity may further support this error in diagnosis. There is a tendency toward fractures. Similar to TRP-I, the Perthes-like picture, as well as the hand anomalies, are present in TRP-II (335).

Both TRP-I and TRP-II are due to mutation or loss of the *TRSP1* gene (307). However, TRP-II is due to a larger loss of the chromosomal region, with loss of the adjacent gene, *EXT-1*, as well. The *EXT-1* gene is one of the genes responsible for hereditary exostoses, and this explains the exostoses associated with TRP-II. The *TRSP1* gene is responsible for the facial malformation and cone epiphyses present in both disorders. Individuals with loss of a large portion of a chromosome are more likely to have mental retardation. This explains the mental retardation in some patients with TRP-II, which is characterized by a larger region of chromosomal deletion. TRP-II is one of the few disorders actually known to be due to two contiguous genes (5).

Radiographically, the hand of a patient with TRP-I or TRP-II shows short fourth and fifth metacarpals, cone epiphyses, a short and broad thumb, and fingers with angled proximal and distal interphalangeal joints (336) (Fig. 8-29). The cone epiphyses, so characteristic of this syndrome, are not seen until after 3 or 4 years of age. The pelvis shows the unilateral or bilateral changes of Perthes in TRP-I and TRP-II, but rather than resolution, the Perthes-like picture persists, evolving into a pattern more like multiple epiphyseal dysplasia with precocious arthritis (Fig. 8-30). Despite the wealth of radiographic abnormalities, the hands rarely have functional disturbances. Osteotomy of the thumb is occasionally needed. If symptomatic, we recommend managing the hips as in symptomatic Perthes, but there is insufficient information available about outcomes. Occasionally, an exostosis may be large or symptomatic enough to require excision.

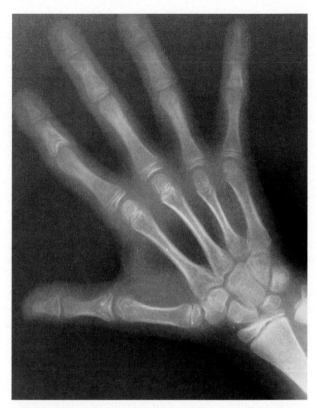

FIGURE 8-29. Trichorhinophalangeal syndrome. This 11-year-old patient has cone- or chevron-shaped epiphyses in the hand, and a broad thumb and distal phalanx.

Prader-Willi Syndrome. Prader-Willi syndrome is characterized by hypotonia, obesity, hypogonadism, short stature, small hands and feet, and mental deficiency (337–339). The incidence is 1 in 5000 births. As newborns, those with Prader-Willi syndrome are floppy babies, having hypotonia, poor feeding, and delayed milestones (340). The symptoms may mimic those of infants with spinal muscular atrophy. Approximately 10% of infants have developmental dysplasia of the hip. The syndrome may be remembered with an "H" mnemonic: hypotonia, hypogonadism, hyperphagia, hypomentation, and small hands, all probably based on a hypothalamic disorder.

After 1 or 2 years of age, a different clinical picture appears (341). A characteristic face of upward-slanting, almond-shaped eyes becomes apparent (Fig. 8-31). Obesity begins, and a Prader-Willi diagnosis is usually suspected because of the onset of a voracious eating disorder. The patient has a preoccupation with food and an insatiable appetite (342, 343). Obesity has a central distribution, sparing the distal limbs. Complex behavioral modification programs are occasionally effective. Affected individuals have short stature, below the 10th percentile, with an ultimate height of 150 cm (59 in.). There is no adolescent growth spurt. The genitalia are hypoplastic, and the patient has small hands and feet (344). Mental retardation is present, but it is extremely variable (342, 345).

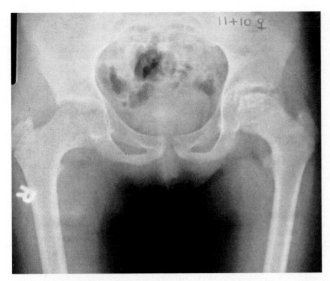

FIGURE 8-30. Trichorhinophalangeal syndrome, type I. The changes mimic Legg-Perthes disease, but by 12 years of age they did not resolve. On the right is a small but spherical epiphysis. On the left, the changes are similar to those seen in Perthes disease and in multiple epiphyseal dysplasia.

Prader-Willi syndrome is caused by a deletion of a small part of chromosome 15 (15q11–13) of paternal origin (346, 347). This is an example of genomic imprinting, because only missing DNA from the father causes the syndrome (348). Genomic imprinting is a process by which genes of maternal origin have different effects from genes

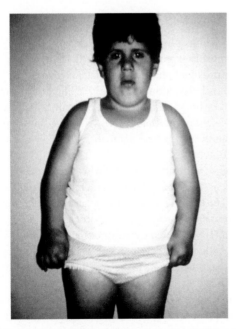

FIGURE 8-31. Prader-Willi syndrome in a 7-year-old patient. The features include truncal obesity and a round face with almond-shaped eyes. (From Goldberg MJ. *The dysmorphic child: an orthopedic perspective.* New York, NY: Raven Press, 1987, with permission.)

of paternal origin. Angelman syndrome, or happy puppet syndrome, is phenotypically dissimilar to Prader-Willi syndrome. Angelman syndrome patients are small and mentally retarded, and they have athetosis and seizures. However, they have the exact chromosome deletion that occurs in Prader-Willi syndrome (15q11–13), except that the deleted DNA is of maternal origin (347).

Several series show that growth hormone improves body composition, fat utilization, and physical strength and agility and as well as growth (286, 349, 350). Despite this information, decisions about the use of growth hormone in this condition are confounded by reports of deaths of children with Prader-Willi syndrome who were given growth hormone. However, it is not known whether these deaths were actually related to growth hormone, or whether the children succumbed to other manifestations of the syndrome (351, 352).

The most significant orthopaedic problem is juvenile-onset scoliosis, which affects roughly half of patients (Fig. 8-32) (353). It is difficult to control with an orthosis because of the truncal fat (354–357). Children with kyphosis associated with scoliosis have a higher change of requiring surgery (353), Those who come to surgery have a higher anesthesia risk because of morbid obesity (358), and there is a higher complication rate to surgery itself (312). While growth hormone was thought to cause worsening of scoliosis progression, a recent randomized trial shows that this is not the case, and as such one should not use the presence of scoliosis as a rationale to avoid growth hormone treatment (286). While a number of other orthopaedic conditions are reported, genu valgum and pes planus are reported most commonly. These have limited or no effect on functional health and physical performance, and as such does not require intervention. While hip dysplasia is present at a higher rate than in the general population, SCFE is not, intriguingly suggesting that endocrinopathy and excess weight alone is not enough to cause a slip of the proximal femoral epiphysis (313).

Rubinstein-Taybi Syndrome. The Rubinstein-Taybi syndrome is characterized by mental retardation associated with characteristic digital changes, consisting mainly of broad thumbs and large toes (359). It is relatively common among mentally retarded persons, with an incidence of 1 in 500 (327). Most cases are sporadic, although there is the possibility of autosomal dominant inheritance (328).

One of the most characteristic clinical features is a Cyrano de Bergerac–like nose with the nasal septum extending below the nostrils (Fig. 8-33). These facial characteristics may change with time, making this a less reliable finding (329). Broad terminal phalanges of the thumb are present in 87% of patients, and the great toe is affected in all patients. One-half of the patients have radially angulated thumbs, and this causes disability. Hallux varus is common, and the physician should consider Rubinstein-Taybi syndrome whenever congenital hallux varus is encountered. Patients have ligamentous laxity and pronated feet, and an increased incidence of fractures (327).

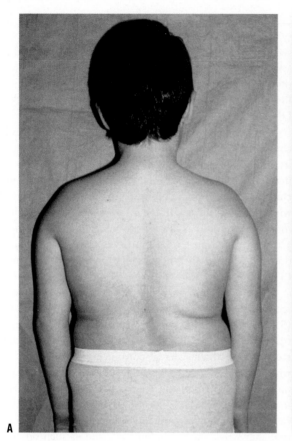 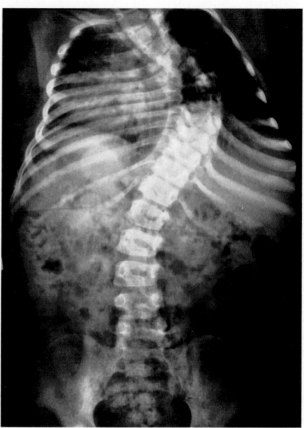

FIGURE 8-32.   Prader-Willi syndrome in a 6-year-old patient. **A:** Scoliosis is difficult to detect because of the truncal obesity. **B:** The roentgenogram of this patient discloses a 50-degree thoracic curve. (**B** from Goldberg MJ. *The dysmorphic child: an orthopedic perspective.* New York, NY: Raven Press, 1987, with permission.)

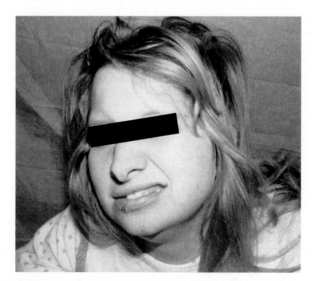

FIGURE 8-33.   Rubinstein-Taybi syndrome. In a 10-year-old girl, the characteristic Cyrano de Bergerac–like nose has a septum that extends below the nostrils.

The radiographs are rather characteristic. The thumb shows a wide distal phalanx, with soft-tissue hypertrophy and a triangular proximal phalanx (i.e., delta phalanx) that accounts for the radial deviation (Fig. 8-34). The toe demonstrates duplicated or broad distal phalanx, but true polydactyly is not part of this syndrome (Fig. 8-34B). There is an assortment of other insignificant skeletal anomalies, many in the axial skeleton (360).

Patients with Rubinstein-Taybi syndrome have been shown to have breakpoints in, and microdeletions of, chromosome 16p13.3. This region contains the gene for CREB-binding protein, a nuclear protein participating as a coactivator in cyclic-AMP–regulated gene expression. This protein plays an important role in the development of the central nervous system, head, and neck, and this explains the facial malformation and mental retardation associated with this syndrome. The propensity to develop tumors in these regions is probably caused by malregulation of cyclic-AMP–regulated gene expression (361).

Birth weight and size are normal, but growth retardation is noticed at the end of the first year, and there is no true pubertal growth spurt (362). The patients are mentally retarded, many with microcephaly. IQ can range from 35 to 80, with a delay in acquiring skills. However, these features vary. Associated

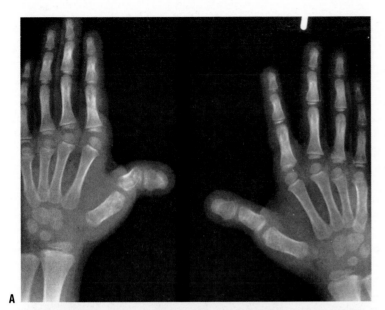

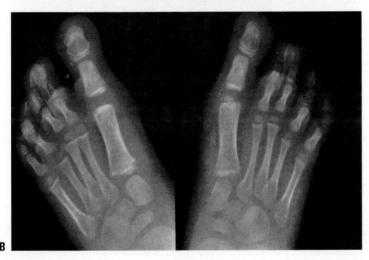

FIGURE 8-34. Rubinstein-Taybi syndrome in a 7-year-old patient. **A:** The thumbs are malformed, with a trapezoid proximal phalanx. The epiphysis extends around the radial side. **B:** The feet are more symmetric. Notice the broadening of the distal phalanx of the great toe. (From Goldberg MJ. *The dysmorphic child: an orthopedic perspective.* New York, NY: Raven Press, 1987, with permission.)

medical problems include visual disturbances, congenital heart disease, and gastrointestinal abnormalities. Later in life, frequent upper respiratory infections are related to abnormal craniofacial features, severe dental caries are common, and other infections lead to morbidity (363–365). Individuals with this syndrome are predisposed to certain types of central nervous system and head and neck tumors (366).

The thumb is treated if the radial deviation interferes with pinch, in which case osteotomy of the proximal phalanx should be performed. The deformity is progressive, and recurrence is common, as with any delta phalanx. The toe rarely requires treatment unless there is a significant congenital hallux varus. Patellar dislocation occurs in this syndrome. Although reports suggest that early surgical intervention might improve function, there are no data comparing early surgical treatment with other managements to support this concept. If surgery is performed, the addition of an extensive quadriceps mobilization seems to decrease the revision rate (367, 368). We reserve surgical intervention for the patella dislocation for symptomatic cases, or for cases in which the dislocation is clearly interfering

with a patient's ability to function. There can be cervical spinal abnormalities, including upper cervical instability and stenosis (322). The mental retardation may mask underlying neurologic problems related to the cervical spine, or to other conditions, such as a tethered cord (323).

Approximately one-third of patients have structural or conductive heart defects. Patients are sensitive to many anesthesia drugs, including neuromuscular blocking agents, which tend to induce arrhythmias and prolong awakening from anesthesia (369, 370). Keloid formation is common (371).

PROTEIN PROCESSING GENES (ENZYMES)

Enzymes modify molecules or other proteins. They often modify substances for degradation, and cause cell dysfunction when mutated because of the accumulation of these substances. Mutations in genes that encode for enzymes can have a wide variety of effects on cells, resulting in a broad range of abnormalities in cell function and a wide range of clinical findings. Many of these disorders result in the excess accumulation of proteins in cells. In these cases, the cells become larger than normal. This results in increased pressure in bones, causing avascular necrosis, and in increased extradural material in the spine, potentially causing paralysis. Multiple systems are almost always involved in these disorders. Medical treatments to replace the defective enzyme have been developed for many of these disorders, and such treatments will often arrest, but not reverse, the skeletal manifestations of the disorder. Early diagnosis and appropriate medical treatment are slowly decreasing the number of these individuals who present to orthopaedists with musculoskeletal problems. Most enzyme disorders are inherited in an autosomal recessive manner.

Mucopolysaccharidoses. This group of genetic disorders is characterized by excretion of mucopolysaccharide in the urine (372). There are at least 13 types (Table 8-4). The mild-to-severe mucopolysaccharidoses (MPS) have similar radiographs and different clinical features, but each produces a particular sugar in the urine because of a specific enzyme defect (372, 373). Changes in the naming and numbering of systems over the years have introduced considerable confusion in understanding the MPS. The incidence is 1 in 10,000.

The patients have somewhat thickened and coarse facial features and short stature, and many develop stiff joints (Fig. 8-35), especially in the hands. Stiffness is postulated to be the result of the deposition of mucopolysaccharide in the capsule and periarticular structures, and is thought to reflect the loss of joint congruity. Radiographs reveal oval vertebral

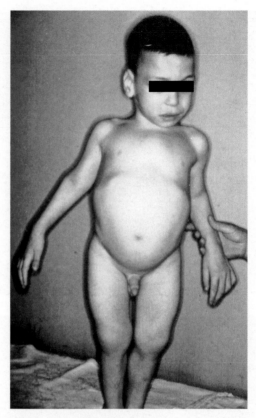

FIGURE 8-35. The classic appearance of a mucopolysaccharidosis in a 3-year-old patient includes facial features that are mildly coarsened, an abdominal protuberance from an enlarged spleen and liver, a short trunk, and stiff interphalangeal joints of the fingers.

TABLE 8-4	Mucopolysaccharidoses				
Designation	**Name**	**Enzyme Defect**	**Stored Substance**	**Inheritance Pattern**
MPS I	Hurler/Scheie	α-L-iduronidase	HS + DS	Autosomal recessive
MPS II	Hunter	Iduronidase-2-sulfatase	HS + DS	X-linked recessive
MPS IIIA	Sanfilippo A	Heparin-sulfatase (sulfamidase)	HS	Autosomal recessive
MPS IIIB	Sanfilippo B	α-N-acetylglucosamidase	HS	Autosomal recessive
MPS IIIC	Sanfilippo C	Acetyl-CoA: α-glucosaminide-N-acetyltransferase	HS	Autosomal recessive
MPS IIID	Sanfilippo D	Glucosamine-6-sulfatase	HS	Autosomal recessive
MPS IVA	Morquio A	N-acetyl galactosamine-6-sulfate sulfatase	KS, CS	Autosomal recessive
MPS IVB	Morquio B	β-D-galactosidase	KS	Autosomal recessive
MPS IVC	Morquio C	Unknown	KS	Autosomal recessive
MPS V	Formerly Scheie disease, no longer used			
MPS VI	Maroteaux-Lamy	Arylsulfatase B, N-acetylgalactosamine-4-sulfatase	DS, CS	Autosomal recessive
MPS VII	Sly	β-D-glucuronidase	CS, HS, DS	Autosomal recessive
MPS VIII		Glucosamine-6-sulfatase	CS, HS	Autosomal recessive

MPS, mucopolysaccharidoses; HS, heparan sulfate; DS, dermatan sulfate; KS, keratin sulfate; CS, chondroitin sulfate.

bodies that are often beaked anteriorly; a pelvis with wide, flat ilia; capacious acetabuli; unossified femoral head cartilage; and coxa valga. The radiographic and clinical features are usually not apparent at birth, but become more apparent as the child gets older. Thus, it may be difficult to diagnose a mucopolysaccharidosis during the first year of life.

All the MPS are autosomal recessive except for mucopolysaccharidosis type II (Hunter syndrome), which is X-linked. The most common MPS are type I (Hurler syndrome) and type IV (Morquio syndrome).

The MPS can be diagnosed by urine screening, using a toluidine blue-spot test. If the initial results are positive, specific blood testing is done for the associated sugar abnormality. Although spot tests are quick and inexpensive, they have high false-positive and high false-negative rates. They are the initial tests that are often obtained before molecular genetic analyses.

The pathobiologic mechanisms are similar for all the MPS. Each has a deficiency of a specific lysosomal enzyme that degrades the sulfated glycosamine glycans: heparan sulfate, dermatan sulfate, keratan sulfate, and chondroitin sulfate. The incomplete degradation product accumulates in the lysozymes themselves. The MPS are part of a larger group of disorders known as the *lysosomal storage diseases*. The incomplete product accumulates in the tissues such as the brain, the viscera, and the joints. This unremitting process leads to the clinical progression of the disease. The child is normal at birth, but a problem may be chemically detectable by 6 to 12 months of age, and clinical progression is apparent by 2 years of age. This accumulation is responsible for the development of avascular necrosis, presumably because of too much material in the intramedullary space, and also contributes to spinal cord compressive symptoms, because of accumulation of material in the spinal canal.

Mucopolysaccharidosis Type I. MPS type I is the clinical prototype. It is characterized by a deficiency of L-iduronidase, the enzyme that degrades dermatan sulfate and heparan sulfate. The Hurler and Scheie forms represent the severe and mild ends of the clinical spectrum in MPS I. Children with the Hurler form have progressive mental retardation, severe, multiple skeletal deformities, and considerable organ and soft-tissue deformities, and die before the age of 10 years. The Scheie form is characterized by stiffness of the joints and corneal clouding, but no mental retardation; the diagnosis is usually made at approximately 15 years of age, and the patient has a normal life expectancy. Many patients with MPS I fall in the middle of this clinical spectrum. The clinical variation is determined by the location and the type of mutation that occurs along the gene for L-iduronidase (374, 375).

Marrow transplantation is used in the treatment of the more severe forms (Hurler syndrome). However, the results on the bones are variable (376), with most children still developing the typical skeletal phenotypic features despite undergoing successful bone marrow transplant (377, 378).

This may be due to the poor penetration of the enzyme derived from the transplanted leukocytes to the osseous cells or to other not completely understood functions of the protein in osteoblasts and chondrocytes (305, 376). There is an initial improvement, or at least an arrest in progression of the nonosseous neurologic manifestations of the disease with marrow transplant. Some longer term studies cast doubt on the long-term effectiveness of marrow transplantation (379). Despite these disappointing longer term reports, marrow transplant may provide short-term improvement, especially in the nonosseous manifestations, and children treated with bone marrow transplantation have a good ambulatory ability (307). It also may be that earlier marrow transplantation will result in better neural function. The musculoskeletal deformities that persist after marrow transplant still require treatment (335).

Malalignment of the limbs can occur, and guided growth techniques, or osteotomies, may be necessary for genu valgum (380). Osteotomies may be associated with recurrence, and as such guided growth approaches are an attractive alternative, however, comparative series are lacking in the literature. Approximately one-fourth of the patients have an abnormality of the upper cervical spine. Odontoid hypoplasia and a soft-tissue mass in the canal can be managed like those in Morquio syndrome (described in the following text). The accumulation of degradation products in closed anatomic spaces, such as the carpal tunnel, causes "triggering" of the fingers and the carpal tunnel syndrome. These can be managed operatively (381, 382).

Mucopolysaccharidosis Type IV. Between 1929 and 1959, there was a miscellany of skeletal diseases described as *Morquio syndrome*, including several types of spondyloepiphyseal dysplasia. Morquio syndrome is an autosomal recessive disorder with an incidence of 3 per 1,000,000 of the population. Three types of Morquio syndrome are classified as subtypes of MPS IV. All are caused by enzyme defects involved in the degradation of keratan sulfate (372–374).

Patients with severe classic MPS IVA are short-trunked dwarfs, although they appear normal at birth. They develop corneal opacities. The bone dysplasia is radiographically obvious, and the final height is <125 cm (50 in.). Patients have abnormal dentition. The deficient enzyme is N-acetylgalactosamine-6-sulfate sulfatase, and the chromosomal defect occurs at 16q24.3 (383). Patients with intermediate MPS IVB have the same but milder phenotypes as those with type IVA. They are taller, with final heights >125 cm (50 in.), and they have normal dentition. Here, the enzyme defect is β-D-galactosidase. Patients with mild MPS IVC have very mild clinical manifestations.

The three forms of Morquio MPS IV can be distinguished by the severity of symptoms and the patient's age at detection. All these patients are normal at birth. For patients with the severe type IVA, the diagnosis is made between 1 and 3 years of age; those with the mild type IVC are diagnosed as teens, and those with the intermediate form (type IVB) are diagnosed somewhere in the middle of this age range. The three forms may also be separated by the severity of the radiographic changes.

Intelligence is normal in patients of all of the MPS IV types, and only rarely are the facial features coarsened. Similarly, all are short-trunked dwarfs with ligamentous laxity; the laxity is rather profound in MPS IVA. The degree of genu valgus is significant, aggravated by the lax ligaments (384–387).

Management of the knee proves difficult because of the osseous malalignment and the lax ligaments. Although it is observed that the fingers and joints are becoming stiff, the medial and lateral instability of the knee remains. Realignment osteotomies can restore plumb alignment, but recurrence may occur, and osteomies may not control the instability during ambulation. The prophylactic use of braces to prevent initial valgus or recurrent deformity after surgery has not been effective (384–387). Guided growth is an attractive alternative to osteomies, avoiding issues of recurrence, but comparative studies are lacking. The hips and knees develop early arthritis. The hips show a progressive acetabular dysplasia. Radiographs may show a small femoral ossific nucleus, but an MRI or arthrogram will show a much larger cartilaginous femoral head. The femoral capital epiphyses are initially advanced for the patient's age, but between 4 and 9 years of age, the femoral heads grow smaller and then disappear altogether (Fig. 8-36). The pathophysiology of the progressive hip disease is not completely understood, and neither medication nor surgery has been shown to improve the prognosis (384–387). Patients may require total joint replacement surgery (388).

Odontoid hypoplasia or aplasia is common, with resultant C1–C2 instability (389–392) (Fig. 8-36). There is a soft-tissue mass in the spinal canal, contributing to cord compression (393, 394). This soft-tissue mass can make the space available for the cord smaller than one would expect on the basis of radiographs alone. Neurologic function, especially upper extremity strength and tone, is probably more important than measuring distances on dynamic cervical spine films. The upper and lower extremity findings are often of flaccidity rather than spasticity. The onset of the myelopathy can occur as early as the first decade of life, progressing as the soft-tissue hypertrophies, with the C1–C2 instabilities aggravating the situation. Sudden deaths of patients with Morquio disease have been reported, and they are typically attributed to the C1–C2 subluxation. C1–C2 fusion before the onset of symptoms is controversial, but promoted by some (393, 395). Others think the best surgery is occipital cervical fusion because it reduces the anterior soft-tissue mass (394, 395). There are no comparative studies evaluating the outcomes of each of the different management approaches. On the basis of the available information, it is reasonable to obtain MRI studies on symptomatic individuals, or on those with radiographic evidence of instability. C1–C2 fusions are recommended for asymptomatic individuals with MRI evidence of cord compression. Symptomatic individuals should have fusions throughout the region of instability and cord

compression. Although decompression is usually performed along with the fusion, anecdotal evidence suggests that fusion alone may be sufficient, resulting in the soft-tissue mass decreasing in size.

Elsewhere in the spine, the vertebrae show a progressive platyspondylia with a thoracic kyphosis. Progressive deformity should be surgically stabilized. Anterior instrumentation is an effective surgical technique (396). Despite these problems, many patients with Morquio disease live for decades. Cardiorespiratory disease is common, but the problems at the upper cervical spine account for most disabilities.

SYNDROMES OF UNKNOWN ETIOLOGY

Hadju-Cheney Syndrome. Hadju-Cheney syndrome, also called *arthrodentosteodysplasia*, consists of acroosteolysis, with osteoporosis and hypoplastic changes in the skull and the mandible. The osteoporosis leads to multiple fractures of the skull, spine, and digits. The cranial sutures persist; wormian bones are seen on the skull radiographs. Basilar impression is a common finding, often requiring operative intervention. The terminal digits exhibit gradual loss of bone mass, sometimes called *pseudoosteolysis*. Patients tend to have deep voices (397–401).

Orthopaedic manifestations include loose-jointedness, patellar dislocations, scoliosis, frequent fractures, and basilar impression (402). The basilar invagination can cause hydrocephalus and an Arnold-Chiari malformation (403). This is usually managed by decompression and an occiput-to-upper-cervical-spine fusion (Fig. 8-37). Not much data are available on the management of other musculoskeletal problems. Scoliosis can be managed as in idiopathic scoliosis, although the underlying osteopenia and associated spinal fractures may make nonoperative management more difficult. The use of bisphosphonate therapy to treat the osteopenia has been reported (404), although it is not known whether this therapy will improve the clinical outcome for children with this disorder.

Polycystic kidney disease and cardiac valvular disease are reported in some Haju-Cheney patients, and thus cardiac and renal functions should be evaluated before placing the patients under anesthesia (405, 406). The disorder can be inherited in an autosomal dominant manner, but the causative gene is unknown.

Progeria. Progeria (Hutchinson-Gilford syndrome) is the best known of many syndromes characterized by premature aging. It is exceedingly rare, with fewer than 30 affected children in North America. The cause is entirely unknown. Autosomal dominant (407) and autosomal recessive (408) inheritance patterns have been proposed, but a sporadic mutation is more likely (409).

These individuals have low levels of growth hormones, and hormone supplementation will increase growth velocity, but not result in improved survival (410). The cause of the

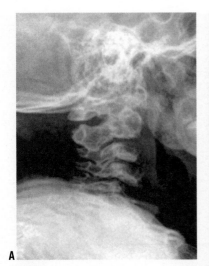

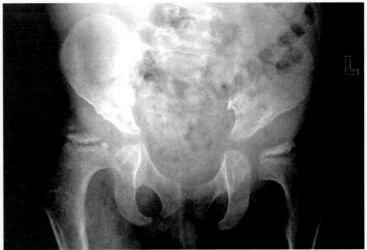

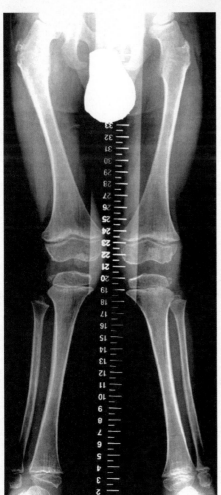

FIGURE 8-36. Morquio syndrome. The radiographic features include an absent odontoid **(A)**, a pelvis with capacious acetabuli and coxa valga **(B)**, and marked platyspondyly **(C)**. It is difficult to imagine that these vertebrae were normal at birth. Genu varum is common.

condition is not known, but a number of reports refer to the use of tissues from these patients in studying the aging process. Fibroblasts from tissue cultures derived from these individuals show a variety of abnormalities, including a decreased ability to clear free radicals (411).

Children with progeria are diagnosed between 1 and 2 years of age by their clinical features alone. There is severe growth retardation and an inability to gain weight. If there is survival to adolescence, there is no pubertal growth spurt. Alopecia and a loss of subcutaneous fat are dramatic, and

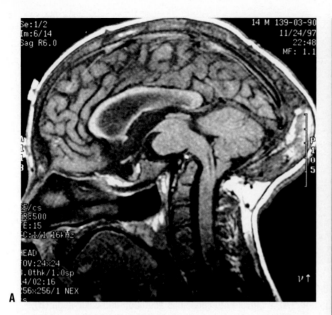

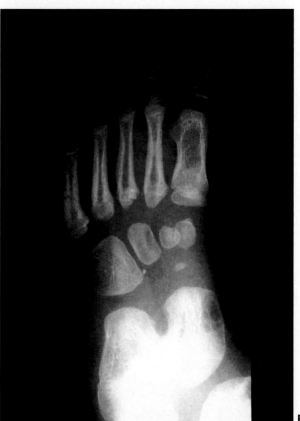

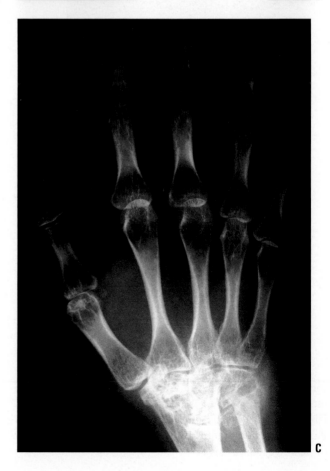

FIGURE 8-37. Hadju-Cheney syndrome. **A:** MRI of the head shows marked basilar invagination with an associated syrinx in the cervical cord. **B:** Radiographs show osteoporosis with pathologic fractures. **C:** Loss of bone mass in the terminal digits, termed *pseudoosteolysis*.

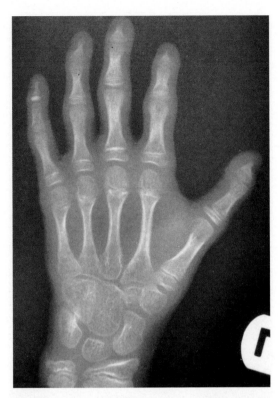

FIGURE 8-38. Progeria. The radiograph shows distal acrolysis, with resorption of the distal phalanges. (From Goldberg MJ. *The dysmorphic child: an orthopedic perspective.* New York, NY: Raven Press, 1987, with permission.)

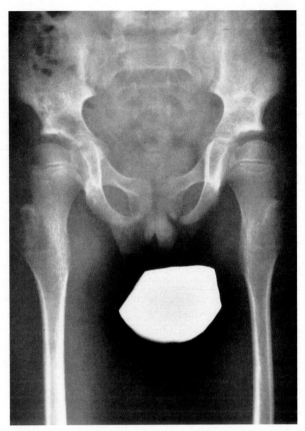

FIGURE 8-39. Progeria in an 11-year-old patient. The radiograph shows a marked degree of coxa valgus and some femoral head uncovering.

account for the distinctive appearance of a skinny old man or woman (412, 413). These patients have stiffness of the joints that is not arthritis, but a periarticular fibrosis. Osteolysis occurs in the fingertips, clavicle, and proximal humerus (407, 414, 415) (Fig. 8-38). The vertebrae may become osteopenic, creating fish-mouth vertebral bodies on radiographs (416–418). Fractures are common, often with delayed union. There is late developmental dysplasia of the hip, and the onset of a rather significant coxa valga (419, 420) (Fig. 8-39). The children do not live long enough to develop arthritis secondary to the acetabular dysplasia. Not all systems age. There are no cataracts; there is no senility. Rather than actually aging, the normal tissues undergo an atrophic or a degenerative change that mimics normal aging. The principal histopathologic atrophic changes occur in the skin, subcutaneous tissue, bone, and cardiovascular system. Atherosclerosis with myocardial infarction by 10 years of age is the rule, and life expectancy rarely exceeds 20 years.

The children show vitality until they are struck down by myocardial infarction. Despite a short life, it is imperative not to permit any suffering. Hip surgery is indicated only if there is a documented functional impairment. Surgery is not indicated to prevent future arthritis. There is no medical treatment for the basic disease process.

CONTRACTURE SYNDROMES

Although contractures are a common feature in a variety of orthopaedic conditions ranging from neuromuscular disorders to the sequelae of injury, there are several disorders in which contractures are the most prominent phenotypic feature. These syndromes are caused by a wide variety of etiologies, including mutations causing developmental problems, mutations dysregulating muscle function, and fetal environmental causes. Many of these are associated with problems in muscle function, as in the case of distal arthrogryposis, which is caused by mutations disrupting fast-twitch muscle fiber activity; there is some overlap in phenotype between these conditions and some of the myopathies. There are many such disorders of different etiologies but, because the management for many of these disorders follows similar guidelines, they are considered together in this chapter.

Arthrogryposis. Arthrogryposis is really a physical finding, not a diagnosis, and represents a large group of disorders, all of which include contractures of joints present at birth. The contracted joints lack skin creases. Since joint creases develop in the intrauterine environment, this clinical finding indicates that a congenital etiology to the contracture. *Arthrogryposis* is used as a noun to describe specific diseases, and as an adjective, *arthrogrypotic* to refer to rigid joint contractures. There are at close to 100 distinct syndromes coded under the term *arthrogryposis* in the OMIM (5), illustrating the large variety of etiologies associated with this term. Most of the syndromes have different clinical courses, prognoses, genetics, causes, and pathologic processes, often making it difficult for the orthopaedist to determine the management of an individual patient (421, 422). A simple way to think about these disorders is to consider them as contracture syndromes, which can be grouped into a few general categories, each of which can be represented by a prototypic disease.

Contracture syndrome groups:

1. Involving all four extremities. This includes arthrogryposis multiplex congenita and Larsen syndrome, with more or less total body involvement.
2. Predominantly or exclusively involving the hands and feet. These are the distal arthrogryposes. Facial involvement can occur with some of these syndromes, and Freeman-Sheldon whistling face is included.
3. Pterygia syndromes in which identifiable skin webs cross the flexion aspects of the knees, elbows, and other joints. Multiple pterygias and popliteal pterygia fit into this group.

Contracture Syndromes Involving All Four Extremities

Arthrogryposis Multiplex Congenita. Arthrogryposis multiplex congenita is the best known of the multiple congenital contracture syndromes (423, 424). Although attempts have been made to change the name *arthrogryposis multiplex congenita* to *multiple congenital contractures* or *amyoplasia* (AMP), the popularity of *arthrogryposis* remains.

The etiology of arthrogryposis multiplex congenita is unknown. It was initially described in 1841 by Adolf Wilhelm Otto, who referred to his patient as a "human wonder with curved limbs" (425). The disorder is sporadic, with affected individuals having reproduced only normal children. Classic arthrogryposis can affect only one of identical twins (426, 427). The development of arthrogryposis may be influenced by an adverse intrauterine factor or the twinning process itself. Teratogens have been suggested, but none are proven, despite the multiple animal models that lend support to that theory (428–432). Some mothers of children with arthrogryposis have serum antibodies that inhibit fetal acetylcholine receptor function. One possibility is that maternal antibodies to these fetal antigens cause the disorder (433).

Histologic analysis discloses a small muscle mass with fibrosis and fat between the muscle fibers. Myopathic and neuropathic features are often found in the same muscle biopsy specimen. The periarticular soft-tissue structures are fibrotic and, in essence, there is a fibrous ankylosis. The number of anterior horn cells in the spinal cord is decreased, without an increase in the number of microglial cells (434–436). The pattern of motor neuron loss in specific spinal cord segments correlates with the peripheral deformities and the affected muscles, suggesting that a primary central nervous system disorder plays an important role in causing this condition (437).

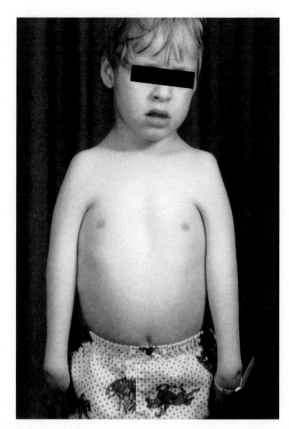

FIGURE 8-40. Arthrogryposis multiplex congenita. The picture shows the classic limb position and fusiform limbs lacking flexion creases.

Clinical examination remains the best way to establish a diagnosis. The limbs are striking in appearance and position (Fig. 8-40). They are featureless and tubular. Normal skin creases are lacking, but there may be deep dimples over the joints. Muscle mass is reduced, although in infancy there is often abundant subcutaneous tissue. Typically, the shoulders are adducted and internally rotated, the elbow more often extended than flexed, and the wrist flexed severely, with ulnar deviation. The fingers are flexed, clutching the thumb. In the lower extremities, the hips are flexed, abducted, and externally rotated; the knees are typically in extension, although flexion is possible; clubfeet are the rule. Motion of the joints is restricted. The condition is pain-free, with a firm, inelastic block to movement beyond a very limited range. In two-thirds of the patients, all four limbs are affected equally, but in one-third, lower limb deformities predominate. Only on rare occasions do the upper extremities predominate. Deformities tend to be more severe and more rigid distally. The hips may be dislocated unilaterally or bilaterally.

The viscera are usually spared from malformations, although gastroschisis has been reported. As a consequence of the general muscle weakness, there is a 15% incidence of inguinal hernia. Major feeding difficulties, caused by a stiff jaw and an immobile tongue, are frequently encountered in infancy, and lead to respiratory infections and failure to thrive (389). The face is not particularly dysmorphic. A few subtle

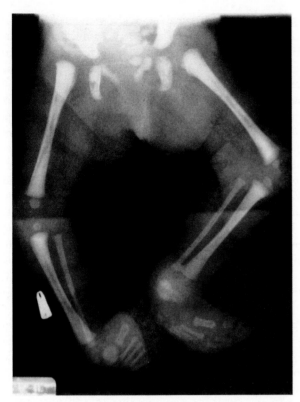

FIGURE 8-41. Arthrogryposis multiplex congenita at birth. Features include clubfeet, knee-flexion deformity, and dislocated right hip. The articular surfaces are normal. Adaptive changes occur as a consequence of the fixed position. (From Goldberg MJ. *The dysmorphic child: an orthopedic perspective.* New York, NY: Raven Press, 1987, with permission.)

features, such as a small jaw, narrowing of the face and, occasionally, limited upward gaze (secondary to ocular muscle involvement). A frontal midline hemangioma may help with the diagnosis (Fig. 8-40).

Radiographs early in life reveal that the joints are normal and that changes are adaptive and acquired over time as a consequence of their fixed position (Fig. 8-41) (390). There is evidence of a loss of subcutaneous fat and tissue. Electromyograms and muscle biopsies are of questionable diagnostic value. A diagnosis of arthrogryposis can be suspected when prenatal ultrasound detects an absence of fetal movement, especially if seen in combination with polyhydramnios (391).

The natural history and long-term outcomes are not well known (392, 438), although children with this condition are substantially less active than others of the same age (439). Some contractures seem to worsen with age, and the joints become stiffer. No new joints become involved. At least 25% of affected patients are nonambulatory, and many others are limited household walkers (440). As a rule, those with arthrogryposis who are very weak as infants stay weak, and those who appear stronger as infants stay strong. The dependency of adults seems to be related to education and coping skills more than to the magnitude of contractures of the joints.

Treatment.   Each of the multiple joints involved presents its own unique opportunities for orthopaedic intervention, but an overview of the total patient must be borne in mind. The overall goals are lower limb alignment and stability for ambulation, and upper extremity motion for self-care (397–399, 421). Outcomes seem better if surgery on joints is done when children are younger, usually before adaptive intra-articular changes occur at ages 4 to 6. Realignment osteotomies, however, are usually performed closer to the completion of growth. Early motion, and avoidance of prolonged casting, may increase joint mobility, thereby improving function. Many children require long-term bracing or other assistive devices (424).

Contractures of the joints make the birthing process difficult, and neonatal fractures may result (400). Physical therapy should not be initiated in the newborn until such fractures are ruled out (401). Mobilization of joints may be accomplished by early and frequent range of motion exercises and splinting of the joint in a position of function with a removable orthotic (401, 424). There are no studies clearly demonstrating that early mobilization improves outcomes in these patients, but such a program may improve the passive range of motion, although the active range of motion does not improve very much (424). In our experience, early mobilization seems to be useful primarily for the upper extremities. Fractures may accompany an overly vigorous range of motion program.

Approximately two-thirds of patients have developmental dysplasia of the hip or frank dislocation (424, 441–443) (Fig. 8-41). At birth, the hips are flexed and abducted. There is considerable controversy about the management of the hips in these children. Closed reduction is rarely, if ever, successful. Operative reduction of a dislocated hip should be performed if it will improve function or decrease pain. Pain is only rarely are a problem with these hips. There is significant variability in functioning ability in these individuals because of the underlying severity of the disease, and this variability makes it difficult to determine any change in function from treating the hips. The range of motion of the hips may be important for functioning, because hip contractures, especially those that cause flexion deformity, adversely affect the gait pattern. Operative procedures to locate dislocated hips, therefore, have the potential to worsen function if they produce significant contractures (442, 444).

Studies of children with untreated dislocated hips concluded that those with bilateral dislocations frequently had satisfactory range of motion; their hips did not prevent them from walking, although rarely around the community, and pain was uncommon (441, 443, 444). Those with unilateral dislocations fared less well. More of them were limited to the household with walkers, and, although scoliosis was present in most patients, it was worse and more frequent in those with unilateral dislocations (424). In both groups, limitation of ambulation resulted more from the severe involvement of all four extremities than from the dislocated hips (424). These data, and case series suggesting little functional improvement with surgery for bilateral hip dislocations, support the concept of leaving bilaterally dislocated hips alone (424, 441, 442, 444). However, in these studies, hip surgery was delayed until the knees were mobilized, and reductions did not occur until at least 1 year of age. This later age at reduction may be associated with higher rates of contractures and worse function. Reports of early open reduction of unilateral and bilateral dislocated hips, with a reduced period of immobilization, show improved postoperative range of motion (335, 416, 443). Hip reduction is unlikely to benefit the child who is not an ambulator; however, there is no way to comfortably predict which children will become ambulators at the age when early surgical treatment is contemplated. Longer term studies show similar results with both operative and non-operative approaches, and a reduced range of motion in hips that have been surgically relocated. However, the numbers of patients reported in these studies were small (388). It therefore seems reasonable to perform early open reduction in most children. The exception may be a child with hips that are quite stiff. Both medial and anterior approaches are advocated for early hip reduction (445–447). More than the specific operative approach, the key factor may be to perform the hip reduction early in life, with minimal immobilization. While this may be accomplished using a medial approach, we feel that the anterior approach gives a more reliable approach in these teratologic dislocations.

Although the classic description of the knees is that they are hyperextended, most are in flexion (390, 424) (Fig. 8-41). The precise plane of motion may be difficult to determine, and although physical therapy is recommended, medial lateral instability may result. Hyperextension deformity responds better to physical therapy and splinting than do flexion deformities. If the flexion deformity remains more than 30 degrees, ambulation is difficult because of the associated relative weakness of the quadriceps in the ability to extend the knee. Sometime before 2 years of age, soft-tissue surgery, including posterior capsulotomy, and realignment of the quadriceps mechanism, should be performed. The actual procedure needs to be individualized, because each knee has a different degree of deformity. While posterior soft-tissue procedures will initially improve the range of motion and function, the contractures usually recur, along with a loss of motion (448). Soft-tissue releases may thus need to be repeated later in life, but before skeletal maturity. Distraction using an external fixator has also been reported, although even with this approach there is recurrence of the contractures (449, 450). Supracondylar osteotomies of the femur are recommended toward the end of growth to correct residual deformity (428, 451–453). Femoral shortening is a useful addition to the osteotomies, especially in cases where the neurovascular structures will be stretched by correcting the deformity. More recently, a guided growth approach at the distal femoral growth plate has been reported to correct flexion deformity of the knee although the ability of this approach to correct the quadriceps mechanism is unclear (454).

Many hyperextension deformities of the knee can be treated without surgery, but quadricepsplasty may be needed in cases with residual lack of motion. Traditional teaching advocates correction of the knee deformity before treating a dislocated hip, in order to allow stretching out of the muscles that cross both joints. However, with early operative intervention, using a short period of immobilization, the hip may be operated upon at the same time as a surgical procedure to correct a hyperextended knee deformity. In this case, the hamstring muscles are relaxed by both procedures, and the knee can be immobilized in a flexed position in the hip spica cast. A flexion deformity of the knee cannot be easily managed at the same time as hip surgery, because it is impossible to appropriately immobilize the hip with the knee held extended. Despite good initial nonoperative results in the hyperextended knee, there may be recurrence of the contracture over time, with surgery often needed later in life. An alternative technique of correction of the knee deformity is by using an external fixator, with gradual correction (448, 449); however, in most cases, an open procedure to release the contracted structures will be adequate, and the deformity may recur after treatment with gradual distraction. Late osteoarthritis seems more common in those with persistent hyperextension contracture.

A severe clubfoot is characteristic (424, 450, 454) (Fig. 8-41). Traditionally, it was felt that treatment using extensive surgery was necessary to correct the deformity; however, using the Ponseti technique with minor modifications seems to work quite well in many cases. A prolonged period of casting and a second tendo Achilles lengthening may be required (417, 455). In cases that do not respond to early manipulative therapy, circumferential releases are usually performed. While surgery for clubfoot is sometimes delayed until 1 year of age or later, as other joints, especially the knees, are attended to first, combined procedures, with minimal immobilization earlier in life, is gaining in popularity. Although primary talectomy has been recommended because of the high incidence of failed soft-tissue surgery (417, 455), most reports show good outcomes with circumferential release alone if performed before 1 year of age (456, 457), and primary talectomy should probably not be used as an initial approach. The positioning of the calcaneus is the key to achieving a good result after talectomy (457). Residual deformity in the teen years can be treated using a triple arthrodesis, or with multiple osteotomies, to maintain motion of the subtalar joints, while producing a plantigrade foot. Gradual correction using an external fixator is also possible (418), but recurrence after gradual distraction is not unusual. A vertical talus is an unusual foot deformity in arthrogryposis multiplex congenita and, if it is encountered, the physician must think of the distal arthrogryposes or pterygia syndromes.

Most patients do not require upper extremity surgical procedures. The physician should never think of an individual joint in the upper extremity but only of the whole arm (458, 459). Analysis needs to include each hand separately and also how the two hands work together as an effective functional unit; that is, a functional assessment should be made before deciding on an operation. Because of this, surgical procedures on the upper extremity are usually delayed until the children are old enough for the surgeon to make such an assessment. There are two key goals in treatment of the upper extremities: self-help skills, such as feeding and toileting; and mobility skills, such as pushing out of a chair and using crutches.

The shoulder is usually satisfactory without treatment. For the elbow, it is ideal to achieve flexion to 90 degrees from the fixed extended position. However, when both elbows are involved, surgery to increase flexion should be done only on one side. Although the fibrotic joint capsule and the weak muscles make the prospect of achieving active elbow flexion difficult, if an extensive release with triceps lengthening is undertaken, successful improvement in the range of motion is possible (456). Passive elbow flexion to a right angle is a prerequisite for considering a tendon transfer for active elbow flexion (402). The triceps brachii and pectoralis have been the most frequently tried muscles. Success is best in children older than 4 years, and who have at least grade four strength of the muscle to be transferred (460–463). Distal humeral osteotomy, designed to place the elbow into flexion and correct some of the shoulder internal rotation deformity, may be performed toward the end of the first decade (444, 459). It is designed to improve hand-to-mouth function. Care must be taken not to externally rotate the distal humerus excessively. The hand and wrist are usually flexed and the ulna deviated, but variations within this pattern exist (403, 404). In general, the ulna-side digits are more involved. Proximal interphalangeal flexion deformities rarely respond to physical therapy or surgery. The thumb is flexed and adducted into the palm, and responds better to surgery than do the other digits.

Approximately one-third of the patients develop scoliosis (405). Curves usually have a C-shaped, neuromuscular pattern. The use of orthoses has been reported (406), although in our experience, these children respond poorly to bracing. Surgery is indicated for progressive curves interfering with balance or function. There are reports of patients regaining their ability to ambulate after surgical correction of large, rigid curves (406); surgery should be considered in patients who lose their ability to ambulate as they develop such curves.

Intelligence is normal, and these children often have a natural ability to learn substitution techniques. There is, however, a strong association between initial feeding difficulties and subsequent language development, which should not be mistaken for retardation (389).

Larsen Syndrome. The essential features of Larsen syndrome are multiple congenital dislocations of large joints, a characteristic flat face, and ligamentous laxity (407) (Fig. 8-42). The cause of the facial flattening is unclear, but it is especially noticeable when observed in profile, and is associated with some hypertelorism and a broad forehead. Dislocation of multiple joints appears in a characteristic pattern that includes bilateral dislocated knees, with the tibia anterior on the femur, bilateral dislocated hips, bilateral dislocated elbows, and bilateral clubfeet (464–468). The physician should think of this syndrome whenever dislocated knees are detected. The ligaments are lax or entirely absent. The ligamentous laxity is often so substantial that Larsen syndrome may be confused with EDS.

Radiographs show that the knees are dislocated, with the tibia anterior to the femur (408). Arthrograms show a small or an absent suprapatellar pouch, absent cruciate ligaments, and a misaligned patella (Fig. 8-43). The elbows have complex radial–humeral, ulnar–humeral, and radial–ulnar dislocations.

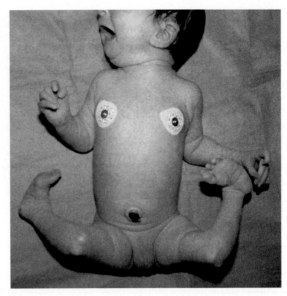

FIGURE 8-42. Larsen syndrome in a 1-week-old patient who has bilateral dislocated knees and clubfeet. (From Goldberg MJ. *The dysmorphic child: an orthopedic perspective*. New York, NY: Raven Press, 1987, with permission.)

Radial–ulnar synostosis is common and usually associated with ulnar–humeral dislocation (Fig. 8-44B). A spheroid ossicle frequently occurs anterior to the elbow joint; its origin is unknown. There are more carpal centers than are normal (Fig. 8-44A), and extra ossification centers in the foot, with a curious double ossification pattern of the calcaneus (Fig. 8-44C). This double ossification pattern can help confirm the diagnosis in cases in which the diagnosis is not clear. Abnormal cervical

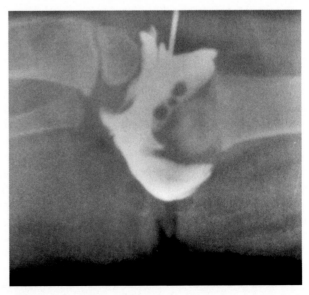

FIGURE 8-43. Larsen syndrome in a 5-month-old patient. The arthrogram of a knee shows anterior dislocation of the tibia on the femur and no suprapatellar pouch.

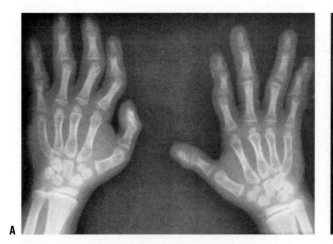

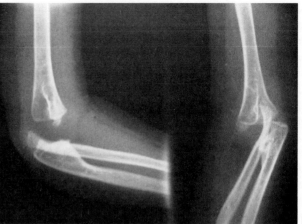

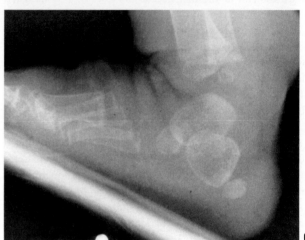

FIGURE 8-44. Characteristic roentgenograms of a 4-year-old patient with Larsen syndrome. **A:** The hands show more carpal centers and interphalangeal joint subluxations than is normal. **B:** The elbow demonstrates total dislocation but full functional ability. **C:** The foot has an abnormal os calcis containing two ossification centers. (A and B from Goldberg MJ. *The dysmorphic child: an orthopedic perspective.* New York, NY: Raven Press, 1987, with permission.)

spine segmentation, with instability, is typical, as is kyphosis, a complication often associated with myelopathy. Some cases are inherited in an autosomal dominant manner, and this aids in the diagnosis.

Both autosomal dominant and recessive inheritances are reported in Larsen syndrome, although many cases are sporadic (409–411). Some autosomal dominant cases are caused by mutations in the gene encoding filamin B (412). This is an intracellular protein that serves as scaffolding on which signaling and protein trafficking pathways are organized. It is expressed in the growth plate and vertebrae, and as such, the mutation likely acts to disrupt normal patterning and development of the joints and vertebral bodies, resulting in the typical phenotypic features. Some recessive cases are due to deficiency carbohydrate sulfotransferase 3, which plays a role in glycosaminoglycan processing, also deregulating joint and spine development (457). There are cases in which only one side of the body has a Larsen syndrome phenotype, suggesting that some cases are due to somatic, or mosaic, mutations (413).

The large numbers of deformities of the lower extremities require treatment in order to achieve stable, located joints. Knee stability is important for ambulation; however, the most important factor is knee stability in extension to allow for optimal quadriceps function. The knee may remain unstable

after reduction because of the lack of stabilizing ligaments, such as the anterior cruciate ligament. Long-term orthoses or anterior cruciate ligament reconstruction may be needed. Extra-articular reconstruction of the anterior cruciate ligament is another approach that maybe required (418). The knee is usually reduced before the hips, although simultaneous procedures are possible (25, 408). Although most knees do not respond to attempts at manipulation and cast correction, traditionally an initial trial of cast treatment is attempted. Too-vigorous manipulations result in distal femoral metaphyseal–physeal fractures. Because manipulation has not been found to be helpful for true dislocations, we believe that it can be abandoned once a dislocation is confirmed. Surgery may be undertaken as early as 3 to 4 months of age. Restoration of the range of motion must be cautious (gaining full extension is often a problem), and a flexion splint or a brace may be required after operative reduction to guard against redislocation.

The hips are dislocated, often despite a rather normal-appearing acetabulum. There is a sense of a good range of motion, although the hip may prove to be irreducible (414). The evolution of hip management in Larsen syndrome mirrors that in arthrogryposis multiplex congenita, and there is a trend toward earlier treatment. The relative rarity of this syndrome, however, accounts for the lack of good comparative data on how best to manage the hip dislocations. Reduction of the hip is associated with a high redislocation rate and revision surgery (408, 414, 415). For this reason, some specialists advocate either leaving bilateral dislocated hips alone, or waiting until after 1 year of age and performing femoral and pelvic osteotomies, along with the open reduction. However, we prefer an approach similar to that in arthrogryposis, with early surgical relocation. Because the knees are hyperextended when dislocated and cast in a flexed position after surgical relocation, both knees and hips can be operated upon at the same time. Secondary osteotomy of the pelvis and femur can be performed later, if necessary.

The clubfeet can be managed in a cast until the knee deformity is corrected. Some feet can be corrected with serial casting (408). The foot may need to be braced to control ankle instability. Despite the dislocations of the elbow or shoulder, the arms remain functional and rarely require treatment. Crutches or walkers can be used despite the dislocations.

The major concern involving the spine is structural abnormalities of the cervical vertebrae (26, 419). This manifestation may occur more frequently than previously recognized, and children should have cervical spine films taken in the first year of life to identify this deformity. Kyphosis is often due to hypoplasia of the vertebral bodies. A combination of cervical kyphosis and forward subluxation may result in quadriplegia and death. Posterior stabilization early (within the first 18 months of life) may prevent the significant problems associated with treatment after myelopathy has occurred and allow for correction of a kyphotic deformity with growth (33). In more severe cases or in the face of myelopathy, anterior and posterior decompression and fusion may be required (458, 459).

Anesthesia complications are common. The mobile infolding arytenoid cartilage creates airway difficulties. The associated tracheomalacia can be especially problematic in the newborn and may delay surgery for the hips and knees (419). The anesthesiologist should be aware of possible cervical spine instability, and a preoperative lateral radiograph is recommended.

The children have normal intelligence. The prognosis is generally good with aggressive orthopaedic treatment if the child survives the first year of life. The mortality figures for the first year may be as high as 40%. During the neonatal period, the cartilage-supporting structure of the larynx and trachea is soft, and there may be alarming elasticity of the thoracic cage at the costochondral junction, leading to respiratory failure and death. Cervical spine problems may also contribute to early mortality. Congenital cardiac septal defects, elongation of the aorta, and acquired lesions of the mitral valve and aorta, similar to those found in Marfan syndrome, further complicate medical and anesthesia management (420, 421).

Contracture Syndromes Involving Predominantly the Hands and Feet

Distal Arthrogryposis. Children with distal arthrogryposis have characteristic fixed hand contractures and foot deformities, but the major large joints of the arms and legs

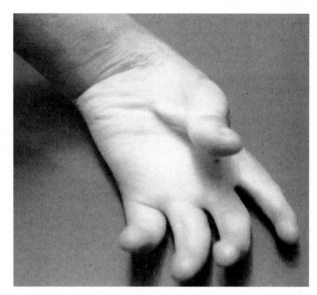

FIGURE 8-45. Distal arthrogryposis. Characteristic hand is the result of ulnar deviation at the metacarpophalangeal joints. Notice the deeply cupped palm and webbing of the MCP joint of the thumb.

are spared (16, 422, 423). Because different craniofacial abnormalities are often associated with distal arthrogryposis, the condition has been categorized as several eponymic syndromes (e.g., Gordon syndrome), a situation that leads to confusion (41). The cardinal features of distal arthrogryposis are the hand deformity with ulnar deviation of the fingers at the metacarpophalangeal (MCP) joint, flexion deformities at the proximal interphalangeal and MCP joints, and a cup-like palm with a single palmar crease (Fig. 8-45). The thumb is flexed and adducted, with a web at its base (424). Distal arthrogryposis is common and is sometimes incorrectly called *multiple camptodactyly*. The inheritance pattern of distal arthrogryposis is autosomal dominant, but there may be considerable variation in families, and this can lead to missing the diagnosis (41, 424–426). Distal arthrogryposis is divided into type I and type II on the basis of the absence or presence of facial findings, respectively.

Some cases of distal arthrogryposis type I are caused by mutations in the *TPM2* gene, which encodes β-tropomyosin, a protein important in fast-twitch muscle fibers (427). Type II distal arthrogryposis (Freeman-Sheldon syndrome) is caused by mutations in an isoform of troponin I that is specific to the troponin-tropomyosin complex of fast-twitch myofibers (427). Both these mutations result in abnormal activity of fast-twitch muscle fibers, suggesting that dysregulation of these muscle fibers is the common pathophysiologic cause of distal arthrogryposis. Because there are a variety of subtypes of distal arthrogryposis, it is likely that a number of causative genes will be identified, and perhaps all of these will play a role in the dysregulation of fast-twitch muscle fibers.

Although the hand deformity is characteristic and constant, the feet may be clubbed, have stiff metatarsus adductus, and have a vertical talus. The major joints in the upper and lower extremities are otherwise normal, although a minor knee-flexion deformity may be found. Intelligence is normal. The associated craniofacial anomalies are cleft lip or cleft palate and, in such patients, the syndrome of distal arthrogryposis may have an eponymous name, such as Gordon syndrome (391, 469). Radiographs show normal bony architecture, and only with persistence of deformities in the hands and feet are articular changes detected. This syndrome can be diagnosed prenatally in the fetus by detecting an unchanged position and lack of motion of the hands in contrast to the normal activity of the large uninvolved joints (42).

Overall, children with distal arthrogryposis have good function. The hands function well because the shoulders, elbows, and wrists are normal. Thumb surgery to lengthen the flexor pollicis longus and rebalance the extensor is the most common surgery (52). The feet more frequently require surgery. Some clubfeet can be corrected with manipulation and serial casts. Most are treated with circumferential releases. The outcome of treatment of clubfoot is better in this syndrome than in other arthrogrypotic clubfeet.

Freeman-Sheldon Syndrome. Freeman-Sheldon syndrome is sometimes called *distal arthrogryposis type II* because the hand and foot deformities are similar to those of distal arthrogryposis. It is recognized by its most characteristic feature, a "whistling face" (Fig. 8-46). The original name, *craniocarpotarsal dystrophy,* is misleading because it does not involve the cranium (53, 470). This syndrome is usually sporadic, although there is evidence of autosomal dominant and autosomal recessive inheritance (428, 433, 434). The eyes are deeply set.

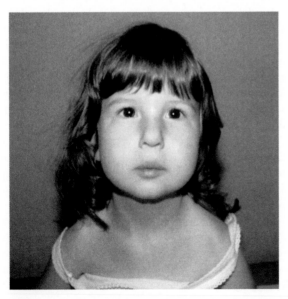

FIGURE 8-46. Freeman-Sheldon syndrome in a 3-year-old patient. Notice the small chin and mouth, long philtrum, puffy cheeks, deeply set eyes, and small chin cleft. (From Goldberg MJ. *The dysmorphic child: an orthopedic perspective.* New York, NY: Raven Press, 1987, with permission.)

The cheeks are fleshy, and pursed lips simulate whistling. There is a small mouth and a curious H-shaped dimple in the chin.

Scoliosis was not initially recognized as a common feature, but it affects more than one-half of the patients. The onset is in the first decade. It is often severe, with a left thoracic pattern reported regularly. The vertebrae are normally shaped. Although the scoliosis can be managed as in idiopathic scoliosis, the curves are more rigid and may not respond well to brace treatment (433, 435).

The hands demonstrate the classic distal arthrogryposis pattern described earlier (433, 435, 436). There are other contractures, including flexion deformities of the elbow and knee, decreased range of motion of the shoulder, decreased range of motion of the neck, and dislocated hips (77). Operative management principles for the upper extremity are similar to those in distal arthrogryposis. The hands are treated with physical and occupational therapy, but there is less improvement than is seen in the other distal arthrogryposis syndromes (437). Most of the other associated contractures can be treated like those in the other arthrogrypotic syndromes.

Clubfoot is the most common foot deformity, with vertical talus being the next most common (Fig. 8-47) (433, 435, 436). Clubfoot and vertical talus deformities are difficult to manage using manipulative techniques, but these should be tried first before using operative techniques.

During infancy, dysphagia and aspiration lead to failure to thrive, and even to death. Surgery to permit adequate mouth opening for feeding may be necessary (76). Children who survive the neonatal period do well and have normal intelligence. Anesthesia complications are common; some are the result of abnormalities related to the laryngeal cartilages (76, 389, 392, 438). The cause is unknown, but the buccinator muscle is hypoplastic, and electromyograms and muscle biopsies are identical to the peripheral muscle studies in classic arthrogryposis multiplex congenita (440), suggesting some similarity in pathophysiology.

Contracture Syndromes with Skin Webs

Pterygia Syndrome. *Pterygium* comes from a Greek word meaning *little wing.* A pterygium is a web. It can be seen as an isolated malformation in some syndromes, such as the pterygium colli in the neck of patients with Klippel-Feil syndrome.

There are two clinically important pterygia syndromes: multiple pterygium syndrome and popliteal pterygia syndrome (397). Several pterygium syndromes are lethal, with the affected patients not surviving the fetal or the newborn period (398, 471). The web syndromes are separated genetically as autosomal recessive (i.e., lethal pterygium syndrome and multiple pterygium) and autosomal dominant (i.e., popliteal pterygium) (422). However, they often overlap. Lethal pterygium syndrome may be diagnosed prenatally by detecting hydrops and cystic hygroma colli (399).

Both popliteal pterygium syndrome and van der Woude syndrome are caused by mutations in the gene encoding interferon regulatory factor-6 (400). Van der Woude syndrome is a

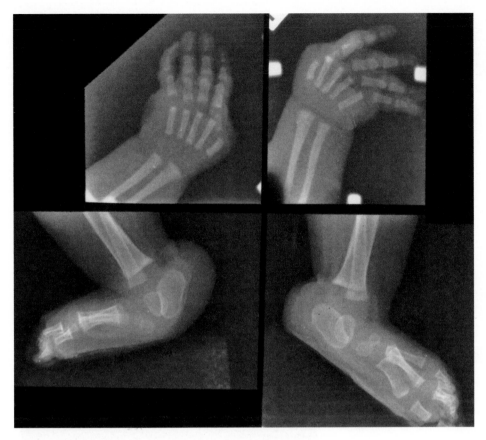

FIGURE 8-47. Freeman-Sheldon syndrome in a 5-year-old patient. Radiographs of the hands demonstrate ulnar deviation at the metacarpophalangeal joint, typical of a distal arthrogryposis syndrome. The feet show bilateral congenital vertical tali. All other joints in this patient were normal. (From Goldberg MJ. *The dysmorphic child: an orthopedic perspective.* New York, NY: Raven Press, 1987, with permission.)

dominantly inherited developmental disorder characterized by pits or sinuses of the lower lip, and cleft lip or cleft palate. It is unclear how a mutation in this interferon regulatory factor causes these seemingly dissimilar syndromes.

Multiple pterygia syndrome (i.e., Escobar syndrome) is characterized by a web across every flexion crease in the extremities, most prominently across the popliteal space, the elbow, and in the axilla (401, 441) (Fig. 8-48). There also are webs across the neck laterally and anteriorly from sternum to chin, drawing the facial features down. The fingers are webbed. The webs can be obvious, but if they are not, the affected children can look very much like those with arthrogryposis multiplex congenita. The two features that differentiate this syndrome from classic arthrogryposis are vertical talus and congenital spine deformity. The vertical talus is fairly constant in multiple pterygium syndrome and can be managed only by surgery. Circumferential release and prolonged protection, as in managing any arthrogrypotic foot deformity, are necessary. The spine deformity is significant, with multiple segmentation abnormalities and lordoscoliosis (442) (Figs. 8-49 and 8-50). The lordoscoliosis may be substantial enough to interfere with trunk and chest growth, leading to respiratory death during the first or second year of life (Fig. 8-50). Mobility depends much on the magnitude of the lower extremity webs and the residual motion of the joints, with many patients limited to wheelchairs for locomotion. The children have normal intelligence, and efforts should be maximized to enable them to function independently. Surgery is rarely needed for the upper extremities.

Popliteal pterygium syndrome (i.e., fascial-genital-popliteal syndrome) has recognizable characteristics in the face, the genitals, and the knee (75, 76, 416, 443, 444). The features include a cleft lip and palate, lip pits, and intraoral adhesions (52, 53). A fibrous band crosses the perineum and distorts the genitalia (23). A popliteal web is usually present bilaterally (76). It runs from ischium to calcaneus, resulting in a severe knee-flexion deformity. Tibia hypoplasia may be associated. Within the popliteal web is a superficial fibrous band, over which lies a tent of muscle running from the os calcis to the ischium, and is known in the older literature as a *calcaneoischiadicus muscle*. The popliteal artery and vein are usually deep, but the sciatic nerve is superficial in the web, just underneath the fibrous band (Fig. 8-51). There is a distinctive foot abnormality in this syndrome: a bifid great toenail and syndactyly of the lesser toes.

Although the original cases of multiple and popliteal pterygium syndromes were clearly defined, there is more phenotypic variation in both than was originally thought. For example, mild webs in joints of the upper extremity may be found in patients with popliteal pterygium syndrome. Adaptive changes in the joints occur over time. On radiographic examination, the patella look elongated, and the femoral condyles flattened, because of knee-flexion deformity.

From a management perspective, the determining factors are the magnitude of scoliosis and the size of the web crossing the knee. The thoracic vertebral dysplasia, thoracic lordosis, and the small chest impair lung development, resulting in

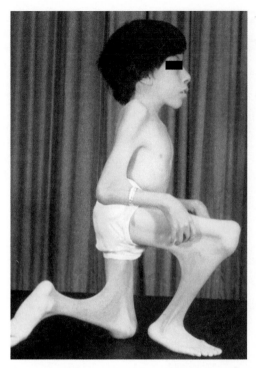

FIGURE 8-48. Multiple pterygium syndrome in a 12-year-old patient. Antecubital webs fix the elbows, and popliteal webs prevent ambulation. The patient had normal intelligence and became a college graduate. (From Goldberg MJ. *The dysmorphic child: an orthopedic perspective.* New York, NY: Raven Press, 1987, with permission.)

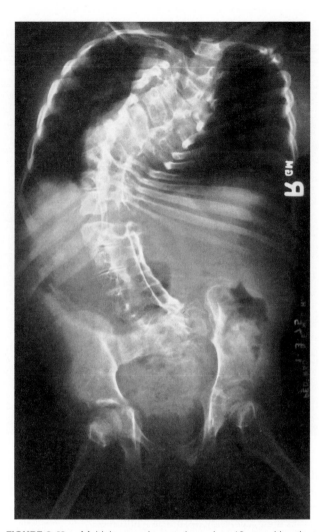

FIGURE 8-49. Multiple pterygium syndrome in a 13-year-old patient. Radiograph shows severe scoliosis, vertebral abnormalities, and an unsegmented bar from T9 to T12 and from L1 to S1, with an apparent gap between the bars. (From Goldberg MJ. *The dysmorphic child: an orthopedic perspective.* New York, NY: Raven Press, 1987, with permission.)

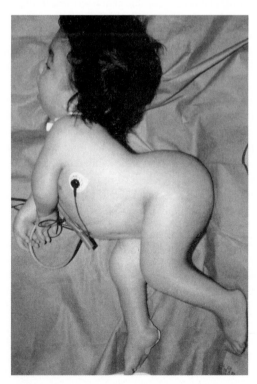

FIGURE 8-50. Multiple pterygium syndrome. Severe limitation of trunk growth was caused by vertebral fusions and lordoscoliosis. Death occurred at 24 months of age because of respiratory failure.

death in the first years of life in those with multiple pterygium syndrome. For the longer term survivors, management of the spine deformity is identical to those with nonsyndromic congenital scoliosis. Preoperative MRI evaluation of intraspinal contents and ultrasound of the kidney are indicated.

The knee is the joint that limits mobility in both syndromes and is the joint that most determines future ambulatory potential (39, 41, 42, 76). Traditionally, treatment of the knee begins with physical therapy, but the effectiveness of this therapy is doubtful. Early popliteal web surgery is recommended before the onset of adaptive changes in the articular surfaces, and before further vascular shortening. The nerve is usually located just under the skin and the web, and care must be taken to avoid nerve damage. The web is resected, and Z-plasty of the skin is performed. There is a high recurrence rate despite use of braces. Femoral shortening with an extension osteotomy is often required. If almost-full knee extension cannot be achieved at surgery, femoral shortening should

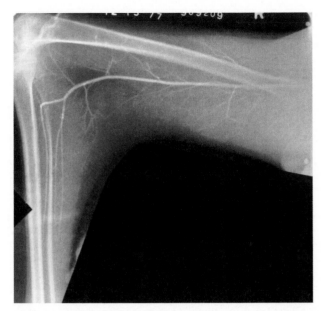

FIGURE 8-51. Popliteal pterygium in a 13-year-old patient. Arteriogram shows that the popliteal artery has been drawn up from its normal position. At the margin of the web is the sciatic nerve. (From Goldberg MJ. *The dysmorphic child: an orthopedic perspective.* New York, NY: Raven Press, 1987, with permission.)

be considered, even if during infancy or childhood (77). Gradual distraction techniques can be used, but an advantage over traditional techniques has not been demonstrated (448). Posterior soft-tissue procedures can be combined with distraction techniques to gradually extend the knee. Femoral shortening techniques are associated with low recurrence rates of the deformity, and have the advantage of reducing tension on the neurovascular structures. These techniques are therefore our treatment of choice.

REFERENCES

1. Goldberg MJ. *The dysmorphic child: an orthopedic perspective.* New York, NY: Raven Press, 1987.
2. Hecht JT, Scott JCI. Genetic study of an orthopedic referral center. *J Pediatr Orthop* 1984;4:208.
3. Jones KL. *Smith's recognizable patterns of human malformation,* 4th ed. Philadelphia, PA: WB Saunders, 1992.
4. Jones KL, Robinson LK. An approach to the child with structural defects. *J Pediatr Orthop* 1983;3:238.
5. Mendelian Inheritance in Man (OMIM). Center for Medical Genetics, Johns Hopkins University and National Center for Biotechnology Information. Bethesda: National Library of Medicine. Available at: http://www.omim.org/
6. Regemorter NV, et al. Congenital malformations in 10,000 consecutive births in a university hospital: need for genetic counseling and prenatal diagnosis. *J Pediatr* 1984;104:386.
7. Alman BA. Genetic etiology does not supplant the need to understand orthopaedic disorders. *Clin Orthop* 2002;401:2–3.
8. Unger S. A genetic approach to the diagnosis of skeletal dysplasia. *Clin Orthop* 2002;401:32–38.
9. Superti-Furga A, Bonafe L, Rimoin DL. Molecular-pathogenetic classification of genetic disorders of the skeleton. *Am J Med Genet* 2001;106(4):282–293.
10. Alman BA. A classification for genetic disorders of interest to orthopaedists. *Clin Orthop* 2002(401):17–26.
11. Pyeritz RE, McKusick VA. The Marfan syndrome. *New Eng J Med* 1979;300:772–777.
12. McKusick VA. Abraham Lincoln and Marfan syndrome. *Nature* 1991;352:280.
13. Pyeritz RE, McKusick VA. The Marfan syndrome: diagnosis and management. *N Engl J Med* 1979;300:772.
14. Parrish JG. Heritable disorders of connective tissue. *Proc R Soc Med* 1960;53:515.
15. Dietz HC, et al. Marfan syndrome caused by a recurrent de novo missense mutation in the fibrillin gene. *Nature* 1991;352:337–339.
16. Habermann CR, et al. MR evaluation of dural ectasia in Marfan syndrome: reassessment of the established criteria in children, adolescents, and young adults. *Radiology* 2005;234(2):535–541.
17. Keech MR, et al. Family studies of the Marfan syndrome. *J Chronic Dis* 1966;19:57.
18. Eldadah ZA, Grifo JA, Dietz HC. Marfan syndrome as a paradigm for transcript-targeted preimplantation diagnosis of heterozygous mutations. *Nature Med* 1995;1:798–803.
19. Pereira L, et al. Targetting of the gene encoding fibrillin-1 recapitulates the vascular aspect of Marfan syndrome. *Nat Genet* 1997;17:218–222.
20. Neptune ER, et al. Dysregulation of TGF-beta activation contributes to pathogenesis in Marfan syndrome. *Nat Genet* 2003;33(3):407–411.
21. Sponseller PD, et al. Results of brace treatment of scoliosis in Marfan syndrome. *Spine* 2000;25(18):2350–2354.
22. Doman I, et al. Subluxation of a lumbar vertebra in a patient with Marfan syndrome. Case report. *J Neurosurg* 2001;94(Suppl 1):154–157.
23. Pearson GD, et al. Report of the National Heart, Lung, and Blood Institute and National Marfan Foundation Working Group on research in Marfan syndrome and related disorders. *Circulation* 2008;118(7):785–791.
24. Ahn NU, et al. Dural ectasia is associated with back pain in Marfan syndrome. *Spine* 2000;25(12):1562–1568.
25. Di Silvestre M, et al. Surgical treatment for scoliosis in Marfan syndrome. *Spine* 2005;30(20):E597–E604.
26. Yang JS, Sponseller PD. Severe cervical kyphosis complicating halo traction in a patient with Marfan syndrome. *Spine* 2009;34(1):E66–E69.
27. McKusick VA. *Heritable disorders of connective tissue,* 4th ed. St. Louis, MO: CV Mosby, 1972.
28. Beighton P, et al. Ehlers-Danlos syndromes: revised nosology. Villefranche 1997. *Am J Med Genet* 1998;77:31–37.
29. Burrows NP, et al. The gene encoding collagen alpha-1(V) (COL5A1) is linked to mixed Ehlers-Danlos syndrome type I/II. *J Invest Derm* 1996;106:1273–1276.
30. Wenstrup RJ, et al. A splice-junction mutation in the region of COL5A1 that codes for the carboxyl propeptide of pro-alpha-1(V) chains results in the gravis form of the Ehlers-Danlos syndrome (type I). *Hum Molec Genet* 1996;5:1733–1736.
31. Barabas AP. Ehlers-Danlos syndrome type IV [Letter]. *New Eng J Med* 2000;343:366.
32. Kaufman A, et al. Osseous destruction by neurofibroma diagnosed in infancy as "desmoplastic fibroma." *J Pediatr Orthop* 1984;4:239.
33. Skaggs DL, et al. Shortening of growing-rod spinal instrumentation reverses cardiac failure in child with Marfan syndrome and scoliosis. A case report. *J Bone Joint Surg Am* 2008;90(12):2745–2750.
34. Wenstrup RJ, et al. Prevalence of aortic root dilation in the Ehlers-Danlos syndrome. *Genet Med* 2002;4:112–117.
35. Kozlowski K, Lipson A. Bony tuberculosis misinterpreted—a cautionary tale. *Aust Radiol* 1993;37:119.
36. Locht RC, Huebert HT, McFarland DF. Subperiosteal hemorrhage and cyst formation in neurofibromatosis: a case report. *Clin Orthop* 1981;155:141.
37. Joseph KN, Bowen JR, MacEwen GD. Unusual orthopedic manifestations of neurofibromatosis. *Clin Orthop Rel Res* 1992;278:17.

38. Riccardo VM. Neurofibromatosis: past, present and future. *N Engl J Med* 1991;324:1285.

39. Sheehan FT, et al. Understanding patellofemoral pain with maltracking in the presence of joint laxity: complete 3D in vivo patellofemoral and tibiofemoral kinematics. *J Orthop Res* 2009;27(5):561–570.

40. Graham PW, Oehlschlaeger FH. *Articulating the elephant man: Joseph Merrick and his interpreters*. Baltimore, MD: Johns Hopkins University Press, 1992.

41. Yang JS, et al. Vascular complications from anterior spine surgery in three patients with Ehlers-Danlos syndrome. *Spine* 2009;34(4):E153–E157.

42. Nematbakhsh A, Crawford AH. Non-adjacent spondylolisthesis in Ehlers-Danlos syndrome. *J Pediatr Orthop B* 2004;13(5):336–339.

43. Xu G, Connell PO, Viskochil D. The neurofibromatosis type 1 gene encodes a protein related to GAP. *Cell* 1990;62:608.

44. Li Y, Bollag G, Clark R. Somatic mutations in the neurofibromatosis 1 gene in human tumors. *Cell* 1992;69:281.

45. The I, Hannigan GE, Cowley GS. Rescue of a *Drosophila* NF1 mutant phenotype by protein kinase A. *Science* 1997;276:794.

46. Gutmann DH, Collins FS. Recent progress toward understanding the molecular biology of von Recklinghausen neurofibromatosis. Brief review. *Ann Neurol* 1992;31:555.

47. Hruban RH, et al. Malignant peripheral nerve sheath tumors of the buttock and lower extremity. A study of 43 cases. *Cancer* 1990;66:1253.

48. Sirois JL III, Drennan JC. Dystrophic spinal deformity in neurofibromatosis. *J Pediatr Orthop* 1990;10:522.

49. Betz RR, et al. Scoliosis surgery in neurofibromatosis. *Clin Orthop Rel Res* 1989;245:53.

50. Khoshhal KI, Ellis RD. Paraparesis after posterior spinal fusion in neurofibromatosis secondary to rib displacement: case report and literature review. *J Pediatr Orthop* 2000;20(6):799–801.

51. Ayral-Kaloustian S, Salaski EJ. Protein farnesyltransferase inhibitors. *Curr Med Chem* 2002;9(10):1003–1032.

52. Korf BR. Statins, bone, and neurofibromatosis type 1. *BMC Med* 2008;6:22.

53. Kolanczyk M, et al. Modelling neurofibromatosis type 1 tibial dysplasia and its treatment with lovastatin. *BMC Med* 2008;6:21.

54. Winter R. Spontaneous dislocation of a vertebra in a patient who had neurofibromatosis: report of a case with dural ectasia. *J Bone Joint Surg Am* 1991;73:1404.

55. Crawford AH, Bagamery JN. Osseous manifestations of neurofibromatosis in childhood. *J Pediatr Orthop* 1986;6:72.

56. Crawford AH. Pitfalls of spinal deformities associated with neurofibromatosis in children. *Clin Orthop Rel Res* 1989;245:29.

57. Funasaki H, et al. Pathophysiology of spinal deformities in neurofibromatosis. An analysis of 71 patients who had curves associated with dystrophic changes. *J Bone Joint Surg Am* 1994;76:692.

58. Winter RB, et al. Spine deformity in neurofibromatosis. A review of one hundred two patients. *J Bone Joint Surg Am* 1979;61:677.

59. Kim HW, Weinstein SL. Spine update. The management of scoliosis in neurofibromatosis. *Spine* 1997;22:2770.

60. Bensaid AH, et al. Neurofibromatosis with dural ectasia and bilateral symmetrical pedicular clefts: report of two cases. *Neuroradiology* 1992;34:107.

61. Ezekowitz RA, Mulliken JB, Folkman J. Interferon alpha-2a therapy for life threatening hemangiomas of infancy. *N Engl J Med* 1992;326:1456.

62. Folkman J. Successful treatment of an angiogenic disease. *N Engl J Med* 1989;320:1211.

63. Brill CB. Neurofibromatosis: clinical overview. *Clin Orthop Rel Res* 1989;245:10.

64. Coleman BG, et al. CT of sarcomatous degeneration in neurofibromatosis. *AJR Am J Roentgenol* 1983;140:383.

65. Gutmann DH, Collins FS. The neurofibromatosis type 1 gene and its protein product, neurofibromin [Review]. *Neuron* 1993;10:335.

66. Meis JM, et al. Malignant peripheral nerve sheath tumors (malignant schwannomas) in children. *Am J Surg Pathol* 1992;16:694.

67. Wanebo JE, et al. Malignant peripheral nerve sheath tumors. A clinicopathologic study of 28 cases. *Cancer* 1993;71:1247.

68. Coleman BG, Arger PH, Dalinka MK. CT of sarcomatous degeneration in neurofibromatosis. *AJR Am J Roentgenol* 1983;140:387.

69. Konishi K, et al. Case report: hypophosphatemic osteomalacia in von Recklinghausen neurofibromatosis. *Am J Med Sci* 1991;301:322.

70. Weinstein RS, Harris RL. Hypercalcemic hyperparathyroidism and hypophosphatemic osteomalacia complicating neurofibromatosis. *Calcif Tissue Int* 1990;46:361.

71. Egelhoff JC, et al. Spinal MR findings in neurofibromatosis types 1 and 2. *Am J Neuroradiol* 1992;13:1071.

72. Habiby R, Silverman B, Listernick R. Precocious puberty in children with neurofibromatosis type 1. *J Pediatr* 1995;126:367.

73. Hofman KJ, Harris EL, Bryan RN. Neurofibromatosis type 1: the cognitive phenotype. *J Pediatr* 1994;124:S8.

74. Ferner RE, Hughes RA, Weinman J. Intellectual impairment in neurofibromatosis 1. *J Neurol Sci* 1996;138:133.

75. Cho TJ, et al. Biologic characteristics of fibrous hamartoma from congenital pseudarthrosis of the tibia associated with neurofibromatosis type 1. *J Bone Joint Surg Am* 2008;90(12):2735–2744.

76. Stevenson DA, et al. Double inactivation of NF1 in tibial pseudarthrosis. *Am J Hum Genet* 2006;79(1):143–148.

77. Durga Nagaraju K, et al. Congenital pseudarthrosis of the ulna. *J Pediatr Orthop B* 2007;16(2):150–152.

78. Shah KJ. Beckwith-Wiedemann syndrome: role of ultrasound in its management. *Clin Radiol* 1983;34:313.

79. Choyke PL, Siegel MJ, Craft AW. Screening for Wilms tumor in children with Beckwith-Wiedemann syndrome or idiopathic hemihypertrophy. *Med Pediatr Oncol* 1999;32:200.

80. Senta H, et al. Cell responses to bone morphogenetic proteins and peptides derived from them: biomedical applications and limitations. *Cytokine Growth Factor Rev* 2009;20(3):213–222.

81. Lee FA. Radiology of the Beckwith-Wiedemann syndrome. *Radiol Clin North Am* 1972;10:261.

82. Angehrn V, Zachmann M, Prader A. Silver-Russell syndrome. Observations in 20 patients. *Helv Paediatr Acta* 1979;34:297.

83. Limbird TJ. Slipped capital femoral epiphysis associated with Russell-Silver syndrome. *South Med J* 1989;82:902.

84. Barkmakian JT, et al. Proteus syndrome. *J Hand Surg* 1992;17:32.

85. Kalen V, Burwell DS, Omer GE. Macrodactyly of the hands and feet. *J Pediatr Orthop* 1988;8:311.

86. Lacombe D, et al. Proteus syndrome in 7 patients: clinical and genetic considerations. *Genet Couns* 1991;2:93.

87. Samn M, Lewis K, Blumberg B. Monozygotic twins discordant for the Russell-Silver syndrome. *Am J Med Genet* 1990;37:543.

88. Dreyer SD, et al. Mutations in LMX1B cause abnormal skeletal patterning and renal dysplasia in nail-patella syndrome. *Nat Genet* 1998;19:47.

89. Loomer RL. Shoulder girdle dysplasia associated with nail-patella syndrome. A case report and literature review. *Clin Orthop Rel Res* 1989;238:112.

90. Jacofsky DJ, Stans AA, Lindor NM. Bilateral hip dislocation and pubic diastasis in familial nail-patella syndrome. *Orthopedics* 2003;26(3):329–330.

91. Lommen EJ, Hamel BC, te Slaa RL. Nephropathy in hereditary osteoonycho dysplasia (HOOD): variable expression or genetic heterogenity. *Prog Clin Biol Res* 1989;305:157.

92. Sherk HH, Whitaker LA, Pasquariello PS. Facial malformations and spinal anomalies. A predictable relationship. *Spine* 1982;7:526.

93. Goodship J, et al. Transmission of Proteus syndrome from father to son? *J Med Genet* 1991;28:781.

94. Wiedemann HR, et al. The Proteus syndrome: partial gigantism of the hands and/or feet, nevi, hemihypertrophy, subcutaneous tumors, macrocephaly or other skull anomalies and possible accelerated growth and visceral affections. *Eur J Pediatr* 1983;140:5.

95. Tibbles JA, Cohen MM. The Proteus syndrome: the Elephant Man diagnosed. *Br Med J* 1986;293:683.

96. Clark RD, et al. Proteus syndrome: an expanded phenotype. *Am J Med* 1987;25:99.

97. Hotamisligil GS. Proteus syndrome and hamartoses with overgrowth. *Dysmorphol Clin Genet* 1990;4:87.

98. Demetriades MD, et al. Proteus syndrome: musculoskeletal manifestations and management: a report of two cases. *J Pediatr Orthop* 1992; 12:106.

99. Stricker S. Musculoskeletal manifestations of Proteus syndrome: report of two cases with literature review. *J Pediatr Orthop* 1992;12:667.

100. Kuroiwa M, et al. Manifestation of alveolar rhabdomyosarcoma as primary cutaneous lesions in a neonate with Beckwith-Wiedemann syndrome. *J Pediatr Surg* 2009;44(3):e31–e35.

101. Azouz EM, Costa T, Fitch N. Radiologic findings in the Proteus syndrome. *Pediatr Radiol* 1987;17:481.

102. Turra S, Santini S, Cagnoni G. Gigantism of the foot: our experience in seven cases. *J Pediatr Orthop* 1998;18:337.

103. Greenberg F, Robinson LK. Mild Brachmann-de Lange syndrome: changes of phenotype with age. *Am J Med Genet* 1989;32:90.

104. Krantz ID, et al. Cornelia de Lange syndrome is caused by mutations in NIPBL, the human homolog of *Drosophila melanogaster* Nipped-B. *Nat Genet* 2004;36:631–635.

105. Beguiristain JL, de Rada PD, Barriga A. Nail-patella syndrome: long term evolution. *J Pediatr Orthop B* 2003;12(1):13–16.

106. Krab LC, et al. Effect of simvastatin on cognitive functioning in children with neurofibromatosis type 1: a randomized controlled trial. *JAMA* 2008;300(3):287–294.

107. Tonkin ET, et al. NIPBL, encoding a homolog of fungal Scc2-type sister chromatid cohesion proteins and fly Nipped-B, is mutated in Cornelia de Lange syndrome. *Nat Genet* 2004;36:636–641.

108. Ireland M, et al. A de novo translocation t(3;17)(q26.a3;q3.1) in a child with Cornelia de Lange syndrome. *J Med Genet* 1991;28:639.

109. Lakshminarayana P, Nallasivam P. Cornelia de Lange syndrome with ring chromosomes 3. *J Med Genet* 1990;27:405.

110. Yakish SD, Fu FH. Long-term follow-up of the treatment of a family with nail-patella syndrome. *J Pediatr Orthop* 1983;3:360.

111. Darlington D, Hawkins CF. Nail-patella syndrome with iliac horns and hereditary nephropathy. Necropsy report and anatomical dissection. *J Bone Joint Surg Br* 1967;49-B:164.

112. Morrison PJ, et al. Cardiovascular abnormalities in the oculo-auriculovertebral spectrum (Goldenhar syndrome). *Am J Med Genet* 1992;44:425.

113. Bever YV, van den Ende JJ, Richieri-Costa A. Oculo-auriculo-vertebral complex and uncommon associated anomalies: report on 9 unrelated Brazilian patients. *Am J Med Genet* 1992;44:683.

114. Kaye CI, et al. Oculoauriculovertebral anomaly: segregation analysis. *Am J Med Genet* 1992;43:913.

115. Darling DB, Feingold M, Berkman M. The roentgenological aspects of Goldenhar's syndrome (oculoauriculovertebral dysplasia). *Radiology* 1968;91:254.

116. Madan R, et al. Goldenhar's syndrome: an analysis of anaesthetic management. A retrospective study of seventeen cases. *Anaesthesia* 1990;45:49.

117. Rodriguez JI, Palacios J, Lapunzina P. Severe axial anomalies in the oculo-auriculo-vertebral (Goldenhar) complex. *Am J Med Genet* 1993; 47(1):69–74.

118. Schrander-Stumpel CT, et al. Oculoauriculovertebral spectrum and cerebral anomalies. *J Med Genet* 1992;29:326.

119. Filippi G. The de Lange syndrome. Report of 15 cases. *Clin Genet* 1989;35:343.

120. Stevens PM, Klatt JB. Guided growth for pathological physes: radiographic improvement during realignment. *J Pediatr Orthop* 2008;28(6):632–639.

121. Die-Smulders CD, et al. On the variable expression of the Brachmann-de Lange syndrome. *Clin Genet* 1992;41:42.

122. Bruner JP, Hsia YE. Prenatal findings in Brachmann-de Lange syndrome. *Obstet Gynecol* 1990;76:966.

123. Drolshagen LF, et al. Prenatal ultrasonographic appearance of "Cornelia de Lange" syndrome. *J Clin Ultrasound* 1992;20:470–474.

124. Condron CJ. Limb anomalies in Cornelia de Lange syndrome infant patient. *Birth Defects* 1969;5:226.

125. Curtis JA, Hara AEO, Carpenter GG. Spurs of the mandible and supracondylar process of the humerus in Cornelia de Lange syndrome. *AJR Am J Roentgenol* 1977;129:156.

126. Filippi G, Renuart AW. Limb anomalies in the Cornelia de Lange syndrome: adult patient. *Birth Defects* 1969;5:228.

127. Halal F, Preus M. The hand profile in de Lange syndrome: diagnostic criteria. *Am J Med Genet* 1979;3:317.

128. Joubin J, Pettrone CF, Pettrone FA. Cornelia de Lange's syndrome. A review article (with emphasis on orthopedic significance). *Clin Orthop* 1982;171:180.

129. Pashayan HM, Fraser FC, Pruzansky S. Variable limb malformations in the Brachmann-Cornelia de Lange syndrome. *Birth Defects* 1975;11:147.

130. Roposch A, et al. Orthopaedic manifestations of Brachmann-de Lange syndrome: a report of 34 patients. *J Pediatr Orthop* 2004;13(2): 118–122.

131. Rosenbach Y, Zahavi I, Dinari G. Gastroesophageal dysfunction in Brachmann-de Lange syndrome. *Am J Med Genet* 1992;42:379.

132. Cates M, et al. Gastroesophageal dysfunction in Cornelia de Lange syndrome. *J Pediatr Surg* 1989;24:248.

133. Fraser WI, Campbell BM. A study of six cases of de Lange Amsterdam dwarf syndrome, with special attention to voice, speech and language characteristics. *Dev Med Child Neurol* 1978;20:189.

134. Dossetor DR, Couryer S, Nicol AR. Massage for very severe self-injurious behaviour in a girl with Cornelia de Lange syndrome. *Dev Med Child Neurol* 1991;33:636.

135. Shear CS, et al. Self-mutilative behavior as a feature of the de Lange syndrome. *J Pediatr* 1971;78:506.

136. Sargent WW. Anesthetic management of a patient with Cornelia de Lange syndrome. *Anesthesiology* 1991;74:1162.

137. Tiet TD, Alman BA. Developmental pathways in musculoskeletal neoplasia: involvement of the Indian Hedgehog-parathyroid hormone-related protein pathway. *Pediatr Res* 2003;53(4):539–543.

138. Tsirikos AI, McMaster MJ. Goldenhar-associated conditions (hemifacial microsomia) and congenital deformities of the spine. *Spine (Phila Pa 1976)* 2006;31(13):E400–E407.

139. Incardona JP, et al. The teratogenic Veratrum alkaloid cyclopamine inhibits sonic hedgehog signal transduction. *Development* 1998; 125(18):3553–3562.

140. Day NL, Richardson GA. Prenatal alcohol exposure: a continuum of effects. *Semin Perinatol* 1991;4:271.

141. Ernhart CB. Clinical correlations between ethanol intake and fetal alcohol syndrome. *Recent Dev Alcohol* 1991;9:127.

142. Knupfer G. Abstaining for foetal health: the fiction that even light drinking is dangerous. *Br J Addiction* 1991;86:1057.

143. Stromland K, et al. Oculo-auriculo-vertebral spectrum: associated anomalies, functional deficits and possible developmental risk factors. *Am J Med Genet A* 2007;143A(12):1317–1325.

144. Rosett HL, et al. Patterns of alcohol consumption and fetal development. *Obstet Gynecol* 1983;61:539.

145. Rosett HL, Weiner L. Prevention of fetal alcohol effects. *Pediatrics* 1982;69:813.

146. Abel EL, Sokol RJ. A revised conservative estimate of the incidence of FAS and its economic impact. *Alcoholism* 1991;15:514.

147. Little RE, Wendt JK. The effects of maternal drinking in the reproductive period: an epidemiologic review. *J Subst Abuse* 1991;3:187.

148. Smith DF, et al. Intrinsic defects in the fetal alcohol syndrome: studies on 76 cases from British Columbia and the Yukon Territory. *Neurobehav Toxicol Teratol* 1981;3:145.

149. Streissguth AP, Clarren SK, Jones KL. Natural history of the fetal alcohol syndrome: a 10-year follow-up of eleven patients. *Lancet* 1985;2:85.

150. Autti-Ramo I, Gaily E, Granstrom ML. Dysmorphic features in offspring of alcoholic mothers. *Arch Dis Child* 1992;67:712.

151. Rost A, et al. Alcohol use in pregnancy, craniofacial features, and fetal growth. *J Epidemiol Commun Health* 1990;44:302.

152. Crain LS, Fitzmaurice NE, Mondry C. Nail dysplasia and fetal alcohol syndrome. *Am J Dis Child* 1983;137:1069.

153. Rensburg LJV. Major skeletal defects in the fetal alcohol syndrome. *J Afr Med J* 1981;59:687.

154. West JR, et al. Polydactyly and polysyndactyly induced by prenatal exposure to ethanol. *Teratology* 1981;24:13.

155. Pazzaglia UE, et al. Bone malformations in Proteus syndrome: an analysis of bone structural changes and their evolution during growth. *Pediatr Radiol* 2007;37(8):829–835.
156. Halmesmaki E, Raivio K, Ylikorkala O. A possible association between maternal drinking and fetal clubfoot. *N Engl J Med* 1985;312:790.
157. Cremin BJ, Jaffer Z. Radiological aspects of the fetal alcohol syndrome. *Pediatr Radiol* 1981;11:151.
158. Lowry RB. The Klippel-Feil anomalad as part of the fetal alcohol syndrome. *Teratology* 1977;16:53.
159. Neidengard L, Carter TE, Smith DW. Klippel-Feil malformation complex in fetal alcohol syndrome. *Am J Dis Child* 1978;132:929.
160. Spiegel PG, et al. The orthopedic aspects of the fetal alcohol syndrome. *Clin Orthop* 1979;139:58.
161. Tredwell SJ, et al. Cervical spine anomalies in fetal alcohol syndrome. *Spine* 1982;7:331.
162. Jaffer Z, Nelson M, Beighton P. Bone fusion in the foetal alcohol syndrome. *J Bone Joint Surg Br* 1981;63:569.
163. Leicher-Duber A, Schumacher R, Spranger J. Stippled epiphyses in fetal alcohol syndrome. *Pediatr Radiol* 1990;20:369.
164. Quan L, Smith DW. The VATER association: vertebral defects, anal atresia, T-E fistula with esophageal atresia, radial and renal dysplasia: a spectrum of associated defects. *J Pediatr* 1973;82:104.
165. Beals RK, Rolfe B. VATER association. A unifying concept of multiple anomalies. *J Bone Joint Surg Am* 1989;71:948.
166. Lawhorn SM, MacEwen GD, Bunnell WP. Orthopaedic aspects of the VATER association. *J Bone Joint Surg Am* 1986;68:424.
167. Wulfsberg EA, Phillips-Dawkins TL, Thomas RL. Vertebral hypersegmentation in a case of the VATER association. *Am J Med Genet* 1992;42:766.
168. Chestnut R, James HE, Jones KL. The VATER association and spinal dysraphia. *Pediatr Neurosurg* 1992;18:144.
169. Raffel C, Litofsky S, McComb JG. Central nervous system malformations and the VATER association. *Pediatr Neurosurg* 1990;16:170.
170. Axelrod FB, Porges RF, Stein ME. Neonatal recognition of familial dysautonomia. *J Pediatr* 1987;110:946.
171. Clayson D, Welton W, Axelrod FB. Personality development and familial dysautonomia. *Pediatrics* 1980;65:274.
172. Axelrod FB, Abularrage JJ. Familial dysautonomia: a prospective study of survival. *J Pediatr* 1982;101:234.
173. Slaugenhaupt SA, et al. Tissue-specific expression of a splicing mutation in the IKBKAP gene causes familial dysautonomia. *Am J Hum Genet* 2001;68:598–605.
174. Anderson SL, et al. Familial dysautonomia is caused by mutations of the IKAP gene. *Am J Hum Genet* 2001;68(3):753–758.
175. Anderson SL, Qiu J, Rubin BY. EGCG corrects aberrant splicing of IKAP mRNA in cells from patients with familial dysautonomia. *Biochem Biophys Res Commun* 2003;310(2):627–633.
176. Anderson SL, Qiu J, Rubin BY. Tocotrienols induce IKBKAP expression: a possible therapy for familial dysautonomia. *Biochem Biophys Res Commun* 2003;306(1):303–309.
177. Pearson J, et al. Quantitative studies of dorsal root ganglia and neuropathologic observations on spinal cords in familial dysautonomia. *J Neurol Sci* 1978;35:77.
178. Albanese SA, Babechko WP. Spine deformity in familial dysautonomia (Riley-Day syndrome). *J Pediatr Orthop* 1979;7:183.
179. Robin GC. Scoliosis in familial dysautonomia. *Bull Hosp Joint Dis Orthop Inst* 1984;44:26.
180. Rubery PT, Speilman JH, Hester P. Scoliosis in familial dysautonomia. *J Bone Joint Surg Am* 1995;77:1369.
181. Guidera KJ, et al. Orthopaedic manifestations in congenitally insensate patients. *J Pediatr Orthop* 1990;10:514.
182. Yoslow W, et al. Orthopaedic defects in familial dysautonomia. A review of sixty-five cases. *J Bone Joint Surg Am* 1971;53:1541.
183. Mitnick JS, et al. Aseptic necrosis in familial dysautonomia. *Radiology* 1982;142:89.
184. Brunt PW. Unusual cause of Charcot joints in early adolescence (Riley-Day syndrome). *Br Med J* 1967;4:277.
185. Axelrod FB, Hilz MJ. Inherited autonomic neuropathies. *Semin Neurol* 2003;23:381–390.
186. Smeets E, et al. Rett syndrome in adolescent and adult females: clinical and molecular genetic findings. *Am J Med Genet* 2003;122A(3):227–233.
187. Leonard H, Thomson M, Bower C. Skeletal abnormalities in Rett syndrome: increasing evidence for dysmorphogenetic defects. *Am J Med Genet* 1995;58:285.
188. Amir RE, et al. Rett syndrome is caused by mutations in X-linked MECP2, encoding methyl-CpG-binding protein 2. *Nat Genet* 1999;23:185.
189. Mo R, et al. Anorectal malformations caused by defects in sonic hedgehog signaling. *Am J Pathol* 2001;159(2):765–774.
190. Coleman M. Is classical Rett syndrome ever present in males? *Brain Dev* 1990;12:32.
191. Armstrong J, et al. Prenatal diagnosis in Rett syndrome. *Fetal Diagn Ther* 2002;17(4):200–204.
192. Kerr AM, et al. Results of surgery for scoliosis in Rett syndrome. *J Child Neurol* 2003;18(10):703–708.
193. Huang TJ, Lubicky JP, Hammerberg KW. Scoliosis in Rett syndrome. *Orthop Rev* 1994;23:937.
194. Guidera KJ, Borrelli J, Raney JE. Orthopaedic manifestations of Rett syndrome. *J Pediatr Orthop* 1991;11:208.
195. Harrison DJ, Webb PJ. Scoliosis in the Rett syndrome: natural history and treatment. *Brain Dev* 1990;12:156.
196. Loder RT, Lee CL, Richards BS. Orthopaedic aspects of Rett syndrome: a multicenter review. *J Pediatr Orthop* 1989;9:562.
197. Roberts AP, Conner AN. Orthopaedic aspects of Rett's syndrome: brief report. *J Bone Joint Surg Br* 1988;70:674.
198. Umansky R, et al. Hand preference, extent of laterality, and functional hand use in Rett syndrome. *J Child Neurol* 2003;18(7):481–487.
199. Gath A. Parental reactions to loss and disappointment: the diagnosis of Down's syndrome. *Dev Med Child Neurol* 1985;27:392.
200. Barden HS. Growth and development of selected hard tissues in Down syndrome: a review. *Hum Biol* 1983;55:539.
201. Caffey J, Ross S. Pelvic bones in infantile mongoloidism: roentgenographic features. *AJR Am J Roentgenol* 1958;80:458.
202. Selby KA, et al. Clinical predictors and radiological reliability in atlantoaxial subluxation in Down's syndrome. *Arch Dis Child* 1991;66:876.
203. Brock DJH. *Molecular genetics for the clinician.* Cambridge, UK: Cambridge University Press, 1993.
204. Tredwell SJ, Newman DE, Lockitch G. Instability of the upper cervical spine in Down syndrome. *J Pediatr Orthop* 1990;10:602.
205. White KS, et al. Evaluation of the craniocervical junction in Down syndrome: correlation of measurements obtained with radiography and MR imaging. *Radiology* 1993;186:377.
206. Gabriel KR, Mason DE, Carango P. Occipito-atlantal translation in Down's syndrome. *Spine* 1990;15:997.
207. Menezes AH, Ryken TC. Craniovertebral abnormalities in Down's syndrome. *Pediatr Neurosurg* 1992;18:24.
208. Stein SM, et al. Atlanto-occipital subluxation in Down syndrome. *Pediatr Radiol* 1991;21:121.
209. Diamond LS, Lynne D, Sigman B. Orthopedic disorders in patients with Down's syndrome. *Orthop Clin North Am* 1981;12:57.
210. Lerman JA, et al. Spinal arthrodesis for scoliosis in Down syndrome. *J Pediatr Orthop* 2003;23(2):159–161.
211. Hresko MT, McCarthy JC, Goldberg MJ. Hip disease in adults with Down syndrome. *J Bone Joint Surg Br* 1993;75:604.
212. Roberts GM, et al. Radiology of the pelvis and hips in adults with Down's syndrome. *Clin Radiol* 1980;31:475.
213. Shaw ED, Beals RK. The hip joint in Down's syndrome. A study of its structure and associated disease. *Clin Orthop Rel Res* 1992;278:101.
214. Greene WB. Closed treatment of hip dislocation in Down syndrome. *J Pediatr Orthop* 1998;18:643.
215. Aprin H, Zink WP, Hall JE. Management of dislocation of the hip in Down syndrome. *J Pediatr Orthop* 1985;5:428.
216. Bennet GC, et al. Dislocation of the hip in trisomy 21. *J Bone Joint Surg Br* 1982;64:289.

217. Ohsawa T, et al. Follow-up study of atlanto-axial instability in Down's syndrome without separate odontoid process. *Spine* 1989;14:1149.

218. Gore DR. Recurrent dislocation of the hip in a child with Down's syndrome. *J Bone Joint Surg Am* 1981;63:823.

219. Nogi J. Hip disorders in children with Down's syndrome. *Dev Med Child Neurol* 1985;27:86.

220. Dugdale TW, Renshaw TS. Instability of the patellofemoral joint in Down syndrome. *J Bone Joint Surg Am* 1986;68:405.

221. Selby-Silverstein L, Hillstrom HJ, Palisano RJ. The effect of foot orthoses on standing foot posture and gait of young children with Down syndrome. *Neurorehabilitation* 2001;16(3):183–193.

222. Cremers MJ, Beijer HJ. No relation between general laxity and atlantoaxial instability in children with Down syndrome. *J Pediatr Orthop* 1993;13:318.

223. Levack B, Roper BA. Dislocation in Down's syndrome. *Dev Med Child Neurol* 1984;26:122.

224. Jacobs PA, et al. A cytogenetic and molecular reappraisal of a series of patients with Turner's syndrome. *Ann Hum Genet* 1990;54:209.

225. Mik G, et al. Down syndrome: orthopedic issues. *Curr Opin Pediatr* 2008;20(1):30–36.

226. Lu DC, Sun PP. Bone morphogenetic protein for salvage fusion in an infant with Down syndrome and craniovertebral instability. Case report. *J Neurosurg* 2007;106(6 Suppl):480–483.

227. Gicquel C, et al. Molecular diagnosis of Turner's syndrome. *J Med Genet* 1992;29:547.

228. Zinn AR, et al. Evidence for a Turner syndrome locus or loci at Xp11.2–p22.1. *Am J Human Genet* 1998;63:1757.

229. Burch M, et al. Myocardial disarray in Noonan syndrome. *Br Heart J* 1992;68:586.

230. Thomson SJ, Tanne NS, Mercer DM. Web neck deformity: anatomical considerations and options in surgical management. *Br J Plast Surg* 1990;43:94.

231. Elder DA, et al. Kyphosis in a Turner syndrome population. *Pediatrics* 2002;109(6):e93.

232. Beals RK. Orthopedic aspects of the XO (Turner's) syndrome. *Clin Orthop* 1973;97:19.

233. Kosowicz J. The deformity of the medial tibial condyle in nineteen cases of gonadal dysgenesis. *J Bone Joint Surg Am* 1960;42:600.

234. Neely EK, et al. Turner syndrome adolescents receiving growth hormone are not osteopenic. *J Clin Endocrinol Metab* 1993;76:861.

235. Matsunaga S, et al. Occult spinal canal stenosis due to C-1 hypoplasia in children with Down syndrome. *J Neurosurg* 2007;107(6 Suppl):457–459.

236. Saggese G, et al. Mineral metabolism in Turner's syndrome: evidence for impaired renal vitamin D metabolism and normal osteoblast function. *J Clin Endocrinol Metab* 1992;75:998.

237. Ross JL, et al. Normal bone density of the wrist and spine and increased wrist fractures in girls with Turner's syndrome. *J Clin Endocrinol Metab* 1991;73:355.

238. Yamazaki M, et al. Abnormal course of the vertebral artery at the craniovertebral junction in patients with Down syndrome visualized by three-dimensional CT angiography. *Neuroradiology* 2008;50(6):485–490.

239. Hata T, Todd MM. Cervical spine considerations when anesthetizing patients with Down syndrome. *Anesthesiology* 2005;102(3):680–685.

240. Rosenfeld RG. Growth hormone therapy in Turner's syndrome: an update on final height. *Acta Paediatr* 1992;383:3.

241. Rosenfeld RG, et al. Six year results of a randomized, prospective trial of human growth hormone and oxandrolone in Turner syndrome. *J Pediatr* 1992;121:49.

242. Bidwell JP, et al. Leg lengthening for short stature in Turner's syndrome. *J Bone Joint Surg Br* 2000;82(8):1174–1176.

243. Bakalov VK, et al. Growth hormone therapy and bone mineral density in Turner syndrome. *J Clin Endocrinol Metab* 2004;89(10):4886–4889.

244. Soriano RM, Weisz I, Houghton GR. Scoliosis in the Prader-Willi syndrome. *Spine* 1988;13:211.

245. Bakalov VK, et al. Bone mineral density and fractures in Turner syndrome. *Am J Med* 2003;115(4):259–264.

246. Mayhew JF, Taylor B. Anaesthetic considerations in the Prader-Willi syndrome. *Can Anaesth Soc J* 1983;30:565.

247. Carrel AL, Myers SE, Whitman BY. Growth hormone improves body composition, fat utilization, physical strength and agility, and growth in Prader-Willi syndrome: a controlled study. *J Pediatr* 1999;134:221.

248. Davies PS, Evans S, Broomhead S. Effect of growth hormone on height, weight, and body composition in Prader-Willi syndrome. *Arch Dis Child* 1998;78:476.

249. Schrander-Stumpel CT, et al. Prader-Willi syndrome: causes of death in an international series of 27 cases. *Am J Med Genet* 2004;124A(4):333–338.

250. Campbell AM, Bousfield JD. Anaesthesia in a patient with Noonan's syndrome and cardiomyopathy. *Anaesthesia* 1992;47:131.

251. Wedge JH, Khalifa MM, Shokeir MHK. Skeletal anomalies in 40 patients with Noonan's syndrome. *Orthop Trans* 1987;11:40.

252. Ogawa M, et al. Clinical evaluation of recombinant human growth hormone in Noonan syndrome. *Endocr J* 2004;51(1):61–68.

253. Tartaglia M, et al. PTPN11 mutations in Noonan syndrome: molecular spectrum, genotype-phenotype correlation, and phenotypic heterogeneity. *Am J Hum Genet* 2002;70:1555–1563.

254. Minguella I, et al. Trichorhinophalangeal syndrome, type I, with avascular necrosis of the femoral head. *Acta Paediatr* 1993;82:329.

255. Ludecke HJ, et al. Molecular definition of the shortest region of deletion overlap in the Langer-Giedion syndrome. *Am J Hum Genet* 1991;49:1197.

256. Guijarro M, et al. Bone mass in young adults with Down syndrome. *J Intellect Disabil Res* 2008;52(pt 3):182–189.

257. Rovet JF. The psychoeducational characteristics of children with Turner syndrome. *J Learn Disabil* 1993;26:333.

258. Gavranich J, Selikowitz M. A survey of 22 individuals with Prader-Willi syndrome in New South Wales. *Aust Paediatr J* 1989;25:43.

259. Curfs LM, Verhulst FC, Fryns JP. Behavioral and emotional problems in youngsters with Prader-Willi syndrome. *Genet Couns* 1991;2:33.

260. Selikowitz M, et al. Fenfluramine in Prader-Willi syndrome: a double blind, placebo controlled trial. *Arch Dis Child* 1990;65:112.

261. Hudgins L, Cassidy SB. Hand and foot length in Prader-Willi syndrome. *Am J Med Genet* 1991;41:5.

262. Waters J, Clarke DJ, Corbett JA. Educational and occupational outcome in Prader-Willi syndrome. *Child Care Health Dev* 1990;16:271.

263. Cassidy SB, ed. *Prader-Willi syndrome and other chromosome 15q deletion disorders.* NATO ASI series H: cell biology, Vol. 61. Heidelberg, Germany: Springer, 1992:265.

264. Knoll JH, Wagstaff J, Lalande M. Cytogenetic and molecular studies in the Prader-Willi and Angelman syndromes: an overview. *Am J Med Genet* 1993;46:2.

265. Nicholls RD. Genomic imprinting and uniparental disomy in Angelman and Prader-Willi syndromes: a review. *Am J Med Genet* 1993;46:16.

266. Gurd AR, Thompson TR. Scoliosis in Prader-Willi syndrome. *J Pediatr Orthop* 1981;1:317.

267. Holm VA, Laurnen EL. Prader-Willi syndrome and scoliosis. *Dev Med Child Neurol* 1981;23:192.

268. Holm VA, et al. Prader-Willi syndrome: consensus diagnostic criteria. *Pediatrics* 1993;91:398.

269. Rees D, et al. Scoliosis surgery in the Prader-Willi syndrome. *J Bone Joint Surg Br* 1989;71:685.

270. Cleeman L, et al. Long term hormone replacement therapy preserves bone mineral density in Turner syndrome. *Eur J Endocrinol* 2009;161(2):251–257.

271. Aycan Z, et al. The effect of growth hormone treatment on bone mineral density in prepubertal girls with Turner syndrome: a multicentre prospective clinical trial. *Clin Endocrinol (Oxf)* 2008;68(5):769–772.

272. Vliet GV, et al. Sudden death in growth hormone-treated children with Prader-Willi syndrome. *J Pediatr* 2004;144(1):129–131.

273. Rubinstein JH. Broad thumb-hallux (Rubinstein-Taybi) syndrome 1957–1988. *Am J Med Genet* 1990;6:3.

274. Hennekam RC, et al. Rubinstein-Taybi syndrome in The Netherlands. *Am J Med Genet* 1990;6:17.

275. Marion RW, Garcia DM, Karasik JB. Apparent dominant transmission of the Rubinstein-Taybi syndrome. *Am J Med Genet* 1993;46:284.

276. Allanson JE. Rubinstein-Taybi syndrome: the changing face. *Am J Med Genet* 1990;6:38.

277. Robson MJ, Brown LM, Sharrad WJW. Cervical spondylolsis syndrome and other skeletal abnormalities in Rubinstein-Taybi syndrome. *J Bone Joint Surg Br* 1980;62:297.

278. Hennekam RC, Doorne JMV. Oral aspects of Rubinstein-Taybi syndrome. *Am J Med Genet* 1990;6:42.

279. Partington MW. Rubinstein-Taybi syndrome: a follow-up study. *Am J Med Genet* 1990;6(Suppl):65.

280. Browd SR, McIntyre JS, Brockmeyer D. Failed age-dependent maturation of the occipital condyle in patients with congenital occipitoatlantal instability and Down syndrome: a preliminary analysis. *J Neurosurg Pediatr* 2008;2(5):359–364.

281. Ali FE, et al. Cervical spine abnormalities associated with Down syndrome. *Int Orthop* 2006;30(4):284–289.

282. Stevens CA, Carey JC, Blackburn BL. Rubinstein-Taybi syndrome: a natural history study. *Am J Med Genet* 1990;6:30.

283. Miller RW, Rubinstein JH. Tumors in Rubinstein-Taybi syndrome. *Am J Med Genet* 1995;56:115.

284. Mehlman CT, Rubinstein JH, Roy DR. Instability of the patellofemoral joint in Rubinstein-Taybi syndrome. *J Pediatr Orthop* 1998;18:511.

285. Stevens JM, et al. The odontoid process in Morquio-Brailsford's disease. The effects of occipitocervical fusion. *J Bone Joint Surg Br* 1991;73:851.

286. de Lind van Wijngaarden RF, et al. Randomized controlled trial to investigate the effects of growth hormone treatment on scoliosis in children with Prader-Willi syndrome. *J Clin Endocrinol Metab* 2009;94(4):1274–1280.

287. Kaplan P, Ramos F, Zackai EH. Cystic kidney disease in Hadju-Cheney syndrome. *Am J Med Genet* 1995;56:30.

288. Abdenur JE, et al. Response to nutritional and growth hormone treatment in progeria. *Metabolism* 1997;46:851.

289. Yan T, et al. Altered levels of primary antioxidant enzymes in progeria skin fibroblasts. *Biochem Biophys Res Commun* 1999;257:163.

290. Badame AJ. Progeria. *Arch Dermatol* 1989;125:540.

291. Gillar PJ, Kaye CI, McCourt JW. Progressive early dermatologic changes in Hutchinson-Gilford progeria syndrome. *Pediatr Dermatol* 1991;8:199.

292. Hopwood JJ, Morris CP. The mucopolysaccharidoses. Diagnosis, molecular genetics and treatment. *Mol Biol Med* 1990;7:381.

293. Scriver CR, et al. *The metabolic basis of inherited disease*, 6th ed. New York, NY: McGraw-Hill, 1989.

294. Fukada S, et al. Mucopolysaccharidosis type IVA. *N*-acetyl galactosamine-6-sulfate sulfatase exonic point mutations in classical Morquio and mild cases. *J Clin Invest* 1992;90:1049.

295. Jin WD, Jackson CE, Desnick RJ. Mucopolysaccharidosis type VI: identification of three mutations in the arylsulfatatase B gene of patients with severe and mild phenotypes provides molecular evidence for genetic heterogeneity. *Am J Hum Genet* 1992;50:795.

296. Field RE, et al. Bone marrow transplantation in Hurler's syndrome. Effect on skeletal development. *J Bone Joint Surg Br* 1994;76:957.

297. Souillet G, et al. Outcome of 27 patients with Hurler's syndrome transplanted from either related or unrelated haematopoietic stem cell sources. *Bone Marrow Transpl* 2003;31(12):1105–1117.

298. Kakkis ED, Muenzer J, Tiller GE. Enzyme replacement therapy in mucopolysaccharidosis I. *N Engl J Med* 2001;344:182–188.

299. Odunusi E, et al. Genu valgum deformity in Hurler syndrome after hematopoietic stem cell transplantation: correction by surgical intervention. *J Pediatr Orthop* 1999;19:270.

300. Haddad FS, Hill RA, Jones DH. Triggering in the mucopolysaccharidoses. *J Pediatr Orthop B* 1998;7:138.

301. Haddad FS, Jones DH, Vellodi A. Carpal tunnel syndrome in the mucopolysaccharidoses and mucopolipidoses. *J Bone Joint Surg Br* 1997;79:576.

302. Baker E, et al. The Morquio A syndrome (mucopolysaccharidosis IVA) gene maps to 16q24.3. *Am J Hum Genet* 1993;52:96.

303. Bassett GS. Orthopaedic aspects of skeletal dysplasias. *Instr Course Lect, AAOS* 1990;39:389.

304. Weleber RG, Beals RK. Hadju-Cheney syndrome: report of 2 cases and review of literature. *J Pediatr* 1976;88:249.

305. Herati RS, et al. Radiographic evaluation of bones and joints in mucopolysaccharidosis I and VII dogs after neonatal gene therapy. *Mol Genet Metab* 2008;95(3):142–151.

306. Quinn CM, Wigglesworth JS, Heckmatt J. Lethal arthrogryposis multiplex congenita: a pathological study of 21 cases. *Histopathology* 1991;19:155.

307. Taylor C, et al. Mobility in Hurler syndrome. *J Pediatr Orthop* 2008;28(2):163–168.

308. Stevens CA. Patellar dislocation in Rubintein-Taybi syndrome. *Am J Med Genet* 1997;72:190.

309. Goldberg MJ. Orthopaedic aspects of bone dysplasia. *Orthop Clin North Am* 1976;7:445.

310. Kopits SE. Orthopaedic complications of dwarfism. *Clin Orthop* 1976;114:153.

311. Nelson J, Thomas PS. Clinical findings in 12 patients with MPS IVA (Morquio's disease): further evidence for heterogeneity. Part III: odontoid dysplasia. *Clin Genet* 1988;33:126.

312. Accadbled F, et al. Complications of scoliosis surgery in Prader-Willi syndrome. *Spine (Phila Pa 1976)* 2008;33(4):394–401.

313. West LA, Ballock RT. High incidence of hip dysplasia but not slipped capital femoral epiphysis in patients with Prader-Willi syndrome. *J Pediatr Orthop* 2004;24(5):565–567.

314. Drake WM, Hiorns MP, Kendler DL. Hadju-Cheney syndrome: response to therapy with bisphosphonates in two patients. *J Bone Miner Res* 2003;18(1):131–133.

315. Kaler SG, Geggel RL, Sadehgi-Nejad A. Hadju-Cheney syndrome associated with severe cardiac valvular and conduction disease. *Am J Med Genet* 1995;56:30.

316. Monu JU, Benka-Coker LB, Fatunde Y. Hutchinson-Gilford progeria syndrome in siblings. Report of three new cases. *Skeletal Radiol* 1990;19:585.

317. Khalifa MM. Hutchinson-Gilford progeria syndrome: report of a Libyan family and evidence of autosomal recessive inheritance. *Clin Genet* 1989;35:125.

318. Brown WT. Progeria: a human-disease model of accelerated aging. *Am J Clin Nutr* 1992;55(Suppl 6):1222S.

319. Moen C. Orthopaedic aspects of progeria. *J Bone Joint Surg Am* 1982;64:542.

320. Reichel W, et al. Radiological findings in progeria. *J Am Geriatr Soc* 1971;19:657.

321. Fernandez-Palazzi F, McLaren AT, Slowie DF. Report on a case of Hutchinson-Gilford progeria, with special reference to orthopedic problems. *Eur J Pediatr Surg* 1992;2:378.

322. Yamamoto T, et al. Congenital anomaly of cervical vertebrae is a major complication of Rubinstein-Taybi syndrome. *Am J Med Genet A* 2005;135(2):130–133.

323. Tanaka T, et al. Rubinstein-Taybi syndrome in children with tethered spinal cord. *J Neurosurg* 2006;105(4 Suppl):261–264.

324. Gamble JG. Hip disease in Hutchinson-Gilford progeria syndrome. *J Pediatr Orthop* 1984;4:585.

325. Hall JG. Genetic aspects of arthrogryposis. *Clin Orthop* 1985;194:44.

326. Hall JG, Reed SD, Driscoll EP. Part I. Amyoplasia: a common, sporadic condition with congenital contractures. *Am J Med Genet* 1983;15:571.

327. Bennet JB, et al. Surgical management of arthrogryposis in the upper extremity. *J Pediatr Orthop* 1985;5:281.

328. Williams PF. Management of upper limb problems in arthrogryposis. *Clin Orthop* 1985;194:60.

329. Doyle JR, et al. Restoration of elbow flexion in arthrogryposis multiplex congenita. *J Hand Surg* 1980;5:149.

330. Sarwark JF, MacEwen GD, Scott CI. Current concepts review. Amyoplasia (a common form of arthrogryposis). *J Bone Joint Surg Am* 1990;72:465.

331. Weston PJ, Ives EJ, Honore RL. Monochromonic diamniotic minimally conjoined twins. *Am J Med Genet* 1990;37:558.

332. Jacobson L, Polizzi A, Morriss-Kay G. Plasma from human mothers of fetuses with severe arthrogryposis multiplex congenita causes deformities in mice. *J Clin Invest* 1999;103:1038.

CHAPTER 8 | SYNDROMES OF ORTHOPAEDIC IMPORTANCE **275**

333. Banker BQ. Neuropathologic aspects of arthrogryposis multiplex congenita. *Clin Orthop* 1985;194:30.

334. Clarren SK, Hall JG. Neuropathologic findings in the spinal cords of 10 infants with arthrogryposis. *J Neurol Sci* 1983;58:89.

335. Malm G, et al. Outcome in six children with mucopolysaccharidosis type IH, Hurler syndrome, after haematopoietic stem cell transplantation (HSCT). *Acta Paediatr* 2008;97(8):1108–1112.

336. Brown LM, Robson MJ, Sharrard WJW. The pathology of arthrogryposis multiplex congenita neurologica. *J Bone Joint Surg Br* 1980;62:291.

337. Robinson RO. Arthrogryposis multiplex congenita: feeding, language and other health problems. *Neuropediatrics* 1990;21:177.

338. Fahy MJ, Hall JG. A retrospective study of pregnancy complications among 828 cases of arthrogryposis. *Genet Couns* 1990;1:3.

339. Carlson WO, et al. Arthrogryposis multiplex congenita. A long-term follow-up study. *Clin Orthop* 1985;194:115.

340. Davidson J, Beighton P. Whence the arthrogrypotics? *J Bone Joint Surg Br* 1976;58:492.

341. Hoffer MM, et al. Ambulation in severe arthrogryposis. *J Pediatr Orthop* 1983;3:293.

342. Hahn G. Arthrogryposis. Pediatric review and rehabilitative aspects. *Clin Orthop* 1985;194:105.

343. Thompson GH, Bilenker RM. Comprehensive management of arthrogryposis multiplex congenita. *Clin Orthop* 1985;194:6.

344. Palmer PM, et al. Passive motion therapy for infants with arthrogryposis. *Clin Orthop* 1985;194:54.

345. Huurman WW, Jacobsen ST. The hip in arthrogryposis multiplex congenita. *Clin Orthop* 1985;194:81.

346. Clair HSS, Zimbler S. A plan of management and treatment results in the arthrogrypotic hip. *Clin Orthop* 1985;194:74.

347. Yau PW, et al. Twenty-year follow-up of hip problems in arthrogryposis multiplex congenita. *J Pediatr Orthop* 2002;22(3):359–363.

348. Guidera JK, et al. Radiographic changes in arthrogrypotic knees. *Skeletal Radiol* 1991;20:193.

349. Zimbler S, Craig CL. The arthrogrypotic foot. Plan of management and results of treatment. *Foot Ankle* 1983;3:211.

350. Green ADL, Fixsen JA, Lloyd-Roberts GC. Talectomy for arthrogryposis multiplex congenita. *J Bone Joint Surg Br* 1984;66:697.

351. Hsu LCS, Jaffray D, Leong JCY. Talectomy for club foot in arthrogryposis. *J Bone Joint Surg Br* 1984;66:694.

352. Niki H, Staheli LT, Mosca VS. Management of clubfoot deformity in amyoplasia. *J Pediatr Orthop* 1997;17:803.

353. Odent T, et al. Scoliosis in patients with Prader-Willi Syndrome. *Pediatrics* 2008;122(2):e499–e503.

354. Sodergard J, Ryoppy S, et al. The knee in arthrogryposis multiplex congenita. *J Pediatr Orthop* 1990;10:177.

355. Thomas B, Schopler S, Wood W. The knee in arthrogryposis. *Clin Orthop* 1985;194:87.

356. Brunner R, Hefti F, Tgetgel JD. Arthrogrypotic joint contracture at the knee and the foot: correction with a circular frame. *J Pediatr Orthop B* 1997;6:192.

357. Mooney JF, Koman LA. Knee flexion contractures: soft tissue correction with monolateral external fixation. *J South Orthop Assoc* 2001;10(1):32–36.

358. Guidera KJ, Drennan JC. Foot and ankle deformities in arthrogryposis multiplex congenita. *Clin Orthop* 1985;194:93.

359. Chang CH, Huang SC. Surgical treatment of clubfoot deformity in arthrogryposis multiplex congenita. *J Formos Med Assoc* 1997;96:30.

360. Bayne LG. Hand assessment and management of arthrogryposis multiplex congenita. *Clin Orthop* 1985;194:68.

361. Yonenobu K, Tada K, Swanson B. Arthrogryposis of the hand. *J Pediatr Orthop* 1984;4:599.

362. Daher YH, et al. Spinal deformities in patients with arthrogryposis. A review of 16 patients. *Spine* 1985;10:608.

363. Yingsakmongkol W, Kumar SJ. Scoliosis in arthrogryposis multiplex congenita: results after nonsurgical and surgical treatment. *J Pediatr Orthop* 200;20(5):656–661.

364. Larsen LJ, Schottstaedt ER, Bost FC. Multiple congenital dislocations associated with characteristic facial abnormality. *J Pediatr* 1950;37:574.

365. Laville JM, Lakermance P, Limouzy F. Larsen's syndrome: review of the literature and analysis of thirty-eight cases. *J Pediatr Orthop* 1994;14:63.

366. Debeer P, et al. Asymmetrical Larsen syndrome in a young girl: a second example of somatic mosaicism in this syndrome. *Genet Couns* 2003;14(1):95–100.

367. Munk S. Early operation of the dislocated knee in Larsen's syndrome. A report of two cases. *Acta Orthop Scand* 1988;59:582.

368. Steel HH, Koh EJ. Multiple dislocations associated with other skeletal anomalies (Larsen's syndrome) in three siblings. *J Bone Joint Surg Am* 1972;54:75.

369. Oki T, et al. Clinical features and treatment of joint dislocations in Larsen's syndrome. Report of three cases in one family. *Clin Orthop* 1976;119:206.

370. Bowen JR, et al. Spinal deformities in Larsen's syndrome. *Clin Orthop* 1985;197:159.

371. Micheli LJ, Hall JE, Watts HG. Spinal instability in Larsen's syndrome. Report of three cases. *J Bone Joint Surg Am* 1976;58:562.

372. Habermann ET, Sterling A, Dennis RI. Larsen's syndrome: a heritable disorder. *J Bone Joint Surg Am* 1976;58:558.

373. Johnston CE, Birch JG, Daniels JL. Cervical kyphosis in patients who have Larsen syndrome. *J Bone Joint Surg Am* 1996;78:545.

374. Stevenson GW, Hall SC, Palmieri J. Anesthetic considerations for patients with Larsen's syndrome. *Anaesthesia* 1991;75:142.

375. Kiel EA, Frias JL, Victorica BE. Cardiovascular manifestations in the Larsen syndrome. *Pediatrics* 1983;71:942.

376. Salis JG, Beighton P. Dominantly inherited digito-talar dysmorphism. *J Bone Joint Surg Br* 1972;54:509.

377. Hall JG, Reed SD, Greene G. The distal arthrogryposes: delineation of new entities—review and nosologic discussion. *Am J Med Genet* 1982;11:185.

378. Zancolli E, Zancolli JE. Congenital ulnar drift of the fingers. Pathogenesis, classification, and surgical management. *Hand Clin* 1985;1:443.

379. Hageman G, et al. The heterogeneity of distal arthrogryposis. *Brain Dev* 198; 6:273.

380. McCormack MK, Coppola-McCormack P, Lee M. Autosomal-dominant inheritance of distal arthrogryposis. *Am J Med Genet* 1980;6:163.

381. Sung SS, et al. Mutations in genes encoding fast-twitch contractile proteins cause distal arthrogryposis syndromes. *Am J Hum Genet* 2003;72:681–690.

382. Robinow M, Johnson GF. The Gordon syndrome: autosomal dominant cleft palate, camptodactyly, and club feet. *Am J Med Genet* 1981;9:139.

383. Rozin MM, Hertz M, Goodman RM. A new syndrome with camptodactyly, joint contractures, facial anomalies, and skeletal defects: a case report and review of syndromes with camptodactyly. *Clin Genet* 1984;26:342.

384. Bui TH, et al. Prenatal diagnosis of distal arthrogryposis type I by ultrasonography. *Prenat Diagn* 1992;12:1047.

385. Malkawi H, Tarawneh M. The whistling face syndrome, or craniocarpal-tarsal dysplasia. Report of two cases in a father and son and review of the literature. *J Pediatr Orthop* 1983;3:364.

386. Wettstein A, et al. A family with whistling face syndrome. *Hum Genet* 1980;55:177.

387. Rinsky LA, Bleck EE. Freeman-Sheldon ("whistling face") syndrome. *J Bone Joint Surg Am* 1976;58:148.

388. Tassinari E, et al. Bilateral total hip arthroplasty in Morquio-Brailsford's syndrome: a report of two cases. *Chir Organi Mov* 2008;92(2):123–126.

389. Matt P, et al. Recent advances in understanding Marfan syndrome: should we now treat surgical patients with losartan? *J Thorac Cardiovasc Surg* 2008;135(2):389–394.

390. Borowski A, et al. Diagnostic imaging of the knee in children with arthrogryposis and knee extension or hyperextension contracture. *J Pediatr Orthop* 2008;28(4):466–470.

391. Hakan T, et al. Spinal schwannomatosis: case report of a rare condition. *Turk Neurosurg* 2008;18(3):320–323.

392. Habashi JP, et al. Losartan, an AT1 antagonist, prevents aortic aneurysm in a mouse model of Marfan syndrome. *Science* 2006;312(5770):117–121.

393. Connell DJO, Hall CM. Cranio-carpo-tarsal dysplasia. A report of seven cases. *Radiology* 1977;123:719.

394. Wenner SM, Shalvoy RM. Two stage correction of thumb adductor contracture in Freeman-Sheldon syndrome. *J Hand Surg* 1989;14:937.

395. Marasovich WA, Mazaheri M, Stool SE. Otolaryngologic findings in whistling face syndrome. *Arch Otolaryngol Head Neck Surg* 1989;115:1373.

396. Duggar RG, DeMars PD, Bolton VE. Whistling face syndrome: general anesthesia and early postoperative caudal analgesia. *Anesthesiology* 1989;70:545.

397. Biesecker L. The challenges of Proteus syndrome: diagnosis and management. *Eur J Hum Genet* 2006;14(11):1151–1157.

398. Doughty KS, Richmond JC. Arthroscopic findings in the knee in nail-patella syndrome: a case report. *Arthroscopy* 2005;21(1):e1–e5.

399. Verona LL, et al. Monozygotic twins discordant for Goldenhar syndrome. *J Pediatr (Rio J)* 2006;82(1):75–78.

400. Boles DJ, Bodurtha J, Nance WE. Goldenhar complex in discordant monozygotic twins: a case report and review of the literature. *Am J Med Genet* 1987;28(1):103–109.

401. Anderson PJ, David DJ. Spinal anomalies in Goldenhar syndrome. *Cleft Palate Craniofac J* 2005;42(5):477–480.

402. Die-Smulders CED, et al. The lethal multiple pterygium syndrome: a nosological approach. *Genet Couns* 1990;1:13.

403. McCall RE, Buddon J. Treatment of multiple pterygium syndrome. *Orthopedics* 1992;15:1417.

404. Penchaszadeh VB, Salszberg B. Multiple pterygium syndrome. *J Med Genet* 1981;18:451.

405. Winter RB. Scoliosis and the multiple pterygium syndrome. *J Pediatr Orthop* 1983;3:125.

406. Escobar V, Weaver D. Popliteal pterygium syndrome. A phenotypic and genetic analysis. *J Med Genet* 1978;15:35.

407. Froster-Iskenns VG. Popliteal pterygium syndrome. *J Med Genet* 1990;27:320.

408. Oppenheim WL, et al. Popliteal pterygium syndrome: an orthopaedic perspective. *J Pediatr Orthop* 1990;10:58.

409. Cunningham LN, et al. Urologic manifestations of the popliteal pterygium syndrome. *J Urol* 1989;141:910.

410. Addison A, Webb PJ. Flexion contractures of the knee associated with popliteal webbing. *J Pediatr Orthop* 1983;3:376.

411. Crawford A. Treatment of popliteal pterygium syndrome. *J Pediatr Orthop* 1982;2:443.

412. Hansson LI, Hansson V, Jonsson K. Popliteal pterygium syndrome in a 74-year-old woman. *Acta Orthop Scand* 1976;47:525.

413. Saleh M, Gibson MF, Sharrard WJ. Femoral shortening in correction of congenital knee flexion deformity with popliteal webbing. *J Pediatr Orthop* 1989;9:609.

414. Wynne JM, Fraser AG, Herman R. Massive oral membrane in the popliteal web syndrome. *J Pediatr Surg* 1982;17:59.

415. Koch H, Grzonka M, Koch J. Popliteal pterygium syndrome with special consideration of the cleft malformation. *Cleft Palate Craniofac J* 1992;29:80.

416. Bertrand J, Floyd LL, Weber MK. Guidelines for identifying and referring persons with fetal alcohol syndrome. *MMWR Recomm Rep* 2005;54(RR-11):1–14.

417. Boehm S, et al. Early results of the Ponseti method for the treatment of clubfoot in distal arthrogryposis. *J Bone Joint Surg Am* 2008;90(7):1501–1507.

418. Johnston DR, et al. Long-term outcome of MacIntosh reconstruction of chronic anterior cruciate ligament insufficiency using fascia lata. *J Orthop Sci* 2003;8(6):789–795.

419. Jones KB, et al. Symposium on the musculoskeletal aspects of Marfan syndrome: meeting report and state of the science. *J Orthop Res* 2007;25(3):413–422.

420. Place HM, Enzenauer RJ. Cervical spine subluxation in Marfan syndrome. A case report. *J Bone Joint Surg Am* 2006;88(11):2479–2482.

421. Van de Velde S, Fillman R, Yandow S. Protrusio acetabuli in Marfan syndrome. History, diagnosis, and treatment. *J Bone Joint Surg Am* 2006;88(3):639–646.

422. Sponseller PD, et al. Protrusio acetabuli in Marfan syndrome: age-related prevalence and associated hip function. *J Bone Joint Surg Am* 2006;88(3):486–495.

423. Van de Velde S, Fillman R, Yandow S. Protrusio acetabuli in Marfan syndrome: indication for surgery in skeletally immature Marfan patients. *J Pediatr Orthop* 2005;25(5):603–606.

424. Stevenson DA, et al. Tibial geometry in individuals with neurofibromatosis type 1 without anterolateral bowing of the lower leg using peripheral quantitative computed tomography. *Bone* 2009;44(4):585–589.

425. Tucker T, et al. Bone health and fracture rate in individuals with NF1. *J Med Genet* 2009;46(4):259–265.

426. Leskela HV, et al. Congenital pseudarthrosis of neurofibromatosis type 1: impaired osteoblast differentiation and function and altered NF1 gene expression. *Bone* 2009;44(2):243–250.

427. Ofluoglu O, Davidson RS, Dormans JP. Prophylactic bypass grafting and long-term bracing in the management of anterolateral bowing of the tibia and neurofibromatosis-1. *J Bone Joint Surg Am* 2008;90(10):2126–2134.

428. Schindeler A, Little DG. Recent insights into bone development, homeostasis, and repair in type 1 neurofibromatosis (NF1). *Bone* 2008;42(4):616–622.

429. Galaini CA, Matt BH. Laryngomalacia and intraneural striated muscle in an infant with Freeman-Sheldon syndrome. *Int J Pediatr Otolaryngol* 1993;25:243.

430. Jones R, Dolcourt JL. Muscle rigidity following halothane in two patients with Freeman-Sheldon. *Anesthesiology* 1992;77:599.

431. Sauk JJ, Delaney JR, Reaume C, et al. Electromyography of oralfacial musculature in craniocarpotarsal dysplasia (Freeman-Sheldon syndrome). *Clin Genet* 1974;6:132.

432. Hall JG, Reed SD, Rosenbaum KN, et al. Limb pterygium syndromes: a review and report of 11 patients. *Am J Med Genet* 1982;12:377.

433. Endo H, et al. Nontraumatic subluxation of the hip after spine surgery for scoliosis in a patient with von Recklinghausen's disease. *J Orthop Sci* 2007;12(5):510–514.

434. Schindeler A, et al. Modeling bone morphogenetic protein and bisphosphonate combination therapy in wild-type and Nf1 haploinsufficient mice. *J Orthop Res* 2008;26(1):65–74.

435. Stevenson DA, et al. The use of anterolateral bowing of the lower leg in the diagnostic criteria for neurofibromatosis type 1. *Genet Med* 2007;9(7):409–412.

436. Dulai S, et al. Decreased bone mineral density in neurofibromatosis type 1: results from a pediatric cohort. *J Pediatr Orthop* 2007;27(4):472–475.

437. Stevenson DA, et al. Bone mineral density in children and adolescents with neurofibromatosis type 1. *J Pediatr* 2007;150(1):83–88.

438. Cytrynbaum CS, et al. Advances in overgrowth syndromes: clinical classification to molecular delineation in Sotos syndrome and Beckwith-Wiedemann syndrome. *Curr Opin Pediatr* 2005;17(6):740–746.

439. Dillon ER, et al. Ambulatory activity in youth with arthrogryposis: a cohort study. *J Pediatr Orthop* 2009;29(2):214–217.

440. Sapp JC, et al. Newly delineated syndrome of congenital lipomatous overgrowth, vascular malformations, and epidermal nevi (CLOVE syndrome) in seven patients. *Am J Med Genet A* 2007;143A(24):2944–2958.

441. Musio A, et al. X-linked Cornelia de Lange syndrome owing to SMC1L1 mutations. *Nat Genet* 2006;38(5):528–530.

442. Tonkin ET, et al. NIPBL, encoding a homolog of fungal Scc2-type sister chromatid cohesion proteins and fly Nipped-B, is mutated in Cornelia de Lange syndrome. *Nat Genet* 2004;36(6):636–641.

443. Ahlgren SC, Thakur V, Bronner-Fraser M. Sonic hedgehog rescues cranial neural crest from cell death induced by ethanol exposure. *Proc Natl Acad Sci U S A* 2002;99(16):10476–10481.

444. Akazawa H, Oda K, Mitani S. Surgical management of hip dislocation in children with arthrogryposis multiplex congenita. *J Bone Joint Surg Br* 1998;80:636.

445. Staheli LT, Chow DE, Elliott JS, et al. Management of hip dislocations in children with arthrogryposis. *J Pediatr Orthop* 1987;7:681.

446. Williams P. The management of arthrogryposis. *Orthop Clin North Am* 1978;9:67.

447. Szoke G, Staheli LT, Jaffer K, et al. Medial-approach open reduction of hip dislocation in amyoplasia-type arthrogryposis. *J Pediatr Orthop* 1996;16:127.

448. Ho CA, Karol LA. The utility of knee releases in arthrogryposis. *J Pediatr Orthop* 2008;28(3):307–313.

449. van Bosse HJ, et al. Treatment of knee flexion contractures in patients with arthrogryposis. *J Pediatr Orthop* 2007;27(8):930–937.

450. Devalia KL, et al. Joint distraction and reconstruction in complex knee contractures. *J Pediatr Orthop* 2007;27(4):402–407.

451. Sodergard J, Ryoppy S. The knee in arthrogryposis multiplex congenita. *J Pediatr Orthop* 1990;10:177.

452. Thomas B, Schopler S, Wood W, et al. The knee in arthrogryposis. *Clin Orthop* 1985;194:87.

453. Murray C, Fixsen JA. Management of knee deformity in classical arthrogryposis multiplex congenita (amyoplasia congenita). *J Pediatr Orthop B* 1997;6:191.

454. Klatt J, Stevens PM. Guided growth for fixed knee flexion deformity. *J Pediatr Orthop* 2008;28(6):626–631.

455. van Bosse HJ, et al. Correction of arthrogrypotic clubfoot with a modified Ponseti technique. *Clin Orthop Relat Res* 2009;467(5):1283–1293.

456. Van Heest A, et al. Posterior elbow capsulotomy with triceps lengthening for treatment of elbow extension contracture in children with arthrogryposis. *J Bone Joint Surg Am* 2008;90(7):1517–1523.

457. Hermanns P, et al. Congenital joint dislocations caused by carbohydrate sulfotransferase 3 deficiency in recessive Larsen syndrome and humerospinal dysostosis. *Am J Hum Genet* 2008;82(6):1368–1374.

458. Madera M, Crawford A, Mangano FT. Management of severe cervical kyphosis in a patient with Larsen syndrome. Case report. *J Neurosurg Pediatr* 2008;1(4):320–324.

459. Sakaura H, et al. Surgical treatment of cervical kyphosis in Larsen syndrome: report of 3 cases and review of the literature. *Spine (Phila Pa 1976)* 2007;32(1):E39–E44.

460. Williams PF. Management of upper limb problems in arthrogryposis. *Clin Orthop* 1985;194:60.

461. Doyle JR, James PM, Larsen W, et al. Restoration of elbow flexion in arthrogryposis multiplex congenita. *J Hand Surg* 1980;5:149.

462. Van Heest A, Waters PM, Simmons BP. Surgical treatment of arthrogryposis of the elbow. *J Hand Surg Am* 1998;23:1063.

463. Axt MW, Niethard FU, Doderlein L. Principles of treatment of the upper extremity in arthrogryposis multiplex congenita type I. *J Pediatr Orthop B* 1997;6:179.

464. Atkins RM, Bell MJ, Sharrard WJW. Pectoralis major transfer for paralysis of elbow flexion in children. *J Bone Joint Surg Br* 1985;67:640.

465. Houston CS, Reed MH, Desautels JEL. Separating Larsen syndrome from the "arthrogryposis basket." *J Can Assoc Radiol* 1981;32:206.

466. Klenn PJ, Iozzo RV. Larsen's syndrome with novel congenital anomalies. *Hum Pathol* 1991;22:1055.

467. Laville JM, Lakermance P, Limouzy F. Larsen's syndrome: review of the literature and analysis of thirty-eight cases. *J Pediatr Orthop* 1994;14:63.

468. Oki T, Terashima Y, Murachi S, et al. Clinical features and treatment of joint dislocations in Larsen's syndrome. Report of three cases in one family. *Clin Orthop* 1976;119:206.

469. Dalainas I. Regarding percutaneous embolization of a lumbar pseudoaneurysm in a patient with type IV Ehlers-Danlos syndrome. *J Vasc Surg* 2008;47(6):1376; author reply 1376.

470. Lampasi M, Greggi T, Sudanese A. Pathological dislocation of the hip in neurofibromatosis: a case report. *Chir Organi Mov* 2008;91(3):163–166.

471. Tsirikos AI, McMaster MJ. Goldenhar-associated conditions (hemifacial microsomia) and congenital deformities of the spine. *Spine* 2006;31(13):E400–E407.

Localized Disorders of Skin and Soft Tissue

This chapter focuses on conditions that have orthopaedic manifestations localized to a particular area or region. It is difficult to classify these conditions under any particular systemic diagnosis or define them as a discrete bone or soft-tissue disease. Some of these conditions are complex and involve multiple organ systems; however, this chapter concentrates primarily on the orthopaedic manifestations and just gives a brief overview on the general condition.

CONGENITAL AND DEVELOPMENTAL DISORDERS

Hemangiomas and Vascular Malformations. Vascular abnormalities are commonly seen in patients and can range in severity from a simple cutaneous hemangioma to a complex arteriovenous malformation in the central nervous system. From an orthopaedic perspective, it is important to recognize which vascular abnormalities give rise to musculoskeletal problems that may require orthopaedic intervention.

The nomenclature for these conditions is historically complex with eponyms such as port wine stains, Sturge-Weber syndrome, Klippel-Trenaunay syndrome, and Proteus syndrome. This has contributed to the confusion in understanding the natural history of these lesions and difficulty in collecting data and developing appropriate treatment strategies. Mulliken and Glowacki (1) simplified our understanding of the underlying pathology and made a distinction between hemangiomas and vascular malformations that forms the basis of their clinical distinction today (1). They based their classification on the clinical presentation and behavior of the lesions and their histology and biochemistry. *Hemangiomas* exhibit cellular proliferation and have rapid growth in infancy and then subsequent regression. *Vascular malformations* on the other hand are composed of malformed vessels that do not exhibit endothelial cell proliferation. They are present at birth, and their growth parallels that of the child. They never regress. Vascular lesions can be arterial, venous, capillary, and lymphatic or a combination of any of these.

This classification was modified slightly in 1996 by the International Society for the Study of Vascular Anomalies (ISSVA) to vascular tumors and vascular malformations (2–4). This allowed the less common tumors of tufted angioma (5) and kaposiform hemangioendothelioma (6) to be included as vascular tumors.

For simplicity, this chapter uses the classification of Mulliken and Glowacki (1).

Hemangiomas and vascular malformations can present in many different ways in infants and young children. The most common presenting complaint is the disfiguration; however, some patients complain of pain, swelling, leg length discrepancy, and occasionally bleeding. The investigations often need to include detailed imaging including magnetic resonance imaging (MRI) and angiography. The nonoperative management is challenging, and the decision for surgical intervention fraught with technical challenges, complications, and variable outcomes. In this respect, it is useful to have a multidisciplinary approach to these patients including ORL, general, orthopaedic, plastic, and vascular surgeons.

Hemangiomas. A hemangioma is a congenital malformation of the local blood vessels. They may be cutaneous, subcutaneous, intramuscular, or visceral. There are many different types of vascular tumors, of which infantile hemangiomas are the most common. Others are rare and include tufted angioma, kaposiform hemangioendothelioma, hemangiopericytoma, and angiosarcoma. Infantile hemangiomas are usually single and occur most commonly in the head and neck region (60%) followed by the trunk and extremities. Internal (cavernous) hemangiomas are more common if there are five or more cutaneous hemangiomas present.

Cutaneous hemangiomas are common. They are present in 1.1% to 2.6% of term neonates and up to 12% of children at 1 year of age (7, 8). They can occur in all races but are more common in white infants. The incidence is three times higher in girls than boys (9). These collection of capillary type vessels appear in the neonatal period often as a small cutaneous mark and will grow disproportionately fast for a few months. The hemangioma is usually a vivid red color with an irregular outline. The lesion does not blanche with direct pressure with the examiner's finger. These lesions were historically referred to as strawberry naevi or capillary hemangioma. The hemangioma has a natural history that can be divided into three phases: proliferative, involuting, and involuted (10). The proliferative phase is characterized by the rapid dividing of the epithelial cells, whereas the involution phase is slower with far less endothelial activity. There is complete regression of the lesions in 70% of the children by 7 years of age (1). Only 50% of children are left with normal skin; the others may have some residual scaring, telangiectasis, or fibrofatty tissue.

Deep hemangiomas usually arise in the dermis or muscle and are not always very visible on the skin. Often the only indication of the underlying hemangioma is a slight "bump" in the skin or bluish discoloration. They used to be called cavernous hemangiomas due to their larger size; however, this nomenclature is no longer used. Deep hemangiomas usually involute like their superficial counterparts. They can be confused with a venous malformation (VM); however, on palpation, the hemangioma is fibrofatty rather than soft and compressible, which is characteristic of a VM. Ultrasound scanning or MRI can easily differentiate between the two if any clinical confusion exists.

Although most hemangiomas resolve, up to 20% can cause significant complications. These mainly occur around the head and neck where there may be direct compression on the eyes, significant vessels, or the airway. High-output cardiac failure can occur if the hemangioma is extremely large. When the gastrointestinal tract is involved, internal bleeding can be significant.

These hemangiomas rarely cause orthopaedic complications; however, knowledge of them is useful as a parent will often ask about these lesions during a consultation. One can usually reassure the family that they will spontaneously resolve; however, if they do not behave in a predictable way, referral to the multidisciplinary vascular clinic is advisable. Occasionally, intralesional or systemic corticosteroids and interferon-α are used for large recalcitrant lesions (8).

Vascular Malformations. Vascular malformations grow "pari passu" with the child, have normal endothelial mitotic activity in the vessel walls, and never regress (1). They are subclassified further according to their flow characteristics.

- Slow flow
  - Capillary malformations (CMs): port wine stains, telangiectasis
  - Venous malformations (VM)
  - Lymphatic malformations (LMs): lymphangiomas and cystic hygromas
- High flow
  - Arterial (AMs) and arterial venous malformations (AVMs)

There are also combined and more complex forms of vascular malformations, for example, Klippel-Trenaunay syndrome, which is a slow-flow lesion that has a combination of CM, VM, and LM. A summary of some more common vascular malformations and their associations is outlined in Table 9-1.

TABLE 9-1	Associations of Vascular Malformations in Children			
Syndrome	Type and Location	Clinical Problems	Orthopaedic Concerns	Mode of Inheritance
Vascular Malformations on Limbs				
Klippel-Trenaunay	Capillary-venous malformation anywhere, arteriovenous malformations in the extremities	Varicose veins, cardiac overload	Limb hypertrophy, macrodactyly	
Blue rubber bleb nevus	Multifocal cutaneous and visceral venous malformations	Gastrointestinal bleeding	Limb hypertrophy, hemarthrosis	Autosomal dominant
Maffucci	Venous malformations in subcutaneous tissue and intraosseous enchondromas	Malignant tumors	Enchondroma with skeletal deformity, overgrowth, and sarcoma	
Central Hemangiomas with Indirect Effects on Skeleton				
Rendu-Osler-Weber (hereditary hemorrhagic telangiectasia)	Capillary malformations on the lips, tongue, mucous membranes, and gastrointestinal and genitourinary systems	Bleeding from all sites, anemia, pulmonary arteriovenous malformations	Skeletal vascular malformations (hands, wrist, axial skeleton)	Autosomal dominant
Sturge-Weber	Capillary malformation on face, vascular malformation on brain	Seizures, mental retardation, glaucoma	Hemiplegia, hemiatrophy (neurogenic)	
Ataxia telangiectasia	Capillary malformations on conjunctivae, face, neck, and arms	Progressive ataxia, sinus and pulmonary infections, lymphomas	Mimics Friedreich ataxia: foot and ankle contractures	Autosomal recessive

Vascular malformations are more relevant to the orthopaedic surgeon than hemangiomas as they often result in altered limb growth. This can be hypertrophy or atrophy.

Slow-Flow Vascular Malformations

A. *Diffuse CM involving an entire limb with congenital hypertrophy of the limb (3).* In this condition, the child is born with an enlarged red limb with the adjacent trunk sometimes involved. There is a sharp midline demarcation. The entire limb is enlarged including the soft tissues and bone. There is no progression in the overgrowth after birth. Doppler ultrasound can be used to exclude any AV malformations. No orthopaedic intervention is required.

B. *Diffuse VM of an extremity.* The limb is usually blue rather than red (capillary) due to the dermal invasion of the large distorted veins. The venous channels also invade the muscles and the joints, which results in amyotrophy and swelling of the limb. MRI is the best investigation as the T2-weighted images clearly show the soft-tissue and joint involvement (Fig. 9-1). The limb may have slight undergrowth that is

usually <2 cm so does not require orthopaedic intervention. Overgrowth is less common and rarely exceeds 2 cm (3). Patients can also get a localized intravascular coagulopathy (LIC) with elevated D-dimer levels and decreased fibrinogen (11). The mainstay of treatment for LIC is low-molecular-weight heparin.

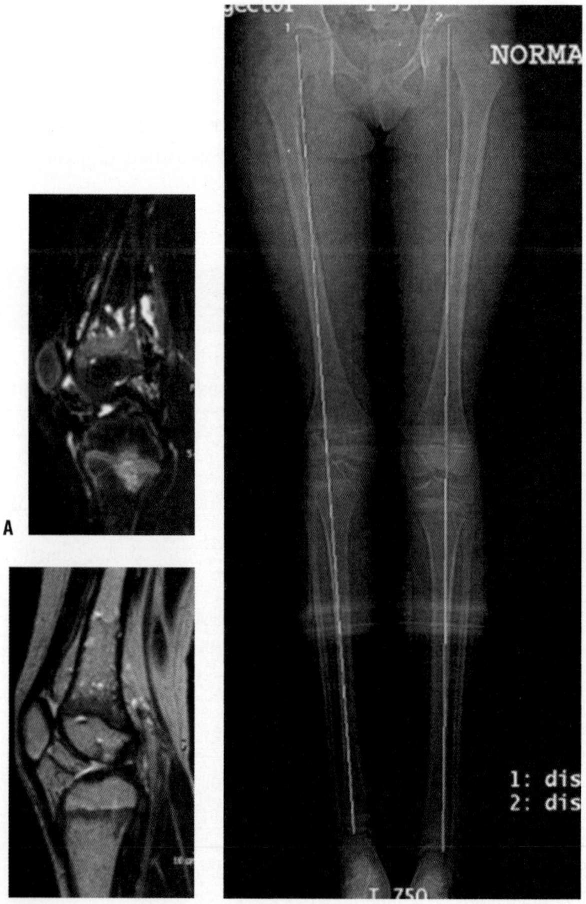

The treatment for these slow-flow vascular lesions is usually nonoperative with the use of elastic garments. As well as decreasing the pain and disfiguration, these garments can help prevent LIC. Surgical excision or sclerotherapy can be used; however, both these techniques can convert LIC to a disseminated intravascular coagulation. Laser treatment is useful only for the diffuse CMs (port wine stains) and not the deeper VMs (12).

Fast-Flow Arteriovenous Malformations. The majority of fast-flow malformations occur in the head and neck region followed by the extremities and then the trunk. They occur equally in males and females. Occasionally, the malformations can be picked up with prenatal ultrasound. The lesions are often difficult to diagnose as there may initially only be subtle discoloration in the skin. Closer examination may reveal increased warmth, a palpable thrill or pulsation, an enlarged extremity, and dilated veins. Enjolras et al. reviewed 200 cases of AVM over a 4-year period and found 40% are present at birth, 35% are detectable during puberty, and 45% are evident in adulthood (13). As the patient grows, changes in the limb can become more pronounced. There is an increase in girth and sometimes length, lymphedema, and skin alteration that includes further discoloration, ulcers, and fibrosis. The bone can also be affected. Bone hypertrophy can occur due to the increased blood supply to the epiphysis. Enjolras also suggests that "hypoxia of the growth cartilage centres" may occur due to the phenomenon known as vascular steal caused by the AVMs (3). Lytic lesions can also occur in the bone and cause pathologic fractures.

Parkes-Weber syndrome is a capillary AVM or a capillary–lymphatic AVM where there is hypertrophy of the limb with increased leg length.

The best investigation for a suspected high-flow malformation is Doppler ultrasound. Arteriography has been used historically; however, this has largely been superseded by MR angiography. Plain radiographs are useful for bone morphology, and serial computed tomography (CT) scanograms are indicated if a leg length discrepancy develops.

The treatment of these malformations is difficult. Initially, elastic stockings are the mainstay as they will help decrease the swelling, minimize vascular steal, and prevent trauma to the skin. Education of foot hygiene and participation in certain sports is also important in preventative care of the limb. Arterial embolization is not a preventative option as there are usually multiple AVMs and it is not possible to embolize them all. It can be used for isolated lesions where there has been a complication, for example, excessive bleeding or a particularly unsightly lesion. There is no role for laser therapy in high-flow AVMs.

FIGURE 9-1.   A–C: Ten-year-old girl with diffuse venous malformation of the right distal thigh with knee joint involvement. The leg is 1.5 cm shorter than the left.

The leg length discrepancy is difficult to manage. Not only is the leg length discrepancy hard to predict but the surgery can be fraught with complications. Enjolras et al. reviewed 17 children with lower extremity Parkes-Weber syndrome. Six of the patients were under 8 years of age and had an average leg length discrepancy of 2.75 cm. The other 11 children were over 10 years of age and had an average discrepancy of 3.26 cm. Nine patients underwent epiphysiodesis and seven children had severe worsening of their vascular and skin lesions with complications, one eventually requiring amputation (3).

A cautious approach needs to be taken to treating the leg length discrepancies in these fast-flow vascular malformations. The use of orthotics should be exhausted before considering surgical intervention. If epiphysiodesis is indicated, it may be advisable to perform a percutaneous drilling rather than an open staple or eight-plate surgery to minimize the surgical trauma to the vascular malformations. Consideration should also be given to shortening or lengthening the contralateral "normal" leg to equalize the leg lengths and thereby avoid the potential complications in the hypertrophied limb.

Complex/Combined Vascular Malformations

Klippel-Trenaunay Syndrome. In 1900, two French physicians Maurice Klippel and Paul Trenaunay described a syndrome that had three components: (a) cutaneous capillary–venous malformations, (b) varicose veins, and (c) hypertrophy of the bones and soft tissues of the limb (14). Much confusion has arisen subsequently with the nomenclature as different physicians have described similar conditions with variations in this triad. Frederick Parkes-Weber described a clinical syndrome in 1918 very similar to Klippel-Trenaunay except that in addition to the slow-flow vascular malformations there were AVMs as well (15). Naturally, there is an overlap between the two syndromes; however, when the AVMs dominate the clinical picture, the term Parkes-Weber syndrome should be used (Fig. 9-2 and Table 9-2). The AVMs in Klippel-Trenaunay are always trivial and of no clinical importance (10).

The cause of Klippel-Trenaunay is largely unknown. There are often other congenital abnormalities associated with the syndrome that make the diagnosis ambiguous at times. (16)

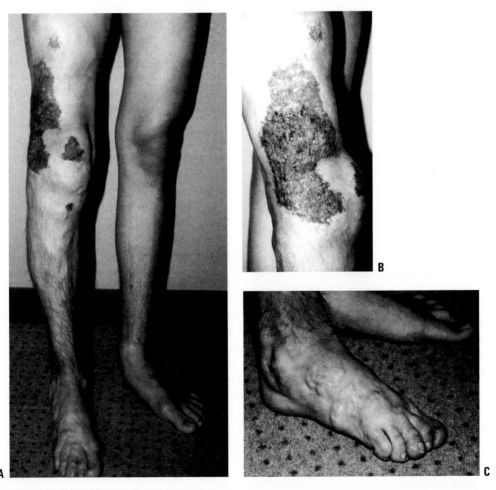

FIGURE 9-2. **A:** A 15-year-old boy with Klippel-Trenaunay syndrome of his right lower extremities with typical findings of hypertrophy, varicosities, and superficial complex, combined vascular malformations. **B,C:** He had aching discomfort from the varicosities, intermittent pain from thrombophlebitis, and drainage from the superficial vascular malformations.

TABLE 9-2	Differences Between Klippel-Trenaunay and Parkes-Weber Syndrome	
Klippel-Trenaunay	**Parkes-Weber**	
Arteriovenous malformations trivial	Arteriovenous malformations significant	
"Port wine" discoloration	Lighter and more diffuse discoloration	
Lymphatic malformation common	Rare lymphatic involvement	
Lateral venous anomaly (with associated venous flares)	No lateral venous anomaly	
Good prognosis	Poorer prognosis	

Lindenauer is the only person to document two siblings as having the syndrome (16). Some authors have suggested the cause of Klippel-Trenaunay syndrome is a mutation in the genes that are involved in angiogenesis and vasculogenesis during embryonic development (17–20). Tian et al. (21) identified a mutant angiogenic factor (Glu133Lys in *VG5Q*) in patients with CMs; however, Boon et al. could not find any of these mutations in bona fide Klippel-Trenaunay patients (10). Translocations (5:11, 8:14) have also been reported as being associated with this syndrome (22). Baskerfield et al. studied 33 patients with Klippel-Trenaunay syndrome and, based on extensive vascular studies, concluded that the syndrome was caused by a mesodermal defect. They felt the persisting vascular malformations were fetal microvascular AV communications (17, 18). Unlike hemihypertrophy, children with Klippel-Trenaunay or Parkes-Weber syndrome do not have an increased incidence of Wilms tumor and therefore do not require abdominal ultrasound screening for this (23, 24).

Pathophysiology. The deep venous system is greatly affected and may even be absent. Rarely a fibrous band can also obstruct the veins (25). There is also an anomalous lateral venous system that can extend from the foot up to the right flank area. Baskerfield et al. found this to be present in 64% of the 33 patients they reviewed. The result of these anomalies in the deep venous system is that blood returns to the heart via the tortuous superficial venous system (17, 18). Another series has found this system to be present in 72% of the patients (26). The venous systems are filled with multiple emboli and the venous stasis contributes to the symptoms the patients complain of.

Surgical specimens in 29 patients were examined by Lie, and he reported the most consistent finding was fibromuscular dysplasia in the venous system (20). The layer in the vein wall that was most affected was the media and it was hypertrophied, irregular, or absent. In the most deficient areas, an aneurysm was often present. He also found that when the deep venous system was sometimes present, there were anomalous valves and that AVMs were uncommon. Other tissues were often hypertrophied; however, the lymphatics were hypoplastic.

Clinical Features. The condition is present from birth; however, the nevus, varicosities, and limb hypertrophy become more evident as the child grows. The lower limb is affected at least 10 times more often than the upper extremities. The affected limb is longer than normal in 90% of the patients (19, 20, 27). The limb girdle and trunk can also be affected and when they are the underlying viscera may also have vascular malformations. The head and neck are rarely involved.

Nevus. This is almost always present at birth but can be difficult to see. Jacob et al. reviewed 252 patients and found that the malformation was present at birth in 98% (26). It is due to the capillary–venous malformation and results in a pink or port wine discoloration. The nevus usually follows a dermatomal distribution, does not cross the midline, and can be on the affected or contralateral limb (28). The size and color of the nevus can change with growth of the child.

Varicosities. Varicose veins are inevitably present at birth and increase in size as the child grows. The extent of the varicosities determines the course of the syndrome. A consistent finding is an anomalous lateral varicosity that extends from the ankle to the flank and is not connected to the hypoplastic deep system. Jacob et al. found this embryonic lateral marginal vein to be present in 72% of the patients in their series (26). In the older child, the resulting stasis can lead to secondary skin changes, ulceration, and thrombophlebitis. Thrombi are usually present in both the deep and superficial venous systems; however, pulmonary emboli rarely occur spontaneously.

When the deep varicosities involve the pelvic organs, erosions can occur giving rise to hematuria, rectal, and vaginal bleeding (29, 30). Rarely, the central nervous system can be involved (31, 32). Scoliosis can occur in approximately 5% of adolescents with Klippel-Trenaunay syndrome; however, it is usually mild and does not require surgical correction (33). When the upper limb is involved, carpal tunnel syndrome has been reported (34). In large malformations, the blood shunting can be so large that the child can suffer from high-output cardiac failure. In such cases, especially in neonates, limb amputation may be life saving (35, 36).

Limb Hypertrophy. Limb overgrowth occurs in both the soft tissues and bone. The increased growth can occur at a distance from the obvious varicosities making the underlying mechanism for this hypertrophy difficult to understand. Sometimes a single digit is involved, part of a limb or half an entire body. Unlike Parkes-Weber syndrome where the degree of AVMs usually determines eventual limb size, the predictability of the hypertrophy in Klippel-Trenaunay is not so straightforward. Not only is there an increase in girth but there is also an increase in length (Fig. 9-2) The girth is very difficult to address surgically; however, surgical correction of the leg length discrepancy is an option especially when a large discrepancy exists. A severe leg length discrepancy is uncommon, and Berry et al. found that only 10% of children will have a discrepancy of >3 cm (19). McCullough and Kenwight even described 2 patients in whom the discrepancy in their leg lengths decreased with growth (37). This shows the importance of following these patients regularly and measuring their leg lengths clinically and radiologically to "best guess" the timing of surgical intervention for this variable pattern of discrepancy (38). The exact aetiology of the limb length overgrowth is not known but was originally thought to be caused by venous hypertension (39). A more recent theory suggests there may be some genetic cause for both the vascular abnormalities and alterations in limb length and girth.

Associated Conditions. Approximately 25% of patients with Klippel-Trenaunay syndrome have anomalies of the fingers and toes (27). These include syndactyly, polydactyly, and clinodactyly. Jacob et al. found that 10 of the 252 patients they reviewed had developmental dysplasia of the hip (26). Other reports have revealed radial head dislocations, melorheostasis, tuberous sclerosis, metatarsus adductus, congenital clubfoot, scoliosis, and Sturge-Weber syndrome (40).

Diagnosis. The diagnosis can usually be made at birth by the clinical appearance of the child. Confirmation of this diagnosis then needs to be made with noninvasive imaging. This is best performed when the child has turned 4 years of age to minimize ambiguous results from the ultrasound due to movement artifact and the small size of the vessels. Doppler ultrasound is very useful especially for differentiating between Klippel-Trenaunay and Parkes-Weber syndrome on the basis of AVMs. MRI, MR angiography, and MR venography are additional imaging studies that can help in the diagnosis and define the extent of the vessel malformation (19, 31, 41–43). More recently, Bastarrika et al. have prospectively imaged 16 patients with Klippel-Trenaunay syndrome using multidetector computed tomography (MDCT) and fast 3-dimensional magnetic resonance imaging (3D-MRI). They found these techniques alone to be adequate in visualizing the deep and superficial venous systems along with other anatomy in order to plan effective treatment strategies (44). Lymphoscintigraphy is also useful if there is considerable limb oedema (19). Plain radiographs are useful to assess the bony involvement, and serial CT scanograms help determine the growth discrepancy that may occur. Arteriography is best reserved for surgical planning. This is especially useful when a hip disarticulation or hemipelvectomy is planned as the network of vessels can be seen and the approach and deep dissection predetermined (45).

Treatment. The treatment for KTS is tailored to the extent of the disease and how the limb changes with increasing age. In the neonatal period, emergency amputation of a limb occasionally needs to be performed to save a child if there is a life-threatening shunt and high-output cardiac failure.

Nonoperative management is the mainstay of treatment. Compressive graduated stockings help reduce the size and pressure in the limb and give symptomatic relief. Nocturnal pneumatic calf pumps can help during the night and the daytime compressive stockings should be applied while the child is still recumbent in bed (26, 46). Good foot hygiene is essential to avoid cellulitis. Although pulmonary embolus is lower than one would expect in this syndrome, it still does occur, so avoiding prolonged sitting and occlusive clothing is important. Young women should probably avoid oral contraceptives.

Surgical intervention is useful in a small number of patients. When a significant leg length discrepancy is present and a shoe lift on the unaffected leg is not tolerated, then an equalization procedure is indicated. This is usually an epiphysiodesis of the affected limb and should be carried out with minimal trauma to the soft tissues (47). The use of eight plates (Orthofix, McKinney, TX) may be useful, so the length can be modulated as it is difficult to predict the eventual discrepancy. At the same time, a "one-off" percutaneous drill epiphysiodesis does the least damage to the soft tissues.

The ability to wear footwear is important for these patients both for a protective function and for cosmesis. Excision of the central metatarsals and epiphysiodesis of the others can help reduce the width and length of the foot (35). Similarly, amputation of an associated large digit will make shoe fitting easier. A Symes amputation is useful for severe foot deformities. Complications from this peripheral surgery are uncommon; however, DVT prophylaxis should be administered (47, 48).

Debulking the soft tissue in the leg is usually unsuccessful with recurrence, swelling, and wound healing problems complicating the surgery. Likewise, varicose vein stripping can result in local symptom relief; however, excessive swelling can occur. The swelling in both cases arises from the inability of the severely deficient deep venous system to function. Selective embolization of vessels can occasionally be successful but often results in early recurrence of the problem (49, 50).

One of the difficult decisions to make is whether to amputate a severely disfiguring or dysfunctional limb or part of the limb. When one considers the multiple operations, unpredictability, and wound healing problems associated with some of the other procedures, amputation sometimes appears the "conservative" option. The difficult decision is often what level to perform the amputation at. This is usually determined by the extent of the VMs as the amputation needs to be made proximal to the severely affected area to minimize complications. Even when an amputation is through an area of "normal" looking soft tissues, there may still be microscopic AVMs or VMs that will be traumatized by the prosthesis. Healing of the stump can be a problem after surgery and Letts had five out of seven children who had an amputation have wound complications (47, 51). All the patients in his study functioned much better after their amputation than before. Pulsed dye laser treatments can be used for treating the cutaneous vascular malformations over limited areas (19).

Proteus Syndrome. Proteus syndrome is a rare condition characterized by skeletal, vascular, and soft-tissue abnormalities that occur in a sporadic fashion. It was originally described in 1979 by Cohen and Hayden; however, it was ascribed the name Proteus syndrome by Wiedermann et al. in 1983 (52). The syndrome was named after the Greek sea god Proteus who was known for his ability to change shape to disguise himself when escaping from his enemies. Proteus syndrome has often been misdiagnosed in the past due to its overlap with a number of other conditions. It can be confused with Klippel-Trenauany syndrome, epidermal nevus syndrome, neurofibromatosis, idiopathic hypertrophy, Maffucci syndrome, isolated macrodactyly, Ollier disease, and many of the lipomatosis syndromes (53).

Etiology. The etiology of Proteus syndrome is still not known. It appears to be a sporadic genetic disorder that results in a hamartomatous growth disorder of the tissues in a mosaic pattern. A number of authors have hypothesized about the possible genetic mutations that may occur (54–56). Others have investigated germ line loss-of-function mutations in the tumor suppression gene *PTEN*, which is found on chromosome 10q23.3. This gene encodes for a dual-specific phosphatize that is involved in various cell-survival pathways. These mutations have been isolated in 20% of patients with Proteus syndrome and 50% of patients with Proteus-like syndromes who also have hamartomatous-like disorders (57, 58). There is only one report of a possible father to son transmission (59).

Clinical Features. Due to the confusion that existed in the diagnosis of Proteus syndrome, a workshop was held in 1998 at the National Institute of Health in Maryland to define the diagnostic criteria (60). Radiographic diagnostic criteria have also been proposed by Jamis-Dow et al. that help in the evaluation of this syndrome (61).

Proteus syndrome is a highly complex variable disorder that involves overgrowth of the skin and subcutaneous tissues, vascular system, bones, and other soft tissues. The histology reveals "hamartomatous mixed connective tissue lesions, benign neoplasms such as lipomata, and lymphatic rich vascular malformations" (62).

Skin and subcutaneous tissue. Almost all patients with Proteus syndrome have at least one skin lesion and these lesions fall into one of two groups: congenital (type 1) or neonatal onset (type 2) (63). The type 1 lesions include the epidermal nevus and vascular malformations that are present at birth and usually do not progress. The type 2 lesions are the lipomas and cerebriform connective tissue nevi that appear after birth and are unpredictable in their progression. The late onset of these lesions often means a diagnosis of Proteus syndrome is not made until late childhood and the child may have already been labeled as having Klippel-Trenaunay syndrome (60). The cerebriform connective tissue nevi are diagnostic of Proteus syndrome and can cause symptoms of pain and pruritus. They can also become infected, bleed, and have a foul odor. Unfortunately, surgery is largely unsuccessful for these nevi and the mainstay of treatment is good skin care and accommodating footwear to minimize skin breakdown (63, 64).

Vascular system. Vascular malformations are not limited to a single limb like Klippel-Trenaunay syndrome but rather can occur randomly anywhere in the body. The cutaneous malformations include vascular tumors, port wine stains, and venous anomalies. Hoeger et al. found these lesions to be present either individually or together in 100% of the 22 patients

with Proteus syndrome they meticulously analyzed (65). They also made the observation that these hemangiomas behave differently in Proteus syndrome. They do not regress spontaneously but rather continue to grow until the child matures around 12 to 14 years of age. The occurrence of thrombosis, thrombocytopenia, and phlebitis is also higher.

Skeletal manifestations. Macrodactyly is probably the most common skeletal manifestation of Proteus syndrome and can occur in the hands or feet and can be independent of the hypertrophied limb (60). The macrodactyly is often not present at birth; however, it can rapidly progress in the first few years of life and then the growth decreases. In the hand, the third and fourth digits are usually affected the most. Macrodactyly can be both disfiguring and functionally limiting. Often partial amputation of a digit is required just to get footwear to fit. A striking finding in the foot is plantar hypertrophy, resulting in cerebriform or gyriform creasing (Fig. 9-3).

Hemihypertrophy is almost as common and can be partial, complete, or crossed. The resulting limb length inequality is unpredictable and can be severe (66). Angular malalignment also occurs in both the upper and lower limb. Surgical attempts to correct the genu valgum often result in recurrence and bracing is ineffectual (66, 67) (Fig. 9-4). Scoliosis and kyphosis occur in approximately 50% of patients with Proteus syndrome (60, 66, 68, 69). Most of these patients who have progressive deformity do not respond to bracing and require spinal fusion. Other spinal deformities include localized spinal overgrowth and infiltration of the spinal canal by angiolipomatous tissue, which can cause both compression of the spinal cord and potential paraplegia (67, 70–73).

Other skeletal manifestations that have been found are hip dysplasia, exostoses that can limit joint movement, hindfoot deformity, and bony protuberances in the skull (61).

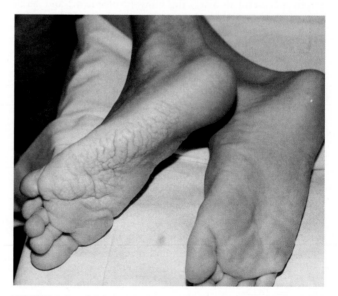

FIGURE 9-3. Adolescent boy with Proteus syndrome with typical gyriform creasing of the sole of his foot.

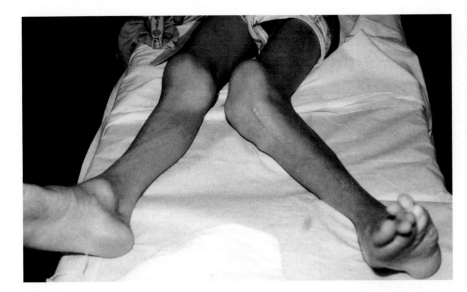

FIGURE 9-4. Adolescent boy with Proteus syndrome with recurrent left genu valgum after a high tibial osteotomy, just prior to repeat osteotomy.

Extraskeletal manifestations. These are far less common than the skeletal and soft-tissue abnormalities. Splenomegaly and nephromegaly can occur along with various abnormalities in the brain (asymmetric megalencephaly and white matter changes) (53, 74, 75). Unusual tumors like ovarian cystadenomas, parotid adenomas, meningiomas, and others have been described but occur rarely (61, 76, 77). Cystic and emphysematous lung changes have also been observed and can be severe. Thromboembolism is more common than in other syndromes with vascular malformations and can lead to sudden death even in children (78, 79).

Treatment. Orthopaedic surgery in patients with Proteus syndrome involves correction of leg length inequality and angular deformity and addressing macrodactyly. The leg length inequality is difficult to predict due to the abnormal growth patterns. Serial clinical and radiologic assessments need to be made to optimize the timing of the epiphysiodesis. The use of eight plates (Orthofix, McKinney, TX) may make this a more forgiving procedure and allow more accurate equalization. Likewise with angular deformity, the use of an eight plate (Orthofix, McKinney, TX) on the convex side will allow growth modulation and eventual correction of the deformity. Surgical correction of macrodactyly is discussed in detail later in this chapter.

When assessing the child with Proteus syndrome for surgery, the anesthetic and surgical team must be cognizant of the associated conditions that may affect surgery. The cystic lung disease, tonsillar hyperplasia, and increased risk of pulmonary embolus may affect the child (80).

Gorham Disease. Gorham disease, sometimes referred to as "disappearing bone disease," is a rare condition that results in massive osteolysis of bone. The cause of the disease is unknown; however, the histology reveals both lymphangiomatosis and hemangiomatosis tissue, which for the purpose of this chapter is classified as a complex combined lymphatic–venous malformation. The first case of spontaneous absorption of bone was reported back in 1838; however, Gorham and Stout (81) and then Gorham (82) described the clinicopathologic features of the disease in the 1950s.

Clinical Presentation. Gorham disease usually occurs in the second or third decade of life; however, case reports have occurred from the neonatal period through to 65 years of age (83–85). There is no familial inheritance pattern of Gorham disease, and there is no greater incidence in either sex or any particular race.

The most commonly involved bones are the maxilla, shoulder girdle, and pelvis although any bone can be involved including the spine (86–89). Gorham disease can present in a number of different ways. It can be recognized on x-rays as an incidental finding following trauma to an area. It can present as a pathologic fracture through an area of osteolysis. Occasionally, there is a history of pain that is not usually severe in the area of underlying osteolysis, and a child can present with some mild deformity of the involved area and some muscle weakness. On rare occasions, the patient may present with symptoms of a chylothorax where the lymphangiomatosis tissue has extended in to the chest from either shoulder girdle or spine involvement. These children usually present with shortness of breath and a chest x-ray will reveal a large pleural effusion (90) (Fig. 9-5). Usually, the disease starts in one bone and can either remain there or spread to adjacent bones with complete disregard for the intervening joint or disc space (91). Other authors have shown that Gorham disease can arise in a multicentric pattern where more than one bone is initially involved but the intervening bone between the lesions is free of disease (92, 93).

Although other causes of osteolytic lesions such as osteomyelitis and metastatic disease can be excluded on the clinical

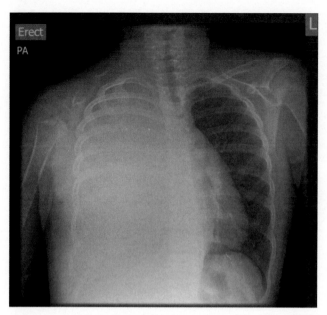

FIGURE 9-5. A 13-year-old girl with Gorham disease who presented with a large right-sided pleural effusion.

findings, other causes of primary osteolytic processes must be considered. Torg et al. described a classification system in 1969, which was further expanded by Macpherson et al. in 1973 and remains the most useful one today (94, 95).

Radiologic Changes. The plain radiographs will reveal either the monostotic involvement or multiostotic disease outlined above. The initial radiographic features were described by Johnson and McClure in 1958 (96). They show that initially there were multiple intramedullary and subcortical radiolucent foci with associated osteoporosis. They then describe an extraosseous stage when the cortex has been disrupted and there is an extension of the pathologic tissue into the adjacent soft tissues. The ends of the tubular bones then taper off to the area of osteolysis and this is thought to be due to compression by the surrounding soft-tissue involvement. One of the characteristic findings, however, is the lack of sclerosis or osteoblastic reaction in the area (97). CT scanning is the next best investigation to look at the bone destruction and absence of any callus formation. An MRI scan, however, is more useful in looking at the soft-tissue extension in the area of osteolysis and beyond (Fig. 9-6). The MRI signal characteristics will change depending on the stage of the disease. Initially, with the neovascularization, there will be increased uptake on the T1 and T2 imaging; however, as the vascular tissue is replaced with fibrous tissue, the T1 and T2 imaging will become increasingly dark (86, 98, 99). Arteriography, venography, and lymphangiography have all been used to help in establishing a diagnosis and investigating the extent of the disease (83, 84, 97). These investigations, however, are rarely required to make the diagnosis and don't usually offer any more information than is attained by the plain radiographs, CT, and MRI scan.

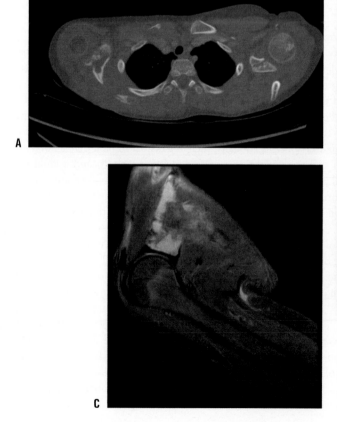

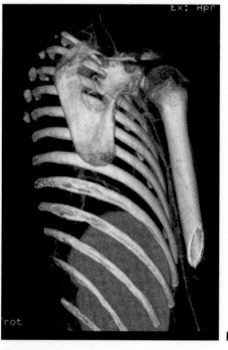

FIGURE 9-6. A 13-year-old girl with CT scan **(A,B)** showing extensive erosion of the scapula. MRI scan **(C)** shows the extraosseous soft-tissue extension.

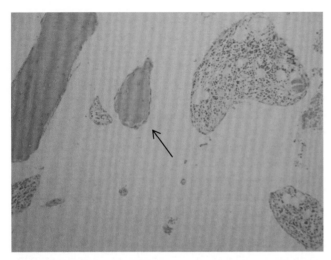

FIGURE 9-7. Histologic slide of a biopsy in Gorham disease showing the thin-walled vessels lined by endothelium cells (*arrow*) and proteinaceous fluid.

Histopathology. The gross finding is of bone that is thin, soft, and spongy in texture. Occasionally, small cysts are also seen with the naked eye (84, 85, 100). Fibrous connective tissue replaces the bone. Histologic examination demonstrates benign endothelial proliferation within the bone. There are numerous thin-walled vessels that are lined by endothelial cells, and these capillaries contain red blood cells and/or proteinaceous fluid (101) (Fig. 9-7). There is no evidence of malignancy or inflammation. The role of osteoclast activity in Gorham disease is somewhat controversial. Some authors have reported the presence of osteoclasts in pathologic specimens (102–104), whereas others have not found any to be present (87, 91, 97, 105). One of the mysteries of Gorham disease is the actual cause of this massive osteolysis. One thought is that the perivascular cells show some characteristics of osteoclast precursors that may form active osteoclasts (87, 106). Other authors have hypothesized that the osteoclast precursors in the area of osteolysis are more sensitive to humeral factors that promote osteoclast formation and bone reabsorption rather than an actual increase in actual osteoclast numbers (107, 108).

Treatment. With no obvious known cause and with such a variable natural history, the treatment of Gorham disease is extremely difficult. Although clinical and radiologic features usually confirm the diagnosis, a biopsy is often performed.

The results of treatment have been particularly difficult to evaluate due to the variable natural history of Gorham disease. Occasionally, the multiple treatment modalities have been used over the years with variable results and still no consensus exists on the most effective treatment strategy. An important prognostic factor is the presence of extraosseous involvement. Guitierez and Spjut reviewed 25 patients with extraosseous involvement and found the mortality rate was higher in this group of patients with Gorham disease (105).

The extraosseous tissue can invade the pleural cavity giving rise to pulmonary complications due to the persistent chylothorax. This can occur when the shoulder girdle is involved or the thoracic or lumbar spine (90, 91, 109). The management of the chylothorax is extremely difficult and usually not successful. Attempts have been made to tie off the thoracic trunk and use different radiation and pleural adhesion therapies (86).

For more straight forward monostotic disease, the treatment has also been variable and disappointing. Spontaneous regression without treatment can occur; however, in the majority of cases, no new bone is ever made. Local excision of the affected bone and soft tissue and bone grafting with or without internal fixation has also been largely unsuccessful (89, 110, 111). Unfortunately, most of the bone grafts are reabsorbed, and this has encouraged some authors to use vascularized fibula grafts to strut the affected area (112). The use of an endoprosthesis to bridge the gap between the so-called "normal bone" can be successful (85, 89, 112, 113). When limb salvage is not possible due to the extent of both the bone and the soft-tissue disease, then amputation is often indicated. In a limb with extensive bone disease and massive soft-tissue involvement, it may be more functional for the patient to have an amputation or limb disarticulation rather than a salvage procedure. Predicting the level of the amputation is difficult as through joint amputation has not always been shown to control the disease process (93, 98, 114).

One can see that not only the type of surgical procedure is a challenge to decide but the timing of the surgical intervention may also be critical. In rapidly evolving disease, it is difficult to know whether to intervene "early" to try and halt the progress or wait until the disease process has slowed down to assess the extent of the reconstruction or amputation. A pathologic fracture through the area of osteolysis has been shown to increase the rapidity of the osteolytic process and Mendez et al. suggest that surgical intervention earlier in this clinical situation may be indicated (115). The management of vertebral Gorham disease is extremely challenging as resection with adequate margins is usually not possible. Spinal bracing is a temporizing treatment; however, definitive surgical intervention is required when there is neural compromise. Anterior and posterior decompression and fusion has been used successfully in this situation at the cervico–thoracic junction (116). In other examples, bone grafting has been useful but has reabsorbed with time (104, 117).

Radiotherapy and chemotherapy have been used in conjunction with surgical treatments to try and arrest the progression of this disease with little to no success (105, 109, 111, 118). Radiation may be an effective adjunct therapy when doses of 30 Gy or more are used (89, 119, 120).

Hemihypertrophy and Hemihypotrophy. Hemihypertrophy and hemihypotrophy are two different conditions that have different clinical manifestations and need to be considered separately. For the purposes of this chapter, the two conditions will be discussed in isolation, but at the same time, they share the same problem of asymmetry between the left and right sides of the body that cannot be attributed to normal variation. In this regard, it is important to explain the nomenclature used in addressing these two conditions.

Nomenclature. Hemihypertrophy is an overgrowth in the size or length of a portion of the body and may involve the extremities, head, trunk, and internal organs. The overgrowth can be limited to an upper or lower limb, head and face, crossed (overgrowth of contralateral limbs) or a full hemihypertrophy where there is overgrowth of the ipsilateral upper and lower limbs.

Hypotrophy is a failure of growth (undergrowth) of a portion of the body and can be classified similarly to hypertrophy above. The term hemiatrophy has been used to describe the same phenomenon; however, it is not used here as this implies a wasting of tissue rather than a failure of growth.

Classification. Hemihypertrophy can be classified as congenital or acquired. Acquired asymmetry can occur secondary to infection, trauma, radiation, or inflammation (121, 122).

Congenital hemihypertrophy is further classified according to the extent of the involvement of the child and whether it is part of a recognized clinical syndrome or not. *Total* forms have involvement of all organ systems, whereas the *limited* forms have only muscular, vascular, skeletal, or neurologic involvement (121). *Limited* forms can be further classified according to the area of their involvement: *Classic* (ipsilateral upper and lower limbs), *segmental* (within a single limb), *facial* (head and face), or *crossed* (contralateral upper and lower limbs) (121–123).

Syndromic hemihypertrophy occurs in conditions like neurofibromatosis, Beckwith-Wiedemann syndrome, Bannayan-Zonana syndrome, Klippel-Trenaunay syndrome, and Proteus syndrome (Table 9-3). *Nonsyndromic* hemihypertrophy

TABLE 9-3 Differential Diagnosis of Hemihypertrophy and Hemihypotrophy

Condition	Features	Growth Pattern	Treatment Implication
Hypertrophy of Normal Tissues			
Idiopathic hemihypertrophy	Increase in length and breadth of one extremity or one-half of body; with or without renal malformation	Proportionate, linear	Monitor for increased risk of Wilms or other neoplasm
Beckwith-Wiedemann syndrome	Large body size, hemihypertrophy of whole body, macroglossia, omphalocele, pancreatic hyperplasia	Irregular	Risk of Wilms or embryonal tumors
Hamartomatous Disorders			
Klippel-Trenaunay syndrome	Limb-length discrepancies; combined, complex vascular malformation (may be on long or short side); varicosities	Often irregular, does not affect all segments equally	Prediction for epiphysiodesis inaccurate; operate for function; amputation sometimes needed; compression therapy
Neurofibromatosis	Cafe-au-lait spots (>5) plus family history of subcutaneous neurofibroma, dystrophic bone changes	Irregular	
Proteus syndrome	Vascular anomalies, asymmetric hypertrophy, macrodactyly, exostoses, subcutaneous masses	Irregular	Valgus often coexists; skeletal age delayed or disassociated
Hemi-3 syndrome	Hemihypertrophy, hemihyperesthesia, hemiareflexia	Hypertrophy of girth, not length	
Undergrowth of Limb			
Idiopathic hemihypotrophy	Greater dysmorphism than in hemihypertrophy, congenital scoliosis, genitourinary malformation	Proportionate	Discrepancy rarely exceeds 2 cm by maturity; treatment rarely indicated
Turner/mosaic (XO/XX)	Short stature, low hairline, peripheral edema, valgus of knees or elbows	Discrepancy accelerated near puberty	Keloids common
Ressell-Silver syndrome	Very short stature (<3%), small, triangular face, one limb or whole side short, developmental dysplasia of the hip, scoliosis, genitourinary anomalies common	Eventual limb-length discrepancy of 1–6 cm	Skeletal age is delayed
Neurogenic (e.g., hemiplegic, polio)	Undergrowth is proportional to weakness	Proportionate, affects weakest limb segments	Lengthening rarely indicated in weak limb
Skeletal dysplasia or dysostoses	Polyostotic fibrous dysplasia, multiple exostoses, multiple enchondromas		

(sometimes referred to as isolated hemihypertrophy) has no other syndromic features; however, along with Beckwith-Wiedemann syndrome is the only type of hemihypertrophy associated with an increased risk of intra-abdominal tumors (52, 124–126).

Both hemihypertrophy and hemihypotrophy become entities when the growth or lack of growth varies from "normal." Although there is no current consensus on what percentage growth difference defines these disorders, the most commonly used reference for normal variation in limb size is a survey from a growth study at Children's Hospital, Boston, by Pappas and Nehme (127). Another reference group of patients used is a series of a thousand United States army recruits reviewed by Rush and Steiner in 1946 (128).

Pappas and Nehme defined abnormal asymmetry as a 5% or greater difference in the length and/or circumference of the involved limb (127). The magnitude of this discrepancy, however, needs to take the age and size of the child into account, and therefore the Anderson and Green growth charts need to be used in combination with the findings of Pappas and Nehme. These measurements are largely academic and necessary only for the more subtle cases. With hemihypertrophy, the overgrowth may be associated with other abnormalities like vascular and digital malformations or macrodactyly. The patient with hypotrophy may have associated mental retardation, muscular wasting, or neurologic symptoms.

The single most important thing for the orthopaedic surgeon to recognize is whether the child or adolescent has hemihypotrophy or hemihypertrophy as the latter is associated with the development of embryonal tumors whereas the former is not.

Hemihypertrophy occurs when one side of the body or limb enlarges asymmetrically both in length and width when compared with the contralateral "normal side." Hemihypertrophy is a rare disease of unknown etiology that affects approximately 1 in 50,000 individuals (121, 123, 127, 129). It is difficult to determine the true prevalence due to the minor asymmetry that can often occur between limbs in normal people (28). Hemihypertrophy is also rarely diagnosed at birth and develops to a variable degree through infancy and early childhood. The asymmetry can also be extremely subtle ranging from an increase in the size of an ear, half the tongue, pupil right up to involvement of abdominal and thoracic organs (122, 124). The skin may be thicker on the involved side and there may be more hair (121). The asymmetrical growth is unpredictable and in some cases can resolve in early childhood or be exaggerated during puberty (130). The total limb inequality rarely exceeds 5 cm by skeletal maturity (124, 127). Approximately two-thirds of the patients will require an equalization procedure for the discrepancy (131). This can be achieved by epiphysiodesis of the contralateral knee epiphyses with a drill technique or staples (124, 127). The use of eight plates (Orthofix, McKinney, TX) to achieve this has become increasingly popular, so the equalization can be modulated if the predictable discrepancy was inaccurate. A nonstructural scoliosis can occur secondary to the leg length discrepancy but usually resolves with correction of the inequality.

Nonsyndromic hemihypertrophy can also have other associated anomalies outside the musculoskeletal system. There is an increased incidence of renal disorders including medullary sponge kidney, renal cysts, and horseshoe kidney. Inguinal hernias and cryptorchidism can also occur (121, 129, 132).

There are a number of theories associated with the etiology of nonsyndromic hemihypertrophy; however, none have been proven. Due to the association with embryonal tumors, abnormal cellular growth control mechanisms have been postulated in these children. Other researchers have suggested that possible chromosomal abnormalities, lesions of the nervous system, or endocrine malfunctions may be a cause of the hypertrophy (121, 125, 126, 133). The malignant tumors that occur with nonsyndromic hemihypertrophy in order of frequency are Wilms tumors, adrenal carcinoma, and hepatoblastoma (134–137). The problem is defining what is the true incidence of these life-threatening conditions and how best to screen for them. One prospective study suggests the incidence of malignancy is approximately 5.9% (133). Many retrospective studies have been performed that calculate the incidence to be slightly lower, around 3% (134, 138, 139). It is difficult to define strict criteria for screening these children for tumors when the incidence is so low, the development of the tumors unpredictable and no studies that show children who have a tumor found on ultrasound screening has any better outcome than a patient who presents with symptoms of the tumor. In some of the prevalence studies, the tumors were diagnosed in 30% of patients before the hemihypertrophy was even recognized (121, 140, 141). It seems intuitive, however, to have a screening program when one recognizes a patient with asymmetry of one side of the body. Initially, the hemihypertrophy needs to be classified accurately as syndromic or nonsyndromic, often with the help of geneticists and pediatricians. The nonsyndromic children and those with Beckwith-Wiedemann syndrome need to have an abdominal ultrasound. Although controversial, these children should have a regular abdominal ultrasound every 3 months up to 7 years of age and then have a physical abdominal examination every 6 months until skeletal maturity (142). Some clinicians recommend no ultrasound screening at all and others ultrasound until skeletal maturity (121).

Hemihypotrophy. Idiopathic hemihypotrophy appears to be approximately one-half as frequent as nonsyndromic hemihypertrophy (123). Hemihypotrophy is more likely to be associated with diffuse skeletal abnormalities when compared to hemihypertrophy (123). There is a higher incidence of other dysmorphic features, including cleft palate and facial malformations, congenital scoliosis, and genitourinary malformations (123, 143). Mental retardation is also more common; however, Wilms tumor and other embryonal tumors are not associated with this condition (28). Unlike hemihypertrophy, the leg length discrepancy is rarely more than 2.5 cm and therefore does not require surgical correction (123, 143).

Hemihypotrophy is classified in the same way as congenital hemihypertrophy as total or limited. The limited forms can therefore be categorized according to the area of involvement: classic, segmental, facial, or crossed (121–123). Undergrowth may also occur as a result of secondary nonsyndromic hypotrophy, mosaicism for Turner syndrome, Russell-Silver syndrome, neurologic asymmetry (cerebral palsy, polio), osteochondromatosis, endochondromatosis, or polyostotic fibrous dysplasia (144).

Russell-Silver syndrome has some features in common with idiopathic hemihypotrophy, but it is characterized by overall short stature, with most patients never exceeding a height of 152 cm. These patients have characteristic small, triangular faces and renal and genital malformations (28). Scoliosis is common and may be congenital or look similar to idiopathic scoliosis. Leg length asymmetry is usually minimal, but as much as 5 cm has been reported (143).

Limb inequalities resulting from neurogenic causes vary in proportion to the asymmetry of the neurologic involvement, rarely exceeding 2.5 cm in the lower extremities in patients with cerebral palsy or 6 cm in patients with polio (145).

It is important for the orthopaedic surgeon to recognize limb overgrowth or undergrowth and therefore classify the deformity accordingly. Although sometimes clinically obvious, growth charts are often required to accurately assess whether the condition is hemihypertrophy or hemihypotrophy. There are different clinical manifestations for each disease as outlined above and different syndromes and clinical features that are associated with the two different conditions. It is not always easy for the orthopaedic surgeon alone to diagnose these conditions and therefore help should often be sought from pediatric and geneticist colleagues.

Macrodactyly. Macrodactyly (also known as localized gigantism) is a rare condition characterized by large digits of the hand and less commonly of the foot that is usually apparent at birth or in early childhood. Usually, the preaxial side of the hand or foot is involved; however, in rare occasions, all the digits or postaxial enlargement can occur (146). Klein described the first case of macrodactyly in 1824 and up until 1999 only 300 cases of macrodactyly of the hand and 60 cases of macrodactyly of the foot had been reported in the literature (147).

Macrodactyly usually occurs as an isolated condition but may also occur in patients with neurofibromatosis, vascular malformations (hemangiomatosis, lymphangiomatosis, or mixed disease), Proteus syndrome, and Klippel-Trenaunay syndrome (148–151). Children with multiple enchondromatosis, Maffucci syndrome, and tuberosclerosis also have enlarged digits. In recognizing macrodactyly, it is therefore important to look for other physical abnormalities that may be present in order to diagnose another underlying disorder. In infancy, cutaneous manifestations of neurofibromatosis or the vascular malformations may not be present making a definitive diagnosis often difficult. Traditionally, it was thought that two types exist: the more common static type, in which the proportion of enlargement remains the same, and the progressive type, in which this proportion or ratio increases with time

(152). These common forms fall under Upton classification of "type 1" and are by far the most common and occur with the most common frequency; however, it is important to consider the other three types so that other disorders are not overlooked.

Type 1: Macrodactyly with nerve-oriented lipofibromatosis
   a. Static subtype
   b. Progressive subtype
Type 2: Macrodactyly with neurofibromatosis
Type 3: Macrodactyly with hyperostosis
Type 4: Macrodactyly with hemihypertrophy

When the cause of type 1 macrodactyly is unknown, it is thought that it may be due to a "neuroinduction" type disorder. This is supported by the clinical findings that the most common distribution of the macrodactyly is along either the median nerve distribution or digital nerve distribution of the digits (151).

Clinical Features. Macrodactyly occurs more commonly in the hand than it does in the foot and is unilateral in 95% of cases (152). The condition occurs slightly more often in men than woman (153). The macrodactyly is commonly seen soon after birth; however, in some cases, it will become more evident as the child grows especially in the type 1b progressive subtype. The second ray is the most commonly enlarged, followed in descending frequency by the third, first, fourth, and fifth rays (Fig. 9-8). Syndactyly may coexist. Usually, the palmar or plantar surfaces are more hypertrophied than the dorsal surface, resulting in hyperextension of the metatarsals or metacarpal phalangeal joints (149, 154) (Fig. 9-9). If two adjacent digits are affected, they usually grow apart from each other. In static macrodactyly, the digits involved are approximately 1.5 times the normal length and width. In the progressive subtype, however, the enlargement can progress well beyond this and can involve tissue more proximal than the digits. As well as the digits, the hand and foot may be involved and even more

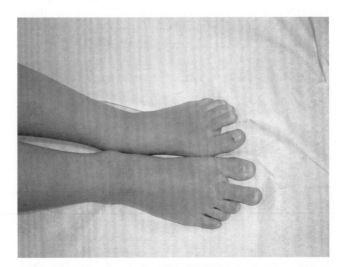

FIGURE 9-8. Macrodactyly of the second toe in a 12-year-old boy. He was asymptomatic and has not required treatment.

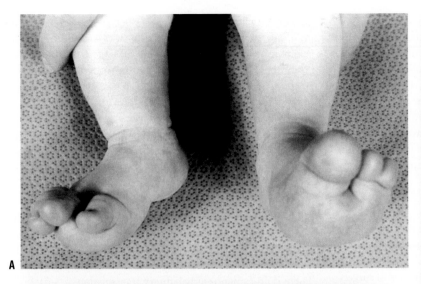

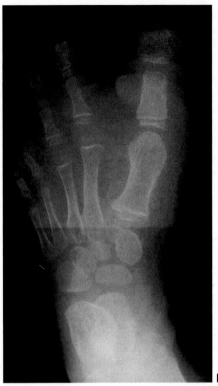

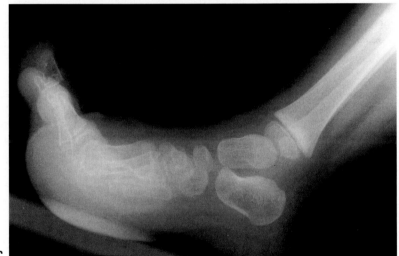

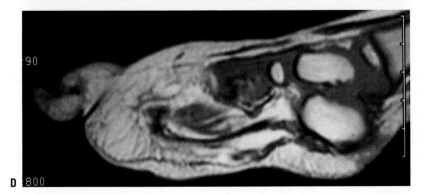

FIGURE 9-9. A 2.5-year-old girl with progressive macrodactyly of both feet, with macrodystrophica-lipomatosa. **A:** There is significant plantar hypertrophy, resulting in hyperextension of the digits, and there is marked asymmetry in the digital enlargement. **B,C:** The plain radiographs demonstrate soft-tissue enlargement, as well as underlying bony enlargement. **D:** The magnetic resonance imaging demonstrates overgrowth of essentially all the elements of the digit, particularly the fibroadipose tissue typically seen in macrodystrophica-lipomatosa.

proximally the whole limb may be slightly increased in length and width (149, 155, 156). When one sees a macrodactyly of a digit, a very careful clinical examination and sometimes radiologic investigation of the whole limb is paramount to assess the extent of the enlargement. This clinical examination will also help in trying to ascertain whether the macrodactyly is associated with any of the other conditions mentioned earlier. The only radiologic investigation required is usually an x-ray.

This is also useful in planning the surgical procedures that may be necessary. The bone age may be advanced in the phalanges involved in the macrodactyly (149, 155).

Pathology. The most consistent finding in macrodactyly is the overgrowth of the fibrofatty tissue but in fact all tissues are enlarged in the involved digit (149, 152, 155). This fibrofatty issue in fact resembles adult subcutaneous tissue rather than children's fat (152). Usually, there is greater involvement of the tissues distally rather than proximally. There is an increase in the amount of fat and fibrous tissue that surrounds the nerves. The perineurium is thickened and there is proliferation of the fibrous tissue in the endoneurium (149, 151, 152, 157). The muscle is infiltrated in a similar way. The bone is increased in both width and length. Ben-Bassat et al. found that there was a proliferation of fibroblasts or osteoblasts between the periosteum and the cortical bone that may account for the phalangeal overgrowth (149, 155). There does not appear to be any pathologic features in the blood vessels.

Treatment. The treatment of macrodactyly is challenging due to the unpredictable progression of the disease that may occur. The patient and family need to be counseled carefully about this before embarking on surgical treatment as sometimes multiple procedures will be necessary. The most important goal of surgery is to improve the function of the involved hand or foot and in most cases to improve the cosmesis. Careful surgical planning is therefore required to maximize the ultimate long-term outcome and especially to improve the function of the limb. A number of factors therefore need to be considered in the treatment of macrodactyly and these include the classification, the age of the patient, the extent of the overgrowth, and which digit/s are involved. The treatment options include debulking of the soft tissue, shortening procedures of the digit, growth modulation of the physeal plate, or amputation. In the static subtype, debulking and shortening procedures including epiphysiodesis or phalangeal resection are usually successful. In the progressive subtype, however, more proximal procedures like ray dissection or even amputations are necessary due to the progressive nature of the disease and the multiple procedures that are often required. Multiple debulking procedures often compromise the blood supply to the area, which can result in wound healing problems.

In mild to moderate macrodactyly, the gigantism can be addressed with soft-tissue debulking and epiphysiodesis (152). The epiphysiodesis needs to be performed before the child is 8 years of age and it must be done on all the involved segments of bone (149, 152, 158, 159). In older children, it is better to perform a phalangeal resection combined with a staged debulking (157, 160, 161). These procedures do not address the increased width that may also be present in the hand or the foot. Increased width is not usually a functional problem in the hand but in the foot it can cause significant problems with shoe wearing. In order to address this increased width in the foot, a ray dissection including one or more metatarsals and a wedge from the tarsal bones is required (151, 153, 162, 163). The minimal numbers of rays to maintain a functional foot is 3. The first ray should never be amputated in isolation because of its importance in weight bearing and balance (164). A metatarsal excision may also be useful in the hand when excessive width is present. Ray resection also prevents "gap formation," which can lead to digit deviation and soft-tissue enlargement. In progressive disease in the foot, a Symes or below knee amputation may be necessary (156). Although there can be a subtle increase in width as the patient matures, there is no increase in

the overall length of the limb and surgery is not required for limb length inequality. The procedures above do improve the function in the involved limb; however, the cosmetic result is often unrewarding. The patient and his or her family need to be counseled about this before surgical correction is carried out so that they are not disappointed by the final result.

Congenital Band Syndrome. Congenital band syndrome is a rare condition that can present with many clinical features, of which the major three components are circumferential transverse bands, acrosyndactyly, and terminal amputations (165–168). The syndrome has been known by a number of other names including amniotic band syndrome, Streeter dysplasia, pseudoainhum, and annular constriction bands to name a few. The reported incidence is 1 in 5000 to 10,000 children and there is no gender difference in the incidence (167, 169). There is no evidence of hereditary transmission.

Clinical Features. The clinical presentation of congenital constriction band varies greatly between patients due to the severity and depth of the constriction. The constrictions can vary from being superficial and incomplete to being deep and circumferential almost causing a congenital amputation (Fig. 9-10). The bands are usually distal in the limb; however, there may be multiple constrictions within the same limb. Involvement of the upper limbs is twice as common as in the lower limb. Patterson has classified congenital constriction band syndrome based on the extent of the banding (170).

1. Simple constriction ring
2. Constriction ring with deformity of the distal part
3. Constriction ring with syndactyly
4. Intrauterine amputation

The extent of the deformity distal to the band usually reflects the depth of the constriction and the subsequent vessels, nerves, and muscle that are compressed. This prevents the normal development of tissue distal to the band and can result in pseudarthrosis of the bone, a paralytic limb, and a devascularized limb. If severe enough, a congenital amputation is the result. The most common part of the limbs involved is the digits particularly the longest central three (165, 167, 169, 171). It seems by being longer increases the risk of these digits in the hand or feet being entangled in a band.

Extremely uncommonly constriction bands can involve the trunk or neck (171a). Craniofacial abnormalities, including cleft lip and palate are seen in 7% of children with constriction band syndrome (168, 169, 172).

The most common component of the syndrome is amputations with normal proximal development to the constriction band (165, 167, 169, 171). These are almost always transverse terminal amputations and on average occur in three digits. They usually occur within the digits at different levels. The next most common anomaly is a fenestrated syndactyly that occurs in approximately half the patients. This unique type of syndactyly occurs when there is a cleft between the two digits both proximally and distally to the constriction band. Nail

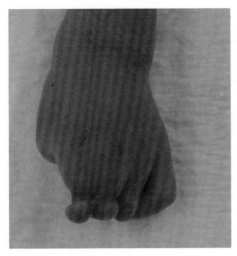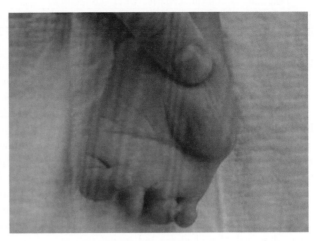

FIGURE 9-10.   An 18-month-old child with congenital amputations of all the digits of the left hand due to constriction band syndrome.

bed deformities are another consistent feature of this syndrome and may signal underlying bony syndactyly (169).

The incidence of clubfoot and constriction band syndrome ranges from 12% to 57% (165, 167–169, 172–174). Cowell and Hessinger (166) were the first to recognize that the clubfoot in association with a congenital constriction band is often paralytic due to the constriction of the peripheral nerves. The clubfeet in this syndrome can be classified as either paralytic or idiopathic like. The idiopathic type clubfeet can be associated with a superficial and often incomplete ipsilateral constriction band or in fact not have an associated band proximal to it. These feet usually respond well to Ponseti manipulations and castings and usually will not require surgical intervention. Paralytic clubfeet, however, are usually more severe and are associated with a deeper circumferential constriction band and these feet often require surgical release. Approximately 30% to 50% of the clubfeet are classified as paralytic (164, 166, 168, 174, 175). In these paralytic feet, the constriction band has caused the deformity by compressing the peripheral nerves, compressed the musculature and may have caused a compartment syndrome. In a recent review by Hennigan and Kuo of 37 clubfeet in 28 patients with congenital constriction band syndrome, they found all the patients who had a neurologic clubfoot had constriction bands that extended down to the deep fascia and were also located between the knee and the ankle (174). These paralytic feet are resistant to nonoperative treatment and usually require multiple surgical procedures to correct the deformity and the constriction band. Bone deformities can occur at the level of the constriction band and distal to it and include pseudarthrosis, angular deformity, and bone dysplasias (170, 176, 177). The pseudarthrosis that can occur due to the constriction can often heal spontaneously. Zion T S et al. (177) suggested that the term "discontinuity" should be used rather than pseudarthrosis because of the excellent prognosis. Likewise, anterolateral bowing that may occur distally can remodel spontaneously, and if a corrective realignment

osteotomy is performed surgically, this usually heals up well unlike what is usually seen in neurofibromatosis (176). Askins and Ger were the first to show an association of leg length discrepancy in some of these patients. Although 39% of the patients had a measurable leg length discrepancy, only a quarter had a discrepancy exceeding 2.5 cm (165). When the lower limb is involved, it is important to clinically assess the leg length discrepancy and monitor it radiologically as an epiphysiodesis may need to be performed before skeletal maturity.

Etiology.   Two schools of thought exist as to whether the etiology of this syndrome is intrinsic or extrinsic to the fetus. The proponents of the intrinsic theory believe that there is defect in germ cell development that results in abnormality of the apical ectodermal ridge (178). There is also evidence that emboli may cause focal necrosis and a subsequent constriction band (34).

Extrinsic (mechanical) theories tend to have the greatest support in the literature. Histologic analysis of the material found deep in the clefts shows pieces of amnion causing the strangulation (179, 180). The cleft lips and palates that can occur are thought to be caused by the swallowing of these mesodermal strings (165). Animal models have been performed to explain this "amniotic band theory." By performing amniocentesis in pregnant rats, researchers have been able to induce excessive uterine contractions with resulting palate and limb defects similar to that seen in congenital constriction band syndrome (167). In a retrospective study of 55 patients with congenital constriction band syndrome, Askins and Ger found a high incidence of prematurity and low birth weight but could not identify any prenatal factors that could be identified as having an association in the etiology of this syndrome (165). Without any definitive intrinsic or extrinsic causes being proven, it may be that a combination of both theories leads to this uncommon condition.

The differential diagnosis includes the "Michelin tire baby syndrome", ainhum and hair/thread constriction.

Treatment. There are 3 clinical scenarios where congenital constriction bands require surgical treatment: acutely in a neonate to salvage a limb or digit, deep bands that are causing vascular and/or neurologic compromise, and cosmetic releases for superficial bands.

Acute release of congenital constriction bands occasionally needs to be performed on a neonate when the limb or digit is severely compromised. This should be performed through a dorsal incision releasing the band rather than a more aggressive Z-plasty or circumferential excision. Often the digit will not be salvageable; however, it will declare itself over time and definitive treatment (often amputation) can then be performed.

Deep constriction bands that extend down to the deep fascia and sometimes beyond can cause vascular and neurologic compromise. The limb distal to the constriction can be very edematous due to the lymphedema and venous engorgement making vascular assessment difficult. Traditionally, the constriction band is released in a staged procedure with a 6- to 12-week interval between the surgeries. This was thought to allow better wound healing and less necrosis of the skin edges because of the poor venous and lymphatic flow (165, 170, 181). Deep constriction bands are now excised and reconstructed as a single procedure (181). Upton and Tan developed a technique of subcutaneous fat advancement flaps as well as multiple Z-plasties to try and prevent the skin indentations that occurs with Z-plasties alone (182). The initial step in the procedure involves excising the band and 1 to 2 mm of adjacent tissue taking care not to divide the underlying neurovascular structures. It is safer to expose these proximally and distal to the band as under the band they are quite deformed. The skin is then undermined with a small amount of subcutaneous tissue and multiple Z-plasties performed at 60 degrees to the excised band. The subcutaneous tissue is then mobilized as described by Upton and Tan so that it can be closed away from the skin incision (182). The peripheral nerves and vascular structures can then be further identified and mobilized.

If a compartment syndrome coexists, a fasciotomy of all the compartments should be performed.

The surgery is easier to perform when the child is older and the fat rolls in their hands have decreased in size. A better cosmetic result may also be achieved if the surgery is performed around 3 to 4 years of age (Fig. 9-11). More expedient surgery is necessary if there is obvious neurologic compromise of the limb due to compression under the band. This is hard to assess in neonates and young children, so careful observation of hand function by the family and surgeon may detect subtle asymmetric changes.

When clubfeet are associated with an ipsilateral constriction band, a staged procedure is usually performed to address the two deformities. These feet are usually neurologic or paralytic and tend to be more severe than clubfeet that are not associated with a neurologic deficit (170, 173, 174). Hennigan and Kuo found in a series of 37 clubfeet in 28 patients with constriction bands that 36% had a neurologic deficit. All the patients who had neurologic involvement had a constriction band that extended down to the deep fascia (grade 3) between the knee and the ankle (Zone 2) (174). Initially, the constriction band is released as described above. The deeper soft tissues can be addressed at the same time if it will help with the foot correction. For example, the tendo Achilles can be lengthened or the posterior tibial talar joint can be released if the constriction band is distal in the leg. For mild clubfoot deformities, serial above knee casting may correct the foot, but usually surgery is required. Soft tissues combined with bone procedures are often necessary as the deformity can be severe. A tibialis tendon transfer to the lateral cuneiform or a split tibialis tendon transfer is commonly needed as the peroneal muscles are usually weak (168, 183). Occasionally, the deformity is so severe that amputation is indicated (174).

Surgical intervention in children with acrosyndactyly is generally performed between the ages of 6 months and 1 year

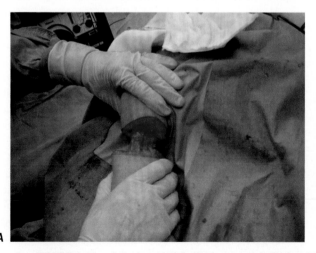 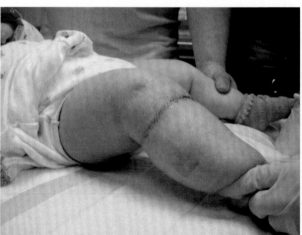

FIGURE 9-11. A 3-year-old girl with deep constriction band in the proximal tibia. This was excised **(A)** and closed without the use of Z-plasties in a single procedure without complication **(B)**. (Courtesy of Dr. Terri Bridwell.)

because of the severity of the deformity and to allow for longitudinal growth and function of the affected digits (171).

DISORDERS INVOLVING JOINT AND BONE

Progressive Diaphyseal Dysplasia.   Progressive diaphyseal dysplasia (PDD) is a rare sclerosing bone disorder characterized by progressive thickening of the diaphysis, bone pain, muscle weakness, and wasting. The disorder was originally described by Camurati in 1922 and again by Engelman in 1929 and has historically been referred to as Camurati-Engelman disease (184, 185).

Etiology.   The disorder is inherited as an autosomal dominant trait caused by mutations in the gene encoding human transforming growth factor-beta 1 (TGF-β1) on chromosome 19q13 (186–188). The molecular mechanisms of this disease have been extensively studied (187). It is a rare condition occurring in approximately one per million and is slightly more common in boys than girls (189).

Clinical Features.   The symptoms of this disease usually occur in the first decade; however, a delay in diagnosis is not uncommon as the symptoms and radiologic findings can be of variable severity. Naveh et al. reviewed 13 affected individuals and the mean age of onset was 15 years and 4 months with a range from 1 to 70 years (189). The main clinical features are limb pain, muscular weakness, and a waddling gait. Other symptoms are loss of appetite, fatigue, and difficulty running (189). Clinical signs also vary and depend on the extent of the disease and the bones involved. These include muscle atrophy, thickening of the long bones, genu valgum, and exophthalmus. With overgrowth of the cranial nerve foramina in the skull, the optic, auditory, and facial nerves can all be compressed. This can lead to hearing loss, visual impairment, and facial muscle paralysis (190). Wallace et al. found cranial nerve compression occurred in 61% of their patients and that raised intracranial pressure can also occur (191).

Systemic manifestations of the disease can also occur. The patient may present with delayed onset of puberty, hypogonadism, anemia, dry skin, and dental caries (192). The condition usually progresses in a slow, unpredictable fashion and in some cases will spontaneously halt (189). Life expectancy is normal.

Laboratory tests are of little use in confirming the diagnosis. The alkaline phosphatase level is elevated in 40% of patients (193). Hernandez et al. evaluated a number of biochemical markers that measure bone turnover and found that they may be useful when analyzed in conjunction with the bone scintigram (194).

Radiographic Features.   The most commonly affected bone is the tibia (90%); however, all long bones of the upper and lower limb can be affected including the clavicle. The initial changes occur in the middle of the diaphysis and progress out toward the metaphyses and epiphysis eventually involving them. The cortex becomes thickened and sclerotic while the medullary canal reduces in width. The cortex may become irregular as the disease progresses. One of the key diagnostic criteria for this dysplasia is that there is symmetrical involvement of the bones (Fig. 9-12). Eventually, other bones become involved including the base of the skull, vertebrae, pelvis, metacarpals, and phalanges (189, 193, 195, 196). Interestingly in the spine, only the posterior elements are involved and this does not cause spinal stenosis (196, 197). The growth plates are not involved as they are products of endochondral bone formation. Valgus deformity of the knee and elbow does occur, however, due to relative overgrowth of the tibia and ulna.

CT scanning shows that the increase in cortical thickness may be focal rather than homogeneous and that endosteal involvement is more extensive than periosteal new bone formation (197). The CT scan is useful for assessing the base of the skull for foraminal stenosis. Technetium-99m bone scans will show increased uptake in the diaphysis often before radiographic changes occur. The bone scans will be negative, however, if the disease is quiescent or has spontaneously resolved. MRI scanning confirms the cortical involvement and sparing of the intramedullary canal and is not a useful investigation.

Pathology.   There are no specific histologic changes pathonemonic for PDD. Rather the findings are what one would expect with increased periosteal and cortical thickness, and a narrow medullary canal that eventually becomes replaced with loose mesenchymal and fibrous tissue. Initially, the changes are typical of recent bone formation with woven bone and lack of Haversian system development. Normal bone remodeling occurs latter in the disease process (190, 192, 195). There is an increase in osteoblast and osteoclast activity with the balance of the two determining the morphology of the involved bone.

Differential Diagnosis.   There are a number of dysplasias that can be considered in the differential diagnosis. Greenspan classified bone dysplasias as to whether they involved enchondral bone formation (e.g., osteopetrosis) or, intramembranous bone formation (e.g., PDD), or both (198). Ribbing disease is a sclerosing dysplasia that has a similar radiologic appearance to PDD; however, it only affects the lower limbs and is not always symmetrical. Cranio diaphyseal dysplasia is inherited by an autosomal recessive pattern and is characterized by early cranial and facial involvement, and the patients usually have mental retardation. Infantile cortical hyperostosis (Caffey disease) is diagnosed earlier than PDD, often in the neonatal period. It is less symmetric; involves predominantly the mandible, ribs, and clavicle; has associated soft-tissue swelling; and usually regresses after infancy.

Osteopetrosis has more extensive bone involvement due to the abnormality in the enchondral bone formation. There is sclerosis throughout the skeleton with both epiphyseal and diaphyseal involvement, and there may be associated pathologic fractures. Other diseases that need to be considered are hyperphosphatasia (markedly elevated alkaline phosphatase level), Hardcastle syndrome (autosomal dominant disorder), juvenile Paget disease, infantile cortical hyperostosis, fibrous dysplasia, and heavy metal poisoning (199).

FIGURE 9-12. **A,B:** A 17-year-old girl with diaphyseal dysplasia. Radiographs demonstrate wide and irregular cortices and marked narrowing of the medullary cavity of the long bones in the upper and lower extremities; the typical finding of genu valgum is demonstrated.

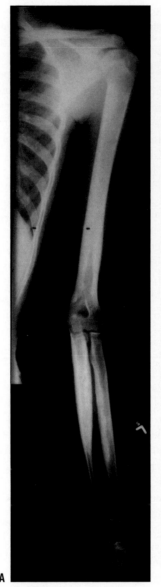
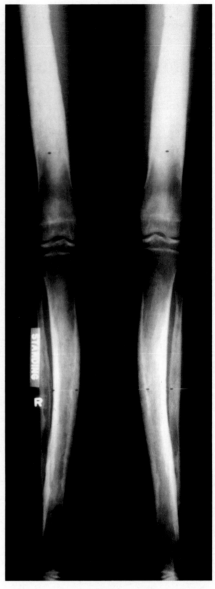

Treatment. There is no cure for PDD, so treatment is aimed at trying to reduce symptoms of bone pain and maximize function. Simple analgesics and anti-inflammatories are used along with an exercise program and physical therapy (PT).

Glucocorticoid treatment has been used effectively for the relief of bone pain. The mechanism of action is not clear. With prolonged use of glucocorticoids, the osteoblast activity is suppressed, and this may decrease the bone pain at the site of sclerosis. Some authors have found that the bone pain is actually relieved very soon after the administration of the glucocorticoid (192). This makes the mechanism of action of the glucosteroids unclear as to exactly how it relieves the bone pain. One of the side effects of prolonged glucocorticoid usage is osteoporosis and this has been found in bone mineral density studies performed on patients with PDD (192, 200, 201). Allen 1970 showed histologically that there is increased bone reabsorption and remodeling with an increase in the osteoclastic activity (202).

Bisphosphonates have also been used in patients with PDD but the results appear quite variable in their ability to reduce the severe skeletal pain. The bisphosphonates, however, may be useful with prolonged therapy with glucocorticoids and the associated osteoporosis that can occur. This combination of therapies has only been reported in one child with PDD (192).

Surgery is rarely required in this disorder; however, corrective osteotomies of the lower limb have been reported (195). These distal femoral and proximal tibia osteotomies were reported to heal well without significant complications. These angular deformities may now be better treated with growth modulation with the use of the eight plates (Orthofix, McKinney, TX).

Osteopoikilosis. Osteopoikilosis, also known as osteopathia condensans disseminate, is a sclerosing bone dysplasia characterized by multiple small foci of increased radio density in cancellous bone. It is an extremely rare disorder that is inherited by an autosomal dominant trait (203).

Clinical Features. This disorder is usually discovered as an incidental radiologic finding as the sclerotic bone lesions themselves are asymptomatic. The disorder develops during childhood; however, the clinical course is quite variable. The lesions may increase or decrease in size and can in fact disappear altogether (204). The children have normal stature with no leg length inequality or angular deformity. Benli et al. reported on 53 patients with osteopoikilosis from 4 families. They found there was no increased likelihood of concurrent pathology in these patients, no increased risk of pathologic fracture, and no malignant change within the lesions (203). Other authors have also found complications of osteopoikilosis to be rare (205, 206). There is one report of an osteosarcoma and one of a chondrosarcoma occurring in two separate patients with osteopoikilosis (207, 208). The true incidence of these malignant changes is unknown as a large number of cases of osteopoikilosis go undiagnosed. No authors recommend routine screening for malignant change once this disorder is detected. Osteopoikilosis is sometimes seen in association with a hereditary dermatologic condition, dermatofibrosis lenticularis disseminata. These papular fibromas are usually asymptomatic and small but can develop into larger dermatofibromas (209). When the two disorders are found together, it is known as Buschke-Ollendorf syndrome. Occasionally, soft-tissue fibrosis and joint contractures can occur that look very similar to melorheostosis. This may be due to the coexistence of these sclerosing conditions, the so-called mixed sclerosing bone dysplasia (210–212). In its "pure form," osteopoikilosis is probably asymptomatic.

Radiographic Features. The osteosclerotic nodules are well-defined, variably shaped radio densities that range in size from 1 to 15 mm in width. They occur in the metaphyses and epiphyses of the long bones and are usually bilateral. They are most commonly found in the bones of the hands and feet followed by the pelvis, femur, and upper limb. The ribs, clavicle, and skull are not involved (203, 204). The cortex is never involved (Fig. 9-13).

A bone scan is not required to make the diagnosis of osteopoikilosis; however, it may be useful when trying to differentiate this condition from metastatic carcinoma. Bone scintigraphy does not have increased uptake in osteopoikilosis but does in metastatic disease (206). Other conditions that should be considered in the differential diagnosis include mastocytosis, melorheostosis, osteopathia striata, and enostosis (bone islands) (198).

Etiology. The etiology of this autosomal dominant disorder is not clear. Lagier et al. postulated that the lesions represent remodeling of cancellous bone secondary to mechanical stress (205). In three unrelated individuals with osteopoikilosis, sequence analysis of LEND 3 gene identified loss of function mutations (213)

Pathology. The sclerotic areas are condensations of compact lamellar bone within the spongiosa (203, 214). This histologic appearance is very similar to what is seen in enostosis (bone islands) (198).

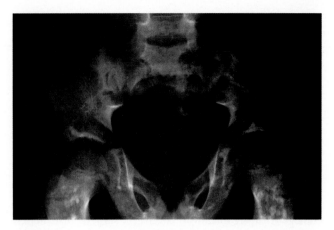

FIGURE 9-13.   A 7-year-old girl with asymptomatic osteopoikilosis.

Treatment. No treatment is required for this benign disorder. In the rare cases where there is associated fibrosis and joint contractures, the management is the same as for melorheostosis.

Melorheostosis.   Melorheostosis is a rare sclerosing skeletal dysplasia that is characterized by soft-tissue contractures in childhood and bone pain in adults (215). The condition was first described by Leri and Joanny in 1922 and the name is derived from the Greek description of the radiologic appearances, "melos" (limb) and "rhein" (flow). Melorheostosis is a nonhereditary disorder occurring equality in both sexes in approximately one per million.

Clinical Features.   Melorheostosis can present at a variable age from 2 to 64 years (216). It usually has a very insidious onset and the symptoms vary according to age. In children, there are usually asymmetric limb contractures that result in leg length inequality. Pain is uncommon in children; however, it develops later in adolescent and early adulthood (217, 218). The lower extremities are more frequently involved than are the upper extremities and the long bones are the most affected. The disease follows a chronic course and can undergo periods of exacerbation and arrest. The progression is often greatest in childhood and can slow down in adulthood (219). The clinical finding is often dependent on how many bones are affected. The condition may affect only one bone (monostotic form), one limb (monomelic form), or multiple bones (polyostotic form). The periarticular ossification can lead to flexion contractures at the knee, hip, ankle, and fingers and can also lead to patella dislocation (218).

The affected limb is usually shorter than the contralateral limb secondary to decreased bone length and further exacerbated by the flexion contractures.

The overlying skin is often tense, shiny, and erythematous with thickened underlying soft tissue (216, 220–222). The affected limb is usually shorter by a mean of 4 cm; however, the occasional patient can have overgrowth of the affected limb (218). There is associated muscular atrophy. Vascular lesions and lymphatic involvement are often associated with cases of melorheostosis. There may be hemangiomas, vascular nevi, varices, AV malformations, lymphedema, and lymphangiectasia (220, 223, 224). Kidney abnormalities, including minimal change nephrotic syndrome and renovascular hypertension secondary to renal artery stenosis, have been described (225–227). Other associated conditions include scleroderma (221, 228–230). There has been reported a slightly increased frequency of soft-tissue tumors, for example, lipoma and desmoid tumors, and osteosarcoma has also been reported (220, 231). Laboratory studies including serum calcium, phosphorous, and alkaline phosphatase levels are all reported to occur within normal limits (219).

Etiology. Melorheostosis is a noninherited disorder and the etiology is largely unknown. Greenspan suggests that there is a disturbance in the processes of intramembranous and endochondral bone formation (198). The distribution of the lesions often corresponds to sclerotomes and this has lead to the hypothesis that an infection similar to herpes zoster may occur resulting in scaring the osseous changes in the distribution of the affected nerve roots (232). This hypothesis could support the monostotic or monomelic distribution of melorheostosis but does not explain the polyostotic form. Kim et al. cultured skin fibroblasts from affected patients and suggested that there is altered expression of several adhesion proteins that may contribute to the development of the hyperostosis and associated soft-tissue abnormalities of melorheostosis (233).

Radiographic Features. The characteristic radiographic appearance of melorheostosis is irregular, asymmetric, osteosclerosis of the long bones of the upper and lower extremities. The osteosclerosis is in a linear pattern that resembles melted wax dripping down one side of a candle (Fig. 9-14).

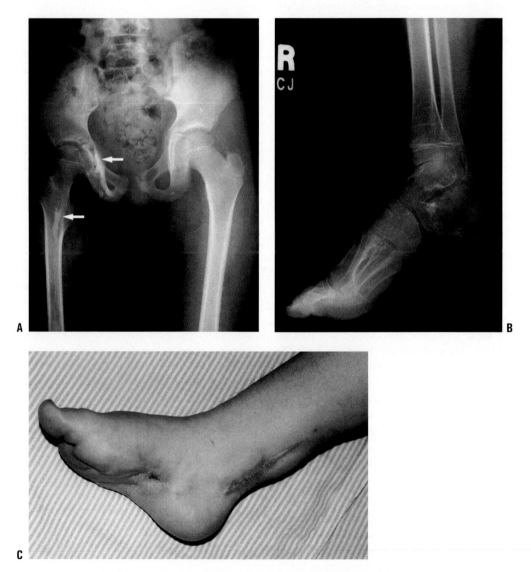

FIGURE 9-14. An 8-year-old with melorheostosis who presented with an equinovarus foot deformity. **A:** The classical findings of irregular linear hyperostosis are seen at the *arrows*. **B:** Patches of hyperostosis are seen in the talus and calcaneus; this is typical of melorheostotic involvement of the tarsals. **C:** There was pain and swelling around the equinovarus foot. Previous surgical releases had resulted in rapid recurrence of the deformity.

This radiographic appearance is a result of the developmental error that has occurred predominantly in intramembranous bone formation (234). In children, the hyperostosis is endosteal, which results in "streakiness" of the long bones and spotting in the phalanges and metacarpals (218). In adults, the hyperostosis is subperiosteal or extracortical, and a distinct demarcation line is seen between the affected and normal bone (219, 234). The axial skeleton is rarely involved (235). Spots or patches of hyperostosis can occur in the epiphyses and in the carpal and tarsal bones, which can often resemble osteopoikilosis. Ossification can also occur in the soft tissue surrounding the larger joints. This is most common posterior to the knee joint and on the medial aspect of the hip joint.

Bone scintigraphy shows increased uptake predominantly in the affected cortex on the side of the bone affected by melorheostosis (206, 236). MRI scanning is not as useful as CT scanning in defining the bony abnormality in melorheostosis. The MRI scan is useful in looking at the surrounding soft-tissue abnormalities; however, it just shows low signal changes in the bone (237).

Histopathology. The histologic features of the hyperostosis include primitive looking bone that is woven or nonlamellar with thickened, sclerotic, and irregular laminae (219). The trabeculae are thickened and there can be increased fibrotic changes within the medullary canal. There can be an abundance of osteoid within mineralization, which indicates the overproduction of bone matrix. Hoshi et al. also found an increase in osteoclasts in the melorheostotic bone indicating increased bone reabsorption (238). They also found an increase in the cytokines TGF-β and fibroblast growth factor, which may play some role in the exuberant bone matrix production and the angiogenesis in the melorheostosis (209).

Differential Diagnosis. The differential diagnosis includes osteomyelitis, osteopetrosis, osteopoikilosis, and osteopathia striata, all of which can have similar radiographic findings. These three disorders are termed "overlap syndromes," which explains some of their similarities and also the fact that two or more of these disorders can sometimes coexist in the same patient (234). The diagnosis of melorheostosis can usually be made, however, by the characteristic appearance on plain radiography and the clinical features discussed earlier. Other conditions that need to be considered in the differential diagnosis include myositis ossificans, osteoma, and parosteal osteosarcoma. Myositis ossificans has a clear zone of demarcation between it and the adjoining cortex and the ossification pattern is quite distinct. Bone scintigraphy usually reveals little or no activity. An osteoma has a smooth surface compared to the irregular surface of the melorheostosis. Parosteal osteosarcomas commonly occur in the posterior aspect of the knee joint and therefore can be confused with melorheostosis. A parosteal osteosarcoma also has an irregular surface and the bone scintigram is very useful in distinguishing between the two. The bone scan in parosteal tumors shows markedly increased uptake within both the extracortical bone and the medullary canal (234). Clinically, focal scleroderma can cause soft-tissue fibrosis and contractures similar to melorheostosis; however, radiographs of the bones are normal (239).

Treatment. The soft-tissue contractures are difficult to manage and in that respect are not dissimilar from those seen in arthrogryposis. Conservative management of these soft-tissue contractures with manipulation, bracing, and serial casting is usually unsuccessful and there is a high rate of recurrence (240). Soft-tissue surgery including releases, tendon lengthening, and capsulotomies also have a higher recurrence rate despite postoperative bracing (218). A closing osteotomy is probably the safest procedure to perform in these children. Young et al. recommended using the principles learned in arthrogryposis in the treatment of severe cases of melorheostosis. The osteotomy should be performed as close to skeletal maturity as possible. The joint should be splinted through periods of rapid growth to minimize contractures. When a soft-tissue procedure is performed, this should involve extensive release with wide capsulotomies and tenotomies accompanied by postoperative bracing (218). Because of the high risk of ischemia with acute corrections of the angular deformities, some authors have recommended both the realignment of the bony abnormalities and soft-tissue contractures with the Illizerov technique (240–244). Complications still occur including pseudarthrosis and ischemia that can lead to amputation of the affected limb (242, 244). This ischemia may be due to too acute correction but may also be secondary to a vascular obstruction and vasculitis, which can occur in the melorheostotic limb (218). Growth plate modulation with the use of an eight plate (Orthofix, McKinney, TX) may have a role in the correction of these deformities as well.

Osteopathia Striata. Osteopathia striata is another of the sclerosing bone dysplasias characterized by dense linear striations in the metaphysis and diaphysis of the long bones (distal femur, proximal tibia, and proximal humerus). The disorder was originally described by Voorhoeve in 1924 and latter named by Fairbank (245).

Clinical Features. Osteopathia striata occurs in less than one per million population. It is probably inherited as an autosomal dominant trait; however, this has not been categorically determined (246, 247). In other cases, when osteopathia striata has been found in association with cranial sclerosis, an X-linked form of the disease has been suggested (248, 249). Similar to the other sclerosing bone dysplasias, osteopathia striata represents a developmental anomaly in enchondral and intramembranous ossification and therefore can "overlap" with osteopoikilosis and melorheostosis.

The diagnosis of this rare condition is usually made on an incidental radiograph as the patient is asymptomatic. There are no physical abnormalities unless there is significant cranial sclerosis that can lead to cranial nerve impingement and resulting abnormalities in vision and hearing. This is a rare syndrome that is also characterized by abnormal facies, macrocephaly, and mental retardation (250, 251). Severe cervical kyphosis has been noted in one patient with this disorder (252).

There are no reports in the literature of any histologic examination of these lesions.

Radiographic Features. The characteristic radiographic findings of this condition are dense linear striations in the tubular and flat bones (Fig. 9-15). The striations that do not change with time are primarily seen in the metaphysis and diaphysis, which are the sites of rapid growth. These striations represent a failure in remodeling of the persistent mature bone (198). The striations may extend into the epiphysis as well. In the iliac wings, the striations form a fan shape reflecting the growth pattern of the pelvis (198). The length of the striations reflects the rate of growth of the particular bone they are seen in. The longest striations therefore are seen in the distal femur (198). The striations are usually symmetric. Once skeletal maturity has been reached, the striations do not change with time. There is no increased uptake on bone scintigraphy (206).

Treatment. No treatment is required for asymptomatic isolated osteopathic striata.

Congenital Pseudarthrosis of the Clavicle. Congenital pseudarthrosis of the clavicle (POC) is a rare disorder where

the clavicle has failed to form normally before birth. The condition almost always occurs on the right hand side and is bilateral in only 10% of cases. The characteristic finding in the neonate is an asymptomatic prominence in the mid-clavicular region with palpable mobility of both ends of the clavicle. The condition is most commonly confused with a fracture following birth trauma or cleidocranial dysostosis. With birth trauma, the clavicle is painful to palpate and there is usually abundant callus on x-ray. With cleidocranial dysostosis, the distance between the clavicular ends is wider; the "lump" smaller, and there is other radiologic changes in the pelvis and skull that are diagnostic.

Etiology. There is some thought that there may be a genetic cause of POC with nine patients in Gibson and Carroll's series having a strong family history (253, 254). This does not explain why the condition predominantly affects the right clavicle, so most authors feel the condition occurs sporadically and that local mechanical or humoral factors are the cause. The other school of thought is that POC is a failure of ossification of the clavicle. The left clavicle is affected only rarely, and when this does occur, there is usually an associated anatomical abnormality, for example, dextrocardia, cervical rib, or elevated ribs (255). These factors are thought to contribute to POC being a predominantly right-sided condition. The subclavian

FIGURE 9-15. Osteopathia striata. The streaking of the proximal femurs did not change much in the patient between the ages of 12 years **(A)** and 25 years **(B)**. Note the flattened femoral epiphysis.

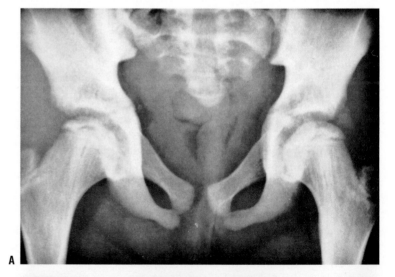

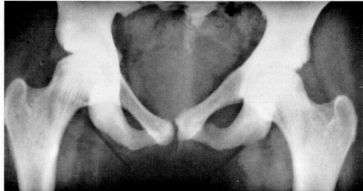

artery passes directly under the pseudarthrosis and the pulsatile pressure of this vessel may cause the defect. With elevated ribs or a cervical rib, this pressure phenomenon is magnified (255).

The intrauterine development of the clavicle has been the subject of debate for many decades. Some authors argue that the clavicle has two centers of ossification and that POC is a result of the two centers not coalescing (256–260). Others have shown that the clavicle develops by endochondral ossification from one center (254, 261).

Clinical Features.
POC is usually diagnosed at birth as a painless lump in the middle third of the right clavicle. The two unfused ends of the clavicle are enlarged and are freely mobile. A radiograph confirms the diagnosis and distinguishes POC from a birth fracture, cleidocranial dysostosis, and neurofibromatosis. The deformity progresses with age and the pseudarthrosis never appears to spontaneously heal. The bone ends continue to enlarge and the shoulder droops making the cosmetic deformity worse. The pseudarthrosis can become mildly painful; however, shoulder function remains normal throughout life (253). There are reports of thoracic outlet syndrome occurring in latter life possibly secondary to POC (254, 257, 259, 260, 262–265).

Radiographic Features.
The radiologic findings in congenital POC are characteristic. The pseudarthrosis always occurs in the middle third of the clavicle with the sternal fragment slightly longer than the acromial fragment. The relationship of the two fragments is always the same with the sternal fragment lying slightly above and in front of the acromial one. The ends of the bones are bulbous due to the cartilage enlargement and there is sclerotic closure of the medullary canal. There is no evidence of callous formation.

Histopathology.
The cartilaginous caps on the ends of both fragments at the pseudarthrosis resemble that of a developing physis. In the intervening gap, there is dense fibrous and fibrocartilaginous tissue with no evidence of synovial tissue (253, 258, 266). In the deep zone of the cartilage, the chondrocytes are arranged in columns with different stages of maturation. By using preoperative tetracycline, Hirata et al. were able to demonstrate new bone formation by endochondral ossification at the bone–cartilage junction (258).

Treatment.
The natural history of POC is for the prominence to become larger and occasionally painful, the shoulder to "droop" but maintain normal function, and rarely thoracic outlet syndrome can develop. For these reasons, most authors recommend surgical treatment of the pseudarthrosis when either the parents are upset with the unsightly appearance or the child becomes symptomatic (254, 258, 262, 263, 265–272). The most commonly recommended surgery is excision of the pseudarthrosis, autologous bone grafting, and fixation with a plate and screws (Fig. 9-16). This is usually performed around 3 to 6 years of age and the fusion rate is excellent (254, 258, 270). Others have used intramedullary fixation successfully (253). Grogan et al. recommended performing the surgery earlier by simply maintaining the periosteal sheath, excising the pseudarthrosis and sclerotic bone, and approximating the bone ends without the use of bone graft (268). They achieved union in all eight patients without the added problem of a secondary operation to remove the metalware.

Dysplasia Epiphysealis Hemimelica.
Dysplasia epiphysealis hemimelica (DEH) is a rare skeletal disorder mainly affecting the lower limb that is characterized by osteochondral overgrowth of one or more epiphysis. It was originally described by Trevor in 1950 who called the condition "tarso-epiphysial aclasis" (273) The dysplasia has also been referred to as "Trevor disease." Fairbank reviewed a further 14 cases and reported these in 1956 (274). He demonstrated that although the tarsus

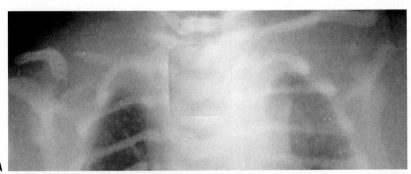
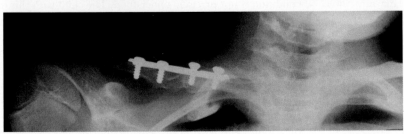

FIGURE 9-16. Pseudarthrosis of the right clavicle. **A:** Congenital pseudarthrosis of the right clavicle. There are no signs of healing. **B:** Radiographic appearance after solid union achieved by open reduction, internal fixation, and autogenous bone grafting in a different 8-year-old boy.

was commonly affected, this disorder was more complex than that originally defined by Trevor and gave it the more descriptive name "dysplasia epiphysealis hemimelica." This name reflects that the whole epiphysis can be involved ("dysplasia"), or just the medial or lateral half of a single limb ("hemimelica").

Etiology. The etiology of DEH is unknown. There is no evidence of a genetic cause for this condition due to an absence of related affected individuals in most studies (275). This is reinforced by Donaldson et al. who studied discordant monozygotic twins with DEH (276). Experimental work on animals led Fairbank to the conclusion that the primary fault lies in the preaxial or postaxial part of the apical cap of a single limb bud (274). The exact timing of this fault is yet to be determined. Trevor postulated an abnormality of cell division at the superficial zone of articular cartilage that leads to delayed maturation and the formation of the large cartilaginous mass (273). Connor et al. suggested that the fundamental defect is an abnormality of the regulation of cartilage proliferation in the affected epiphysis, which results in the cartilaginous exostoses and cartilage nests that can be seen in the adjacent metaphysis (275).

Clinical Features. The disorder is uncommon and occurs in approximately one per million people (277). The diagnosis is usually made between the ages of 2 and 14 years and it is more common in males than females with a ratio of 3:1 (275, 278). It occurs in white children more often than black children (279). The lower limb is almost exclusively involved; however, there are a few reports of upper limb involvement (282, 283). The dysplasia is initially asymptomatic; however, with time, the resulting overgrowth causes localized pain, swelling, and joint stiffness. There is secondary wasting of the muscles in the affected limb. In adulthood, secondary degenerative changes have been reported in the affected joints of some individuals; however, the incidence appears lower than was predicted by Fairbank (274, 275). The most common anatomical sites involved are the distal femur, distal tibia, and talus (273, 274, 279, 280). Other areas reported in the literature include the femoral head, acetabulum, sacroiliac joint, wrist, and shoulder (115, 281–286). The local pain occurs for a number of reasons. The soft tissues are altered by the osteocartilaginous enlargement, and ligaments are stretched and tendons become inflamed when they are displaced from their normal positions. There are altered stresses across the joint that result in subchondral edema and bone pain. The asymmetric growth of the epiphysis can result in malalignment of the lower limb and a small leg length discrepancy. The medial side of the epiphysis is the most commonly involved, so the angulation is usually valgus (274). Azouz et al. classified the dysplasia into three categories: (a) localized (solitary involvement of an epiphysis), (b) classical (multiple epiphyses of a single limb), and (c) generalized (whole lower limb involvement from pelvis to foot) (287). The classical form is the most common, and when more than one epiphysis is affected, either the medial or lateral side is exclusively involved. There are cases, however, where the medial side of one epiphysis is affected and the lateral side of another in the same limb (275).

Radiographic Features. The most characteristic findings on plain radiographs are an irregular enlargement of one side of the epiphysis with a number of small irregular centers of ossification separate to the main epiphysis (Fig. 9-17). These secondary centers can fuse with each other and then with the main epiphysis or can remain as a separate entity once maturation is complete. The lesion enlarges with skeletal growth and the opposing epiphysis may have secondary deformation. The cartilaginous overgrowths can remain contiguous with the epiphysis or they can fragment and become detached. The affected epiphysis may ossify earlier and end up larger than the unaffected contralateral side (278, 288, 289). Although the term "hemimelica" is used, the entire epiphysis can be affected or the opposite halves of different epiphyses in the same limb can be involved (275). The metaphysis is occasionally affected as well (278, 279, 284). CT scanning has been useful in defining the bony anatomy especially with skeletal maturity; however, MRI scanning has become a more useful investigation with its ability to image the cartilaginous growth and soft-tissue involvement (Fig. 9-18). Peduto et al. performed MRI scans on 10 patients with DEH and were able to show muscle, tendon, ligament, and cartilage abnormalities (290). There were less predictable ligament insertion sites, bony fragments, chronic tendonitis, articular cartilage deformation and thinning, and bone edema on both sides of the joint. The plain radiographs often show the overgrowth in only one plane, whereas the MRI defines the position of bony or cartilaginous fragments more accurately and often reveals that the anatomy is more complex than originally thought. Surgical planning is easier when the MRI has defined the cleavage plane between the overgrowth and "normal" epiphysis (279, 290–292).

Histopathology. The outgrowth looks very similar to an epiphysis with "glistening bluish cartilage" and a smooth surface (274). Sometimes the surface can be slightly irregular and a groove of variable depth can sometimes be seen between the epiphysis and the outgrowth. Microscopically a thick zone of hyperplastic cartilage is distinguishable from the rest of the cartilaginous epiphysis only by some irregularity in the size and distribution of the chondrocytes (274, 278). There is a cartilage boundary between the lesion and the epiphysis. When the fragment has separated, fibrous bands are present as well. These findings are not dissimilar to those seen in an osteochondroma; however, DEH does not become pedunculated. Malignant transformation has not been reported.

Treatment. The majority of reported cases of DEH have been treated surgically and therefore the natural history of this condition is not precisely understood. The child with this disorder should be treated for symptoms arising from the overgrowth rather than prophylactically and care should be taken to preserve as much of the joint surface as possible. There has been no reported malignant change in these lesions. An MRI scan is very useful in the preoperative planning as the scan will usually define the cleavage plain between the over growth and their normal epiphysis as well as defining the extent of the lesion. The MRI scan helps define the lesions as either

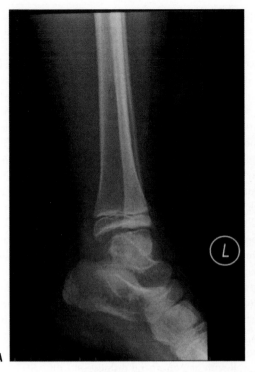

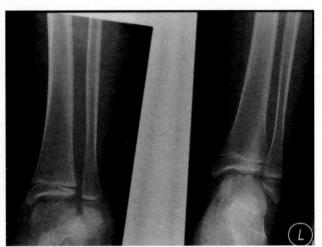

FIGURE 9-17.   A,B: An 8-year-old girl with dysplasia epiphysealis hemimelica of the talus.

juxta-articular or intra-articular. Juxta-articular lesions can be relatively easily excised surgically with few complications. If the lesion is excised prior to skeletal maturity, there is an increased risk of recurrence (280, 281). The treatment of the articular lesions, however, remains more controversial. Kuo

et al. treated three patients with partial excision of the articular lesions and had two fair and one poor result (280). They do not recommend excision of an articular lesion unless it has become an obvious loose body. Keret et al. performed extra-articular osteotomies to correct the angular deformity rather

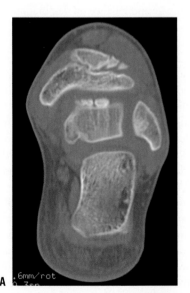

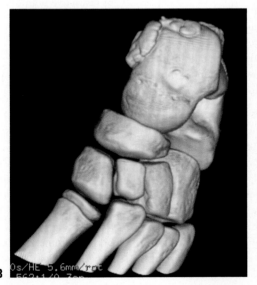

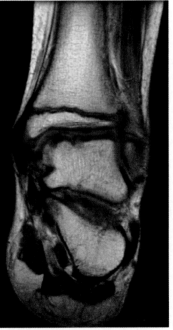

FIGURE 9-18.   CT **(A,B)** and MRI **(C)** scan of an 8-year-old girl with dysplasia epiphysealis hemimelica of the talus showing the asymmetric growth medially.

than excise an intra-articular overgrowth. They confirmed that they had a congruent joint space by arthrogram and MRI scan before doing this. If the osteotomy is performed before skeletal maturity, however, they had an increased recurrence of the deformity (279). Despite surgical intervention, a number of patients will still go on to develop early degenerative changes in the affected joint (275, 279, 280).

Fibrodysplasia Ossificans Progressiva.

Fibrodysplasia ossificans progressiva (FOP) is a rare genetic disorder of connective tissue characterized by a short valgus great toe and predictable progressive ossification of tendons, ligaments, striated muscles, and fascia. It occurs in one per million people, and although inherited as an autosomal dominant trait, the majority of cases are sporadic mutations (275, 293, 294).

Etiology. Researchers have shown that an overexpression of bone morphogenetic protein 4 (BMP 4), its messenger ribonucleic acid (mRNA), and elevated steady-state levels of BMP 4 receptor mRNA are present in affected and nonaffected tissue from patients with FOP (113, 295, 296). The BMP 4 gene, however, is not mutated, but an underexpression of a BMP-antagonist response (reduced negative feedback mechanism) may mean the loss of normal morphogenetic regulation and hence excessive ossification (297, 298). Recent research has revealed that all individuals with a definite diagnosis of fibrodysplasia ossificans progressive have a mutation in the ACVR1 gene that provides instructions for producing BMP type I receptors. The ACVR1 protein is found in many tissues of the body and helps to control the growth and development of the bones and muscles, including the ossification process that occurs in normal skeletal maturation. A mutation in the ACVR1 gene may change the shape of the receptor under certain conditions and disrupt mechanisms that control the receptor's activity. As a result, the receptor may be constantly activated causing overgrowth of bone and cartilage as one sees in FOP (299–301). Other theories have also been postulated for the genetic cause of FOP and because of its heterogeneity, there may well be a number of factors contributing to the clinical scenario one sees (302–304). A better understanding of the molecular pathology of this condition will help in the prevention or treatment of this debilitating disease.

Clinical Features. The condition is recognizable at birth due to the abnormal great toes. Connor and Evans classified the great toe deformities into four subtypes (305). The majority were type 1 where the toe was short, lacked a skin crease due to only a single phalanx, and had valgus alignment. The child may also have short thumbs and clinodactyly of the little finger. Often these abnormalities are subtle and are not recognized in the neonatal period and it is not until heterotopic ossification occurs that FOP is diagnosed. Heterotopic ossification occurs at a mean age of 5 years; however, it can occur at birth or as late as the third decade. The ossification usually begins in the neck region, followed by the spine and shoulder girdle. It can arise spontaneously or as a result of even minor trauma. The spread of heterotopic ossification is predictable from axial

to appendicular, cranial to caudal, and finally proximal to distal (76). The hip, knee, elbow, and wrist are other sites commonly involved but latter in the disease process. The dorsal surface is usually involved before the ventral surface. Kaplan et al. described three stages in the process of progressive ossification (294). The first stage is the appearance of an erythematous, subfascial nodule on the back of the neck or spine (early lesion). This lesion is painful, warm, and swollen and often resembles an infectious process. If it occurs in the limbs, there can be quite extreme swelling probably due to the angiogenesis occurring at this time. A few weeks later, the swelling and pain subside; however, there is an increase in induration of the soft tissues (intermediate lesion). The late lesion is usually present by 12 weeks and consists of a hard, painless lump that can also be seen radiographically. This process of soft-tissue nodules becoming calcified and then forming mature bone is characteristic of endochondral ossification.

This progressive heterotopic ossification leads to the ankylosis of the major joints. This occurs initially in the neck and back and then spreads to the shoulder girdles, hips, and then along the appendicular skeleton. This can result in the spine becoming ankylosed to the pelvis or the shoulder girdle to the chest wall with glenohumeral dislocation (306, 307). The rate of disease progression varies amongst individuals; however, most patients are wheelchair bound by the third or fourth decade of life. The heterotopic ossification can be stimulated by any form of trauma to the soft tissues including immunization, dental injections, soft-tissue surgery (including biopsies), and even viral illnesses (305). Eventually, the temporomandibular joint is involved and ankylosis can lead to difficulties with eating and poor nutrition. The restricted joint movement and bony prominences result in pressure sores if preventative care is not undertaken. Eventually, the severely involved patient succumbs to cardiopulmonary complications. The heart muscle is not involved; however, the spinal and chest wall ankylosis leads to restrictive pulmonary disease and reliance on diaphragmatic breathing (76, 308).

Radiographic Features. Radiographs of the great toe show shortening of the first ray, a delta-shaped proximal phalanges, interphalangeal joint fusion, and a resulting valgus deformity (305). Radiographs of the hands may also show short first metacarpals and fifth finger clinodactyly in almost half the patients with this disorder. Other radiologic changes include short broad femoral necks, abnormal cervical vertebrae with small bodies, large pedicles, and large spinous processes and exostoses in the proximal tibia (305) (Fig. 9-19).

The abnormal areas of heterotopic ossification are initially similar in appearance to myositis ossificans with diffuse calcification that develops into peripheral maturation. These areas of heterotopic ossification demonstrate features of normal bone remodeling, and over time will resemble normal bone. The bone forms along striated muscles, fascia, tendons, and ligaments, which results in ankylosis of the adjacent joints. The heterotopic bone is subject to the same mechanical stresses as the rest of the skeleton and will exhibit hypertrophy or osteopenia

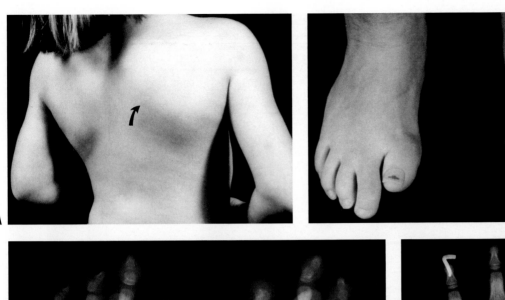

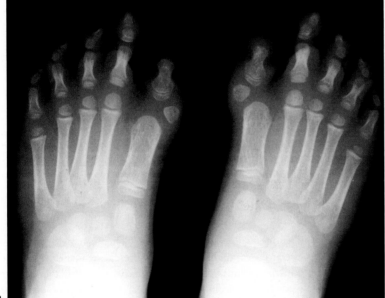

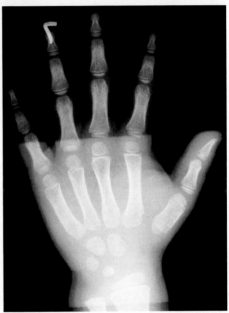

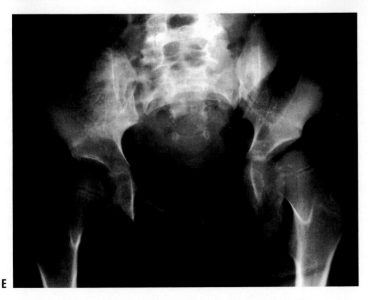

FIGURE 9-19. Fibrodysplasia ossificans progressive. A 4-year-old girl at the time of presentation. She complained of right periscapular swelling, warmth, and tenderness. **A:** Clinical photograph demonstrating the area of right periscapular involvement (*arrow*). **B:** Characteristic great toe morphology, demonstrating shortening of the great toes bilaterally. **C:** Bilateral radiograph of the feet demonstrating shortened great toes, with bilateral delta phalanges and shortened first metatarsals. **D:** Anteroposterior radiograph of the hand, demonstrating characteristic shortening of the thumb metacarpal. **E:** Anteroposterior radiograph of the pelvis, demonstrating short, broad femoral necks, and exostoses.

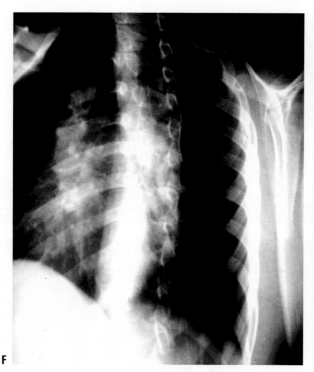
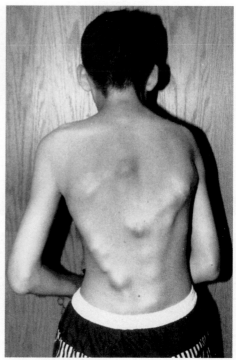

FIGURE 9-19. (*continued*) **F:** Early spontaneous fusion along the posterior elements and lateral masses is demonstrated. **G:** Clinical appearance of an older individual with advanced subcutaneous ossification and characteristic dorsal-to-ventral pattern.

dependent on how much loading occurs across the bone. Fractures through the areas of heterotopic bone heal normally.

Histopathology. A limited amount of biopsy material has been available for analysis with this condition as the trauma of performing the biopsy can precipitate further ossification. Histologic evaluation of the tissue at different stages, however, has revealed that the bone forms by the process of endochondral ossification. This proceeds through the three standard phases with the early infiltration of loose myxoid fibrous tissue and chondroblastic cells. As the endochondral ossification becomes more organized, mature lamella bone is laid down with normal marrow tissue that can support ectopic hematopoiesis (76). Kaplan et al. reviewed the biopsies from eleven patients with biologic features of FOP and found that the tissue is S-100 antigen positive before the tissue demonstrates differentiated osteochondral tissue. They found that six children had been misinterpreted as having a diagnosis of fibromatosis or sarcoma based on the biopsy before there was radiographic evidence of heterotopic ossification (309) Gannon et al. have shown that the first changes in FOP are an intense perivascular lymphocytic infiltration into normal appearing skeletal muscle. They also showed that inflammatory mast cells are present at every stage in the development of the lesions but are present in highest concentration in this early vascular fibroproliferative stage (310, 311). There are no reports of late sarcomatous changes in these areas of heterotopic ossification.

Treatment Recommendations. There are still no known effective treatments for FOP. At present, management of these patients includes the early diagnosis, the avoidance of iatrogenic harm (vaccinations, biopsies), the prevention of falls and pressure sores, and the symptomatic treatment of painful flare-ups. Surgical excision of areas of heterotopic bone should be avoided as this will only stimulate more proliferative heterotopic ossification (305). The more severely affected patients with FOP will require a wheelchair by their third or fourth decade. This needs to be well padded and accommodating for the skeletal deformities so that pressure sores do not occur.

Medical therapy has been attempted to try and influence the development of the heterotopic ossification. The use of high doses or oral bisphosphonates and corticosteroids has been shown to ameliorate the local pain and swelling in patients but had no effect on the subsequent progression of the early fibrovascular lesions to ossification. Consideration has to be given to the side effects of these medications as well on the normal bone. Isotretinoin (an inhibitor of metacymal tissue differentiation into cartilage and bone) has also been used to try and prevent the progression of the lesions through the endochondral process. Zasloff et al. performed a prospective study in 21 patients but were unable to determine whether this medication was effective in preventing disease flare-ups (312). Effective therapies for the treatment of FOP will be based around the recent discovery of the FOP gene. By possibly blocking the activin-like kinase-2 receptor, pharmacological agents may be able to alter the BMP signaling pathway and therefore either prevent or modify this devastating disorder (313).

ACQUIRED DISORDERS

Myositis Ossificans. Myositis ossificans refers to the presence of benign heterotopic ossification in the soft tissues (usually skeletal muscle) typically as a result of localized trauma. The precise molecular mechanism that initiates the hematoma to turn into bone is still unknown. When trauma has not been involved, it has been called pseudomalignant myositis ossificans or myositis ossificans circumscripta (314). The condition is most common in adolescent boys; however, it is also reported in infants (315).

Etiology. Trauma is the precipitating event in approximately 70% of children who develop myositis ossificans (316). The trauma can vary from a direct blow to the soft tissues, an elbow dislocation, repetitive microtrauma, or even from a vaccination injection. Myositis ossificans can also occur in some neurologic conditions, spinal cord injury, or following severe head injury (317–320). Patients with Guillain-Barré syndrome, poliomyositis, and acquired immunodeficiency syndrome encephalopathy have been reported to form heterotopic ossification (321–323). Attempts to isolate any local or systemic inductive factors that cause ossification in these conditions has been unsuccessful (298). Thermal injuries and total joint replacement surgery are other conditions where myositis ossificans is seen (324–326).

The pathogenesis of heterotopic ossification in this condition is not well understood. Kaplan et al. have summarized that three requisite components are necessary: "inductive signaling pathways, inducible osteoprogenitor cells, and a heterotopic

environment conductive to osteogenesis" (298). With a recent greater understanding of the genetic and molecular processes involved in fibrodysplasia ossificans progressiva and progressive osseous heteroplasia, the pathogenesis of the heterotopic ossification in myositis ossificans may be easier to unravel (299–301, 327, 328). This will then allow for more effective prevention and treatment regimens.

Clinical Features. Localized pain, swelling, joint "stiffness," and a palpable mass 1 to 3 weeks following trauma are the most common presenting complaints. The areas most affected are the quadriceps muscle in the lower limb and the brachialis muscle in the upper limb. The patient with myositis ossificans occasionally has a fever, and the affected area can also feel warm, which mimics musculoskeletal infection (314). The pain usually reduces over an 8- to 12-week time period as the ossification matures, and during this time, contractures can develop in the adjacent joints. Laboratory investigations are not required to make the diagnosis. The serum calcium and phosphorus levels are normal and the alkaline phosphatase level is only elevated early in the ossification process and then quickly returns to normal as maturation proceeds (298).

Radiographic Features. The initial radiographs, within a couple of weeks of the injury, will show subtle changes of soft-tissue swelling and small flecks of calcification in the affected muscle, usually in the diaphyseal region of the limb. With time, the calcification increases and the floccular calcifications coalesce to form an obvious area of heterotopic calcification (Fig. 9-20). Characteristically, the peripheral calcification undergoes osseous maturation first leaving a central lucent zone in the lesion. This is opposite to what happens in an osteosarcoma where the tumor grows centripetally (central to peripheral). The mass is usually separated from the periosteum

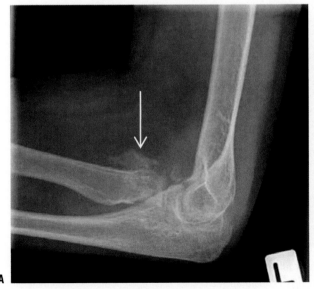
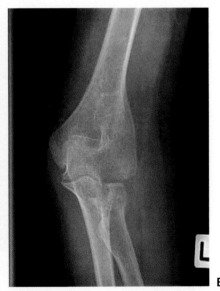

FIGURE 9-20.   **A,B:** Heterotopic bone formation after a closed elbow injury treated in a cast.

by a thin lucent line on the radiograph; however, in some cases, there is a connection by a thin stalk, and in others, the mass can be adherent to the diaphysis with a broad base (329, 330). Over a 5- to 6-month period, the mature bone is quite evident and the lesion may start decreasing in size. Radionucleotide bone scans are very sensitive to heterotopic new bone formation and are positive before the lesions can be seen on plain radiographs. As the bone matures, there is less uptake of technetium-99m, and the scans become less sensitive. Unfortunately, the bone scans have little specificity, so they do not help in differentiating tumor from heterotopic ossification. Ultrasonography can also identify early myositis ossificans as a focal hypoechoic mass within the area of traumatized muscle. The CT scan is more useful as it clearly shows the zonal maturation within the lesion and its relationship to the nearby bone (316, 331) (Fig. 9-21). MRI scans are not necessary to help with the diagnosis when there is a clear history of trauma and plain radiographs or CT scans have been performed. The MRI will show well-defined lesions that are inhomogeneous. The histologic stage of the lesion correlates well with the MRI findings (332).

Histopathology. The lesions occur predominantly in muscle; however, they can also occur in tendons and subcutaneous fat. The histopathology of myositis ossificans is characterized by four histologic zones that were described by Ackerman in 1958 (333): (a) a central (inner) zone of undifferentiated cells and atypical mitotic figures, (b) adjacent (middle) zone of well-orientated osteoid formation in a nonneoplastic stroma, (c) new bone formation, and (d) a peripheral (outer) zone of well-organized lamellar bone, clearly demarcated from the surrounding tissue (333). A biopsy is rarely required for diagnosis and can

in fact stimulate more aggressive heterotopic ossification especially in fibrodysplasia ossificans progressive. If a biopsy is performed, a specimen large enough to show all these zones should be taken to help differentiate it from a sarcoma whose leading edge will be more cellular and contain many mitotic figures.

Treatment. The basis for the prevention and treatment of myositis ossificans is in the modification of the inductive signaling pathways, the osteoprogenitor cells, and the angiogenesis in the involved muscle. The signaling pathways have been altered clinically by the use of nonsteroidal anti-inflammatory drugs (NSAIDs) especially in patients undergoing total joint replacement. A review of the literature, however, shows the difficulty in choosing the correct agent, dose, and duration of treatment. The local population of osteoprogenitor cells can probably be reduced or altered by radiation therapy. This has been used therapeutically again in total joint replacement patients and pelvic fractures but would be inappropriate in children due to the potential side effects. Modification of the local environment (injured skeletal muscle) is the area where most research has been carried out in children. Many authors have devised protocols involving rest, ice, compressive bandaging, stretching, and graduated passive exercises to try and prevent heterotopic ossification (334–337). None of these papers, however, give any clear evidence that such measures prevent or decrease the severity of the myositis ossificans. Surgical excision of the heterotopic ossification is reserved for patients with functional limitations due to the size of position of the mass. Surgery should not be undertaken until the lesion has fully matured into bone on the plain radiographs, and the bone scan shows normal uptake of technetium-99m, which is usually 12 to 18 months after the injury. Spontaneous resorption of

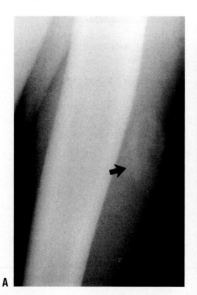
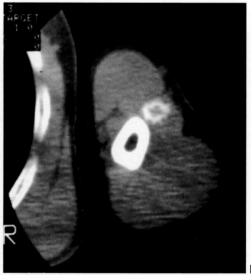

FIGURE 9-21. Myositis ossificans. **A:** Anteroposterior radiograph demonstrating myositis ossificans in the left upper arm (*arrow*). **B:** CT scan of the same patient, delineating peripheral maturation and clear separation of the lesion from the underlying cortex of the humerus.

the myositis ossificans can occur and therefore waiting as long as possible before excising is preferable (330, 338).

The Osteochondroses.

Osteochondrosis is a common localized disorder that affects the epiphysis of many different bones. The exact etiology is not clear; however, there is a disturbance in the endochondral ossification that results in altered growth of the epiphysis, apophysis, and physis. There is an alteration of both chondrogenesis and osteogenesis that occurs in an epiphysis that was previously growing in a normal way (339). There have been many attempts at trying to classify the osteochondroses based on anatomical location, etiology, or whether they involve the epiphysis, physeal epiphysis, or are extra-articular (340–345). The various osteochondroses have been given eponyms depending on their region of occurrence (Table 9-4). They generally have well-defined natural histories with predictable outcomes (345). The more clinically significant osteochondroses are described throughout this textbook according to anatomic region, but are highlighted here because they include features of localized disorders of bone and cartilage.

Etiology.

The etiology of osteochondroses is multifactorial, and there is no one single factor that can account for all aspects of the disease (346, 347). The primary process in the development of osteochondroses has mainly been researched in animals. The different factors involved in this include the anatomy of the affected area, vascular events, trauma, heredity (species of animal), a period of rapid growth, and perhaps diet (347). The underlying pathogenesis that most authors agree on is that there is a disruption to the vascular supply of the involved area of epiphyseal cartilage. This may result from anatomically fragile or small vessels, repetitive microtrauma to the vessels, or occlusion secondary to infection or major trauma.

TABLE 9-4	Examples of Osteochondroses by Region

Upper extremity
  Capitellum (Panner)
  Carpal navicular (Keinboch)
  Phalangeal epiphysis (Theemann)
  Distal radial epiphysis (Madelung)
Vertebral end plates
  Scheuermann
Lower extremity
  Capital femoral epiphysis (Legg-Perthes)
  Proximal tibial physis (Blount)
  Tibial tubercle (Osgood-Schlatter)
  Calcaneal apophysis (Sever)
  Tarsal navicular (Kohler)
  Metatarsal heads, 2, 3, 4 (Freiberg)
General
  Osteochondritis dissecans, especially knee, ankle, elbow

The resulting focal ischemia leads to failure in the endochondral ossification and an abnormal epiphysis (339, 348). The pathogenesis of osteochondritis dissecans may be slightly different as the segmental epiphyseal necrosis involves both the subchondral bone and the overlying articular cartilage. It is not clear whether the vascular necrosis precedes or follows necrosis of the cartilage. The osteochondroses that affect nonarticular cartilage (traction apophysitis) may be related to mechanical disruption of the endochondral mechanism from longitudinally directed shear forces along tendonous or ligamentous attachments.

Clinical Features.

The clinical features of the different osteochondroses vary and are largely dependent on the joint that is affected and the stage of the disease. Early in the disease process, there might only be mild pain and a small effusion. The joint may move through a full range of motion. This is typical of a lesion in the elbow (Panner disease), which may be seen incidentally on a radiograph. On the other hand, long-standing osteochondroses of the proximal tibia (Blount disease) may lead to obvious varus alignment of the lower limb and significant pain.

Radiographic Features.

The radiologic features are characteristic for each anatomic site; however, they all share certain general features as the lesion goes through its stages of maturation. Initially, there is an arrest in ossification of the involved epiphysis, so it will often appear smaller on plain radiographs. During the revascularization phase, there is bony resorption that can resemble cystic type lesions in the subchondral bone. The reossification phase follows and the result can be either a normal looking epiphysis or one with an altered shape. This reossification phase is usually complete by skeletal maturity. Delay in complete revascularization of a fragmented necrotic centrum may result in separation of a nonunited segment, as in osteochondritis dissecans. Some of these radiologic features, however, are seen in different anatomical sites during normal growth. A fragmented calcaneal apophysis or tibial tubercle is a common finding on radiographs of a young adolescent but does not mean they have osteochondritis. Siffert preferred to call the osteochondroses a "syndrome" rather than a disease, implying that there need to be clinical features consistent with the radiologic findings (339).

Histopathology.

There has been very little pathologic material analyzed from humans as it is rarely necessary to operate on most of these patients. What has been analyzed has shown changes of segmental or focal necrosis, revascularization, granulation tissue invasion, osteoclast resorption of necrotic material, and reparative osteogenesis (339). The pathologic sequence of soft-tissue change, irregularity (necrosis) of the epiphysis, and repair can take as long as 6 years; however, the patient may only experience symptoms for a fraction of this time (349). Interestingly, the subchondral bone in some excised lesions of osteochondritis dissecans of the knee revealed viable bone rather than necrotic fragments (350).

Treatment Recommendations. The natural history for most of the osteochondroses is that they are self-limiting (350–352). Knowing this, it is important to help the child symptomatically and educate them and their family of the usually favorable outcome. Initially, the treatment involves rest, ice, stretching, simple analgesics, and anti-inflammatories. Immobilization is rarely required; however, it can be useful for short periods of time to completely rest the joint or apophysis. With time the child can be encouraged back into some sports with pain being the main factor that will determine their participation. Unfortunately, this condition can remain symptomatic for 12 to 18 months, so a lot of reassurance needs to be given to the patient and family that the "syndrome" will eventually resolve. Surgery is occasionally required in Blount disease to realign a severely varus tibia and in osteochondritis dissecans of the knee or ankle to remove or repair a loose body.

Infantile Quadriceps Fibrosis.
Infantile quadriceps fibrosis is a condition where there is progressive fibrosis and contracture of the extensor mechanism of the knee with resulting limitation of flexion and associated lateral patella dislocation.

The condition can be present at birth but usually occurs in the first few years of life. There have been a number of names used for the same condition including *congenital fibrosis* and *progressive fibrosis of quadriceps*. It is important not to confuse this condition with congenital dislocation of the knee or patella that has quadriceps contractures as a secondary phenomenon rather than the primary cause of the deformity (353–355).

Etiology. Many theories exist as to the cause of this progressive fibrosis in the quadriceps mechanism including a congenital muscular dysplasia, a "torticollis type" lesion similar to that seen in the sternocleidomastoid, localized arthrogryposis, and repeated intramuscular injections (353, 356, 357). Gunn was the first to publish on the role of intramuscular injections in causing this fibrosis in 1964 (357). Others have confirmed his findings that repeated injections of sufficient volume of "noxious" agents into the lateral quadriceps of an infant can damage the muscle sufficiently with resulting fibrosis (345, 358–361).

Pathology. Histologic examination of the muscle tissue reveals an excess of adipose and fibrous tissue both within and between the muscle fibers (356). The vastus intermedius is the most commonly affected muscle followed by the vastus lateralis and rectus femoris (353, 356, 357). The middle and distal muscle fibers are more affected than the proximal muscle. Changes in the iliotibial tract are probably secondary to the quadriceps fibrosis and resulting contracture rather than due to any direct injury or congenital malformation.

Clinical Features. The characteristic clinical findings are quadriceps muscle atrophy, genu valgum, patella alta, and limitation of knee flexion (353, 354, 357). The skin can be adherent to the underlying muscle where the injections have

been inserted. This sometimes results in a small dimple that is made more prominent with flexion of the knee. The child can present in one of four different ways: (a) a stiff hyperextended knee at birth, (b) progressive loss of knee flexion in infancy, (c) habitual dislocation of the patella in childhood, and (d) a painful knee in adolescence secondary to the above factors (362). The extension contracture and range of motion varies between affected children. When the examiner or patient dislocates the patella laterally, further knee flexion is possible (357). The condition is more common in girls than boys. There is usually a history of repeated injections into the thigh during infancy for prolonged illness (339, 348, 357).

Treatment Recommendations. Nonoperative management with PT, manipulation, and splinting is usually tried initially with this condition but is rarely successful in preventing surgery (353, 363). A number of surgical approaches have been used to address the fibrotic quadriceps muscle once conservative management has failed. In younger children, a proximal quadriceps release through a small subtrochanteric incision can be successful (345). Sasaki et al. operated on 65 patients with 3 different soft-tissue releases and found the best results occurred when the area of fibrosis was released (364). The iliotibial band is usually tight and needs to be released or lengthened at the same time. In older children, with more severe deformity, a distal lengthening of the quadriceps muscle is required with a V–Y plasty, and a lateral release of the tight retinacular fibers (353, 354, 357, 362). This distal release often results in an extensor lag that improves with time; however, full extension may not return in some children. In untreated adolescent children with progressive quadriceps fibrosis, secondary skeletal changes including genu valgum, irreducible patella dislocation, and extension of the distal femur may occur. In these cases, soft-tissue rebalancing alone may not be sufficient to correct the deformity and corrective osteotomies will need to be performed.

Complex Regional Pain Syndrome.
This syndrome previously known by a variety of names including reflex sympathetic dystrophy (RSD), causalgia, and Sudeck atrophy is a devastating painful disorder that can occur following operative or nonoperative management of an injury in an adult or child. Complex regional pain syndrome (CRPS) type 1 is diagnosed when there is severe pain present out of proportion to the severity of the injury. The pain is difficult to control even with oral narcotics. Light touch will often stimulate an unusual pain response accompanied by allodynia. The limb clinically demonstrates the signs of autonomic dysfunction including edema. CRPS type 2 has similar symptoms and signs to the above; however, there is a known peripheral nerve injury. Although CRPS type 1 was initially thought to be rare in children, the condition is now being increasingly recognized (365, 366).

Clinical Features. CRPS occurs most commonly in girls with the incidence peaking at or just before puberty (367). The condition is also more common in white children (366, 368).

The pain that the child experiences is usually severe and of longer duration than one would expect in the clinical context of the injury. The distribution of the pain is also variable and often not localized and in extreme cases may involve the whole limb. Associated with the chronic pain is a dysfunction of the autonomic nervous system. On examination of the limb, there will be mottling of the skin, altered skin temperature, hyperhydrosis, and altered hair and nail growth. Dietz et al. reviewed 80 patients with CRPS and described a sign of autonomic dysfunction they called *tache cerebrale*. This sign is an erythematous line that develops 10 to 15 seconds after stroking the skin with a blunt object and may last for 10 to 15 minutes. It was present in all their patients (369). Edema of the limb can occur early in the process. Through disuse of the limb muscle will atrophy. Chronic trophic changes are not as common in children as adults. Bernstein et al. reported no patients with trophic changes whereas Wilder et al. reported a 15% incidence (366, 368). There is a marked preponderance of lower extremity cases in children compared to adults (367). Wilder et al. reviewed 70 children (average age 12.5 years) with RSD and 87% had injuries to the lower limb. Eighty-four percent of their patients were girls and on average the time from injury to a diagnosis of RSD had taken 12 months to make (366). Despite multidisciplinary treatments, 54% of patients still had persistent symptoms of RSD at 3 years after diagnosis. They emphasized that CRPS has a different disease course in children when compared with adults and needs to be treated appropriately.

Plain radiographs can be normal or they can demonstrate progressive osteopenia (369). Radioisotope bone scans and MRI have been used in an attempt to help make the diagnosis of CRPS. Bone scans can have variable uptake at different stages of the disease process that do not necessarily correlate with the child's symptoms (369, 370). The sensitivity and specificity therefore are not good enough to advocate the routine use of bone scans to diagnose CRPS (370, 371). MRI scans can show bone and soft-tissue changes in CRPS. Edema can be present in the bone marrow early in the disease process but is rarely seen in the dystrophic phase (372). Occult fractures not seen on plain radiographs can also be picked up on MRI. Soft-tissue changes seen on MRI are variable but include skin thickening or thinning, edema, muscle atrophy, joint effusions, and synovial thickening (372, 373). Although the diagnosis of CRPS is usually made clinically, the different radiology modalities can be useful in looking for underlying pathologies that can be causing the pain. Often a negative finding is reassuring for the patient and their family and may help them psychologically to deal with their painful condition.

Treatment Recommendations   Most tertiary children's hospitals now have multidisciplinary pain teams that treat CRPS. These comprise a physician (anesthetist or pediatrician), a psychiatrist or clinical psychologist, physiotherapists, and sometimes an occupational therapist. The child initially undergoes a multidisciplinary assessment that involves both the schooling and social circumstances. The physiotherapist carries out a thorough functional assessment. It used to be thought that the child with CRPS had a psychological profile that predisposed them to developing this condition; however, the literature does not support this. The child may be undergoing a "stressful" time in their life or be an "overachiever"; however, the profile of these children is really no different to others of similar age without CRPS (374–376). Although psychological therapy has been successful for treating CRPS in some case reports, it is not the primary treatment for this condition (366, 377, 378).

The goal of treatment is to reduce the pain and improve function. Therefore, extensive PT is performed initially as a number of studies have found that PT alone can cure a high percentage of children with CRPS (376, 379, 380). The length and intensity of treatment is not well defined; however, a recent randomized prospective study by Lee et al. found no significant difference between once-weekly or three-times-weekly outpatient PT (377). Analgesics often need to be used to facilitate PT and include antinflammatories, antidepressants (amitriptyline), steroids, and anticonvulsants (gabapentin) (381–383). These medications need to be monitored closely to avoid unwanted side effects. TENS machines have also been used to help with pain relief; however, their efficacy has not been proven in a prospective study (367). Occasionally, in severe cases, regional blocks need to be used to control the pain (366). These sympathetic blocks help define the pain that is sympathetically mediated but do not cure the condition or contribute to making the diagnosis of CRPS. These regional blocks can be used in severe cases of CRPS to enable PT to be carried out when simple analgesics have not been effective. The child is admitted to the hospital or rehabilitation center and an indwelling catheter is inserted under sedation or general anesthetic. A combination of opioids, clonidine, and local anesthetic can be infused to achieve the appropriate sensory and motor block that will allow adequate pain relief but still allow the child to participate with inpatient PT (366, 377, 384). Children appear to respond to PT better than adults and they require less medication and fewer invasive procedures. On the other hand, the recurrence rate of CRPS is higher in children; however, they respond well to the reinitiation of treatment (367, 376, 377, 385). Occasionally, the patient will require inpatient care. During this time, the child's behavior can be observed over prolonged periods and intensive functional therapy can be instituted.

REFERENCES

1. Mulliken JB, Glowacki J. Hemangiomas and vascular malformations in infants and children: a classification based on endothelial characteristics. *Plast Reconstr Surg* 1982;69(3):412–422.
2. Browllard P, Vikkula M. Vascular malformations: localised defects in vascular morphogenesis. *Clin Genet* 2003;63(5) May:340–351.
3. Enjolras O, Chapot R, et al. Vascular anomalies and the growth of limbs: a review. *J Pediatr Orthop B* 2004;13(6):349–357.

4. Enjolras O, Mulliken JB. Vascular tumors and vascular malformations. *Adv Dermatol* 1998;13:375–422.

5. Jones EW, Orkin M. Tufted angioma (angioblastoma). A benign progressive angioma, not to be confused with Kaposi's sarcoma or low-grade angiosarcoma. *J Am Acad Dermatol* 1989;20(2 Pt 1):214–225.

6. Bischoff J. Monoclonal expansion of endothelial cells in hemangioma: an intrinsic defect with extrinsic consequences? *Trends Cardiovasc Med* 2002;12(5):220–224.

7. Chapas AM, Geronemus RG. Our approach to pediatric dermatologic laser surgery. *Lasers Surg Med* 2005;37(4):255–263.

8. Fishman SJ, Mulliken JB. Vascular anomalies. A primer for pediatricians. *Pediatr Clin North Am* 1998;45(6):1455–1477.

9. Huikeshoven M, Koster PH, et al. Redarkening of port-wine stains 10 years after pulsed-dye-laser treatment. *N Engl J Med* 2007;356(12):1235–1240.

10. Cohen MM Jr. Vascular update: morphogenesis, tumors, malformations, and molecular dimensions. *Am J Med Genet A* 2006;140(19):2013–2038.

11. Marchuk DA, Srinivasan S, et al. Vascular morphogenesis: tales of two syndromes. *Hum Mol Genet* 2003;12(Spec No. 1): R97–R112.

12. Stier MF, Glick SA, et al. Laser treatment of pediatric vascular lesions: port wine stains and hemangiomas. *J Am Acad Dermatol* 2008;58(2):261–285.

13. Enjolras O, Logeart I, et al. Arteriovenous malformations: a study of 200 cases. *Ann Dermatol Venereol* 2000;127(1):17–22.

14. Klippel M, Trenaunay P. Du naevus variquex osteohypertrophique. *Arch Gen Med* 1993;185:641.

15. Parkes-Weber F. Haemangiectac hypertrophy of limbs—congenital phlebactenectasis and so-called congenital varicose veins *Br J Child Dis* 1918;15:13.

16. Lindenauer SM. The Klippel-Trenaunay syndrome: varicosity, hypertrophy and hemangioma with no arteriovenous fistula. *Ann Surg* 1965;162:303–314.

17. Baskerville PA, Ackroyd JS, et al. The etiology of the Klippel-Trenaunay syndrome. *Ann Surg* 1985a;202(5):624–627.

18. Baskerville PA, Ackroyd JS, et al. The Klippel-Trenaunay syndrome: clinical, radiological and haemodynamic features and management. *Br J Surg* 1985b;72(3):232–236.

19. Berry SA, Peterson C, et al. Klippel-Trenaunay syndrome. *Am J Med Genet* 1998;79(4):319–326.

20. Lie JT. Pathology of angiodysplasia in Klippel-Trenaunay syndrome. *Pathol Res Pract* 1988;183(6):747–755.

21. Tian J, Gong H, et al. Accurate multiplex gene synthesis from programmable DNA microchips. *Nature* 2004;432(7020):1050–1054.

22. Whelan AJ, Watson MS, et al. Klippel-Trenaunay-Weber syndrome associated with a 5:11 balanced translocation. *Am J Med Genet* 1995;59(4):492–494.

23. Greene AK, Kieran M, et al. Wilms tumor screening is unnecessary in Klippel-Trenaunay syndrome. *Pediatrics* 2004;113(4): e326–e329.

24. Kundu RV, Frieden IJ. Presence of vascular anomalies with congenital hemihypertrophy and Wilms tumor: an evidence-based evaluation. *Pediatr Dermatol* 2003;20(3):199–206.

25. Servelle M, Bastin R, et al. Hematuria and rectal bleeding in the child with Klippel and Trenaunay syndrome. *Ann Surg* 1976;183(4):418–428.

26. Jacob AG, Driscoll DJ, et al. Klippel-Trenaunay syndrome: spectrum and management. *Mayo Clin Proc* 1998;73(1):28–36.

27. Moor JT, Warren FH, et al. Klippel-Trenaunay syndrome: rarely a surgical disease. *South Med J* 1988;81(1):83–85.

28. Goldberg M. *Hemangioma syndromes. The dysmorphic child.* New York, NY: Raven Press, 1987.

29. Furness PD III, Barqawi AZ, et al. Klippel-Trenaunay syndrome: 2 case reports and a review of genitourinary manifestations. *J Urol* 2001;166(4):1418–1420.

30. Wilson CL, Song LM, et al. Bleeding from cavernous angiomatosis of the rectum in Klippel-Trenaunay syndrome: report of three cases and literature review. *Am J Gastroenterol* 2001;96(9):2783–2788.

31. D'Costa H, Hunter JD, et al. Magnetic resonance imaging in macromelia and macrodactyly. *Br J Radiol* 1996;69(822):502–507.

32. Oyesiku NM, Gahm NH, et al. Cerebral arteriovenous fistula in the Klippel-Trenaunay-Weber syndrome. *Dev Med Child Neurol* 1988; 30(2):245–248.

33. Arai Y, Takagi T, et al. Myelopathy due to scoliosis with vertebral hypertrophy in Klippel-Trenaunay-Weber syndrome. *Arch Orthop Trauma Surg* 2002;122(2):120–122.

34. Van Allen MI, Siegel-Bartelt J, et al. Constriction bands and limb reduction defects in two newborns with fetal ultrasound evidence for vascular disruption. *Am J Med Genet* 1992;44(5):598–604.

35. Letts RM. Orthopaedic treatment of hemangiomatous hypertrophy of the lower extremity. *J Bone Joint Surg Am* 1977;59(6):777–783.

36. Lindenauer SM. Congenital arteriovenous fistula and the Klippel-Trenaunay syndrome. *Ann Surg* 1971;174(2):248–263.

37. McCullough CJ, Kenwright J. The prognosis in congenital lower limb hypertrophy. *Acta Orthop Scand* 1979;50(3):307–313.

38. Peixinho M, Arakaki T, et al. Correction of leg inequality in the Klippel-Trenaunay-Weber syndrome. *Int Orthop* 1982;6(1):45–47.

39. Bircher AJ, Koo JY, et al. Angiodysplastic syndrome with capillary and venous malformation associated with soft tissue hypotrophy. *Dermatology* 1994;189(3):292–296.

40. Troost BT, Savino PJ, et al. Tuberous sclerosis and Klippel-Trenaunay-Weber syndromes. Association of two complete phakomatoses in a single individual. *J Neurol Neurosurg Psychiatry* 1975;38(5):500–504.

41. Laor T, Hoffer FA, et al. MR lymphangiography in infants, children, and young adults. *AJR Am J Roentgenol* 1998;171(4):1111–1117.

42. Mandell GA, Alexander MA, et al. A multiscintigraphic approach to imaging of lymphedema and other causes of the congenitally enlarged extremity. *Semin Nucl Med* 1993;23(4):334–346.

43. McCarthy RE, Lytle JO, et al. The use of total circulatory arrest in the surgery of giant hemangioma and Klippel-Trenaunay syndrome in neonates. *Clin Orthop Relat Res* 1993;289:237–242.

44. Bastarrika G, Redondo P, et al. New techniques for the evaluation and therapeutic planning of patients with Klippel-Trenaunay syndrome. *J Am Acad Dermatol* 2007;56(2):242–249.

45. Yousem DM, Scott WW Jr, et al. Case report 440: Klippel-Trenaunay syndrome of right lower extremity. *Skeletal Radiol* 1987;16(8):652–656.

46. Stringel G, Dastous J. Klippel-Trenaunay syndrome and other cases of lower limb hypertrophy: pediatric surgical implications. *J Pediatr Surg* 1987;22(7):645–650.

47. Gates PE, Drvaric DM, et al. Wound healing in orthopaedic procedures for Klippel-Trenaunay syndrome. *J Pediatr Orthop* 1996;16(6):723–726.

48. Guidera KJ, Brinker MR, et al. Overgrowth management in Klippel-Trenaunay-Weber and Proteus syndromes. *J Pediatr Orthop* 1993;13(4):459–466.

49. Joyce PF, Sundaram M, et al. Embolization of extensive peripheral angiodysplasias. The alternative to radical surgery. *Arch Surg* 1980;115(5):665–668.

50. Stanley RJ, Cubillo E. Nonsurgical treatment of arteriovenous malformations of the trunk and limb by transcatheter arterial embolization. *Radiology* 1975;115(3):609–612.

51. Letts M, Pang E, et al. Parosteal fasciitis in children. *Am J Orthop* 1995;24(2):119–127.

52. Wiedemann H. Tumors and hemihypertrophy associated with Wiedemann-Beckwith syndrome. *Eur J Pediatr* 1983;141:129.

53. Biesecker LG, Peters KF, et al. Clinical differentiation between Proteus syndrome and hemihyperplasia: description of a distinct form of hemihyperplasia. *Am J Med Genet* 1998;79(4):311–318.

54. Aylsworth CF. Effects of lipids on gap junctionally-mediated intercellular communication: possible role in the promotion of tumorigenesis by dietary fat. *Prog Clin Biol Res* 1986;222:607–622.

55. Happle R. Lethal genes surviving by mosaicism: a possible explanation for sporadic birth defects involving the skin. *J Am Acad Dermatol* 1987;16(4):899–906.

56. Sakuntabhai A, Dhitavat J, et al. Mosaicism for ATP2A2 mutations causes segmental Darier's disease. *J Invest Dermatol* 2000;115(6):1144–1147.

57. Eng C. PTEN: one gene, many syndromes. *Hum Mutat* 2003;22(3):183–198.

58. Zhou XP, Marsh DJ, et al. Germline and germline mosaic PTEN mutations associated with a Proteus-like syndrome of hemihypertrophy, lower

limb asymmetry, arteriovenous malformations and lipomatosis. *Hum Mol Genet* 2000;9(5):765–768.

59. Goodship J, Redfearn A, et al. Transmission of Proteus syndrome from father to son? *J Med Genet* 1991;28(11):781–785.

60. Biesecker LG, Happle R, et al. Proteus syndrome: diagnostic criteria, differential diagnosis, and patient evaluation. *Am J Med Genet* 1999; 84(5):389–395.

61. Jamis-Dow CA, Turner J, et al. Radiologic manifestations of Proteus syndrome. *Radiographics* 2004;24(4):1051–1068.

62. Hoey SE, Eastwood D, et al. Histopathological features of Proteus syndrome. *Clin Exp Dermatol* 2008;33(3):234–238.

63. Twede JV, Turner JT, et al. Evolution of skin lesions in Proteus syndrome. *J Am Acad Dermatol* 2005;52(5):834–838.

64. Nguyen D, Turner JT, et al. Cutaneous manifestations of proteus syndrome: correlations with general clinical severity. *Arch Dermatol* 2004;140(8):947–953.

65. Hoeger PH, Martinez A, et al. Vascular anomalies in Proteus syndrome. *Clin Exp Dermatol* 2004;29(3):222–230.

66. Demetriades D, Hager J, et al. Proteus syndrome: musculoskeletal manifestations and management: a report of two cases. *J Pediatr Orthop* 1992;12(1):106–113.

67. Stricker S. Musculoskeletal manifestations of Proteus syndrome: report of two cases with literature review. *J Pediatr Orthop* 1992;12(5):667–674.

68. Samlaska CP, Levin SW, et al. Proteus syndrome. *Arch Dermatol* 1989;125(8):1109–1014.

69. Wiedemann HR, Burgio GR, et al. The proteus syndrome. Partial gigantism of the hands and/or feet, nevi, hemihypertrophy, subcutaneous tumors, macrocephaly or other skull anomalies and possible accelerated growth and visceral affections. *Eur J Pediatr* 1983;140(1):5–12.

70. Ring D, Snyder B. Spinal canal compromise in Proteus syndrome: case report and review of the literature. *Am J Orthop* 1997;26(4):275–278.

71. Skovby F, Graham JM Jr, et al. Compromise of the spinal canal in Proteus syndrome. *Am J Med Genet* 1993;47(5):656–659.

72. Takebayashi T, Yamashita T, et al. Scoliosis in Proteus syndrome: case report. *Spine* 2001;26(17): E395–E398.

73. Whitley JM, Flannery AM. Lymphangiolipoma of the thoracic spine in a pediatric patient with Proteus syndrome. *Childs Nerv Syst* 1996;12(4):224–227.

74. Dietrich RB, Glidden DE, et al. The Proteus syndrome: CNS manifestations. *AJNR Am J Neuroradiol* 1998;19(5):987–990.

75. Sheard RM, Pope FM, et al. A novel ophthalmic presentation of the Proteus syndrome. *Ophthalmology* 2002;109(6):1192–1195.

76. Cohen RB, Hahn GV, et al. The natural history of heterotopic ossification in patients who have fibrodysplasia ossificans progressiva. A study of forty-four patients. *J Bone Joint Surg Am* 1993;75(2):215–219.

77. Gordon PL, Wilroy RS, et al. Neoplasms in Proteus syndrome. *Am J Med Genet* 1995;57(1):74–78.

78. Eberhard DA. Two-year-old boy with Proteus syndrome and fatal pulmonary thromboembolism. *Pediatr Pathol* 1994;14(5):771–779.

79. Newman B, Urbach AH, et al. Proteus syndrome: emphasis on the pulmonary manifestations. *Pediatr Radiol* 1994;24(3):189–193.

80. Lublin M, Schwartzentruber DJ, et al. Principles for the surgical management of patients with Proteus syndrome and patients with overgrowth not meeting Proteus criteria. *J Pediatr Surg* 2002;37(7):1013–1020.

81. Gorham LW, Stout AP. Massive osteolysis (acute spontaneous absorption of bone, phantom bone, disappearing bone); its relation to hemangiomatosis. *J Bone Joint Surg Am* 1955;37-A(5):985–1004.

82. Gorham LW. Circulatory changes associated with osteolytic and osteoblastic reactions in bone. The possible mechanism involved in massive osteolysis an experimental study. *Arch Intern Med* 1960;105:199–216.

83. Abrahams J, Ganick D, et al. Massive osteolysis in an infant. *AJR Am J Roentgenol* 1980;135(5):1084–1086.

84. Bullough PG. Massive osteolysis. *N Y State J Med* 1971;71(19): 2267–2278.

85. Ross JL, Schinella R, et al. Massive osteolysis. An unusual cause of bone destruction. *Am J Med* 1978;65(2):367–372.

86. Aoki M, Kato F, et al. Successful treatment of chylothorax by bleomycin for Gorham's disease. *Clin Orthop Relat Res* 1996;330:193–197.

87. Heyden G, Kindblom LG, et al. Disappearing bone disease. A clinical and histological study. *J Bone Joint Surg Am* 1977;59(1):57–61.

88. Mendez AA, Keret D, et al. Massive osteolysis of the femur (Gorham's disease): a case report and review of the literature. *J Pediatr Orthop* 1989;9(5):604–608.

89. Shives TC, Beabout JW, et al. Massive osteolysis. *Clin Orthop Relat Res* 1993;294:267–276.

90. Miller GG. Treatment of chylothorax in Gorham's disease: case report and literature review. *Can J Surg* 2002;45(5):381–382.

91. Hambach R, Pujman J, et al. Massive osteolysis due to hemangiomatosis; report of a case of Gorham's disease with autopsy. *Radiology* 1958;71(1):43–47.

92. Enneking WF. *Musculoskeletal tumour surgery.* New York, NY: Churchill Livingstone; 1983:105.

93. Fornasier VL. Haemangiomatosis with massive osteolysis. *J Bone Joint Surg Br* 1970;52(3):444–451.

94. Macpherson RI, Reed MH, et al. Intrathoracic gastrogenic cysts: a cause of lethal pulmonary hemorrhage in infants. *J Can Assoc Radiol* 1973;24(4):362–369.

95. Torg JS, DiGeorge AM, et al. Hereditary multicentric osteolysis with recessive transmission: a new syndrome. *J Pediatr* 1969;75(2):243–252.

96. Johnson PM, McClure CJ. Observations on massive osteolysis; a review of the literature and report of a case. *Radiology* 1958;71(1):28–42.

97. Sage MR, Allen PW. Massive osteolysis. Report of a case. *J Bone Joint Surg Br* 1974;56(1):130–135.

98. Remia LF, Richolt J, et al. Pain and weakness of the shoulder in a 16-year-old boy. *Clin Orthop Relat Res* 1998;347:268–271, 287–290.

99. Yoo SY, Hong SH, et al. MRI of Gorham's disease: findings in two cases. *Skeletal Radiol* 2002;31(5):301–306.

100. Singh R, Grewal DS, et al. Haemangiomatosis of the skeleton. Report of a case. *J Bone Joint Surg Br* 1974;56(1):136–138.

101. Joseph J, Bartal E. Disappearing bone disease: a case report and review of the literature. *J Pediatr Orthop* 1987;7(5):584–588.

102. Gorham LW, Wright AW, et al. Disappearing bones: a rare form of massive osteolysis; report of two cases, one with autopsy findings. *Am J Med* 1954;17(5):674–682.

103. Milner SM, Baker SL. Disappearing bones. *J Bone Joint Surg Br* 1958;40-B(3):502–513.

104. Woodward HR, Chan DP, et al. Massive osteolysis of the cervical spine. A case report of bone graft failure. *Spine (Phila Pa 1976)* 1981;6(6):545–549.

105. Gutierrez RM, Spjut HJ. Skeletal angiomatosis: report of three cases and review of the literature. *Clin Orthop Relat Res* 1972;85:82–97.

106. Bonucci E. New knowledge on the origin, function and fate of osteoclasts. *Clin Orthop Relat Res* 1981;158:252–269.

107. Devlin RD, Bone HG III, et al. Interleukin-6: a potential mediator of the massive osteolysis in patients with Gorham-Stout disease. *J Clin Endocrinol Metab* 1996;81(5):1893–1897.

108. Hirayama T, Sabokbar A, et al. Cellular and humoral mechanisms of osteoclast formation and bone resorption in Gorham-Stout disease. *J Pathol* 2001;195(5):624–630.

109. Koblenzer PJ, Bukowski MJ. Angiomatosis (hamartomatous hemlymphangiomatosis). Report of a case with diffuse involvement. *Pediatrics* 1961;28:65–76.

110. Aston JN. A case of massive osteolysis of the femur. *J Bone Joint Surg Br* 1958;40-B(3):514–518.

111. Halliday DR, Dahlin DC, et al. Massive osteolysis and angiomatosis. *Radiology* 1964;82:637–644.

112. Picault C, Comtet J, et al. Surgical repair of the extensive idiopathic osteolysis of the pelvic girdle. *J Bone Joint Surg [Br]* 1968;50-B:158–159.

113. Shafritz AB, Shore EM, et al. Overexpression of an osteogenic morphogen in fibrodysplasia ossificans progressiva. *N Engl J Med* 1996;335(8): 555–561.

114. Sato K, Sugiura H, et al. Gorham massive osteolysis. *Arch Orthop Trauma Surg* 1997;116(8):510–513.

115. Mendez AA, Keret D, et al. Isolated dysplasia epiphysealis hemimelica of the hip joint. A case report. *J Bone Joint Surg Am* 1988;70(6): 921–925.

116. Watkins RGt, Reynolds RA, et al. Lymphangiomatosis of the spine: two cases requiring surgical intervention. *Spine* 2003;28(3):E45–E50.

117. Choma ND, Biscotti CV, et al. Gorham's syndrome: a case report and review of the literature. *Am J Med* 1987;83(6):1151–1156.

118. Edwards WH Jr, Thompson RC Jr, et al. Lymphangiomatosis and massive osteolysis of the cervical spine. A case report and review of the literature. *Clin Orthop Relat Res* 1983;177:222–229.

119. Dunbar SF, Rosenberg A, et al. Gorham's massive osteolysis: the role of radiation therapy and a review of the literature. *Int J Radiat Oncol Biol Phys* 1993;26(3):491–497.

120. McNeil KD, Fong KM, et al. Gorham's syndrome: a usually fatal cause of pleural effusion treated successfully with radiotherapy. *Thorax* 1996;51(12):1275–1276.

121. Ballock RT, Wiesner GL, et al. Hemihypertrophy. Concepts and controversies. *J Bone Joint Surg Am* 1997;79(11):1731–1738.

122. Ward J, Lerner HH. A review of the subject of congenital hemihypertrophyand a complete case report. *J Pediatr* 1947;31(4):403–414.

123. Beals RK. Hemihypertrophy and hemihypotrophy. *Clin Orthop Relat Res* 1982;166:199–203.

124. MacEwen GD, Case JL. Congenital hemihypertrophy. A review of 32 cases. *Clin Orthop Relat Res* 1967;50:147–150.

125. Ringrose RE, Jabbour JT, et al. Hemihypertrophy. *Pediatrics* 1965; 36(3):434–448.

126. Sotelo-Avila C, Gooch WM III. Neoplasms associated with the Beckwith-Wiedemann syndrome. *Perspect Pediatr Pathol* 1976;3: 255–272.

127. Pappas AM, Nehme AM. Leg length discrepancy associated with hypertrophy. *Clin Orthop Relat Res* 1979;144:198–211.

128. Rush WA, Steiner HA. A study of lower extremity length. *AJR Am J Roentgrnol* 1946;56:616–623.

129. Viljoen D, Pearn J, et al. Manifestations and natural history of idiopathic hemihypertrophy: a review of eleven cases. *Clin Genet* 1984;26(2): 81–86.

130. Nudleman K, Andermann E, et al. The hemi 3 syndrome. Hemihypertrophy, hemihypaesthesia, hemiareflexia and scoliosis. *Brain* 1984; 107 (Pt 2):533–546.

131. Cavaliere RG, McElgun TM. Macrodactyly and hemihypertrophy: a new surgical procedure. *J Foot Surg* 1988;27(3):226–235.

132. Harris RE, Fuchs EF, et al. Medullary sponge kidney and congenital hemihypertrophy: case report and literature review. *J Urol* 1981;126(5):676–678.

133. Hoyme HE, Seaver LH, et al. Isolated hemihyperplasia (hemihypertrophy): report of a prospective multicenter study of the incidence of neoplasia and review. *Am J Med Genet* 1998;79(4):274–278.

134. Fraumeni JF Jr, Miller RW. Adrenocortical neoplasms with hemihypertrophy, brain tumors, and other disorders. *J Pediatr* 1967;70(1):129–138.

135. Fraumeni JF Jr, Miller RW, et al. Primary carcinoma of the liver in childhood: an epidemiologic study. *J Natl Cancer Inst* 1968;40(5): 1087–1099.

136. Parker DA, Skalko RG. Congenital asymmetry: report of 10 cases with associated developmental abnormalities. *Pediatrics* 1969;44(4):584–589.

137. Parker L, Kollin J, et al. Hemihypertrophy as possible sign of renal cell carcinoma. *Urology* 1992;40(3):286–288.

138. Miller RW, Fraumeni JF Jr, et al. Association of Wilms's tumor with aniridia, hemihypertrophy and other congenital malformations. *N Engl J Med* 1964;270:922–927.

139. Pendergrass TW. Congenital anomalies in children with Wilms' tumor: a new survey. *Cancer* 1976;37(1):403–408.

140. Green DM, Breslow NE, et al. Screening of children with hemihypertrophy, aniridia, and Beckwith-Wiedemann syndrome in patients with Wilms tumor: a report from the National Wilms Tumor Study. *Med Pediatr Oncol* 1993;21(3):188–192.

141. Janik JS, Seeler RA. Delayed onset of hemihypertrophy in Wilms' tumor. *J Pediatr Surg* 1976;11(4):581–582.

142. Clericuzio CL, Johnson C. Screening for Wilms tumor in high-risk individuals. *Hematol Oncol Clin North Am* 1995;9(6):1253–1265.

143. Finch GD, Dawe CJ. Hemiatrophy. *J Pediatr Orthop* 2003;23(1):99–101.

144. Phelan EM, Carty HM, et al. Generalised enchondromatosis associated with haemangiomas, soft-tissue calcifications and hemihypertrophy. *Br J Radiol* 1986;59(697):69–74.

145. Shapiro F. Developmental patterns in lower-extremity length discrepancies. *J Bone Joint Surg Am* 1982;64(5):639–651.

146. Bhat AK, Bhaskaranand K, et al. Bilateral macrodactyl of the hands and feet with post-axial involvement—a case report. *J Hand Surg [Br]* 2005;30(6):618–620.

147. Wood V. Macrodactyly. In: Green DM, Hotchkiss R, Pederson W, eds. *Operative hand surgery*, Vol 1. Philadelphia, PA: Churchill Livingstone. 1999:533–544.

148. Ackland MK, Uhthoff HK. Idiopathic localized gigantism: a 26-year follow-up. *J Pediatr Orthop* 1986;6(5):618–621.

149. Dennyson WG, Bear JN, et al. Macrodactyly in the foot. *J Bone Joint Surg Br* 1977;59(3):355–359.

150. Miura H, Uchida Y, et al. Macrodactyly in Proteus syndrome. *J Hand Surg [Br]* 1993;18(3):308–309.

151. Turra S, Santini S, et al. Gigantism of the foot: our experience in seven cases. *J Pediatr Orthop* 1998;18(3):337–345.

152. Barsky AJ. Macrodactyly. *J Bone Joint Surg Am* 1967;49(7):1255–1266.

153. Kalen V, Burwell DS, et al. Macrodactyly of the hands and feet. *J Pediatr Orthop* 1988;8(3):311–315.

154. Stevens P. Toe deformities. In: Drennan J, ed. *The child's foot and ankle*. New York, NY: Raven Press, 1984.

155. Ben-Bassat M, Casper J, et al. Congenital macrodactyly. A case report with a three-year follow-up. *J Bone Joint Surg Br* 1966;48(2):359–364.

156. Herring JA, Tolo VT. Macrodactyly. *J Pediatr Orthop* 1984;4(4): 503–506.

157. Tsuge K. Treatment of macrodactyly. *Plast Reconstr Surg* 1967;39(6): 590–599.

158. Jones KG. Megalodactylism. Case report of a child treated by epiphyseal resection. *J Bone Joint Surg Am* 1963;45:1704–1708.

159. Topoleski TA, Ganel A, et al. Effect of proximal phalangeal epiphysiodesis in the treatment of macrodactyly. *Foot Ankle Int* 1997;18(8): 500–503.

160. Kotwal PP, Farooque M. Macrodactyly. *J Bone Joint Surg Br* 1998; 80(4):651–653.

161. Tan O, Atik B, et al. Middle phalangectomy: a functional and aesthetic cure for macrodactyly. *Scand J Plast Reconstr Surg Hand Surg* 2006;40(6):362–365.

162. Dedrick D, Kling TJ. Ray resection in the treatment of macrodactyl of the foot in children. *Orthop Trans* 1985;9:145.

163. Grogan DP, Bernstein RM, et al. Congenital lipofibromatosis associated with macrodactyly of the foot. *Foot Ankle* 1991;12(1):40–46.

164. Chang CH, Kumar SJ, et al. Macrodactyly of the foot. *J Bone Joint Surg Am* 2002;84-A(7):1189–1194.

165. Askins G, Ger E. Congenital constriction band syndrome. *J Pediatr Orthop* 1988;8(4):461–466.

166. Cowell H, Hensinger R. The relationship of clubfoot to congenital annular bands. In: Bademan JE, ed. *Foot science*. Philadelphia, PA: WB Saunders, 1976.

167. Kino Y. Clinical and experimental studies of the congenital constriction band syndrome, with an emphasis on its etiology. *J Bone Joint Surg Am* 1975;57(5):636–643.

168. Tada K, Yonenobu K, et al. Congenital constriction band syndrome. *J Pediatr Orthop* 1984;4(6):726–730.

169. Moses JM, Flatt AE, et al. Annular constricting bands. *J Bone Joint Surg Am* 1979;61(4):562–565.

170. Patterson TJ. Congenital ring-constrictions. *Br J Plast Surg* 1961;14:1–31.

171. Wiedrich TA. Congenital constriction band syndrome. *Hand Clin* 1998;14(1):29–38.

171a. Gupta ML. Congenital annular defects of the extremities and trunk. *J Bone Joint Surg Am* 1963;45(3):571–622.

172. Coady MS, Moore MH, et al. Amniotic band syndrome: the association between rare facial clefts and limb ring constrictions. *Plast Reconstr Surg* 1998;101(3):640–649.

173. Allington NJ, Kumar SJ, et al. Clubfeet associated with congenital constriction bands of the ipsilateral lower extremity. *J Pediatr Orthop* 1995;15(5):599–603.

174. Hennigan SP, Kuo KN. Resistant talipes equinovarus associated with congenital constriction band syndrome. *J Pediatr Orthop* 2000;20(2):240–245.

175. Gomez VR. Clubfeet in congenital annular constricting bands. *Clin Orthop Relat Res* 1996;323:155–162.

176. Bourne MH, Klassen RA. Congenital annular constricting bands: review of the literature and a case report. *J Pediatr Orthop* 1987;7(2):218–221.

177. Zionts LE, Osterkamp JA, et al. Congenital annular bands in identical twins. A case report. *J Bone Joint Surg Am* 1984;66(3):450–453.

178. Streeter G. Focal deficiencies in fetal tissues and their relation to intra-uterine amputations. *Contrib Embryol Carnegie Inst* 1930;22:1–46.

179. Torpin R. Amniochorionic mesoblastic fibrous strings and amnionic bands: associated constricting fetal malformations or fetal death. *Am J Obstet Gynecol* 1965;91:65–75.

180. Torpin R. *Fetal malformations caused by amnion rupture during gestation.* Springfield, IL: Thomas; 1968.

181. Greene WB. One-stage release of congenital circumferential constriction bands. *J Bone Joint Surg Am* 1993;75(5):650–655.

182. Upton J, Tan C. Correction of constriction rings. *J Hand Surg Am* 1991;16(5):947–953.

183. Chang CH, Huang SC. Clubfoot deformity in congenital constriction band syndrome: manifestations and treatment. *J Formos Med Assoc* 1998;97(5):328–334.

184. Camurati M. Dilulraro caso di osteite simmetrica erditaria degli arti inferriori. *Chir Organi Mov* 1922;6:622.

185. Engelmann G. Osteopathia hyperostotica (sclerotisans) multiplex infantilis. *Fortschritte Rontgenstr* 1929;39:1101.

186. Ghadami M, Makita Y, et al. Genetic mapping of the Camurati-Engelmann disease locus to chromosome 19q13.1–q13.3. *Am J Hum Genet* 2000;66(1):143–147.

187. Janssens K, Gershoni-Baruch R, et al. Localisation of the gene causing diaphyseal dysplasia Camurati-Engelmann to chromosome 19q13. *J Med Genet* 2000;37(4):245–249.

188. Kinoshita A, Saito T, et al. Domain-specific mutations in TGFB1 result in Camurati-Engelmann disease. *Nat Genet* 2000;26(1):19–20.

189. Naveh Y, Kaftori JK, et al. Progressive diaphyseal dysplasia: genetics and clinical and radiologic manifestations. *Pediatrics* 1984;74(3):399–405.

190. Saraiva JM. Progressive diaphyseal dysplasia: a three-generation family with markedly variable expressivity. *Am J Med Genet* 1997;71(3):348–352.

191. Wallace SE, Lachman RS, et al. Marked phenotypic variability in progressive diaphyseal dysplasia (Camurati-Engelmann disease): report of a four-generation pedigree, identification of a mutation in TGFB1, and review. *Am J Med Genet A* 2004;129A(3):235–247.

192. Bondestam J, Mayranpaa MK, et al. Bone biopsy and densitometry findings in a child with Camurati-Engelmann disease. *Clin Rheumatol* 2007;26(10):1773–1777.

193. Hundley JD, Wilson FC. Progressive diaphyseal dysplasia. Review of the literature and report of seven cases in one family. *J Bone Joint Surg Am* 1973;55(3):461–474.

194. Hernandez MV, Peris P, et al. Biochemical markers of bone turnover in Camurati-Engelmann disease: a report on four cases in one family. *Calcif Tissue Int* 1997;61(1):48–51.

195. Clawson DK, Loop JW. Progressive diaphyseal dysplasia (Engelmann's disease). *J Bone Joint Surg Am* 1964;46:143–150.

196. Grey AC, Wallace R, et al. Engelmann's disease: a 45-year follow-up. *J Bone Joint Surg Br* 1996;78(3):488–491.

197. Kaftori JK, Kleinhaus U, et al. Progressive diaphyseal dysplasia (Camurati-Engelmann): radiographic follow-up and CT findings. *Radiology* 1987;164(3):777–782.

198. Greenspan A. Sclerosing bone dysplasias—a target-site approach. *Skeletal Radiol* 1991;20(8):561–583.

199. Norton KI, Wagreich JM et al. Diaphyseal medullary stenosis (sclerosis) with bone malignancy (malignant fibrous histiocytoma): Hardcastle syndrome. *Pediatr Radiol* 1996;26(9):675–677.

200. Bas F, Darendeliler F, et al. Deflazacort treatment in progressive diaphyseal dysplasia (Camurati-Engelmann disease). *J Paediatr Child Health* 1999;35(4):401–405.

201. Heymans O, Gebhart M, et al. Camurati-Engelmann disease. Effects of corticosteroids. *Acta clinica Belgica* 1998;53(3):189–192.

202. Allen DT, Saunders AM, et al. Corticosteroids in the treatment of Engelmann's disease: progressive diaphyseal dysplasia. *Pediatrics* 1970;46(4):523–531.

203. Benli IT, Akalin S, et al. Epidemiological, clinical and radiological aspects of osteopoikilosis. *J Bone Joint Surg Br* 1992;74(4):504–506.

204. Chigira M, Kato K, et al. Symmetry of bone lesions in osteopoikilosis. Report of 4 cases. *Acta Orthop Scand* 1991;62(5):495–496.

205. Lagier R, Mbakop A, et al. Osteopoikilosis: a radiological and pathological study. *Skeletal Radiol* 1984;11(3):161–168.

206. Whyte MP, Murphy WA, et al. 99mTc-pyrophosphate bone imaging in osteopoikilosis, osteopathia striata, and melorheostosis. *Radiology* 1978;127(2):439–443.

207. Grimer RJ, Davies AM, et al. Chondrosarcoma in a patient with osteopoikilosis. Apropos of a case. *Rev Chir Orthop Reparatrice Appar Mot* 1989;75(3):188–190.

208. Mindell ER, Northup CS, et al. Osteosarcoma associated with osteopoikilosis. *J Bone Joint Surg Am* 1978;60(3):406–408.

209. Walpole IR, Manners PJ. Clinical considerations in Buschke-Ollendorff syndrome. *Clin Genet* 1990;37(1):59–63.

210. Butkus CE, Michels VV, et al. Melorheostosis in a patient with familial osteopoikilosis. *Am J Med Genet* 1997;72(1):43–46.

211. Debeer P, Pykels E, et al. Melorheostosis in a family with autosomal dominant osteopoikilosis: report of a third family. *Am J Med Genet A* 2003;119A(2):188–193.

212. Nevin NC, Thomas PS, et al. Melorheostosis in a family with autosomal dominant osteopoikilosis. *Am J Med Genet* 1999;82(5):409–414.

213. Ben-Asher E, Zelzer E, et al. LEMD3: the gene responsible for bone density disorders (osteopoikilosis). *Isr Med Assoc J* 2005;7(4):273–274.

214. Walker GF. Mixed sclerosing bone dystrophies. Two case reports. *J Bone Joint Surg Br* 1964;46:546–552.

215. Leri A, Joanny J. Une affection non décrite des os; hyperostose 'en coulée' sur toute la longueur d'une membre ou 'mélorhéostose'. *Bul Mem Soc Hop Paris* 1922;46:1141–1145.

216. Fryns JP, Pedersen JC, et al. Melorheostosis in a 3-year-old girl. *Acta paediatrica Belgica* 1980;33(3):185–187.

217. Rozencwaig R, Wilson MR, et al. Melorheostosis. *Am J Orthop* 1997;26(2):83–89.

218. Younge D, Drummond D, et al. Melorheostosis in children. Clinical features and natural history. *J Bone Joint Surg Br* 1979;61-B(4):415–418.

219. Campbell CJ, Papademetriou T, et al. Melorheostosis. A report of the clinical, roentgenographic, and pathological findings in fourteen cases. *J Bone Joint Surg Am* 1968;50(7):1281–1304.

220. Ippolito V, Mirra JM, et al. Case report 771: Melorheostosis in association with desmoid tumor. *Skeletal Radiol* 1993;22(4):284–288.

221. Moreno Alvarez MJ, Lazaro MA, et al. Linear scleroderma and melorheostosis: case presentation and literature review. *Clin Rheumatol* 1996;15(4):389–393.

222. Morris JM, Samilson RL, et al. Melorheostosis. Review of the literature and report of an interesting case with a nineteen-year follow-up. *J Bone Joint Surg Am* 1963;45:1191–1206.

223. Kessler HB, Recht MP, et al. Vascular anomalies in association with osteodystrophies—a spectrum. *Skeletal Radiol* 1983;10(2):95–101.

224. Soffa DJ, Sire DJ, et al. Melorheostosis with linear sclerodermatous skin changes. *Radiology* 1975;114(3):577–578.

225. de Goede E, Fagard R, et al. Unique cause of renovascular hypertension: melorheostosis associated with a malformation of the renal arteries. *J Hum Hypertens* 1996;10(1):57–59.

226. Iglesias JH, Stocks AL, et al. Renal artery stenosis associated with melorheostosis. *Pediatr Nephrol* 1994;8(4):441–443.

227. Roger D, Bonnetblanc JM, et al. Melorheostosis with associated minimal change nephrotic syndrome, mesenteric fibromatosis and capillary haemangiomas. *Dermatology* 1994;188(2):166–168.

228. Siegel A, Williams H. Linear scleroderma and melorheostosis. *Br J Radiol* 1992;65(771):266–268.

229. Thompson NM, Allen CE, et al. Scleroderma and melorheostosis; report of a case. *J Bone Joint Surg Br* 1951;33-B(3):430–433.

230. Todesco S, Bedendo A, et al. Melorheostosis and rheumatoid arthritis. *Clin Exp Rheumatol* 1983;1(4):349–352.

231. Baer SC, Ayala AG, et al. Case report 843. Malignant fibrous histiocytoma of the femur arising in melorheostosis. *Skeletal Radiol* 1994;23(4):310–314.

232. Murray RO, McCredie J. Melorheostosis and the sclerotomes: a radiological correlation. *Skeletal Radiol* 1979;4(2):57–71.

233. Kim JE, Kim EH, et al. A TGF-beta-inducible cell adhesion molecule, betaig-h3, is downregulated in melorheostosis and involved in osteogenesis. *J Cell Biochem* 2000;77(2):169–178.

234. Greenspan AE, Azouz M. Bone dysplasia series. Melorheostosis: review and update. *Can Assoc Radiol J* 1999;50(5):324–330.

235. Garver P, Resnick D, et al. Melorheostosis of the axial skeleton with associated fibrolipomatous lesions. *Skeletal Radiol* 1982;9(1):41–44.

236. Spieth ME, Greenspan A, et al. Radionuclide imaging in forme fruste of melorheostosis. *Clin Nucl Med* 1994;19(6):512–515.

237. Osgood GM, Lee FY, et al. Magnetic resonance imaging depiction of tight iliotibial band in melorheostosis associated with severe external rotation deformity, limb shortening and patellar dislocation in planning surgical correction. *Skeletal Radiol* 2002;31(1):49–52.

238. Hoshi K, Amizuka N, et al. Histopathological characterization of melorheostosis. *Orthopedics* 2001;24(3):273–277.

239. Buckley SL, Skinner S, et al. Focal scleroderma in children: an orthopaedic perspective. *J Pediatr Orthop* 1993;13(6):784–790.

240. Atar D, Lehman WB, et al. The Ilizarov apparatus for treatment of melorheostosis. Case report and review of the literature. *Clin Orthop Relat Res* 1992;281:163–167.

241. Choi ML, Wey PD, et al. Pediatric peripheral neuropathy in proteus syndrome. *Annals of plastic surgery* 1998;40(5):528–532.

242. Griffet J, el Hayek T, et al. Melorheostosis: complications of a tibial lengthening with the Ilizarov apparatus. *Eur J Pediatr Surg* 1998;8(3):186–189.

243. Marshall JH, Bradish CF. Callotasis in melorheostosis: a case report. *J Bone Joint Surg* Br 1993;75(1):155.

244. Naudie D, Hamdy RC, et al. Complications of limb-lengthening in children who have an underlying bone disorder. *J Bone Joint Surg Am* 1998;80(1):18–24.

245. Fairbank H. Osteopathia striata *J Bone Joint Surg Br* 1950;32B(1):117–125.

246. Horan FT, Beighton PH. Osteopathia striata with cranial sclerosis. An autosomal dominant entity. *Clin Genet* 1978;13(2):201–206.

247. Schnyder PA. Osseous changes of osteopathia striata associated with cranial sclerosis. An autosomal dominant entity. *Skeletal Radiol* 1980;5(1):19–22.

248. Behninger C, Rott HD. Osteopathia striata with cranial sclerosis: literature reappraisal argues for X-linked inheritance. *Genet Couns* 2000;11(2):157–167.

249. Pellegrino JE, McDonald-McGinn DM, et al. Further clinical delineation and increased morbidity in males with osteopathia striata with cranial sclerosis: an X-linked disorder? *Am J Med Genet* 1997;70(2):159–165.

250. Rott HD, Krieg P, et al. Multiple malformations in a male and maternal osteopathia strata with cranial sclerosis (OSCS). *Genet Couns* 2003;14(3):281–288.

251. Viot G, Lacombe D, et al. Osteopathia striata cranial sclerosis: nonrandom X-inactivation suggestive of X-linked dominant inheritance. *Am J Med Genet* 2002;107(1):1–4.

252. Kondoh T, Yoshinaga M, et al. Severe cervical kyphosis in osteopathia striata with cranial sclerosis: case report. *Pediatr Radiol* 2001;31(9):659–662.

253. Cadilhac C, Fenoll B, et al. Congenital pseudarthrosis of the clavicle: 25 childhood cases. *Rev Chir Orthop Reparatrice Appar Mot* 2000;86(6):575–580.

254. Gibson DA, Carroll N. Congenital pseudarthrosis of the clavicle. *J Bone Joint Surg Br* 1970;52(4):629–643.

255. Lloyd-Roberts GC, Apley AG, et al. Reflections upon the aetiology of congenital pseudarthrosis of the clavicle. With a note on cranio-cleido dysostosis. *J Bone Joint Surg Br* 1975;57(1):24–29.

256. Alldred AJ. Congenital pseudarthrosis of the clavicle. *J Bone Joint Surg Br* 1963;45-B:312–319.

257. Gardner E. The embryology of the clavicle. *Clin Orthop Relat Res* 1968;58:9–16.

258. Hirata S, Miya H, et al. Congenital pseudarthrosis of the clavicle. Histologic examination for the etiology of the disease. *Clin Orthop Relat Res* 1995;315:242–245.

259. Lombard JJ. Pseudarthrosis of the clavicle. A case report. *S Afr Med J* 1984;66(4):151–153.

260. Mall F. On ossification centers in human embryos less than one hundred days old. *Am J Anat* 1906;5(8):433–458.

261. Koch AR. The early development of the clavicle in man. *Acta Anat (Basel)* 1960;42:177–212.

262. Bargar WL, Marcus RE, et al. Late thoracic outlet syndrome secondary to pseudarthrosis of the clavicle. *J Trauma* 1984;24(9):857–859.

263. Hahn K, Shah R, et al. Congenital clavicular pseudoarthrosis associated with vascular thoracic outlet syndrome: case presentation and review of the literature. *Cathet Cardiovasc Diagn* 1995;35(4):321–327.

264. Ogunbiyi AO, Adewole IO, et al. Focal dermal hypoplasia: a case report and review of literature. *West Afr J Med* 2003;22(4):346–349.

265. Sales de Gauzy J, Baunin C, et al. Congenital pseudarthrosis of the clavicle and thoracic outlet syndrome in adolescence. *J Pediatr Orthop B* 1999;8(4):299–301.

266. Behringer BR, Wilson FC. Congenital pseudarthrosis of the clavicle. *Am J Dis Child* 1972;123(5):511–517.

267. Garnier D, Chevalier J, et al. Arterial complications of thoracic outlet syndrome and pseudarthrosis of the clavicle: three patients. *J Mal Vasc* 2003;28(2):79–84.

268. Grogan DP, Love SM, et al. Operative treatment of congenital pseudarthrosis of the clavicle. *J Pediatr Orthop* 1991;11(2):176–180.

269. Lozano P, Doaz M, et al. Venous thoracic outlet syndrome secondary to congenital pseudoarthrosis of the clavicle. Presentation in the fourth decade of life. *Eur J Vasc Endovasc Surg* 2003;25(6):592–593.

270. Schnall SB, King JD, et al. Congenital pseudarthrosis of the clavicle: a review of the literature and surgical results of six cases. *J Pediatr Orthop* 1988;8(3):316–321.

271. Schoenecker PL, Johnson GE, et al. Congenital pseudarthrosis. *Orthop Rev* 1992;21(7):855–860.

272. Young MC, Richards RR, et al. Thoracic outlet syndrome with congenital pseudarthrosis of the clavicle: treatment by brachial plexus decompression, plate fixation and bone grafting. *Can J Surg* 1988;31(2):131–133.

273. Trevor D. Tarso-epiphysial aclasis; a congenital error of epiphysial development. *J Bone Joint Surg Br* 1950;32-B(2):204–213.

274. Fairbank TJ. Dysplasia epiphysialis hemimelica (tarso-epiphysial aclasis). *J Bone Joint Surg Br* 1956;38-B(1):237–257.

275. Connor JM, Horan FT, et al. Dysplasia epiphysialis hemimelica. A clinical and genetic study. *J Bone Joint Surg Br* 1983;65(3):350–354.

276. Donaldson JS, Sankey HH, et al. Osteochondroma of the distal femoral epiphysis. *J Pediatr* 1953;43(2):212–216.

277. Wynne-Davies R. Dysplasia epiphysealis hemimelica. In: *Atlas of skeletal dysplasias.* Edinburgh: Churchill-Livingstone, 1985:539–543.

278. Kettelkamp DB, Campbell CJ, et al. Dysplasia epiphysealis hemimelica. A report of fifteen cases and a review of the literature. *J Bone Joint Surg Am* 1966;48(4):746–765; discussion 765–766.

279. Keret D, Spatz DK, et al. Dysplasia epiphysealis hemimelica: diagnosis and treatment. *J Pediatr Orthop* 1992;12(3):365–372.

280. Kuo RS, Bellemore MC, et al. Dysplasia epiphysealis hemimelica: clinical features and management. *J Pediatr Orthop* 1998;18(4):543–548.

281. Graves SC, Kuester DJ, et al. Dysplasia epiphysealis hemimelica (Trevor disease) presenting as peroneal spastic flatfoot deformity: a case report. *Foot Ankle* 1991;12(1):55–58.

282. Levi N, Ostgaard SE, et al. Dysplasia epiphysealis hemimelica (Trevor's disease) of the distal radius. *Acta Orthop Belg* 1998;64(1):104–106.

283. Maylack FH, Manske PR, et al. Dysplasia epiphysealis hemimelica at the metacarpophalangeal joint. *J Hand Surg [Am]* 1988;13(6):916–920.

284. Saxton HM, Wilkinson JA. Hemimelic skeletal dysplasia. *J Bone Joint Surg Br* 1964;46:608–613.

285. Segal LS, Vrahas MS, et al. Dysplasia epiphysealis hemimelica of the sacroiliac joint: a case report. *Clin Orthop Relat Res* 1996;333:202–207.

286. Tschauner C, Roth-Schiffl E, et al. Early loss of hip containment in a child with dysplasia epiphysealis hemimelica. *Clin Orthop Relat Res* 2004;427:213–219.

287. Azouz EM, Slomic AM, et al. The variable manifestations of dysplasia epiphysealis hemimelica. *Pediatr Radiol* 1985;15(1):44–49.

288. Bigliani LU, Neer CS II, et al. Dysplasia epiphysealis hemimelica of the scapula. A case report. *J Bone Joint Surg Am* 1980;62(2):292–294.

289. Silverman FN. Dysplasia epiphysealis hemimelica. *Semin Roentgenol* 1989;24(4):246–258.

290. Peduto AJ, Frawley KJ, et al. MR imaging of dysplasia epiphysealis hemimelica: bony and soft-tissue abnormalities. *AJR Am J Roentgenol* 1999;172(3):819–823.

291. Iwasawa T, Aida N, et al. MRI findings of dysplasia epiphysealis hemimelica. *Pediatr Radiol* 1996;26(1):65–67.

292. Lang IM, Azouz EM. MRI appearances of dysplasia epiphysealis hemimelica of the knee. *Skeletal Radiol* 1997;26(4):226–229.

293. Delatycki M, Rogers JG. The genetics of fibrodysplasia ossificans progressiva. *Clin Orthop Relat Res* 1998;346:15–18.

294. Kaplan FS, McCluskey W, et al. Genetic transmission of fibrodysplasia ossificans progressiva. Report of a family. *J Bone Joint Surg Am* 1993;75(8):1214–1220.

295. Lanchoney TF, Olmsted EA, et al. Characterization of bone morphogenetic protein 4 receptor in fibrodysplasia ossificans progressiva. *Clin Orthop Relat Res* 1998;346:38–45.

296. Olmsted EA, Gannon FH, et al. Embryonic overexpression of the c-Fos protooncogene. A murine stem cell chimera applicable to the study of fibrodysplasia ossificans progressiva in humans. *Clin Orthop Relat Res* 1998;346:81–94.

297. Ahn J, Serrano de la Pena L, et al. Paresis of a bone morphogenetic protein-antagonist response in a genetic disorder of heterotopic skeletogenesis. *J Bone Joint Surg Am* 2003;85-A(4):667–674.

298. Kaplan FS, Glaser DL, et al. Heterotopic ossification. *J Am Acad Orthop Surg* 2004;12(2):116–125.

299. Groppe JC, Shore EM, et al. Functional modeling of the ACVR1 (R206H) mutation in FOP. *Clin Orthop Relat Res* 2007;462:87–92.

300. Nakajima M, Haga N, et al. The ACVR1 617G>A mutation is also recurrent in three Japanese patients with fibrodysplasia ossificans progressiva. *J Hum Genet* 2007;52(5):473–475.

301. Shore EM, Xu M, et al. A recurrent mutation in the BMP type I receptor ACVR1 causes inherited and sporadic fibrodysplasia ossificans progressiva. *Nat Genet* 2006;38(5):525–527.

302. Feldman G, Li M, et al. Fibrodysplasia ossificans progressiva, a heritable disorder of severe heterotopic ossification, maps to human chromosome 4q27–31. *Am J Hum Genet* 2000;66(1):128–135.

303. Lucotte G, Bathelier C, et al. Localization of the gene for fibrodysplasia ossificans progressiva (FOP) to chromosome 17q21–22. *Genet Couns* 2000;11(4):329–334.

304. Virdi AS, Shore EM, et al. Phenotypic and molecular heterogeneity in fibrodysplasia ossificans progressiva. *Calcif Tissue Int* 1999;65(3):250–255.

305. Connor JM, Evans DA. Fibrodysplasia ossificans progressiva. The clinical features and natural history of 34 patients. *J Bone Joint Surg Br* 1982;64(1):76–83.

306. Sawyer JR, Klimkiewicz JJ, et al. Mechanism for superior subluxation of the glenohumeral joint in fibrodysplasia ossificans progressiva. *Clin Orthop Relat Res* 1998;346:130–133.

307. Shah PB, Zasloff MA, et al. Spinal deformity in patients who have fibrodysplasia ossificans progressiva. *J Bone Joint Surg Am* 1994;76(10):1442–1450.

308. Connor JM, Evans CC, et al. Cardiopulmonary function in fibrodysplasia ossificans progressiva. *Thorax* 1981;36(6):419–423.

309. Kaplan FS, Tabas JA, et al. The histopathology of fibrodysplasia ossificans progressiva. An endochondral process. *J Bone Joint Surg Am* 1993;75(2):220–230.

310. Gannon FH, Glaser D, et al. Mast cell involvement in fibrodysplasia ossificans progressiva. *Hum Pathol* 2001;32(8):842–848.

311. Gannon FH, Valentine BA, et al. Acute lymphocytic infiltration in an extremely early lesion of fibrodysplasia ossificans progressiva. *Clin Orthop Relat Res* 1998;346:19–25.

312. Zasloff MA, Rocke DM, et al. Treatment of patients who have fibrodysplasia ossificans progressiva with isotretinoin. *Clin Orthop Relat Res* 1998;346:121–129.

313. Kaplan FS, Glaser DL, et al. A new era for fibrodysplasia ossificans progressiva: a druggable target for the second skeleton. *Expert Opin Biol Ther* 2007;7(5):705–712.

314. Merkow SJ, St Clair HS, et al. Myositis ossificans masquerading as sepsis. *J Pediatr Orthop* 1985;5(5):601–604.

315. Howard CB, Porat S, et al. Traumatic myositis ossificans of the quadriceps in infants. *J Pediatr Orthop B* 1998;7(1):80–82.

316. Cushner FD, Morwessel RM. Myositis ossificans traumatica. *Orthop Rev* 1992;21(11):1319–1326.

317. Damanski M. Heterotopic ossification in paraplegia. *J Bone Joint Surg Br* 1961;43B(2):286–299.

318. Garland DE, Blum CE, et al. Periarticular heterotopic ossification in head-injured adults. Incidence and location. *J Bone Joint Surg Am* 1980;62(7):1143–1146.

319. Hardy A, Dickson J. Pathological ossification in traumatic paraplegia. *J Bone Joint Surg Br* 1963;45B(1):76–87.

320. Wharton GW, Morgan TH. Ankylosis in the paralyzed patient. *J Bone Joint Surg Am* 1970;52(1):105–112.

321. Costello FV, Brown A. Myositis ossificans complicating anterior poliomyelitis. *J Bone Joint Surg Br* 1951;33-B(4):594–597.

322. Drane WE, Tipler BM. Heterotopic ossification (myositis ossificans) in acquired immune deficiency syndrome. Detection by gallium scintigraphy. *Clin Nucl Med* 1987;12(6):433–435.

323. Hung JC, Appleton RE, et al. Myositis ossificans complicating severe Guillain-Barre syndrome. *Dev Med Child Neurol* 1997;39(11):775–776.

324. Ahrengart L. Periarticular heterotopic ossification after total hip arthroplasty. Risk factors and consequences. *Clin Orthop Relat Res* 1991;263:49–58.

325. Evans EB. Orthopaedic measures in the treatment of severe burns. *J Bone Joint Surg Am* 1966;48(4):643–669.

326. Ritter MA, Vaughan RB. Ectopic ossification after total hip arthroplasty. Predisposing factors, frequency, and effect on results. *J Bone Joint Surg Am* 1977;59(3):345–351.

327. Illes T, Dubousset J, et al. Characterization of bone forming cells in posttraumatic myositis ossificans by lectins. *Pathol Res Pract* 1992;188(1–2):172–176.

328. Reilly TM, Seldes R, et al. Similarities in the phenotypic expression of pericytes and bone cells. *Clin Orthop Relat Res* 1998;346:95–103.

329. Beiner JM, Jokl P. Muscle contusion injuries: current treatment options. *J Am Acad Orthop Surg* 2001;9(4):227–237.

330. Ogilvie-Harris, DJ, Fornasier VL. Pseudomalignant myositis ossificans: heterotopic new-bone formation without a history of trauma. *J Bone Joint Surg Am* 1980;62(8):1274–1283.

331. Amendola MA, Glazer GM, et al. Myositis ossificans circumscripta: computed tomographic diagnosis. *Radiology* 1983;149(3):775–779.

332. Kransdorf MJ, Meis JM, et al. Myositis ossificans: MR appearance with radiologic-pathologic correlation. *AJR Am J Roentgenol* 1991;157(6):1243–1248.

333. Ackerman LV. Extra-osseous localized non-neoplastic bone and cartilage formation (so-called myositis ossificans): clinical and pathological confusion with malignant neoplasms. *J Bone Joint Surg Am* 1958;40-A(2):279–298.

334. Hughston JC, Whatley GS, et al. Myositis ossificans traumatica (myoosteosis). *South Med J* 1962;55:1167–1170.

335. Jackson DW, Feagin JA. Quadriceps contusions in young athletes. Relation of severity of injury to treatment and prognosis. *J Bone Joint Surg Am* 1973;55(1):95–105.

336. Ryan JB, Wheeler JH, et al. Quadriceps contusions. West Point update. *Am J Sports Med* 1991;19(3):299–304.

337. Thorndike A. Myositis ossificans traumatica. *J Bone Joint Surg* 1940; 22:315–323.

338. Spencer JD, Missen GA. Pseudomalignant heterotopic ossification (myositis ossificans). Recurrence after excision with subsequent resorption. *J Bone Joint Surg Br* 1989;71(2):317–319.

339. Siffert RS. Classification of the osteochondroses. *Clin Orthop Relat Res* 1981;158:10–18.

340. Bradford DS. Vertebral osteochondrosis (Scheuermann's kyphosis). *Clin Orthop Relat Res* 1981;158:83–90.

341. Katz JF. Nonarticular osteochondroses. *Clin Orthop Relat Res* 1981; 158:70–76.

342. Langenskiold A. Tibia vara: osteochondrosis deformans tibiae. Blount's disease. *Clin Orthop Relat Res* 1981;158:77–82.

343. Omer GE Jr. Primary articular osteochondroses. *Clin Orthop Relat Res* 1981;158:33–40.

344. Pappas AM. Osteochondrosis dissecans. *Clin Orthop Relat Res* 1981; 158:59–69.

345. Sengupta S. Pathogenesis of infantile quadriceps fibrosis and its correction by proximal release. *J Pediatr Orthop* 1985;5(2):187–191.

346. Schenck RC Jr, Goodnight JM. Osteochondritis dissecans. *J Bone Joint Surg Am* 1996;78(3):439–456.

347. Ytrehus B, Carlson CS, et al. Etiology and pathogenesis of osteochondrosis. *Vet Pathol* 2007;44(4):429–448.

348. Carlson CS, Meuten DJ, et al. Ischemic necrosis of cartilage in spontaneous and experimental lesions of osteochondrosis. *J Orthop Res* 1991; 9(3):317–329.

349. Pappas AM. The osteochondroses. *Pediatr Clin North Am* 1967; 14(3):549–570.

350. Chiroff RT, Cooke CP III. Osteochondritis dissecans: a histologic and microradiographic analysis of surgically excised lesions. *J Trauma* 1975;15(8):689–696.

351. Borges JL, Guille JT, et al. Kohler's bone disease of the tarsal navicular. *J Pediatr Orthop* 1995;15(5):596–598.

352. Green W, Banks H. Osteochondritis dissecans in children. *J Bone Joint Surg* 1953;35-A:26–47.

353. Hnvkovsk O. Progressive fibrosis of the vastus intermedius muscle in children: a cause of limited knee flexion and elevation of the patella. *J Bone Joint Surg Br* 1961;43-B:318–325.

354. Karlen A. Congenital fibrosis of the vastus intermedius muscle. *J Bone Joint Surg Br* 1964;46:488–491.

355. Uhthoff HK, Ogata S. Early intrauterine presence of congenital dislocation of the knee. *J Pediatr Orthop* 1994;14(2):254–257.

356. Fairbank TJ, Barrett AM. Vastus intermedius contracture in early childhood. *J Bone Joint Surg* 1961;43:326.

357. Gunn DR. Contracture of the quadriceps muscle. A discussion on the etiology and relationship to recurrent dislocation of the patella. *J Bone Joint Surg Br* 1964;46:492–497.

358. Hollaert P, Adijns P, et al. Review of the literature on quadriceps fibrosis and study of 11 cases. *Acta Orthop Belg* 1975;41(3):255–258.

359. Makhani JS. Quadriceps fibrosis. A complication of intra-muscular injections in the thigh. *Indian J Pediatr* 1971;38(277):54–60.

360. Shanmugasundaram TK. Post-injection fibrosis of skeletal muscle: a clinical problem. A personal series of 169 cases. *Int Orthop* 1980;4(1): 31–37.

361. Valdiserri L, Andrisano A, et al. Post-injective quadriceps contracture. *Ital J Orthop Traumatol* 1989;15(3):267–272.

362. Williams PF. Quadriceps contracture. *J Bone Joint Surg Br* 1968; 50(2):278–284.

363. Lloyd-Roberts GC, Thomas TG. The etiology of quadriceps contracture in children. *J Bone Joint Surg Br* 1964;46:498–517.

364. Sasaki T, Fukuhara H, et al. Postoperative evaluation of quadriceps contracture in children: comparison of three different procedures. *J Pediatr Orthop* 1985;5(6):702–707.

365. Cimaz R, Matucci-Cerinic M, et al. Reflex sympathetic dystrophy in children. *J Child Neurol* 1999;14(6):363–367.

366. Wilder RT, Berde CB, et al. 1992. Reflex sympathetic dystrophy in children. Clinical characteristics and follow-up of seventy patients. *J Bone Joint Surg Am* 74(6):910–919.

367. Wilder RT. 2006. Management of pediatric patients with complex regional pain syndrome. *Clin J Pain* 22(5):443–448.

368. Bernstein BH, Singsen BH, et al. Reflex neurovascular dystrophy in childhood. *J Pediatr* 1978;93(2):211–215.

369. Dietz FR, Mathews KD, et al. Reflex sympathetic dystrophy in children. *Clin Orthop Relat Res* 1990;258:225–231.

370. Laxer RM, Allen RC, et al. Technetium 99 m-methylene diphosphonate bone scans in children with reflex neurovascular dystrophy. *J Pediatr* 1985;106(3):437–440.

371. Figuerola Mde L, Levin G, et al. Normal sympathetic nervous system response in reflex sympathetic dystrophy. *Funct Neurol* 2002;17(2):77–81.

372. Crozier F, Champsaur P, et al. Magnetic resonance imaging in reflex sympathetic dystrophy syndrome of the foot. *Joint Bone Spine* 70(6):503–508, 2003.

373. Schweitzer ME, Mandel S, et al. Reflex sympathetic dystrophy revisited: MR imaging findings before and after infusion of contrast material. *Radiology* 1995;195(1):211–214.

374. Bruehl S, Husfeldt B, et al. Psychological differences between reflex sympathetic dystrophy and non-RSD chronic pain patients. *Pain* 1996;67(1):107–114.

375. Ciccone DS, Bandilla EB, et al. Psychological dysfunction in patients with reflex sympathetic dystrophy. *Pain* 1997;71(3):323–333.

376. Sherry DD, Weisman R. Psychologic aspects of childhood reflex neurovascular dystrophy. *Pediatrics* 1988;81(4):572–578.

377. Lee BH, Scharff L, et al. Physical therapy and cognitive-behavioral treatment for complex regional pain syndromes. *J Pediatr* 2002;141(1): 135–140.

378. Stanton RP, Malcolm JR, et al. Reflex sympathetic dystrophy in children: an orthopedic perspective. *Orthopedics* 1993;16(7):773–779; discussion 779–780.

379. Murray CS, Cohen A, et al. Morbidity in reflex sympathetic dystrophy. *Arch Dis Child* 2000;82(3):231–233.

380. Stanton-Hicks M, Baron R, et al. Complex regional pain syndromes: guidelines for therapy. *Clin J Pain* 1998;14(2):155–166.

381. Christensen K, Jensen EM, et al. The reflex dystrophy syndrome response to treatment with systemic corticosteroids. *Acta Chir Scand* 1982;148(8):653–655.

382. Ruggeri SB, Athreya BH, et al. Reflex sympathetic dystrophy in children. *Clin Orthop Relat Res* 1982;163:225–230.

383. Wheeler DS, Vaux KK, et al. Use of gabapentin in the treatment of childhood reflex sympathetic dystrophy. *Pediatric neurology* 2000;22(3):220–221.

384. Matsui M, Ito M, et al. Complex regional pain syndrome in childhood: report of three cases. *Brain Dev* 2000;22(7):445–448.

385. Veldman PH, Reynen HM, et al. Signs and symptoms of reflex sympathetic dystrophy: prospective study of 829 patients. *Lancet* 1993;342(8878):1012–1016.

Diseases of the Hematopoietic System

Diseases of the hematopoietic system can profoundly affect musculoskeletal form and function. The hematopoietic system consists of the cellular elements in circulating blood, bone marrow, spleen, lymph nodes, and the reticuloendothelial system. This chapter discusses the diseases of the hematopoietic system that have musculoskeletal features that a pediatric orthopaedist would be expected to diagnose and treat. Such diseases can be divided into (a) disorders of the bone marrow, where most of the cells of this system are produced; (b) disorders of erythrocytes/hemoglobin, predominantly involving abnormalities in hemoglobin synthesis or erythrocyte production; (c) disorders of neutrophils and lymphocytes, with accompanying immune deficiencies; (d) disorders of monocytes and macrophages, with abnormalities of metabolism and proliferation; (e) disorders of hemostasis, causing abnormal bleeding or thrombosis; and (f) hematologic malignancies. The orthopaedic evaluation and management are discussed for each disorder, along with recent advances in pathophysiology, molecular genetics, treatment, and prognosis.

BONE MARROW FAILURE DISORDERS

The cellular elements of the hematopoietic system are produced in the bone marrow. Bone marrow failure is characterized by deficient production of one or more cell lines in the bone marrow. Disorders characterized by bone marrow failure can cause anemia, thrombocytopenia, leukopenia, or pancytopenia, depending on which hematopoietic precursors are affected and at what stage of stem cell differentiation the abnormality occurs. There are many bone marrow failure disorders with musculoskeletal manifestations, the most common of which include Fanconi anemia (FA), thrombocytopenia with absent radius (TAR) syndrome, Diamond-Blackfan anemia (DBA), Schwachman-Diamond syndrome (SDS), and cartilage-hair hypoplasia (CHH). The orthopaedist should be familiar with these disorders, because the musculoskeletal manifestations

that can cause significant functional disabilities and cosmetic problems may be their first clinically apparent signs.

Fanconi Anemia. FA is an autosomal recessive disorder characterized by bone marrow failure, physical anomalies, and predisposition to malignancies. The disorder is uncommon, with an incidence of <1 per 100,000 live births (1). The disorder has a slight male predominance 1.3:1(2) and shows no clear racial dependence (3). Multiple genes have been implicated in FA, the most common of which FANCA is located on chromosome 16q24.3 (4). While the exact function of FA proteins is unclear, they likely lead to defects in apoptosis of hematopoietic progenitors (5). Patients with FA show increased chromosomal breakage especially when exposed to DNA crosslinking agents. As skeletal anomalies are the most obvious clinical manifestations of FA apparent at birth, the orthopaedist may be the first physician consulted. Nearly 60% of patients exhibit short stature while nearly 50% manifest upper limb anomalies. The hand and forearm are the sites most often affected, with a variety of radial ray differences (6–8). Thumb hypoplasia or absence is common, although thumb duplication and triphalangeal thumb may also be seen. The radius is typically either hypoplastic or absent. It is important to distinguish FA from TAR syndrome. In FA, if the radius is affected, the thumb is also abnormal, while in TAR, if the radius is absent, the thumb is always present. Although radial ray differences are a common manifestation of FA, they are not pathognomonic (9). Nonetheless, any child with a radial ray deficiency should be referred to genetic specialists and/or hematologists for evaluation of the possibility of an underlying hematologic problem. Because 20% of patients with FA have no clinically apparent anomalies at birth, the diagnosis may be delayed.

Other skeletal anomalies such as congenital hip dislocation, spina bifida, and scoliosis have been reported in patients with FA, but not often enough to be considered an integral feature of the disorder. Patients tend to have a variety of facial abnormalities including micrognathia, epicanthal folds, and a broad nasal bridge. Skin pigmentation anomalies, including *café-au-lait* spots, are common. As the child grows, growth retardation becomes apparent in approximately 80% of patients (6), often associated with endocrinopathies (10). Renal anomalies are present in approximately one-third of patients with FA, although the exact prevalence is likely underestimated because not all patients in large series have undergone renal diagnostic imaging (11). Cardiovascular and gastrointestinal anomalies can be found in 15% to 30% of patients. The central nervous system is often affected, with microcephaly, hearing loss, eye anomalies, and mental retardation apparent in up to 37% of patients (6).

Bone marrow failure occurs in 90% of patients and while it may begin with one cell line often progresses to profound decreases in all cell lines (1). The pancytopenia typical of FA does not typically appear until age 7 or 8 years (12), although it can occur at any age (1). Because patients with FA have increased susceptibility to DNA breakage, the incidence of solid tumors and leukemia is increased in patients with FA. One-fourth of patients with FA have at least one malignancy, and in one-fourth of these patients, the finding of malignancy preceded the diagnosis of FA. The treatment of the upper extremity anomalies is covered elsewhere in this text.

Thrombocytopenia with Absent Radius Syndrome.

TAR syndrome is a rare autosomal recessive disorder characterized by marked thrombocytopenia and absent radii. The radial absence is complete and almost always bilateral (13). The radial clubhands seen in TAR syndrome differ from those in FA in that the thumbs are present in TAR syndrome but are absent in FA if the radii are absent (Fig. 10-1). (See Table 10-1 for a comparison of FA and TAR syndrome.) The thumbs are hypoplastic in about half of patients with TAR syndrome. Thumb and finger function is impaired to varying degrees, and wrist function is abnormal owing to the lack of radius and abnormal carpal bones and musculature. Typically, the ulna is hypoplastic and bowed, as in other causes of radial clubhand. In approximately 40% of the patients, the humerus is hypoplastic or absent, and the shoulder girdle is abnormal in one-third of the patients (14). Major intercalary transverse deficiencies may exist, with hands arising directly from the shoulder girdle (14, 15).

Lower extremity deformities are also common in TAR syndrome, despite the name of the disorder. In the original description of 40 patients by Hall et al. (14), 40% had lower-extremity deformities. More recent series have estimated an 80% prevalence of lower extremity deformities (16, 17). The severity of upper extremity involvement seems to correlate with the presence and severity of lower extremity involvement (15). As with the fingers, all five toes are typically preserved, even with fibular hemimelia or other lower extremity deformities (15). Knee abnormalities have been studied in detail in 21 patients by Schoenecker et al. (16). Genu varum was present in 18 patients and was apparent at birth in 12 of them. The genu

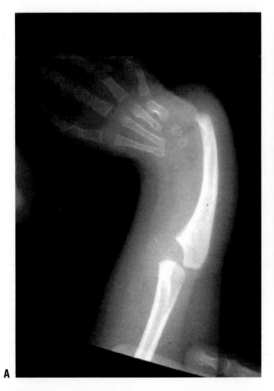
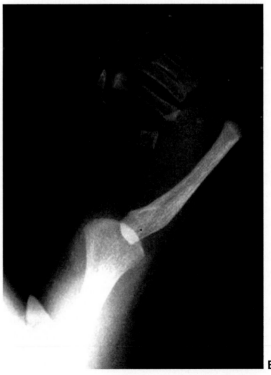

A   B

FIGURE 10-1. Forearm and hand radiographs in (**A**) Fanconi anemia and (**B**) TAR syndrome. Note the absence of a thumb in the child with Fanconi anemia, as is the case when the radius is completely absent. However, note the presence of the thumb in the child with TAR syndrome, despite complete absence of the radius.

TABLE 10-1   Clinical Features of Fanconi Anemia and TAR Syndrome

	Fanconi Anemia	TAR Syndrome
Radius	Hypoplastic or absent	Absent bilaterally
Thumb	Hypoplastic or absent (always absent when radius absent)	Always present, often hypoplastic
Other upper extremity anomalies	Ulnar bowing	Ulnar bowing, humerus can be hypoplastic or absent
Lower extremity involvement	Hip dislocations in 10%	Common, including genu varum, medial femoral condyle anomalies
Hematologic manifestations	Pancytopenia at age 7–8 yr	Thrombocytopenia severe during first year of life
Hematologic course	Progressive and fatal without bone marrow transplant	Spontaneous resolution after 1 yr of age
Cancer risk	Malignancies in 20%–25%	No increased risk

varum was usually associated with varus laxity of the knee joint rather than a fixed bony deformity. Intra-articular pathology was found to be extensive at surgery in six patients, including concave medial femoral condyles. Internal rotation of the tibia was also common. Patellar anomalies included hypoplasia, instability, and total absence. The deformities tended to progress as the children grew, requiring bracing. Lower extremity deformities usually recurred following corrective osteotomies, although some have reported success in correcting a fixed knee deformity with osteotomy (18). Anomalies of other systems, including cardiac, neurologic, and genitourinary, are reported in one-third of patients (14).

The hematologic manifestation of TAR syndrome is a profound thrombocytopenia that can cause serious bleeding within the first few months of life (14). Bone marrow examination typically reveals infrequent or absent megakaryocytes, but the cause of this is unknown. Viral illnesses can exacerbate the thrombocytopenia, and patients should be kept relatively isolated in the early months to avoid undue viral challenges. Bone marrow transplant is rarely indicated, as most patients resume platelet production spontaneously (19). Elective surgery should be avoided in the first year of life if thrombocytopenia is present. The radial clubhands should initially be splinted and reconstructive procedures performed later.

Diamond-Blackfan Anemia.
DBA is a rare congenital hypoplastic anemia affecting only the erythropoietic cell line and associated with hand and other skeletal anomalies. Approximately 4 in 1 million live births are affected by DBA (20). Typically, the disorder occurs sporadically, but up to 45% of cases are familial. The first identified DBA gene (ribosomal protein RPS19) is located at 19q13. and is thought to have a role in ribosome biogenesis 2 (12, 21, 22). Approximately 30% of patients have associated skeletal anomalies (12). Among upper limb differences, triphalangeal or hypoplastic thumbs are the most common features (12). Radial hypoplasia is uncommon in DBA (23). Patients with

DBA also have urogenital anomalies, and cardiac anomalies such as atrial or ventricular septal defects.

Whereas the skeletal anomalies are apparent at birth, the signs of severe anemia do not usually develop until later in infancy. The anemia is typically normochromic and macrocytic, with most patients being identified before 1 year of age. The exact cause of DBA is unknown, and the features of the disorder are highly variable. Bone marrow examination reveals an isolated deficiency of erythroid precursors (12). A predisposition to malignancies may exist in patients with DBA, but as no known impairment exists in DNA repair mechanisms, the predisposition is slight compared to that of FA.

Treatment is evolving (24). Corticosteroids remain the mainstay of treatment in most patients; however, side effects of long-term steroid use is common. For those who do not respond to corticosteroids, treatment options include chronic transfusion therapy, hematopoietic growth factors such as erythropoietin, interleukin-3 (IL-3), and stem cell factor, cyclosporin A, or metaclopromide. Bone marrow transplantation from human leukocyte antigen–matched donors has been utilized (25). Gene therapy has met with some clinical success in a small number of patients (26).

Schwachman-Diamond Syndrome.
SDS is an autosomal recessive disorder causing pancreatic insufficiency, bone marrow hypoplasia, metaphyseal dyschondroplasia, and growth retardation. Patients can appear normal at birth, but typically have low birth weights (27). The first signs of the disorder are attributable to malabsorption, including failure to thrive, growth retardation, and steatorrhea. Severe respiratory infections also occur in the first year of life. Few patients have an uneventful neonatal period.

Patients with SDS are referred to the orthopaedist because of skeletal abnormalities contributing to delayed growth and deformity. Metaphyseal chondrodysplasia occurs in approximately 62% of patients, usually in the proximal femur (27). This lesion in the proximal femur can cause coxa vara, coxa magna, pathologic femoral neck fracture, or pseudoarthrosis (27, 28). Other common sites for chondrodysplasia include the knees, wrists, spine, and ribs (27, 28). Spinal deformity can include kyphosis and scoliosis. Ribs are typically short and anteriorly flared. Long bone bowing is a common finding and can recur following osteotomies. Clinodactyly was reported in almost half of the patients in one series (27).

Bone marrow failure in SDS causes neutropenia in 95% to 100%, thrombocytopenia in 66% to 70%, and anemia in 24% to 50% (27, 29). All three cell lines are affected in 25% of patients (19). Myelodysplasia was found in 7 of 21 patients in one series, and 5 of these developed acute myelogenous leukemia (29). Laboratory studies reveal that the pancreatic insufficiency gives rise to enzymatic abnormalities, including the absence of trypsin, lipase, and amylase in the stool. SDS can be differentiated from cystic fibrosis by a normal sweat chloride test. Hepatic, respiratory, and renal dysfunction also occurs. Neurologic development is usually delayed.

Early mortality is usually from infections. Overall, half of the patients with SDS will live to the age of 35 years, but survival is reduced to 24 years for patients with pancytopenia and to 10 years for patients with leukemia. Early treatment includes oral administration of pancreatic enzymes and aggressive antibiotic treatment of infections. The bone marrow failure may respond to growth factors and androgens, although these treatments are only temporarily effective (19). Bone marrow transplantation with reduced intensity conditioning regimens have shown great promise in curing this disorder (30).

Cartilage-Hair Hypoplasia.

CHH is a rare autosomal recessive disorder characterized by disproportionate, short-limbed dwarfism, thin, sparse hair, and cellular immunodeficiency. The skeletal manifestations of this condition are covered in detail elsewhere in this text.

The hematologic manifestations of CHH include cellular immunodeficiency and anemia. The degree of immunodeficiency varies greatly (31). Recurrent respiratory tract infections may occur in these patients, and serious illness can result from vaccinations with live viruses. The immunodeficiency is usually due to diminished numbers of T lymphocytes. The anemia of CHH is an integral feature, occurring in 73% of patients (32). Anemia may be severe in infancy, but tends to improve with growth (32).

For patients who have no increased susceptibility to infection and have only mild anemia, often no treatment is required. For more severe immunodeficiency with anemia, bone marrow transplantation may be needed. Bone marrow transplantation can correct the immunodeficiency (33, 34) but not the chondrodysplasia (35).

DISORDERS OF HEMOGLOBIN

Erythrocytes in circulating blood carry oxygen to tissues. Hemoglobin carries the oxygen in erythrocytes. Mutations in the genes that encode for protein synthesis can cause abnormal hemoglobin molecules that affect the form and function of erythrocytes. Iron deficiency and chronic inflammation can also diminish production of hemoglobin, resulting in anemia. Disorders in number, form, or function of erythrocytes can cause significant musculoskeletal pathology, and can complicate the treatment of other musculoskeletal conditions.

Sickle Cell Disease.

Sickle cell disease (SCD) is an inherited disorder of hemoglobin synthesis. The protein component of hemoglobin is composed of four globin chains: two α-globin chains and two β-globin chains. Hemoglobin S refers to hemoglobin containing abnormal β-globin produced by a single base change mutation (GAT to GTT) in the sixth codon of exon 1 in the β-globin gene on chromosome 11 (36). As a result, the molecule polymerizes upon (37) deoxygenation, causing distortion or "sickling" of the erythrocytes that contain the abnormal hemoglobin. Hemoglobin C contains β-globin chains with a glutamic acid-to-lysine substitution at the same position.

Four major types of SCD are recognized, according to the genotype of the β-globin gene and the resulting proportion of hemoglobin S. (a) SS disease results from homozygous inheritance of the hemoglobin S mutation. All hemoglobin is hemoglobin S and the sickling is severe. (b) SC disease results from inheritance of one hemoglobin S allele and one hemoglobin C allele. None of the hemoglobin is normal, but the tendency to sickle is tempered by the presence of hemoglobin C. (c) $S\beta^+$ disease results from inheritance of one hemoglobin S allele and an allele with a β-thalassemia mutation that causes slightly reduced β-globin synthesis. Some normal β-globin is produced, and sickling is less severe. (d) $S\beta^0$ disease results from inheritance of one hemoglobin S allele and an allele with a β-thalassemia mutation that causes greatly reduced β-globin synthesis. Very little normal β-globin is produced, leading to a preponderance of hemoglobin S and severe sickling.

Marrow hyperplasia can lead to osteopenia, biconcave vertebrae, and medullary expansion and cortical thinning due to marrow (38) (Fig. 10-2).

Vascular occlusion causes most of the clinical manifestations of SCD. Several factors cause sickle cells to occlude the microvasculature, including abnormal cell shape, cellular dehydration, and increased cellular adhesion to vascular endothelium. Sickling of erythrocytes is thought to confer resistance to infection by *Plasmodium falciparum* malaria, contributing to the high prevalence in populations where malaria is common. In the United States, SCD affects 1 in 300 to 1 in 600 African Americans (39, 40). Screening facilitates early diagnosis and treatment, which can improve the clinical course (41).

Vaso-occlusive pain events, or pain crises involving the extremities and the back, are common manifestations of SCD (42). Pain crises are commonly associated with infarcts in the humerus, tibia, and femur (43), although infarcts can occur in any bone in the body. Patients presenting with pain crises rarely have striking findings on physical examination. Swelling and decreased range of motion are usually not present. Fever is variably present. Peripheral leukocytosis and erythrocyte morphology on peripheral blood smears have no diagnostic use in a pain crisis (44). Analgesia is the cornerstone of treatment for

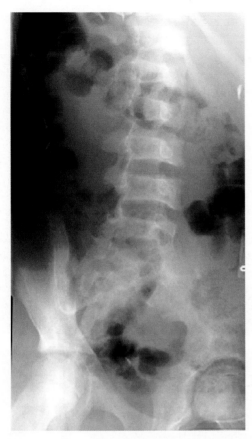

FIGURE 10-2. Oblique radiograph of the spine in a patient with SCD. Note biconcave vertebral bodies.

a pain crisis. Hydration is an important adjunct to analgesics. Oxygen supplementation has no proven benefit in a patient who is not hypoxic (45).

Dactylitis, a painful swelling of fingers or toes, occurs in early childhood and is often the first clinical manifestation of SCD and is typically seen in children under the age of 6 years. Onset of dactylitis before the age of 1 year has been suggested to predict a more severe case of SCD (46). The rarity of dactylitis in older children is thought to result from a shift in hematopoiesis from distal sites such as fingers and toes in infants to more central sites in older children (45). Radiographs are initially normal, but may progress to demonstrate periosteal elevation and osteolysis, mimicking osteomyelitis. Cultures of bone aspirates can help in making a diagnosis by differentiating between the two disorders. The pain associated with dactylitis is often mild and is relieved by nonsteroidal anti-inflammatory drugs (NSAIDs) in infants, but can be severe in older children.

Osteomyelitis occurs in patients with SCD and can be difficult to differentiate from a pain crisis. Osteomyelitis is much less common than pain crises; in one study, only 1.6% of patients admitted to the hospital for severe musculoskeletal pain had osteomyelitis (47). Although patients with SCD experience higher rates of *Salmonella* osteomyelitis than patients without SCD, *Staphylococcus aureus* is still the most common bacterial pathogen (48–50). As microvascular

occlusion in the spleen causes repeated splenic infarcts, patients become functionally asplenic and susceptible to infections with encapsulated bacteria such as *Streptococcus pneumoniae*, *Salmonella*, and *Haemophilus* (51–53). Intestinal infarcts with translocation of gut bacteria are thought to be responsible for the high rate of infection from *Salmonella* and other enteric bacteria. Prompt recognition and treatment of osteomyelitis is important. However, it is difficult to differentiate between painful bone infarcts and osteomyelitis, and, therefore, the diagnosis of osteomyelitis is often delayed (54–57). The history and physical examination findings are similar in the two conditions. Also laboratory values such as white blood cell count, erythrocyte sedimentation rate, and C-reactive protein are also similar. Imaging is often inconclusive. Plain films are rarely diagnostic. Ultrasound is occasionally effective in detecting subperiosteal fluid collections. Technetium-99m sulfur colloid bone marrow scan followed by technetium-99m methylene diphosphonate bone scan has been reported to differentiate between the two conditions (58), but without proven consistency. Magnetic resonance imaging (MRI) cannot reliably differentiate between sickle infarct and osteomyelitis. The bone marrow manifestations of SCD are primarily related to the hematopoietic marrow hyperplasia, infarction, and perivascular fibrosis. Findings of acute marrow infarction are present in only one-third of cases. Conversely, similar findings on MIR often occur in the absence of clinical symptoms, probably as a result of subclinical (59) infarcts. Gadolinium-enhanced MRI can be useful in distinguishing vascularized inflammatory tissue from abscess, thus guiding aspiration for fluid collection.

The clinical response is important for differentiating between painful crisis and osteomyelitis in patients with SCD. In a painful crisis, symptoms should abate within 24 to 48 hours with hydration and analgesics. If the patient fails to improve, MRI is typically the next step. MRI evidence of intraosseous, subperiosteal, or soft-tissue fluid collection warrants aspiration or surgical drainage.

Septic arthritis is less common than osteomyelitis (57, 60). As opposed to osteomyelitis, septic arthritis is not caused by unusual organisms such as *Salmonella* (57, 60). The treatment of septic arthritis in patients with SCD follows the principles outlined elsewhere in this text.

Osteonecrosis (ON) of the femoral and the humeral heads is common in patients with SCD (Fig. 10-3). ON of the femoral head is slightly more common than that of the humeral head. The development of ON is related to age and genotype (61, 62). By age 45, nearly one-third of patients have femoral head ON, and nearly one-fourth have humeral head ON. Femoral head ON is bilateral in 54% of the patients, and humeral head ON is bilateral in 67% of the patients. Concomitant femoral and humeral head ON occurs in three-fourths of the patients. The genotype affects the prevalence of ON. As with other manifestations of the disease, patients with SS or Sβ^0 disease have a higher incidence of ON than do those with SC or Sβ^+ disease (61, 62).

ON may be asymptomatic in the hips and shoulders of children. Abnormalities may show up on radiographs several

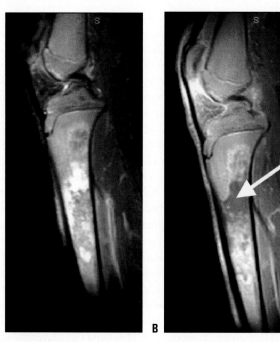
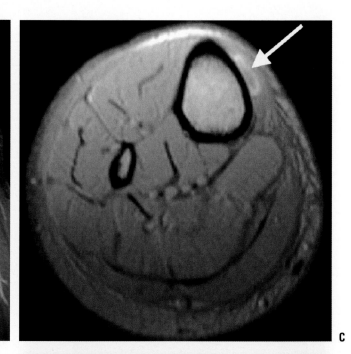
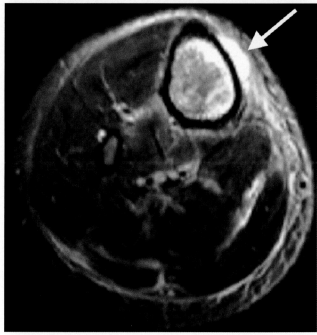

FIGURE 10-3. A 17-year-old boy with SCD presented with symptoms of a painful crisis in his leg. Plain radiographs of his tibia revealed no abnormalities. Failure to respond to hydration after 2 days, along with elevated peripheral white blood cell count and C-reactive protein, prompted investigation with MRI. Sagittal T1-weighted images before (**A**) and after (**B**) gadolinium injection demonstrate heterogeneous enhancement throughout a large area of abnormal signal intensity in the marrow of the tibia. An intraosseous fluid collection can be seen (*arrow*). Axial T1-weighted (**C**) and T2-weighted (**D**) images without gadolinium demonstrate an extraosseous fluid collection (*arrows*) with surrounding edema. Operative corticotomy yielded purulent material.

years before symptoms appear, and the prognosis is worse in SCD than other causes of femoral head necrosis (61, 63, 64). The age at onset of ON of the femoral head has been reported to correlate with outcome (65), and there may be an impairment of the fibrinolytic pathway in some individuals predisposing them to a worse outcome (66). Plain radiographs and MRI are used for evaluating ON. MRI can delineate the extent and stages of involvement (67, 68). Improving the prognosis and outcomes of ON of the femoral head in patients with SCD is difficult, so the treatment is controversial (69, 70). It roughly parallels that in patients without SCD, as covered elsewhere in this text. Containment and physical therapy may be

sufficient in young children with limited involvement of the femoral head. Non–weight-bearing therapy, core decompression, femoral osteotomies, total joint replacement all become options in older and more severely involved hips (71–76).

Any surgery in patients with SCD should be accompanied by adequate hydration, maintenance of blood volume and oxygenation, and prevention of hypothermia. The use of a tourniquet is allowed, as it does not induce sickling (77). Transfusions are typically given perioperatively to keep the total hemoglobin around 10 g/dL (78).

Pathologic fractures occur in approximately 10% of patients with SCD, usually complicating osteomyelitis (55, 79, 80).

One series (79) found that delayed union, malunion, and joint stiffness complicate 10% to 15% of fractures. However, fractures are not a prominent feature of SCD.

Many other organ systems are affected by SCD. Anemia in SCD is related to erythrocyte fragility and hemolysis. The chronic baseline anemia is generally mild and well tolerated in childhood. However, anemia can be worsened acutely by splenic sequestration, a sudden increase in splenic hemolysis that can be fatal, and by aplastic anemia, a temporary marrow suppression often triggered by parvovirus B19 infection.

Acute chest syndrome (ACS) refers to any new pulmonary infiltrate seen on a chest radiograph in conjunction with fever and chest pain or respiratory symptoms and can be fatal (81). ACS can result from a wide variety of infectious or noninfectious causes, including rib infarcts (82).

SCD also causes genitourinary problems, including enuresis and priapism. Cholelithiasis is common in patients with SCD because of ongoing hemolysis and buildup of bilirubin. Stroke is a common and potentially devastating result of cerebral vasoocclusion or hemorrhage. Infections are a significant risk in infancy and early childhood. Sepsis used to be a major cause of mortality in this age group. The widespread use of penicillin prophylaxis and pneumococcal vaccination in children younger than 5 years reduces the incidence of pneumococcal bacteremia by 84% (83).

Medical treatment of SCD has advanced considerably in recent decades. Hydroxyurea, a chemotherapeutic agent, causes increased formation of hemoglobin F and has been found to reduce the incidence of painful crises and ACS, as well as to reduce the requirement for transfusion in adults (84). Several studies have proven similar efficacy of this drug in children as young as 2 years, although the U.S. Food and Drug Administration (FDA) has not yet approved this drug for use in children. Many other drugs are currently under investigation. Most children now receive pneumococcal vaccine, and it should be highly considered in children with SCD. Bone marrow transplantation has been used in approximately 150 children with severe SCD worldwide, with 92% to 94% survival and 75% to 84% event-free survival (85).

Thalassemia. The thalassemias are a heterogeneous group of autosomal recessive inherited disorders of hemoglobin synthesis. Together, they represent the most common inherited diseases worldwide (86). The diseases and their treatments can cause an array of alterations in skeletal dynamics that the orthopaedist should be able to recognize.

The many kinds of mutations that are responsible for thalassemia cause deficient or nil production of either α- or β-globin chains. Alpha thalassemia results from mutations in one or more of the four copies of the α-globin gene. One mutation results in a silent carrier state. Mutation of two genes causes a thalassemia trait, characterized by mild normocytic or microcytic anemia. Mutation of three genes causes substantially diminished α-globin production and hemoglobin H disease (named for the stable tetramer formed by the remaining β chains) with moderate hemolytic anemia. Mutation of all four

α-globin genes causes hydrops fetalis, which is usually fatal *in utero*. Beta thalassemia results from mutations in the β-globin gene and is classified as (a) β^+ thalassemia, with reduced synthesis of β-globin or (b) β^0 thalassemia, with absent β-globin synthesis. An alternate classification of thalassemia is based entirely on clinical severity. *Thalassemia major* refers to severe disease, *thalassemia intermedia* refers to moderate disease, and *thalassemia minor* refers to mild disease.

Among the α thalassemias, hemoglobin H disease is the most often seen clinically. Children generally present with moderately severe anemia, splenomegaly, and cholelithiasis, which may occur in response to oxidative stress caused by infections, fever, or certain medications (87). Patients with thalassemia major (homozygous β thalassemia) develop severe anemia, with hemoglobin in the 3 to 4 g/dL range within the first 6 months of life, as fetal hemoglobin production wanes. Thalassemia major requires frequent transfusions in order to maintain health and prolong life expectancy beyond 5 years of age. Transfusions are generally started when the anemia becomes clinically detrimental and are aimed at keeping hemoglobin levels more than 9.5 to 10.5 g/dL. Thalassemia intermedia typically presents in the second year of life with a less profound anemia (86).

The skeletal manifestations of the thalassemias, which may occur as a result of both the anemia and its treatments, include marrow hyperplasia, short stature, skeletal dysplasia, and osteopenia. Without transfusions to correct the severe anemia in thalassemia major, erythropoietin secretion increases. The resulting marrow hyperplasia causes widening of the medullary cavities and thinning of the cortices of long bones (Fig. 10-4). This process is initially apparent in the hands and feet, where the tubular bones become rectangular and then convex. Premature closure of physes, especially in the proximal humerus, can also occur (88). Marrow hyperplasia can cause dramatic expansion of calvarial bones (89). Marrow hyperplasia in the spine is associated with back pain in adults with thalassemia who started transfusions after 3 years of age (90). Extramedullary hematopoiesis commonly occurs in the liver, spleen, and chest. Extramedullary hematopoiesis in the paravertebral space can cause spinal cord compression (91–94). MRI is helpful in detecting and evaluating this process in the spine. Surgical decompression, radiation therapy, and transfusions are treatment options. Marrow hyperplasia from severe anemia is not often seen today, because of the use of maintenance transfusions.

Growth disturbance can result from the effects of transfusion-induced iron overload on the anterior pituitary gland and hypothalamus. Endocrinopathies resulting from iron overload include decreased growth hormone (GH) release or GH resistance (95), delayed puberty and hypogonadism (96), and hypoparathyroidism. In one series of transfusion-dependent patients with thalassemia major (97), 8% of boys aged 7 to 8 years had short stature (less than third percentile), as well as 12% and 15% of older boys and girls, respectively. The short stature tends to be disproportionate, with a relatively short trunk (98). The correction of GH deficiency and the

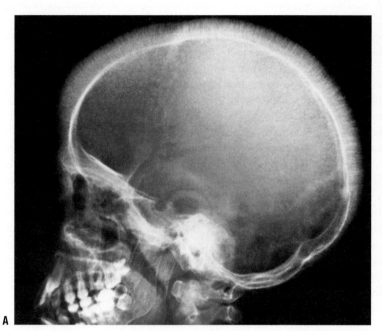
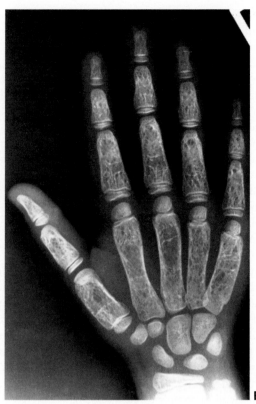

FIGURE 10-4.   A: Lateral radiograph of the skull in a 11-year-old boy with thalassemia major. Note radial striations in the calvarium. **B:** Radiograph of the hand of the same patient. Note widened marrow cavities, thinned cortices, and osteoporosis.

induction of puberty with gonadotropins partially correct this growth disturbance (96, 98).

The skeletal dysplasia of thalassemia is related to iron chelation treatment. Iron chelation with desferrioxamine or oral deferasirox to prevent iron overload has dramatically impacted the health status of patients who require transfusions for thalassemia major (99–101). Desferrioxamine, although essential in prolonging survival among transfusion-dependent patients, causes significant skeletal dysplasia in approximately 50% of cases (102). The findings include a slowing of spinal growth, biconcave vertebrae that progress to platyspondyly in some cases, and physeal widening at the wrist and knee that, in some patients, were severe enough to resemble rickets. Biopsies from patients with desferrioxamine-induced dysplasia show reduced and irregular bone mineralization as well as significant alterations in cartilage histology (103, 104). The spinal deformities are typically progressive, but metaphyseal lesions may heal with reduction of the desferrioxamine dose or following a switch to other iron chelators (105, 106). Skeletal dysplasias have not been reported with the newer oral iron chelator deferasirox (99, 107).

Osteopenia is a major skeletal manifestation of thalassemia major, occurring in more than 90% of patients despite optimal transfusion and chelation (108). Bone mineral density is lower in patients who have delayed puberty or amenorrhea (109, 110), indicating a possible role for endocrinopathy in the pathogenesis of osteopenia. Decreased bone density in

patients with thalassemia is predominantly trabecular and associated with iron deposition (111). Consistent biochemical alterations in bone turnover have not been found (112). In patients with impaired sexual maturation, bone mineral density increases in response to hormone replacement therapy (113). In GH-deficient patients, GH administration can normalize markers of bone turnover but does not increase bone density (114). Bisphosphonates were ineffective in increasing bone mineral density in two placebo-controlled trials (115, 116).

Fractures are common in patients with thalassemia major, although they occur less often since the widespread use of young-onset transfusions began. The 40% to 50% incidence of fractures reported in some early series (117–119) has decreased to 13% to 21% in recent series (120–122). However, a multicenter review (121) found fractures to be often multiple or recurrent. The orthopaedist treating a fracture in a child with thalassemia should consider the problems of multiple fractures, weakened bone, high refracture risk, and clinically significant anemia.

The problems associated with transfusions and chelation have led to a search for alternative medical treatments for the thalassemias. Hydroxyurea, which stimulates hemoglobin F production, may prove effective (123), although at the time of writing this chapter, it has not been approved by the U.S. FDA for children with thalassemia. Bone marrow transplantation has been used successfully in several centers for the treatment of severe thalassemia (124–126), but it has not been shown to prevent osteopenia (109). Stem cell transplantation from umbilical cord blood of related donors has also been used with some success (127). Despite success in a mouse model (128), gene therapy for thalassemia is not yet a clinical reality.

DISORDERS OF NEUTROPHILS AND LYMPHOCYTES

The major cellular components of the immune system include neutrophils, lymphocytes, monocytes, and macrophages. Neutrophils serve as a first line of defense against bacterial and fungal diseases. Neutrophils circulate in the peripheral blood and, through a complex chemotactic process, migrate to sites of infection where they recognize, phagocytose, and kill pathogenic microorganisms. Lymphocytes are classified as B cells derived from bone marrow and T cells derived from the thymus. B cells control humoral immunity and T cells control cellular immunity. The complex interaction of the cells of the immune system is mediated largely through cytokines, and a discussion of this process is beyond the scope of this chapter. This section will discuss disorders of neutrophils [chronic granulomatous disease (CGD)], B cells [X-linked agammaglobulinemia (XLA)], and T cells (acquired immunodeficiency syndrome) that are relevant to the pediatric orthopaedist.

Chronic Granulomatous Disease.
CGD commonly causes recurrent, deep, bacterial or fungal infections of the musculoskeletal system, including osteomyelitis. Therefore, despite being a rare disease, CGD should enter the orthopaedist's mind in the setting of atypical, unusually severe, or difficult-to-treat infections.

CGD is the most common congenital disorder affecting neutrophils, and occurs in approximately 1 in 200,000 to 1 in 500,000 live births (129). The disorder can be inherited in an X-linked recessive or autosomal recessive fashion. A key component of neutrophil function is the respiratory burst. After phagocytosis, creation of hydrogen peroxide and hypochlorous acid in the phagosome allows optimal killing of ingested pathogenic microorganisms. The creation of these oxidants is dependent on nicotinamide adenine dinucleotide phosphate (NADPH) oxidase. CGD is a group of disorders characterized by a variety of mutations of any of the NADPH component genes, transmitted in X-linked or autosomal patterns (130). The mean age at diagnosis depends on the type of CGD. X-linked CGD presents at a mean age of 3 years, whereas the autosomal recessive types typically present at 7 to 8 years (129). The diagnosis of CGD is made by detecting *in vitro* dysfunction of the respiratory burst (130).

The respiratory burst is particularly important in the killing of catalase-positive microorganisms. Catalase-positive organisms commonly encountered in infections in patients with CGD include *S. aureus*, gram-negative enteric bacteria, *Burkholderia* spp., *Nocardia* spp., and *Aspergillus* spp. (129).

Infections with catalase-negative organisms such as *S. pneumoniae* and *Haemophilus influenzae* are uncommon because such organisms produce hydrogen peroxide that can be used by the neutrophil for killing when NADPH oxidase is ineffective.

Children with CGD typically present with recurrent bacterial and fungal infections (131). These infections can be superficial, such as lymphadenitis, infectious dermatitis, and perirectal abscesses, or deep, such as pneumonia, liver abscesses, and osteomyelitis. Also, the lack of the oxidant products of the respiratory burst, which would have acted to mediate or suppress further neutrophil chemotaxis, allows continued recruitment of neutrophils and the formation of granulomata.

Osteomyelitis occurs in approximately 25% of patients with CGD, according to a review of 368 patients in a national registry (129). Common sites include the hands and feet (132), as well as the spine and ribs (133). *Aspergillus* infections of the spine are typically difficult to treat. Some experts recommend surgical debridement with the wound left open to heal secondarily (133), although others have reported successful medical cure of spinal *Aspergillus* osteomyelitis using interferon-γ and antifungals (134–136). One child with tibial *Aspergillus* osteomyelitis was successfully treated with interferon-γ and antifungals after failure of surgical debridement (137).

The treatment of established infections should be aggressive, with early surgical debridement and liberal use of antibiotics. Accurate cultures are essential, because pathogens uncommonly encountered in the general pediatric population are common causes of infection in patients with CGD. The possibility of fungal infection should always be specifically investigated with fungal smears and cultures.

Prophylaxis against infection is important in the treatment of children with CGD. Routine preventative measures such as hand-washing and good hygiene assume paramount importance in these individuals. Prophylactic administration of interferon-γ (138), itraconazole (139), or Bactrim helps to prevent infections.

Until recently, fewer than 50% of patients lived beyond the second decade of life (129); however, the long-term prognosis for children with CGD seems to be improving (140). Stem cell transplantation has been used with some success to "cure" CGD (141). Gene therapy has shown promise, but has yet to show lasting clinical efficacy (142). Bone marrow transplantation may soon have a role as well (143).

X-Linked Agammaglobulinemia.
XLA, an inherited defect in B cell maturation and function, may present to the orthopaedist as a clinical picture of arthritis. Arthritis occurs in XLA for unclear reasons and may be an initial presenting symptom in children at an average age of 2 years (144). Fifteen of sixty-nine patients in one series had arthritis at initial presentation; only four of these cases were due to infection (145). The arthritis of XLA most often affects the knees, wrists, ankles, and fingers, and may be polyarticular in presentation (146). The clinical picture may closely resemble juvenile rheumatoid arthritis (147). Synovitis is present, and the synovial tissue has a large number of suppressor

T lymphocytes, differentiating it pathologically from that of juvenile rheumatoid arthritis (148). Septic arthritis must be ruled out in both acute and chronic presentations because mycoplasmal infection was the leading cause of chronic arthritis in a series of 358 patients with XLA (149). The arthritis, if aseptic, usually responds to immune globulin treatment and anti-inflammatory medication (146). A knowledge of the clinical picture and consequences of XLA will allow the orthopaedist to appropriately refer patients for further evaluation and treatment.

Initially reported by Bruton in 1953 as the first recognized primary immunodeficiency, XLA is otherwise known as *Bruton agammaglobulinemia* (150). XLA results from one of more than 750 possible mutations in the gene for B-lymphocyte tyrosine kinase, which is necessary for B cell maturation (151). The immunologic abnormality of XLA therefore consists of very low numbers of mature B cells and profoundly decreased production of all three major immunoglobulin classes (152). The number and function of T cells are usually normal.

Individuals with XLA are normal at birth, but as maternal IgG levels begin to decline in the first few months, recurrent infections begin to appear (153). Respiratory infections are common and are typically caused by organisms such as *Streptococcus* spp. and *H. influenzae* (144). Infections are usually severe enough to require hospitalization before a diagnosis of XLA is made (154). Therefore, the orthopaedist who is evaluating a child with unexplained arthritis should inquire about past history of hospitalization for respiratory or other infections. Infectious disease consultation should be obtained if an infection history accompanies a clinical picture of arthritis in young children.

The diagnosis of XLA is presumed in the setting of hypogammaglobulinemia and very low numbers of circulating B-lymphocytes. Treatment of XLA consists of immune globulin replacement and aggressive treatment of infections. Immune globulin, given as a regular prophylaxis, can lower the incidence of respiratory infections or other systemic infection and thereby prolong life (155). Recurrent respiratory infections lead to chronic lung disease, and respiratory failure is a major cause of mortality (153).

DISORDERS OF THE MONOCYTE–MACROPHAGE SYSTEM

The monocyte–macrophage system is a group of cell types derived from a common bone marrow precursor that provides important immune functions in various parts of the body. Macrophages ingest cellular debris, pathogens, and foreign bodies, and are particularly abundant in the spleen, liver, lymph nodes, lungs, and bone. Osteoclasts are a specialized form of macrophage, derived from the same precursor. Dendritic cells are nonphagocytic antigen-presenting cells that are thought to arise from the monocyte-macrophage stem cell. A wide variety of diseases affect the monocyte-macrophage system. Two diseases with musculoskeletal manifestations discussed in this chapter are Gaucher disease, which is a lysosomal storage disease, and Langerhans cell histiocytosis (LCH), which is a dendritic cell proliferative disorder.

Gaucher Disease. Lysosomal storage disorders involve deficiencies of catabolic enzymes that allow toxic accumulation of metabolic pathway products. A variety of enzyme deficiencies lead to a variety of diseases with different manifestations. The most common lysosomal storage disease is Gaucher disease, and this example will be discussed in detail in this chapter. Gaucher disease has significant skeletal manifestations, and can require orthopaedic attention for bone pain, osteomyelitis, osteopenia, pathologic fractures, and ON.

In his doctoral thesis in 1882, Phillipe Charles Ernest Gaucher described a disease that causes splenic enlargement (156). The cause of the disease was not identified until 1965, when Brady et al. (157) linked it to a deficiency of glucocerebrosidase, a membrane-bound enzyme responsible for cleaving glucocerebroside. The lipid glucocerebroside accumulates in macrophages, and such lipid-laden macrophages are termed *Gaucher cells*. The clinical manifestations of Gaucher disease are caused by the accumulation of these cells in organs, resulting in organ dysfunction.

Gaucher disease is the most common inherited lysosomal storage disease, with an autosomal recessive inheritance pattern and a prevalence of 1 in 40,000 in the general population and 1 in 400 to 1 in 600 among Ashkenazi Jews (158–161). Three forms of Gaucher disease are recognized: type 1 (nonneuronopathic), type 2 (acute neuronopathic), and type 3 (subacute neuronopathic). Type 1 is by far the most common form and is characterized by hepatosplenomegaly, pancytopenia, and predominant skeletal manifestations. Type 2 is a rare form that involves the central nervous system and cranial nerves and usually causes death by apnea or aspiration before the age of 2 years (162). Type 3 disease is characterized by neurologic symptoms, including seizures, that begin during adolescence (163). More than 100 disease-producing mutations of the *glucocerebrosidase* gene, which is located on the short arm of chromosome 1, have been identified (163), and some mutations predict the phenotype (164). The detection of glucocerebroside in blood and urine confirms the diagnosis of Gaucher disease.

The age at onset and clinical presentation depend upon the genotype and clinical type. In a series of 53 patients, Zimran et al. (165) found that the average age at diagnosis was 25 years (range, 8 months to 70 years). Another series (164) of 34 children and adolescents with type 1 disease found that most of them presented before the age of 10 years. A patient with Gaucher disease may present initially to the orthopaedist with musculoskeletal symptoms. Bone pain or fracture is the reason for presentation in 13% to 60% of patients (165, 166). Growth retardation is also a common musculoskeletal presenting symptom, with 26% and 30% of patients presenting with less than the third percentile of normal values for weight and height, respectively (164). Skeletal abnormalities are detected radiographically in 88% to 94% of patients at presentation (164, 166).

The clinical manifestations of Gaucher disease depend on which organs are affected by accumulated Gaucher cells. Splenic involvement causes splenomegaly and can cause hypersplenism, leading to anemia, thrombocytopenia, or pancytopenia. Liver involvement can cause mild liver dysfunction. Impaired hepatic synthesis of clotting factors may compound the thrombocytopenia, causing clinically significant coagulopathy.

Skeletal involvement is a prominent feature in Gaucher disease and substantially impacts the quality of life (165, 167). In a review of 602 patients with type 1 Gaucher disease from the Gaucher registry, 21% were found to have some form of disability in mobility related to skeletal involvement (168). Skeletal manifestations include pain, deformity, osteopenia, ON, osteomyelitis, pathologic fracture, and vertebral collapse (167). Gaucher disease is associated with a classic abnormality that shows up on radiographs as an "Erlenmeyer flask" deformity of the distal femur and proximal tibia, representing impairment of remodeling (Fig. 10-5). However, this finding is not pathognomonic for Gaucher disease and occurs only in 56% to 70% of patients with known Gaucher disease (165, 166).

Bone crises are a common symptom of skeletal involvement. Bone crises are thought to be related to intramedullary or subperiosteal hemorrhage (169, 170) made possible by thrombocytopenia and deficient clotting factor synthesis. Bone crises are episodes of acute bone pain accompanied by fever, leukocytosis, and elevated erythrocyte sedimentation rate. Because of this clinical picture, bone crises are also known as *pseudo-osteomyelitis*. Blood cultures may help differentiate between bone crisis and osteomyelitis. Further differentiation is difficult, as in SCD, and imaging studies may not be helpful. Early in bone crises, plain radiographs are normal, but may progress to show periosteal reaction and areas of radiolucency (171, 172). Radionuclide bone scans may show an area of decreased uptake early in the course of the process (173) and increased uptake

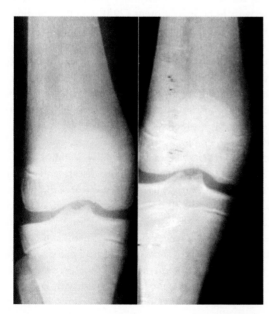

FIGURE 10-5. Radiographs of the knee in a child with Gaucher disease. Note the typical flaring of the distal femoral metaphysis, or Erlenmeyer flask deformity. (Photo courtesy of Henry J. Mankin, MD.)

around a photopenic area later in the course (174). MRI shows marrow edema on T2-weighted images, with or without signs of hemorrhage (168, 170). Periosteal fluid accumulation seen on MRI may indicate infection and should be aspirated for culture under sterile conditions and radiographic guidance.

Treatment of bone crises is supportive. Severe pain early in the course usually requires opioid analgesics, which can be augmented with high-dose prednisolone (175). The symptoms gradually abate over 2 to 4 weeks. Failure of the symptoms to improve should warrant further investigation into the possibility of osteomyelitis. Bone aspiration in an operating room setting may be required. Osteomyelitis can follow a bone crisis, often with anaerobic organisms, suggesting that there has been a period of ischemia (176). Treatment of osteomyelitis in Gaucher disease parallels that in SCD as discussed earlier, although attention should be paid to the altered structural integrity of bone and increased bleeding risk when surgical debridement is considered in a patient with Gaucher disease. ON can follow a bone crisis, so routine radiographic evaluation of an affected area is necessary even after the crisis resolves.

Chronic bone pain varies in severity and does not correlate well with other signs of skeletal involvement. Back pain is common in children with spinal involvement (177). Chronic back pain may be severe enough to require bracing.

ON occurs in 12% to 34% of patients with Gaucher disease (165, 166, 168). The common sites are the femoral head, femoral condyles, tibial plateau, and humeral head (167, 172). Despite poor radiographic findings following ON, total joint arthroplasty is not often required (178). Of the 1476 patients in the Gaucher Registry, 79% of whom were adults, total joint arthroplasty had been performed in only 13% (168). The possibility that thrombosis plays a role in the pathogenesis of ON is supported by elevated D-dimer levels in patients with Gaucher disease and ON compared to those without ON (179).

Pathologic fractures are not uncommon in patients with Gaucher disease. Fractures occurred in 23% of 1476 patients in the Gaucher Registry (168). The common sites of fracture are the distal femur, proximal tibia, and femoral neck, and 65% of the fractures occur at the site of a prior bone crisis (180). Fractures at the base of the femoral neck occur in young children and can be complicated by coxa vara, pseudoarthrosis, and ON. Vertebral compression fractures occur with spinal involvement and can lead to severe kyphosis and spinal cord compromise on rare occasions (177, 181). Fracture healing is impaired in patients with untreated Gaucher disease, and delayed union and nonunion are common.

Osteopenia is nearly universal in Gaucher disease in children (167). Osteopenia can affect trabecular and cortical bone and present as a focal or diffuse process (168). Osteopenia in Gaucher disease can be quantified by dual-energy x-ray absorptiometry (DEXA) (182, 183) or broadband ultrasound attenuation of the calcaneus (182). Quantitative computed tomography (CT) can also accurately measure bone mineral density, but is not recommended in children because of the very high radiation doses involved (184). Chemical markers of bone turnover are also abnormal in Gaucher disease. When compared with a

control group, patients with Gaucher disease had elevated urinary excretion of pyridinoline and deoxypyridinoline (182), as
well as elevated serum levels of carboxy terminal telopeptide of
type I collagen (185), all of which are markers of bone resorption. Serum levels of carboxyterminal propeptide of type I collagen, a marker of bone formation, are significantly lower in
patients with Gaucher disease than in the controls (185).

Infiltration of bone marrow by Gaucher cells can be quantified. Quantitative chemical shift imaging (QCSI) is an MR
spectroscopic technique that utilizes the difference in resonance
between fat and water in bone marrow to quantify the reduction in fat fraction that occurs in Gaucher disease (186, 187).
Marrow infiltration in vertebral bodies measured by QCSI correlates well with disease severity (187), and the technique is reproducible (188). A bone marrow burden score has recently been
developed to allow quantification of marrow infiltration using
standard MRI (189), with high inter- and intrarater reliability
and sensitivity only slightly less than that of QCSI. Several other
semiquantitative techniques using standard MRI have been
developed and are currently under investigation (184, 190).

Because Gaucher disease is a deficiency of a specific
enzyme, enzyme replacement therapy (ERT) is the cornerstone
of treatment. In fact, replacement of macrophage-directed glucocerebrosidase has become standard medical treatment for
type 1 Gaucher disease (164, 191–193). Given intravenously at
2-week intervals, ERT reliably reverses anemia, thrombocytopenia, and splenomegaly with a dose-dependent (194) relationship. Although marrow infiltration responds more variably and
more slowly (195–197), bone mineral density and bone pain
improve with ERT (198, 199). Children tend to respond more
quickly and reliably than adults (199). Enzyme replacement,
if started early in life, can prevent skeletal deformity and allow
normal skeletal development and growth (200, 201). A decrease
in the incidence of fractures has also been observed (202). Bone
marrow transplantation has been used in patients with a variety
of lysosomal storage diseases, including Gaucher disease (203).
Also, because the pathogenesis of Gaucher disease involves an
accumulation of glucocerebroside, efforts to decrease production of this molecule may prove effective in treating the disease
(204). Gene therapy is not yet routinely available.

Langerhans Cell Histiocytosis. LCH refers to a disease
complex characterized by abnormal proliferation of a marrow-
derived histiocytic cell initially described by Langerhans in 1868
(205). The skeletal manifestations of LCH were not described in
detail in the literature until a report by Fraser in 1935 (205). In
1940, Lichtenstein and Jaffe coined the term *eosinophilic granuloma of bone* (205). One year later, Farber argued that eosinophilic granuloma of bone belonged to the same spectrum as
Hand-Schüller-Christian disease and Letterer-Siwe disease. Later
Lichtenstein grouped all three conditions under the term *histiocytosis X* (205). In 1961, Birbeck used electron microscopy to
detect the oblong granules in Langerhans cells (205), but it was
not until 1973 that Nezelof identified these granules in specimens of histiocytosis X and recognized the disease as a proliferation of Langerhans cells (206). Today, the term LCH is the
preferred name of the spectrum of conditions.

Approximately two to five cases of LCH are diagnosed
per million persons per year (207, 208). The median age at
diagnosis is between 1 and 3 years, but the diagnosis can be
made at any age from infancy to over 80 years (209). There
is a slight male preponderance in the occurrence of the condition (210, 211). Bone involvement is found in 80% to 97%
of patients with LCH (208, 210–215). The skull is the most
often affected bone, followed by the femur, spine, ribs, mandible, and pelvis (216–218). Bone involvement in the hands
and feet is uncommon (219, 220). Widespread involvement of
multiple organ systems can occur and carries a worse prognosis
than isolated bone involvement (221). This chapter will discuss in detail the evaluation and management of bone lesions
only, whether solitary or multiple.

The most common pattern of LCH at presentation in children is a solitary bone lesion without a soft-tissue mass (108,
213–215). Polyostotic involvement is seen at presentation in
10% of cases (222). Presentation with a solitary bone lesion
carries a favorable prognosis, and no deaths have been reported
in this group (208, 213, 214, 223, 224). It is uncommon for
patients who present with solitary bone lesions to develop secondary bone lesions. However, a series with 52 patients found
that 30% of them developed secondary bone lesions, half of
which were asymptomatic; the lesions were detected during routine skeletal surveys (215). The prognosis in patients with multiple bone involvement without soft-tissue lesions is still favorable,
with death occurring in 1 of 22 patients in one series (208).

The most common symptoms of LCH of bone are pain,
swelling, or limping. The pain is usually of <2 months' duration. Symptoms such as lethargy, cough, dyspnea, and failure
to thrive are uncommon, and may indicate widespread
involvement. Because diabetes insipidus is the most common extraskeletal abnormality that develops in patients presenting with bone involvement (225), specific questioning is
required regarding polyuria and polydipsia. Skin rash, jaundice, hepatosplenomegaly, tachypnea, exophthalmos, hearing
difficulties, and poor growth are important signs of widespread
involvement. Physical examination may reveal a tender mass
associated with a bone lesion in the skull, jaw, or extremities.
Torticollis, scoliosis, kyphosis, and neurologic impairment
may accompany a spine lesion (226–230).

Plain radiographs are the first step in evaluating LCH
of bone (Fig. 10-6). The radiographic appearance of LCH of
bone depends upon the phase of the disease and the site of
occurrence. In the early phase of the disease, the lesion may
appear aggressive, with a permeative pattern of osteolysis
and laminated periosteal reaction mimicking Ewing sarcoma
(231–233). Later in the course of the disease, the lesion
appears less aggressive, with well-defined margins, a narrow
zone of transition, and mature or absent periosteal reaction
(220). Widening of the medullary cavity with cortical thinning, scalloping, or penetration are also common findings in
long bone lesions (220). In the long bones, the lesion typically
exists in the diaphysis or metaphysis. Epiphyseal involvement
is uncommon (220, 234, 235). In the skull, LCH may give rise
to a lesion that appears round, radiolucent, and "punched-out"
when viewed on plain radiographs (Fig. 10-7).

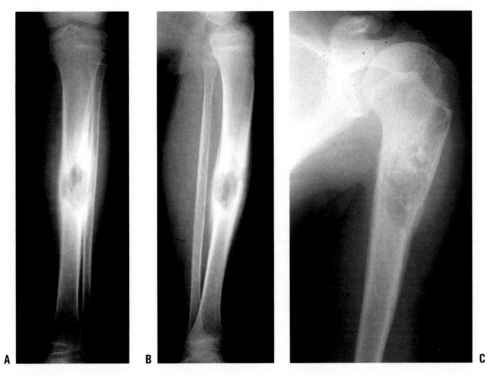

FIGURE 10-6. Langerhans cell histiocytosis of the tibia (**A, B**) and of the proximal humerus (**C**) in two children. In both cases, the lesions healed following biopsy, both symptomatically and by radiographic findings.

The classic manifestation of LCH in the spine is *vertebra plana*. The vertebral body is markedly flattened, but the posterior elements are usually spared. In contrast to osteomyelitis, the disc spaces are preserved in LCH. The thoracic vertebrae are affected in more than half of the patients. Cervical spine involvement is uncommon (220), but involvement of the posterior elements in the cervical spine has been reported (236, 237), as has cervical vertebral body involvement without vertebra plana (238).

Skeletal surveys or bone scans should be performed in the diagnostic workup of any patient with a radiographic lesion resembling LCH. In fact, one should consider obtaining results from both studies, as neither is wholly sensitive: in one series of 42 patients who were studied with both modalities, bone scans missed 36 of 191 lesions (19%), and skeletal surveys missed 55 (29%) (239). Bone scans were more effective at detecting lesions in locations that are difficult to view clearly on plain radiographs, such as the ribs, spine, and pelvis. CT can demonstrate the extent of bony destruction. MRI is helpful in evaluating the extent of the lesion, soft-tissue involvement, and marrow edema. A high-intensity signal is seen on T2-weighted images within and around the lesion (231). MRIs may be normal initially but progress to markedly abnormal within a few weeks (240). Because many patients present with a lesion that radiographically resembles a sarcoma of bone, MRI is essential for ruling out the soft-tissue mass that often accompanies a sarcoma.

Laboratory evaluation of patients with suspected LCH should include a complete blood count, liver function tests,

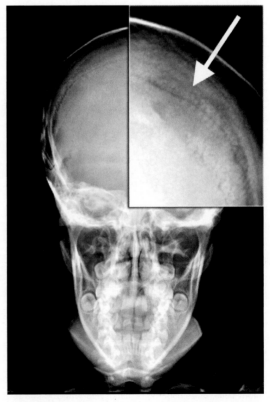

FIGURE 10-7. Langerhans cell histiocytosis lesion in the skull (*arrow*, **inset**).

and serum and urine osmolality if history suggests diabetes insipidus. A hematology/oncology consultation is essential for all patients with suspected LCH. For patients with evidence of multiple organ involvement or for patients younger than 3 years with multiple bone lesions, investigations such as arterial blood gas; bone marrow aspirate; CT of the chest; abdominal ultrasonography; and audiology, dental, and immunologic assessments may be obtained as indicated in coordination with the oncology team (215).

The diagnosis of LCH depends on histopathology. Skin biopsies are easy to perform and are recommended when skin involvement is present. In the absence of skin involvement, bone lesions, preferably the most easily accessible, should be biopsied. Biopsies can be performed either open or by CT-guided needle aspiration. Some experts have reported an accuracy of as high as 90% to 100% for needle aspiration (241, 242). Biopsies of suspicious lesions must be sent as fresh specimens, because immunohistochemical tests for α-D-mannosidase and CD1a are not possible with paraffin-embedded tissue.

Histologically, the Langerhans cell is a large, mononuclear cell with a grooved nucleus and characteristic racket-shaped organelles (Birbeck granules) in the cytoplasm. Langerhans cells are considered to be antigen-presenting cells that are members of the dendritic cell family (243, 244). Pathologic Langerhans cells (LCH cells) phenotypically represent Langerhans cells arrested at an early stage of maturation, in that they lack certain differentiated features of dendritic cells (245). The exact pathogenesis of LCH is unknown, and theories of viral, reactive, and neoplastic etiologies have been put forth with variable supporting evidence. Langerhans cells are not the only cells in an LCH lesion, and are accompanied by T cells, eosinophils, and macrophages (246) (Fig. 10-8).

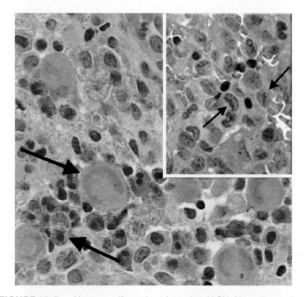

FIGURE 10-8. Hematoxylin and eosin stain of LCH. Note the eosinophils, giant cells, and Langerhans histiocytes with the coffee bean–shaped nucleus showing a central groove (*arrows*, **inset**).

The typical natural tendency of bone lesions, especially in the absence of systemic involvement, is toward resolution, irrespective of whether or not the lesions were treated (236, 247). Most lesions will resolve following biopsy alone. One series (236) found that of 26 patients with solitary lesions, 25 showed partial or complete healing after a mean of 4 years, despite the fact that only 4 were treated in any way. Also, two of the four treated patients suffered treatment-related complications. Reappearance of a trabecular pattern is seen in bone lesions 6 to 10 weeks after diagnosis, and complete healing is seen at 36 to 40 weeks on radiographic investigation (248). Failure to heal after approximately 4 months of observation may indicate the need for intervention.

Treatment of LCH of bone is generally limited to lesions that cause substantial pain or threaten pathologic fracture. There are several treatment options for bone (249) lesions. Curettage with or without bone grafting hastens the healing process (250). Intralesional injection of steroids relieves the pain of bone lesions (251, 252). Indomethacin has been used successfully in treating the symptoms of LCH in 8 of 10 children in one series (253). Low-dose radiotherapy is effective in widespread disease (254); however, the risk of secondary malignancy (215, 255) probably outweighs the advantages of radiation for solitary bone lesions.

Skeletal surveys assist in localizing multiple lesions, and MRI can identify a soft-tissue mass that would raise the suspicion of a sarcoma. We prefer an open biopsy with intraoperative frozen section. Sufficient tissue is needed for histology, immunohistochemistry, cultures, and occasionally electron microscopy or molecular genetics studies. Intraoperative frozen section confirms the acquisition of lesional tissue and can support the diagnosis of LCH.

For symptomatic spine involvement, short-term immobilization with casts or braces can provide relief (256). Vertebral height typically reconstitutes. Neurologic dysfunction is uncommon with spine involvement (230, 257). MRI is required whenever there is neurologic dysfunction, and can differentiate between nerve root and spinal cord compression. Surgical decompression and stabilization are indicated for spinal cord compression, whereas bedrest with systemic or injected corticosteroids can effectively treat nerve root compression. In the absence of nerve root or cord compression, long-term back and neck problems from spine LCH are uncommon (257).

Widespread, multiorgan LCH carries a poor prognosis. Chemotherapy, interferon, and bone marrow transplantation have been used with some success.

DISORDERS OF HEMOSTASIS

Hemostasis involves a complex interaction between elements of the circulatory and hematopoietic systems. Normal hemostasis begins with vascular injury. Injury to a blood vessel causes vasoconstriction, helping to stem blood loss. Disruption of the endothelium allows interaction between vessel wall components and circulating platelets and plasma components.

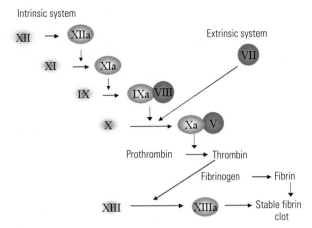

FIGURE 10-9. Schematic depiction of the intrinsic and extrinsic pathways of the clotting cascade. See text for details.

Platelet aggregation occurs in response to the injury in the endothelium and, with the assistance of the von Willebrand factor (vWF), begins the process of thrombus formation. In the plasma, coagulation factors interact to form fibrin, which completes the thrombogenic process.

The process by which plasma-clotting factors contribute to thrombogenesis is termed the *clotting cascade* (Fig. 10-9). The intrinsic pathway is stimulated by collagen exposure and the extrinsic pathway by tissue thromboplastin. Both pathways result in activation of factor X, which combines with activated factor V to convert prothrombin into thrombin, which in turn converts fibrinogen into fibrin. Of particular relevance to disorders of hemostasis are factors VIII and IX, which combine to activate factor X in the intrinsic pathway. Intrinsic pathway function is measured in the laboratory by the activated partial thromboplastin time (aPTT), and extrinsic pathway function by the prothrombin time (PT). The functions of specific factors can be assessed by quantifying their activity levels. Disorders of platelet function are evaluated by platelet aggregation and release assays.

Hemophilia. Hemophilia is a disorder of hemostasis caused by a deficiency of clotting factor. Hemophilia A is a deficiency of factor VIII, whereas hemophilia B, or Christmas disease, is a deficiency of factor IX. In a large surveillance study in the United States, the incidence of hemophilia was found to be 1 in 5032 live male births, with an age-adjusted prevalence of 13.4 per 100,000 among the male sex (258). Seventy-nine percent of these had hemophilia A. Extrapolation of the prevalence data from the six states represented in the United States study estimated that, in 1994, there were approximately 16,000 persons with hemophilia nationwide (258).

Both forms of hemophilia are typically transmitted in a sex-linked recessive pattern, largely limiting the disorder to the male sex. Female carriers may also be symptomatic, despite the recessive nature of the gene. Skewed random inactivation of the normal X chromosome may result in reduced levels of clotting factor and a consequent bleeding diathesis in these girls and women (259).

Deficiencies in factors VIII and IX are clinically indistinguishable. The clinical manifestations of hemophilia depend on its severity. Severe clotting factor deficiency (<1% factor activity) leads to spontaneous joint and soft-tissue bleeds. In moderate hemophilia (1% to 5% factor activity), spontaneous bleeds are uncommon, but excessive bleeding and hemarthroses can occur following minor trauma. In mild hemophilia (5% to 40% factor activity), abnormal bleeding is typically seen only following major trauma or surgery. According to surveillance data, hemophilia is severe in 43% of patients, moderate in 26%, and mild in 31% (258).

Hemarthroses and muscle hematomas are common in hemophilia and comprise most of the pathology that the orthopaedist sees. The knee, elbow, and ankle are the most commonly affected joints (260–262). The shoulder, hip, and wrist are less often affected. An acute hemarthrosis causes pain, warmth, and swelling in the affected joint; these symptoms abate over a period of a few days if properly treated. Hemophilic arthropathy is a degeneration of joints following recurrent hemarthroses, and can be quite destructive and debilitating. Muscle hematomas usually occur in the pelvis, thigh, buttocks and arm. These hematomas cause pain, swelling, and muscle spasm, and may also induce compartment syndrome or nerve palsies. Recurrent intramuscular bleeding, particularly if inadequately treated, can lead to the development of pseudotumors, or "blood cysts," in the extremities and pelvis. Hematuria and bleeding from mucosal surfaces in the mouth and nose also occur to a variable extent but will not be discussed in this chapter. Other serious consequences include airway compromise from neck hematomas and neurologic compromise from intracranial bleeding.

Hemophilia is suspected in infants who have a positive family history, excessive bleeding from circumcision, or easy bruising from minor trauma or immunizations. A single swollen joint from minor trauma can also be a presenting sign of hemophilia (263). In a recent study of children with severe hemophilia, the first clue that pointed toward the diagnosis was hematoma in 47%, family history in 24%, and excessive bleeding after an operation in 14% (264). Mouth, joint, and muscle bleeds prompted the diagnosis in 5% each. All the children were diagnosed prior to 2 years of age, with 81% being diagnosed during the first year of life and 38% in the first month of life. However, others have found a higher prevalence of mild and moderate hemophilia in the 5- to 14-year-old age group than in the 1- to 4-year-old age group, suggesting a delay in diagnosis of milder forms of hemophilia (258).

Measuring the activity of the clotting factors makes the diagnosis of hemophilia; hemophilia exists if factor activity is <40% of normal. The aPTT is typically prolonged because the deficient factors affect the intrinsic coagulation pathway. The PT and the platelet count are normal.

The administration of factor is the first step in the acute treatment of any bleeding episode in a patient with hemophilia, especially prior to any necessary emergent surgical intervention. Factor replacement should be administered prior to elective invasive procedures, even those as simple as injections, radiographic studies, and suturing of lacerations. Many different formulations of factor VIII and IX replacement concentrates are available, and each has its own limitations. The discovery of cryoprecipitate and concentrated clotting factors in the 1960s (265–267) made the replacement of deficient factors realizable for patients with hemophilia. However, such preparations of factor were derived from pooled sources of human blood and therefore had the potential to transmit disease. Exposure to hepatitis B or C was found in up to 85% of patients with severe hemophilia in the 1980s (268–270). HIV was found to infect 70% of stored hemophilic blood samples that were collected in 1982 (271), and by June 1991, 91% of the cases of HIV infection that were reported to the Center for Disease Control and Prevention were in patients with hemophilia (272). The heat treatment of factor concentrates, instituted in 1984, has effectively eliminated the transmission of HIV, and newer forms of virus inactivation have essentially eliminated the transmission of hepatitis. Factors VIII and IX are mostly now derived from recombinant DNA techniques, virtually eliminating the risk of disease transmission. Such products are now considered the replacement factors of choice (273), despite their higher initial cost.

Patients with hemophilia can develop antibodies to exogenous factor VIII, or rarely factor IX, and if these antibodies deactivate the exogenous factor they are termed *inhibitors*. Inhibitors to factor VIII have been reported in 3.6% to 52% of patients with hemophilia (274). Once a patient develops an inhibitor, exogenous factor replacement no longer corrects their coagulation deficit. Although bleeds do not increase in frequency, they are harder to treat. Patients with low titers of inhibitors can often be treated simply with higher doses of factor replacement. Patients with high titers, however, typically cannot be adequately treated with any exogenous human form of factor VIII. Bleeds in these patients require treatment with bypassing agents such as recombinant activated factor VII (rFVIIa) or activated prothrombin complex concentrates.

Hemophilic Arthropathy.   Degenerative joint disease due to recurrent hemarthrosis is the single largest preventable cause of morbidity for patients with hemophilia A and B. Recurrent spontaneous or trauma induced joint bleeding is often seen in children and adults with severe hemophilia. The impact of hemophilic arthropathy is wide ranging. Many patients miss school or work and require assistive devices for ambulation or completion of activities of daily living (275). The pathogenesis of the resultant arthropathy is multifactorial; however, iron is the most likely culprit triggering the degenerative changes. While any joint can become involved, the ankles are most commonly involved, followed by elbows, knees, and shoulders. Occasionally, the first metatarsal phalangeal joint, wrist, and others are affected.

Two scoring systems exist for evaluating joint deterioration from plain radiographs of patients with hemophilia. The Arnold-Hilgartner score (Table 10-2) was developed based

TABLE 10-2	Arnold-Hilgartner Hemophilic Joint Staging System
Stage I	No skeletal abnormalities visible on the roentgenograms, but there is soft-tissue swelling secondary to the hemarthrosis or bleeding into the soft tissues around the joint
Stage II	There is osteoporosis particularly in the epiphyses as well as overgrowth of the epiphyses. The integrity of the joint is maintained with no narrowing of the joint space or bone cysts
Stage III	The synovium may be opacified with hemosiderin deposits. The intercondylar notch of the knee and intertrochlear notch of the ulna are widened. There may be squaring of the patella. Bony cysts may be present. The joint space is preserved.
Stage IV	Stage III findings are more pronounced and joint space narrowing/cartilage destruction is present.
Stage V	Fibrous joint contracture is present along with loss of joint space, extensive enlargement of the epiphyses and substantial disorganization of the joint structures

Adapted from Arnold WD, Higartner MW. Hemophilic arthropathy. *J Bone Joint Surg Am* 1977;59(3).

upon the theory that blood-induced joint damage occurs in a progressive manner: from early soft-tissue changes to later bony changes (276). The Pettersson scale was developed with the assumption that these changes are additive in nature and can occur concomitantly (277) (Table 10-3). While neither scale has been validated in clinical trials, the Pettersson scale was adopted by the World Federation of Hemophilia, and current evidence suggests that the additive approach is likely to be more valid than the progressive approach (278). Unfortunately, physical findings are often subtle in the early stages of joint disease, and plain radiographs do not adequately evaluate soft-tissue changes. Therefore, investigation with MRI may be required to demonstrate hemosiderin deposition and or hypertrophic synovium. To that end, two MRI scoring systems were proposed. The Denver scale was a progressive scale, while the European scale relied on an additive approach (279, 280). Subsequently, the scales have been merged into a validated compatible scale (281). It remains to be seen if MRI can be used in a predictive manner.

Hemophilic Synovitis.   Similar to inflammatory arthritis, the disease in hemophilia begins with synovitis. A normal synovial lining is thin, consisting of only one to two cell layers. After repeated bleeds, the synovium hypertrophies and becomes villous with intense neovascularization (282, 283). Histologic examination shows iron deposits within the synovium and in subsynovial areas (284). Diffuse lymphocyte and macrophage infiltrates are observed particularly in areas of iron deposition (283, 284). Additionally, hemophilic synovial tissue produces more inflammatory cytokines (IL-1β, IL-6, and tumor necrosis factor alpha) than nonhemophilic synovium (284). Angiogenic

TABLE 10-3	Radiographic/Pettersson (0–13)	
Osteoporosis	Absent	0
	Present	1
Enlarged epiphysis	Absent	0
	Present	1
Irregular subchondral bone	Absent	0
	Partly involved	1
	Totally involved	2
Narrowing of joint space	Absent	0
	Joint space >1 mm	1
	Joint space <1 mm	2
Subchondral cyst formation	Absent	0
	1 cyst	1
	>1 cyst	2
Erosions at joint margins	Absent	0
	Present	1
Incongruence of joint surfaces	Absent	0
	Slight	1
	Pronounced	2
Joint deformity (angulation and/or displacement between the articulating bony ends)	Absent	0
	Slight	1
	Pronounced	2

factors also seem to play a role in hemophilic synovitis. The relative roles of angiogenesis, inflammatory cytokines, and protooncogene influence on the initiation and propagation of the synovial changes seen in hemophilic joint disease are not known. Clinically, however, joints with hypertrophic synovium are predisposed to recurrent bleeding and rapidly progressive joint damage. Decreased use of these abnormal joints leads to progressive muscular atrophy, stiffness, osteoporosis, and a self-perpetuating destruction of the joints. Following effective treatment, the symptoms of joint pain, swelling, stiffness, and warmth should abate over a few days. Factor replacement is continued for the duration of symptoms. In some cases, signs of inflammation persist despite control of the bleeding. Oral corticosteroids have been used in these situations; however, their benefits have not been clearly defined (285, 279).

Articular Cartilage Destruction. As the synovitis persists, articular cartilage begins to suffer. Articular cartilage consists of chondrocytes in an extracellular matrix of collagen fibrils and proteoglycans. Supernatants of cultured hemosiderotic synovial tissue produce inhibition of proteoglycan synthesis relative to nonhemosiderotic synovium from the same hemophilic patient. However, the mechanism of inhibition is not known (284). *In vitro* exposure of normal human or canine cartilage to homologous whole blood showed >98% inhibition of proteoglycan synthesis after 4 days of exposure. This inhibition was still present 2, 5, and 10 weeks (286). In an *in vivo* dog model, proteoglycan synthesis was inhibited by 22%, and proteoglycan content was decreased by 18% 4 days after one injection of autologous blood into the knee joint.

IL-1β is an important mediator in osteoarthritis and rheumatoid arthritis (287). Production of IL-1β appears to be from the mononuclear cells and not from chondrocytes (287). The combination of an iron source from lysed red blood cells (RBCs) and IL-1β causes significant inhibition of proteoglycan synthesis (286). The combination of iron from lysed RBCs and IL-1β from mononuclear cells may also stimulate hydrogen peroxide from within chondrocytes and lead to free radical damage of chondrocytes. Age of cartilage may also be a factor in blood-induced changes. After autologous blood injection into the knee, proteoglycan synthesis is significantly reduced in skeletally immature canine cartilage compared to mature animals (288). Weight bearing after hemarthrosis may be detrimental to articular cartilage. Forced joint loading in combination with joint hemorrhage in this dog model resulted in more pronounced histologically observed cartilage changes compared to joint hemorrhage without forced loading (288). Analysis of human cartilage after exposure to whole blood revealed a significant increase in apoptotic chondrocytes (289).

Authors' Preferred Method of Treatment. Patients with hemophilia benefit from multidisciplinary care in comprehensive hemophilia treatment centers. The treatment of bleeding in hemophilia centers on replacement of the deficient factor via intermittent intravenous infusions. Recommended treatment for common bleeding events is demonstrated in Table 10-4. Most patients or parents of children with hemophilia under routine care for hemophilia are taught to self-administer factor replacement, so treatment often begins at home.

Factor infusions can either be delivered in response to bleeding episodes "demand therapy" or to prevent bleeding "prophylaxis." To prevent or minimize long-term sequela, demand therapy should be given as soon as possible after a bleeding episode is recognized. Because the need for urgent treatment is so important, many patients affected by hemophilia are educated in home infusion techniques. In the emergency department or an office setting, factor replacement therapy should never be delayed to perform imaging or laboratory studies. Demand therapy can be utilized to effectively treat bleeding episodes; however, it is not effective in preventing the most common complication of hemophilia, which is blood-induced joint disease (290).

In developed countries, prophylactic therapy delivered one to four times per week dosed to keep trough levels above 1% is considered standard of care. If prophylactic infusions are started at a young age prior to the development of arthropathy, it is termed primary prophylaxis and is the only therapy proven to prevent the long-term complication of degenerative joint disease (278). While there is no universally accepted starting age, dose or frequency of infusions for primary prophylaxis, it is common practice to begin prophylaxis prior to the onset of recurrent joint bleeding. This is because the risk of irreversible joint damage increases if the onset of prophylaxis is delayed (290a). Secondary prophylaxis refers to long-term factor replacement after a hemophilia complication has been

TABLE 10-4	Suggested Approach to Treatment of Bleeding Episodes in Hemophilia		
Bleed Site	**Desired Factor Level**	**Length of Therapy**	**Considerations**
Central nervous system	100%	7–14 d then prophylaxis for ≥6 mo	Continuous infusion factor Antiepileptic prophylaxis Surgical decompression
Persistent oral/mucosal	30%–60%	3–7 d	Antifibrinolytic therapy Custom mouthpiece Topical thrombin powder
Retropharyngeal	80%–100%	7–14 d	Continuous infusion factor Antifibrinolytic therapy
Nose	30%–60%	1–3 d	Packing, cautery Saline nose spray/gel Nasal vasoconstrictor spray Antifibrinolytic therapy
Gastrointestinal	40%–80%	3–7 d	Antifibrinolytic therapy Endoscopy with cautery
Persistent gross urinary	40%–60%	1–3 d	Vigorous hydration Evaluation for stones/UTI Avoid antifibrinolytic agents Glucocorticoids
Muscle	40%–80%	Every other day until pain free	"RICE" Physical therapy
Iliopsoas	80%–100%	Until radiographic resolution	Continuous infusion factor Bedrest Physical therapy
Joint	40%–80%	1–2 d	"RICE" Physical therapy
Target joint	80% day 1 40% day 2 and 4	3–4 d	"RICE" Physical therapy

"RICE," rest, ice, compression, elevation.
Adapted with permission From Dunn et al Rudolphs Textbook of Pediatrics.

experienced. This practice is commonly utilized after intracranial hemorrhage or once joint disease has become established. While secondary prophylaxis effectively reduces the frequency of bleeding episodes, it has not been shown to halt the progression of joint disease (291, 292).

The dose and frequency of factor delivery are calculated based upon the ½ life of the product (typically 10 to 12 hours for FVIII and 20 to 24 hours for FIX), the intravascular volume of distribution (1 international unit (IU) of FVIII per kilogram raises the plasma concentration by about 2%, and one IU of FIX per kilogram raises the plasma concentration by about 1%,), and the desired clotting factor activity. For example, to raise the factor level of a 30-kilogram child with severe hemophilia A to 100%, the dose should be 30 kg × 50 IU = 1500 IU. Forty percent activity is considered hemostatic in most cases; however, in the setting of surgery or life/limb-threatening hemorrhage, higher levels are necessary. Ancillary measures such as compressive dressings, cautery, packing, and splinting should also be implemented when appropriate. Agents that affect platelet function should be avoided. Table 10-4 illustrates an approach to factor replacement therapy of commonly encountered bleeding events (293).

Desmopressin or DDAVP (1-deamino-8-D-arginine vasopressin) is a synthetic form of the hormone vasopressin. DDAVP causes release of FVIII and vWF from storage sites along the endothelium and within platelet storage granules (294). Patients with mild or moderate hemophilia A can be tested with this product, and their response (rise in FVIII level) can be measured. If patients show a response by manifesting hemostatic levels of FVIII, this product is often sufficient to treat mild bleeding symptoms. FVIII storage pools become depleted after multiple doses, so this treatment is not adequate for lengthy therapy. Additionally, fluid intake must be monitored closely as severe hyponatremia may result (295). In most cases, life- or limb-threatening bleeding episodes require exogenous factor replacement. Antifibrinolytic therapy to stabilize the fibrin clot is particularly useful in diminishing bleeding symptoms in locations with prominent fibrinolytic activity such as the mouth, gastrointestinal tract, and uterus.

Recurrent hemarthroses are common and can lead to progressive joint damage. Prompt treatment of these hemarthroses is therefore essential. Aspiration of a hemarthrosis is rarely helpful. The most important aspect in treatment of an acute hemarthrosis is factor replacement. Factor activity levels should be increased to 50% to 100% of normal until the joint has returned to baseline. Because of the variable preferences for and responses to specific factor formulations among patients with hemophilia, the choice of the factor replacement product should be left to the patient, the patient's hematologist, and the hemophilia treatment center that is coordinating the patient's care.

Nonsteroidal anti-inflammatory medications are typically avoided in these patients because of their tendency toward bleeding complications, so pain control is usually achieved with opioid analgesics. Cyclooxygenase 2–specific inhibitors however can be safely utilized in this population. Ice packs may help alleviate pain and swelling. Immobilization can be helpful for significantly painful hemarthroses, but should be limited to 1 or 2 days, because stiffness following a hemarthrosis can be problematic. Although rest is encouraged when the inflammation is acute, weight bearing is generally allowed as tolerated.

Arthroscopic synovectomy has been utilized in children with hemophilia to remove abnormal synovium and thereby reduce the ill effects of a persistent synovitis. These procedures can be done on an outpatient basis and are highly effective at reducing synovitis and recurrent bleeding. Early intervention, as early as 3 years of age, seems to be key, being associated with better results and fewer complications. Lost motion is the most common complication; joints with narrowed cartilage and significant contractures are at greatest risk and constitute a relative contraindication to surgery. Consistent and effective factor replacement and physical therapy are key to success (296). Articular changes can continue if significant cartilage damage was present at the time of the procedure, and it is yet to be proven how much the synovectomy benefits the articular cartilage over time (297).

Radionuclide synovectomy/synoviorthosis has also been employed with good results to address recurrent bleeding in affected joints. In this procedure, a radioactive compound is injected into the joint and leads to subsequent synovial sclerosis. Multiple agents with different characteristics have been utilized with similar results (298, 299). This procedure is less expensive than arthroscopic synovectomy but has the additional risk of radiation exposure. Two cases of leukemia have been reported in hemophilia patients who had this procedure, but causality is unclear (299a). Our primary indication for choosing radionuclide synovectomy over an arthroscopic synovectomy has been the inhibitor patient for whom clotting management during and following surgery can be extremely difficult and expensive.

von Willebrand Disease.   von Willebrand disease (vWD) is a disorder of hemostasis caused by deficient production or ineffective functioning of vWF, a high-molecular-weight glycoprotein that promotes platelet aggregation in the early phases of hemostasis. vWF also serves as a carrier protein for factor VIII in plasma, and therefore plays an important role in intrinsic coagulation. vWD is the most common inherited bleeding disorder,

affecting 1% to 2% of children in various populations (300, 301). The disorder can be broadly classified into three types: Type 1 vWD refers to a partial quantitative deficiency of vWF; type 2 is a qualitative (functional) deficiency of vWF; type 3 refers to the virtually complete absence of vWF.

Type 1 vWD is the most common form of vWD, accounting for 60% to 80% of cases (302). It is inherited in an autosomal dominant fashion in most cases. Patients typically present with signs and symptoms of a mild coagulopathy, such as easy bruising, prolonged nosebleeds, or abnormal bleeding from surgical or dental procedures (303). In postmenarchal girls, heavy menses are a common finding (304). Diagnosis of type 1 vWD is made by bleeding history, family history, and low plasma levels of vWF antigen, ristocetin cofactor, and factor VIII. Type 2 vWD comprises 15% to 30% of cases of vWD (302). A wide variety of mutations, inherited in a variety of patterns, accounts for several subtypes of type 2 vWD. The clinical presentation is similar to that of type 1 vWD in most subtypes, although some subtypes may have a presentation similar to hemophilia A because of factor VIII deficiency caused by dysfunctional stabilization by the abnormal vWD. Type 3 vWD is the least common major type, accounting for approximately 5% of patients. Synthesis of vWF is impaired, and vWF is virtually undetectable in the plasma. Because of increased proteolysis, Factor VIII levels are typically 1% to 5% of normal, making type 3 vWD clinically indistinguishable from moderate hemophilia A.

The treatment of vWD, as with hemophilia, focuses on correcting the coagulation deficiency. The bleeding diathesis should be corrected prior to any orthopaedic surgery or procedure likely to cause bleeding, including injection and fracture manipulation. In most type 1 and some type 2 patients, desmopressin (1-deamino-8-D-arginine vasopressin; DDAVP), a synthetic analog of vasopressin that increases vWF and factor VIII levels (305), is effective when given intravenously, intranasally, or subcutaneously. Repeated infusions can cause hyponatremia in children if given within a short period of time or if fluid restrictions are not followed (306). Antifibrinolytic agents such as aminocaproic acid and tranexamic acid can be used as adjuncts to DDAVP, and can be given orally, topically, or intravenously. For patients with Type 3 vWD or those otherwise unresponsive to DDAVP, transfusion of vWF containing factor concentrates is the optimal way to achieve and maintain hemostasis. Orthopaedic manifestations of vWD are largely limited to types 2 and 3. Apart from the differences in factor replacement, the treatment of muscle and joint hemorrhages and all resulting complications in type 3 vWD parallels that in hemophilia.

Thrombophilia.   Hemostasis involves an intricate balance between thrombotic and antithrombotic mechanisms. Thrombophilia refers to any condition that predisposes the individual to abnormally increased thrombosis. Venous thromboembolic disease is a common concern in adults, especially following prolonged immobilization or major orthopaedic, abdominal, or pelvic surgery. Pathologic thrombosis in children is uncommon, carrying with it a risk of venous thromboembolism that is one-tenth of the risk in adults (307). Nonetheless, children may have several inherited conditions that cause pathologic thrombosis, the most common of which are (a) protein C deficiency, (b) protein S deficiency, (c) antithrombin deficiency, (d) mutation of factor V (factor V Leiden), and (e) mutation of prothrombin (G20210A prothrombin).

Protein C is a 62-kDa double-chain glycoprotein synthesized by the liver in a vitamin K–dependent fashion. Protein C activation is mediated by thrombin. Activated protein C (APC) exerts two antithrombotic effects: first, APC proteolytically inactivates coagulation factors VIIIa and Va; second, it exerts a fibrinolytic effect by inactivating plasminogen activator inhibitor-1. Deficient production of protein C can result from one of over 150 mutations of the protein C gene, located on chromosome 2 (308). These mutations typically reduce APC activity to approximately 50% of normal, and increase the risk of a venous thromboembolic event (VTE) 10-fold (309). Approximately 1 in 350 individuals (0.3%) are affected (310).

Protein S is a single-chain protein also synthesized in the liver in a vitamin K–dependent fashion. Protein S circulates in the blood, mostly bound to complement factor C4b-binding protein (60%). Free protein S (40%) inhibits thrombogenesis primarily by serving as an APC cofactor. Over 30 mutations in the protein S gene located on chromosome 3 have been found, any of which may cause protein S deficiency (308). As with protein C, protein S mutations reduce activity to 50% of normal and increase thrombotic risk 10-fold (309). Protein S deficiency is estimated to be about as prevalent as protein C deficiency (309). Inflammatory states that increase circulating levels of C4b-binding protein can also increase the bound fraction of protein S, thereby effectively reducing protein S activity.

Antithrombin is also synthesized in the liver and inhibits factors IIa, Xa, IXa, XIa, and XIIa. The activity of antithrombin is markedly increased by heparin. More than 50 mutations of the antithrombin gene, located on chromosome 1, have been identified (307). Antithrombin activity can be reduced by either diminished production of normal protein or normal production of a dysfunctional protein. Activity is typically reduced to 50% of normal, thereby increasing the thrombotic risk 20-fold. Approximately 1 in 2500 individuals are affected (311).

Factor V Leiden is an abnormal factor V that contains a Gln to Arg substitution at position 506 resulting from a point mutation in the factor V gene on chromosome 1. Factor Va is normally inactivated by APC by cleavage at one of several sites, including Arg 506. Factor Va with the factor V Leiden mutation is resistant to cleavage by protein C, and individuals with factor V Leiden are said to have APC resistance. Factor V Leiden is found in approximately 4% of Caucasians, although its prevalence is highly variable among nationalities (309). Heterozygosity for the factor V Leiden gene increases thrombotic risk fourfold. Homozygosity for factor V Leiden is found in approximately 1 in 2000 whites and increases thrombotic risk 50-fold (312).

The prothrombin G20210A mutation in the prothrombin gene on chromosome 2 elevates prothrombin levels by 25%. This mutation occurs in approximately 2% of Caucasians and carries with it a twofold-to-threefold increase in the risk for VTE (313).

Management of thrombotic events in children with thrombophilia consists of anticoagulation. The low rate of occurrence of unprovoked VTE in children with known thrombophilia does not generally warrant primary prophylaxis with anticoagulation (309). However, the risk of thrombosis is higher than normal following surgery, so perioperative prophylaxis with low-molecular-weight heparin may be recommended in high-risk patients in some situations. In patients with antithrombin deficiency, antithrombin concentrates have been used effectively (314). If a VTE occurs following surgery in a patient with thrombophilia, anticoagulation should be administered acutely if the risk of surgical related bleeding is low and continued until resolution of the thrombus, typically 6 months (309).

Consumptive Coagulopathy. Abnormalities in hemostasis may follow the depletion of circulating procoagulant and anticoagulant factors. Two instances in which this process may become apparent in the practice of pediatric orthopaedics are disseminated intravascular coagulation (DIC) and dilutional coagulopathy following transfusions for massive traumatic or operative hemorrhage. The prevention, recognition, and treatment of these states of abnormal hemostasis are essential, as they complicate already serious illness or injury.

DIC, as its name implies, begins with thrombosis throughout the vascular system following serious infection or trauma. The coagulation is typically a result of stimulation of thrombogenesis and impairment of fibrinolysis and is largely mediated by cytokines (315). Cytokines that are expressed during a state of widespread inflammation stimulate expression of tissue factor by endothelial cells, circulating neutrophils, and monocytes. Tissue factor then activates factor VII, setting off the intrinsic arm of the clotting cascade that ultimately converts fibrinogen to fibrin (316). In DIC, the thrombosis progresses unchecked because the inflammatory state also impairs natural antithrombotic mechanisms (317). After thrombosis has begun in DIC, fibrinolysis to remove the coagulation is initially upregulated but ultimately impaired (318). Widespread thrombosis causes organ damage by occluding microcirculation, particularly in the kidneys, heart, lungs, and central nervous system (319). Bleeding then follows the widespread thrombosis as clotting factors are consumed. Because mucosal and skin hemorrhages are easily detectable, bleeding manifestations of DIC are detected more often than thrombotic manifestations (320–322).

Most children with DIC have underlying problems such as congenital anomalies, prematurity, malignancy, sepsis, or hematologic abnormalities. DIC can also follow severe head trauma in children (323).

The laboratory evaluation of DIC reveals many abnormalities of hemostasis. Anemia and RBC fragmentation due to hemolysis are present in 50% to 90% (322, 324), and thrombocytopenia is apparent in 86% (322). The bleeding time, PT, and PTT are prolonged because of the consumption of platelets and clotting factors from all pathways. D-dimer, a fibrin degradation product, can be reliably measured and serve as indicators of fibrinolysis. Abnormalities in all these tests can support the diagnosis of DIC, but none is pathognomonic.

DIC is difficult to treat. Sometimes adequate treatment of the underlying pathology can remove the trigger for inflammation and coagulation and obviate the need for treatment of the DIC. Heparin or low-molecular-weight heparin can be used to counteract the thrombotic tendency, but studies have shown highly variable results (325, 326). The use of fresh frozen plasma or cryoprecipitate to counteract bleeding or to prepare for an invasive procedure is equally risky and controversial, as it may stimulate further thrombosis and end-organ damage (309). Antithrombin can prevent disseminated coagulation without increasing the bleeding risk, but has shown conflicting results in clinical series in patients with DIC, sepsis, and antithrombin deficits (327, 328).

The prognosis of DIC is difficult to ascertain, as it occurs in the setting of otherwise potentially life-threatening illness and injury. A 42% mortality rate was found in a series of 100 patients (322). Multiorgan dysfunction causes most of the morbidity and mortality following DIC (320, 321).

Dilutional Coagulopathy. Coagulopathy can also result from dilution of clotting factors and platelets following fluid and blood resuscitation for massive bleeding. Hemorrhage is a major cause of death in severely injured patients who present to trauma centers (329). Coagulopathy develops in these patients by several mechanisms: hypothermia, acidosis, DIC from vascular injury and inflammation, and dilution of coagulation factors and platelets during fluid and blood resuscitation (330). Hypothermia accompanies major trauma, often as a result of decreased motor activity, exposure during evaluation and resuscitation, and rapid administration of unwarmed intravenous fluids. For every degree Celsius of hypothermia, enzymatic activity in the coagulation cascade decreases 10% (331). Coagulopathy becomes quite severe at below 34°C and virtually irreversible at below 32°C (332). Acidosis, which also accompanies tissue trauma and hypoperfusion, directly reduces coagulation activity and platelet function (333). Brain injury can release tissue factor, thereby causing DIC, and liver injury may impair synthesis of clotting factors.

Dilution of clotting factors and platelets following hemorrhage begins with the shift of interstitial water into the intravascular space because of the blood pressure dropping less than the colloid osmotic pressure. This dilution increases with administration of crystalloid solutions to restore blood pressure. Administration of pRBCs further increases dilution. A unit of pRBCs contains no functional platelets and only 35 mL of plasma. Factors V and VIII are labile and do not survive the processing of RBCs. Therefore, after transfusion of 10 U of pRBCs, it is estimated that 70% of plasma has been lost and only 10% has been replaced, leading to detectable abnormalities in the PT and PTT (333, 334). A recent mathematical model of blood loss and hemodilution predicted the PT to be the earliest and most sensitive indicator of coagulopathy arising from hemodilution during hemorrhage (335).

Platelets, many of which are adherent to vessel walls or sequestered in the spleen, are lost more slowly. Platelet counts may remain at more than 100,000 per μL even after transfusion of 20 U of pRBCs (333).

Prevention and treatment of dilutional coagulopathy are essential. The most important first step is to control the hemorrhage by surgical means. Aggressive fluid resuscitation prior to surgical control of bleeding increases mortality (336). If, despite surgical attempts to control hemorrhage, large-scale transfusions are required, platelets and plasma should be coadministered. Various recommendations have been made regarding the ratios and timing of administration of blood products. The American Society of Anesthesiologists recommends transfusion of blood products in the trauma setting to maintain the PT and PTT at <1.5 times normal, the platelet count at >50 × 10^9 per L, coagulation factor activity levels at >30% of normal, and fibrinogen at >0.8 g/dL (337). These values are unlikely to be reached until the loss and replacement of more than 150% of total blood volume (338). Others recommend prophylactic administration of platelets and plasma prior to detectable coagulopathy. Some physicians transfuse 1 U of plasma for every unit of pRBCs over 10 U transfused, and 1 U of platelets for every unit of pRBCs over 20 U transfused (333). They recognize, however, that variability exists between patients, and no routine algorithm will be universally successful. According to a mathematical model, the optimal ratio of product transfusion (in units) to prevent dilutional coagulopathy is 2:3 for plasma:pRBCs and 8:10 for platelet:pRBCs (335). If plasma and platelet transfusions were to be delayed, respectively, until after transfusion of 3 and 10 U of pRBCs, coagulopathy would ensue.

It may also be beneficial to administer purified clotting factors, especially when patients cannot tolerate the osmotic load of fresh frozen plasma. Showing particular promise in small series is recombinant factor VIIa, initially designed for use in patients with hemophilia and high-titer inhibitors to factor VIII. The administration of factor VIIa bypasses deficiencies in the intrinsic and extrinsic pathways and has been shown to rapidly decrease microvascular bleeding and save lives following dilutional coagulopathy (333).

Further confusing the picture is that most studies have been performed in adults, and extrapolation to children is difficult. Nonetheless, the orthopaedist faced with severe traumatic or surgical hemorrhage in a child should be aware of the possibility of dilutional coagulopathy and work with the anesthesiologist and critical care specialists to prevent, recognize, and treat this potentially fatal event.

HEMATOLOGIC MALIGNANCY

Acute Leukemia. The skeletal manifestations of acute leukemia are important to recognize, as they may be the presenting signs and symptoms and may be first seen by an orthopaedist. Musculoskeletal pain is common early in the course of acute leukemia, and is a presenting complaint in 40% to 62% of patients (339, 340). Pain in an extremity at presentation is seen more often in acute lymphoblastic leukemia (ALL) than in leukocytosis (340). Almost 50% of patients in one series had gait abnormalities or refusal to walk at presentation (341). Back pain is common at presentation and can be associated with pathologic fractures of the vertebral bodies in the setting of severe osteoporosis (342–346). The diagnosis of acute leukemia should be entertained for any child with unexplained musculoskeletal pain together with constitutional symptoms, or with unusual abnormalities as seen on radiographic examination.

Pain and swelling in the joints, resembling juvenile rheumatoid arthritis, is present in 11% to 13% of patients with ALL at presentation (340, 347–349). Typically, more than one joint is involved, with knees, ankles, and elbows being most commonly affected (340). The clinical picture of involvement of the joints can resemble septic arthritis, and the diagnosis may be further confused by a mild leukocytosis (350). These children may have constitutional symptoms such as listlessness, poor appetite, and low-grade fevers, which should raise suspicion of leukemia when they occur in conjunction with back or joint pain.

An increased risk of fracture is seen in leukemia and is likely related to osteoporosis (351). Most fractures occurred in the extremities following trauma. The incidence of fractures in ALL patients is as high as 12% to 38%, especially during chemotherapy treatment (343, 351, 352). Osteopenia is a common radiographic finding in acute leukemia. In prospective studies, 21% to 30% of patients with ALL have bone mineral density Z-scores below −1.645 SD (fifth percentile) as determined by DEXA scans at the time of diagnosis (351, 353). Abnormalities in bone metabolism may account for the osteoporosis induced by leukemia (353). Bone mineral density decreases further during the initial phase of intense chemotherapy (351–353).

Acute leukemia is the most common nonsolid cancer in children. Approximately 3250 cases are diagnosed annually in children and adolescents, and the incidence is increasing (www.seer.cancer.gov) (354, 355). Approximately 80% of childhood acute leukemia is ALL, and 20% is acute nonlymphoblastic leukemia. The peak age at diagnosis is between 2 and 4 years. The pathogenesis of childhood leukemia is multifactorial. A variety of genetic mutations and chromosomal rearrangements have been shown to be associated with acute leukemia, and these have been correlated with immunologic type and clinical course. The Philadelphia chromosome, t(9;22)(934;q11), is associated with an especially poor prognosis (356).

Advances in chemotherapy have greatly improved survival rates for children with ALL. In developed countries, current cure rates for ALL approach or exceed 80%, depending upon the cell type, genotype, and in some cases, the race of the patient (357–359).

Routine laboratory studies may show normal results in the early stages of leukemia, even after skeletal involvement has begun. Peripheral leukocytosis may not exist at the time of presentation. Anemia is often present in early ALL and can provide a clue to the diagnosis of leukemia. Platelets are decreased in two-thirds of the time at presentation of ALL; they are typically increased in musculoskeletal sepsis. The erythrocyte sedimentation rate may be elevated, but this result is also not specific.

Imaging studies can give clues leading to the diagnosis of leukemia in a child with unexplained back or extremity pain. Radiolucent metaphyseal bands are a common and early radiographic finding in acute leukemia, and are thought to represent abnormal mineralization of metaphyseal bone rather than infiltration of leukemia cells (360). Periosteal new bone formation along the diaphyses of long bones is also common. Radiolucent lesions in cortical bone are also found, and most likely represent bone destruction from leukemic infiltrates (360). These lesions can be found in the small bones of the hands and feet, metaphyses of long bones of the extremities, or skull. The prognostic significance of skeletal lesions in leukemia is unclear. Abnormalities in marrow signal on MRI may also be present (361), and MRI may be a valuable tool in evaluating a child with early skeletal changes suggestive of leukemia in the setting of a normal peripheral hematologic profile. The diagnosis of leukemia is made by flow cytometric evidence of a clonal population. Flow cytometry can be obtained from peripheral blood or bone marrow specimens.

ON can complicate the treatment of leukemia. Symptomatic ON was diagnosed in 15 of 1421 patients treated with intensive chemotherapy for childhood ALL in one series (362). Most patients had multiple sites of ON, with the femoral head being the most common site. Most cases of ON are attributed to the high doses of corticosteroids used in chemotherapy, or to bone marrow transplantation.

The neutropenia associated with chemotherapy and bone marrow transplantation places children with acute leukemia at high risk for fungal infections. Cutaneous infection with fungi from the genus *Aspergillus*, which can be fatal (363), may come to the attention of an orthopaedist as a suspected abscess or cellulitis. The lesion typically consists of a well-defined area of skin necrosis surrounded by erythema and swelling, often at the prior site of a venous access catheter. No purulent drainage is emitted. Diagnosis is made by KOH preparations of smears from the margin of the lesion. Treatment consists of wide excision followed by systemic antifungal treatment under the guidance of an infectious diseases specialist. Simple incision and drainage of a lesion is not only ineffective, but may allow the fungal hyphae to spread into the microvasculature, thereby contributing to widespread disease.

REFERENCES

1. Kutler DI, Singh B, Satagopan B, et al. A 20-year perspective on the International Fanconi Anemia Registry (IFAR). *Blood* 2003; 101:1249.
2. Alter B. Inherited bone marrow failure. In: Nathan DG, Orkin SH, Ginsberg D, et al. eds. *Nathan and Oski's hematology of infancy and childhood*, 6th ed. Philadelphia, PA: WB Saunders, 2003:280.

3. Macdougall LG, Rosendorff J, Poole JE, et al. Comparative study of Fanconi anemia in children of different ethnic origin in South Africa. *Am J Med Genet* 1994;52:279.

4. Tischkowitz MD, Hodgson SV. Fanconi anaemia. *J Med Genet* 2003; 40(1):1–10.

5. Lieberman L, Dror Y. Advances in understanding the genetic basis for bone-marrow failure. *Curr Opin Pediatr* 2006;18(1):15–21.

6. Glanz A, Fraser FC. Spectrum of anomalies in Fanconi anaemia. *J Med Genet* 1982;19:412.

7. Giampietro PF, Adler-Brecher B, Verlander PC, et al. The need for more accurate and timely diagnosis in Fanconi anemia: a report from the International Fanconi Anemia Registry. *Pediatrics* 1993;91:1116.

8. Alter BP. Arm anomalies and bone marrow failure may go hand in hand. *J Hand Surg Am* 1992;17:566.

9. Cox H, Viljoen D, Versfeld G, et al. Radial ray defects and associated anomalies. *Clin Genet* 1989;35:322.

10. Wajnrajch MP, Gertner JM, Huma Z, et al. Evaluation of growth and hormonal status in patients referred to the International Fanconi Anemia Registry. *Pediatrics* 2001;107:744.

11. De Kerviler E, Guermazi A, Zagdanski AM, et al. The clinical and radiological features of Fanconi's anaemia. *Clin Radiol* 2000;55:340.

12. Alter BP, Young NS. The bone marrow failure syndromes. In: Nathan DG, Oski SH, eds. *Hematology of infancy and childhood*, 5th ed. Philadelphia, PA: WB Saunders, 1998:237.

13. Hedberg VA, Lipton JM. Thrombocytopenia with absent radii. A review of 100 cases. *Am J Pediatr Hematol Oncol* 1988;10:51.

14. Hall JG, Levin J, Kuhn JP, et al. Thrombocytopenia with absent radius (TAR). *Medicine* 1969;48:411.

15. Hall JG. Thrombocytopenia and absent radius (TAR) syndrome. *J Med Genet* 1987;24:79.

16. Schoenecker PL, Cohn AK, Sedgwick WG, et al. Dysplasia of the knee associated with the syndrome of thrombocytopenia and absent radius. *J Bone Joint Surg Am* 1984;66:421.

17. Christensen CP, Ferguson RL. Lower extremity deformities associated with thrombocytopenia and absent radius syndrome. *Clin Orthop Relat R* 2000;375:202.

18. Moir JS, Scotland T. Thrombocytopenia absent radius syndrome and knee deformity. *J Pediatr Orthop B* 1995;4:222.

19. Alter BP. Arms and the man or hands and the child: congenital anomalies and hematologic syndromes. *J Pediatr Hematol Oncol* 1997;19:287.

20. Ball SE, McGuckin CP, Jenkins G. et al. Diamond-Blackfan anaemia in the U.K.: analysis of 80 cases from a 20-year birth cohort. *Br J Haematol* 1996;94:645.

21. Dokal I, Vulliamy T. Inherited aplastic anemias/bone marrow failure. *Blood Rev* 2008;22(3):141–153.

22. Vlachos A, Lipton JM. Bone marrow failure in children. *Curr Opin Pediatr* 1996;8:33.

23. Hurst JA, Baraitser M, Wonke B. Autosomal dominant transmission of congenital erythroid hypoplastic anemia with radial abnormalities. *Am J Med Genet* 1991;40:482.

24. Vlachos A, Ball S, Dahl N, et al. Diagnosing and treating Diamond Blackfan anemia: results of an International Clinical Consensus Conference. *Br J Haematol* 2008;142(6): 859–876.

25. Mugishima H, Gale RP, Rowlings PA, et al. Bone marrow transplantation for Diamond-Blackfan anemia. *Bone Marrow Transpl* 1995;15:55.

26. Hamaguchi I, Ooka A, Brun A, et al. Gene transfer improves erythroid development in ribosomal protein S19-deficient Diamond-Blackfan anemia. *Blood* 2002;1000:2727.

27. Aggett PJ, Cavanagh NP, Matthew DJ, et al. Shwachman's syndrome. A review of 21 cases. *Arch Dis Child* 1980;55:331.

28. Dhar S, Anderton JM. Orthopaedic features of Shwachman syndrome. A report of two cases. *J Bone Joint Surg Am* 1994;76:278.

29. Smith OP, Hann IM, Chessells JM, et al. Haematological abnormalities in Shwachman-Diamond syndrome. *Br J Haematol* 1996;94:279.

30. Myers KC, Davies SM. Hematopoietic stem cell transplantation for bone marrow failure syndromes in children. *Biol Blood Marrow Transplant* 2009;3(15):279–292.

31. Makitie O, Kaitila I. Cartilage-hair hypoplasia—clinical manifestations in 108 Finnish patients. *Eur J Pediatr* 1993;152:211.

32. Makitie O, Juvonen E, Dunkel L, et al. Anemia in children with cartilage-hair hypoplasia is related to body growth and to the insulin-like growth factor system. *J Clin Endocrinol Metab* 2000;85:563.

33. Williams MS, Ettinger RS, Hermanns P, et al. The natural history of severe anemia in cartilage-hair hypoplasia. *Am J Med Genet A* 2005; 138(1):35–40.

34. Guggenheim R, Somech R, Grunebaum E, et al. Bone marrow transplantation for cartilage-hair-hypoplasia. *Bone Marrow Transplant* 2006; 38(11):751–756. Epub 2006 Oct 16.

35. Berthet F, Siegrist CA, Ozsahin H, et al. Bone marrow transplantation in cartilage-hair hypoplasia: correction of the immuno-deficiency but not of the chondrodysplasia. *Eur J Pediatr* 1996;155:286.

36. Ingram VM. Gene mutations in human haemoglobin: the chemical difference between normal and sickle cell haemoglobin. *Nature* 1957; 180:326.

37. Ejindu VC, Hine AL, Mashayekhi M, et al. Musculoskeletal manifestations of sickle cell disease. *Radiographics* 2007;27(4):1005–1021.

38. Huo MH, Friedlaender GE, Marsh JS. Orthopaedic manifestations of sickle-cell disease. *Yale J Biol Med* 1990;63:195.

39. Motulsky AG. Frequency of sickling disorders in U.S. blacks. *N Engl J Med* 1973;288:31.

40. Schneider RG, Hightower B, Hosty TS, et al. Abnormal hemoglobins in a quarter million people. *Blood* 1976;48:629.

41. Badakjian-Michlau J, Gilloud-Bataile M, Maier-Redelsperger M, et al. Decreased morbidity in homozygus sickle cell disease detected at birth. *Hemoglobin* 2002;26:211.

42. Platt OS, Thorington RD, Brambilla DJ, et al. Pain in sickle cell disease: rates and risk factors [Comment]. *N Engl J Med* 1991;325:11.

43. Keeley K, Buchanan GR. Acute infarction of long bones in children with sickle cell anemia. *J Pediatr* 1982;101:170.

44. Ballas SK, Larner J, Smith ED, et al. Rheologic predictors of the severity of the painful sickle cell crisis. *Blood* 1988;72:1216.

45. Fixler J, Styles L. Sickle cell disease. *Pediatr Clin North Am* 2002;49:1193.

46. Miller ST, Sleeper LA, Pegelow CH. Prediction of adverse outcomes in children with sickle cell disease. *N Engl J Med* 2000;342:83–89.

47. Dalton GP, Drummond DS, Davidson RS, et al. Bone infarction versus infection in sickle cell disease in children. *J Pediatr Orthop* 1996;16:540.

48. Burnett MW, Bass JW, Cook BA. Etiology of osteomyelitis complicating sickle cell disease. *Pediatrics* 1998;101:296.

49. Sadat-Ali M, Sankaran K, Kannan K. Recent observations on osteomyelitis in sickle-cell disease. *Int Orthop* 1985;9:97.

50. Sadat-Ali M. The status of acute osteomyelitis in sickle cell disease. A 15-year review. *Int Surg* 1998;83:84.

51. Pearson HA, Gallagher D, Chilcote R, et al. Developmental pattern of splenic dysfunction in sickle cell disorders. *Pediatrics* 1985;76:392.

52. Wright J, Thomas P, Serjeant GR. Septicemia caused by *Salmonella* infection: an overlooked complication of sickle cell disease [Comment]. *J Pediatr* 1997;130:394.

53. Gill FM, Sleeper LA, Weiner SJ, et al. Clinical events in the first decade in a cohort of infants with sickle cell disease. Cooperative Study of Sickle Cell Disease [Comment]. *Blood* 1995;86:776.

54. Greene WB, McMillan CW. *Salmonella* osteomyelitis and hand-foot syndrome in a child with sickle cell anemia. *J Pediatr Orthop* 1987;7:716.

55. Epps CH Jr, Bryant III DD, Coles MJ et al. Osteomyelitis in patients who have sickle-cell disease. Diagnosis and management. *J Bone Joint Surg Am* 1991;73:1281.

56. Bennett OM, Namnyak SS. Bone and joint manifestations of sickle cell anaemia. *J Bone Joint Surg Br* 1990;72:494.

57. Chambers JB, Forsythe DA, Bertrand SL, et al. Retrospective review of osteoarticular infections in a pediatric sickle cell age group. *J Pediatr Orthop* 2000;20:682.

58. Skaggs DL, Kim SK, Greene NW, et al. Differentiation between bone infarction and acute osteomyelitis in children with sickle-cell disease with use of sequential radionuclide bone-marrow and bone scans. *J Bone Joint Surg Am* 2001;83-A:1810.

59. Almeida A, Roberts I. Bone involvement in sickle cell disease. *Br J Haematol* 2005;129(4):482–490.

60. Syrogiannopoulos GA, McCracken GH Jr, Nelson JD. Osteoarticular infections in children with sickle cell disease. *Pediatrics* 1986;78:1090.

61. Milner PF, Kraus AP, Sebes JI, et al. Sickle cell disease as a cause of osteonecrosis of the femoral head. *N Engl J Med* 1991;325:1476.

62. Milner PF, Kraus AP, Sebes JI, et al. Osteonecrosis of the humeral head in sickle cell disease. *Clin Orthop Relat R* 1993;289:136.

63. Mont MA, Zywiel MG, Marker DR, et al. The natural history of untreated asymptomatic osteonecrosis of the femoral head: a systematic literature review. *J Bone Joint Surg Am* 2010;92(12):2165–2170.

64. Hernigou P, Habibi A, Bachir D, et al. The natural history of asymptomatic osteonecrosis of the femoral head in adults with sickle cell disease. *J Bone Joint Surg Am* 2006;88(12):2565–2572.

65. Akinyoola AL, Adediran IA, Asaleye CM, et al. Risk factors for osteonecrosis of the femoral head in patients with sickle cell disease. *Int Orthop* 2009;33(4):923–926.

66. Hernigou P, Galacteros F, Bachir D, et al. Deformities of the hip in adults who have sickle-cell disease and had avascular necrosis in childhood. A natural history of fifty-two patients. *J Bone Joint Surg Am* 1991;73:81.

67. Ware HE, Brooks AP, Toye R, et al. Sickle cell disease and silent avascular necrosis of the hip. *J Bone Joint Surg Br* 1991;73:947.

68. Rao VM, Mitchell DG, Steiner RM, et al. Femoral head avascular necrosis in sickle cell anemia: MR characteristics. *Magn Reson Imaging* 1988;6:661.

69. Marti-Carvajal, Solà I, Agreda-Pérez LH. Treatment for avascular necrosis of bone in people with sickle cell disease. *Cochrane Database Syst Rev* 2009;(3):CD004344.

70. Neumayr LD, Aguilar C, Earles AN, et al; National Osteonecrosis Trial in Sickle Cell Anemia Study Group. Physical therapy alone compared with core decompression and physical therapy for femoral head osteonecrosis in sickle cell disease. Results of a multicenter study at a mean of three years after treatment. *J Bone Joint Surg Am* 2006;88(12):2573–2582.

71. Mukisi-Mukaza M, Manicom O, Alexis C, et al. Treatment of sickle cell disease's hip necrosis by core decompression: a prospective case-control study. *Orthop Traumatol Surg Res* 2009;95(7):498–504.

72. Acurio MT, Friedman RJ. Hip arthroplasty in patients with sickle-cell haemoglobinopathy. *J Bone Joint Surg Br* 1992;74:367.

73. Bishop AR, Roberson JR, Eckman JR, et al. Total hip arthroplasty in patients who have sickle-cell hemoglobinopathy. *J Bone Joint Surg Am* 1988;70:853.

74. Booz MM, Hariharan V, Aradi AJ, et al. The value of ultrasound and aspiration in differentiating vaso-occlusive crisis and osteomyelitis in sickle cell disease patients. *Clin Radiol* 1999;54:636.

75. Vichinsky EP, Neumayr LD, Haberkern C, et al. The perioperative complication rate of orthopedic surgery in sickle cell disease: report of the National Sickle Cell Surgery Study Group. *Am J Hematol* 1999;62:129.

76. Garden MS, Grant RE, Jebraili S. Perioperative complications in patients with sickle cell disease. An orthopedic perspective. *Am J Orthop (Chatham, NJ)* 1996;25:353.

77. Stein RE, Urbaniak J. Use of the tourniquet during surgery in patients with sickle cell hemoglobinopathies. *Clin Orthop Relat R* 1980;151:231.

78. Vichinsky EP, Haberkern CM, Neumayr L, et al. A comparison of conservative and aggressive transfusion regimens in the perioperative management of sickle cell disease. The Preoperative Transfusion in Sickle Cell Disease Study Group [Comment]. *N Engl J Med* 1995;333:206.

79. Anand AJ, Glatt AE. Salmonella osteomyelitis and arthritis in sickle cell disease. *Semin Arthritis Rheu* 1994;24:211.

80. Ebong WW. Pathological fracture complicating long bone osteomyelitis in patients with sickle cell disease. *J Pediatr Orthop* 1986;6:177.

81. Vichinsky EP, Styles LA, Colangelo LH, et al. Acute chest syndrome in sickle cell disease: clinical presentation and course. Cooperative Study of Sickle Cell Disease. *Blood* 1997;89:1787.

82. Rucknagel DL. The role of rib infarcts in the acute chest syndrome of sickle cell diseases. *Pediatr Pathol Mol Med* 2001;20:137.

83. Riddington C, Owusu-Ofori S. Prophylactic antibiotics for preventing pneumococcal infection in children with sickle cell disease. *Cochrane Database Syst Rev* 2002;(3):CD003427.

84. Charache S, Terrin ML, Moore RD, et al. Effect of hydroxyurea on the frequency of painful crises in sickle cell anemia. Investigators of the Multicenter Study of Hydroxyurea in Sickle Cell Anemia [Comment]. *N Engl J Med* 1995;332:1317.

85. Amrolia PJ, Almeida A, Halsey C, et al. Therapeutic challenges in childhood sickle cell disease. Part 1: current and future treatment options. *Br J Haematol* 2003;120:725.

86. Lo L, Singer ST. Thalassemia: current approach to an old disease. *Pediatr Clin North Am* 2002;49:1165.

87. Wongchanchailert M, Laosombat V, Maipang M. Hemoglobin H disease in children. *J Med Assoc Thai* 1992;75:611.

88. Colavita N, Orazi C, Danza SM, et al. Premature epiphyseal fusion and extramedullary hematopoiesis in thalassemia. *Skeletal Radiol* 1987;16:533.

89. Parano E, Pavone V, Gregorio FD, et al. Extraordinary intrathecal bone reaction in beta-thalassaemia intermedia [Comment]. *Lancet* 1999;354:922.

90. Angastiniotis M, Pavlides N, Aristidou K, et al. Bone pain in thalassaemia: assessment of DEXA and MRI findings. *J Pediatr Endocrinol Metab* 1998;11(Suppl 3):779.

91. Aydingoz U, Oto A, Cila A. Spinal cord compression due to epidural extramedullary haematopoiesis in thalassaemia: MRI. *Neuroradiology* 1997;39:870.

92. Coskun E, Keskin A, Suzer T, et al. Spinal cord compression secondary to extramedullary hematopoiesis in thalassemia intermedia. *Eur Spine J* 1998;7:501.

93. Lau SK, Chan CK, Chow YY. Cord compression due to extramedullary hemopoiesis in a patient with thalassemia. *Spine* 1994;19:2467.

94. Chourmouzi D, Pistevou-Gompaki K, Plataniotis G, et al. MRI findings of extramedullary haematopoiesis. *Eur Radiol* 2001;11:1803.

95. Roth C, Pekrun A, Bartz M, et al. Short stature and failure of pubertal development in thalassaemia major: evidence for hypothalamic neurosecretory dysfunction of growth hormone secretion and defective pituitary gonadotropin secretion. *Eur J Pediatr* 1997;156:777.

96. De Sanctis V. Growth and puberty and its management in thalassaemia. *Horm Res* 2002;58(Suppl 1):72.

97. Theodoridis C, Ladis V, Papatheodorou A, et al. Growth and management of short stature in thalassaemia major. *J Pediatr Endocrinol Metab* 1998;11(Suppl 3):835.

98. Filosa A, Di Maio S, Baron I, et al. Final height and body disproportion in thalassaemic boys and girls with spontaneous or induced puberty. *Acta Paediatr* 2000;89:1295.

99. Voskaridou E, Plata E, Maroussa D, et al. Treatment with deferasirox (Exjade) effectively decreases iron burden in patients with thalassaemia intermedia: results of a pilot study. *Br J Haematol* 2010;148(2):332–334.

100. Olivieri NF, Nathan DG, MacMillan JH, et al. Survival in medically treated patients with homozygous beta-thalassemia [Comment]. *N Engl J Med* 1994;331:574.

101. Giardina PJ, Grady RW. Chelation therapy in beta-thalassemia: the benefits and limitations of desferrioxamine. *Semin Hematol* 1995;32:304.

102. Chan YL, Pang LM, Chik KW, et al. Patterns of bone diseases in transfusion-dependent homozygous thalassaemia major: predominance of osteoporosis and desferrioxamine-induced bone dysplasia. *Pediatr Radiol* 2002;32:492.

103. de Sanctis V, Savarino L, Stea S, et al. Microstructural analysis of severe bone lesions in seven thalassemic patients treated with deferoxamine. *Calcif Tissue Int* 2000;67:128.

104. de Sanctis V, Stea S, Savarino L, et al. Osteochondrodystrophic lesions in chelated thalassemic patients: an histological analysis. *Calcif Tissue Int* 2000;67:134.

105. Naselli A, Vignolo M, Battista ED, et al. Long-term follow-up of skeletal dysplasia in thalassaemia major. *J Pediatr Endocrinol Metab* 1998;11(Suppl 3):817.

106. Mangiagli A, De Sanctis V, Campisi S, et al. Treatment with deferiprone (L1) in a thalassemic patient with bone lesions due to desferrioxamine. *J Pediatr Endocrinol Metab* 2000;13:677.

107. Cappellini MD, Taher A. Deferasirox (Exjade) for the treatment of iron overload. *Acta Haematol* 2009;122:165–173.

108. Jensen CE, Tuck SM, Agnew JE, et al. High prevalence of low bone mass in thalassaemia major. *Br J Haematol* 1998;103:911.

109. Bielinski BK, Darbyshire PJ, Mathers L, et al. Impact of disordered puberty on bone density in beta-thalassaemia major. *Br J Haematol* 2003;120:353.

110. Pafumi C, Roccasalva L, Pernicone G, et al. Osteopenia in female beta-thalassemic patients. *J Pediatr Endocrinol Metab* 1998;11(Suppl 3):989.

111. Domrongkitchaiporn S, Sirikulchayanonta V, Angchaisuksiri P, et al. Abnormalities in bone mineral density and bone histology in thalassemia. *J Bone Miner Res* 2003;18:1682.

112. Lala R, Chiabotto P, Stefano MD, et al. Bone density and metabolism in thalassaemia. *J Pediatr Endocrinol Metab* 1998;11(Suppl 3):785.

113. Molyvda-Athanasopoulou E, Sioundas A, Karatzas N, et al. Bone mineral density of patients with thalassemia major: four-year follow-up. *Calcif Tissue Int* 1999;64:481.

114. Sartorio A, Conte G, Conti A, et al. Effects of 12 months rec-GH therapy on bone and collagen turnover and bone mineral density in GH deficient children with thalassaemia major. *J Endocrinol Invest* 2000;23:356.

115. Morabito N, Lasco A, Gaudio A, et al. Bisphosphonates in the treatment of thalassemia-induced osteoporosis. *Osteoporos Int* 2002;13:644.

116. Pennisi P, Pizzarelli G, Spina M, et al. Quantitative ultrasound of bone and clodronate effects in thalassemia-induced osteoporosis. *J Bone Miner Metab* 2003;21:402.

117. Dines DM, Canale VC, Arnold WD. Fractures in thalassemia. *J Bone Joint Surg Am* 1976;58:662–666.

118. Exarchou E, Politou C, Vretou E, et al. Fractures and epiphyseal deformities in beta-thalassemia. *Clin Orthop Relat Res* 1984;189:229.

119. Finsterbush, A, Farber I, Mogle P, et al. Fracture patterns in thalassemia. *Clin Orthop Relat R* 1985;192:132.

120. Michelson J, Cohen A. Incidence and treatment of fractures in thalassemia. *J Orthop Trauma* 1988;2:29.

121. Ruggiero L, De Sanctis V. Multicentre study on prevalence of fractures in transfusion-dependent thalassaemic patients. *J Pediatr Endocrinol Metab* 1998;11(Suppl 3):773.

122. Basanagoudar PL, Gill SS, Dhillon MS, et al. Fractures in transfusion dependent beta thalassemia—an Indian study. *Singapore Med J* 2001;42:196.

123. Bradai M, Abad MT, Pissard S, et al. Hydroxyurea can eliminate transfusion requirements in children with severe beta-thalassemia. *Blood* 2003;102:1529.

124. Lawson SE, Roberts IA, Amrolia P, et al. Bone marrow transplantation for beta-thalassaemia major: the UK experience in two paediatric centres. *Br J Haematol* 2003;120:289.

125. Ball LM, Lankester AC, Giordano PC, et al. Paediatric allogeneic bone marrow transplantation for homozygous beta-thalassaemia: the Dutch experience. *Bone Marrow Transpl* 2003;31:1081.

126. Mentzer WC, Cowan MJ, Bone marrow transplantation for beta-thalassemia: the University of California San Francisco experience. *J Pediatr Hematol Oncol* 2000;22:598.

127. Locatelli F, Rocha V, Reed W, et al. Related umbilical cord blood transplantation in patients with thalassemia and sickle cell disease. *Blood* 2003;101:2137.

128. May C, Rivella S, Chadburn A, et al. Successful treatment of murine beta-thalassemia intermedia by transfer of the human beta-globin gene. *Blood* 2002;99:1902.

129. Winkelstein JA, Marino MC, Johnston Jr RB, et al. Chronic granulomatous disease. Report on a national registry of 368 patients. *Medicine* 2000;79:155.

130. Lakshman R, Finn A. Neutrophil disorders and their management. *J Clin Pathol* 2001;54:7.

131. Johnston RB, Newman SL. Chronic granulomatous disease. *Pediatr Clin North Am* 1977;24:365.

132. Wolfson JJ, Kane WJ, Laxdal SD, et al. Bone findings in chronic granulomatous disease of childhood. A genetic abnormality of leukocyte function. *J Bone Joint Surg Am* 1969;51:1573.

133. Sponseller PD, Malech HL, McCarthy EF Jr, et al. Skeletal involvement in children who have chronic granulomatous disease. *J Bone Joint Surg Am* 1991;73:37.

134. Heinrich SD, Finney T, Craver R, et al. Aspergillus osteomyelitis in patients who have chronic granulomatous disease. Case report. *J Bone Joint Surg Am* 1991;73:456.

135. Kline MW, Bocobo FC, Paul ME, et al. Successful medical therapy of Aspergillus osteomyelitis of the spine in an 11-year-old boy with chronic granulomatous disease. *Pediatrics* 1994;93:830.

136. Pasic S, Abinun M, Pistignjat B, et al. *Aspergillus osteomyelitis* in chronic granulomatous disease: treatment with recombinant gamma-interferon and itraconazole. *Pediatr Infect Dis J* 1996;15:833.

137. Tsumura N, Akasu Y, Yamane H, et al. *Aspergillus osteomyelitis* in a child who has p67-phox-deficient chronic granulomatous disease. *Kurume Med J* 1999;46:87.

138. The International Chronic Granulomatous Disease Cooperative Study Group. A controlled trial of interferon gamma to prevent infection in chronic granulomatous disease [Comment]. *N Engl J Med* 1991;324:509.

139. Gallin JI, Alling DW, Malech HL, et al. Itraconazole to prevent fungal infections in chronic granulomatous disease [Comment]. *N Engl J Med* 2003;348:2416.

140. Kang EM, Malech HL. Advances in treatment for chronic granulomatous disease. *Immunol Res* 2009;43(1–3):77–84.

141. Del Giudice I, Iori AP, Mengarelli A, et al. Allogeneic stem cell transplant from HLA-identical sibling for chronic granulomatous disease and review of the literature. *Ann Hematol* 2003;82:189.

142. Qasim W, Gaspar HB, Thrasher AJ. Progress and prospects: gene therapy for inherited immunodeficiencies. *Gene Ther* 2009;16(11): 1285–1291. Epub 2009 Sep 24.

143. Leung T, Chik K, Li C, et al. Bone marrow transplantation for chronic granulomatous disease: long-term follow-up and review of literature. *Bone Marrow Transplant* 1999;24(5):567–570.

144. Plebani A, Soresina A, Rondelli R, et al. Clinical, immunological, and molecular analysis in a large cohort of patients with X-linked agammaglobulinemia: an Italian Multicenter Study [Comment]. *Clin Immunol* 2002;104:221.

145. Hansel TT, Haeney MR, Thompson RA. Primary hypogammaglobulinaemia and arthritis. *Br Med J (Clin Res Ed)* 1987;295:174.

146. Lee AH, Levinson AI, Schumacher HR Jr. Hypogammaglobulinemia and rheumatic disease. *Semin Arthritis Rheum* 1993;22:252.

147. Fu JL, Shyur SD, Lin HY, et al. X-linked agammaglobulinemia presenting as juvenile chronic arthritis: report of one case. *Acta Paediatr Taiwan* 1999;40:280.

148. Chattopadhyay C, Natvig JB, Chattopadhyay H. Excessive suppressor T-cell activity of the rheumatoid synovial tissue in X-linked hypogammaglobulinaemia. *Scand J Immunol* 1980;11:455.

149. Franz A, Webster AD, Furr PM, et al. Mycoplasmal arthritis in patients with primary immunoglobulin deficiency: clinical features and outcome in 18 patients. *Br J Rheumatol* 1997;36:661.

150. Bruton OC. Agammaglobulinemia (congenital absence of gamma globulin); report of a case. *Med Ann Dist Columbia* 1953;22:648.

151. http://bioinf.uta.fi/BTKbase/index.html, accessed December 20, 2003.

152. Pearl ER, Vogler LB, Okos AJ, et al. B lymphocyte precursors in human bone marrow: an analysis of normal individuals and patients with antibody-deficiency states. *J Immunol* 1978;120:1169.

153. Lederman HM, Winkelstein JA. X-linked agammaglobulinemia: an analysis of 96 patients. *Medicine* 1985;64:145.

154. Conley ME, Howard V. Clinical findings leading to the diagnosis of X-linked agammaglobulinemia. *J Pediatr* 2002;141:566.

155. Quartier P, Debre M, De Blic J, et al. Early and prolonged intravenous immunoglobulin replacement therapy in childhood agammaglobulinemia: a retrospective survey of 31 patients. *J Pediatr* 1999;134:589.

156. Gaucher PCE. De l'epithelioma primitif de la rate, hypertophie idiopathique de la rate sans leucemie. Thesis. Paris, 1882.

157. Brady RO, Kanfer JN, Bradley RM, et al. Demonstration of a deficiency of glucocerebroside-cleaving enzyme in Gaucher's disease. *J Clin Invest* 1966;45:1112.

158. Meikle PJ, Hopwood JJ, Clague AE, et al. Prevalence of lysosomal storage disorders. *JAMA* 1999;281:249.

159. Cox TM, Schofield JP. Gaucher's disease: clinical features and natural history. *Bailliere Clin Haem* 1997;10:657.

160. Dionisi-Vici C, Rizzo C, Burlina AB, et al. Inborn errors of metabolism in the Italian pediatric population: a national retrospective survey. *J Pediatr* 2002;140:321.

161. Beutler E, Nguyen NJ, Henneberger MW, et al. Gaucher disease: gene frequencies in the Ashkenazi Jewish population. *Am J Hum Genet* 1993;52:85.

162. Tayebi N, Stone DL, Sidransky E. Type 2 Gaucher disease: an expanding phenotype. *Mol Genet Metab* 1999;68:209.

163. Brady RO, Barton NW, Grabowski GA. The role of neurogenetics in Gaucher disease. *Arch Neurol* 1993;50:1212.

164. Zevin S, Abrahamov A, Hadas-Halpern I, et al. Adult-type Gaucher disease in children: genetics, clinical features and enzyme replacement therapy. *Q J Med* 1993;86:565.

165. Zimran A, Kay A, Gelbart T, et al. Gaucher disease. Clinical, laboratory, radiologic, and genetic features of 53 patients. *Medicine* 1992;71:337.

166. Charrow J, Andersson HC, Kaplan P, et al. The Gaucher registry: demographics and disease characteristics of 1698 patients with Gaucher disease. *Arch Intern Med* 2000;160:2835.

167. Stowens DW, Teitelbaum SL, Kahn AJ, et al. Skeletal complications of Gaucher disease. *Medicine* 1985;64:310.

168. Wenstrup RJ, Roca-Espiau M, Weinreb NJ, et al. Skeletal aspects of Gaucher disease: a review. *Brit J Radiol* 2002;75(Suppl 1):A2.

169. Hermann G, Shapiro RS, Abdelwahab IF, et al. MR imaging in adults with Gaucher disease type I: evaluation of marrow involvement and disease activity. *Skeletal Radiol* 1993;22:247.

170. Horev G, Kornreich L, Hadar H, et al. Hemorrhage associated with "bone crisis" in Gaucher's disease identified by magnetic resonance imaging. *Skeletal Radiol* 1991;20:479.

171. Hermann G, Pastores GM, Abdelwahab IF, et al. Gaucher disease: assessment of skeletal involvement and therapeutic responses to enzyme replacement. *Skeletal Radiol* 1997;26:687.

172. Amstutz HC, Carey EJ. Skeletal manifestations and treatment of Gaucher's disease: review of twenty cases. *J Bone Joint Surg Am* 1966;48:670.

173. Bilchik TR, Heyman S. Skeletal scintigraphy of pseudoosteomyelitis in Gaucher's disease. Two case reports and a review of the literature. *Clin Nucl Med* 1992;17:279.

174. Katz K, Mechlis-Frish S, Cohen IJ, et al. Bone scans in the diagnosis of bone crisis in patients who have Gaucher disease. *J Bone Joint Surg Am* 1991;73(5):513 [erratum appears in *J Bone Joint Surg Am* 1991;73(5):791].

175. Cohen IJ, Kornreich L, Mekhmandarov S, et al. Effective treatment of painful bone crises in type I Gaucher's disease with high dose prednisolone. *Arch Dis Child* 1996;75:218.

176. Bell RS, Mankin HJ, Doppelt SH. Osteomyelitis in Gaucher disease. *J Bone Joint Surg Am* 1986;68:1380.

177. Katz K, Sabato S, Horev G, et al. Spinal involvement in children and adolescents with Gaucher disease. *Spine* 1993;18:332.

178. Katz K, Horev G, Grunebaum M, et al. The natural history of osteonecrosis of the femoral head in children and adolescents who have Gaucher disease. *J Bone Joint Surg Am* 1996;78:14.

179. Shitrit D, Rudensky B, Zimran A, et al. D-dimer assay in Gaucher disease: correlation with severity of bone and lung involvement. *Am J Hematol* 2003;73:236.

180. Katz K, Cohen IJ, Ziv N, et al. Fractures in children who have Gaucher disease. *J Bone Joint Surg Am* 1987;69:1361.

181. Wiesner L, Niggemeyer O, Kothe R, et al. Severe pathologic compression of three consecutive vertebrae in Gaucher's disease: a case report and review of the literature. *Eur Spine J* 2003;12:97.

182. Fiore CE, Barone R, Pennisi P, et al. Bone ultrasonometry, bone density, and turnover markers in type 1 Gaucher disease. *J Bone Miner Metab* 2002;20:34.

183. Pastores GM, Wallenstein S, Desnick RJ, et al. Bone density in Type 1 Gaucher disease. *J Bone Miner Res* 1996;11:1801.

184. Maas M, Poll LW, Terk MR. Imaging and quantifying skeletal involvement in Gaucher disease. *Brit J Radiol* 2002;75(Suppl 1):A13.

185. Ciana G, Martini C, Leopaldi A, et al. Bone marker alterations in patients with type 1 Gaucher disease. *Calcif Tissue Int* 2003;72:185.

186. Rosenthal DI, Barton NW, McKusick KA, et al. Quantitative imaging of Gaucher disease. *Radiology* 1992;185:841.

187. Johnson LA, Hoppel BE, Gerard EL, et al. Quantitative chemical shift imaging of vertebral bone marrow in patients with Gaucher disease. *Radiology* 1992;182:451.

188. Maas M, Akkerman EM, Venema HW, et al. Dixon quantitative chemical shift MRI for bone marrow evaluation in the lumbar spine: a reproducibility study in healthy volunteers. *J Comput Assist Tomogr* 2001;25:691.

189. Maas M, van Kuijk C, Stoker J, et al. Quantification of bone involvement in Gaucher disease: MR imaging bone marrow burden score as an alternative to Dixon quantitative chemical shift MR imaging—initial experience. *Radiology* 2003;229:554.

190. Vlieger EJ, Maas M, Akkerman EM, et al. Vertebra disc ratio as a parameter for bone marrow involvement and its application in Gaucher disease. *J Comput Assist Tomogr* 2002;26:843.

191. Zimran A, Elstein D, Levy-Lahad E, et al. Replacement therapy with imiglucerase for type 1 Gaucher's disease [Comment]. *Lancet* 1995;345:1479.

192. Barton NW, Brady RO, Dambrosia JM, et al. Replacement therapy for inherited enzyme deficiency—macrophage-targeted glucocerebrosidase for Gaucher's disease [Comment]. *N Engl J Med* 1991;324:1464.

193. Altarescu G, Schiffmann R, Parker CC, et al. Comparative efficacy of dose regimens in enzyme replacement therapy of type I Gaucher disease [Comment]. *Blood Cells Mol Dis* 2000;26:285.

194. Grabowski GA, Kacena KC, Hollak JA, et al. Dose-response relationships for enzyme replacement therapy with imiglucerase.alglucerase in patients with Gaucher disease type 1. *Genet Med* 2009;11:92–100.

195. Rudzki Z, Okon K, Machaczka M, et al. Enzyme replacement therapy reduces Gaucher cell burden but may accelerate osteopenia in patients with type I disease—a histological study. *Eur J Haematol* 2003;70:273.

196. Poll LW, Koch JA, vom Dahl S, et al. Magnetic resonance imaging of bone marrow changes in Gaucher disease during enzyme replacement therapy: first German long-term results. *Skeletal Radiol* 2001;30:496.

197. Terk MR, Dardashti S, Liebman HA. Bone marrow response in treated patients with Gaucher disease: evaluation by T1-weighted magnetic resonance images and correlation with reduction in liver and spleen volume. *Skeletal Radiol* 2000;29:563.

198. Bembi B, Ciana G, Mengel E, et al. Bone complications in children with Gaucher disease. *Brit J Radiol* 2002;75(Suppl 1):A37.

199. Poll LW, Maas M, Terk MR, et al. Response of Gaucher bone disease to enzyme replacement therapy. *Brit J Radiol* 2002;75(Suppl 1):A25.

200. Altarescu G, Hill S, Wiggs E, et al. The efficacy of enzyme replacement therapy in patients with chronic neuronopathic Gaucher's disease. *J Pediatr* 2001;138:539.

201. Kaplan P, Mazur A, Manor O, et al. Acceleration of retarded growth in children with Gaucher disease after treatment with alglucerase. *J Pediatr* 1996;129:149.

202. Cohen IJ, Katz K, Kornreich L, et al. Low-dose high-frequency enzyme replacement therapy prevents fractures without complete suppression of painful bone crises in patients with severe juvenile onset type I Gaucher disease [Comment]. *Blood Cells Mol Dis* 1998;24:296.

203. Krivit W, Peters C, Shapiro EG. Bone marrow transplantation as effective treatment of central nervous system disease in globoid cell leukodystrophy, metachromatic leukodystrophy, adrenoleukodystrophy, mannosidosis, fucosidosis, aspartylglucosaminuria, Hurler, Maroteaux-Lamy, and Sly syndromes, and Gaucher disease type III. *Curr Opin Neurol* 1999;12:167.

204. Platt FM, Jeyakumar M, Andersson U, et al. Inhibition of substrate synthesis as a strategy for glycolipid lysosomal storage disease therapy. *J Inherit Metab Dis* 2001;24:275.

205. Coppes-Zantinga A, Egeler RM. The Langerhans cell histiocytosis X files revealed. *Br J Haematol* 2002;116:3.

206. Nezelof C, Basset F, Rousseau MF. Histiocytosis X histogenetic arguments for a Langerhans cell origin. *Biomedicine* 1973;18:365.

207. Nicholson HS, Egeler RM, Nesbit ME. The epidemiology of Langerhans cell histiocytosis. *Hematol Oncol Clin North Am* 1998;12:379.

208. Raney RB, D'Angio GJ Jr. Langerhans' cell histiocytosis (histiocytosis X): experience at the Children's Hospital of Philadelphia, 1970–1984. *Med Pediatr Oncol* 1989;17:20.

209. Arico M, Girschikofsky M, Genereau T, et al. Langerhans cell histiocytosis in adults. Report from the International Registry of the Histiocyte Society. *Eur J Cancer* 2003;39:2341.

210. Broadbent V, Egeler RM, Nesbit ME Jr. Langerhans cell histiocytosis—clinical and epidemiological aspects. *Br J Cancer Suppl* 1994;23:S11.

211. Meyer JS, Harty MP, Mahboubi S, et al. Langerhans cell histiocytosis: presentation and evolution of radiologic findings with clinical correlation. *Radiographics* 1995;15:1135.

212. Broadbent V. Favourable prognostic features in histiocytosis X: bone involvement and absence of skin disease. *Arch Dis Child* 1986;61:1219.

213. Leavey P, Varughese M, Breatnach F, et al. Langerhans cell histiocytosis—a 31 year review. *Ir J Med Sci* 1991;160:271.

214. Bollini G, Jouve JL, Gentet JC, et al. Bone lesions in histiocytosis X. *J Pediatr Orthop* 1991;11:469.

215. Dimentberg RA, Brown KL. Diagnostic evaluation of patients with histiocytosis X. *J Pediatr Orthop* 1990;10:733.

216. Egeler RM, Nesbit ME. Langerhans cell histiocytosis and other disorders of monocyte-histiocyte lineage. *Crit Rev Oncol Hematol* 1995;18:9.

217. Levine SE, Dormans JP, Meyer JS, et al. Langerhans' cell histiocytosis of the spine in children. *Clin Orthop* 1996;323:288.

218. Greis PE, Hankin FM. Eosinophilic granuloma. The management of solitary lesions of bone. *Clin Orthop* 1990;257:204.

219. Demiral AN, Ozdemir O, Coskunol E, et al. Solitary eosinophilic granuloma of the third metacarpal at pediatric age. *Pediatr Hematol Oncol* 2003;20:589.

220. David R, Oria RA, Kumar R, et al. Radiologic features of eosinophilic granuloma of bone. *AJR Am J Roentgenol* 1989;153:1021.

221. Lahey E. Histiocytosis X—an analysis of prognostic factors. *J Pediatr* 1975;87:184.

222. Lieberman PH, Jones CR, Steinman RM, et al. Langerhans cell (eosinophilic) granulomatosis. A clinicopathologic study encompassing 50 years. *Am J Surg Pathol* 1996;20:519.

223. Berry DH, Gresik MV, Humphrey GB, et al. Natural history of histiocytosis X: a Pediatric Oncology Group Study. *Med Pediatr Oncol* 1986;14:1.

224. Fiorillo A, Sadile F, De Chiara C, et al. Bone lesions in Langerhans cell histiocytosis. *Clin Pediatr (Phila)* 1993;32:118.

225. Grois NG, Favara BE, Mostbeck GH, et al. Central nervous system disease in Langerhans cell histiocytosis. *Hematol Oncol Clin North Am* 1998;12:287.

226. Green NE, Robertson Jr WW, Kilroy AW. Eosinophilic granuloma of the spine with associated neural deficit. Report of three cases. *J Bone Joint Surg Am* 1980;62:1198.

227. Kanterewicz E, Condom E, Canete JD, et al. Spinal cord compression by a unifocal eosinophilic granuloma: a case report of an adult with unusual roentgenological features. *Neurosurgery* 1988;23:666.

228. Kerr R. Radiologic case study. Eosinophilic granuloma of the spine causing neurologic deficit. *Orthopedics* 1989;12:309.

229. Kumar A. Eosinophilic granuloma of the spine with neurological deficit. *Orthopedics* 1990;13:1310.

230. Alley RM, Sussman MD. Rapidly progressive eosinophilic granuloma. A case report. *Spine* 1992;17:1517.

231. Kilborn TN, Teh J, Goodman TR. Paediatric manifestations of Langerhans cell histiocytosis: a review of the clinical and radiological findings. *Clin Radiol* 2003;58:269.

232. Kozlowski K, Diard F, Padovani J, et al. Unilateral mid-femoral periosteal new bone of varying aetiology in children. Radiographic analysis of 25 cases. *Pediatr Radiol* 1986;16:475.

233. Meyer JS, De Camargo B. The role of radiology in the diagnosis and follow-up of Langerhans cell histiocytosis. *Hematol Oncol Clin North Am* 1998;12:307.

234. Gardner DJ, Azouz EM, Derbekyan V. Solitary lucent epiphyseal lesions in children. Radiological case of the month. Solitary costal eosinophilic granuloma. *Skeletal Radiol* 1988;17:497.

235. Leeson MC, Smith A, Carter JR, et al. Eosinophilic granuloma of bone in the growing epiphysis. *J Pediatr Orthop* 1985;5:147.

236. Ghanem I, Tolo VT, D'Ambra PD, et al. Langerhans cell histiocytosis of bone in children and adolescents. *J Pediatr Orthop* 2003;23:124.

237. Garg S, Mehta S, Dormans JP. An atypical presentation of Langerhans cell histiocytosis of the cervical spine in a child. *Spine* 2003;28:E445.

238. Baber WW, Numaguchi Y, Nadell JM, et al. Eosinophilic granuloma of the cervical spine without vertebrae plana. *J Comput Tomogr* 1987;11:346.

239. Dogan AS, Conway JJ, Miller JH, et al. Detection of bone lesions in Langerhans cell histiocytosis: complementary roles of scintigraphy and conventional radiography. *J Pediatr Hematol Oncol* 1996;18:51.

240. Hung PC, Wang HS, Jaing TH, et al. From normal to abnormal MR findings within three weeks in a solitary pelvic Langerhans histiocytosis. *Skeletal Radiol* 2003;32:481.

241. Elsheikh T, Silverman JF, Wakely PE Jr, et al. Fine-needle aspiration cytology of Langerhans' cell histiocytosis (eosinophilic granuloma) of bone in children. *Diagn Cytopathol* 1991;7:261.

242. Yasko AW, Fanning CV, Ayala AG, et al. Percutaneous techniques for the diagnosis and treatment of localized Langerhans-cell histiocytosis (eosinophilic granuloma of bone). *J Bone Joint Surg Am* 1998;80:219.

243. Favara BE, Feller AC, Pauli M, et al. Contemporary classification of histiocytic disorders. The WHO Committee on Histiocytic/Reticulum Cell Proliferations. Reclassification Working Group of the Histiocyte Society. *Med Pediatr Oncol* 1997;29:157.

244. Pileri SA, Grogan TM, Harris NL, et al. Tumours of histiocytes and accessory dendritic cells: an immunohistochemical approach to classification from the International Lymphoma Study Group based on 61 cases. *Histopathology* 2002;41:1.

245. Laman JD, Leenen PJ, Annels NE, et al. Langerhans-cell histiocytosis "insight into DC biology." *Trends Immunol* 2003;24:190.

246. Schmitz L, Favara BE. Nosology pathology of Langerhans cell histiocytosis. *Hematol Oncol Clin North Am* 1998;12:221.

247. Womer RB, Raney RB, Jr, D'Angio GJ. Healing rates of treated and untreated bone lesions in histiocytosis X. *Pediatrics* 1985;76:286.

248. Alexander JE, Seibert JJ, Berry DH, et al. Prognostic factors for healing of bone lesions in histiocytosis X. *Pediatr Radiol* 1988;18:326.

249. Han I, Suh ES, Lee S-H, et al. Management of eosinophilic granuloma occurring in the appendicular skeleton in children. *Clin Orthop Surg* 2009;1(2):63–67.

250. Broadbent V, Gadner H. Current therapy for Langerhans cell histiocytosis. *Hematol Oncol Clin North Am* 1998;12:327.

251. Egeler RM, Thompson RC Jr, Voute PA, et al. Intralesional infiltration of corticosteroids in localized Langerhans' cell histiocytosis. *J Pediatr Orthop* 1992;12:811.

252. Platt FM, Jeyakumar M, Andersson U, et al. Inhibition of substrate synthesis as a strategy for glycolipid lysosomal storage disease therapy. *J Inherit Metab Dis* 2001;24:275.

253. Munn SE, Olliver L, Broadbent V, et al. Use of indomethacin in Langerhans cell histiocytosis [Comment]. *Med Pediatr Oncol* 1999;32:247.

254. Seegenschmiedt HM, Micke O, Olschewski T, et al. Radiotherapy is effective in symptomatic Langerhans Cell Histiocytosis (LCH): long-term results of a multicenter study in 63 patients. *Int J Radiat Oncol Biol Phys* 2003;57:S251.

255. Greenberger JS, Crocker AC, Vawter G, et al. Results of treatment of 127 patients with systemic histiocytosis. *Medicine* 1981;60:311.

256. Mammano S, Candiotto S, Balsano M. Cast and brace treatment of eosinophilic granuloma of the spine: long-term follow-up. *J Pediatr Orthop* 1997;17:821.

257. Robert H, Dubousset J, Miladi L. Histiocytosis X in the juvenile spine. *Spine* 1987;12:167.

258. Soucie JM, Evatt B, Jackson D. Occurrence of hemophilia in the United States. The Hemophilia Surveillance System Project Investigators. *Am J Hematol* 1998;59:288.

259. Favier R, Lavergne JM, Costa JM, et al. Unbalanced X-chromosome inactivation with a novel FVIII gene mutation resulting in severe hemophilia A in a female. *Blood* 2000;96:4373.

260. Aronstam A, Rainsford SG, Painter MJ. Patterns of bleeding in adolescents with severe haemophilia A. *Br Med J* 1979;1:469.

261. Gamble JG, Bellah J, Rinsky LA, et al. Arthropathy of the ankle in hemophilia. *J Bone Joint Surg Am* 1991;73:1008.

262. Houghton GR, Duthie RB. Orthopedic problems in hemophilia. *Clin Orthop* 1979;138:197.

263. Nolan B, Vidler V, Vora A, et al. Unsuspected haemophilia in children with a single swollen joint. *Brit Med J* 2003;326:151.

264. Pollmann H, Richter H, Ringkamp H, et al. When are children diagnosed as having severe haemophilia and when do they start to bleed? A 10-year single-centre PUP study. *Eur J Pediatr* 1999;158 (Suppl 3):S166.

265. Pool JG, Shannon AE. Production of high-potency concentrates of antihemophilic globulin in a closed-bag system. *N Engl J Med* 1965;273:1443.

266. Brinkhous KM, Shanbrom E, Roberts HR, et al. A new high-potency glycine-precipitated antihemophilic factor (AHF) concentrate. Treatment of classical hemophilia and hemophilia with inhibitors. *JAMA* 1968;205:613.

267. Wagner BH, McLester WD, Smith M, et al. Purification of antihemophilic factor (factor VIII) by amino acid precipitation. *Thromb Diath Haemorrh* 1964;11:64.

268. Aledort LM, Levine PH, Hilgartner M, et al. A study of liver biopsies and liver disease among hemophiliacs. *Blood* 1985;66:367.

269. Bianchi L, Desmet VJ, Popper H, et al. Histologic patterns of liver disease in hemophiliacs, with special reference to morphologic characteristics of non-A, non-B hepatitis. *Semin Liver Dis* 1987;7:203.

270. Kernoff PB. Hepatitis and factor VIII concentrates. *Semin Hematol* 1988;25:8.

271. Eyster ME, Gail MH, Ballard JO, et al. Natural history of human immunodeficiency virus infections in hemophiliacs: effects of T-cell subsets, platelet counts, and age. *Ann Intern Med* 1987;107:1.

272. Telfer MC. Clinical spectrum of viral infections in hemophilic patients. *Hematol Oncol Clin North Am* 1992;6:1047.

273. United Kingdom Haemophelia Centre Doctors' Organisation. Guidelines on the selection and use of therapeutic products to treat haemophilia and other hereditary bleeding disorders. *Haemophilia* 2003;9:1.

274. Scharrer I, Neutzling O. Incidence of inhibitors in haemophiliacs. A review of the literature. *Blood Coagul Fibrin* 1993;4:753.

275. Soucie JM, Cianfrini C, Janco RL, et al. Joint range-of-motion limitations among young males with hemophilia: prevalence and risk factors. *Blood* 2004;103(7):2467–2473.

276. Arnold WD, Hilgartner MW. Hemophilic arthropathy. Current concepts of pathogenesis and management. *J Bone Joint Surg Am* 1977;59(3):287–305.

277. Pettersson H, Nilsson IM, Hedner U, et al. Radiologic evaluation of prophylaxis in severe haemophilia. *Acta Paediatr Scand* 1981;70(4):565–570.

278. Manco-Johnson MJ, Abshire TC, Shapiro AD, et al. Prophylaxis versus episodic treatment to prevent joint disease in boys with severe hemophilia [see comment]. *N Engl J Med* 2007;357(6):535–544.

279. Lundin B, Pettersson H, Ljung R. A new magnetic resonance imaging scoring method for assessment of haemophilic arthropathy. *Haemophilia* 2004;10(4):383–389.

280. Kilcoyne RF, Nuss R. Radiological assessment of haemophilic arthropathy with emphasis on MRI findings. [Review] [26 refs]. *Haemophilia* 2003;9(Suppl 1):57–63; discussion–4.

281. Lundin B, Babyn P, Doria AS, et al. Compatible scales for progressive and additive MRI assessments of haemophilic arthropathy [see comment]. *Haemophilia* 2005;11(2):109–115.

282. Valentino LA, Hakobyan N, Kazarian T, et al. Experimental haemophilic synovitis: rationale and development of a murine model of human factor VIII deficiency. *Haemophilia* 2004;10(3):280–287.

283. Acharya SS, MacDonald DD, DiMichele DM, et al. A role for angiogenesis in hemophilic synovitis. *ASH Annu Meeting Abstr* 2004;104(11):42.

284. Roosendaal G, Vianen ME, Wenting MJ, et al. Iron deposits and catabolic properties of synovial tissue from patients with haemophilia. *J Bone Joint Surg Br* 1998;80(3):540–545.

285. Medeiros D, Laufenberg JA, Miller KL, et al. Short-term oral corticosteroid therapy for acute haemarthrosis in haemophilia patients with high-titre inhibitors. *Haemophilia* 2007;13(1):85–89.

286. Roosendaal G, Lafeber FP. Blood-induced joint damage in hemophilia. *Semin Thromb Hemost* 2003;29(1):37–42.

287. Hooiveld MJ, Roosendaal G, van den Berg HM, et al. Haemoglobin-derived iron-dependent hydroxyl radical formation in blood-induced joint damage: an in vitro study. *Rheumatology (Oxford)* 2003;42(6):784–790.

288. Hooiveld MJ, Roosendaal G, Vianen ME, et al. Immature articular cartilage is more susceptible to blood-induced damage than mature articular cartilage: an in vivo animal study. *Arthritis Rheum* 2003;48(2):396–403.

289. Hooiveld M, Roosendaal G, Wenting M, et al. Short-term exposure of cartilage to blood results in chondrocyte apoptosis. *Am J Pathol* 2003;162(3):943–951.

290. Aledort LM, Haschmeyer RH, Pettersson H. A longitudinal study of orthopaedic outcomes for severe factor-VIII-deficient haemophiliacs. The Orthopaedic Outcome Study Group. *J Intern Med* 1994;236(4):391–399.

290a. Fischer K, van Hout BA, van der Bom JG, et al. Association between joint bleeds and Pettersson scores in severe haemophilia. *Acta Radiol* 2002;43(5):528–532.

291. Fischer K, Astermark J, van der Bom JG, et al. Prophylactic treatment for severe haemophilia: comparison of an intermediate-dose to a high-dose regimen. *Haemophilia* 2002;8(6):753–760.

292. van den Berg HM, Fischer K, van der Bom JG. Comparing outcomes of different treatment regimens for severe haemophilia. *Haemophilia* 2003;9(Suppl 1):27–31; discussion 31.

293. Dunn AL, Abshire TC. Recent advances in the management of the child who has hemophilia. [Review] [141 refs]. *Hematol Oncol Clin North Am* 2004;18(6):1249–1276, viii.

294. Mannucci PM. Desmopressin (DDAVP) in the treatment of bleeding disorders: the first twenty years. *Haemophilia* 2000;6(Suppl 1):60–67.

295. Franchini M. The use of desmopressin as a hemostatic agent: a concise review. [Review] [74 refs]. *Am J Hematol* 2007;82(8):731–735.

296. Journeycake JM, Miller KL, Anderson AM, et al. Arthroscopic synovectomy in children and adolescents with hemophilia. *J Pediatr Hematol Oncol* 2003;25(9):726–731.

297. Dunn AL, Busch MT, Wyly JB, et al. Arthroscopic synovectomy for hemophilic joint disease in a pediatric population. *J Pediatr Orthop* 2004;24(4):414–426.

298. Silva M, Luck JV Jr, Siegel ME. 32P chromic phosphate radiosynovectomy for chronic haemophilic synovitis. *Haemophilia* 2001;7(Suppl 2):40–49.

299. Dunn AL, Busch MT, Wyly JB, et al. Radionuclide synovectomy for hemophilic arthropathy: a comprehensive review of safety and efficacy and recommendation for a standardized treatment protocol. [Review] [104 refs]. *Thromb Haemost* 2002;87(3):383–393.

299a. Dunn AL, Manco JM, Busch MT, et al. Leukemia and P32 radionuclide synovectomy for hemophilic arthropathy. *J Thromb Haemost* 2005;3(7):1541–1542.

300. Rodeghiero F, Castaman G, Dini E. Epidemiological investigation of the prevalence of von Willebrand's disease. *Blood* 1987;69:454.

301. Werner EJ, Broxson EH, Tucker EL, et al. Prevalence of von Willebrand disease in children: a multiethnic study. *J Pediatr* 1993;123:893.

302. Lenk H, Nilsson IM, Holmberg L, et al. Frequency of different types of von Willebrand's disease in the GDR. *Acta Med Scand* 1988;224:275.

303. Cohen AJ, Kessler CM, Ewenstein BM. Management of von Willebrand disease: a survey on current clinical practice from the Haemophilia Centres of North America. *Haemophilia* 2001;7:235.

304. Kadir RA, Economides DL, Sabin CA, et al. Assessment of menstrual blood loss and gynaecological problems in patients with inherited bleeding disorders. *Haemophilia* 1999;5:40.

305. Cash JD, Gader AM, da Costa J. Proceedings: The release of plasminogen activator and factor VIII to lysine vasopressin, arginine vasopressin, I-desamino-8-d-arginine vasopressin, angiotensin and oxytocin in man. *Br J Haematol* 1974;27:363.

306. Smith TJ, Gill JC, Ambruso DR, et al. Hyponatremia and seizures in young children given DDAVP. *Am J Hematol* 1989;31:199.

307. Andrew M, David M, Adams M, et al. Venous thromboembolic complications (VTE) in children: first analyses of the Canadian registry of VTE. *Blood* 1994;83:1251.

308. Lane DA, Mannucci PM, Bauer KA, et al. Inherited thrombophilia: Part 1. *Thromb Haemost* 1996;76:651.

309. Kearon C, Crowther M, Hirsh J. Management of patients with hereditary hypercoagulable disorders. *Annu Rev Med* 2000;51:169.

310. Tait RC, Walker ID, Reitsma PH, et al. Prevalence of protein C deficiency in the healthy population. *Thromb Haemost* 1995;73:87.

311. Tait RC, Walker ID, Perry DJ, et al. Prevalence of antithrombin deficiency in the healthy population. *Br J Haematol* 1994;87:106.

312. Rosendaal FR, Koster T, Vandenbroucke JP, et al. High risk of thrombosis in patients homozygous for factor V Leiden (activated protein C resistance). *Blood* 1995;85:1504.

313. Poort SR, Rosendaal FR, Reitsma PH, et al. A common genetic variation in the region of the prothrombin gene is associated with elevated plasma prothrombin levels and an increase in venous thrombosis. *Blood* 1996;88:3698.

314. Bauer KA. Management of thrombophilia. *J Thromb Haemost* 2003;1:1429.

315. Levi M, van der Poll T, ten Cate H, et al. The cytokine-mediated imbalance between coagulant and anticoagulant mechanisms in sepsis and endotoxaemia. *Eur J Clin Invest* 1997;27:3.

316. Osterud B, Bjorklid E. The tissue factor pathway in disseminated intravascular coagulation. *Semin Thromb Hemost* 2001;27:605.

317. Levi M, Keller TT, van Gorp E, et al. Infection and inflammation and the coagulation system. *Cardiovasc Res* 2003;60:26.

318. Schleef RR, Bevilacqua MP, Sawdey M, et al. Cytokine activation of vascular endothelium. Effects on tissue-type plasminogen activator and type 1 plasminogen activator inhibitor. *J Biol Chem* 1988;263:5797.

319. Bakhshi S, Arya LS. Diagnosis and treatment of disseminated intravascular coagulation. *Indian Pediatr* 2003;40:721.

320. Bick RL. Disseminated intravascular coagulation and related syndromes: a clinical review. *Semin Thromb Hemost* 1988;14:299.

321. Baker WF Jr. Clinical aspects of disseminated intravascular coagulation: a clinician's point of view. *Semin Thromb Hemost* 1989;15:1.

322. Chuansumrit A, Hotrakitya S, Sirinavin S, et al. Disseminated intravascular coagulation findings in 100 patients. *J Med Assoc Thai* 1999;82(Suppl 1):S63.

323. Becker S, Schneider W, Kreuz W, et al. Post-trauma coagulation and fibrinolysis in children suffering from severe cerebro-cranial trauma. *Eur J Pediatr* 1999;158(Suppl 3):S197.

324. Bull BS, Rubenberg ML, Dacie JV, et al. Microangiopathic haemolytic anaemia: mechanisms of red-cell fragmentation: in vitro studies. *Br J Haematol* 1968;14:643.

325. Hoyle CF, Swirsky DM, Freedman L, et al. Beneficial effect of heparin in the management of patients with APL. *Br J Haematol* 1988;68:283.

326. Sakuragawa N, Hasegawa H, Maki M, et al. Clinical evaluation of low-molecular-weight heparin (FR-860) on disseminated intravascular coagulation (DIC)—a multicenter cooperative double-blind trial in comparison with heparin. *Thromb Res* 1993;72:475.

327. Fourrier F, Chopin C, Huart JJ, et al. Double-blind, placebo-controlled trial of antithrombin III concentrates in septic shock with disseminated intravascular coagulation. *Chest* 1993;104:882.

328. Eisele B, Lamy M. Clinical experience with antithrombin III concentrates in critically ill patients with sepsis and multiple organ failure. *Semin Thromb Hemost* 1998;24:71.

329. Sauaia A, Moore FA, Moore EE, et al. Epidemiology of trauma deaths: a reassessment. *J Trauma* 1995;38:185.

330. Cosgriff N, Moore EE, Sauaia A, et al. Predicting life-threatening coagulopathy in the massively transfused trauma patient: hypothermia and acidoses revisited. *J Trauma* 1997;42:857.

331. Watts DD, Trask A, Soeken K, et al. Hypothermic coagulopathy in trauma: effect of varying levels of hypothermia on enzyme speed, platelet function, and fibrinolytic activity. *J Trauma* 1998;44:846.

332. Jurkovich GJ, Greiser WB, Luterman A, et al. Hypothermia in trauma victims: an ominous predictor of survival. *J Trauma* 1987;27:1019.

333. Armand R, Hess JR. Treating coagulopathy in trauma patients. *Transfus Med Rev* 2003;17:223.

334. Reiss RF. Hemostatic defects in massive transfusion: rapid diagnosis and management. *Am J Crit Care* 2000;9:158.

335. Hirshberg A, Dugas M, Banez EI, et al. Minimizing dilutional coagulopathy in exsanguinating hemorrhage: a computer simulation. *J Trauma* 2003;54:454.

336. Bickell WH, Wall MJ Jr, Pepe PE, et al. Immediate versus delayed fluid resuscitation for hypotensive patients with penetrating torso injuries. *N Engl J Med* 1994;331:1105.

337. Anesthesiologists" ASo. Practice guidelines for blood component therapy: A report by the American Society of Anesthesiologists Task Force on Blood Component Therapy. *Anesthesiology* 1996;84:732.

338. Hiippala ST, Myllyla GJ, Vahtera EM. Hemostatic factors and replacement of major blood loss with plasma-poor red cell concentrates. *Anesth Analg* 1995;81:360.

339. Jonsson OG, Sartain P, Ducore JM, et al. Bone pain as an initial symptom of childhood acute lymphoblastic leukemia: association with nearly normal hematologic indexes. *J Pediatr* 1990;117:233.

340. Barbosa CM, Nakamura C, Terreri MT, et al. Musculoskeletal manifestations the onset of acute leukemias in childhood. *J Pediatr (Rio J)* 2002; 78:481.

341. Halton JM, Atkinson SA, Fraher L, et al. Mineral homeostasis and bone mass at diagnosis in children with acute lymphoblastic leukemia. *J Pediatr* 1995;126:557.

342. Heinrich SD, Gallagher D, Warrior R, et al. The prognostic significance of the skeletal manifestations of acute lymphoblastic leukemia of childhood. *J Pediatr Orthop* 1994;14:105.

343. Rogalsky RJ, Black GB, Reed MH. Orthopaedic manifestations of leukemia in children. *J Bone Joint Surg Am* 1986;68:494.

344. Santangelo JR, Thomson JD. Childhood leukemia presenting with back pain and vertebral compression fractures. *Am J Orthop* 1999;28:257.

345. Bertuna G, Fama P, Nigro LL, et al. Marked osteoporosis and spontaneous vertebral fractures in children: don't forget, it could be leukemia. *Med Pediatr Oncol* 2003;41:450.

346. Meehan PL, Viroslav S, Schmitt EW Jr. Vertebral collapse in childhood leukemia. *J Pediatr Orthop* 1995;15:592.

347. Ostrov BE, Goldsmith DP, Athreya BH. Differentiation of systemic juvenile rheumatoid arthritis from acute leukemia near the onset of disease. *J Pediatr* 1993;122:595.

348. Saulsbury FT, Sabio H. Acute leukemia presenting as arthritis in children. *Clin Pediatr (Phila)* 1985;24:625.

349. Appell RG, Buhler T, Willich E, et al. Absence of prognostic significance of skeletal involvement in acute lymphocytic leukemia and non-Hodgkin lymphoma in children. *Pediatr Radiol* 1985;15:245.

350. Kumar R, Walsh A, Khalilullah K, et al. An unusual orthopaedic presentation of acute lymphoblastic leukemia. *J Pediatr Orthop B* 2003;12:292.

351. van der Sluis IM, van den Heuvel-Eibrink MM, Hahlen K, et al. Altered bone mineral density and body composition, and increased fracture risk in childhood acute lymphoblastic leukemia. *J Pediatr* 2002;141:204.

352. Atkinson SA, Halton JM, Bradley C, et al. Bone and mineral abnormalities in childhood acute lymphoblastic leukemia: influence of disease, drugs and nutrition. *Int J Cancer Suppl* 1998;11:35.

353. Swiatkiewicz V, Wysocki M, Odrowaz-Sypniewska G, et al. Bone mass and bone mineral metabolism at diagnosis and after intensive treatment in children with acute lymphoblastic leukemia. *Med Pediatr Oncol* 2003; 41:578.

354. Ravindranath Y. Recent advances in pediatric acute lymphoblastic and myeloid leukemia. *Curr Opin Oncol* 2003;15:23.

355. McNeil DE, Cote TR, Clegg L, et al. SEER update of incidence and trends in pediatric malignancies: acute lymphoblastic leukemia. *Med Pediatr Oncol* 2002;39:554.

356. Uckun FM, Nachman JB, Sather HN, et al. Clinical significance of Philadelphia chromosome positive pediatric acute lymphoblastic leukemia in the context of contemporary intensive therapies: a report from the Children's Cancer Group. *Cancer* 1998;83:2030.

357. Arnold WD, Hilgartner MW. Hemophilic arthropathy. Current concepts of pathogenesis and management. *J Bone Joint Surg Am* 1977;59:287.

358. Goldberg JM, Silverman LB, Levy DE, et al. Childhood T-cell acute lymphoblastic leukemia: the Dana-Farber Cancer Institute Acute Lymphoblastic Leukemia Consortium Experience. *J Clin Oncol* 2003;21:3616.

359. Pui CH, Sandlund JT, Pei D, et al. Results of therapy for acute lymphoblastic leukemia in black and white children. *JAMA* 2003;290:2001.

360. Gallagher DJ, Phillips DJ, Heinrich SD. Orthopedic manifestations of acute pediatric leukemia. *Orthop Clin North Am* 1996;27:635.

361. Lu CS, Huang IA, Wang CJ, et al. Magnetic resonance abnormalities of bone marrow in a case of acute lymphoblastic leukemia. *Acta Paediatr Taiwan* 2003;44:109.

362. Arico M, Boccalatte MF, Silvestri D, et al. Osteonecrosis: an emerging complication of intensive chemotherapy for childhood acute lymphoblastic leukemia. *Haematologica* 2003;88:747.

363. D'Antonio D, Pagano L, Girmenia C, et al. Cutaneous aspergillosis in patients with haematological malignancies. *Eur J Clin Microbiol Infect Dis* 2000;19:362.

CHAPTER 11

Pamela F. Weiss

Juvenile Idiopathic Arthritis

OVERVIEW OF PEDIATRIC RHEUMATIC DISEASE ENCOUNTERED BY THE PEDIATRIC ORTHOPAEDIC SURGEON

Joint pain is a common childhood complaint. Each year, as many as 1% of all children will be evaluated by a physician for joint pain (1). Approximately 15% of healthy children reported on a health questionnaire that they had episodes of musculoskeletal pain (2). Further, healthy children in day care centers have approximately one painful episode every 3 hours, arising from play, disciplining, or interaction with peers (3). The orthopaedic surgeon is often the first specialist to encounter the child with joint, limb, or back pain. In a study of subspecialty referrals of juvenile arthritis, most children with pauciarticular juvenile rheumatoid arthritis (JRA) (62%) were referred to orthopaedic surgeons prior to referral to pediatric rheumatology care (4). Among children who are evaluated by a physician for pain in the joints, only 1 in 100 will eventually be diagnosed as having arthritis, but among those who present to an orthopaedist, the frequency of arthritis is surely higher. Accordingly, it is important that the orthopaedic surgeon be able to identify the most likely cause of the pain and either initiate treatment or refer the patient to an appropriate medical specialist.

The purpose of this chapter is to provide the orthopaedic surgeon with an in-depth understanding of the presentation, differential diagnosis, and management of children with arthritis. With this framework, the orthopaedic specialist should be able to identify children with juvenile arthritis and to differentiate arthritis from benign pains of childhood, psychogenic pain syndromes, benign musculoskeletal back pain, infection, malignancy, or other systemic autoimmune diseases (lupus, dermatomyositis, and vasculitis). Infectious, malignant, congenital, mechanical, or traumatic causes of arthralgias and arthritis are presented in order to contrast the symptoms with those of juvenile arthritis; detailed presentations on these conditions can be found elsewhere in this text.

CLASSIFICATION OF JUVENILE ARTHRITIS

Juvenile arthritis is a term for persistent arthritis lasting >6 weeks of unclear etiology. A diagnosis of juvenile arthritis is made by taking a thorough history, performing a skilled and comprehensive physical examination, utilizing directed laboratory tests and imaging procedures, and following the child over time.

Over the past several decades, there have been three sets of criteria utilized for the diagnosis and classification of juvenile arthritis (Table 11-1). The first set of criteria was proposed in 1972 by the American College of Rheumatology (ACR) and defined three major categories of JRA: oligoarticular (pauciarticular), polyarticular, and systemic (5). The ACR JRA criteria exclude other causes of juvenile arthritis, such as spondyloarthropathies [JAS, inflammatory bowel disease (IBD)-associated arthritis, and related diseases], juvenile psoriatic arthritis, arthritis associated with other systemic inflammatory diseases [systemic lupus erythematosus (SLE), dermatomyositis, sarcoidosis, etc.], and infectious or neoplastic disorders. The second set of criteria was formulated in 1977 by the European League Against Rheumatism (EULAR) and coined the term juvenile chronic arthritis (JCA) (6). JCA is differentiated into the following subtypes: pauciarticular, polyarticular, juvenile rheumatoid [positive rheumatoid factor (RF)], systemic, juvenile ankylosing spondylitis (JAS), and juvenile psoriatic arthritis. The ACR and EULAR criteria, although similar, do not identify identical populations or spectra of disease. However, they have often been used interchangeably, leading to confusion in the interpretation of studies relating to the epidemiology, treatment, and outcome of juvenile arthritis.

In 1993, The International League of Associations of Rheumatologists (ILAR) proposed (7) and revised (8) criteria for the diagnosis and classification of juvenile arthritis (Table 11-2). The term juvenile idiopathic arthritis (JIA) has been proposed as a replacement for both JRA and JCA. The

TABLE 11-1	Comparison of JRA, JCA, and JIA Classifications		
	JRA	**JCA**	**JIA**
Committee	ACR	EULAR	ILAR
Age at onset	<16 yr	<16 yr	<16 yr
Disease duration	>6 wk	>3 mo	>6 wk
Onset types	Pauciarticular	Pauciarticular	Oligoarticular, persistent
	Polyarticular	Polyarticular RF-negative	Oligoarticular, extended
	Systemic	Juvenile rheumatoid arthritis	Polyarticular RF-negative
		Systemic	Polyarticular RF-positive
		Juvenile psoriatic arthritis	Systemic
		Juvenile ankylosing spondylitis	Psoriatic arthritis
			Enthesitis-related arthritis
Exclusions	Juvenile psoriatic arthritis	Other forms of juvenile arthritis	Other forms of juvenile arthritis
	Juvenile ankylosing spondylitis		
	Inflammatory bowel disease		
	Other forms of juvenile arthritis		

RF, rheumatoid factor.

TABLE 11-2	Criteria for Classification of JIA	
JIA Subtype	**Exclusions[a]**	**Inclusion Criteria[b]**
Oligoarthritis	1–5	
Persistent		≤4 joints during disease course
Extended		>4 joints after the first 6 mo
Polyarthritis RF-negative	1–5	Arthritis affecting ≥5 joints during the first 6 mo
Polyarthritis RF-positive	1–3, 5	Arthritis affecting ≥5 joints during the first 6 mo, plus RF positivity on two occasions more than 3 mo apart
Systemic	1–4	Arthritis with or preceded by daily fever of at least 2 weeks' duration, accompanied by one or more of the following: Evanescent, nonfixed erythematous rash; Generalized adenopathy; Hepatomegaly or splenomegaly; Serositis
Psoriatic	2–5	Arthritis and psoriasis, or arthritis and at least two of the following: a. Dactylitis; b. Nail abnormalities (pitting or onycholysis); c. Family history of psoriasis in a first-degree relative
Enthesitis-related	1, 4, 5	Arthritis and enthesitis, or arthritis or enthesitis with at least two of the following: 1. SI joint tenderness and/or inflammatory spinal pain; 2. Presence of HLA-B27; 3. Family history of HLA-B27–associated disease in a first-degree relative; 4. Onset of arthritis in a male after the age of 6 yr
Undifferentiated		Children with arthritis of unknown cause that persists ≥6 wk; Does not fulfill criteria for any of the other categories; Fulfills criteria for ≥1 of the other categories

[a]Exclusions: 1, psoriasis in the patient or a first-degree relative; 2, arthritis in an HLA-B27 positive male beginning after the sixth birthday; 3, ankylosing spondylitis, enthesitis-related arthritis, sacroiliitis with IBD, Reiter syndrome, or acute anterior uveitis in a first-degree relative; 4, IgM RF on at least two occasions more than 3 mo apart; 5, presence of systemic JIA.
[b]Inclusion criteria for all subtypes: 1, age at onset <16 yr; 2, arthritis in one or more joints; 3, duration of disease is at least 6 wk.
From Petty RE, et al. International League of Associations for Rheumatology classification of juvenile idiopathic arthritis: second revision, Edmonton, 2001. *J Rheumatol* 2004;31(2):390–392.

ILAR criteria allow for uniform interpretation of clinical and therapeutic data. Recent validation of the ILAR classification criteria has found that 80% to 88% of children could be classified, and 12% to 20% were classified as "Undifferentiated" because they either did not fit into any category or fulfilled the criteria under two categories (9–12). As genetic risk factors and specific triggers of juvenile arthritis are identified, modifications to the criteria can be made. In the remaining sections of this chapter, the emphasis will be on the JIA classification scheme. The terms JRA and JCA will be used only when referring to specific epidemiologic, therapeutic, or outcome data.

Oligoarthritis

Definition.   Oligoarthritis is the most common subtype of JIA and is defined by arthritis in four or fewer joints during the first 6 months of disease. Oligoarticular JIA is further divided into persistent and extended course. Persistent oligoarthritis affects a maximum of four joints throughout the disease course. Extended oligoarthritis affects a total of more than four joints after the first 6 months of disease. Exclusions to a diagnosis of oligoarticular JIA include the following: (a) psoriasis or a history of psoriasis in a first-degree relative; (b) arthritis in a first-degree relative after the age of 6 years; (c) ankylosing spondylitis (AS), enthesitis-related arthritis sacroiliitis with IBD, reactive arthritis, or acute anterior uveitis, or a history of one of these in a first-degree relative; (d) presence of IgM RF on at least two occasions, measured 3 months apart; and (e) systemic JIA (8).

Epidemiology.   Most children with oligoarthritis present before 4 years of age and girls outnumber boys by a ratio of 4 to 1. Whites are affected more often than other races. It is the most frequent subtype of JIA, accounting for up to 40% of cases (13, 14). Prevalence is estimated at 60 per 100,000 children (15).

Etiology.   The etiology of oligoarticular JIA is unknown, but associations with HLA-A2, DRB1*01, DRB1*08, DRB1*11, DRB1*13, DPB1*02, DQA1*04, and DQB1*04 have been reported (14, 16). Oligoarticular JIA is rarely familial. Approximately 70% of oligoarticular JIA patients are positive for antinuclear antibodies (ANA).

Clinical Features.   Approximately 50% of children with oligoarticular JIA present with a single affected joint, most commonly the knee, followed by ankles and small joints of the hands. The hips and shoulders are rarely affected. Early wrist involvement is uncommon and may portend progression to a polyarticular or extended oligoarticular course. At presentation, the majority of children have morning stiffness, gelling, and pain. However, up to 25% of children have painless arthritis at presentation (17).

Most children with oligoarticular JIA have a mild and remitting course. However, in untreated children with long-standing unilateral knee arthritis, there can be overgrowth of the affected limb, resulting in a marked leg-length discrepancy (18, 19). Temporomandibular joint (TMJ) arthritis is present in a majority of children at disease onset (20) and if untreated, may cause localized growth disturbances, micrognathia, malocclusion, and chewing difficulties (21–23). Chronic uveitis is the most common extra-articular complication seen in oligoarthritis, is associated with ANA positivity, and occurs in approximately 20% of children. Periodic screening for uveitis is necessary as the inflammation is typically asymptomatic and unable to be detected without the use of a slit lamp. Untreated uveitis may result in cataracts, band keratopathy, secondary glaucoma, and blindness.

Long-term, children with oligoarticular JIA have the greatest likelihood of remission of all JIA subtypes. In one study, 68% of persistent and 31% of extended oligoarticular JIA patients achieved long-term clinical remission off medication (24).

Polyarticular Arthritis

Definition.   Polyarticular JIA is defined by arthritis in five or more joints during the first 6 months of disease. Polyarticular JIA is further divided into RF-positive and -negative disease. RF positivity is defined as the presence of IgM RF on at least two occasions, measured at least 3 months apart. Exclusions to a diagnosis of polyarticular JIA include the following: (a) psoriasis or a history of psoriasis in a first-degree relative; (b) arthritis in a first-degree relative after the age of 6 years; (c) AS, enthesitis-related arthritis sacroiliitis with IBD, reactive arthritis, or acute anterior uveitis; (d) or a history of one of these in a first-degree relative; and (e) systemic JIA (8).

Epidemiology.   RF-negative polyarthritis can occur at any age, with the median age of onset at 6.5 years (25), with girls outnumbering boys by a ratio of 3:1. RF-positive polyarticular JIA occurs most frequently in adolescent girls and is indistinguishable from adult rheumatoid arthritis (RA). Polyarticular JIA is the second most frequent subtype of JIA, accounting for up to 22% of cases (13, 14). Prevalence is estimated at 40 and 10 per 100,000 children for RF-negative and RF-positive subtypes, respectively (15).

Etiology.   The etiology of polyarticular JIA is unknown. Multiple studies have examined the association of HLA genes and disease. RF-negative polyarticular JIA has been associated with HLA-A2, DRB1*08, DQA1*04, and DPB1*03. Associations of RF-positive polyarticular JIA with HLA-DQA1*03, DQB1*03, and DRB1*04, a gene also associated with adult RA, have been reported (14).

Clinical Features.   Polyarticular-onset JIA is characterized by the insidious, but occasionally acute, onset of symmetric arthritis in five or more joints. It can involve both large and small joints and frequently affects the cervical spine and TMJs. Mild systemic features such as low-grade fever, lymphadenopathy, and hepatosplenomegaly may be present at diagnosis. The fevers are not typically the high quotidian temperature spikes that are diagnostic of systemic arthritis, and rash is rarely seen (26).

This RF-negative subgroup may be ANA positive (40% to 50%), and this is associated with an increased incidence of uveitis (5%) (27). Children with RF-positive polyarticular JIA are more likely to have a symmetric small-joint arthritis, rheumatoid nodules, and early erosive synovitis with a chronic course. However, these children rarely develop chronic uveitis.

Children with RF-positive polyarticular JIA are at risk for a prolonged and destructive course. These children are typically older girls with involvement of multiple joints (20 or more) including the small joints of the hands and feet, early erosions, and rheumatoid nodules. The presence of hip arthritis has been shown to be a poor prognostic sign and may lead to destruction of the femoral heads (28). If polyarthritis persists longer than 7 years, remission is unlikely. In a recent study, only 5% of RF-positive and 30% of RF-negative polyarticular JIA patients achieved long-term remission off medication (24).

Systemic Arthritis

Definition. Systemic-onset juvenile arthritis (29) was first completely described by Still in 1897, and is therefore often referred to as *Still disease*. Systemic JIA is defined by arthritis in at least one joint, fever of at least 2 weeks' duration that is documented to be quotidian for at least 3 days, and at least one of the following: (a) evanescent and erythematosus rash (Fig. 11-1); (b) generalized lymphadenopathy; (c) hepatosplenomegaly; and (d) serositis. Exclusions to a diagnosis of systemic JIA include

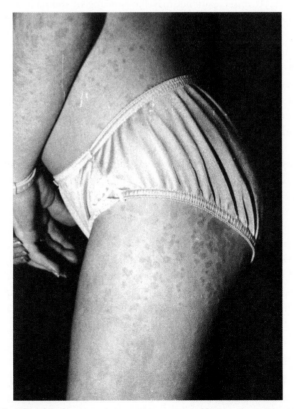

FIGURE 11-1. Rash associated with systemic-onset juvenile idiopathic arthritis.

the following: (a) psoriasis or a history of psoriasis in a first-degree relative; (b) arthritis in a first-degree relative after the age of 6 years; (c) AS, enthesitis-related arthritis sacroiliitis with IBD, reactive arthritis, or acute anterior uveitis, or a history of one of these in a first-degree relative; and (d) presence of IgM RF on at least two occasions, measured 3 months apart (8).

Epidemiology. Systemic JIA is one of the least common JIA subtypes, accounting for approximately 10% of all JIA cases (13). Onset can occur at anytime during childhood but peaks between 1 and 5 years of age (25). Boys and girls are affected equally. Prevalence of systemic JIA is estimated at 10 per 10,000 children (15).

Etiology. Etiology of systemic JIA is unknown. HLA associations that have been reported include DRB1*04, DRB1*11, and DQA1*05 (14). Non-HLA genetic associations have been found with macrophage migration inhibitory factor (30) and a variant of the interleukin-6 (IL-6) gene (8).

Clinical Features. The fever of systemic JIA is typically daily or twice-daily, usually to 39°C or higher (31). In between fever spikes, the temperature is often below normal. Children frequently appear quite ill while febrile but recover in between fevers. The fever often responds poorly to nonsteroidal anti-inflammatory drugs (NSAIDs) but will typically respond well to corticosteroids. In most children, the fever is accompanied by a characteristic rash that consists of discrete, transient, non-pruritic erythematous macules (Fig. 11-2) (32). The rash is typically more pronounced on the trunk but may occur on the extremities and the face. The most commonly involved joints are the knee, wrist, and ankle (33). Many children with systemic JIA will have extra-articular manifestations, including hepatosplenomegaly, pericarditis, pleuritis, lymphadenopathy, and abdominal pain. The extra-articular features may be present for weeks, months, and, occasionally, years prior to the onset of arthritis. Usually, the extra-articular manifestations of systemic JIA are self-limiting and will resolve spontaneously or with corticosteroid therapy. Occasionally, the pericarditis can result in tamponade.

The prognosis of systemic JIA is determined predominantly by the course of arthritis. Approximately 50% of children with systemic arthritis will have a mild oligoarticular course, and in most of these children, the arthritis will ultimately remit. The remaining half of the children with systemic onset will develop a polyarticular arthritis that can remit, but progresses in approximately 50% of the cases (25% of all systemic-onset JIA) to a severe, unrelenting, and destructive course despite all currently available therapeutic interventions (34). Chronic anterior uveitis is extremely rare in systemic arthritis. Systemic amyloidosis, usually presenting with the onset of proteinuria and hypertension, can occur as a result of any chronic inflammatory disease. Approximately 8% of European children with systemic JIA have been shown to develop this life-threatening complication (35). The incidence of amyloidosis in North America is significantly lower

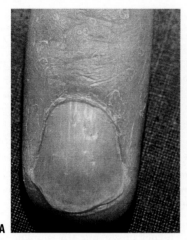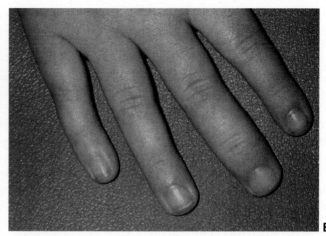

FIGURE 11-2.   Juvenile psoriatic arthritis. **A:** Nail pitting associated with psoriasis. **B:** Swelling of a single DIP joint in a child with juvenile psoriatic arthritis.

than that seen in Europe. The reason for this discrepancy remains unclear.

Macrophage activation syndrome (MAS), also termed *hemophagocytic lymphohistiocytosis*, is a severe, potentially life-threatening complication seen nearly exclusively in systemic arthritis. It is characterized by macrophage activation with hemophagocytosis and is associated with hepatic dysfunction, disseminated intravascular coagulation with a precipitous fall in the erythrocyte sedimentation rate (ESR) secondary to hypofibrinogenemia, and encephalopathy (36). It has been suggested that anti-inflammatory medications and viral infections can induce this syndrome. High-dose corticosteroids, cyclosporine A, and IL-1 inhibition have been shown to improve the outcome of MAS (37–39).

Psoriatic Arthritis

Definition.   Psoriatic arthritis is defined as the presence of arthritis and psoriasis, or arthritis and at least two of the following: (a) dactylitis, (b) nail pitting or onycholysis (Fig. 11-2), and (c) psoriasis in a first-degree relative. Exclusions to a diagnosis of psoriatic JIA include the following: (a) arthritis in a first-degree relative after the age of 6 years; (b) AS, enthesitis-related arthritis sacroiliitis with IBD, reactive arthritis, or acute anterior uveitis, or a history of one of these in a first-degree relative; (c) presence of IgM RF on at least two occasions, measured 3 months apart; and (d) systemic JIA (8).

Epidemiology.   Psoriasis occurs in approximately 0.5% of the population (40), 20% to 30% of whom have associated arthritis (41, 42). There is a bimodal distribution of age of onset with a peak in the preschool years and again around 10 years of age. Girls are slightly more affected than boys. Psoriasis often begins after the onset of arthritis, usually within 2 years. The prevalence of psoriatic JIA is estimated at 15 per 100,000 children (15). Psoriatic arthritis accounts for 5% to 7% of JIA (13).

Etiology.   The etiology of psoriatic arthritis is unknown but genetic associations with HLA-Cw6, DRB1*01, and DQA1*0101 have been demonstrated (14, 43). There is often a strong family history of psoriasis or psoriatic arthritis in affected children.

Clinical Features.   The arthritis in psoriatic JIA is often an asymmetric mono- or polyarthritis affecting both large and small joints. At onset, patients may have pitting of the nails (67%) (Fig. 11-2) and a family history of psoriasis (69%) or dactylitis (39%), while less than one-half of the children have the rash of psoriasis (13% to 43%) (25, 44, 45). JIA criteria do not require the development of psoriasis to confirm a diagnosis of psoriatic arthritis (Table 11-2) (46). In children younger than 5 years, the presentation is often characterized by the involvement of a small number of fingers or toes that are relatively asymptomatic, but leading to marked overgrowth of the digit(s).

Children with psoriatic arthritis may have chronic life-long arthritis that follows a relapsing and remitting course. Arthritis mutilans and severe distal interphalangeal (DIP) joint disease are unusual. However, many of the children will have prolonged polyarthritis that may result in irreversible joint damage (47). Amyloidosis has been reported in the European literature as having resulted in the deaths of at least three children (47, 48). Chronic anterior uveitis has been observed in up to 17% of the children (44, 45) and is associated with a positive ANA titer; the uveitis associated with psoriatic JIA is clinically indistinguishable from the uveitis in oligoarticular and polyarticular JIA.

Enthesitis-Related Arthritis

Definition.   The JIA criteria for classification of ERA describe a group of arthritides that includes undifferentiated spondyloarthritis, JAS, and IBD-associated arthritis. The JIA criteria include many of the children who were previously diagnosed with a syndrome of seronegativity, enthesopathy, and arthropathy (SEA syndrome) who were shown to be at increased risk for development of classic spondyloarthritis or JAS (49, 50). ERA is defined as arthritis and enthesitis or arthritis or enthesitis with at least two of the following: (a) the presence or a history of sacroiliac (SI) tenderness or lumbosacral pain; (b) HLA-B27 antigen positivity; (c) onset of arthritis in a male after age of 6 years; (d) acute anterior uveitis; and (e) history of AS, ERA, sacroiliitis with IBD, reactive arthritis, or acute anterior uveitis in a first-degree relative. Exclusions for a diagnosis of ERA include (a) psoriasis or a history of psoriasis in the patient or a first-degree relative; (b) presence of IgM RF on at least two occasions, measured 3 months apart; and (c) systemic JIA.

Epidemiology. Unlike the other subtypes of JIA, ERA is more common in boys. Disease onset is typically after the age of 6 years. Prevalence is estimated at 50 per 100,000 children (15).

Etiology. The presence of HLA-B27 is part of the diagnostic criteria for ERA. In these children, molecular mimicry is thought to contribute to the pathogenesis. Other HLA genetic associations that have been found are HLA-DRB1*01, DQA1*0101, and DQB1*05 (14).

Clinical Features. ERA is often associated with enthesitis and arthralgias or arthritis long before any axial skeletal involvement is identified (50). Enthesitis is identified when marked tenderness is noted at the 6, 10, and 2 o'clock positions on the patella, at the tibial tuberosity, iliac crest, or the attachments of the Achilles tendon or plantar fascia (Fig. 11-3) (51). However, in ERA not all entheses are created equal; some entheses are more prone to trauma and mechanical damage such as in Sinding-Larsen-Johansson syndrome while other entheses are frequently tender in normal children such as the

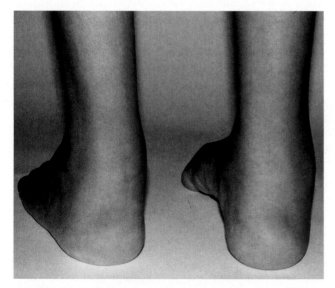

FIGURE 11-3. Achilles tendonitis and enthesitis in a child with enthesitis-related arthritis. (Courtesy of Dr. Ruben Burgos-Vargas.)

plantar fascia insertion into the metatarsal heads. One study suggested that "pathologic" enthesitis be defined as the presence of three tender entheses at the following sites: SI joints, inferior patellar pole, Achilles tendon insertion, and plantar fascia insertion into the calcaneus (52).

The primary extra-articular manifestation of ERA is acute anterior uveitis, which can occur in up to 27% of children with AS (53). The uveitis is manifested by an acute, painful, red, photophobic eye. ERA-associated uveitis may resolve with no ocular residua, but some of the children will have a persistent uveitis that is relatively resistant to therapy and can result in blindness (54, 55).

Juvenile Ankylosing Spondylitis

Definition. The definition of ERA overlaps with that of spondyloarthropathies, a group of conditions that includes JAS and reactive arthritis. Radiographic evidence of bilateral sacroiliitis is necessary to fulfill the New York criteria for AS (Table 11-3).

Epidemiology. JAS most often presents in late childhood or adolescence. Boys outnumber girls by a ratio of 6 to 1 (56). There is a high frequency of JAS in Pacific Canada Indians (57) and a low incidence in African Americans (58).

Etiology. The similarities between JAS and reactive arthritis, in which gastrointestinal and genitourinary infections trigger disease, suggest a role for infection. There is a strong genetic component to disease as AS occurs up to 16 times more frequently in HLA-B27–positive family members of patients with AS than in HLA-B27–positive individuals in the population at large (59). Further, children with JAS and SI involvement are frequently HLA-B27 positive (82% to 95%) (56).

Clinical Course. Children with early JAS often fulfill the diagnostic criteria for ERA. Episodic arthritis of the lower extremity large joints, enthesitis, and tarsitis within 1 year of symptom onset predicts of progression to JAS (60). The presentation of JAS is most remarkable for the absence of axial involvement. Only 12% to 24% of children with JAS have pain, stiffness, or limitation of motion of the SI or lumbosacral spine at disease onset. A peripheral arthropathy or enthesopathy,

TABLE 11-3	New York Criteria for AS
Clinical criteria	Limited lumbar motion in all three planes
	History or presence of lumbar spinal pain
	≤2.5 cm of chest expansion at the 4th intercostal space
Definite AS	Grade 3 or 4 bilateral radiographic SI changes plus at least 1 clinical criterion
	Grade 3 or 4 unilateral or grade 2 bilateral radiographic SI changes plus clinical criterion 1 or criteria 2 and 3
Probable AS	Grade 3 or 4 bilateral radiographic SI changes without any clinical criteria

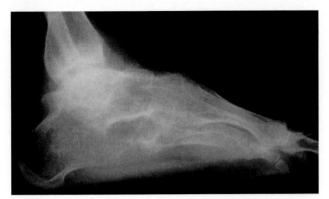

FIGURE 11-4. Ankylosing tarsitis, a complex disorder resulting in ankylosis of the foot in a child with JAS. (Courtesy of Dr. Ruben Burgos-Vargas.)

affecting predominantly the lower limb joints and entheses, is seen in 79% to 89.4%. These children tend to have fewer than 5 joints involved and rarely more than 10. At presentation, the pattern of involvement of the joints is usually asymmetric (61). Small joints of the toes are commonly involved in JAS but are seldom affected in other forms of JIA, with the exception of psoriatic arthritis. However, polyarticular and axial disease are usually evident after the 3rd year of illness (61). Children with long-standing JAS have been shown to develop tarsal bone coalition that has been termed *ankylosing tarsitis* (Fig. 11-4) (62).

Outcome data for JAS are incomplete and at times contradictory. The prognosis of JAS has been reported as being worse according to some studies, and better according to others, than adult-onset AS (63, 64). Hip disease has been associated with a poor functional outcome (63, 65) and may require total hip arthroplasty.

Inflammatory Bowel Disease–Associated Arthritis

The frequency of arthritis in children with IBD has been reported to be 7% to 21%, and it usually occurs after the diagnosis of the bowel disease (66–68). Two different patterns of arthritis are seen (51). The most common type is oligo- or polyarticular

arthritis of the lower limbs. This group is less likely to meet the criteria for ERA. This arthritis is often episodic, with exacerbation lasting 4 to 6 weeks or, rarely, for months. The activity of the peripheral arthritis is often related to the underlying bowel disease activity. The less common type of IBD-associated arthritis is an HLA-B27–associated oligoarticular arthritis of the lower limbs, with sacroiliitis and enthesitis, and no relationship to bowel inflammation (51). This form is more likely to persist and progress despite adequate control of the bowel disease. The clinical course is similar to that in other children with ERA.

DIFFERENTIAL DIAGNOSIS OF PAIN AND SWELLING IN THE JOINTS IN CHILDREN

A comprehensive differential diagnosis of arthritis in childhood is beyond the scope of this chapter as there are over 100 disorders in which arthritis may be a significant manifestation (69). The most common classes of disorders that must be considered in the differential diagnosis of JIA include infection, postinfectious phenomenon, inflammatory arthropathies, systemic autoimmune disease, mechanical or orthopaedic conditions, trauma, and pain disorders. Often, the differential diagnosis will be determined by whether the presentation is acute, subacute, or chronic, whether the child has monoarticular or polyarticular arthritis, and whether there are systemic signs such as fever (Table 11-4).

Infection-Related Arthritis

Septic Arthritis. Septic arthritis generally affects a single joint and is associated with fever, elevated neutrophil count, ESR, C-reactive protein (CRP), and extreme pain. Synovial fluid analysis typically reveals white cell counts of >50,000 (70), neutrophil predominance, low glucose (<30 mg/dL), and a positive Gram stain. Oligoarticular JIA, in contrast, is seldom associated with systemic inflammation and joint effusions are often out of proportion to the reported pain. The most commonly infected joints in children are the knees, hips, ankles, and elbows. Gonococcal arthritis may present in a

TABLE 11-4	Differential Diagnosis of JIA	
Monoarticular Arthritis	**Polyarticular Arthritis**	**Febrile Syndromes**
Oligoarthritis	Polyarthritis	Systemic arthritis
Psoriatic arthritis	Psoriatic arthritis	Malignancy:
Enthesitis-related arthritis	Enthesitis-related arthritis	Lymphoid
Sarcoidosis	Sarcoidosis	Neuroblastoma
Transient synovitis of the hip	Systemic lupus erythematosus	Systemic lupus erythematosus
Trauma	Juvenile dermatomyositis	Juvenile dermatomyositis
Hemophilia	Systemic vasculitis	Systemic vasculitis
Pigmented villonodular synovitis	Scleroderma	Infection (viral or bacterial)
Septic arthritis	Gonococcal septic arthritis	Inflammatory bowel disease
Reactive arthritis	Reactive arthritis	Reactive arthritis

sexually active adolescent as an oligoarticular, polyarticular, or migratory arthritis with significant tenosynovitis.

Lyme Arthritis.

Lyme arthritis may occur weeks to months after infection with the tick-borne spirochete *Borrelia burgdorferi*. Up to 60% of patients with untreated disease develop arthritis, which may be manifested by intermittent or continuous swelling (71). Many patients with untreated Lyme disease complain of migratory arthralgias or arthritis (72). In a recent retrospective study of 90 children with Lyme arthritis, Gerber et al. (73) noted that the majority (63%) had monoarticular disease, but no child had more than four joints involved. The knee was affected most often (90%), followed by hip (14%), ankle (10%), wrist (9%), and elbow (7%), whereas small joints were rarely involved. Most children with Lyme arthritis do not recall a tick bite or erythema migrans (73, 74). Lyme arthritis is typically an inflammatory synovitis with a very large and relatively painless joint effusion (Fig. 11-5). The ESR can be normal or elevated (73). The diagnosis should be confirmed with serologic testing, which includes an enzyme-linked immunosorbent assay (ELISA) and Western blot. There is a high rate of false-positives with ELISA testing, so if the ELISA is positive, then a confirmatory Western blot should be performed. If the ELISA is negative, no further testing is needed. Synovial fluid analysis typically reveals white cell counts of 10,000 to 25,000. A small percentage of children may develop a persistent arthritis despite multiple courses of oral and/or intravenous antibiotics; persistence of swelling is associated with *HLA-DR4* and *HLA-DR2* alleles (75). In these patients, intra-articular corticosteroid injections are often helpful. Detection of *Borrelia burgdorferi* in the synovial fluid using polymerase chain reaction (PCR) can be confirmatory in seropositive patients. However, a positive PCR in the setting of negative serologies is likely to be a false-positive (76). Further a positive PCR is not proof of active infection as remnant DNA may persist for some time after *Borrelia burgdorferi* killing has occurred (76).

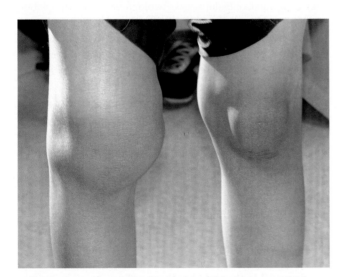

FIGURE 11-5. Right knee effusion in a child with Lyme arthritis.

Postinfectious Arthritis.

Postinfectious or reactive arthritis results in a sterile synovitis that is an immune response to a nonarticular infection. In most children, the reactive arthritis occurs after upper respiratory or gastrointestinal infections, whereas in adult patients it is more likely to occur following a genitourinary infection (77–79). The classic presentation of reactive arthritis is the triad of conjunctivitis, urethritis, and arthritis. The complete triad of reactive arthritis is very uncommon in childhood. The ratio of boys to girls is 4 to 1 (79, 80). Most patients with reactive arthritis carry the *HLA-B27* allele (79, 81).

Transient Synovitis of the Hip.

Transient synovitis of the hip is a self-limiting, postinfectious, inflammatory arthritis. Transient synovitis of the hip has a peak incidence, predominantly in boys (70%), at between 3 and 10 years of age. It is an idiopathic disorder often preceded by a nonspecific upper respiratory tract infection (82). The onset of pain is often gradual, is rarely bilateral, and lasts for an average of 6 days. There is often low-grade fever and mild elevation of inflammatory markers (83). With rest and NSAIDs, most children will have complete resolution of symptoms within 2 weeks. Most children with transient synovitis of the hip will have only a single event; however, 4% to 17% have a recurrence within 6 months (84).

Acute Rheumatic Fever.

Acute rheumatic fever (ARF) is a postinfectious reaction to an untreated group A β-hemolytic streptococcus infection of the pharynx (85). Arthritis, which is the most common but least specific ARF manifestation, classically appears 2 to 3 weeks after the streptococcal infection. The classic arthritis of ARF is a migratory polyarthritis. The affected joints are erythematous, swollen, and extremely painful. The joint pain is exquisitely responsive to aspirin or NSAIDs; dramatic relief is often obtained within several hours after the first dose. Since children with ARF are at an increased risk for rheumatic carditis, streptococcal prophylaxis is recommended until age 21. The diagnosis can be confirmed by the presence of the other major JONES criteria (Table 11-5), which include carditis, migratory subcutaneous nodules, chorea, and erythema marginatum.

TABLE 11-5	Modified Jones Criteria for Acute Rheumatic Fever
Major Manifestations	**Minor Manifestations**
Carditis	Fever
Polyarthritis	Arthralgia
Subcutaneous nodules	Prolonged PR interval
Erythema marginatum	Increased ESR or CRP
Chorea	

Diagnosis requires the presence of two major criteria, or one major and two minor criteria, with supporting evidence of a preceding streptococcal infection (rising streptococcal antibody titers, positive throat culture, or rapid streptococcal antigen test).
ESR, erythrocyte sedimentation rate; CRP, C-reactive protein.

Poststreptococcal Arthritis. Poststreptococcal-reactive arthritis is a postinfectious reaction to a streptococcal infection that does not fulfill ARF criteria. It typically presents as a nonmigratory oligo- or polyarthritis. Unlike ARF, it is poorly responsive to aspirin or other nonsteroidal drugs. Limited studies have suggested that further episodes of streptococcal pharyngitis lead to an increased risk for ARF and rheumatic carditis and that streptococcal prophylaxis is indicated for 1 to 2 years (86, 87).

Serum Sickness. Serum sickness is a clinical syndrome resulting from an adverse immunologic response to foreign antigens mediated by the deposition of immune complexes. The most common culprits are antibiotics (penicillins and sulfonamides) and infections (88–90). Serum sickness is characterized by fever, arthralgia or arthritis, lymphadenopathy, cutaneous eruptions (urticarial or morbilliform), and angioedema. Both serum sickness and allergic angioedema can be mistaken for acute-onset JIA. However, most children with serum sickness will spontaneously improve within a few weeks. For mild disease, removal of the offending antigen and treatment with antihistamines and nonsteroidal anti-inflammatory medications is sufficient. In severe cases, a several-week course of corticosteroids may be required.

Other Inflammatory Arthropathies

Gout. Gouty arthritis is characterized by hyperuricemia and deposition of monosodium urate crystals into the joint. The major clinical manifestations include acute mono- or oligoarthritis, frequently involving the first metatarsophalangeal joint. Gout may result from either increased production or decreased excretion of uric acid. Gout is extremely rare in children (91). The diagnosis can be confirmed by demonstration of negatively birefringent, monosodium urate crystals in the synovial fluid. Acute gout is treated with nonsteroidal anti-inflammatory medications, colchicine, and occasionally prednisone. After the acute event has subsided, allopurinol is utilized to prevent recurrences. The use of allopurinol is not recommended during the acute phase of gout.

Cystic Fibrosis–Associated Arthritis. Cystic fibrosis (CF)-associated arthritis (92) is an episodic transient arthritis often associated with pulmonary exacerbations (93–97). The joint symptoms typically last for 1 to 10 days and may be associated with a pruritic and nodular rash. Additionally, CF patients have a higher-than-expected occurrence of RF-positive polyarticular JIA or adult RA (98). Some children with CF may develop secondary hypertrophic osteoarthropathy, demonstrable on radiographs (99, 100).

Systemic Autoimmune Diseases. Many of the systemic autoimmune diseases can cause acute or chronic arthritis. There are often signs, symptoms, or laboratory abnormalities that will aid in the diagnosis of these conditions. For a thorough discussion of these diseases in children, several excellent texts and reviews are available (51, 69, 101).

SLE is an episodic, autoimmune inflammatory disease characterized by multiorgan system inflammation. Arthralgia and arthritis affect 75% of the children with SLE. It is usually polyarticular, and the joint pain is often out of proportion to the physical findings. Typically, the arthritis responds readily to corticosteroids, is rarely erosive (102), and does not result in deformity.

Sarcoidosis is uncommon in childhood (103). However, arthritis is frequent in childhood-onset sarcoidosis, and typically presents as an oligoarthritis affecting the knees, ankles, and/or elbows. Large and boggy effusions with minimal discomfort characterize the arthritis. A synovial biopsy is often diagnostic, showing the presence of noncaseating granulomas.

Vasculitis in childhood may be associated with arthritis. The disease most likely to be seen by the orthopaedic surgeon is Henoch-Schönlein purpura (HSP). HSP is the most common vasculitic syndrome in childhood, occurring in slightly more than 1 in 10,000 children per year (104). The classic manifestations of HSP are nonthrombocytopenic palpable purpura, arthritis, abdominal pain, gastrointestinal hemorrhage, and glomerulonephritis. In the complete syndrome, the diagnosis is often clear. However, the arthritis can precede the appearance of the rash, and the rash may be unrecognized if a comprehensive skin examination is not done. The rash of HSP often begins on the lower extremities as an urticarial eruption, followed by petechiae and purpura, which are most often concentrated on the buttocks and lower extremities. The arthritis of HSP presents as a periarticular swelling and tenderness, most commonly of large joints, with severe pain and limitation of motion. The younger child will often refuse to use the affected joint. The arthritis is usually transient, and resolves without sequelae in a few days to weeks.

Foreign Body Synovitis. Plant thorns and wood splinters in the joint space can cause a chronic synovitis or tendonitis (105). Typically, the injury has been long forgotten, because many months may pass between entry of the thorn into the skin and passage into the joint. Surgical removal of the splinter and synovectomy are the only effective treatments.

Coagulopathies and Hemoglobinopathies. Children with congenital coagulopathies (hemophilia) and hemoglobinopathies (sickle cell disease) will present with acute pain and swelling in the joints, resulting from hemarthrosis and localized ischemia, respectively. A comprehensive discussion of these conditions is found in Chapter 11.

Malignancy. It is not uncommon for malignancies such as childhood leukemia to present as musculoskeletal pain and joint swelling. Often these symptoms present before blasts are detectable in the peripheral blood, making diagnosis challenging (106). In a recent study of 277 children ultimately diagnosed with either JIA or acute lymphocytic leukemia (ALL), the features that best predicted a diagnosis of ALL were leukopenia ($<4 \times 10^9$/L), borderline low platelet count ($150–200 \times 10^9$/L), and a history of nighttime pain (106). Plain radiographs may show subperiosteal elevation, osteolytic reaction, or metaphyseal rarefaction.

Pigmented Villonodular Synovitis. Pigmented villonodular synovitis (PVNS) is a benign tumor of the synovium.

PVNS is a rare cause of episodic joint effusions (107, 108). The effusions are minimally painful and cause progressive cartilage destruction and bone erosions (Fig. 11-6A). Synovial aspirates that are very bloody should arouse suspicion of the diagnosis. Magnetic resonance imaging (MRI) can be helpful, but confirmation of the diagnosis is made by synovial biopsy showing nodular hypertrophy, with proliferating fibroblasts and synovial cells, and hemosiderin-laden macrophages (Fig. 11-6B). Treatment consists of surgical excision. However, recurrence is frequent and multifocal disease can occur.

Benign Nocturnal Pains of Childhood.

Growing pains, or benign nocturnal pains of childhood, are common and may affect up to 20% of all children (109). These pains typically occur in school-age children. The pain typically affects the lower extremities symmetrically. Characteristically, the pain occurs in the early evening or at night and often awakens the child from sleep. The pains are always resolved by the morning and respond well to massage or analgesics. The physical examination and laboratory studies are always normal. Children with recurring nighttime pains often have significant relief from a single bedtime dose of acetaminophen, ibuprofen, or naproxen.

Reflex Sympathetic Dystrophy.

Reflex sympathetic dystrophy (RSD) is likely underrecognized in children (110–113). The onset of RSD often occurs after minor trauma or after a fracture has healed and the cast has been removed. There is an initial pain that causes the child to stop using the affected limb. The disuse perpetuates the pain and the extremity involved becomes painful to light touch (allodynia), swollen, cold, and discolored. Plain radiographs of the affected limb may show soft-tissue swelling and, after 6 to 8 weeks, a generalized osteoporosis. Technetium-99m bone scans may show either a diffuse increase (early) or decrease (late) in uptake of isotope (Fig. 11-7). The most effective treatment for RSD is vigorous physical therapy and careful attention to the underlying psychosocial stressors (110, 111, 114). The affected limb should never be immobilized, because this will uniformly cause a worsening of the pain during or after the period of immobilization.

RADIOGRAPHIC FEATURES OF JIA

Plain radiographs are useful in the initial evaluation of children with pain and/or swelling in the joints, predominantly for identifying periarticular osteopenia, fractures, or other bony lesions. Radiographic features associated with JIA include the following, in order of appearance: (a) soft-tissue swelling and widening of the joint space, (b) generalized osteoporosis, (c) joint space narrowing, (d) erosions, (e) subluxation, and (f) ankylosis (Figs. 11-8 and 11-9). However, the diagnosis of JIA is often made before radiographic changes are detectable. Erosive changes, with the exception of the TMJs, are uncommon before 2 years of active disease. Children with chronic polyarthritis may develop bony ankylosis of the carpal and tarsal joints, and in the cervical spine. Radiologic abnormalities of the cervical spine (Fig. 11-10) can result from apophyseal joint inflammation and bony fusion, often initially at the C2–C3 level. Atlantoaxial instability, which is not uncommon with cervical disease, is identified when the atlanto-odontoid space is >4 mm. If instability is identified, special care should be used if intubation is required for a surgical procedure.

Children with AS will develop radiographically visible changes in the SI joints, but this may not occur for 1 to 15 (average 6.5) years after diagnosis (53). These findings can include pseudo-widening caused by erosions, sclerosis, and fusion (Fig. 11-11). Radiologic changes in the lumbosacral spine occur later in the course of JAS and are less frequent (115). Chronic enthesitis, particularly at the calcaneus, can result in erosion at the insertion of the Achilles tendon or plantar fascia.

Other imaging modalities that are useful in the evaluation of JIA include ultrasound, Tc-99m scintography, and MRI (116). Ultrasound is a rapid, inexpensive, and noninvasive way to identify an intra-articular effusion. Radionucleotide imaging with Tc-99m (bone scan) is helpful to screen for osteomyelitis, malignancy, and joints with subclinical inflammation. MRI (116) is the most sensitive technique for detecting early articular changes in JIA and is the imaging technique of choice for evaluation of TMJ arthritis (20, 117–119).

OTHER DIAGNOSTIC STUDIES FOR JIA

Laboratory Tests.

There are no diagnostic laboratory tests for JIA. The selection of specific laboratory evaluations should be guided by the history and physical examination. A complete blood count with differential, CRP, and ESR should be part of the initial evaluation of any child with joint swelling. These tests will help to identify hematologic abnormalities suggesting malignancy, and to document the presence or absence of systemic inflammation. Systemic JIA, malignancies, systemic autoimmune diseases, and infections typically have an elevated ESR, often >100 mm/hour. However, most children with oligoarticular and some with polyarticular JIA will have a normal ESR and CRP. The addition of a CRP test can be helpful in situations in which infection is strongly suspected, because the short half-life of this acute-phase protein results in a rapid decline in concentration with effective antibiotic treatment, whereas the ESR may continue to rise. In addition, serologic testing for Lyme is appropriate in the setting of monoarthritis if the patient is from a Lyme endemic area.

The ANA titer is a measure of serum antibodies that can bind to one of many potential antigens present in the nucleus of normal human cells. ANA titer at a dilution of >1 to 40 is considered positive. The presence of an elevated ANA is not diagnostic of JIA and should not be used as a screening test for arthritis. ANA can be positive in up to 20% of the normal population and may be induced by illness or be present in first- or second-degree relatives with SLE (120, 121). Unless there is a high index of suspicion of JIA, a positive ANA test results in unnecessary subspecialty referrals and parental anxiety.

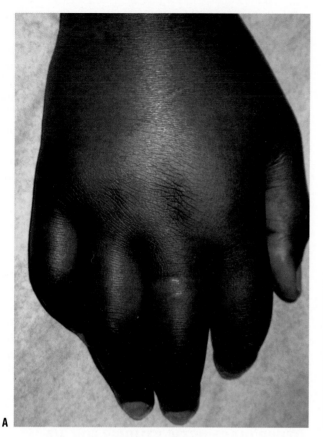

A

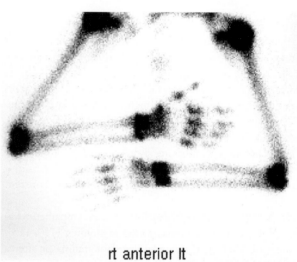

rt anterior lt   B

FIGURE 11-6. Reflex sympathetic dystrophy in a child with a 1 month history of hand swelling and pain. **A:** Right hand after 1 month of symptoms. **B:** Technetium-99m bone scan showing diffuse increased isotope uptake in the affected hand. **C:** Right hand after 3 weeks of intensive physical therapy and psychotherapy.

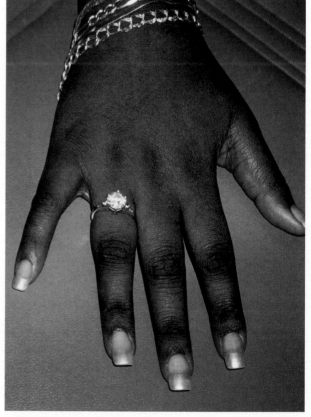

C

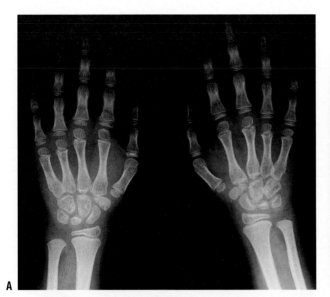
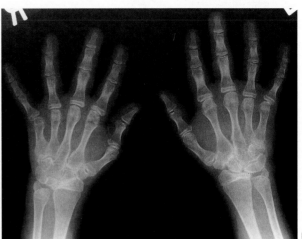

A

B

FIGURE 11-7. Polyarticular JIA with wrist and finger involvement. **A:** At 6 years of age, there is periarticular osteopenia and diffuse swelling of the wrist and fingers. **B:** At 20 years of age there is significant carpal and carpometacarpal fusion.

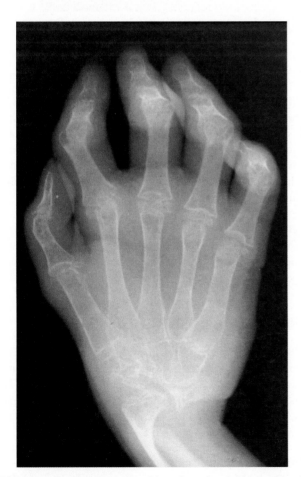

FIGURE 11-8. Systemic JIA with prolonged arthritis resulting in severe osteopenia and destructive changes in the hand and wrist, with severe ulnar deviation.

Children who have a positive ANA in the absence of systemic inflammation and arthritis are unlikely to subsequently develop a significant autoimmune disease (120, 122). In children with an established JIA diagnosis, the frequency of ANA positivity is greatest in young girls with oligoarticular disease, and represents an increased risk for anterior uveitis (123). If JIA is suspected on the basis of a history and physical exam, positive ANA should prompt an immediate referral to an ophthalmologist for a slit-lamp examination to evaluate for the presence of uveitis.

The RF is an autoreactive IgM, anti-IgG that is commonly used to help diagnose adult RA. In contrast to adults with RA, RF positivity is infrequent in children with JIA. Therefore, like the ANA, RF is not a good screening test for JIA. When present, it is most commonly associated with polyarticular JIA. RF is associated with a higher frequency of erosive synovitis and a poorer prognosis (124, 125).

Anti-citrullinated cyclic peptide (anti-CCP) antibodies have a sensitivity and specificity of 48% and 98%, respectively, for adult RA (126). Additionally, adult CCP-positive RA patients have a more aggressive disease course manifested by joint erosions and destruction (127, 128). Anti-CCP antibodies are mainly detected in polyarticular RF-positive JIA patients and are of limited diagnostic value. However, in a child with established polyarticular disease, seropositivity for anti-CCP antibodies may portend a more destructive disease course and, therefore, help to identify patients who might benefit from more aggressive therapy at diagnosis.

The presence of HLA-B27 is strongly associated with transient reactive arthritis, IBD, and ERA. The high familial occurrence of AS is directly related to the presence of HLA-B27 (129). Although HLA-B27 is found in approximately 8% of the white population, it can be useful in the diagnosis of

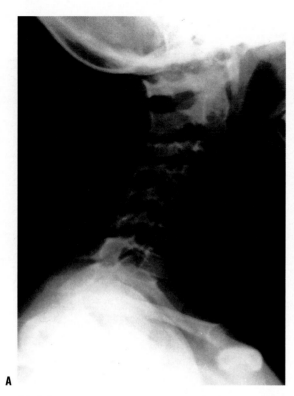 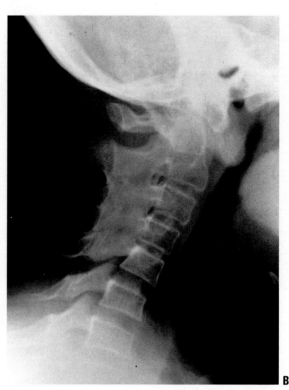

FIGURE 11-9. The cervical spine in a child with polyarticular JIA. **A.** At 6 years of age, there are no radiographic abnormalities. **B.** At 21 years of age there is ankylosis of C2–C5.

ERA. It is especially important in boys above the age of 6, where there is a family history of HLA-B27–associated illness, or SI joint or spinal inflammatory pain.

Synovial Fluid Analysis. Arthrocentesis with synovial fluid analysis and culture should be performed in all children

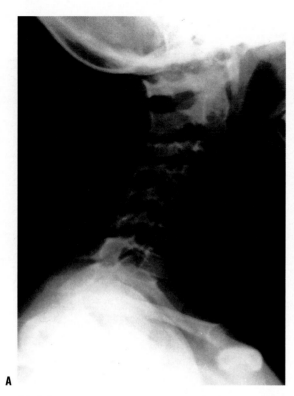

FIGURE 11-10. CT scan of SI joints in a child with JAS showing erosions and sclerosis of the SI joints. (Courtesy of D. Ruben Burgos-Vargas.)

with an acute arthritis accompanied by fever or in children for whom the diagnosis is unclear. In JIA, synovial fluid is type II, or inflammatory. The appearance is typically yellow and cloudy with decreased viscosity. Leukocyte counts are generally between 15 and 20,000 cells/mm^3; however, they may range as high as 100,000 cells/mm^3 (130–132). There is typically a neutrophil predominance (130).

Synovial Biopsy. A synovial biopsy should be performed if the diagnosis remains unclear after laboratories, imaging, and synovial fluid analysis. Biopsy is particularly helpful if a diagnosis of tuberculosis, PVNS, or sarcoidosis is being considered.

TREATMENT RECOMMENDATIONS

Medications. The fundamental purpose of pharmacologic therapy is to achieve pain control, decrease inflammation, prevent joint destruction, and to maintain remission. The medications used are individualized for each patient, depending on their subtype of arthritis, degree of inflammation, and previous pharmacologic response.

Nonsteroidal Anti-Inflammatory Drugs. NSAIDs are the initial therapeutic intervention in many children with JIA. NSAIDs provide both analgesia and anti-inflammatory effects. NSAIDs affect the biosynthesis of prostaglandins by direct inhibition of cyclo-oxygenase (COX) (133). There are two isoforms

rare (134). Gastroduodenal injury is more frequent in children who are receiving high doses, or more than one NSAID at a time (135). The use of aspirin in JIA is no longer recommended because of the risk of Reye syndrome.

In the United States, the most commonly used NSAID for JIA is naproxen (10 to 20 mg/kg/d). In children with fevers, serositis, or pericarditis associated with systemic arthritis, reactive arthritis, or JAS, indomethacin is often the most effective NSAID (51).

The doses of NSAIDs in children are based on body weight, and are often proportionally greater than in adult rheumatic diseases (Table 11-6). Preparations that come in a liquid form and have once- or twice-daily dosing are preferred. Children on long-term NSAID therapy should have a complete blood count, renal and liver function tests, and urine analysis at baseline, within 6 weeks of therapy initiation, and every 6 to 12 months thereafter. The average time required for a therapeutic response to NSAIDs is 2 to 12 weeks (136). Therefore, an NSAID is usually tried for several weeks before another is substituted. Approximately 50% of children respond to the first NSAID; of those who do not respond, 50% respond to an alternate NSAID (137). Nearly two-thirds of children with juvenile arthritis are inadequately treated with NSAIDs alone (138). These children require additional pharmacologic interventions.

Corticosteroids. Intra-articular corticosteroid injections have been shown to be safe and effective in controlling the synovitis in JIA (139, 140). A recent decision analysis reported that initial intra-articular injection, rather than a trial of NSAIDs, is the optimal treatment for monoarthritis (141). In order to avoid a singled intra-articular injection, 3.8 children need to be treated with an initial trial of NSAIDs; the cost of initial therapy with NSAIDs was an expected additional

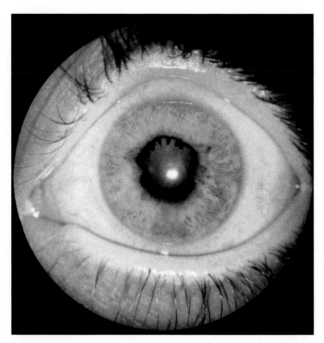

FIGURE 11-11. Iritis in oligoarticular JIA. Posterior synechiae with an irregular pupil.

of the COX enzyme. COX-1 is constitutively expressed and is involved in gastric cytoprotection, maintenance of renal perfusion, and platelet aggregation. COX-2 is upregulated at sites of inflammation. Most NSAIDs inhibit both COX isoforms, with consequential side effects such as GI toxicity or renal hypoperfusion. NSAIDs are generally safe and well tolerated in most children. Abdominal pain, nausea, and vomiting are the most common side effects, and gastrointestinal hemorrhage is

TABLE 11-6	**NSAIDs for the Treatment of JIA**	
Drug	**Dosage (mg/kg/d)**	**Maximum Daily Dose (mg)**
TID medications		
Indomethacin (Indocin)[a,b]	2–3	200
Salicylsalicylic acid (Aspirin)[b]	80–100	5200
Ibuprofen (Motrin, Advil, etc.)[a,b]	45	3200
Tolmetin (Tolectin)[b]	30–40	1800
BID medications		
Sulindac (Clinoril)	4–6	400
Choline magnesium trisalicylate (Trilisate)[a]	50–65	4500
Naproxen (Naprosyn)[a,b]	15–20	1000
Diclofenac sodium (Voltaren)	2–3	150
Celecoxib (Celebrex)[b]	4–6	400
Daily medications		
Nabumetone (Relafen)	20–30	2000
Meloxicam (Mobic)[a,b]	0.25	15
Feldene	0.25–0.4	20

[a]Liquid preparation available.
[b]U.S. Food and Drug Administration (FDA)-labeled for use in children.

6.7 months of active arthritis (141). Further, early intra-articular corticosteroid injections are associated with less leg-length discrepancy (LLD) in young children with oligoarthritis (142).

Triamcinolone hexacetonide (1 mg/kg for large joints and 0.5 mg/kg for medium joints) is the most commonly used agent and often provides long-term control of inflammation. The most frequent adverse consequence of intra-articular corticosteroids is the development of subcutaneous atrophy at the site of injection. Other side effects of intra-articular injections include infection, chemical irritation, and periarticular calcifications.

Systemic corticosteroids can be used for rapid control of severe arthritis. However, long-term use should be restricted to those children who have severe arthritis or systemic features that do not respond to other interventions.

Methotrexate.

The efficacy of methotrexate in JIA is well established (143, 144). It is a folic aid analogue, a competitive inhibitor of dihydrofolate reductase, and an inhibitor of purine biosynthesis.

Methotrexate is typically given at a dosage of 0.5 to 1 mg/kg/wk or 15 mg/m^2/wk (with a maximum of 25 mg) once weekly, either orally or by subcutaneous injection (145, 146). The most common side effects of methotrexate are nausea, fatigue, and liver transaminitis. Supplementation with folic acid (1 mg/d) can usually prevent gastrointestinal complications. Subcutaneous methotrexate should be considered for children who require doses >20 mg or who have significant gastrointestinal toxicity with the oral formulation. The average timecourse for clinical response to methotrexate is 6 to 8 weeks. Children on methotrexate should have a complete blood count and liver function tests at baseline, within 6 weeks of therapy initiation and then every 2 to 3 months thereafter.

Antitumor Necrosis Factor Agents.

Although the etiology and pathogenesis of juvenile arthritis are still unclear, macrophage-derived cytokines, such as tumor necrosis factor-α, appear to play a critical role in the induction and perpetuation of the chronic inflammatory process in JIA. Etanercept (Enbrel) is a soluble protein containing the extracellular domains of a p75 human TNF receptor attached to the Fc portion of a type 1 human immunoglobulin. Etanercept binds TNF-α in circulation and prevents subsequent cell activation. A multicenter placebo-controlled, double-blinded trial showed it to be effective in the treatment of juvenile arthritis that was resistant to initial therapy with methotrexate (147, 148). Further, the safety and efficacy of etanercept is maintained for up to 8 years (149). Etanercept is given subcutaneously at a dose of 0.8 mg/kg/wk.

Infliximab (Remicade) is a chimeric, monoclonal anti–TNF-α antibody that binds both soluble and membrane-bound TNF-α. Infliximab has been shown to be efficacious in combination with methotrexate for the treatment of refractory juvenile arthritis (150) and chronic inflammatory uveitis (151). However, recently, a double-blinded, randomized trial did not show a statistically significant difference between children treated with methotrexate plus placebo versus methotrexate plus infliximab (149). Infliximab is given intravenously at a dosage

of 3 to 10 mg/kg/dose; higher doses are often used for the treatment of refractory uveitis. Higher doses (≥6 mg/kg/dose) are also associated with less frequent adverse events, infusion reactions, and induced antibodies to the drug itself, ANA and double-stranded DNA (149).

Adalimumab (Humira) is a fully human monoclonal anti–TNF-α antibody that binds soluble and membrane-bound TNF-α. Adalimumab alone or in combination with methotrexate was well tolerated and effective in treatment-refractory RA (152), juvenile arthritis (153), and treatment-refractory JIA-associated uveitis (154). Adalimumab is given subcutaneously at a dose of 24 mg/m^2 (maximum dose 40 mg) every other week (153).

The major adverse events associated with the use of anti–TNF-α agents are an increased risk of infection, coccidiomycosis, and reactivation of latent tuberculosis (155). Prior to the onset of therapy, patients should have a documented negative PPD.

Sulfasalazine.

Sulfasalazine has been used extensively in Europe, and increasingly in North America for the treatment of JIA. It was developed on the idea that RA was caused by an infection; therefore, it has both antibacterial and anti-inflammatory properties. A randomized, double-blind, placebo-controlled trial showed that sulfasalazine is both safe and effective for the treatment of oligo- and polyarticular juvenile arthritis (156).

It is typically given in an enteric-coated form at a dose of 50 mg/kg/d in two divided doses. Serious side effects have been noted in children with systemic arthritis, and the routine use of sulfasalazine is not recommended for this subgroup (157, 158). Side effects occur in up to 30% of patients (159) and include cytopenias, severe allergic reactions such as Stevens Johnson syndrome, hypogammaglobulinemia, and IgA deficiency. Children taking sulfasalazine should have a complete blood count, liver function tests, and urinalysis at baseline and every 2 to 3 months thereafter. Immunoglobulin levels should be monitored every 6 months.

Abatacept.

Abatacept (Orencia) is a fully human monoclonal antibody (MRA) that consists of the extracellular domain of the CTLA-4 receptor attached to the Fc portion of the immunoglobulin receptor. CTLA-4 competitively binds CD-80/86 and blocks T-cell co-stimulation. Abatacept is efficacious and safe in TNF-resistant adult RA (160). In a double-blinded, randomized controlled trial, children with methotrexate-resistant or TNF-resistant JIA who were treated with abatacept had a statistically significant decrease in the occurrence of and increased time to disease flare (161).

Abatacept is given at a dose of 10 mg/kg every 4 weeks. The major adverse events are infusion reactions and infection (161).

Anti-Interleukin 1 Agents.

Anakinra (kineret) is an IL-1 receptor antagonist. It has been shown to be safe and efficacious in combination with methotrexate for adult RA (162). A recent randomized, placebo-controlled trial showed that anakinra was safe and well tolerated at a dose of

1 mg/kg/d (maximum 100 mg) but did not significantly reduce disease flares in children with polyarticular JIA (163). In JIA, it has been anecdotally used for systemic JIA, although there are no randomized controlled trials published at this time. The major side effects of anakinra are injection site reactions and infection.

Anti-Interleukin 6 Agents.

IL-6 is a key inflammatory cytokine in RA and JIA. Anti–IL-6 receptor MRA has been studied for the treatment of systemic JIA in open label phase II trials. These preliminary trials have demonstrated that MRA is safe, well tolerated, and resulted in improvement in symptoms and inflammatory markers (164, 165). Tocilizumab (RoActemra or Actemra) is a recombinant humanized MRA that acts as an IL-6 receptor antagonist. A recent double-blinded trial demonstrated that Tocilizumab monotherapy was superior to methotrexate monotherapy in RA, with a rapid improvement in symptoms and a favorable safety profile (166). Tocilizumab trials in children have not been published yet.

PHYSICAL AND OCCUPATIONAL THERAPY

All children with prolonged arthritis should be evaluated by a physical and/or occupational therapist to provide an appropriate teaching and treatment program. Most treatment programs for JIA will include active and passive range-of-motion exercises, strengthening, and other modalities such as use of hot paraffin for relief of hand stiffness. Swimming has the advantage of providing muscle strengthening and active range of motion without significant weight bearing. Splinting may be used for maintaining alignment, providing rest, and reducing flexion contractures. For children with severe flexion contractures, a dynamic tension splint or serial casting can be used to correct the contracture. Physical therapy for range of motion in JAS is primarily to prevent loss of mobility and poor functional positioning.

Surgical Interventions.

For most children with JIA, orthopaedic surgery has a limited role in the management plan. With early detection and aggressive medical management, the majority of children with JIA have a satisfactory outcome without significant disability. However, for those children with persistent arthritis despite medical therapy, continued pain, or progressive leg-length discrepancy, there is often significant benefit from individualized orthopaedic surgical intervention. Surgical intervention in JIA presents unique challenges to the management team. The small size of children and their growth potential must be taken into consideration. Also, in the postsurgical period, prolonged immobilization can lead to decreased strength and range of motion. Intensive physical therapy is frequently required during the recovery period. There is no universal agreement about which procedures are indicated for the treatment of complications of JIA. However, the overall goal is to provide symptomatic relief and improved functioning.

Synovectomy.

Synovectomy may be indicated in JIA for relief of persistent joint pain, swelling, and loss of range of motion related to synovial hypertrophy. Several recent studies suggest that arthroscopic synovectomy for treatment-refractory monoarthritis only partially effective JRA and that recurrence was common (167, 168). In one study, two-thirds of children relapsed within 24 months of the procedure (167), and in a second study, 67%, 95%, and 100% of children with oligo-, poly-, and psoriatic JIA relapsed after an average of 1 year (168). Predictors of a good response were normal inflammatory markers and short disease duration at the time of the procedure (167).

Soft-Tissue Release.

Soft-tissue release may be useful in a child with a severe contracture of the knee or hip that is resistant to splinting or serial casting. Reports have demonstrated various results. The most recent publications have shown only a modest benefit (169, 170).

Arthrodesis.

Arthrodesis may be indicated for severe joint destruction of the ankles or cervical spine secondary to prolonged synovitis. After puberty, a fixed and painful deformity of the ankle may be corrected by a triple arthrodesis. Occasionally, in children with isolated damage of the subtalar or talonavicular joint, a single joint fusion may be appropriate (171). Although many children with JIA have cervical spine arthritis and atlantoaxial instability, there is no consensus on the indications for prophylactic fusion. In many cases, a simple cervical orthosis may stabilize the neck and prevent further subluxation. However, fusion of the cervical spine (C1–C2) is indicated in children who have progressive neurologic involvement (172, 173).

Epiphysiodesis.

An appropriately timed epiphysiodesis can be successfully used to correct leg-length discrepancies in oligoarticular JIA (174, 175). The discrepancy can be predicted using the method of Moseley (92). Simon et al. (175) reported that 15 such patients were followed up to skeletal maturity and showed satisfactory results.

Total Joint Arthroplasty.

Total joint arthroplasty is indicated for children with JIA who have severe destructive joint changes with functional impairment. The most common joints replaced are the hip and knee, followed by the shoulder and elbow.

Cemented hip replacements may reduce pain and improve functional ability; however, there is a significant rate of loosening and need for subsequent revision (176, 177). A recent study has suggested that bipolar hemiarthroplasty of the hip, with a 79% 10-year survival, may be an alternative to conventional joint arthroplasty (178).

Results of total knee arthroplasty in JIA have been encouraging, with few revisions required (179–183). Cementless total knee arthroplasty has been used in selected cases (184). Recent studies have confirmed the efficacy of the procedure by reporting an overall 99% survival for nonconstrained anatomically graduated components prosthesis with cementless fixation (183).

In a recent review, Connor and Morrey (185) evaluated the long-term outcome for 19 children (23 elbows) who had been managed with total elbow arthroplasty and followed up for at least 2 years. Only three (13%) had poor results caused by late complications: aseptic loosening, instability, and worn bushings (185).

COMPLICATIONS

Uveitis.   Uveitis is one of the most severe extra-articular complications of JIA. It is often asymptomatic and, if untreated, can lead to synechiae, cataracts, glaucoma, retinal detachment, and visual loss (Fig. 11-11). Significant predictors of ocular inflammation include JIA subtype, younger age at disease onset, and ANA positivity (186). Oligoarticular JIA has the highest cumulative incidence of uveitis, occurring in up to 25% and 16% of children with extended and persistent courses, respectively (186). Uveitis is much less frequent in polyarticular and systemic JIA patients, 4% and 1%, respectively. In ERA, ocular inflammation occurs in up to 7% of children; in two-thirds of children, it is manifested by pain, photophobia, and conjunctival erythema (186). Uveitis is present in up to 10% of psoriatic JIA patients and is typically asymptomatic (186). Although the overall incidence and severity of uveitis seem to be decreasing (187, 188), even a low-grade chronic uveitis can result in a poor visual outcome (189). Current guidelines for ophthalmologic examination are based on age, ANA status, and type of JIA onset (190) (Table 11-7).

Growth Retardation.   Chronic inflammation and corticosteroid therapy adversely impact the growth of children with

JIA (Fig. 11-9A,B). Growth failure, as defined by at least two of the following, is present in up to 19% of children with JIA (191): (a) less than the 3rd percentile height for age, (b) growth velocity less than the 3rd percentile for age >6 months, and (c) crossing two or more percentiles on the height for age growth chart. Once remission is achieved and corticosteroid therapy is discontinued, as much as 70% have catch-up growth; however, the remaining 30% may have persistent growth retardation (192). Preliminary results of recombinant growth hormone look promising (193); however, use of growth hormone in the JIA population is not part of currently recommended routine therapy.

Osteoporosis.   Risk factors for osteoporosis in JIA include chronic corticosteroid use, physical inactivity, delayed puberty, and malnutrition (194). Recent studies have demonstrated that children with chronic arthritis are at risk for low volumetric bone mineral density and bone strength (195). Furthermore, a recent population-based study demonstrated an elevated risk of fracture in children with chronic arthritis (196). Careful attention to calcium and 25-OH vitamin D status may help minimize osteoporosis in the JIA population.

Leg-Length Discrepancy.   Increased blood flow to inflamed joints also results in increased nutrient delivery to adjacent growth plates, resulting in increased bone growth. If arthritis is asymmetric in the lower extremities, this may result in LLD over time. LLD < 1 cm are probably clinically insignificant and may be a variant of normal. LLD > 1 cm, however, may result in strain on the shorter leg and back. Early treatment of arthritis may prevent LLD. One study showed that early and continued use of intra-articular corticosteroid injections help prevent LLD and decrease the need for shoe lifts (142).

PEARLS AND PITFALLS

- JIA has been proposed as a replacement for both JCA and JRA.
- Oligoarthritis is the most common subtype of JIA.
- Only 5% of RF-positive and 30% of RF-negative polyarticular JIA patients achieve long-term remission off medication.
- Less than one-fourth of children with JAS have pain, stiffness, or limitation of motion of the SI or lumbosacral spine at disease onset.
- Small joints of the toes are commonly involved in JAS and are seldom affected in other forms of JIA, with the exception of psoriatic arthritis.
- Initial laboratory evaluation of arthritis should include a CBC, ESR, and CRP. Lyme ELISA should also be considered if living in a Lyme endemic area.
- RF and ANA positivity are not diagnostic of JIA
- Plain radiographs are useful in the initial evaluation for identifying osteopenia, fractures, or other bony lesions.
- Radiographic features associated with JIA include soft-tissue swelling and widening of the joint space, generalized

TABLE 11-7	Guidelines for Initial Frequency of Screening Eye Exams in JIA	
	Minimum Screening Frequency	
	Age at Onset	
JIA Onset Type	**<7 yr**	**≥7 yr**
Oligoarticular		
ANA+	3 mo	6 mo
ANA–	6 mo	6 mo
Polyarticular		
ANA+	3–4 mo	6 mo
ANA–	6 mo	6 mo
Systemic	1 yr	1 yr
Psoriatic		
ANA+	3 mo	6 mo
ANA–	6 mo	6 mo
Enthesitis-related arthritis	1 yr	1 yr

All patients with an irregular iris, or an acute red, painful, or photophobic eye, should be examined immediately.
ANA, antinuclear antibodies.

osteoporosis, joint space narrowing, erosions, subluxation, and ankylosis.
- Screening flexion and extension films are recommended prior to anesthesia if cervical disease is suspected.
- ANA positivity is a marker of risk for JIA-associated uveitis.
- All children with JIA should be evaluated for uveitis at diagnosis and routinely thereafter.
- JIA patients are at risk for growth failure, osteoporosis, and LLD.

REFERENCES

1. Kunnamo I, Kallio P, Pelkonen P. Incidence of arthritis in urban Finnish children: a prospective study. *Arthritis Rheum* 1986;29:2132.
2. Goodman J, McGraft P. The epidemiology of pain in children and adolescents: a review. *Pain* 1991;46:247.
3. McGrath P, McAlpine L. Psychologic perspectives on pediatric pain. *J Pediatr* 1993;122:52.
4. Cuesta I, Kerr K, Simpson P. Subspecialty referrals for pauciarticular juvenile rheumatoid arthritis. *Arch Pediatr Adolesc Med* 2000;154(2):122.
5. Brewer E, Bass J, Cassidy J. Criteria for the classification of juvenile rheumatoid arthritis. *Bull Rheum Dis* 1972;23:712–719.
6. Bulletin 4. *Nomenclature and classification of arthritis in children.* Basel, Switzerland: National Zeitung AG, 1977.
7. Fink C. Proposal for the development of classification criteria for idiopathic arthritides of childhood. *J Rheumatol* 1995;22:1566.
8. Petty RE, et al. International League of Associations for Rheumatology classification of juvenile idiopathic arthritis: second revision, Edmonton, 2001. *J Rheumatol* 2004;31(2):390–392.
9. Foeldvari I, Bidde M. Validation of the proposed ILAR classification criteria for juvenile idiopathic arthritis. International League of Associations for Rheumatology. *J Rheumatol* 2000;27(4):1069.
10. Ramsey S, Bolaria R, Cabral D. Comparison of criteria for the classification of childhood arthritis. *J Rheumatol* 2000;27(5):1283.
11. Hofer M, Mouy R, Prieur A. Juvenile idiopathic arthritides evaluated prospectively in a single center according to the Durban criteria. *J Rheumatol* 2001;28(5):1083.
12. Krumrey-Langkammerer M, Hafner R. Evaluation of the ILAR criteria for juvenile idiopathic arthritis. *J Rheumatol* 2001;28(11):2544.
13. Danner S, et al. Epidemiology of juvenile idiopathic arthritis in Alsace, France. *J Rheumatol* 2006;33(7):1377–1381.
14. Prahalad S. Genetics of juvenile idiopathic arthritis: an update. *Curr Opin Rheumatol* 2004;16(5):588–594.
15. Woo P, Laxer R, Sherry D. *Pediatric rheumatology in clinical practice.* London, UK: Springer, 2007.
16. Morling N, et al. DNA polymorphism of HLA class II genes in pauciarticular juvenile rheumatoid arthritis. *Tissue Antigens* 1991;38(1):16–23.
17. Sherry DD, et al. Painless juvenile rheumatoid arthritis. *J Pediatr* 1990;116(6):921–923.
18. Bunger C, Bulow J, Tondebold E. Microcirculation of the juvenile knee in chronic arthritis. *Clin Orthop* 1986;204:294.
19. Vostrejs M, Hollister J. Muscle atrophy and leg length discrepancies in pauciarticular juvenile rheumatoid arthritis. *Am J Dis Child* 1988;142:343.
20. Weiss PF, et al. High prevalence of temporomandibular joint arthritis at disease onset in children with juvenile idiopathic arthritis, as detected by magnetic resonance imaging but not by ultrasound. *Arthritis Rheum* 2008;58(4):1189–1196.
21. Twilt, M, et al. Temporomandibular involvement in juvenile idiopathic arthritis. *J Rheumatol* 2004;31(7):1418–1422.
22. Bakke M, et al. Orofacial pain, jaw function, and temporomandibular disorders in women with a history of juvenile chronic arthritis or persistent juvenile chronic arthritis. *Oral Surg Oral Med Oral Pathol Oral Radiol Endod* 2001;92(4):406–414.
23. Karhulahti T, Ronning O, Jamsa T. Mandibular condyle lesions, jaw movements, and occlusal status in 15-year-old children with juvenile rheumatoid arthritis. *Scand J Dent Res* 1990;98(1):17–26.
24. Wallace CA, et al. Patterns of clinical remission in select categories of juvenile idiopathic arthritis. *Arthritis Rheum* 2005;52(11):3554–3562.
25. Symmons D, Jones M, Osborne J. Pediatric rheumatology in the United Kingdom: data from the British Pediatric Rheumatology Group National Diagnostic Register. *J Rheumatol* 1996;23:1975.
26. Cassidy J, Levinson J, Bass J. A study of classification criteria for a diagnosis of juvenile rheumatoid arthritis. *Arthritis Rheum* 1986;29:274.
27. Kanski J. Uveitis in juvenile chronic arthritis. *Eye* 1988;2:641.
28. Blane C, Ragsdale C, Hensinger R. Late effects of JRA on the hip. *J Pediatr Orthop* 1987;7:677.
29. Schneider R, Laxer R. Systemic onset juvenile rheumatoid arthritis. *Baillieres Clin Rheum* 1998;12:245.
30. De Benedetti F, et al. Functional and prognostic relevance of the −173 polymorphism of the macrophage migration inhibitory factor gene in systemic-onset juvenile idiopathic arthritis. *Arthritis Rheum* 2003;48(5):1398–1407.
31. Calabro J, Marchesano J. Fever associated with juvenile rheumatoid arthritis. *N Engl J Med* 1967;276:11.
32. Calabro J, Marchesano J. Rash associated with juvenile rheumatoid arthritis. *J Pediatr* 1968;72:611.
33. Behrens EM, et al. Evaluation of the presentation of systemic onset juvenile rheumatoid arthritis: data from the Pennsylvania Systemic Onset Juvenile Arthritis Registry (PASOJAR). *J Rheumatol* 2008;35(2):343–348.
34. Schneider R, Lang B, Reilly B. Prognostic indicators of joint destruction in systemic-onset juvenile rheumatoid arthritis. *J Pediatr* 1992;120:200.
35. David J, Vouyiouka O, Ansell B. Amyloidosis in juvenile chronic arthritis: a morbidity and mortality study. *Clin Exp Rheumatol* 1993;11:85.
36. Prieur A, Stephan J. Macrophage activation syndrome in children with joint diseases. *Rev Rheum Engl Ed* 1994;61:385.
37. Ravelli A, Benedetti FD, Viola S. Macrophage activation syndrome in systemic juvenile rheumatoid arthritis successfully treated with cyclosporine. *J Pediatr* 1996;128:275.
38. Mouy R, Stephan J, Pillet P. Efficacy of cyclosporine A in the treatment of macrophage activation syndrome in juvenile arthritis: report of five cases. *J Pediatr* 1996;129:750.
39. Pascual V, et al. Role of interleukin-1 (IL-1) in the pathogenesis of systemic onset juvenile idiopathic arthritis and clinical response to IL-1 blockade. *J Exp Med* 2005;201(9):1479–1486.
40. Church R. The prospect of psoriasis. *Br J Dermatol* 1958;70(4):139–145.
41. Baker H. Epidemiological aspects of psoriasis and arthritis. *Br J Dermatol* 1966;78(5):249–261.
42. Green L, et al. Arthritis in psoriasis. *Ann Rheum Dis* 1981;40(4):366–369.
43. Ho PY, et al. HLA-Cw6 and HLA-DRB1*07 together are associated with less severe joint disease in psoriatic arthritis. *Ann Rheum Dis* 2007;66(6):807–811.
44. Southwood T, Petty R, Malleson P. Psoriatic arthritis in children. *Arthritis Rheum* 1989;32:1007.
45. Roberton D, Cabral D, Malleson P. Juvenile psoriatic arthritis: follow-up and evaluation of diagnostic criteria. *J Rheumatol* 1996;23:166.
46. Petty R, Southwood T, Baum J. Revision of the proposed classification criteria for juvenile idiopathic arthritis: Durban, 1997. *J Rheumatol* 1998;25:1991.
47. Shore A, Ansell B. Juvenile psoriatic arthritis: an analysis of 60 cases. *J Pediatr* 1982;100:529.
48. Wesolowska H. Clinical course of psoriatic arthropathy in children. *Mater Med Pol* 1985;55:185.
49. Rosenberg A, Petty R. A syndrome of seronegative enthesopathy and arthropathy in children. *Arthritis Rheum* 1982;25:1041.
50. Cabral D, Oen K, Petty R. SEA syndrome revisited: a long-term followup of children with a syndrome of seronegative enthesopathy and arthropathy. *J Rheumatol* 1992;19:1282.

51. Cassidy J, Petty R. *Textbook of pediatric rheumatology*, 3rd ed. Philadelphia, PA: WB Saunders, 1995.

52. Sherry DD, Sapp LR. Enthesalgia in childhood: site-specific tenderness in healthy subjects and in patients with seronegative enthesopathic arthropathy. *J Rheumatol* 2003;30(6):1335–1340.

53. Ansell B. Ankylosing spondylitis. In: Moll JMH, ed. *Juvenile spondylitis and related disorders.* Edinburgh, UK: Churchill Livingstone, 1980:120.

54. Rosenbaum J. Acute anterior uveitis and spondyloarthropathies. *Rheum Dis Clin North Am* 1992;18:143.

55. Power W, Rodriguez A, Pedroza-Seres M. Outcomes in anterior uveitis associated with the HLA-B27 haplotype. *Ophthalmology* 1998; 105:1646.

56. Cabral D, Malleson P, Petty R. Spondyloarthropathies of childhood. *Pediatr Clin North Am* 1995;42:1051.

57. Gofton JP, Robinson HS, Trueman GE. Ankylosing spondylitis in a Canadian Indian population. *Ann Rheum Dis* 1966;25(6):525–527.

58. Baum J, Ziff M. The rarity of ankylosing spondylitis in the black race. *Arthritis Rheum* 1971;14(1):12–18.

59. van der Linden SM, et al. The risk of developing ankylosing spondylitis in HLA-B27 positive individuals. A comparison of relatives of spondylitis patients with the general population. *Arthritis Rheum* 1984;27(3): 241–249.

60. Burgos-Vargas R, Vazquez-Mellado J. The early clinical recognition of juvenile-onset ankylosing spondylitis and its differentiation from juvenile rheumatoid arthritis. *Arthritis Rheum* 1995;38:835.

61. Burgos-Vargas R, Petty R. Juvenile ankylosing spondylitis. *Rheum Dis Clin North Am* 1992;18:123.

62. Burgos-Vargas R. Spondyloarthropathies and psoriatic arthritis in children. *Curr Opin Rheumatol* 1993;5:634.

63. Garcia-Morteo O, Maldonado-Cocco J, Suarez-Almazor M. Ankylosing spondylitis of juvenile onset: comparison with adult onset disease. *Stand J Rheumatol* 1983;12:246.

64. Calin A, Elswood J. The natural history of juvenile-onset ankylosing spondylitis: a 24-year retrospective case-control study. *Br J Rheumatol* 1988;27:91.

65. Marks S, Barnett M, Calin A. A case-control study of juvenile- and adult-onset ankylosing spondylitis. *J Rheumatol* 1982;9:739.

66. Farmer R, Michener W. Prognosis of Crohn's disease with onset in childhood and adolescence. *Dig Dis Sci* 1979;24:752.

67. Lindsley C, Schaller J. Arthritis associated with inflammatory bowel disease in children. *J Pediatr* 1974;84:16.

68. Hamilton J, Bruce M, Abdourhamam M. Inflammatory bowel disease in children and adolescents. *Adv Pediatr* 1979;26:311.

69. Klippel J, Weyand C, Wortmann R. *Primer on the rheumatic diseases*, 11th ed. Atlanta, GA: Arthritis Foundation, 1997:1.

70. Speiser JC, et al. Changing trends in pediatric septic arthritis. *Semin Arthritis Rheum* 1985;15(2):132–138.

71. Steere AC, Schoen RT, Taylor E. The clinical evolution of Lyme arthritis. *Ann Intern Med* 1987;107(5):725–731.

72. Steere A, Schoen R, Taylor E. The clinical evolution of Lyme arthritis. *Ann Intern Med* 1987;107:725.

73. Gerber M, Zemel L, Shapiro E. Lyme arthritis in children: clinical epidemiology and long-term outcomes. *Pediatrics* 1998;102:905.

74. Huppertz H, Karch H, Suschke H. Lyme arthritis in European children and adolescents. *Arthritis Rheum* 1995;38:361.

75. Steere A, Dwyer E, Winchester R. Association of chronic Lyme arthritis with HLA-DR4 and HLA-DR2 alleles. *N Engl J Med* 1990;323:219.

76. Sigal LH. The polymerase chain reaction assay for Borrelia burgdorferi in the diagnosis of Lyme disease. *Ann Intern Med* 1994;120(6):520–521.

77. Cuttica J, Schenines E, Garay S. Juvenile onset Reiter's syndrome: a retrospective study of 26 patients. *Clin Exp Rheumatol* 1992;10:285.

78. Smith R. Evidence for *Chlamydia trachomatis* and *Ureaplasma urealyticum* in a patient with Reiter's disease. *J Adolesc Health Care* 1989;10:155.

79. Rosenberg A, Petty R. Reiter's disease in children. *Am J Dis Child* 1979;133:394.

80. Wright V, Reiter's disease. In: Scott JT, ed. *Copeman's textbook of the rheumatic diseases.* London, UK: Longmans Green, 1978:549.

81. Keat A, Maini R, Pegrum G. The clinical features and HLA associations of reactive arthritis associated with nongonococcal urethritis. *Q J Med* 1979;190:323.

82. Harrersen D, Weiner D, Weiner S. The characterization of "transient synovitis of the hip" in children. *J Pediatr Orthop* 1986;6:11.

83. Wingstrand H. Transient synovitis of the hip in the child. *Acta Orthop Scand* 1986;57:219.

84. Koop S, Quanbeck D. Three common causes of childhood hip pain. *Pediatr Clin North Am* 1996;43:1053.

85. Pineda Marfa M. Neurological involvement in rheumatic disorders and vasculitis in childhood. *Rev Neurol* 2002;35(3):290–296.

86. Schaffer F, Agarwal R, Helm J. Post-streptococcal-reactive arthritis and silent carditis: a case report and review of the literature. *Pediatrics* 1994;93:837.

87. Cunto CD. Prognosis of children with poststreptococcal reactive arthritis. *Pediatr Infect Dis J* 1988;7:683.

88. Beilory L. Human serum sickness: a prospective analysis of 35 patients treated with equine anti-thymocyte globulin for bone marrow failure. *Medicine* 1988;67:40.

89. Weston W, Brice S, Jester J. Herpes simplex virus in childhood erythema multiforme. *Pediatrics* 1992;89:32.

90. Erffmeyer J. Serum sickness. *Ann Allergy* 1986;56:105.

91. Howell R. Juvenile gouty arthritis. *Am J Dis Child* 1985;139:547.

92. Moseley C. A straight line graph for leg length discrepancies. *J Bone Joint Surg Am* 1977;59:174.

93. Schidlow D, Goldsmith D, Palmer J. Arthritis in cystic fibrosis. *Arch Dis Child* 1984;59:377.

94. Summers G, Webley M. Episodic arthritis in cystic fibrosis: a case report. *Br J Rheumatol* 1986;31:535.

95. Pertuiset E, Menkes C, Lenoi G. Cystic fibrosis arthritis. A report of five cases. *Br J Rheumatol* 1992;28:341.

96. Newman A, Ansell B. Episodic arthritis in children with cystic fibrosis. *J Pediatr* 1979;94:594.

97. Dixey J, Redington A, Butler R. The arthropathy of cystic fibrosis. *Ann Rheum Dis* 1988;47:218.

98. Sagransky D, Greenwald R. Seropositive rheumatoid arthritis in a patient with cystic fibrosis. *Am J Dis Child* 1980;129:634.

99. Nathanson I, Riddlesberger M. Pulmonary hypertrophic osteoarthropathy in cystic fibrosis. *Radiology* 1980;135:649.

100. Athreya B, Borns P, Roselund M. Cystic fibrosis and hypertrophic osteoarthropathy in children. *Am J Dis Child* 1973;129:634.

101. Isenberg DA, Miller JJ, eds. *Adolescent rheumatology.* London, UK: Martin Dunitz, 1999.

102. Ragsdale C, Petty R, Cassidy J. The clinical progression of apparent juvenile rheumatoid arthritis to systemic lupus erythematosus. *J Rheumatol* 1980;17:777.

103. Pattishall E, Strope G, Spinola A. Childhood sarcoidosis. *J Pediatr* 1986;108:169.

104. Steward M, Savage J, Bell B. Long term renal prognosis of Henoch-Schonlein purpura in an unselected childhood population. *Eur J Pediatr* 1988;147:113.

105. Barton L, Saied K. Thorn-induced arthritis. *J Pediatr* 1978;93:322.

106. Jones OY, et al. A multicenter case-control study on predictive factors distinguishing childhood leukemia from juvenile rheumatoid arthritis. *Pediatrics* 2006;117(5):e840–e844.

107. Flandry F, Hughston J. Pigmented villonodular synovitis. *J Bone Joint Surg Am* 1987;69:942.

108. Walls J, Nogi J. Multifocal pigmented villonodular synovitis in a child. *J Pediatr Orthop* 1985;5:229.

109. Peterson H. Growing pains. *Pediatr Clin North Am* 1986;33:1356.

110. Sherry D, McGuire T, Mellins E. Psychosomatic musculoskeletal pain in childhood: clinical and psychological analyses of 100 children. *Pediatrics* 1991;88:1093.

111. Bernstein B, Singsen B, Kent J. Reflex neurovascular dystrophy in childhood. *J Pediatr* 1978;93:211.

112. Wilder R, Berde C, Wolohan M. Reflex sympathetic dystrophy in children. Clinical characteristics and follow-up of seventy patients. *J Bone Joint Surg Am* 1992;74:910.

113. Silber T, Majd M. Reflex sympathetic dystrophy syndrome in children and adolescents. Report of 18 cases and review of the literature. *Am J Dis Child* 1988;142:1325.

114. Sherry D, Weisman R. Psychologic aspects of childhood reflex neurovascular dystrophy. *Pediatrics* 1988;81:572.

115. Ladd J, Cassidy J, Martel W. Juvenile ankylosing spondylitis. *Arthritis Rheum* 1971;14:579.

116. Rahimtoola Z, Finger S, Imrie S. Outcome of total hip arthroplasty in small-proportioned patients. *J Arthroplasty* 2000;15(1):27.

117. Senac M, Deutsch D, Bernstein B. MR imaging in juvenile rheumatoid arthritis. *AJR Am J Roentgenol* 1988;150:873.

118. Verbruggen L, Shahabpour M, Roy PV. Magnetic resonance imaging of articular destruction in juvenile rheumatoid arthritis. *Arthritis Rheum* 1990;33:1426.

119. Yulish B, Lieberman J, Newman A. Juvenile rheumatoid arthritis: assessment with MR imaging. *Radiology* 1987;165:149.

120. Cabral D, Petty R, Fung M. Persistent antinuclear antibodies in children without identifiable inflammatory, rheumatic or autoimmune disease. *Pediatrics* 1992;89:441.

121. Allen R, Dewez P, Stuart L. Antinuclear antibodies using HEp-2 cells in normal children and in children with common infections. *J Paediatr Child Health* 1991;27:39.

122. Deane P, Liard G, Siegel D. The outcome of children referred to a pediatric rheumatology clinic with a positive antinuclear antibody test but without an autoimmune disease. *Pediatrics* 1995;95:892.

123. Rosenberg A. Uveitis associated with juvenile rheumatoid arthritis. *Semin Arthritis Rheum* 1987;16:158.

124. Stillman J, Barry P. Juvenile rheumatoid arthritis: series 2. *Arthritis Rheum* 1977;20:171.

125. Schaller J. Juvenile rheumatoid arthritis: series 1. *Arthritis Rheum* 1977; 20:165.

126. Schellekens GA, et al. The diagnostic properties of rheumatoid arthritis antibodies recognizing a cyclic citrullinated peptide. *Arthritis Rheum* 2000;43(1):155–163.

127. Kroot EJ, et al. The prognostic value of anti-cyclic citrullinated peptide antibody in patients with recent-onset rheumatoid arthritis. *Arthritis Rheum* 2000;43(8):1831–1835.

128. van Jaarsveld CH, et al. The prognostic value of the antiperinuclear factor, anti-citrullinated peptide antibodies and rheumatoid factor in early rheumatoid arthritis. *Clin Exp Rheumatol* 1999;17(6):689–697.

129. Petty R. HLA-B27 and rheumatic diseases of childhood. *J Rheumatol* 1990;17:7.

130. Cassidy J, Brody G, Martel W. Monoarticular juvenile rheumatoid arthritis. *J Pediatr* 1967;70:867.

131. Baldassare A, Chang F, Zuckner J. Markedly raised synovial fluid leukocyte counts not associated with infectious arthritis in children. *Ann Rheum Dis* 1978;37:404.

132. Zuckner J, Baldassare A, Chang F. High synovial fluid leukocyte counts of noninfectious etiology. *Arthritis Rheum* 1977;20:270.

133. Vane J. Inhibition of prostaglandin synthesis as a mechanism of action for aspirin-like drugs. *Nat New Biol* 1971;231:232.

134. Lindsley C. Uses of nonsteroidal anti-inflammatory drugs in pediatrics. *Am J Dis Child* 1993;147:229.

135. Mulberg A, Linz C, Bern E. Identification of nonsteroidal antiinflammatory drug-induced gastroduodenal injury in children with juvenile rheumatoid arthritis. *J Pediatr* 1993;122:647.

136. Lovell D, Giannini E, Brewer E. Time course of response to nonsteroidal anti-inflammatory drugs in patients with juvenile rheumatoid arthritis. *Arthritis Rheum* 1984;27:1433.

137. Skeith KJ, Jamali F. Clinical pharmacokinetics of drugs used in juvenile arthritis. *Clin Pharmacokinet* 1991;21(2):129–149.

138. Giannini E, Cawkwell G. Drug treatment in children with juvenile rheumatoid arthritis. Past, present, and future. *Pediatr Clin North Am* 1995;42:1099.

139. Huppertz H, Tschammler A, Horwitz A. Intraarticular corticosteroids for chronic arthritis in children: efficacy and effects on cartilage and growth. *J Pediatr* 1995;127:317.

140. Padeh S, Passwell J. Intraarticular corticosteroid injection in the management of children with chronic arthritis. *Arthritis Rheum* 1998;41:1210.

141. Beukelman T, Guevara JP, Albert DA. Optimal treatment of knee monarthritis in juvenile idiopathic arthritis: a decision analysis. *Arthritis Rheum* 2008;59(11):1580–1588.

142. Sherry DD, et al. Prevention of leg length discrepancy in young children with pauciarticular juvenile rheumatoid arthritis by treatment with intraarticular steroids. *Arthritis Rheum* 1999;42(11):2330–2334.

143. Giannini EH, et al. Methotrexate in resistant juvenile rheumatoid arthritis. Results of the U.S.A.-U.S.S.R. double-blind, placebo-controlled trial. The Pediatric Rheumatology Collaborative Study Group and The Cooperative Children's Study Group. *N Engl J Med* 1992;326(16):1043–1049.

144. Woo P, et al. Randomized, placebo-controlled, crossover trial of low-dose oral methotrexate in children with extended oligoarticular or systemic arthritis. *Arthritis Rheum* 2000;43(8):1849–1857.

145. Ruperto N, et al. A randomized trial of parenteral methotrexate comparing an intermediate dose with a higher dose in children with juvenile idiopathic arthritis who failed to respond to standard doses of methotrexate. *Arthritis Rheum* 2004;50(7):2191–2201.

146. Wallace CA, Sherry DD. Preliminary report of higher dose methotrexate treatment in juvenile rheumatoid arthritis. *J Rheumatol* 1992; 19(10):1604–1607.

147. Lovell DJ, et al. Etanercept in children with polyarticular juvenile rheumatoid arthritis. Pediatric Rheumatology Collaborative Study Group. *N Engl J Med* 2000;342(11):763–769.

148. Lovell D, Giannini E, Reiff A. Long-term efficacy and safety of etanercept in children with polyarticular-course juvenile rheumatoid arthritis: interim results from an ongoing multicenter, open-label, extended treatment trial. *Arthritis Rheum* 2003;48(1):218.

149. Lovell DJ, et al. Safety and efficacy of up to eight years of continuous etanercept therapy in patients with juvenile rheumatoid arthritis. *Arthritis Rheum* 2008;58(5):1496–1504.

150. Gerloni V, Lurati A, Gattinara M. Efficacy of infusions of an anti TNF-α antibody (infliximab) in persistently active refractory juvenile idiopathic arthritis. Results of a two years open label prospective study. *Arthritis Rheum* 2003;48(9):S92.

151. Ardoin S, Rabinovich E, Jaffe G. Infliximab to treat pediatric chronic inflammatory uveitis. *Arthritis Rheum* 2003;48(9):S93.

152. Burmester GR, et al. Adalimumab alone and in combination with disease-modifying antirheumatic drugs for the treatment of rheumatoid arthritis in clinical practice: the Research in Active Rheumatoid Arthritis (ReAct) trial. *Ann Rheum Dis* 2007;66(6):732–739.

153. Lovell DJ, et al. Adalimumab with or without methotrexate in juvenile rheumatoid arthritis. *N Engl J Med* 2008;359(8):810–820.

154. Foeldvari I, et al. Tumor necrosis factor-alpha blocker in treatment of juvenile idiopathic arthritis-associated uveitis refractory to second-line agents: results of a multinational survey. *J Rheumatol* 2007;34(5):1146–1150.

155. Wallis R, Broder M, Wong J. Granulomatous infectious diseases associated with tumor necrosis factor antagonists. *Clin Infect Dis* 2004;38:1261.

156. Van Rossum MA, Fiselier T, Franssen M. Sulfasalazine in the treatment of juvenile chronic arthritis: a randomized, double-blind, placebo-controlled, multicenter study. Dutch Juvenile Chronic Arthritis Study Group. *Arthritis Rheum* 1998;41:808.

157. Ansell B, Hall M, Loftus J. A multicenter pilot study of sulphasalazine in juvenile chronic arthritis. *Clin Exp Rheumatol* 1991;9:201.

158. Hertzberger-ten Cate R, Cats A. Toxicity of sulfasalazine in systemic juvenile chronic arthritis. *Clin Exp Rheumatol* 1991;9:85.

159. van Rossum MA, et al. Sulfasalazine in the treatment of juvenile chronic arthritis: a randomized, double-blind, placebo-controlled, multicenter study. Dutch Juvenile Chronic Arthritis Study Group. *Arthritis Rheum* 1998;41(5):808–816.

160. Genovese MC, et al. Abatacept for rheumatoid arthritis refractory to tumor necrosis factor alpha inhibition. *N Engl J Med* 2005;353(11): 1114–1123.

161. Ruperto N, et al. Abatacept in children with juvenile idiopathic arthritis: a randomised, double-blind, placebo-controlled withdrawal trial. *Lancet* 2008;372(9636):383–391.

162. Cohen SB, et al. A multicentre, double blind, randomised, placebo controlled trial of anakinra (Kineret), a recombinant interleukin 1 receptor antagonist, in patients with rheumatoid arthritis treated with background methotrexate. *Ann Rheum Dis* 2004;63(9):1062–1068.

163. Ilowite N, et al. Anakinra in the treatment of polyarticular-course juvenile rheumatoid arthritis: safety and preliminary efficacy results of a randomized multicenter study. *Clin Rheumatol* 2009;28(2):129–137.

164. Woo P, et al. Open label phase II trial of single, ascending doses of MRA in Caucasian children with severe systemic juvenile idiopathic arthritis: proof of principle of the efficacy of IL-6 receptor blockade in this type of arthritis and demonstration of prolonged clinical improvement. *Arthritis Res Ther* 2005;7(6):R1281–R1288.

165. Yokota S, et al. Therapeutic efficacy of humanized recombinant anti-interleukin-6 receptor antibody in children with systemic-onset juvenile idiopathic arthritis. *Arthritis Rheum* 2005;52(3):818–825.

166. Jones G, et al. Comparison of tocilizumab monotherapy versus methotrexate monotherapy in patients with moderate to severe rheumatoid arthritis: the AMBITION study. *Ann Rheum Dis* 2009.

167. Toledo MM, et al. Is there a role for arthroscopic synovectomy in oligoarticular juvenile idiopathic arthritis? *J Rheumatol* 2006;33(9):1868–1872.

168. Dell'Era L, Facchini R, Corona F. Knee synovectomy in children with juvenile idiopathic arthritis. *J Pediatr Orthop B* 2008;17(3):128–130.

169. Rydholm U, Brattstrom H, Lidgren L. Soft tissue release for knee flexion contracture in juvenile chronic arthritis. *J Pediatr Orthop* 1986;6:448.

170. Swann M, Ansell B. Soft-tissue release of the hips in children with juvenile chronic arthritis. *J Bone Joint Surg Br* 1986;68:404.

171. Sammarco G, Tablante E. Subtalar arthrodesis. *Clin Orthop Rel Res* 1998;349:73.

172. Hensinger R, Devito P, Ragsdale C. Changes in the cervical spine in juvenile rheumatoid arthritis. *J Bone Joint Surg Am* 1986;68:189.

173. Fried J, Athreya B, Gregg J. The cervical spine in juvenile rheumatoid arthritis. *Clin Orthop* 1983;179:102.

174. Rydholm U, Brattstrom H, Bylander B. Stapling of the knee in juvenile chronic arthritis. *J Pediatr Orthop* 1987;7:63.

175. Simon S, Whiffen J, Shapiro F. Leg-length discrepancies in monoarticular and pauciarticular juvenile rheumatoid arthritis. *J Bone Joint Surg Am* 1981;63:209.

176. Chmell M, Scott R, Thomas W. Total hip arthroplasty with cement for juvenile rheumatoid arthritis. Results at a minimum of ten years in patients less than thirty years old. *J Bone Joint Surg Am* 1997;79:44.

177. Witt J, Swann M, Ansell B. Total hip replacement for juvenile chronic arthritis. *J Bone Joint Surg Br* 1991;73:770.

178. Yun A, Martin S, Zurakowski D. Bipolar hemiarthroplasty in juvenile rheumatoid arthritis: long-term survivorship and outcomes. *J Arthroplasty* 2002;17(8):978.

179. Carmichael E, Chaplin D. Total knee arthroplasty in juvenile rheumatoid arthritis. A seven-year follow-up study. *Clin Orthop* 1986;210:192.

180. Sarokhan A, Scott R, Thomas W. Total knee arthroplasty in juvenile rheumatoid arthritis. *J Bone Joint Surg Am* 1983;65:1071.

181. Stuart M, Rand J. Total knee arthroplasty in young adults who have rheumatoid arthritis. *J Bone Joint Surg Am* 1988;70:84.

182. Dalury D, Ewald F, Christie M. Total knee arthroplasty in a group of patients less than 45 years of age. *J Arthroplasty* 1995;10:598.

183. Lyback C, Belt E, Hamalainen M. Survivorship of AGC knee replacement in juvenile chronic arthritis: 13-year follow-up of 77 knees. *J Arthroplasty* 2000;15(2):166.

184. Boublik M, Tsahakis P, Scott R. Cementless total knee arthroplasty in juvenile onset rheumatoid arthritis. *Clin Orthop* 1993;286:88.

185. Connor, P. and B. Morrey. Total elbow arthroplasty in patients who have juvenile rheumatoid arthritis. *J Bone Joint Surg Am* 1998;80:678.

186. Heiligenhaus A, et al. Prevalence and complications of uveitis in juvenile idiopathic arthritis in a population-based nation-wide study in Germany: suggested modification of the current screening guidelines. *Rheumatology* (*Oxford*) 2007;46(6):1015–1019.

187. Sherry D, Mellins E, Wedgewood R. Decreasing severity of chronic uveitis in children with pauciarticular arthritis. *Am J Dis Child* 1991; 145:1026.

188. Chalom E, Goldsmith D, Koehler M. Prevalence and outcome of uveitis in a regional cohort of patients with juvenile rheumatoid arthritis. *J Rheumatol* 1997;24:2031.

189. Nguyen Q, Foster S. Saving the vision of children with juvenile rheumatoid arthritis-associated uveitis. *JAMA* 1998;280:1133.

190. Guidelines for ophthalmologic examinations in children with juvenile rheumatoid arthritis. *Pediatrics* 1993;92:295.

191. Solari N, et al. Assessing current outcomes of juvenile idiopathic arthritis: a cross-sectional study in a tertiary center sample. *Arthritis Rheum* 2008;59(11):1571–1579.

192. Simon D, et al. Linear growth in children suffering from juvenile idiopathic arthritis requiring steroid therapy: natural history and effects of growth hormone treatment on linear growth. *J Pediatr Endocrinol Metab* 2001;14(Suppl 6):1483–1486.

193. Simon D, et al. Early recombinant human growth hormone treatment in glucocorticoid-treated children with juvenile idiopathic arthritis: a 3-year randomized study. *J Clin Endocrinol Metab* 2007;92(7): 2567–2573.

194. Burnham JM, Leonard MB. Bone disease in pediatric rheumatologic disorders. *Curr Rheumatol Rep* 2004;6(1):70–78.

195. Burnham JM, et al. Bone density, structure, and strength in juvenile idiopathic arthritis: importance of disease severity and muscle deficits. *Arthritis Rheum* 2008;58(8):2518–2527.

196. Burnham JM, et al. Childhood onset arthritis is associated with an increased risk of fracture: a population based study using the General Practice Research Database. *Ann Rheum Dis* 2006;65(8): 1074–1079.

Musculoskeletal Infection

Musculoskeletal infection may present in a myriad of clinical situations in all regions of the musculoskeletal system. Bone and joint infection may cause rapid destruction and permanent impairment if not treated urgently, so prompt diagnosis is imperative. Unfortunately, there is not a single clinical finding or a test that consistently allows rapid diagnosis. Trauma, neoplasm, inflammatory arthropathy, or synovitis may all present with a clinical picture similar to infection. In 20% or more of musculoskeletal infection cases, no organism is identified, making diagnosis and even definition challenging (1). To complicate the situation further, as a disease entity, musculoskeletal infection is continually changing. Over relatively short time periods, as immunization, antibiotics, and living conditions change, new infectious organisms causing clinically significant disease arise, and organisms previously responsible for infection become less prevalent. The most important recent change in musculoskeletal infection is the emergence of community-acquired methicillin-resistant *Staphylococcus aureus* (MRSA) infection in pediatric and adolescent patients, which is discussed in detail later in the chapter.

All of this would be of little interest to the orthopaedic surgeon if musculoskeletal infection in children was a rare condition, but, in fact, it is a relatively common disorder. These varied factors ensure that musculoskeletal infection will remain an important and a challenging pediatric orthopaedic disorder.

DEFINITION

Defining musculoskeletal infection is difficult because it is not possible to identify a causative organism in a significant percentage of patients with this medical condition. As a consequence, the presence of an identifiable organism cannot be an essential criterion for definition and diagnosis of the disease. Morrey and Peterson (2) proposed a definition that classified osteomyelitis as being definite, probable, or likely. Definite osteomyelitis is present when an organism is recovered from bone or adjacent soft tissue or when there is histologic evidence of infection. Osteomyelitis is probable when there is a positive blood culture in addition to clinical and radiographic features of osteomyelitis, and osteomyelitis is likely to be present when there are typical clinical and radiographic features of osteomyelitis along with a response to antibiotics in the absence of a positive culture. Peltola and Vahvanen (3) have suggested a definition of osteomyelitis considering the diagnosis to be firm when two of the following four criteria are present: pus aspirated from bone; positive bone or blood culture; classic symptoms of localized pain, swelling, warmth, and limited range of motion (ROM) of the adjacent joint; and radiographic changes typical of osteomyelitis.

Compared with osteomyelitis patients, an even higher percentage of patients with septic arthritis have negative cultures, and therefore it is also important to establish diagnostic criteria for septic arthritis that do not mandate positive cultures. Morrey et al. (4) included patients with negative cultures who experience five of the following six criteria: temperature >38.3°C, pain in the affected joint made worse by motion, swelling of the affected joint, systemic symptoms, absence of other pathologic processes, and satisfactory response to antibiotic therapy.

Musculoskeletal infection can be classified by patient's age, causative organism, duration of symptoms, and route of infection. Infection in the neonate has distinct characteristics that differ from childhood osteomyelitis, which in turn differs from osteomyelitis in the adult population. Pyogenic organisms are the most common causative organisms, but granulomatous infection is being encountered more frequently with increased international travel and immigration. The most common route of infection is hematogenous, but direct inoculation is frequently the route of infection in the foot.

EPIDEMIOLOGY

Osteomyelitis is neither common nor rare, with the annual rate of acute hematogenous osteomyelitis (AHO) in children younger than 13 years estimated to be 1 in 5000 in the United States (5). Worldwide incidence estimates range from 1 in 1000 to 1 in 20,000 (6), and half of all cases of osteomyelitis occur in children younger than age 5 (7, 8). In childhood, septic arthritis occurs about twice as often as osteomyelitis and also tends to have its peak incidence in the early years of the first decade (9).

The epidemiologic patterns of musculoskeletal infection are continually changing. Atypical forms of infection such as subacute osteomyelitis are becoming more common, but several studies have suggested that the overall incidence of musculoskeletal infection may be declining (10, 11). These changes may be due to a variety of factors including immunization patterns and modification of clinical disease by antibiotics. At the Royal Hospital for Sick Children in Glasgow, Scotland, researchers noted a 44% decline in incidences of AHO when the period from 1970 to 1990 was compared to the period from 1990 to 1997 (12). Annual incidence dropped to a rate of 2.9 new cases per 100,000 population per year. *Staphylococcus aureus* remains the most common causative organism, occurring in 40% to 90% of cases of musculoskeletal infection (12–17). Other organisms commonly causing osteomyelitis or septic arthritis include coagulase-negative *Staphylococcus*, group A β-hemolytic *Streptococcus, Streptococcus pneumoniae*, and group B *Streptococcus* (17).

Since the development of routine vaccinations of infants against *Haemophilus influenza*, the incidence of musculoskeletal infection caused by *H. influenza* has dramatically decreased. In 1982, the University of Helsinki organized a prospective multicenter study of orthopaedic infection. In 1986, Finland began a large-scale immunization program against *H. influenza*. From 1982 to 1988, 36% of orthopaedic infections treated by the study group were caused by *H. influenza*, whereas from 1988 to 1998, there was not a single orthopaedic case of *H. influenza* infection, and the total number of childhood septic arthritis cases decreased by 30% (15). This change in epidemiology has resulted in modification of initial empiric antimicrobial therapy recommendations to cover primarily gram-positive cocci. Howard et al. (18) reported similar results following immunization for *H. influenza* in eastern Ontario, where *H. influenza* septic arthritis dropped from 41% of cases to 0% of cases following initiation of an *H. influenza* immunization program. Dramatic reduction in *H. influenza* infection following immunization has been confirmed by authors at other centers from around the world (13, 19).

Other organisms, such as *Kingella kingae*, are now recognized as being responsible for a greater percentage of musculoskeletal infections. In a study by Yagupsky and Dagan, *K. kingae* was the most common organism responsible for septic arthritis in children younger than 24 months (20). *K. kingae* is a fastidious, gram-negative bacillus that until relatively recently was thought to rarely cause clinical infection

in children. Residing in the oropharynx of young children, *K. kingae* appears to be an opportunistic pathogen that gains access to the bloodstream during the course of upper respiratory infection. Kingella is transmitted from child to child and has been associated with outbreaks among day care attendees (21, 22).

Once in the bloodstream, *K. kingae* has a predilection for the heart and musculoskeletal system. Our greater appreciation of *K. kingae* as a clinically significant causative organism for musculoskeletal infection may in part be due to our improved understanding of how to culture this organism. Inoculation of a specimen into enriched blood culture media has considerably improved recovery rate (23–26). *K. kingae* is often resistant to Vancomycin and Clindamycin but sensitive to β-lactum antibiotics and typically responds well to appropriate antibiotic treatment with few sequelae (26, 27).

Musculoskeletal infection is much more likely to affect the lower extremity than the upper extremity or axial skeleton. In a recent study performed in Taiwan, 90% of septic arthritis cases occurred in the lower extremity. The hip was the most commonly involved joint, occurring in 54% of patients (17). Newton et al. (28) reported the hip and knee to be the joints most commonly affected in their series of 186 patients with septic arthritis. In a study by Khachatourians et al. (14) of 50 patients with septic arthritis and/or osteomyelitis, 70% of infections occurred in the lower extremities. Peltola et al. (29) reported 72% of osteomyelitis cases in their series to occur in the lower extremities.

Osteomyelitis and septic arthritis may occur simultaneously. Patients younger than 18 months have a blood supply to the chondroepiphysis, which predisposes infants to develop osteomyelitis and septic arthritis. These diseases can also occur in four locations in older children where the metaphysis lies within the joint: in the proximal femur, proximal humerus, distal lateral tibia, and proximal radius. Septic arthritis results when bacteria breach the metaphyseal periosteum and enter the joint. Perlman et al. (30) reported that signs of adjacent joint septic arthritis may be as high as 40%, and therefore careful evaluation of neighboring joints is important.

The most ominous change in musculoskeletal infection epidemiology is the emergence of MRSA. In a study of musculoskeletal infection treated at the University of Texas Southwestern, Gafur et al. (31) compared patients treated from 2002 to 2004, with patients treated at the same institution and reported in 1982. MRSA was isolated as the causative organism in 30% of children treated from 2002 to 2004 compared to no patient treated 20 years earlier.

ETIOLOGY

Bacteria travel through the circulatory and musculoskeletal systems daily and yet rarely cause clinical infection. For musculoskeletal infection to occur, several circumstances must be present. A virulent organism capable of causing infection is necessary, sufficient numbers of that organism for multiplying and reaching a critical mass must be present, and the species and the number of bacteria present must overwhelm host defenses in the particular anatomic site in question. Although random chance may have a role in determining where and when bone and joint infection occurs, specific patterns of infection have been observed that can lead to no other conclusion than that specific factors influence where and in whom musculoskeletal infection occurs.

Metaphyseal bone adjacent to the physis is the most common site for AHO to develop. Hobo (32) described vascular loops present in the long bone metaphysis that take sharp bends and empty into venous lakes, creating areas of turbulence where bacteria accumulate and cause infection. Relative absence of tissue macrophages in metaphyseal bone adjacent to the physis appears to contribute to the predilection of osteomyelitis for this location. Others have suggested that gaps in the endothelium of growing metaphyseal vessels allow passage of bacteria (33) that may adhere to type I collagen in the hypertrophic zone of the physis. *S. aureus* surface antigens may play a key role in this local adherence (34).

Among factors that have been implicated as contributing to the development of infection, none is as common as trauma (Fig. 12-1). Local trauma has been associated with AHO in 30% to 50% of reported cases (35–39). The best evidence confirming the role of trauma has been established in an animal model by Morrissy and Haynes, who noted that intravenous injection of *S. aureus* caused infection in the metaphysis of an injured rabbit (40, 41). Interestingly, infection did not develop in fractures of the fibula diaphysis, indicating that fracture hematoma cannot be the explanation. Although rare, acute infection of fracture hematoma has occurred clinically. There are no similar clinical data for septic arthritis, but experimental models demonstrate the role of trauma in the production of the disease (42, 43). Therefore, the precise mechanism by which trauma reduces local host defenses and predisposes a particular location for infection has not been conclusively determined.

Naturally occurring situations confirm the importance of host defense mechanisms preventing bone and joint infection. Patients with conditions associated with decreased or altered immune response, such as the neonate, are known to be susceptible to infection. Varicella infection provides a portal for bacteria to enter the musculoskeletal system and also lowers the host immune system, making the host more susceptible to infection (44, 45). Other aspects of musculoskeletal infection etiology, such as the predilection for men and the lower extremity and peak age incidence, are less well understood and are yet to be explained.

PATHOPHYSIOLOGY

Osteomyelitis. Knowledge of normal pediatric bone physiology facilitates better understanding of osteomyelitis pathophysiology. The diaphyseal region of long bones consists of a dense lamellar cortex, which is relatively acellular, and a medullary cavity, which contains little bone but is filled with a rich reticuloendothelial system. In contrast, the metaphyseal region is composed of a cortex that is little more than compact cancellous bone and a medullary cavity that has greater bone content arranged in a trabecular pattern but relatively few reticuloendothelial cells. Covering metaphyseal and diaphyseal cortical bone is the periosteum, which in children is thick, easily separated from bone, but not easily penetrated. Periosteal blood supply comes from the outside so that it remains viable, producing osteoid and bone even when elevated off of the bone surface.

In a classic article, Hobo (32) described his experiments on the localization of both India ink particles and bacteria in bone after intravenous injection. Hobo noted that although most bacteria lodged in the diaphyseal medullary cavity, they were rapidly phagocytosed and no infection resulted. In contrast, relatively few bacteria were localized to the area beneath the epiphyseal plate, but because of the absence of phagocytic cells in this region of the bone, infection subsequently developed. Hobo proposed that the vessels beneath the physeal plate were small arterial loops that emptied into venous sinusoids and that the resulting turbulence was the cause of localization. Subsequently, electron microscopic studies have shown these to be small terminal branches (46). In addition, it has been demonstrated that the endothelial wall of new metaphyseal capillaries have gaps that allow the passage of blood cells and, presumably, bacteria (33).

Hematogenous osteomyelitis has a strong predilection for the most rapidly growing end of the large long bones, especially those of the lower extremity. This predilection may be explained by the observation that in rapidly growing bones, there is greater distance between bacteria being deposited in new bone being formed by the epiphyseal plate and phagocytic cells that are moving in from the diaphysis. Therefore, the immune system response takes longer to reach the bacteria, allowing a clinical infection to become established.

Once bacteria begin to multiply in the metaphysis adjacent to the physis, a process of net bone resorption begins. Osteoblasts die and bone trabeculae are resorbed by numerous osteoclasts within 12 to 18 hours. Lymphocytes may release osteoclastic-activating factor, and macrophages, monocytes, and vascular endothelial cells may all directly resorb both the crystalline and matrix components of bone. In response to toxins and bacterial antigens, interleukin-1 is produced by macrophages and polymorphonuclear leukocytes (47). Prostaglandin E_2 is also produced, which stimulates further bone resorption (48). These stimuli cause inflammatory cells to migrate and accumulate in the area of bacterial localization beneath the physis. As inflammatory cells migrate to the site of accumulating bacteria, bone in the path of this migration is resorbed.

The accumulation of bacteria and inflammatory cells causes thrombosis of medullary vessels, further reducing the host's ability to fight infection. A purulent exudate is formed that may exit the porous metaphyseal cortex to create a subperiosteal abscess. As the periosteum is elevated, the cortical bone is deprived of its blood supply and may become necrotic,

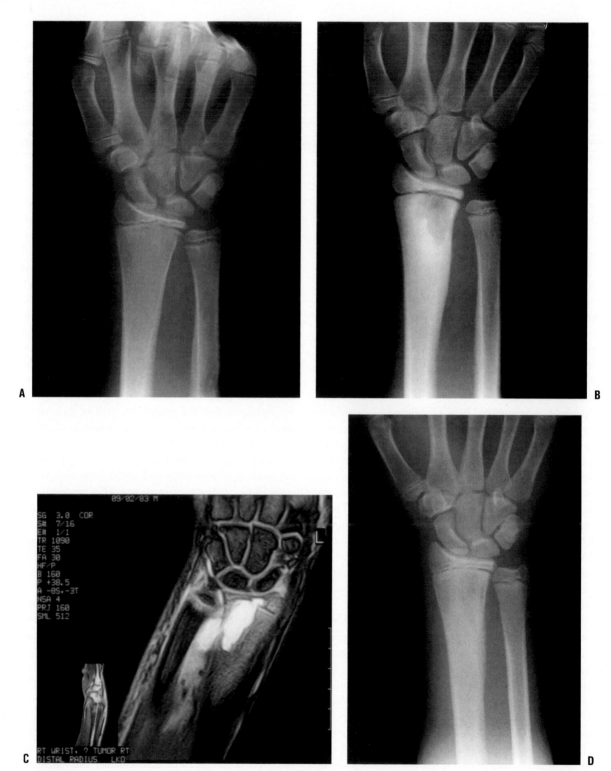

FIGURE 12-1.   A: 12-year-old boy was struck in the distal radius by a hockey puck. Initial radiographs were negative, and the patient's symptoms completely resolved over 2 weeks. **B:** Two months later, the patient experienced increasing pain and swelling. Radiographs were repeated and demonstrated a lytic lesion with a sclerotic margin that appeared to cross the physis consistent with osteomyelitis. **C:** T2-weighted MRI confirms the processes crosses the distal radial physis with cortical breach and adjacent soft-tissue abscess. **D:** Irrigation and debridement of purulent material was performed, and cultures obtained at surgery confirmed *S. aureus* osteomyelitis. To reduce risk of persistent infection and to reduce the likelihood of physeal arrest, no bone graft was placed. Two years after surgery, the bone defect has healed, there is no evidence of infection, and the distal radial physis is growing normally.

forming a sequestrum. Because the periosteum retains its blood supply, it remains viable and produces osteoid. The new bone forming around the necrotic sequestrum is known as *involucrum*. If the metaphysis is intra-articular at the site where infection breaches the metaphyseal cortex, septic arthritis results. Infection generally does not spread down the medullary cavity because the well-developed reticuloendothelial system of the diaphysis is able to prevent its expansion in this direction.

Because of the unique and changing anatomy of the interosseous blood supply, osteomyelitis pathophysiology in the infant may vary from the pattern described in preceding text. Trueta first noted that before the ossific nucleus forms, the vessels from the metaphysis penetrate directly into the cartilaginous physis analog (49) [see also Trueta (248)]. Because of this blood supply pattern, the initial bacterial localization may occur in the cartilage epiphysis precursor. Infection of the epiphysis precursor may spread to the joint, causing septic arthritis as well as physeal injury and growth alteration. As the ossific nucleus develops, a separate blood supply to this epiphysis develops and the metaphyseal vessels crossing the developing physeal plate disappear. When the physeal plate is fully formed, it acts as a barrier to intraosseous blood flow between the metaphysis and the epiphysis.

Septic Arthritis. Distinct anatomic and histologic characteristics of a synovial joint affect the pathophysiology of septic arthritis. Joint synovium is a unique tissue that does not have a basement membrane and secretes fluid that is essentially a transudate of serum. Just as in bone, it is likely that transient bacteremia results in bacteria entering the joint, but, in almost all cases, the joint has the ability to clear itself of bacteria and avoid infection (50). Bactericidal properties of joint fluid may help prevent septic arthritis. Gruber et al. (51) compared growth of bacteria inoculated onto culture media containing synovial fluid with growth of bacteria inoculated onto culture media alone Fluid was plated and incubated, and colonies were counted after 1, 4, and 24 hours to determine bacterial growth. Statistically significant differences in bacterial counts were found between control and experimental groups at 0, 4, and 24 hours. Bacterial counts in the control specimens demonstrated exponential growth over 24 hours as would be expected in the absence of growth inhibition. In contrast, bacterial counts in all of the synovial fluid specimens decreased steadily over 24 hours. These results demonstrate synovial fluid possesses potent bactericidal activity against the most common gram-positive pathogens responsible for septic arthritis.

However, when the inoculum is large, or when virulent pathologic bacteria such as *S. aureus* are less effectively cleared, clinical infection may result. The precise pathophysiology by which septic arthritis occurs is less well understood than for osteomyelitis. Although trauma has been implicated as a causative factor (43), trauma cannot completely explain the tendency for infection to involve large joints and those of the lower extremities. What is known is that when septic arthritis occurs, bacteria rapidly gain access to the joint cavity and within a matter of hours cause synovitis and formation of fibrinous exudate followed by areas of synovial necrosis.

The main goal of the treating physician is to interrupt and reverse the process of articular cartilage destruction, and an understanding of this process will facilitate optimal treatment. Proteases, peptidases, and collagenases are released from leukocytes, synovial cells, and cartilage. These enzymes catalyze reactions that break down the cellular and extracellular structure of cartilage (50, 52–57). The loss of glycosaminoglycans is the first measurable change in articular cartilage, occurring as early as 8 hours after bacteria are introduced into the joint (58). Loss of glycosaminoglycans softens the cartilage and may cause it to be susceptible to increased wear. Collagen destruction follows and is responsible for visible change in cartilage appearance (59–61). Chronic changes occur in the synovium as well, including neovascularization and cell proliferation, accompanied by persistent bacterial colonization and heterogeneous inflammatory infiltration (62). Once catalytic enzymes are released into the joint, the presence of living bacteria is not necessary for cartilage destruction to continue.

CLINICAL FEATURES

History. A detailed history provides important information critical to the diagnosis of musculoskeletal infection in children. Pain is the most common symptom in patients with bone or joint sepsis (63, 64), but children are not always able to verbalize this common symptom. Instead, children may refuse to walk, refuse to bear weight, limp, or refuse to use or move a limb. Frequently, the physician obtains the history indirectly from a parent or caregiver instead of obtaining it directly from the patient. Careful questioning can provide important information about the infection location, likely causative organisms, and the duration of the infectious process.

A toddler who refuses to walk, but does crawl, is willing to bear weight on the thigh, and the clinician can focus on the leg distal to the knee as the possible infection location. Patient age, recent activity, and exposure can all provide clues to the causative organism; the neonate is more likely to have infection caused by group B *Streptococcus* or gram-negative rods, and patients with sickle cell disease are predisposed to *Salmonella* infection.

Fever, malaise, anorexia, and night pain are common symptoms of musculoskeletal infection but are not always present. Temperature >38°C has been reported to occur in only 36% to 74% of patients (17, 64, 65). Few patients fit the stereotype of an ill-appearing child who has experienced symptoms for a week and who presents with an obviously infected bone or joint. More frequently, children may present within 12 hours of onset of limp, with normal or mildly elevated laboratory values.

Recent antibiotic use may blunt symptoms of musculoskeletal infection or may affect the type of musculoskeletal infection present. A history of recent antibiotic use should cause the treating physician to maintain greater vigilance for subacute osteomyelitis.

A history of recent or concurrent illness is important information to consider when evaluating a patient for possible musculoskeletal infection, and such illness may be present in one-third to one-half of patients. Recent upper respiratory symptoms may suggest a noninfectious cause for patient symptoms such as toxic synovitis or poststreptococcal reactive arthritis (PSRA). Rashes or swollen lymph nodes are important for their association with conditions such as Lyme disease, cat-scratch disease, rheumatoid arthritis, and leukemia. Concurrent chickenpox is notable for creating a portal of entry into the circulatory system as well as for lowering host immunity, predisposing a patient to musculoskeletal infection caused by group A *Streptococcus* in particular.

Patients with musculoskeletal infection frequently present with a history of local trauma, and, as noted previously, local trauma can contribute to the development of bone or joint sepsis. The crucial and difficult issue for the clinician to determine is whether a patient's pain is caused by trauma or by infection. Close attention to the clinical course following a traumatic event is very helpful; symptoms caused by trauma tend to improve, whereas symptoms caused by sepsis generally worsen.

Examination.   Much helpful information can be obtained while simply observing the child in the examination room while obtaining the history as part of the evaluation. If the child does not appear acutely ill or moribund, encourage the child to play independently while you are interviewing the parent. Unaware that he or she is being observed, the young child will often be more active than later in the structured segment of the physical examination. Refusal to bear weight on a lower extremity, a limp, or the disuse of an upper extremity gives important clues about the location of pathology.

Bone pain in a febrile child is osteomyelitis until proven otherwise. The importance of palpable bone pain in establishing the diagnosis of osteomyelitis cannot be overemphasized. Gentle, systematic palpation is often the best means available on physical examination to localize pathology in an irritable, uncooperative 2-year-old child who refuses to use an extremity. Allowing the child to remain in the arms of the parent and watching the child's face, not the limb, while systematically palpating the limb often reveals the location of pathology. In the case of small children who cry at the mere presence of a stranger and panic at being touched, it is often beneficial to instruct the parent how to elicit the tender area. After showing the parent how to palpate the area, the physician should leave the room and allow the parent to first examine the unaffected part, then the affected part, and report the results.

In addition to establishing pain, the physician closely examines for increased warmth, erythema, or other skin changes. Erythema and swelling may appear as early as 24 to 36 hours following onset of pain and can progress rapidly. Skin changes are detectable earliest in bones or joints that are not covered by muscle. Visual comparison of the normal and affected limbs, symmetrically positioned, should always be done. Loss of normal concavities, contours, and normal skin wrinkles are other subtle clues that may be present. Severe limb swelling may indicate extensive underlying infection or deep venous thrombosis (DVT) (66).

Sympathetic joint effusion may occur adjacent to osteomyelitis but should not cause substantial joint irritability. Pain with passive joint motion is a hallmark sign of septic arthritis and is usually associated with decreased ROM as well. Palpation of joints often elicits tenderness, and joint effusion can frequently be demonstrated in joints that are not covered by large amounts of tissue. Joints of the axial skeleton, including the spine and pelvis, are less accessible for examination, and diagnosis is more dependent on findings such as pain with motion, percussion, and compression. The hip joint is also inaccessible to direct observation, but noting the position of thigh relative to the pelvis may be helpful. The patient often lies with the hip flexed, abducted, and externally rotated because internal rotation, extension, and adduction all tighten the hip capsule, causing pain in a distended and inflamed joint.

Other diagnoses included in the differential can also present with similar signs, but knowledge of characteristic patterns is helpful in establishing a diagnosis. Rheumatoid arthritis often presents as a joint that looks worse than it feels. The joint may be warm and markedly swollen with inflamed synovium and effusion but not be especially painful. Rheumatic fever has a tendency to appear just the opposite, with exquisite pain and markedly restricted motion in a joint having minimal effusion or swelling.

Laboratory.   Laboratory testing for suspected musculoskeletal infection should include complete blood count (CBC) with differential, blood culture, erythrocyte sedimentation rate (ESR), and C-reactive protein (CRP). None of these tests are specific for musculoskeletal infection. White blood cell (WBC) count is the least sensitive, being elevated in 25% to 73% of patients with osteomyelitis (2, 17, 29, 64, 67). Similar sensitivity has been reported for patients with septic arthritis (4, 35, 63, 64). Occasionally, patients with apparent AHO will have a low WBC or platelet count, which may indicate systemic sepsis or leukemia. If the diagnosis of musculoskeletal infection is in question, a manual differential count should be performed to look for atypical leukocytes and leukemia. In patients presenting with a clinical picture less clearly suggestive of bacterial sepsis, Lyme disease titer, antinuclear antibodies (ANAs), rheumatoid factor, and HLA-B27 antigen should also be considered.

The ESR and CRP are the two most common tests used to measure acute-phase response and are more useful than CBC. Acute-phase response is the increase or decrease in the levels of a variety of plasma proteins in response to cytokine production that occurs in acute or chronic inflammation. These proteins are responsible for many of the systemic symptoms seen in infection, such as fever, anorexia, lethargy, and anemia, and an increase in the levels of many of these proteins can be measured in the blood.

ESR is a nonspecific test that measures the rate at which an erythrocyte falls through plasma and is dependent on the concentration of fibrinogen. The ESR result can be affected by the size, shape, and number of erythrocytes present, as well as by other proteins in plasma. Therefore, the ESR is less reliable in the neonate, in the presence of anemia, in patients with sickle cell disease, or when the patient is taking steroids (64, 65).

The ESR typically becomes elevated within 48 to 72 hours of the onset of infection and returns to normal over a period of 2 to 4 weeks after elimination of infection. The ESR is less reliable in the first 48 hours of infection than after 48 hours. Clinicians can expect the ESR to be elevated in 85% to 95% of cases of septic arthritis (4, 14, 17) and in 90% to 95% of osteomyelitis cases (63, 64). Although noted to be elevated just as often in patients with osteomyelitis, the ESR has been noted to be significantly higher in patients with septic arthritis (4).

One problem with the clinical usefulness of the ESR is that it continues to rise for 3 to 5 days after institution of successful therapy. Although a continuing rise beyond the 4th to 5th day of treatment can be an indication of treatment failure, it is because of this delayed response that the ESR is not a good means of assessing the resolution of sepsis during the first week of treatment (68).

The CRP is a substance found in the serum in response to inflammation and also trauma. The CRP may begin to rise within 6 hours of the triggering stimulus and then increases several hundredfold, reaching a peak within 36 to 50 hours. Because of the short half-life of the protein (47 hours), it also falls quickly to normal with successful treatment, in contrast to the ESR. This makes the CRP of greater value than the ESR, not only for earlier diagnosis of infection but also for determining resolution of the inflammation (69).

CRP is perhaps the most helpful laboratory test in the evaluation of musculoskeletal infection, its level being elevated in as many as 98% of patients with osteomyelitis compared to 92% of patients having elevated ESR (70). Peak CRP is typically noted on day 2 compared to peak ESR measured on days 3 through 5 (Fig. 12-2). Following initiation of treatment, it may take the ESR approximately 3 weeks to normalize, whereas the CRP typically returns to normal within 1 week. Failure of the CRP to rapidly normalize after initiation of treatment has been predictive of long-term sequelae (71). Therefore, the CRP is more likely to be helpful in diagnosing an early case of infection and is more useful in monitoring its resolution.

A CRP within the normal range is also a strong indicator that a patient does not have musculoskeletal infection. Levine et al. (72) reported that if the CRP is <1.0 mg/dL, the probability that a patient does not have septic arthritis is 87%. The presence of both osteomyelitis and adjacent septic arthritis also increases the likelihood that serologic testing will be abnormal. Khachatourians et al. (14) reported the ESR and CRP being elevated 100% of the time and the WBC count being elevated in 87% of patients with both septic arthritis and adjacent osteomyelitis.

As expected, the peak and the normalization of ESR and CRP are also affected by surgery (14). Khachatourians et al. (14) reviewed 50 patients with septic arthritis, osteomyelitis, or both. Twenty-five patients were treated with surgery, and

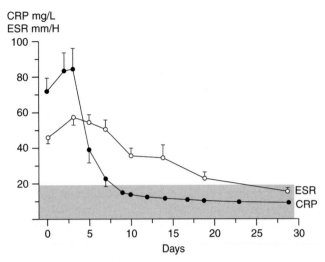

FIGURE 12-2.   CRP reaches a peak value more precipitously and has a more rapid return to normal than does the ESR. The stippled area denotes the normal range of values. (Adapted from Unkila-Kallio L, Kallio MJT, Eskola J, et al. Serum C-reactive protein, erythrocyte sedimentation rate, and white blood cell count in acute hematogenous osteomyelitis of children. *Pediatrics* 1994;93:59–62.)

25 patients were treated with antibiotics alone. In the surgery group, it took twice as long for the CRP and ESR to reach peak values and then twice as long to normalize after initiation of treatment.

The question is often raised as to whether or not the CRP is useful in separating a musculoskeletal infection from an otitis media, which is commonly seen in children. Elevated CRP values are reported in 22% of patients with a bacterial otitis media and in 65% of those with a viral otitis media (73). Therefore, it would seem that CRP cannot reliably differentiate between musculoskeletal infection and otitis media.

The relatively low yield and delay in species identification associated with standard bacterial cultures has stimulated significant interest in molecular techniques for detection and speciation of bacterial and viral infections (16, 74). Molecular testing is appealing because it can be performed in an hour, does not depend on the presence of live bacteria for culture, and test results should not be affected if antibiotic treatment has already begun. Molecular testing techniques fall into two broad categories: nonamplified and amplified. In nonamplified techniques, direct binding of a target molecule is done with a labeled oligonucleotide probe or a monoclonal antibody, followed by the detection of the probe agent with radiolabeling, enzyme-linked immunosorbent assay (ELISA), or chemoluminescence.

When using amplification techniques, geometric amplification of a target molecule is achieved through enzyme-driven reactions. The most common technique is polymerase chain reaction (PCR). A target segment of bacterial DNA or RNA is chosen that is not present in human cells. A probe or primer specific to that segment of DNA or RNA is introduced, which promotes binding of a polymerase that replicates the target segment in a series of temperature-dependent cycles. The amplification products are then identified by gel electrophoresis. PCR has produced some promising results in the diagnosis of periprosthetic infections and septic arthritis, but a high false-positive rate has been reported (75). Recently, success has been reported performing molecular diagnosis of musculoskeletal *K. kingae* infection by specific, real-time PCR assay (76–78). These authors report the *K. kingae* PCR assays to be reliable and especially helpful in identifying infection caused by this fastidious organism.

Blood cultures should always be included in the initial battery of tests obtained when one suspects musculoskeletal infection because, in both osteomyelitis and septic arthritis, blood cultures yield organisms in 30% to 60% of patients (5, 13, 64), allowing organism identification and facilitating optimal antibiotic therapy. The yield from both blood culture and aspirated material decreases with previous antibiotic therapy (4). Even with previous antibiotic treatment, however, the chances of obtaining positive cultures, when all sources (i.e., blood, bone, and joint fluid) are cultured, remain high (64).

Radiologic Features

Standard Radiographs.

Imaging should begin with standard radiographs (79); the sensitivity and specificity of radiographs range from 43% to 75% and from 75% to 83%, respectively (80). The role of radiography in the diagnosis of early bone and joint sepsis is often undervalued because clinicians often look only for changes seen in bone. Plain radiographs may show soft-tissue swelling and loss of tissue planes within 3 days of infection onset, whereas bone changes may not appear for 7 days or more (67, 81). Because the inflammation in the bone or joint produces edema in the soft tissues adjacent to the area of inflammation, there is swelling in this region, and enlargement of this muscle layer is detectable on the radiograph. Radiographs to detect deep soft-tissue swelling are of most value in suspected sepsis of the long bones. Symmetrically positioned views of the contralateral extremity may be helpful for comparison.

Septic arthritis may cause a large effusion that is most easily seen in peripheral joints such as the knee or elbow. At the hip, there may be asymmetric widening of the joint space compared to the uninvolved hip (Fig. 12-3). Although this may be seen frequently in the neonate, hip joint space widening is often lacking in older children. It is a late sign, and its absence is not to be interpreted as lack of sepsis (82). Untreated septic arthritis may result in joint destruction, narrowing of the joint space, or pathologic bone changes on both sides of the joint. Additional sequelae such as osteonecrosis of the femoral head may also be seen.

The time required before bone changes become visible on plain radiographs suggests that by the time bone changes are seen, osteomyelitis is already well established. While not entirely reliable, it is fair to suggest that when radiographic changes are present, surgical treatment of osteomyelitis is more likely to be necessary than if radiographic changes are not present. Although infection can appear in any bone and in any location, the most common radiographic presentation for osteomyelitis is a destructive, lytic, eccentric metaphyseal lesion, often associated with periosteal elevation and new bone formation. Bone destruction caused by osteomyelitis may appear aggressive, infiltrative, and ominous in appearance and may be mistaken for neoplasm (83–85).

Bone Scan.

Radionucleotide technetium-99m diphosphonate bone scanning is an excellent test for localizing suspected musculoskeletal infection, with reported sensitivity of 89% to 94% and specificity of 94%, with overall accuracy of approximately 92% (13, 86). The bone scan consists of three phases: an angiogram, performed immediately after injection; immediately followed by the second or "blood pool" phase; and 2 to 3 hours later, the mineral phase, which reflects uptake in the bone. All three phases are helpful, especially in distinguishing cellulitis from osteomyelitis. The mechanism by which technetium-99 m bone scanning works is isotope uptake, which depends on vascularity and calcium phosphate deposition (87).

To obtain the highest quality and most sensitive images, the bladder should be empty at the time of the scan to prevent accumulated isotope from obstructing the sacrum and sacroiliac (SI) joints. Symmetrically positioned views of both sides should be obtained. Technetium scanning using pinhole-collimated views and single-photon emission computerized tomography can increase both sensitivity and specificity (88). Because most AHO occurs in the metaphysis adjacent to the physeal plate, such views are necessary to separate early metaphyseal changes from the large amount of uptake found in the physeal plate. These images are time consuming to obtain and may require that the child be sedated. It is therefore important that the physician communicate the desired areas of interest to the radiologist.

Technetium-99m scanning is most helpful when examining patients in whom the site of suspected musculoskeletal infection is unclear (Fig. 12-4) or when looking for multiple foci of bone involvement (89). Bone aspiration and initiation of treatment should not be delayed for fear of affecting bone scan results. Using an animal model, Canale et al. (90) demonstrated that if a bone scan is performed within 48 hours after bone aspiration, the bone aspiration does not cause a false-positive scan result.

Whereas typically a bone scan is suggestive of osteomyelitis when "hot" or showing increased uptake, a "cold" bone scan may provide evidence of severe osteomyelitis and has been reported to have a positive predictive value of 100% (88, 91, 92) A "cold" scan results from infection causing an area of bone ischemia. Pennington et al. (93) at the Medical College of Wisconsin reviewed 81 patients evaluated with technetium bone scan for osteomyelitis. Seven of the 81 patients had a photopenic region defect, or cold scan, consistent with osteomyelitis. A control group of matched patients with hot scan osteomyelitis was compared to the cold scan group. Patients with cold scan osteomyelitis had statistically increased

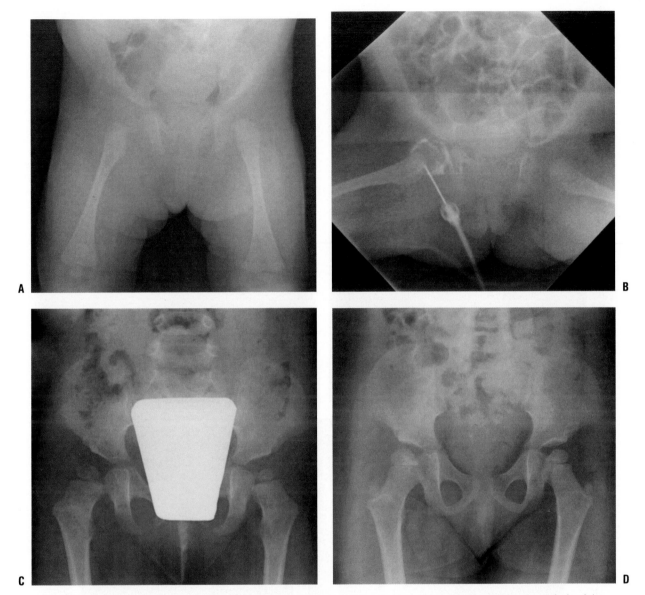

FIGURE 12-3. **A:** A 2-month-old infant presents following 3 days of increasing irritability, fever, and pseudoparalysis of the right leg. Anteroposterior pelvis radiograph demonstrates widening of the right hip joint space. **B:** The patient was brought emergently to the operating room, where the right hip was aspirated and an arthrogram was performed to document intra-articular position of the needle. Cell count of the hip joint aspirate was 65,000 per mL; open joint irrigation and debridement of septic arthritis were performed. Cultures later confirm group A *Streptococcus* infection. **C:** Two years following open surgical irrigation and drainage, the patient is asymptomatic but A-P pelvis radiograph demonstrates mild hip dysplasia on the right with acetabular index of 25 degrees compared to 22 degrees on the left, 50% femoral head coverage on the right compared to 70% coverage on the left, and widening of the right femoral neck. **D:** Four years following irrigation and debridement, the right hip dysplasia has improved, with the right acetabular index now measuring 21 degrees and with a femoral head coverage of 70%. Mild coxa magna and femoral neck widening persists.

temperature, resting pulse rate, ESR, length of hospital stay, and rate of surgical intervention compared to patients with hot scan osteomyelitis.

Septic arthritis is suggested by equally increased uptake on both sides of a joint. Although bone scanning may correctly identify the site of joint sepsis in approximately 90% of infected joints, it does not separate bone from joint sepsis or differentiate infectious from noninfectious arthritis (86, 94). This is a particular problem in the hip, in which the differential diagnoses may include transient synovitis, septic arthritis, or osteomyelitis of the femoral neck.

Technetium-99m bone scanning does have its limitations. Technetium scanning is relatively nonspecific, and increased uptake may be caused by any process that increases vascularity

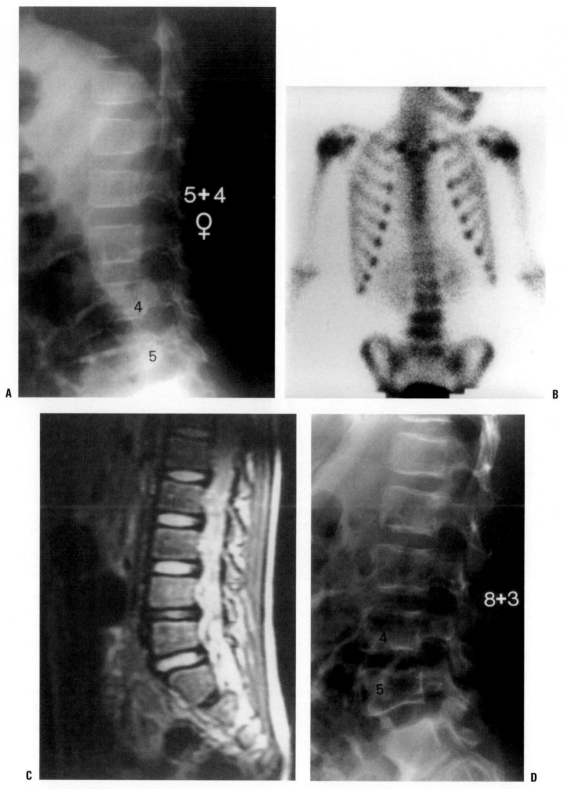

FIGURE 12-4.   A 5-year-old child presents with an increasing limp over 48 hours and with suspected musculoskeletal infection. History and physical examination do not localize the process. ESR and CRP are elevated. **A:** The lateral (as well as the antero-posterior) radiograph of the spine is normal. **B:** Technetium bone scan shows increased isotope uptake in the L4 and L5 vertebral bodies suggestive of discitis, but neoplasm cannot be excluded. **C:** T2-weighted MRI helps confirm the diagnosis of discitis, demonstrating that the process is centered in the L4–L5 disc with no evidence of neoplasm, bone, soft tissue, or epidural abscess. Intravenous followed by oral antibiotic treatment was initiated, with complete resolution of symptoms after antibiotic therapy duration of 3 weeks. **D:** Final follow-up 3 years later demonstrates a normal lumbar spine radiograph in the asymptomatic patient.

or deposition of calcium phosphate. Tumor, trauma, and bone resorption due to disuse may cause increased uptake. The scans may be negative in the first 24 hours of infection before stimulation of bone turnover, and there may be a 4% to 20% false-negative rate with technetium scanning (64). In neonatal infection, the reported sensitivity for technetium scanning has ranged from 30% to 86%, and standard radiography may be more helpful (6, 7, 95). Overall specificity and sensitivity are improved when the scan is interpreted with knowledge of the clinical findings and initial laboratory studies, compared to when the interpretation was a blind reading of the scan (96).

Other radionucleotide imaging techniques have been less helpful in evaluating osteomyelitis in children. Gallium-67 citrate and indium-labeled leukocytes are more expensive, result in more radiation exposure, take longer to complete, and are not often useful in the evaluation of musculoskeletal infection in children (10). Indium-111–labeled WBC scanning may be helpful in the rare circumstance when infection is suspected but the technetium scan is normal. However, indium scanning requires preparation time and may take as long as 24 hours to perform (16). Granulocyte scintigraphy is an imaging technique performed with a technetium-99m–labeled monoclonal murine antibody (MoAb) against granulocytes and has been shown to be an effective and a specific method of imaging infection in adults. Unfortunately, in children, the same imaging technique was neither sensitive nor specific (97).

Magnetic Resonance Imaging. magnetic resonance imaging (MRI) is an increasingly valuable imaging tool used to evaluate musculoskeletal infection, with reported sensitivity ranging from 88% to 100%, specificity from 75% to 100%, and a positive predictive value of 85% (98–100). MRI provides better soft-tissue resolution and can be used to identify abscesses as well as to help differentiate cellulitis from osteomyelitis. MRI is useful in visualizing marrow involvement and differentiating between malignant neoplasm and infection (Figs. 12-5 and 12-6). MRI findings of osteomyelitis include a decrease in the normally high marrow signal intensity on T1-weighted images caused by replacement of marrow fat by inflammatory cells and edema. The inflammatory cells and the edema appear as increased signal intensity on T2-weighted images (10). Grey has described a high signal intensity feature of the thin layer of granulation tissue that lines the abscess cavity on T1-weighted magnetic resonance (MR) images, calling it the "Penumbra Sign." Subsequent authors have confirmed its value in differentiating osteomyelitis from neoplasm with a sensitivity of 73.3% and specificity of 99.1% for osteomyelitis (101).

Administration of gadolinium provides further assistance in differentiating infection from other pathologic processes such as neoplasm, fracture, or bone infarct. Acute bone infarcts demonstrated thin, linear rim contrast enhancement, whereas osteomyelitis caused more geographic and irregular marrow enhancement (102). Osteomyelitis cases may also demonstrate subtle cortical defects with abnormal signal crossing marrow and soft tissue.

Invasive community-acquired *S. aureus* musculoskeletal infection has been associated with a high incidence of extraosseous infection and other complications such as DVT that are effectively detected by MRI. In a series of 199 children with community-acquired *S. aureus* osteomyelitis treated at Texas Children's Hospital, MRI was compared with bone scintigraphy (103). The sensitivity of MRI and bone scintigraphy for osteomyelitis was 98% and 53%, respectively. In all discordant cases, MRI was correct compared to bone scintigraphy. Extraosseous complications of community-acquired *S. aureus* osteomyelitis detected only by MRI included subperiosteal abscesses (*n* = 77), pyomyositis (*n* = 43), septic arthritis (*n* = 31), and DVT (*n* = 12). Therefore, MRI is the preferred imaging modality for the investigation of severe, pediatric community-acquired musculoskeletal infection because it offers superior sensitivity for osteomyelitis compared to bone scintigraphy and detects extraosseous complications that occur in a substantial proportion of patients.

MRI is very helpful when evaluating suspected sepsis involving the hip and axial skeleton. Yang et al. (104) used MRI when trying to differentiate between transient synovitis and septic arthritis. Septic arthritis was statistically more likely to have signal intensity abnormalities in adjacent bone marrow and contrast enhancement within surrounding soft tissue, while toxic synovitis was more likely to be associated with contralateral hip effusion. Karmazyn et al. (105) reported the utility of MRI when differentiating conditions such as pyomyositis, and sacroiliitis from septic arthritis of the hip, while McPhee et al. (106) reported the value of MRI when localizing infection in complex pelvis anatomy. MRI of suspected spinal infection allows visualization of pathology such as epidural or paraspinal abscesses as well as detection of the presence of soft-tissue masses that would be suggestive of neoplasm.

Whole-body MRI has recently been reported as a possible screening study that could be used to localize musculoskeletal infection in a manner similar to scintigraphy but with several potential advantages (107). Use of a moving tabletop and automatic direct realignment of the images after acquisition make whole-body MRI possible. The scan plane is coronal with additional planes being added depending on the indication and findings. Whole-body MRI is targeted for maximum coverage of the body within the shortest possible time using the minimum number of sequences. The evaluation of the bone marrow has been the primary indication, and, therefore, inversion recovery sequences like STIR or TIRM are typically used with the T1-weighted sequence being added variably. If an area of pathology is detected, then imaging technique can be changed from a screening protocol to an imaging regimen designed to provide detailed information on the specific region in question. Whole-body MRI may be especially helpful in neonates where multifocal infection is common, scintigraphy is relatively insensitive, and patient size is small.

Two recent studies have been reported on the use of MRI in postsurgical patients. Kan and coauthors at Vanderbilt University evaluated the diagnostic efficacy and the impact of emergent MRI after recent surgical intervention in children

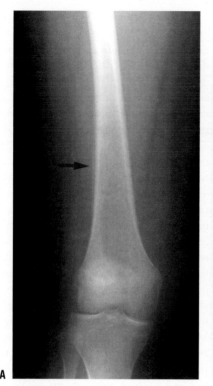
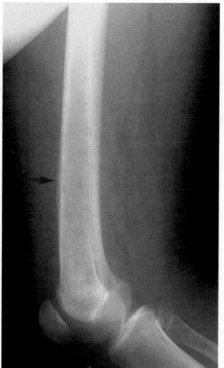

A

B

FIGURE 12-5. MRI may be very helpful when differentiating between osteomyelitis and primary bone malignancy. **A,B:** This 12-year-old female patient was referred for evaluation of femoral osteosarcoma. The standard anteroposterior and lateral radiograph shows periosteal reaction along the distal one-third of the femur, consistent with primary bone sarcoma or osteomyelitis (*arrows*). **C:** T2-weighted MRI without contrast demonstrates preservation of some normal marrow fat within the intramedullary canal and a fluid-filled abscess cavity diagnostic of osteomyelitis. Diffuse inflammation is present in adjacent soft tissues without a discrete soft-tissue mass. Osteomyelitis was confirmed at surgery.

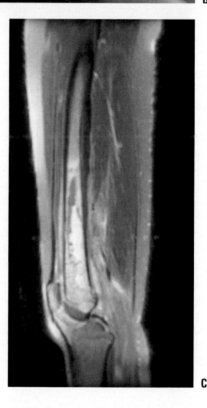

C

with suspected osteomyelitis or septic arthritis and found that iatrogenic soft tissue and bone edema related to recent surgery in children with suspected osteomyelitis or septic arthritis has minimal effect on diagnostic accuracy of MRI (108). Spiegel et al. (109) at Children's Hospital of Philadelphia evaluated the usefulness of MRI as a routine follow-up test used to assess surgical treatment of musculoskeletal infection and noted that if patients'

clinical course was unremarkable, MRI did not add clinically significant additional information. From these two studies, we can conclude that if patients demonstrate clinical improvement with treatment, then routine follow-up MRI is not necessary, but if the treatment course is complicated by clinical evidence of persistent or recurrent infection, then MRI can provide helpful, reliable information that is not degraded by previous surgery.

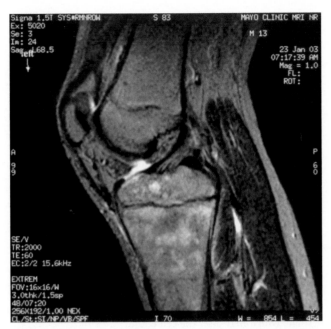

FIGURE 12-6. This 13-year-old male presents with a 4-month history of proximal tibial pain and normal plain film radiographs. Lateral T2 MRI without contrast lacks the high signal intensity associated with marrow edema caused by osteomyelitis and suggests a more indolent cause. MRI is the only imaging modality that can provide such detailed information. Biopsy established the diagnosis of a diffuse, large B-cell lymphoma.

Disadvantages of MRI scanning include its cost and the frequent necessity for sedation or general anesthesia in small children. When making the decision whether or not to evaluate presumed musculoskeletal infection with MRI, in each clinical circumstance one must weigh these disadvantages against the helpful information and benefit provided.

Computed Tomography. Computed tomography (CT) is helpful to determine the extent of bone destruction as well as to detect soft-tissue abnormalities and is the most sensitive imaging study for detecting gas in soft tissues (16, 89). Especially when evaluating infection of the axial skeleton such as the spine and pelvis, CT is very helpful in localizing the infection and can assist in planning the surgical approach if debridement is indicated. CT scanning can be used to guide needle localization prior to surgical biopsy or debridement, to direct aspiration of bone or soft tissue, or to guide percutaneous placement of drainage tubes. Compared to MRI, its advantages include its greater availability and lower cost, which must be considered along with the disadvantages of being unable to detect changes within the marrow in early cases and being less sensitive at detecting soft-tissue changes.

Ultrasonography. The utility of ultrasonography in the evaluation of musculoskeletal infection has been studied extensively, especially with regard to septic arthritis of the hip. Ultrasonography is attractive because of its low cost, relative availability, noninvasive nature, absence of ionizing radiation,

and the lack of need for sedation. However, ultrasound as a noninvasive means of evaluating musculoskeletal infection has been disappointing. The lack of specificity, the dependence on operator skill, and the inability to image marrow or show cortical detail have limited ultrasound's usefulness.

Gordon et al. (110) reviewed hip ultrasound results in 132 patients being evaluated for hip pain during an 18-month period. They found a false-negative rate of 5% in patients who were determined by ultrasonography to have no effusion but were subsequently diagnosed with septic arthritis. Children with onset of symptoms <24 hours prior to hip ultrasonography and children who had bilateral hip effusions were more likely to have a false-negative result. Zamzan reported similar findings noting a positive predictive value of ultrasound for the diagnosis of septic arthritis to be 87.9% and concluding that ultrasound cannot be used safely to distinguish between pediatric septic arthritis and transient synovitis.

Benign conditions such as toxic synovitis cannot be reliably differentiated from septic arthritis by ultrasound alone. Toxic synovitis may have a higher incidence of bilateral hip effusions than septic arthritis, and late septic arthritis may have an effusion that is more echo dense and appears fibrinous compared to toxic synovitis, but these findings are not accurate enough to be diagnostic (111, 112). Ultrasonography may be used to guide hip aspiration when performed for patients where septic arthritis is suspected.

Ultrasonography has been used to evaluate osteomyelitis, primarily on the basis of detection of subperiosteal abscess, thickening of the periosteum, and changes in the surrounding soft tissues (113). Sadat-Ali et al. (114) recently reported that ultrasonography can be helpful when differentiating between vasoocclusive crisis and osteomyelitis in patients with sickle cell disease. Ultrasonography scan showed that six patients had periosteal thickening and elevation with hypoechogenic regions, eight had abscesses, and three patients had cortical destruction. All patients were found at surgery to have osteomyelitis. These changes are all relatively late findings of osteomyelitis. Ultrasonography is of limited value when attempting to detect early changes within bone.

Author's Preferred Treatment. A 5-year-old child with a 48-hour history of increasing limp and suspected musculoskeletal infection presents an imaging dilemma that illustrates the importance of all four components of patient evaluation for infection: history, examination, laboratory evaluation, and imaging studies. If the 5-year-old can localize the source of pain, and localization is confirmed by physical exam, then plain film radiographs, CBC, ESR, and CRP are initial appropriate diagnostic tests. If examination is not suggestive of septic arthritis, plain film radiographs are normal, and all laboratory values are normal, then close observation with reexamination in 1 to 3 days is appropriate. If history and examination suggest a localized process, laboratory values suggest infection, and plain film radiographs are normal, then aspiration and culture of the localized bone and/or joint is appropriate. If clinical evaluation suggests infection but does not allow localization of the process, then technetium bone scintigraphy is an appropriate next imaging study (Fig. 12-4). If additional imaging is needed to establish a diagnosis or characterize a pathologic process once the process has been localized, then MRI is the imaging study of choice to provide maximal information about the bone and soft-tissue pathology. For straightforward musculoskeletal infection in the appendicular skeleton, MRI is often not necessary; but for patients whose history, examination, laboratory evaluation, and plain film radiographs are not concordant, or for patients with suspected infection of the pelvis or axial skeleton, MRI is a very helpful imaging study.

Aspiration. Aspiration of bone or joint should be performed whenever possible and as soon as possible when musculoskeletal infection is suspected, because it serves two important purposes: (a) aspiration may confirm the presence of a bone/subperiosteal abscess or septic joint that requires urgent surgical drainage and (b) aspiration often allows identification of the specific bacteria responsible for infection. Whenever possible and when safe to do so, initiation of antibiotic treatment should be held until initial cultures are obtained.

The fact that metaphyseal bone is the most common location for osteomyelitis is fortuitous and makes bone aspiration a relatively easy task to accomplish in the emergency department. Depending on the age and cooperation of the child, sedation may be beneficial. Fluoroscopy is not necessary for bone or joint aspiration in the appendicular skeleton but is now available in many emergency departments and can be helpful in guiding and documenting needle placement. At the point of maximal tenderness, the skin is sterilely prepped. Avoidance of cellulitic skin when possible is desirable but not mandatory; aspiration of bone through cellulitis has not been shown to cause osteomyelitis, and direct culture of cellulitic areas yields a positive culture in <10% of cases (115). Local anesthetic is used to anesthetize the skin and the underlying periosteum with its abundant nerve supply. Using a large-bore trocar needle, such as an 18- or 20-gauge spinal needle, the area at and beneath the periosteum is aspirated for possible subperiosteal abscess.

If no purulent material is aspirated at the periosteum, the needle is passed through the thin metaphyseal cortex by rotating the needle back and forth with gentle pressure directed toward the center of the bone. A spinal needle with its solid trocar facilitates passage through bone and prevents the needle lumen from being plugged with bone fragments. Once inside the cortex, aspiration may yield purulent material but, more commonly, and especially in early osteomyelitis, sanguinous fluid returns. The purulent or sanguinous fluid is then placed in appropriate media and sent for aerobic and anaerobic culture as well as for microscopic Gram stain analysis. Depending on the clinical situation, the aspirate may be sent for fungal and mycobacterial culture. Sending bone aspirate for cell count is less helpful than sending joint fluid, but if adequate aspirate fluid is available, elevated WBC count can support the diagnosis of infection. Bone aspirate cultures yield organisms in 50% to 85% of patients with osteomyelitis (13, 16, 64, 68).

Joint aspiration also offers the opportunity to gather critically important clinical information. Using an 18- or 20-gauge needle, the joint is aspirated and fluid is placed in appropriate culture media and tubes for fluid analysis. Hip aspiration should typically be performed under general anesthesia in the operating room using a spinal needle and accompanied by an arthrogram to document the presence of the needle within the hip joint (Fig. 12-3). Depending on the facility, hip aspiration may be performed under conscious sedation using ultrasound guidance in the emergency or radiology departments. The most important tests for joint fluid aspirate are Gram stain, culture, leukocyte count, and determination of the percentage of polymorphonuclear cells. If Lyme disease is suspected, synovial fluid should be sent for PCR testing as well. Routine use of other synovial fluid tests is of little value (116, 117). Because fluid from an infected joint frequently clots, it may be helpful to rinse the syringe with heparin before aspirating the joint. Often, only a small amount of fluid is obtained, and care must be taken not to leave any significant volume of heparin in the syringe, which may alter the cell count.

Much emphasis has been given to the presence of a joint aspirate cell count >50,000 per mL. Although the most likely cause for a joint aspirate cell count to be >50,000 per mL is bacterial septic arthritis, it is neither 100% sensitive nor 100% specific (Table 12-1). In a series of 126 bacteriologically proven cases of septic arthritis, Fink and Nelson (116) found leukocyte counts of 50,000 per mL or less in 55%, with 34% having counts <25,000 per mL. At the same time, inflammatory diseases (e.g., rheumatoid arthritis) may have counts in excess of 80,000 per mL (69). Joint fluid WBC differential provides very helpful additional information because a percentage of polymorphonuclear cells >75% is highly suggestive of joint sepsis (118).

Atypical organisms are less likely to cause joint fluid aspirate cell count to approach 50,000 per mL. Nine patients with brucellar arthritis treated at Ben-Gurion University had a median synovial fluid cell count of 9500 WBC per mm^3 (range: 300 to 61,500 WBC per mm^3), and only one patient

TABLE 12-1	Synovial Fluid Analysis	
Disease	**Leukocyte[a] Cells/mL**	**Polymorphs[a] (%)**
Normal	<200	<25
Traumatic effusion	<5000 with many erythrocytes	<25
Toxic synovitis	5000–15,000	<25
Acute rheumatic fever	10,000–15,000	50
JRA	15,000–80,000	75
Septic arthritis	>50,000	>75

[a]The leukocyte count and the percentage of polymorphs can vary in most diseases, depending on the severity and duration of the process. Overlap greater than shown in these averages is possible.
From Morrissy RT, Shore S. Septic arthritis in children. In: Gustilo RB, Gruninger RP, Tsukayama DT, eds. *Orthopaedic infection: diagnosis and treatment*. Philadelphia, PA: WB Saunders, 1989:261–270, with permission.

had a cell count of >50,000 per mL. *Brucella melitensis* was recovered from the synovial fluid culture in all patients (119).

As in osteomyelitis, the frequency of positive cultures seems to be slightly higher with open biopsy than with needle biopsy, but the difference is not great. In addition, the positive yields are generally not as high as in osteomyelitis, ranging in various reports from 30% to 80% (63, 68, 120). The importance of obtaining material from blood and bone or joint aspiration is emphasized in a report by Vaughan et al. (121), in which many children with osteomyelitis had only positive blood cultures, whereas other patients had only positive bone cultures.

Gram staining is the only opportunity for presumptive identification of the organism within a few hours of initial patient contact and is therefore a valuable test that should not be ignored. It appears from reports of both septic arthritis and osteomyelitis that the Gram stain demonstrates an organism in about one-third of the bone or joint aspirates (63, 64, 116).

Most bacterial cultures will yield results within 48 hours of specimen collection. However, fastidious organisms may take as long as 7 days to become positive. *S. aureus* remains the most common causative organism, causing musculoskeletal infection in 60% to 90% of patients (67, 122). Streptococci, pneumococci, *K. kingae*, and gram-negative bacteria are also potential causative organisms.

Several authors have questioned a distinction between culture-positive and culture-negative septic arthritis. Lyon and Evanich reviewed 76 children treated at Medical College of Wisconsin and Children's Hospital of Wisconsin for isolated joint infection between 1990 and 1997 (123). All patients underwent joint aspiration with fluid analysis, including culture, and a causative organism was identified in only 30% of cases. There were no significant clinical or laboratory differences between the culture-positive and culture-negative groups, and all patients were treated similarly with joint drainage and antibiotic therapy. All patients had complete resolution of infection following treatment. Lyon and Evanich concluded that, with regard to clinical presentation and response to treatment, culture-negative septic arthritis did not differ significantly from culture-positive septic arthritis and therefore warranted a similar diagnostic and treatment approach.

Investigators from LSU Health Sciences Center did note several differences in the clinical presentation of culture-positive septic arthritis compared to culture-negative arthritis (1). Patients whose cultures were positive were more likely to have antecedent trauma, overlying skin changes, and a shorter duration of symptoms prior to diagnosis. However, treatment and treatment results did not differ significantly between groups. In summary, culture-negative septic arthritis can be treated empirically as presumed staphylococcal disease, perhaps with slightly broadened antibiotic coverage, with excellent long-term results.

DIFFERENTIAL DIAGNOSIS

Osteomyelitis. Trauma and neoplasm are conditions that may present with characteristics similar to osteomyelitis, and they may be mistaken for infection. Trauma is the most common and made more confusing because trauma can predispose patients to develop osteomyelitis. Similar features are typically present, including pain, tenderness, swelling, and soft-tissue swelling on radiographs. However, several distinguishing features may be present. Traumatic symptoms are usually sudden in onset with gradual improvement, compared to symptoms of infection, which are more likely to be gradual in onset and progressive in nature. Trauma may be associated with elevation of the CRP but not the ESR, whereas both are usually elevated in osteomyelitis.

More difficult is distinguishing osteomyelitis from neoplasia (84, 85). The most common malignancy in children is leukemia, and approximately 30% of these children present with bone pain (124). Approximately 40% of children with leukemia present with constitutional symptoms such as lethargy, 18% present with fever, and 60% have an elevated leukocyte count and elevated ESR (125). Although lucent metaphyseal bands are said to be characteristic of leukemia, other bone changes are also seen. One study found lytic lesions in 19%, sclerotic lesions in 4%, and periosteal new bone in 2% (125). A purely lytic lesion without uptake on bone scan is also characteristic of leukemia as well as eosinophilic granuloma (126). Bleeding, bone pain in multiple sites, and easy bruising should raise suspicion of leukemia. A low leukocyte count may be present in 35% of patients with leukemia, although this can also be a sign of serious systemic sepsis. Anemia and an abnormally low platelet count should also raise suspicion. Abnormal WBC forms seen on manual differential is often diagnostic.

Other less common neoplasms may mimic osteomyelitis (83–85). In the young child, metastatic neuroblastoma or eosinophilic granuloma should be considered. Older children are more likely to have Ewing or osteogenic sarcoma. Lymphoma may also occasionally arise primarily from bone (Fig. 12-6). These lesions should be approached as a malignancy with complete staging studies and diagnosis confirmed by biopsy using an approach that will not jeopardize limb salvage surgery. The adage "culture the tumor and biopsy the infection" is wise advice to follow.

Septic Arthritis. Establishing the diagnosis of septic arthritis may be more challenging than for osteomyelitis for several reasons. There is greater urgency because septic arthritis can cause permanent articular cartilage changes within 8 hours if untreated (58), and for septic arthritis there are more diagnostic alternatives than for osteomyelitis. Interestingly, specific joints appear to be especially susceptible to permanent injury following septic arthritis. For example, the hip is more likely than the knee to progress to joint destruction following septic arthritis. The physician should always consider what must be diagnosed today, what can be diagnosed tomorrow, and what can be diagnosed next week. For example, septic arthritis, particularly of the hip, should be diagnosed as soon as possible, whereas there is little harm to the patient if juvenile rheumatoid arthritis (JRA) is diagnosed next week.

One of the most difficult and yet important differentials is between septic arthritis of the hip and toxic synovitis, a condition thought to be a postinfectious arthritis. Both may present with a history of a few to several days of hip pain and with limp progressing to the inability to walk. The physical signs are similar in both, with limited and painful internal rotation, abduction, and extension. A longer history of symptoms, with cyclic improvement and worsening, suggests toxic synovitis. The pain is usually worse and the motion more restricted in septic arthritis.

Kocher et al. (127) reviewed the cases of all children treated at Boston Children's Hospital from 1979 to 1996 for an acutely irritable hip and developed a clinical prediction algorithm to differentiate between septic arthritis and toxic synovitis. Although several variables differed significantly between septic arthritis and toxic synovitis, there was considerable overlap, making diagnosis based on individual variables alone difficult. However, four independent multivariate clinical predictors—history of fever, non–weight bearing, ESR of at least 40, and serum WBC count of more than 12,000 per mL—were identified that, when combined, improved diagnostic accuracy. The predicted probability of septic arthritis was 3.0% if one predictor was present, 40% for two predictors, 93.1% for three predictors, and 99.6% if all four predictors were present. Although the presence of three or more predictors was very specific for septic arthritis, it was not highly sensitive.

Two follow-up studies have subsequently been published attempting to validate the clinical algorithm proposed by Kocher et al. At the same institution where the clinical algorithm was initially formulated, Kocher et al. (128) prospectively applied the algorithm to children presenting with acute hip irritably. The predicted probability of septic arthritis in the follow-up study was 9.5% if one predictor was present, 35.0% for two predictors, 72.8% for three predictors, and 93.0% if all four predictors were present. The authors concluded that the four clinical predictors of septic arthritis demonstrated diminished, but nevertheless good, diagnostic performance in a new patient population. At a different institution, Luhmann et al. (129) applied Kocher's clinical algorithm retrospectively to 163 patients who presented with an acutely irritable hip and found that if all four of the clinical variables in the algorithm were present, the predicted probability of their patients having septic arthritis was 59%, in contrast to the 99.6% predicted probability reported in Kocher's original article. Most recently, a group from Children's Hospital of Philadelphia analyzed factors associated with septic arthritis in 53 patients undergoing hip aspiration for presumed septic arthritis, reporting that the presence of five factors (oral temperature >38.5°C, elevated CRP, elevated sedimentation rate, elevated WBC, and refusal to bear weight) was associated with a 98% chance of having septic arthritis, while those with four factors had a 93% chance (130). Although the proposed algorithms may be helpful, differentiating between septic arthritis and toxic synovitis of the hip in an acutely ill child will continue to depend on the clinical acumen of the orthopaedist.

JRA is frequently considered in the differential diagnosis with septic arthritis, but several clinical features may be used to distinguish between the two disorders. The hip joint is rarely the initial joint affected in JRA. Symptoms in JRA are typically more gradual in onset than septic arthritis, and the patient almost always remains ambulatory. A joint affected by JRA typically looks worse than it functions, with relatively good motion and modest pain despite the large amount of swelling and synovitis that is typically present. Initial laboratory values are often of little help in distinguishing between septic arthritis and JRA. Joint fluid cell count typically contains fewer than 100,000 leukocytes per mL in JRA, but leukocyte counts of >100,000 per mL have been reported (131). In such cases, the treating physician has little choice but to begin treatment of septic arthritis while continuing to work to determine the diagnosis.

Rheumatic fever has a distinctly different clinical appearance than JRA, typically causing exquisite joint pain that seems out of proportion to the normal-appearing joint. A sequela of group A streptococcal infection, rheumatic fever most often causes pain in the knees, ankles, elbow, and wrists that is evanescent and migratory. Detailed questioning of the patient may unearth a history of untreated pharyngitis, febrile illness, or rash caused by group A *Streptococcus* approximately 2 weeks before onset of symptoms. Involvement of multiple joints strongly directs the investigator away from septic arthritis. Diagnosis of rheumatic fever is based on the Jones criteria. Major criteria include carditis, arthritis, chorea, subcutaneous nodules, and erythema marginatum. The minor criteria are arthralgia, elevated ESR or CRP, heart block on electrocardiogram, and a history of previous rheumatic fever. The diagnosis is made when a patient has two major criteria, or one major and two minor criteria.

For patients who have a documented history of recent group A *Streptococcus* exposure, do not meet the Jones criteria, but have significant arthralgia without other identifiable cause, the diagnosis of PSRA has been used (132, 133). A recent streptococcal infection may be documented by the presence of an antibody response to group A *Streptococcus* or positive throat culture. Patients with acute rheumatic fever are treated with long-term prophylactic antibiotics to prevent recurrent rheumatic fever and associated carditis. The risk of carditis to children with PSRA is unclear but felt to be low, and the role of long-term prophylactic antibiotics following PSRA is controversial but not typically recommended.

Cat-scratch disease is a clinical syndrome associated with *Bartonella henselae* that has been reported to be associated with arthropathy in approximately 3% of cases (134). Knee, wrist, ankle, and elbow joints are most frequently affected. The arthropathy is typically self-limited, resolving on its own at a median of 6 weeks. However, a small percentage can develop a severely painful arthropathy that can persist as long as 50 months.

Other disorders that may cause acute arthritis and can mimic septic arthritis include Henoch-Schönlein purpura and enteroarthritis secondary to *Salmonella* or *Yersinia* infection. Kawasaki disease and serum sickness are two additional conditions also characterized by a rash and arthritis. Although the joint symptoms do not require treatment and usually disappear within days, patients with any of these conditions may require medical management for the other, sometimes more serious, manifestations of the disease.

TREATMENT RECOMMENDATIONS

Treatment options available for the eradication of musculoskeletal infection consist of antibiotics and surgery. The goal of treatment should be to select the safest, least morbid, and most cost-effective treatment that provides the highest likelihood for complete and permanent elimination of infection without sequelae. The treatment best able to accomplish this goal depends on multiple factors, including whether the infection is septic arthritis or osteomyelitis, its location, the extent of involvement, the duration of symptoms, and the specific causative organism.

Osteomyelitis

Nonsurgical. A distinction must be made between acute and chronic osteomyelitis. Acute osteomyelitis without abscess formation can typically be managed successfully with antibiotics alone (135), whereas chronic osteomyelitis is typically most appropriately treated with surgical debridement. Although there is not any absolute or uniformly accepted definition, it is reasonable to consider osteomyelitis chronic if the patient has been experiencing symptoms more than 3 weeks or there is radiographic evidence of long-standing infection.

In the absence of a known source of infection, focal point tenderness over bone in a febrile child should be considered AHO until proven otherwise. Blood cultures and appropriate lab tests should be obtained and bone aspiration performed urgently. If subperiosteal or bone abscess is encountered during bone aspiration, then surgical debridement is typically indicated. As soon as cultures are obtained, empiric high-dose intravenous antibiotic treatment should be initiated with the antibiotic choice based on patient age and clinical circumstances (Table 12-2). The most common organism causing AHO in patients of all ages is *S. aureus*, which must be adequately covered. For neonatal osteomyelitis, treatment targeting group B streptococci and gram-negative rods should be added. Children younger than 4 years should be covered for *H. influenza* type b if not immunized. Fully immunized children are most likely infected by *Staphylococcus aureus*, *Streptococcus pyogenes*, and *Streptococcus pneumoniae* (16). Ibia compared osteomyelitis caused by *Staphylococcus aureus*, *Streptococcus pyogenes*, and *Streptococcus pneumoniae*, reporting several helpful differences between bacteria (136). Median age at the time

of infection was 13.7 months for *Streptococcus pneumoniae*, 36.0 months for *Streptococcus pyogenes*, and 96 months for *Staphylococcus aureus*. At presentation, both *Streptococcus* species had a significantly elevated mean temperature of 38.9°C and elevated WBC count of 17,000 compared to a mean temperature of 38.1°C and WBC count of 10,600 for *S. aureus*. If bone aspirate or blood cultures are positive for a specific bacteria, the antibiotic choice is adjusted accordingly. Table 12-3 lists antibiotics and dosages commonly used in the treatment of pediatric osteomyelitis.

There has been a recent series of papers describing osteomyelitis associated with cat-scratch disease (137–140). It is unclear if this represents a true change in the epidemiology of osteomyelitis or simply a greater awareness of osteomyelitis caused by *Bartonella hensea*. Typically a self-limiting condition characterized by chronic lymphadenopathy in children or adolescents having a history of cat contact, in separate reports the authors above describe a series of children ages 6 to 12 years experiencing osteomyelitis associated with cat-scratch disease. MRI was the study most helpful when imaging a localized lesion, while bone scan was very useful when disseminated disease was suspected. The diagnosis was usually confirmed by serologic and PCR testing. Osteomyelitis had a predilection for the shoulder girdle region and axial skeleton including the spine and pelvis. In virtually all cases, the *B. hensea* osteomyelitis was eradicated with antibiotic treatment alone. A variety of antibiotics were used with apparent success including rifampin, clindamycin, azithromycin, and trimethoprim-sulfamethoxazole.

For *S. aureus* osteomyelitis, if a patient is not allergic to penicillin, a β-lactamase–resistant semisynthetic penicillin may be chosen. Methicillin may cause interstitial nephritis, and nafcillin may cause skin sloughing if subcutaneous infiltration occurs, so oxacillin is a good initial choice. Cefazolin is also an excellent option and has the advantage of being administered three times per day instead of the four times daily required by oxacillin. At the time of conversion to an appropriate oral antibiotic, an acceptable choice would be cephalexin at a dose of 100 to 150 mg/kg/d or dicloxacillin at 100 mg/kg/d divided q.i.d. For patients allergic to penicillin, clindamycin is an appropriate oral antibiotic choice, and vancomycin is an

TABLE 12-2	Empiric Antibiotic Treatment Recommendations for Musculoskeletal Infection	
Age group	**Probably organism**	**Initial antibiotic**
Penicillin allergy or area endemic with MRSA	MRSA, MSSA	Vancomycin or Clindamycin
Neonate	Group B Streptococcus, gram-negative bacilli, *S. aureus*	Oxacillin and Cefotaxmine or Oxacillin and Gentamycin or Ceftriaxone
Infants and children 3 mo to 4 yr	*Staphylococcus aureus, K. kingae, Streptococcus pneumoniae*, group A *Streptococcus, H. influenza* (if not vaccinated)	Oxacillin, Nafcillin, Cefazolin, or Clindamycin
Children older than 4 yr	*S. aureus*	Nafcillin, Cefazolin, Clindamycin, or Vancomycin

TABLE 12-3 Antibiotics Commonly Used in the Treatment of Bone and Joint Sepsis

	Route	Dosage[b,c]	Comments
Amoxicillin	Oral	80–100 mg/kg/d q8h	
Ampicillin	IV, IM	100–400 mg/kg/d q6h	
Dicloxacillin	Oral	100 mg/kg/d q6h	
Nafcillin	IV, IM	150 mg/kg/d q6h	
Penicillin G[a]	IV	150,000–250,000 U/kg/d q4–6h	
Penicillin V[a]	Oral	100 mg/kg/d q6h	
Oxacillin	IV, IM	150–200 mg/kg/d q6h	
Cefazolin (Ancef, Kefzol)	IV, IM	100 mg/kg/d q8h	Max dose 6 g/d
Cephalexin (Keflex)	Oral	100–150 mg/kg/d q8h	
Cefotaxime (Claforan)	IV, IM	150 mg/kg/d q6–8h	
Ceftazidime (Fortaz)	IV, IM	100–200 mg/kg/d q8h	Max dose 8 g/d
Ceftriaxone (Rocephin)	IV, IM	50–75 mg/kg/d q12–24h	Max dose 2 g/d
Cefuroxime (Zinacef)	IV, IM	100–150 mg/kg/d q8h	
Cefuroxime axetil (Ceftin)	Oral	60 mg/kg/d q12h	
Ciprofloxacin[d] (Cipro)	IV	30 mg/kg/d q12h	Max 800 mg/d
	Oral	30 mg/kg/d q12h	Max 1500 mg/d Not approved for patients less than age 18 yr
Azithromycin	IV, PO	5–10 mg/kg/d q12h	
Linezolid	IV, PO	20–30-mg/kg/d q12h	
Rifampin	IV, PO	10–20 mg/kg/d	
Clindamycin	IV, oral	25–40 mg/kg/d q6–8h	
Gentamicin	IV, IM	7.5 mg/kg/d q8h	Monitor peak and trough, start at third dose
Vancomycin	IV	40 mg/kg/d q6h	Administer over 1 h, monitor peak and trough, start at fourth dose
Metronidazole	IV	30 mg/kg/d q6h	
	Oral	15–35 mg/kg/d q8h	
Trimethoprim/sulfamethoxazole (Bactrim)	IV, oral	10 mg/kg/d (of trimethoprim component) b.i.d.	

[a]CBC should be monitored weekly for neutropenia or anemia in any patient on high-dose IV penicillin or cephalosporin therapy. It should be monitored monthly on high-dose oral therapy.
[b]Doses recommended are for normal children with normal renal function for the treatment of bone and joint infections. Recommended doses for the treatment of other conditions may be lower or higher.
[c]For doses in the neonatal period see Nelson JD. *Pocket book of pediatric antimicrobial therapy*, 17th ed. Baltimore, MD: Lippincott Williams & Wilkins, 2009.
[d]Not approved for children; used only when antibiotic susceptibility, resistance, or allergy necessitates.

appropriate intravenous antibiotic. Similar to the antibiotic treatment of septic arthritis, the administration route and the duration of treatment of AHO are controversial and depend upon the clinical situation of each patient. At one time, nearly all children with AHO were routinely treated with 6 weeks of intravenous antibiotics as a hospital inpatient. Over the last two decades, several trends have developed: (a) treatment has moved from inpatient to an outpatient setting and (b) treatment has shifted from entirely parenteral to a parenteral then oral antibiotic regimen. Intravenous therapy is initiated in the hospital setting, but once therapeutic response to treatment is confirmed, conversion to oral antibiotic treatment is made and continued on an outpatient basis.

The optimal duration of antibiotic treatment of AHO is not known and varies with clinical circumstances. Previous authors have reported that total treatment duration of <3 weeks is associated with an increased likelihood of recurrence

(35), and antibiotic treatment of at least 3 weeks has now become accepted (13, 29, 64, 70). The route and duration of antibiotic treatment are individualized for each patient, considering factors such as the age and overall health of the patient, duration of infection, whether a bacterial organism has been isolated, the susceptibility of the organism, the amount of tissue destruction present, previous surgery, adequacy of debridement, and the site of involvement. If a susceptible organism is cultured and the patient experiences a good clinical response to treatment, then conversion to an appropriate high-dose oral antibiotic as early as 3 to 5 days after initiating treatment is appropriate. If there is no clinical response to medical management within approximately 48 hours, the presence of an abscess becomes a possibility. Reevaluation of the patient with consideration of additional imaging studies such as CT or MRI and contemplation of surgical treatment is appropriate.

Favorable clinical response to antibiotic treatment is the most important factor to consider when making the decision to convert to oral antibiotics; it may be defined as the absence of fever with improvement in symptoms such as tenderness, limp, malaise, anorexia, and night pain, and reduction in CRP. Ultimately, it is the antibiotic serum concentration rather than the route administration that correlates with treatment success (141). To achieve adequate serum antibiotic levels with oral therapy, several prerequisites have been suggested including the patient's ability to swallow and absorb oral antibiotics, the ability to follow serum bactericidal levels, and the resistance or susceptibility of the organism to available oral antibiotics. (67, 141). Peak antibiotic serum levels are obtained by drawing a blood sample 1 hour after oral administration of the drug. A bactericidal level of 1:8 has been recommended (122). Recent literature suggests that if high recommended dosages are followed, monitoring bactericidal levels is not necessary to achieve excellent treatment results (29). More chronic infections caused by virulent or resistant organisms in patients experiencing a slow clinical response warrant a longer duration of intravenous antibiotics.

In addition to clinical response to treatment, previous authors have suggested that treatment continue until ESR normalization (141). Because ESR may require 4 to 8 weeks before normalization, antibiotic therapy may be unnecessarily prolonged if ESR normalization is a prerequisite for discontinuation of antibiotic therapy. Peltola and the Finnish Study Group discontinued antibiotic therapy before ESR normalized with no increase in infection recurrence rate (29).

Song and Sloboda recommend a protocol in which empiric treatment is begun using intravenous cefazolin at a dose of 100 to 150 mg/kg/d divided every 8 hours, after obtaining local bone and blood cultures (16). Serial values for CRP are monitored daily (or every other day) and in uncomplicated AHO should normalize within 5 to 7 days following initiation of parenteral treatment. Good clinical response, as demonstrated by absence of fever, lack of tenderness, improvement in swelling, resolution of limp, return of appetite, and absence of night or rest pain, should coincide with normalization of CRP. Once CRP normalizes and clinical improvement is seen, oral cephalexin therapy is begun at a dosage of 150 mg/kg/d divided every 6 hours. For uncomplicated AHO that responds rapidly to the regimen described in preceding text, a total duration of 3 weeks of antibiotic therapy is appropriate. Additional authors have similarly demonstrated a high level of efficacy with low rates of failure or complication after early conversion to oral antibiotics (142, 143).

Whether the patient is on parenteral or oral outpatient therapy, we recommend weekly laboratory testing, including CBC, ESR, CRP, aspartate aminotransferase (AST), and alanine aminotransferase (ALT), to monitor for continued response to treatment and antibiotic-related side effects such as neutropenia or alteration in liver function tests.

Surgical. The primary indication for surgical treatment of AHO is the presence of an abscess within bone (10, 16, 135). Surgery for osteomyelitis should remove the purulent material as well as necrotic or avascular bone and all possible grossly infected and nonviable soft tissue. When the bacterial mass and the necrotic tissue are dramatically reduced, host defense mechanisms work more effectively and antibiotic delivery to the region is facilitated. When possible, surgical debridement is performed before antibiotics are administered, and bone cultures taken at the time of surgery provide another opportunity to identify the causative organism.

Specimens should also be sent for routine histology. The importance of routine histologic examination of material from the bone is twofold. Some tumors have a tendency to become necrotic and, when surgically explored, may look similar to pus; the most common is metastatic neuroblastoma, followed by Ewing sarcoma. In addition, if positive identification of the organism is not obtained, it is reassuring to have a histologic diagnosis of osteomyelitis.

Failure to respond to appropriate high-dose, parenteral antibiotic therapy is a second and important indication for surgical treatment of acute osteomyelitis. Before proceeding immediately to surgical exploration and debridement, the treating physician should evaluate more carefully why antibiotic treatment alone was not sufficient. The most likely causative organism should be reexamined, antibiotic choice and dose reviewed, possible alternative source of infection considered, and evaluation for bone or soft-tissue abscess performed. If no explanation other than insufficiently treated local musculoskeletal infection can be found, local imaging with CT or MRI is often helpful to identify possible abscess and to plan surgical debridement. Because it provides the greatest soft-tissue detail and marrow edema imaging, MRI is becoming the study of choice if readily available.

Surgical debridement of AHO can usually be closed primarily over drains. Intravenous antibiotic treatment is initiated immediately after cultures are obtained, and conversion to oral antibiotics is made after clinical response to treatment has been documented.

In contrast to AHO, osteomyelitis is defined as being chronic if the patient has been experiencing symptoms for more than 3 weeks or there is radiographic evidence of long-standing infection. Aggressive osseous debridement is the most important aspect of chronic osteomyelitis surgical treatment (10). Whether to perform a single debridement or multiple debridements is a decision made based on clinical circumstances and surgeon judgment at the time of the operation. A small area of infection that is aggressively debrided can be closed primarily over drains. Whenever in doubt, the safe course is to return for a second look with repeat debridement 2 to 3 days later. A common mistake and natural tendency is to perform inadequate debridement. The status of the periosteum overlying infected bone is significant (144). The presence of an involucrum confirms periosteum viability and its ability to form new bone. Involucra form when infection elevates the periosteum off of underlying infected bone, and the periosteum begins to form bone in its new position. Infected, with its periosteal blood supply no longer intact, the underlying cortical bone quickly becomes a necrotic sequestrum. A valuable general treatment principle is to aggressively debride the necrotic sequestrum but to leave in place the viable involucrum.

The ability to form bone in young children is truly remarkable, such that large defects created by debridement will reossify without bone grafting. Unfortunately, older patients are less able to reossify extensive bone defects created by chronic osteomyelitis and debridement. Depending on the size and location of the lesion, children younger than 10 years will occasionally benefit from bone grafting, children between ages 10 and 15 will often require bone grafting, and patients 16 years and older will almost always benefit from bone grafting, especially in weight-bearing bones. The timing and source of bone graft are a matter for discussion. Bone grafting at the time of initial debridement risks persistent infection by placing nonviable tissue into an area where high bacteria counts are known to exist. Primary bone grafting may be acceptable in situations where radical debridement of infection caused by a susceptible organism is performed. In most situations, bone grafting is best performed at a second operation. In favorable clinical situations, bone grafting may be done 2 to 3 days following the initial debridement.

The issue of whether to use autologous bone graft, allogenic bone graft, or another material to stimulate bone formation in large osseous defects continues to evolve and is beyond the scope of this chapter. Factors that should be considered when choosing a material include safety, effectiveness, availability, and cost. Unfortunately, there currently is no manufactured substance that clearly surpasses autologous or allograft bone material, and therefore bone grafting remains the most appropriate means of filling large osseous defects following osteomyelitis debridement. Powdered antibiotic such as tobramycin, gentamicin, or vancomycin may be mixed with bone at the time of grafting.

In less favorable situations, bone grafting may be delayed a full month while clinical and laboratory parameters confirm successful treatment by continued parenteral antibiotics. If delayed bone grafting is anticipated, placement of antibiotic-impregnated polymethylmethacrylate (PMMA) at the conclusion of the initial series of debridements may be considered. The antibiotic-impregnated PMMA is removed at the time of bone grafting.

Indications for the use of antibiotic-impregnated PMMA have not been clearly established, but the use of antibiotic-impregnated PMMA is increasing. Antibiotic-impregnated PMMA should not be used for uncomplicated metaphyseal osteomyelitis. Adequate surgical debridement and appropriate parenteral and/or oral antibiotic therapy has such a high success rate that antibiotic-impregnated PMMA adds no significant benefit. Relative indications for antibiotic-impregnated PMMA include

1. Recurrent/persistent infection despite a course of reasonable and appropriate treatment
2. Extensive chronic infection that cannot be completely débrided surgically
3. Extensive osseous defects and dead space to be treated by delayed bone grafting (Fig. 12-7)

Antibiotic-impregnated PMMA does allow delivery of very high concentrations of antibiotic locally while maintaining low systemic levels. An acceptable antibiotic cement mixture consists of 4.8 g of gentamicin (1.2 g per vial) or 4.8 g of tobramycin (1.2 g per vial), 4.0 g of vancomycin (1.0 g per vial), and one full batch of PMMA. Methylene blue may be added to facilitate mixing the large volume of powdered antibiotic and PMMA as well as to aid in visualization of PMMA at the time of removal. In situations where antibiotic-impregnated PMMA is used, patients typically receive 6 to 8 weeks of parenteral antibiotics. A reasonable protocol is to place antibiotic-impregnated PMMA into the infection bed at the time of initial closure. Four weeks after closure, the PMMA is removed, and bone grafting is performed if necessary. This protocol allows for 2 to 4 weeks of parenteral antibiotics to continue after antibiotic PMMA removal.

Distraction osteogenesis has also been used successfully to treat large osseous defects. Kucukkaya et al. (145) used the Ilizarov method in seven children, aged 6 to 8, with tibial defects averaging 7.4 cm in length following osteomyelitis debridement. All patients had complete healing without bone grafting.

Unfortunately infection, including chronic osteomyelitis, remains one of the most common musculoskeletal disorders in the underdeveloped world. The principle of debridement of severe, chronic osteomyelitis remains true, but in resource-poor circumstances, where drains and appropriate antibiotic may not be available, wound closure by dressing changes and secondary intention has been shown to be more effective than primary closure at successfully eradicating chronic osteomyelitis (146).

Septic Arthritis

Nonsurgical. Empiric antibiotic therapy should begin immediately following blood culture and culture of bone or joint. Understanding the relative incidence of causative organisms in particular clinical situations is very important because it allows for selection of an effective antibiotic before an organism is positively identified by culture (Table 12-2). Neonates are at risk for septic arthritis caused by group B *Streptococcus*, gonococci, *S. aureus*, and coliform bacteria; thus, initial therapy should consist of ceftriaxone or cefotaxime and oxacillin. For unimmunized infants younger than 2 years, *H. influenzae*, group A *Streptococcus*, *K. kingae*, and *S. aureus* are likely pathogens, and initial therapy should consist of cefuroxime, ceftriaxone or cefotaxime, and oxacillin. Septic arthritis in immunized infants and older children is most likely caused by *Staphylococcus*, pneumococcus, or group A *Streptococcus* species and can be treated initially with oxacillin or cefazolin. Table 12-3 lists antibiotics and dosages commonly used in the treatment of pediatric bone and joint sepsis.

Initial therapy should be intravenous, resulting in immediate and elevated serum antibiotic levels. The timing for transition to oral medication remains controversial. Ampicillin, cephalexin, cloxacillin, dicloxacillin, and penicillin G all penetrate into pus and synovial fluid in children with septic arthritis in concentrations several times greater than the mean inhibitory and mean bactericidal concentrations for *S. aureus* (147). However, because toxic products of septic arthritis may cause irreversible damage to articular cartilage within 8 hours of infection onset, septic arthritis should be treated with joint irrigation and debridement in addition to antibiotic treatment.

Long-term parenteral antibiotic has been the gold standard for treatment of musculoskeletal infection. Although parenteral administration of antibiotics ensures an immediate and high serum concentration, this is achieved with some risk, inconvenience, and expense. Outpatient parenteral antibiotic therapy (OPAT) has reduced hospital stays and expense, but not without potential problems (148). In a study of 184 patients with musculoskeletal infection treated using OPAT, investigators at the University of Florida Health Science Center identified several difficulties associated with OPAT (149). Only 64% of patients completed their OPAT course without interruption, and rehospitalization occurred in 26% of patients. Early discontinuation of parenteral antibiotics because of adverse drug reactions occurred in 24% of patients. There were 128 complications, approximately half of which were related to catheter malfunction, and catheter malfunction was more common in peripheral intravenous central catheters (PICCs) than in central catheters.

As an alternative to parenteral antibiotics, clinicians have examined the efficacy of oral antibiotic therapy. In the 1970s, Nelson and others demonstrated that adequate bactericidal activity in bone and joint tissue of children could be obtained using oral antibiotics (141, 147). The ability to confirm adequate serum antibiotic concentrations has led many physicians to use high-dose oral therapy following initial intravenous antibiotic therapy as standard practice, with excellent results.

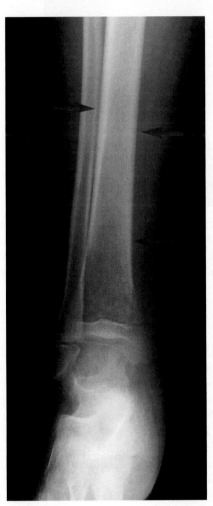

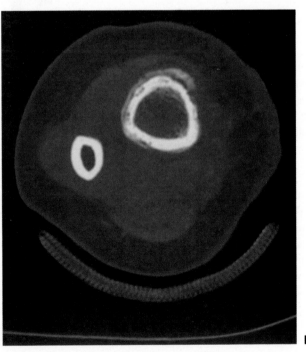

FIGURE 12-7. **A:** An 8-year-old girl is placed in a cast after an ankle sprain. Multiple trips to the local emergency department for increasing pain were treated with narcotic pain medication. Three weeks following the injury, the cast was removed to reveal a swollen, erythematous leg. The anteroposterior radiograph demonstrates an infiltrative, destructive process in the distal tibial metaphysis suggestive of osteomyelitis. Periosteal reaction can be seen over the distal half of the tibia (*arrows*). **B:** A CT image at the metaphyseal–diaphyseal junction shows the infection eroding through the cortex and elevating the periosteum. The elevated periosteum forms an involucrum as the distal tibia becomes a sequestrum.

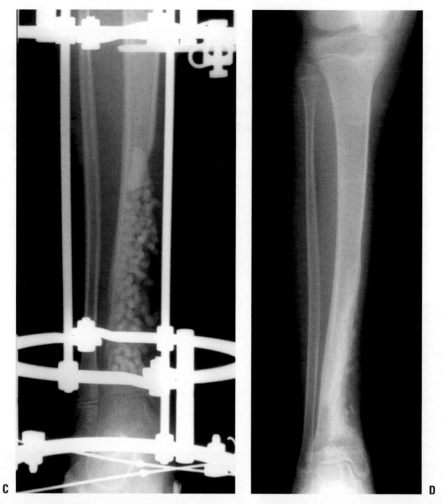

FIGURE 12-7. (*continued*) **C:** Thorough debridement of osteomyelitis created a very large segmental defect that was filled with antibiotic-impregnated PMMA beads to deliver local antibiotics, fill dead space, and prepare for future bone grafting. A circular fixator was placed to maintain stability, length, and alignment. **D:** One year after initial debridement, the patient is free from evidence of infection, and bone graft continues to consolidate, but varus deformity of the distal tibia caused by partial physeal arrest is present.

Investigators at San Diego Children's Hospital and Case Western Reserve in Cleveland reviewed records of 186 children treated for septic arthritis with parenteral followed by oral antibiotics (28). Initial parenteral therapy consisted of cefazolin administered at 75 to 100 mg/kg/d divided every 8 hours. Children who demonstrated clear improvement on parenteral therapy—decreased swelling, tenderness, and erythema and decreasing or absent fever—and who had families judged to be compliant with oral therapy were placed on an oral antibiotic. Children with sterile cultures or whose cultures were positive for staphylococci were administered cephalexin or cloxacillin at a dose of 100 to 150 mg/kg/d or dicloxacillin at 75 to 100 mg kg/d divided q.i.d. For streptococcal or pneumococcal infections, penicillin V or amoxicillin at 75 to 100 mg/kg/d was used. Bactericidal titers were drawn 60 to 90 minutes following the second or third oral dose of antibiotic. If the titer

was <1:8, the oral dose of the β-lactum antibiotic was increased to a maximum of 150 mg/kg/d, and repeat bactericidal testing was performed to ensure that a titer of at least 1:4 to 1:8 was achieved. Using this protocol, no child required readmission for parenteral therapy due to inadequate serum bactericidal activity. Average total duration of therapy was 30 days, with normalization of ESR at a mean of 33 days. Infection was eradicated without sequelae in all except one patient for a recurrence rate of 0.5%. Additional authors report similar results with conversion to oral antibiotic after clinical response to a short duration of parenteral antibiotics in the treatment of acute septic arthritis or acute osteomyelitis (150–152).

Peltola et al. (29) questioned the need for peak bactericidal titers in the treatment of musculoskeletal infection. In a prospective study of acute *S. aureus* osteomyelitis performed at eight tertiary pediatric hospitals in Finland, peak bactericidal titers were not measured, instead utilizing empiric high-dose clindamycin or cephalosporin and monitoring clinical response to treatment, leukocyte count, ESR, and CRP. All patients received initial parenteral antibiotic therapy and switched to high-dose oral therapy within 5 days. No treatment failures were detected at 1-year follow-up, suggesting that early conversion to oral antibiotic treatment without monitoring serum bactericidal levels can simplify treatment and reduce laboratory costs.

The serum level of other antibiotics (e.g., gentamicin and vancomycin) can and should be monitored in all cases. These antibiotics can be measured directly in the blood. Not only does the blood level of these intravenous antibiotics vary significantly between individuals, but their toxic side effects are significant. Both the peak and the trough levels need to be measured and monitored. For gentamicin, blood is drawn approximately 30 minutes after administration and just before the next dose. The peak level should be between 5 and 10 µg/mL, and the trough should be 1.9 µg/mL or less. For vancomycin, blood is drawn 1 hour after administration and just before the next dose. The peak level should vary between 20 and 40 µg/mL and the trough between 5 and 10 µg/mL.

Generally, blood levels of gentamicin or vancomycin should be measured every 3 to 4 days, as should the levels of blood urea nitrogen and creatinine. For prolonged (longer than 3 weeks) or recurrent therapy with these drugs, it is wise also to monitor the patient for ototoxicity. Vancomycin should be infused over no <1 hour to avoid the release of histamine by the drug (red man syndrome) or serious hypotension. If a rash occurs, it usually can be circumvented by administering the drug over 90 to 120 minutes or by the use of intravenous diphenhydramine (Benadryl) 1 mg/kg (total dose not to exceed 50 mg) just before the infusion.

Recent reports have focused on reducing variability and cost while maintaining a high treatment success rate for patients with septic arthritis. Utilizing early conversion to oral antibiotics, Kocher et al. (153) created a clinical practice guideline for treatment of septic arthritis (see Appendix). Thirty consecutive patients with septic arthritis of the hip managed before utilization of the guideline were compared with 30 consecutive patients treated according to the guideline. There were several statistically significant differences noted between groups. Patients treated according to the guideline were much more likely to have a follow-up CRP performed, had a lower rate of initial bone scanning, a lower rate of presumptive surgical hip drainage, a greater compliance with recommended antibiotic therapy, a faster change to oral antibiotics, and a shorter hospital stay. There were no significant differences with regard to outcome variables, including readmission to the hospital, recurrent infection, recurrent drainage, development of osteomyelitis or septic osteonecrosis, and limitation of motion. Patients treated according to the clinical practice guideline had less variation in the process of care and improved efficiency of care without adverse outcome.

MRSA is becoming increasingly prevalent among pediatric and adolescent patients and will be discussed in greater detail later in the chapter (154, 155). Musculoskeletal infection caused by MRSA has been associated with a significantly increased risk of sequelae (17). The choice of antibiotics for treatment of MRSA is critical and limited. Vancomycin and clindamycin have been the antibiotics of choice for MRSA. Martinez-Aguilar et al. (155) examined the effectiveness of clindamycin treatment in 46 children with MRSA infection of bone, joint, and sites outside the musculoskeletal system. No significant difference could be detected between the patients with MRSA infection and the group of patients with methicillin-sensitive *S. aureus* (MSSA) infection, with successful eradication of infection in all groups allowing the authors to conclude that clindamycin is an acceptable antibiotic choice for the treatment of MRSA. Emergence of vancomycin-resistant *S. aureus* in Japan and in parts of the United States has raised the possibility of musculoskeletal infection caused by bacteria for which there is no known effective antibiotic treatment (156). Continued development of new antibiotics such as linezolid offers hope that effective antibiotic options will continue to be available in the future (157). Linezolid is the first of a new class of antibiotic agents, the oxazolidinones, and is particularly effective against gram-positive infections. Little resistance has been reported even among methicillin- and vancomycin-resistant bacteria (158).

Antibiotic treatment does have several potential harmful side effects. Pancytopenia, leukopenia, impaired liver function, or impaired renal function may occur and should be monitored by weekly determination of levels of creatinine, ALT, AST, and CBC. ESR and CRP should also be checked weekly to monitor response to treatment. Antibiotic choice and dosage are adjusted on the basis of side effects that may arise.

Surgical. Despite our ability to deliver antibiotics to the site of infection and to achieve serum concentrations that should be sufficient to kill bacteria, antibiotic treatment alone is not sufficient. Factors that may reduce antibiotics' effectiveness include possible interference by purulent material from gram-negative organisms with the action of certain antibiotics (159, 160), as well as the production of large amounts of β-lactamase by bacteria, rendering semisynthetic penicillins and cephalosporins ineffective (161–163). These factors suggest that the local environment is important to the effective action of the antibiotic. It makes sense, then, that altering the local environment by irrigation and debridement improves antibiotic effectiveness.

Surgery is indicated for culture and biopsy, for evacuation and elimination of bone or joint abscess, and for stopping tissue destruction. Antibiotic therapy is always used in addition to surgery when musculoskeletal infection is confirmed. By eliminating dead space, nonviable tissue, and bacterial and host by-products, abscess debridement and evacuation facilitates antibiotic delivery and effectiveness. By removing harmful bacterial and host by-products, debridement prevents further cartilage and tissue damage as well (164–166).

In experimental staphylococcal septic arthritis in rabbits that were treated with antibiotics, the beneficial effect of surgical lavage has been demonstrated (61). During the first arthrotomy at 4 days, the material generated by infection in the knee could be washed out; at 7 days, it had to be removed manually. All cultures were negative at 7 days. Both the surgically treated and the nonsurgically treated animals showed loss of glycosaminoglycan. There was no collagen degradation in those treated by surgical lavage, however. A similar study has shown that arthrotomy and irrigation may be more effective than repeated aspirations (167).

The stakes are high, risking life-long arthritis in a child or an adolescent. Erring on the side of surgical joint debridement is appropriate. At the time the decision is made whether or not to treat septic arthritis, culture results are rarely available. The decision to treat (and usually to operate) is based primarily on history, examination, and several laboratory tests, as discussed in preceding text. The most helpful test is synovial fluid cell count (Table 12-1). Although rheumatoid arthritis may cause a WBC count to become elevated to more than 50,000 per mL, in most patients a synovial fluid WBC of more than 50,000 per mL is caused by septic arthritis and warrants irrigation and debridement.

ANTERIOR DRAINAGE OF THE SEPTIC HIP (FIGS.12-8 TO 12-12)

In most situations, bacterial septic arthritis is an urgent indication for surgery, and in septic arthritis of the hip, a true surgical emergency. Once the decision has been made to surgically drain and débride the hip, a second question arises as to whether the hip should be approached anteriorly or posteriorly. There are several reasons to prefer an anterior approach, although a posterior approach may also be used. The transverse anterior skin incision is cosmetically superior to a posterior incision. The anterior approach provides a distinct anatomic landmark—the anterosuperior iliac spine—which is not the case in the chubby buttocks of an infant with a septic hip. Throughout the anterior hip dissection, there are distinct anatomic intervals to facilitate the surgical approach. Perhaps most importantly, the incision for hip drainage should be placed in the anterior capsule. Septic arthritis is a recognized risk factor causing hip instability, and a posterior capsular incision may contribute further to instability. Finally, a closed suction drainage catheter should be placed within the hip joint at the time of closure, exiting laterally and percutaneously through the skin.

Postoperative Care. There are many options for care after hip drainage and debridement, depending on the surgeon's preferences and the circumstances of the case. Closed suction drainage should be maintained for 24 to 48 hours following surgery or until drainage subsides. Suction

drainage provides continuous decompression of the joint. Spica casting, split Russell traction, pediatric hip abduction pillow, or no immobilization at all may be used following surgery. The decision whether or not to immobilize the patient following surgical drainage is based on the perceived risk of hip instability. If the hip is subluxated or dislocated, it is often desirable to achieve a closed reduction at the time of wound closure and to place the patient directly into a spica cast. Many surgeons prefer to treat all children with septic arthritis of the hip with a single-leg spica cast for 2 to 3 weeks to avoid late subluxation secondary to capsular laxity. If the cast is not applied at the time of surgery, it may be applied before discharge. If the septic arthritis is acute and the hip is stable during intraoperative exam, then no immobilization is necessary.

Open surgical debridement remains the gold standard for treatment of septic arthritis. It is a procedure with which most orthopaedists are familiar and that can be performed on short notice, in a short amount of time, through a small incision with little specialized equipment, yielding a high success rate. Debridement of all nonviable, grossly infected tissue is indicated. Acute septic arthritis does not require synovectomy and often can be closed over drains after a single surgical procedure, whereas more chronic infections may benefit from serial debridement. Gordon et al. (168) in St Louis performed a retrospective analysis comparing primary closure with delayed closure in patients having septic arthritis, finding a similar failure rate in both groups. Surgical treatment failure was associated with patient age >7 years, with a polymorphonuclear leukocyte count in the synovial fluid >100,000, and with osteomyelitis adjacent to the joint. Chronic infection or recurrent septic arthritis may result in a thick rind of tissue that lines the joint cavity and must be removed. Several tissue cultures should be sent during surgery before antibiotics are administered. Sending specimens to pathology for microscopic examination may also be helpful in establishing a diagnosis, especially if all cultures turn out to be negative.

There have been several recent reports of successful arthroscopic joint debridement for septic arthritis of the knee, hip, and shoulder (144, 145, 169–171). The specific joint involved, chronicity of the infection, experience of the surgeon, and experience of the allied health staff available at the time of surgery should be considered before deciding to perform arthroscopic joint debridement. In the hands of an experienced arthroscopist, debridement of relatively inaccessible areas such as the posterior compartment of the knee can be performed, and the joint can be irrigated with a very large volume of fluid. One distinct disadvantage of arthroscopic debridement is that because the arthroscope is looking out from the inside of the joint, it may be very difficult to accurately assess the depth of the purulent material and the extent of infection, especially in chronic cases. This may lead to inadequate debridement and persistent infection.

Most recently, in a randomized prospective study of culture positive acute septic arthritis in children, Peltola et al.

Text continued on page 395

Anterior Drainage of the Septic Hip (Figs. 12-8 to 12-12)

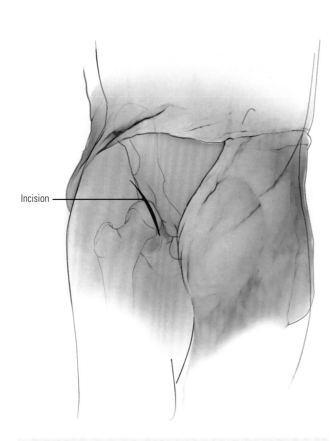

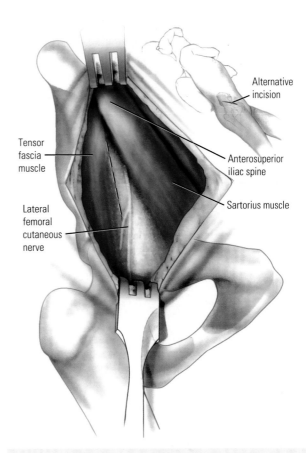

FIGURE 12-8. Anterior Drainage of the Septic Hip. The patient is positioned supine with a generous bump placed beneath the affected hemipelvis to elevate the hemipelvis and hip 30 to 45 degrees from the table. Prepping and draping the entire leg and buttocks into the surgical field allows full movement of the hip intraoperatively to thoroughly débride and irrigate the hip. The incision, placed about a finger breadth beneath the anterosuperior iliac spine, can be transverse or oblique and can be smaller than an incision used for other major hip procedures because it is not necessary to expose the outer table of the ilium.

FIGURE 12-9.   The interval between the sartorius and the tensor muscles is identified and separated up to the anterosuperior iliac spine. If necessary, the periosteum can be elevated from the outer table of the ilium in the region of the anterosuperior iliac spine; however, after some experience with this approach, this step is usually not required.

FIGURE 12-10. At the base of the exposure between the sartorius and the tensor muscles is the rectus femoris muscle. In this area, close to the anteroinferior iliac spine, its tendinous portion can be identified. A periosteal elevator can be used to separate the fatty tissue covering this tendon. The lateral border of this tendon with its muscular origin is freed and retracted medially.

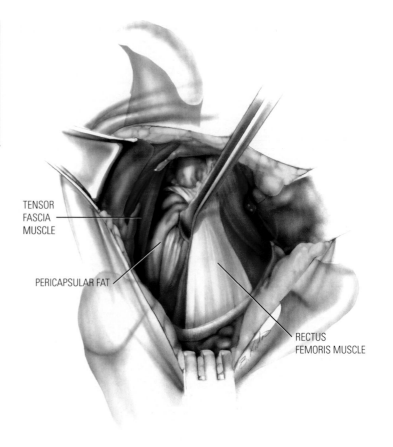

FIGURE 12-11. The hip capsule now lies in the base of the field. It is covered by the precapsular fatty tissue, which may be thick and edematous in the septic hip. This can also be separated with a periosteal elevator, scissors, or scalpel to expose the hip capsule, and the capsule is then incised. A cruciate incision has been used with good effect, but the author prefers to excise a window of capsule to allow free and unhindered drainage. Whether a cruciate incision or a capsular window is used, care must be exercised to incise the capsule over the anterior femoral neck and the base of the femoral head, avoiding vessels that supply the epiphysis as they ascend along the superior aspect of the femoral neck. To prevent instability, excessive capsular and/or labral incision must be avoided

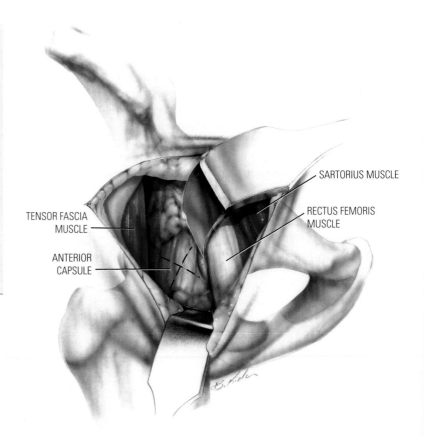

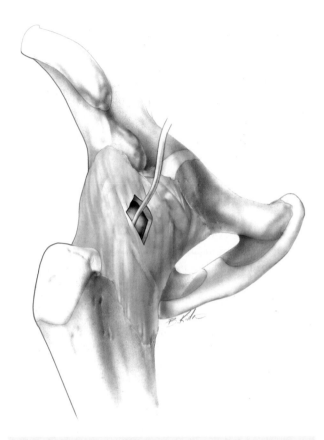

FIGURE 12-12. A small red rubber catheter, with multiple perforations cut into the tip, may be passed around the femoral neck and into the various recesses of the joint to provide thorough irrigation. Pulsatile lavage while moving the hip through full ROM is also effective. Inspection should ensure that no fibrinous clots of inflammatory material remain in the joint. Often these have to be removed with a forceps. After complete irrigation and debridement, a drainage catheter is place inside the hip joint, exiting the patient percutaneously through the hip abductors and the skin anterolaterally. The muscles are allowed to fall back together and the deep fascia and skin are closed.

(172) evaluated whether surgery is necessary in all patients. Patients were randomized to receive clindamycin or a first-generation cephalosporin for 10 or 30 days (intravenously for the first 2 to 4 days), and monitored for clinical response to treatment. All patients underwent an initial joint aspiration, but only 12% required subsequent surgical debridement after failing to improve with antibiotic treatment. All patients recovered uneventfully, and there was no difference between the 10- and the 30-day treatment group. This study is provocative and should stimulate further research to analyze when acute septic arthritis may be effectively and safely managed by aspiration and antibiotics alone.

Whether irrigation and debridement is performed with open surgery or arthroscopically, drains should be placed at the conclusion of the procedure and appropriate empiric parenteral antibiotic therapy initiated.

AUTHOR'S PREFERRED TREATMENT RECOMMENDATIONS

Acute septic arthritis: The author recommends open surgical debridement and initial parenteral antibiotics with conversion to oral antibiotics after favorable treatment response. Total treatment duration of approximately 3 weeks is appropriate, depending on clinical and laboratory response to treatment.

AHO: Bone aspiration and culture should be performed. If no abscess is present, then surgical debridement is not indicated. Parenteral antibiotics should be initiated, with conversion to oral antibiotics after favorable clinical response for total treatment duration of approximately 3 weeks, depending on clinical and laboratory response to treatment.

AHO with abscess: If the patient presents with a history of acute infection (e.g., 4 days of increasing symptoms) and aspiration demonstrates subperiosteal or bone abscess, then surgical debridement of the abscess is indicated. Closure over drains and initiation of parenteral, then oral, antibiotic treatment for AHO, as described, is appropriate.

Chronic hematogenous osteomyelitis: When symptoms have been present for more than 3 weeks, in association with bone abscess or destruction, surgical debridement is indicated. Both preoperative MRI and CT are often helpful for determining the extent of infection and planning surgical debridement. Tissue cultures are obtained at surgery, and depending on culture results, extent of infection, and response to treatment, a long-term course of parenteral antibiotics for 6 to 8 weeks is often appropriate. If the infection is recurrent or cannot be completely debrided, the use of antibiotic-impregnated PMMA is acceptable. Bone grafting or bone transport may be used to fill large bone defects and can be performed 3 to 4 weeks after initiating parenteral antibiotic treatment.

COMPLICATIONS

The predilection of osteomyelitis for metaphyseal bone places infection in close proximity to the physis. Physeal involvement by osteomyelitis may injure a region of the physis or destroy the physis completely, causing growth inhibition and angular deformity or limb-length discrepancy. Prompt, appropriate treatment of infection and avoidance of bone grafting across the physis may prevent growth disturbance (Fig. 12-1). Children who experience systemic sepsis such as meningococcemia or purpura fulminans may develop multiple physeal arrests and extensive soft-tissue injury with distressing consequences. Failure to completely eradicate osteomyelitis may result in chronic pain or draining sinus tract.

Sequelae of septic arthritis include permanent joint destruction, joint contracture, gait abnormality, and abnormalities of bone growth. Avascular or osseous necrosis of the femoral head is a known complication of hip septic arthritis. Most likely caused by occlusion of intracapsular ascending vessels by increased intracapsular pressure or involvement by infection itself, osseous necrosis of the femoral head can be a devastating complication for which there is no good treatment. Femoral head osseous necrosis typically results in collapse, fragmentation, and growth retardation of the femoral head. Both the femoral head and the acetabulum may become dysplastic with subluxation and dislocation possible. These events lead to limb-length discrepancy, stiffness, and end-stage joint destruction.

Complications associated with antibiotic treatment are typically minor and treatable when appropriate monitoring is performed (16). Diarrhea, nausea, rash, thrombocytopenia, transient changes in liver enzymes, and antibiotic-induced neutropenia have been observed (141). Checking weekly ESR, CRP, CBC, and liver function tests ALT and AST can monitor for adequate response to treatment and for adverse side effects associated with antibiotic treatment. Long-term intravenous antibiotic treatment has been associated with a higher complication rate than long-term oral antibiotic treatment (143, 173, 174), including additional procedures required to replace catheters that have become obstructed or infected.

Musculoskeletal infection caused by drug-resistant organisms has resulted in increased use of new antibiotics, such as Linezolid, which come with their own potential problems and complications. Although very effective against gram-positive, antibiotic-resistant organisms, Linezolid has been associated with bone marrow suppression and optic neuropathy (158, 175). Flucloxacillin has been linked with the development of neutropenia (176), and Ciprofloxicillin has been associated with cartilage abnormality in a skeletally immature animal model, but its clinical significance in children has been questioned.

Invasive strains of MSSA and MRSA have emerged. In addition to significantly increased local tissue destruction, these aggressive bacteria have been associated with complications including septic emboli, DVT, empyema, and pneumonia (177–180). At Texas Children's hospital in Houston, Texas, nine children with DVT associated with musculoskeletal infection were studied (179). Seven of the nine children had infection caused by community-acquired MRSA carrying the Panton-Valentine leukocidin (PVL) gene and seven of nine children belonged to the same clonal group, USA300. Their findings strongly suggest that bacteria from specific genetic strains have a unique propensity to cause DVT in association with musculoskeletal infection.

Osteomyelitis of the proximal upper or lower extremity, pelvis, and vertebral osteomyelitis are locations that have been associated with increased risk of DVT. The DVT typically (but not always) occurs adjacent to the site of infection (177, 179). Central access catheters are often necessary for antibiotic administration in patients with musculoskeletal infection and have also been identified as a risk factor for DVT formation (179). Clinicians should consider vascular thrombosis in children with musculoskeletal sepsis who experience severe limb swelling, axial skeleton osteomyelitis of the proximal upper or lower extremity MRSA or invasive MSSA associated with the PVL antigen and/or the USA300 genetic strain.

SPECIAL CONDITIONS

Methicillin-Resistant *S. aureus.* The most important recent development in pediatric and adolescent musculoskeletal infection has been the emergence of community-acquired MRSA. In a study performed at University of Texas Southwest Medical Center, in Dallas, Texas, all children admitted with acute osteomyelitis between January 1999 and December 2003 were reviewed (181). A dramatic increase occurred in the percentage of children admitted with MRSA from 6% during time period from January 1999 to June 2001, to 31% during time period from July 2001 to December 2003, and virtually identical findings have been reported by other authors (182, 183). MRSA musculoskeletal infections have been reported on all continents (except Antarctica) (155, 184–188) and in patients of all ages from neonates (189) to adults.

The genetic basis for methicillin resistance arises from the *mecA* gene, which confers methicillin resistance by encoding penicillin-binding protein PBP2a (184, 190). The *mecA* gene is contained within a mobile genetic element called the staphylococcal chromosome cassette (SCC*mec*). SCCmec has 5 subtypes, I to V. Hospital-acquired MRSA is typically caused by SCCmec subtypes I to III. SCCmec subtypes I to III usually contain multiple genes that mediate resistance to nonlactam antibiotics and confer Clindamycin and Erythromycin resistance through the *erm* gene. Community-acquired MRSA infection is typically caused by SCCmec types IV and V, which lack additional antibiotic resistance genes and therefore are usually Clindamycin sensitive. The *erm* gene is large and not translocatable, but antibiotic pressure can cause SCCmec types IV and V to take up *erm* containing plasmids, thereby inducing Clindamycin resistance in community-acquired MRSA.

Compared with most MSSA strains, a very important distinction between MSSA and MRSA is the tendency for MRSA to cause more aggressive and fulminant infection. This is evidenced by significantly greater degree and duration of elevated temperature, elevated acute-phase reactants (WBC, ESR, and CRP), increased length of hospital stay, increased duration of antibiotic therapy, increased number of septic foci, increased number of surgical intervention, increased rate of complications, and worse clinical outcomes (181, 182) (Fig. 12-13). Failure to resolve after routine surgical debridement and the occurrence of septic emboli resulting in necrotizing pneumonia, which can be lethal in otherwise healthy children, are additional characteristics of community-acquired MRSA. DVT associated with MRSA infection is much more common as well (191).

Invasive MRSA infections are typically caused by bacteria sharing specific genetic characteristics including the USA300 genetic strain and the PVL gene (192). These same genetic elements can be found in aggressive MSSA infections as well. PVL is a pore-forming cytolytic toxin with an affinity for leukocytes that causes the release of inflammatory mediators that cause severe tissue damage. In a study of 85 patients with acute, community-acquired *S. aureus* osteomyelitis, Bocchini and coauthors found that all MRSA patients were

PVL positive (56 out of 56 MRSA patients) and that a small minority of MSSA patients were also PVL positive (3 of 29 MSSA patients). MSSA patients who were PVL positive had the same virulent infection characteristics as MRSA patients. Independent of whether patients were MRSA or MSSA, the presence of the PVL antigen was associated with increased ESR

and CRP levels, increased likelihood of having positive blood cultures, and a greater chance of having myositis or pyomyositis associate with osteomyelitis (193). In France, where only a minority of PVL-positive cases are associated with MRSA, infection severity has been linked to PVL secretion rather than antibiotic resistance (184).

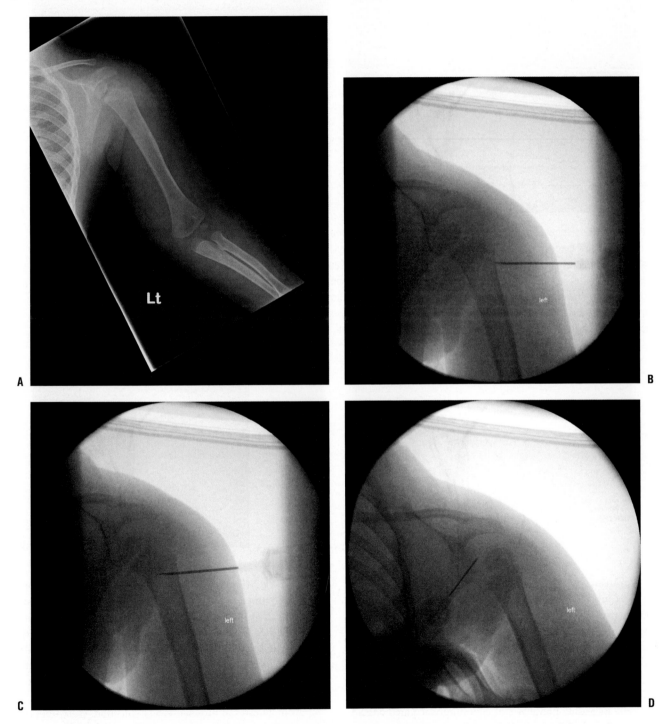

FIGURE 12-13. **A:** A 2-year-old child presents to the emergency department with a 3-day history of increasing left arm pain and swelling, fever to 39.5, WBC count of 17,000, ESR of 95 and CRP of 37 and normal standard radiographs. **B–D:** Based on the physical exam and the laboratory evaluation, the patient was brought emergently to the operating room where aspiration revealed the presence of a subperiosteal abscess **B**, and intraosseous abscess **C**, but negative shoulder joint aspiration **D**.

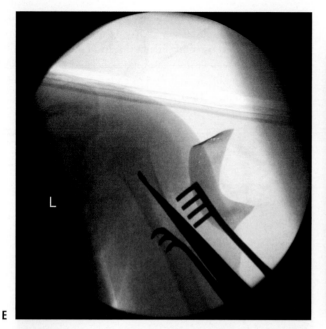

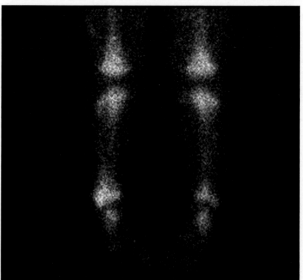

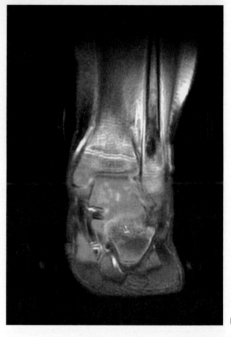

FIGURE 12-13. (*continued*) **E:** The abscesses were drained and a trough was created in cortex to allow curettage decompression of the intramedullary cavity. Pulsavac lavage was used to irrigate the bone and the surrounding soft tissues. **F:** Blood and bone cultures grew MRSA. After initial improvement, the patient clinically worsened 48 hours after wound closure. Bone scan performed to search for other foci of infection demonstrates increased uptake in the distal left fibula. **G:** MRI scan confirms the presence of a second focus of osteomyelitis that was treated with irrigation and debridement.

In Australia, MRSA cases occurring in the Western region of the country have been mainly caused by PVL-negative strains, while PVL-positive strains have predominated in the east (187). Thirty separate MRSA genetic clones have been identified, typically causing skin and soft-tissue infections, except PVL-positive strains that have a predilection for causing furunculosis, necrotizing pneumonia, and osteomyelitis, occasionally being lethal in healthy children.

The increasing prevalence of community-acquired MRSA has necessitated a change in empiric antibiotic treatment recommendations. In the past, a synthetic penicillin or first-generation cephalosporin has been recommended for initial parenteral treatment for suspected musculoskeletal infection, but this has resulted in a delay of appropriate therapy when infection is caused by MRSA strains (188). The two antibiotics commonly recommended for suspected MRSA are Clindamycin and Vancomycin (155, 181, 184, 188). There is some controversy as to whether Clindamycin or Vancomycin is the best initial choice. Clindamycin resistance has been reported in up to 10% of MRSA infections (188). The use of newer antibiotics such as linezolid and daptomycin holds promise for the treatment of MRSA but requires further study (194).

As in all cases of musculoskeletal infection, every opportunity should be taken to culture an organism from blood, joint fluid, and/or bone. In cases of suspected MRSA or invasive MSSA, obtaining an MRI scan early in the evaluation is very helpful to determine the precise location of the infection, to determine the extent of the infection in bone and surrounding soft tissues, as well as to detect other associated consequences within the region such as DVT (195). If septic arthritis, bone abscess, or soft-tissue abscess is detected, then urgent surgical irrigation and debridement is recommended. In cases of aggressive infection, packing the wound open decompresses the infected area and returning in 1 to 3 days permits a second thorough irrigation and debridement. Fluoroscopic guidance is helpful to ensure adequate debridement of the infected region as demonstrated on preoperative MRI and to avoid injury to the adjacent physis during debridement. Closure over drains is important to prevent abscess recurrence. Drains that are properly placed and managed may function as long as 7 to 10 days until output is minimal and clinical improvement has been demonstrated.

Failure to improve following treatment warrants careful reexamination of the patient and reevaluation of the treatment regimen. Inspection and palpation of the patient from head to toe may demonstrate a previously undetected focus of infection. If Clindamycin is being used, consider the possibility of antibiotic resistance and changing to Vancomycin. Check Vancomycin peak and trough levels to ensure therapeutic blood levels are present. Bone scan may be helpful to identify a second or third infection site (Fig. 12-13). Consider reimaging the known focus of infection with MRI for possible abscess formation. Chest x-ray or Chest CT should be performed in all patients with pulmonary symptoms to evaluate for lung involvement. Obtain duplex ultrasound to evaluate for DVT in patients with significant persistent limb swelling, especially in children older than age 8 years (180).

The duration of antibiotic treatment for MRSA should be longer than for uncomplicated musculoskeletal infection. In general, osteomyelitis should be treated for 4 to 6 weeks, septic arthritis for 3 to 4 weeks, and pyomyositis for 2 to 3 weeks. Although one appealing aspect of Clindamycin treatment is the ability to convert to high-dose oral administration, it is common for the entire course of antibiotic treatment to be administered intravenously via PICC or central line. Once sustained clinical improvement occurs with convincing downward trend in CRP and absence of fever above 38.5°C, antibiotic treatment may be continued as an outpatient. Following discharge from the hospital, weekly laboratory testing is imperative to monitor for side effects from the antibiotic and to confirm favorable response to treatment. Regular outpatient follow-up should occur approximately every other week to permit physical examination and confirm compliance with antibiotic treatment. Plain radiographs should be obtained at the conclusion of antibiotic treatment and as clinically indicated to monitor for the sequelae if infection such as chondrolysis, osteonecrosis, or physeal arrest.

Author's Recommendations. For all patients presenting with symptoms of musculoskeletal infection, assess very thoroughly for MRSA or PVL-positive MSSA infection. Carefully examine and palpate all extremities and the axial skeleton looking for multiple infection sites. Obtain laboratory tests including CBC with differential, CRP and ESR, looking carefully for marked elevation in the values. Culture

blood and aspirate all suspected foci of infection as well as the adjacent bone or joint whenever possible. If no septic arthritis, bone or soft-tissue abscess is encountered, begin Vancomycin immediately at a dose of 40 mg/kg/d divided every 6 hours, adjusting dose as necessary based on the peak and trough results. Clindamycin is an acceptable second choice. If an abscess is strongly suspected but not clinically apparent, or if the axial skeleton is involved, obtain an MRI of the affected region but do not delay antibiotic administration. If aspiration or MRI confirms the presence of an abscess, urgently surgically debride the region of infection. During surgery, if the septic joint or the musculoskeletal abscess appears extensive or aggressively involved, pack the wound open and return 1 to 2 days later for repeat irrigation and debridement. Follow the patient carefully while on IV antibiotics and if there is evidence of persistent infection as suggested by persistent elevated temperature, increased CRP, repeatedly positive blood cultures or persistent malaise, anorexia or night pain, obtain a technitium bone scan to look for undetected foci of infection. Evaluate the lungs by chest x-ray or CT for septic emboli or pneumonia if pulmonary symptoms are present. Consider mechanical DVT prophylaxis for MRSA infection of the lower extremity or pelvis and evaluate using Doppler ultrasound when clinical suspicion for venous thrombosis exists. For confirmed MRSA infection, continue parenteral Vancomycin or Clindamycin for 4 to 6 weeks depending on the severity of infection and patient clinical response.

Axial Skeleton. Infection of the spine and pelvis presents unique diagnostic and treatment challenges (196). Discitis, a relatively uncommon infection in adults, is the most common spinal infection in children (197). Over the past several decades, various descriptions in the literature of vertebral osteomyelitis and discitis reflect the uncertainty that these are indeed two separate conditions (198, 199). Modern imaging modalities, such as scintigraphy, CT, and MRI, have helped resolve the confusion by demonstrating evidence of bone involvement in children with the clinical presentation of discitis (200, 201). It therefore appears that both vertebral osteomyelitis and discitis are the result of a hematogenous infection beginning in the bone adjacent to the cartilaginous vertebral end plate.

Studies of vertebral body and disc vascular anatomy have demonstrated that the blood supply to the disc comes from the contiguous bone of the vertebral bodies (202–205). In the young child, vessels can be identified traversing the cartilaginous vertebral endplate and entering the annulus. By the age of 8, these vessels have largely disappeared. It is likely that discitis and vertebral osteomyelitis represent two slightly different clinical manifestations of a similar disease process affected by changes in vascular anatomy with growth and development. Immature vertebral endplate and disc-space vascular anatomy result in a clinical focus of infection within the discs of young children, whereas older children are more likely to have a primary focus of infection within the vertebral body. This is consistent with the observation that the average age at onset in patients with discitis is 2.5 years compared to the mean age at presentation for vertebral osteomyelitis, which is 7.5 years of age (206).

Children with discitis infrequently present with systemic signs of illness such as fever, malaise, anorexia, or sleep disturbance (207). Patients often refuse to walk but have a normal lower extremity exam. Frequently, children will refuse to bend forward to pick up a toy or an object from the floor. Back pain or abdominal pain may, or may not, also be present. Spine exam frequently demonstrates decreased ROM and discomfort to palpation and percussion. Laboratory parameters, including ESR and CRP, are usually, but not always, elevated. Plain film radiographs are typically normal but may show subtle vertebral endplate irregularity and, later, slight reduction in disc height at the suspected level. In confusing clinical situations, bone scan is often the most helpful test to localize infection of the axial skeleton (Fig. 12-4). If the clinical situation strongly suggests a pathologic process of the spine, but additional imaging is necessary to confirm the diagnosis, MRI is recommended as it provides the greatest amount of information in a single imaging study (200, 201).

There is no complete agreement as to whether discitis is the result of bacterial infection. Blood cultures are usually negative, disc aspiration and culture are rarely performed, and there have been several reports of patients recovering completely after treatment with immobilization alone. When positive, the biopsy results show a preponderance of *S. aureus* as the causative organism (207–210). Most agree that discitis is a bacterial infection that is best treated with high-dose intravenous followed by oral antibiotics and immobilization as necessary to control symptoms. Empiric intravenous antibiotic therapy is directed at the most common offending organism, *S. aureus*. Following clinical response to treatment, transition to an appropriate oral antibiotic is made, and treatment is continued for approximately 3 to 5 weeks. Weekly lab testing is performed to monitor for antibiotic side effects and response to treatment.

Resolution of symptoms usually occurs within the first 72 hours. If this is not the case, the physician should begin to question the diagnosis or the specific bacterial etiology. Further imaging studies, such as CT or MRI, may be justified in such circumstances to search for tumor or abscess formation. Biopsy may be indicated in a patient who fails to respond to antibiotics and bed rest and is indicated in any child whose imaging studies suggest a diagnosis other than typical discitis.

In contrast to discitis, vertebral osteomyelitis is less common in children than in adults (211). Compared to discitis, children with osteomyelitis are older, are more often febrile and ill-appearing, and have a longer symptom duration (206). Standard radiographs are often normal during the first few weeks of symptoms in patients with vertebral osteomyelitis, and either bone scan or MRI is often helpful in establishing the diagnosis. The abundant vertebral blood supply provides outstanding antibiotic delivery. Vertebral osteomyelitis can almost always be eradicated by antibiotics alone unless abscess formation occurs.

Epidural abscess is a rare but very serious spinal infection (197). Usually presenting with back pain, patients can present with neurologic deficit. MRI is the preferred imaging modality for evaluation of suspected epidural abscess. When present and correlative with neurologic deficit, emergent decompression of the epidural abscess is indicated. If there is no neurologic deficit or displacement of the spinal cord caused by the epidural abscess, antibiotic treatment alone can be effective.

Patients with osteomyelitis of the pelvis may present with vague hip or back pain and have difficulty localizing their symptoms. Their physical exam is often nonspecific, often resulting in a delay in diagnosis (212). Nonarticular pelvic abscess or SI joint infection may present with symptoms suggesting septic arthritis of the hip or appendicitis (196, 213). Pelvic osteomyelitis and SI joint infection are generally seen in older children (214, 215) with the mean age of 10 years, whereas septic hip is more common in the younger child. Despite complaints of pain around the hip, children with SI joint infection often remain ambulatory. SI joint infection patients often have relatively pain-free internal rotation of the hip and have increased pain with external hip rotation. This is in contrast to patients with septic arthritis of the hip who typically have greater discomfort with internal hip rotation than external hip rotation. If the FABER test (flexion, abduction, external rotation) is performed, it usually elicits pain in the presence of SI joint sepsis, as does compression of the pelvis (Gaenslen test). Tenderness almost always is found over the SI joint, if sought. Other areas (e.g., the ischium, pubis, ilium) should always be palpated for tenderness in children with gait disturbance or hip pain.

Standard imaging studies may not be helpful. In most cases of SI joint infection or pelvic osteomyelitis, the initial radiographs are normal. This is especially true when symptoms have been present for fewer than 1 or 2 weeks. The earliest sign of infection on the radiograph is disappearance of the subchondral margins and erosion; however, this should be considered to be a late finding. If radiographic changes are present within <1 week of symptoms, careful consideration should be given to other disorders, such as tumor or chronic inflammatory SI disease. Radionucleotide bone scan may be helpful in localizing the infection. Because of the complicated three-dimensional pelvic anatomy, CT or MRI should be performed in all patients with pelvic osteomyelitis to determine the extent of bone and soft-tissue involvement as well as to detect possible abscess formation (Fig. 12-8). MRI is coming to the forefront as the imaging modality of choice for suspected musculoskeletal infection of the pelvis because of its ability to better demonstrate the extent of bone involvement early in the course of infection, before abnormality is visible on CT (216, 217).

Schaad et al. (214) reported that the bacterial etiology was established in 57% of the pelvic osteomyelitis cases they studied from their own patients and in a literature review. In most cases, *S. aureus* is the organism that is cultured from blood, direct aspiration, or biopsy (218–222), while *Streptococcus* species *K. kingae, Pseudomonas aeruginosa, Enterobacter cloacae,* and *Salmonella* species have also been reported (212, 214, 222–224).

Reports in the literature demonstrate that surgical debridement of pelvic osteomyelitis or soft-tissue abscess about the pelvis is usually unnecessary (215, 223, 225, 226). Complex anatomy often makes surgical approach and debridement difficult. In a comprehensive recent review, Davidson et al. (227) described the most frequent locations for osteomyelitis to occur within the pelvis and reported treatment results in 62 children. The most common pelvic sites of infection were the ilium in 21 and the acetabulum in 20 patients, followed by the pubis and ischium in 11 and 10, respectively. Osteomyelitis typically involved the metaphyseal equivalent sites within the pelvis. Fifty-seven patients were treated with antibiotics alone, and five were treated with antibiotics and surgical debridement, suggesting that surgery is indicated in a minority of patients with pelvic osteomyelitis. Indications for surgery include the need for biopsy in the case of suspected tumor, an unusual presentation, or failure to respond to appropriate antibiotic treatment in a reasonable period of time. Pyomyositis and abscess formation may accompany pelvic osteomyelitis (216, 217). Abscess drainage can often be performed percutaneously under image guidance, with a reported success rate in children of 85% to 90% (33, 228).

Initial antibiotic therapy should be with an intravenous semisynthetic penicillin or first-generation cephalosporin, as used in the treatment of AHO (Table 12-2). If MRSA is suspected, Vancomycin or Clindamycin are preferred. If symptoms resolve and the CRP begins to fall, the patient may be switched to high-dose oral antibiotics in 5 to 7 days. Initial and subsequent antibiotics should be adjusted to reflect information from blood and tissue cultures as well as from biopsy material if that has been obtained.

Author's Preferred Treatment.

When treating patients with suspected infection of the axial skeleton, we recommend a three-step approach:

1. Localize the infection. If history, exam, and standard radiographs do not allow localization of the infection, technetium bone scan should be performed.
2. Determine the extent of infection. Once localized, CT or MRI should be performed in virtually all patients with suspected osteomyelitis of the pelvis or spine. Discussion with your radiologist is often helpful when making the decision whether to use MRI or CT. MRI provides the greatest amount of information regarding bone and soft-tissue pathology, but it may require general anesthesia for young children, is more expensive than CT, and is not as readily available as CT is at some institutions. CT may allow aspiration or placement of percutaneous drains under image guidance.
3. Treat the infection. Although epidural abscess with neurologic compromise or large abscess with systemic sepsis requires immediate surgical treatment, almost all other infection of the axial skeleton can be treated effectively with parenteral antibiotics. Failure to respond to parenteral antibiotic therapy warrants abscess drainage. This may be performed percutaneously or surgically, depending on abscess size, location, and availability of interventional radiology.

Foot. Simply because the foot is where we come into contact with the earth, it is susceptible to trauma and puncture that can result in infection (Fig. 12-14). The foot is more likely to be inoculated with bacteria from the local environment and therefore is more likely to have infection caused by a spectrum of bacteria different from those causing the hematogenous osteomyelitis seen in long bones. Since Johanson's 1968 report, orthopaedic surgeons have become increasingly aware of the association between puncture wounds of the foot and *P. aeruginosa* as the causative organism of deep infections that follow (229). It was subsequently demonstrated that *Pseudomonas* can be recovered from the inner spongy sole of nearly all well-worn tennis shoes (230). *P. aeruginosa* is a gram-negative aerobic organism with anaerobic tolerance, which is found widely in soil, water, and on the skin. As a human pathogen seen in orthopaedic conditions, it seems to have an affinity for cartilage.

Despite the relative increased prevalence of *Pseudomonas* from the foot environment and from puncture wounds of the foot, it is important to remember that *S. aureus* is still the most common soft-tissue infection following a puncture wound. In addition, *Aeromonas hydrophilia* is common when puncture wounds or lacerations occur in fresh water, for example, ponds (231).

Fortunately, most children who sustain puncture wounds to the foot do not develop bone or joint infection. Fitzgerald and Cowan (232) reviewed records of children younger than age 15 who presented to the emergency department for evaluation of a puncture wounds to the foot. Only 0.6% of those who were presenting for initial evaluation subsequently developed osteomyelitis. Of 132 patients seen with soft-tissue infection after puncture wound of the foot, 112 had a prompt response to soaks, rest, elevation, and antibiotics.

Given the low incidence of osteomyelitis and serious soft-tissue infection, a conservative approach to the initial management of a puncture wound is warranted. Superficial cleaning and debridement of the skin and inspection for a foreign body is appropriate. Tetanus prophylaxis is important. There does not seem to be any solid evidence either for or against the routine use of antibiotics in the initial management. Treatment with soaks, elevation, and an oral antistaphylococcal antibiotic is warranted and if the patient has cellulitis, this regimen usually results in a cure.

Significant persistence of pain and swelling despite soaks, rest, elevation, and oral antibiotic treatments suggests the presence of septic arthritis, osteomyelitis, or retained foreign body (233). Careful clinical examination is helpful in establishing the presence and location of infection. Comparison with the contralateral foot is helpful, looking for focal swelling, skin changes, or tenderness on palpation. Pain on motion of a specific metatarsophalangeal joint is usually indicative of a septic arthritis in that joint. Dorsal swelling on the forefoot, or swelling laterally and medially around the heel, is often an additional sign of a serious deep infection.

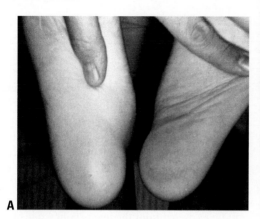
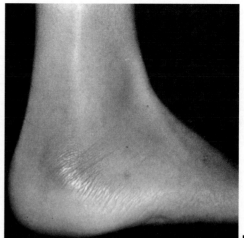
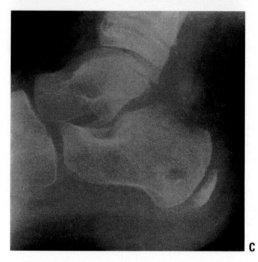

FIGURE 12-14. This patient was seen with pain 2 weeks after a puncture wound of the heel. He initially came to the emergency department 3 days after the puncture wound because of increasing pain and swelling. Therapy was begun with a first-generation cephalosporin antibiotic. He experienced temporary improvement, but later the pain became worse. **A:** Note the swelling of the affected heel, compared with the opposite contralateral heel side. **B:** The swelling and erythema on the lateral side of the heel indicate deep infection. **C:** A radiograph demonstrates a lytic lesion of the heel, in addition to the soft-tissue swelling. *P. aeruginosa* was cultured from the infected site.

Plain radiographs are rarely helpful in detecting early osteomyelitis or septic arthritis, but should be obtained to look for bone changes or a metallic foreign body. MRI may be the most cost-effective way of identifying deep infection of the foot following puncture wounds (234). If deep infection is identified, surgical debridement is indicated to evacuate infected material and search for a foreign body.

Pseudomonas infection of a bone or joint is a surgical disease; the failure of antibiotics alone to resolve these infections has been adequately demonstrated (235). The surgical approach may be either dorsal or volar but must give adequate access to both the bones and the joints in the region of the puncture, because *P. aeruginosa* is a cartilage-seeking organism. Some surgeons believe that the volar approach leaves a potentially painful scar. When properly placed, however, this should not be the case. This approach has the advantage of directly exposing the puncture track, which is an essential part of the surgery, because of the high incidence of foreign material found at surgical debridement (232, 236). The dorsal approach allows direct access to the joints and bones through a more anatomic and extensile approach and can be combined with a limited debridement of the volar puncture wound. The calcaneus should be approached from a medial or lateral incision, or from both.

Infections due to puncture wounds are often caused by multiple organisms. For this reason, it makes sense to begin antibiotic therapy with a combination of antibiotics effective against both gram-positive organisms and gram-negative organisms, including *P. aeruginosa*. An initial choice may be ceftazidime (Fortaz) and gentamicin or oxacillin and gentamicin (Table 12-3). Jacobs et al. (235, 236) suggest that 7 days of intravenous antibiotics after adequate surgical debridement is sufficient, although others recommend longer treatment, from 10 days to 2 weeks.

Ciprofloxacin is antibiotic that is effective against *Pseudomonas*. However, its use in children has been limited by reports of interfering with the growth plate in animal studies. Despite this, it has been used in cystic fibrosis and in other serious infections in children, without reports of ill effects on cartilage or growth.

In addition to puncture wounds, AHO can occur in the foot as well and may have a predilection for the calcaneus. Puffinbarger et al. (237) reported a series of 11 cases of osteomyelitis of the calcaneus and noted that cases of hematogenous osteomyelitis were most commonly caused by *S. aureus*, whereas all puncture-related cases were positive for *P. aeruginosa*. Several factors make treatment of calcaneal osteomyelitis especially challenging. The calcaneus does not have investing musculature to provide blood supply and antibiotic delivery or to provide soft-tissue coverage following surgery. Eggshell-like bone and limited ability to regenerate itself following debridement limit surgical options for calcaneus debridement. These factors do not limit what needs to be done but may cause increased morbidity with surgery.

Prompt diagnosis and treatment of calcaneal osteomyelitis allows effective treatment with antibiotics alone. Jaakkola and Kehl (238) reported successful antibiotic treatment of hematogenous calcaneal osteomyelitis without surgical intervention. If the diagnosis of calcaneal osteomyelitis is delayed, significant complications may result including shortening of the foot, tarsal bone fusion, adjacent bone osteomyelitis, and avascular necrosis that can require radical surgery such as calcanectomy (239–241).

Neonate. The neonate, defined for our purposes as any child up to 8 weeks of age, is susceptible to a variety of musculoskeletal infections unique to this age group. Their immature immune system makes neonates susceptible to a wide range of organisms that are less virulent under normal circumstances and prevents them from expressing symptoms and signs that allow early diagnosis. Metaphyseal and epiphyseal vascular anatomy of the neonate is unique resulting in frequent involvement of the physis and adjacent joint, and multiple distant sites are often involved.

Two types of infection typically appear in the neonate: infection recognized in the hospital often occurring in premature infants and infection that becomes apparent after discharge from the nursery in otherwise healthy, full-term neonates. The type manifest in the hospital usually occurs in premature infants undergoing invasive monitoring. These neonates remain in the intensive care unit in the presence of nosocomial pathogens, coupled with invasive monitoring, intravenous feeding, drug administration, and blood sampling. Indwelling vascular catheters, particularly those in the umbilical vessels, have long been recognized as one of the main sources of infection (242). These neonates are more likely to have infection caused by *S. aureus* or gram-negative organisms and more than 40% have more than one site of involvement (243, 244).

The other type is usually manifest between 2 and 4 weeks of life (sometimes as late as 8 weeks), in infants who are not systemically ill and are developing and feeding normally. These infections are more likely to be due to group B *Streptococcus* and involve a single site. Infants delivered by vaginal delivery are exposed to potential pathogenic bacteria during delivery. Before vaginal delivery, women undergo culture of the birth canal for group B *Streptococcus*. If positive, women are treated prophylactically with antibiotic coverage at the time of delivery to prevent transmission of group B *Streptococcus* infection to the newborn. Should transmission of group B *Streptococcus*

to the newborn occur, the newborn is at risk of developing osteomyelitis or septic arthritis.

The most common cause of sepsis in the neonate is still *S. aureus*. In addition to group B *Streptococcus*, group A *Streptococcus*, *Streptococcus pneumoniae*, *Escherichia coli*, and *Staphylococcus aureus*, gram-negative bacilli and *Streptococcus pneumonia* also may cause musculoskeletal infection in neonates (245, 246).

In the neonate, before the secondary centers of ossification appear, metaphyseal vessels penetrate directly into the chondroepiphysis. Osteomyelitis originating in the metaphysis can spread into the epiphysis and joint, with a reported association as high as 76% (243, 244). The transphyseal vessels persist until 6 to 18 months of age, when secondary ossification centers begin to form and the physis becomes a mechanical barrier to infection. Permanent growth arrest, physeal injury, and joint destruction can result. The lesson for the physician is that when a septic joint is diagnosed in the neonate, a thorough search for osteomyelitis in an adjacent metaphysis or epiphysis is mandatory.

The neonate cannot mount a normal immune response to infection, so typical symptoms, signs, and laboratory indicators of infection are often absent, and multiple sites of infection are common. Physical examination often demonstrates swelling and pain or irritability with movement, but findings are often unremarkable, compared to what they would be in an older child. The leukocyte count and the differential leukocyte count are not reliably elevated, and patients may present with leukopenia (246). The blood cultures are positive in approximately 50% of patients with proven infection. In a study by Klein examining the sensitivity of objective parameters in patients with septic arthritis of the hips, none of the neonates in the study group were febrile or had an elevated leukocyte count, but all did have an elevated ESR (65).

Technetium bone scans may be helpful in detecting multiple sites of infection, but false-negative studies often occur, and bone scan may not reveal all infected sites. The literature varies as to the sensitivity of technetium-99 scanning in neonates. In one report on the value of bone scintigraphy in detection of neonatal osteomyelitis, the sensitivity for diagnosing focal disease by clinical findings was 20%, radiography 65%, and bone scintigraphy 90% (247), but other investigators have found the bone scan to be less sensitive. Ash and Gilday (249) found that only 32% of proven sites of osteomyelitis in 10 neonates were positive on bone scan. Higher resolution scintigraphy equipment and magnification views of all suspected areas appear to provide improved results (249).

Aspiration of all suspected sites of bone or joint sepsis should be performed, and fluid aspirate sent for analysis including Gram stain and culture. One can make a strong case for aspirating both hips in any neonate with known osteomyelitis or septic arthritis because

- Multiple sites of involvement are common.
- The proximal femur and the hip joint are frequently involved.

- Symptoms and signs are often subtle or lacking.
- The hip is the most difficult joint to examine.
- The window of opportunity for effective treatment is small.
- The hip joint is the most frequent site of permanent sequelae.

Treatment varies slightly from that in older children and should be managed in conjunction with a neonatologist or a pediatric infectious disease consultant whenever possible. Most importantly, initial antibiotic selection must cover bacteria unique to neonatal musculoskeletal infection (Table 12-2). In this age group, choices may include oxacillin along with gentamicin or a third-generation cephalosporin such as cefotaxime (Claforan). Ceftriaxone (Rocephin) is also a good choice in a child without jaundice. Because neonates are more prone to generalized sepsis, have less consistent oral antibiotic absorption, and have less predictable radiographic and serologic response to treatment, it has been generally recommended that the entire course of treatment be intravenous (16, 95).

Surgical debridement of septic arthritis and bone abscess is appropriate. To reduce the risk of permanent growth alteration or joint abnormality, cautious debridement of the chondroepiphysis is indicated.

Gonococcal Arthritis. Gonococcal arthritis is usually a sexually transmitted disease caused by the gram-negative diplococcus *Neisseria gonorrhoeae*. In the newborn, the disease is contracted from the mother during passage through the birth canal and results most commonly in conjunctivitis and scalp abscesses (250, 251). Gonococcal infection is also frequently seen in the adolescent age group. Although gonococcal infection can take many forms, the orthopaedist is most likely to encounter this infection as septic arthritis following dissemination of genitourinary disease. The delay between the genitourinary infection and the arthritis is variable, ranging from a few days to several weeks (252).

When the disease is noted after the newborn period, before puberty, and in sexually inactive adolescents, sexual abuse should be suspected. Sexual abuse may occur in as many as 10% of all abuse cases, and it is estimated that between 5% and 20% of sexually abused children have a sexually transmitted disease, most commonly gonococcal infection (253, 254). Children who are identified with or suspected of having a gonococcal infection should have cultures of all mucous membranes, including pharynx, vagina, and rectum, before the administration of antibiotics. These cultures should be handled in a manner that permits them to be used as evidence in court. In addition, reporting of suspected cases is mandated by the Child Abuse Reporting Law. For all of these reasons, the orthopaedist should involve a knowledgeable pediatrician in the evaluation of these patients.

The initial skin lesion seen in gonococcal infection is a small erythematous macule present on the genitalia. This may disappear or develop a small vesicle, followed by a necrotic center that may form a pustule. Approximately one-third of patients develop a distinctive rash that is the result of gonococcal

septicemia. Additional associated systemic symptoms include fever, tenosynovitis, and migratory polyarthralgia (255).

Joint involvement is polyarticular in 80% of cases. The knee is most often affected, but it is important to remember that any joint, large or small, can be involved. The size of the effusion may vary widely and may even be absent. The involved joints are usually painful. The nature of the arthritis does not appear to have changed over the past several decades, although treatment with antibiotics has resulted in the virtual elimination of joint destruction (256–260). Osteomyelitis still may be seen as an occasional complication (261).

Culture is the only way to confirm the diagnosis. Culture and Gram staining of joint fluid, and of the cervix of post-pubertal girls and the vagina of prepubertal girls, should be performed. Any urethral or prostatic discharge in boys should also be cultured and examined by Gram staining. Blood cultures should be routine. The organism may occasionally be isolated from skin lesions, but Gram staining gives a higher yield.

N. gonorrhoeae is a difficult organism to grow, and special care is needed in the handling of the material for culture. Because the organism is sensitive to cold, material for culture should be plated directly onto a warm medium whenever possible (262). Special culture tubes for transport of gonococcal cultures are available and should be used; specimens should be delivered promptly to the bacteriology laboratory when direct plating is not feasible. Cultures from sterile sites (e.g., blood, synovial fluid) are plated on chocolate blood agar. Cultures from nonsterile sites (e.g., the vagina, skin lesions) should be plated on selective media (e.g., Thayer-Martin agar) that contains antibiotics to inhibit the growth of other organisms. Cultures are grown in a 5% to 10% CO_2 atmosphere.

Increasing resistance of *N. gonorrhoeae* to penicillin and tetracycline makes parenteral administration of a third-generation cephalosporin (e.g., ceftriaxone, 50 mg/kg/d intramuscularly or intravenously, once daily) the initial drug of choice (262) (Table 12-2). If the organism is demonstrated to be sensitive to it, penicillin can be used. Involvement of the hip joint requires surgical drainage. Recommendations for drainage of other joints remain variable. In other large joints with large amounts of purulent fluid, surgical drainage may be preferable to repeated needle aspiration. If surgical drainage is used, it is wise to leave a closed suction drain in the joint, because the tendency to reaccumulate fluid in gonococcal infection is greater than with other forms of septic arthritis.

Human Immunodeficiency Virus. Children with human immunodeficiency virus (HIV) infection have a propensity for infection by *S. pneumoniae* (16). Fortunately, there is no information to date suggesting that the presenting signs or symptoms or recovery from infection are affected by HIV coinfection; however, broad-spectrum antibiotic coverage is recommended due to the wide range of causative organisms that have been reported in children with HIV infection (6). HIV infection can have several musculoskeletal manifestations. Patients may experience rheumatologic manifestations of HIV as well as susceptibility to atypical musculoskeletal infection (263). Rheumatologic manifestations including Raynaud phenomenon, vasculitis, and arthralgia were identified by Martinez-Rojano in 5 of 26 HIV-infected children (263, 264). All rheumatologic changes were seen in advanced stages of HIV disease.

Lyme Disease. Lyme disease is an atypical infection caused by the organism *Borrelia burgdorferi*. The organism is spread to humans through the bite of the deer tick, endemic to northern states in the upper Midwest and New England. The hallmark clinical feature of Lyme disease is the appearance of single or multiple expanding skin lesions, erythema migrans, which expand to at least 5 cm and may have partial central clearing. The most common orthopaedic manifestation caused by *B. burgdorferi* is an intermittent reactive arthritis that does not cause the joint destruction seen in bacterial septic arthritis but causes recurrent intermittent swelling, stiffness, and pain. Arthralgia can occur in the acute or late phases of Lyme disease and typically affects the knee (265). The clinical picture is often more similar to JRA than to bacterial septic arthritis, with swelling and stiffness but less severe pain. When compared to patients with septic arthritis, Lyme arthritis patients are less likely to have a history of elevated temperature, and tend to have a lower ESR and lower CRP (266).

Standard anteroposterior and lateral plain film radiographs are appropriate as part of the routine evaluation of joint pain. MRI is not routinely indicated, but when performed, three features have been suggested to differentiate Lyme arthritis from acute septic arthritis: the presence of myositis, adenopathy, and the lack of subcutaneous edema (267).

The diagnosis of reactive Lyme disease arthropathy is most often made by positive blood serology in a patient with a history of possible exposure and in whom other causes have been excluded. Almost all untreated patients have high levels of serum immunoglobulin G antibodies and sometimes low levels of immunoglobulin M antibodies to *B. burgdorferi*. At many centers, screening is done by ELISA and confirmed by Western blot. Serologic immunoglobins may persist after effective antibiotic treatment and do not accurately distinguish between active or past infection. Joint aspirate fluid can also be tested for Lyme disease but is not necessary to make the diagnosis. Treatment in children is simply amoxicillin 25 to 50 mg/kg/d divided b.i.d. for 3 weeks and is very effective at completely eliminating the organism and all musculoskeletal symptoms (268). A small percentage of patients have persistent knee synovitis that may be caused by intrasynovial autoimmunity (265).

Occasionally, patients may present with acute arthritis that mimics septic arthritis. Willis et al. (267) reported a series of 10 cases in which Lyme arthritis presented as acute painful arthritis. None of these 10 patients had a known history of a tick bite or had evidence of erythema migrans. Five patients were febrile at presentation, and all patients had limited joint motion with pain at motion endpoints. All the patients were able to ambulate independently at home, although two patients refused to bear weight at initial presentation to the orthopaedic surgeon. One-third of patients had an elevated serum WBC, but only one had a

significant left shift. The ESR was elevated beyond 40 mm/hour in 60% of the cases and beyond normal (20 mm/hour) in 90% of cases. The CRP was elevated in 9 of 10 patients.

Joint aspiration was performed in all cases and sent for cell count and differential as well as culture. The joint WBC count in this series of 10 patients with Lyme arthritis averaged 82,900 cells per mm^3 (range: 40,900 to 140,500), and 60% of the aspirates had more than 80,000 cells per mm^3. In all patients, the percentage of polymorphonuclear cells was more than 80%. All patients had positive screening and confirmatory serologic testing for *B. burgdorferi*. Based on initial history, examination, and laboratory and joint aspirate data, seven patients underwent surgical joint irrigation. The factors that best differentiated cases of Lyme arthritis from septic arthritis in this series were the ability to ambulate and normal serum polymorphonuclear cell count. Rapid 1-hour Lyme immunoassays are now becoming available, which will greatly facilitate prompt diagnosis.

Because Lyme arthritis shares features with both septic and nonseptic, non-Lyme arthritis, and because there is considerable overlap between septic, nonseptic, and Lyme arthritis, a clinically useful predictive model for Lyme arthritis has not been developed. Therefore, in endemic areas, Lyme testing should be performed on all patients presenting with acute monoarticular arthritis (266). If the patient is ambulatory and has a normal serum WBC and differential, and the rapid Lyme enzyme immunoassay (EIA) results are available and positive, the physician may choose to initiate Lyme-specific antibiotic therapy while awaiting final joint aspiration cultures and confirmatory Lyme Western blot serologic testing. However, if rapid Lyme EIA results are not available or if there remains significant clinical suspicion regarding the diagnosis of septic arthritis, we recommend proceeding with immediate irrigation and debridement of the affected joint, and later altering the treatment regimen appropriately based on the final results of preoperatively obtained bacterial cultures and two-stage Lyme serology.

Varicella. Varicella zoster has been associated with significant musculoskeletal infection in children, most frequently caused by group A *β-hemolytic Streptococcus* (270–273). Group A *β*-hemolytic *Streptococcus* may have a selective advantage in patients who have varicella because of its ability to gain access to deeper tissue through the varicella vesicle itself. The vesicle is created by a split in the epidermis that fills with a proteinaceous fluid. This may provide a route from the surface of the skin to the subcutaneous tissues, with subsequent bacteremia, or local spread, and musculoskeletal infection. Trauma to the skin from scratching may contribute to bacterial contamination of the varicella vesicle. Group A *β*-hemolytic *Streptococcus* possesses tissue-dissolving enzymes such as hyaluronidase and streptolysin, which facilitate penetration of the tissue. In addition to local factors, varicella appears to cause a transient systemic suppression of immunity, making patients susceptible to infection (274).

Recent availability and use of a vaccine against varicella may lead to a decrease in musculoskeletal infection associated with varicella, but no studies have been published to confirm this hypothesis. Physicians should have a high level of suspicion of musculoskeletal infection when examining children with varicella who have localized warmth and erythema, swelling, or pain or who refuse to bear weight. Prompt evaluation, appropriate operative intervention, and adjunctive systemic antibiotic therapy may prevent the spread of infection and the loss of life or limb. Because of transient immune suppression and susceptibility to infection, it is prudent to avoid elective surgery within 1 month of varicella infection or definite exposure.

Sickle Cell Disease. Patients with sickle cell disease demonstrate a unique predilection for *Salmonella* osteomyelitis, and multiple sites may be involved (275–279). Patients with sickle cell disease have significant impairment in splenic function and are also at increased risk for infection caused by encapsulated organisms such as *H. influenzae* and *S. pneumoniae*. Musculoskeletal infection caused by such encapsulated organisms, however, is not as prevalent as *Salmonella* infection and typically occurs in children younger than 3 years compared with infection caused by *Salmonella*, which has a peak onset between 5 and 10 years of age (274, 277, 278). In addition to osteomyelitis, patients with sickle cell anemia are also at increased risk of developing septic arthritis, but *Salmonella* is not the most common causative organism. Staphylococcus species are the most common cause of septic arthritis in patients with sickle cell disease.

Why patients with sickle cell anemia are predisposed to *Salmonella* infections has not been conclusively determined. Infarction of intestinal mucosa may facilitate entry of *Salmonella* into the circulatory system. Impaired splenic function and decreased specific antibiotic production may contribute to susceptibility. Preceding episodes of bone avascular necrosis have been found to be more frequent in patients with osteomyelitis, suggesting that ischemic bone may provide a favorable environment for localized infection (280). Despite these clues, there is not a clear understanding why sickle cell disease causes susceptibility to *Salmonella* infection.

The incidence of osteomyelitis in patients with sickle cell anemia in the United States is low, despite the attention it receives in the literature. In 1971, Specht (281) found only 82 cases in the literature, and the relatively few cases reported over several years in other large centers attest to the infrequent occurrence (282, 283). This low incidence is important to the orthopaedist when considered relative to the number of admissions for sickle cell crisis (283, 284). It is important to remember that patients presenting with sickle cell ischemic crisis outnumber those with osteomyelitis associated with sickle cell disease 50:1.

Patients with sickle cell disease present a challenging diagnostic and treatment dilemma. Sickle cell disease causes patients to experience vasoocclusive crises and predisposes patients to musculoskeletal infection. Bone infarction and bone infection may have identical clinical presentations but are treated with very different therapy; vasoocclusive crisis is treated with hydration and analgesia, whereas musculoskeletal infection requires antibiotics and occasionally emergent surgical debridement.

Considerable effort has been expended to develop a reliable means of differentiating between these two events. Clinical examination provides little help in differentiating between infarction and infection, because both patient groups tend to present with focal tenderness to palpation, swelling, and severe limp. Fever, elevated ESR, and elevated CRP are also commonly found with both conditions.

Thoughtful consideration of sickle cell disease pathophysiology may be the most powerful tool in helping to differentiate between infarction and infection. Clinically, the exquisite pain of ischemia associated with fever, swelling, and limp may show signs of improvement within 48 hours of initiating hydration therapy and appropriate analgesia, whereas clinical symptoms may continue to worsen, and ESR and CRP continue to rise, if the patient is experiencing musculoskeletal infection.

Technetium bone scan is typically cold in the very early ischemic phase of a sickle cell crisis, whereas osteomyelitis is much more likely to immediately show increased uptake in the early stages of infection. As the sickle cell crisis evolves and local inflammation surrounds the area of infarction, bone scanning will show increased uptake within 36 to 48 hours, making serial scanning more helpful than a single isolated scan.

MRI is emerging as the preferred imaging study used to differentiate between vasoocclusive crises and acute osteomyelitis (285, 286). MRI findings of cortical defects, fluid collections in adjacent soft tissue, and bone marrow enhancement are suggestive of infection over infarction. Unfortunately, marrow and soft-tissue changes seen with sepsis are not always reliably differentiated from ischemia on MRI (102, 287). As our knowledge and interpretation skills improve, MRI has the greatest promise to allow early identification of osteomyelitis in patients with sickle cell disease.

Several investigators have found ultrasonography to be useful in differentiating vasoocclusive crises from osteomyelitis (114, 288). Ultrasonographic scans in patients with vasoocclusive disease were totally normal, whereas those with osteomyelitis showed a variety of changes such as periosteal elevation, subperiosteal or intramedullary abscess, and cortical erosions. However, these are relatively late changes caused by osteomyelitis, and ultrasound may be less helpful in the early stages of infection. Ultrasonography is attractive because of its availability, relatively low cost, safety, and the short time needed to complete the evaluation.

A unique manifestation of this disorder is a condition known as sickle cell dactylitis, or hand–foot syndrome (39, 289). The condition occurs in infants and young children, usually those younger than 4 years. No case of a child older than 7 years has been reported. It may precede the diagnosis of sickle cell disease. The actual incidence is probably between 10% and 20% of children with sickle cell disease, and it seems to be more common in Africa. Patients present with acute, painful swelling of the hands and feet. Although sickle cell dactylitis is considered to be a benign condition requiring no further evaluation (289), *Salmonella* osteomyelitis has been associated with this condition (290, 291). Laboratory tests do not help in the differential diagnosis. Radiographic findings in the hand–foot syndrome at first demonstrate only soft-tissue swelling, but after 7 to 14 days, periosteal new bone formation is visible, followed by medullary resorption, coarsening of trabeculae, and cortical thinning. The changes revert to normal in weeks to months. Chronic radiographic changes associated with sickle cell disease include biconcave deformity of the vertebral end plates and avascular necrosis of the femoral and humeral heads.

With so few objective findings and tests to help differentiate between bone infarction and osteomyelitis, the ability to isolate a causative organism and confirm the diagnosis of infection becomes of great importance. Blood cultures should always be obtained, and aspiration of bone should be performed whenever infection is suspected. Because sickle cell osteomyelitis has a predilection for diaphyseal location, it requires aspiration through cortical bone, which is a difficult procedure best performed in the operating room under sterile conditions.

In the literature, recommendations for or against surgical debridement are variable: some believe it to be the best treatment (292), some believe that patients do well without surgery (293–295), and others report surgery without specific indications (294, 295). A close look at the outcomes and complications of this disease leads the modern orthopaedist to conclude that the most predictable treatment with highest likelihood of rapid and complete eradication of infection and the lowest chance of late sequelae utilizes surgical drainage in addition to antibiotic therapy. Early diagnosis and prompt drainage of an abscess, especially in an area of infarction, may result in outcomes comparable with normal children having the usual course of pyogenic osteomyelitis.

The question of using a tourniquet in patients with sickle cell disease who are undergoing extremity surgery is frequently raised because of the possibility that the ischemia may provoke thrombosis. This does not seem to be a problem; when the patient is properly prepared for surgery, no complications from the use of a tourniquet should result (296, 297). Appropriate precautions to reduce the incidence of vasoocclusive events include adequate preoperative hydration, avoidance of intraoperative hypothermia, and maintenance of adequate blood volume and oxygenation. Recent evidence suggests that preoperative transfusion to achieve a hemoglobin of at least 10 g/dL is recommended and is as effective at preventing vasoocclusive events as more aggressive exchange transfusion protocols that attempt to lower the sickle cell hemoglobin to a specific percentage (298).

The literature is contradictory as to whether *S. aureus* or *Salmonella* is the more common infectious agent in patients with sickle cell anemia (293, 294, 297), but this question has little clinical significance because both organisms must be covered by antibiotic therapy. An article reviewing the world literature since 1959 found *Salmonella* to be the most common (299). Initial antibiotic choices are cefotaxime (Claforan) or ceftriaxone (Rocephin), each of which covers both *S. aureus* and *Salmonella* species, including those *Salmonella* resistant to ampicillin, chloramphenicol, or trimethoprim-sulfamethoxazole (Bactrim) (Table 12-3). Initial antibiotics are administered intravenously, and conversion to oral antibiotic is made after

clinical and laboratory signs of effective treatment response for a total duration of therapy of approximately 4 to 6 weeks.

Arthritis may be seen in various forms in patients with sickle cell disease (300). The most common is an aseptic arthritis, most likely due to the sickle cell disease. It may be seen during crisis but is more often a transient synovitis, usually involving the knee, which resolves within 5 days (301, 302). A second form of aseptic arthritis is that associated with a remote *Salmonella* infection. This may be seen with other organisms, and the exact mechanism is not clear. Finally, the patient with sickle cell disease may have a septic arthritis. When this is the case, *Salmonella* is not the most likely organism. *Salmonella* is a rare organism in septic arthritis (302); when it occurs, it is most often in patients without sickle cell disease. When *Salmonella* septic arthritis occurs in patients with sickle cell anemia, it is most often from contiguous spread of osteomyelitis. More likely organisms in septic arthritis are *Staphylococcus* species (292, 303). As with osteomyelitis, there is a difference of opinion on the advisability of arthrotomy for drainage (292, 303).

Author's Preferred Treatment.   A 10-year-old child with known sickle cell disease presents following 24 hours of severe increasing bone pain.

The initial evaluation in the emergency department should include CBC with differential, ESR, CRP, blood cultures, plain film radiographs, technetium bone scan, and MRI. Admission to the hospital is recommended with initiation of hydration therapy, appropriate analgesia, and transfusion if necessary to achieve a hemoglobin of 10 g/dL. If the patient's symptoms improve significantly with initial therapy, management of the ischemic episode is continued. If symptoms are unchanged or worsen, laboratory studies, technetium bone scan, and MRI are repeated approximately 48 hours after admission. If laboratory values or imaging studies are equivocal or suggest osteomyelitis, bone aspiration for culture and Gram stain is performed. Bone aspiration is performed in the operating room because it is very difficult to aspirate through diaphyseal bone where osteomyelitis associated with sickle cell disease is most likely to reside. Empiric antibiotic therapy covering *Salmonella* and *S. aureus* is initiated and continued until culture results are available. If subperiosteal or bone abscess is encountered, surgical debridement is performed with wound closure over drains.

Tuberculosis.   Endemic in developing countries, there has been a recent resurgence of musculoskeletal infection caused by tuberculosis in developed countries as well (304). These data, which include patients of all ages, found 1985 to be the year with the lowest number of reported tuberculosis cases since the reporting began in 1953. However, since 1985, the incidence of tuberculosis has risen sharply. The largest increase has been reported for patients born outside of the United States and its territories. In 1993, these patients comprised almost 30% of the reported cases. California, New York, and Texas saw the largest increases. The increased incidence has been accompanied by HIV infection and multidrug-resistant organisms.

Because extrapulmonary tuberculosis is more common among children, particularly those younger than 5 years, the orthopaedic surgeon must again become aware of this possibility when evaluating chronic joint inflammation or chronic bone lesions. Patients who are exposed to tuberculosis may or may not become infected, and those who are infected may or may not become diseased. There is a time lag between infection and diagnosis of the extrapulmonary disease of approximately 1 year.

Most patients are infected by human contact following the inhalation of droplets containing *Mycobacterium tuberculosis*. In developing countries, bovine tuberculosis may occur following the ingestion of unpasteurized milk. The tubercle bacilli may disseminate to bones or joints during the lymphatic and hematogenous spread of the initial infection. If the initial lung infection remains untreated, involvement of the bones and/or joints occurs in 5% to 10% of children (304, 305). The development of the lesions in bone is time- and location-related. Dactylitis may occur within a few months in younger children. Long-bone involvement may occur in 1 to 3 years.

Compared with bacterial osteomyelitis, patients experiencing tuberculous osteomyelitis have a less acute onset with less severe symptoms, and delayed diagnosis is common. Patients with tuberculosis osteomyelitis are typically afebrile, have less pain, and may have normal laboratory values. Patients often experience local swelling, and initial radiographs may be normal (306). Osteolytic lesions develop with the focus of osteomyelitis usually in the metaphysis, occasionally in the epiphysis, and rarely in the diaphysis of long bones. Involvement of virtually any bone can occur (240, 307).

As the osteomyelitis develops, it enlarges the area of bone destruction in a centrifugal fashion, producing a characteristic round lytic lesion with ill-defined margins. These lesions are filled with an inflammatory granulation tissue, creating a reactive hyperemia, which produces a wide area of osteopenia surrounding the lesion. This process is almost purely destructive or lytic, with little or no bone reaction, no sclerotic margins, and no periosteal response. Because of the chronicity and hyperemia, widening and accelerated growth of the epiphysis may be seen. Similar to pyogenic infection, the physeal plate offers little resistance to the spread of the infection.

Skeletal tuberculosis most often affects the spine (308), usually in the anterior third of a vertebral body in the lower thoracic or the upper lumbar spine. The first lumbar vertebra is most commonly involved, whereas T10 infection is most commonly associated with neurologic deficit (309). Paravertebral abscess formation is characteristic, and calcification developing within the abscess is almost diagnostic of a tuberculous abscess. The discs become involved when two adjacent vertebral bodies are affected. The bone lesions in the vertebral bodies are mainly destructive. This frequently leads to kyphotic deformity, which becomes rigid when chronic. Patients with significant kyphosis often present with neurologic deficit (310).

Tuberculous arthritis usually affects the major joints, particularly the hip and knee (Fig. 12-10). Involvement of the hip may be especially debilitating (311). Isolated joint infections, unusual in childhood, are initially characterized by effusion in addition to synovial proliferation and thickening. In the early stages, there are no radiographic characteristics that separate tuberculous arthritis from any chronic inflammation of the joint. As with the bone lesions, the hyperemia causes widespread osteopenia and may cause overgrowth of the epiphyses. The infection proceeds both by pannus formation over the articular cartilage and by erosion of the subchondral bone, beginning at the synovial margins (312, 313). The result is joint space narrowing and subchondral cystic erosion. MRI may demonstrate central and peripheral erosions, active and chronic pannus, abscess, bone chips, and synovial changes (314).

As the infection continues untreated, large amounts of caseous material and pus accumulate and dissect along normal tissue planes. Eventually, a sinus track to the surface is formed—a hallmark of a long-standing neglected case. The abscess formed by tuberculous infection is called a *cold abscess* because of the lack of any signs of acute inflammation.

Two other presentations occur in childhood. The first, tuberculous dactylitis, may resemble sickle cell dactylitis, with swelling of the phalanges, metacarpals, and metatarsals. Tuberculous dactylitis is usually not very painful, however, and onset is usually consecutive rather than simultaneous. Before the availability of radiographs, this was called *spina* (Latin for "a short bone") *ventosa* (meaning "inflated with air"). The radiographs show a cyst-like expansion of the tubular bones, with thinning of the cortex (315). A second presentation is with multifocal cystic involvement of the bone. This is characterized by areas of simultaneous destruction in the shafts of long bones and in flat bones, with a strong tendency to symmetry (316).

The first and most important step in the diagnosis of tuberculous infection of the bone or joint is to consider it as a possibility. In addition, when tuberculosis is diagnosed, underlying HIV infection must also be considered. Tuberculosis should be considered whenever a chronic-appearing bone lesion is encountered. Early diagnosis is important to prevent spread to a contiguous joint. The clinical picture is variable, depending on the location and the stage of the disease. It is characterized by its insidious onset; lack of characteristic inflammatory features, such as erythema; and bone destruction or joint involvement greater than the symptoms would suggest.

Laboratory studies usually show a normal leukocyte count and an elevated ESR (311). The purified protein derivative skin test usually is positive. Radiographic changes are usually present at the time of presentation. The diagnosis depends on the identification of the organism *M. tuberculosis*. Positive cultures are obtained in 85.5% of patients who have both pulmonary and extrapulmonary diseases, in 83.5% of those with only pulmonary disease, and in 76.5% of those who have only extrapulmonary disease (317). *M. tuberculosis* is one organism that can be reliably diagnosed by PCR (318–320), and tissue should be sent for PCR testing whenever possible.

Tuberculosis produces a widespread synovial inflammation, which may lead the surgeon to obtain biopsy material that does not contain mycobacteria and results in negative cultures. In tuberculosis arthritis without bone involvement, the biopsy should be taken from the peripheral junction of the synovium with the bone, or preferably from the junction of the synovium with a cyst (321). In cases with bone lesions, the granulation tissue filling the destructive bone lesion is the best material for biopsy.

The treatment of skeletal tuberculosis is medical. Surgical debridement of the bone lesions is not necessary for a cure, although drainage of large abscesses often improves the patient's overall constitutional symptoms (316, 321, 322). In addition, open surgical biopsy is often necessary. Surgical treatment of the knee for early disease has been reported to achieve favorable results (323), whereas later-stage disease with joint space narrowing at presentation did not benefit from surgical treatment. Because of the effectiveness of drug therapy, there is little chance that surgical biopsy will lead to sinus formation. It is important to always be aware that superinfection with pyogenic organisms can occur, and this may be a reason for apparent treatment failure with antitubercular drugs. This is particularly true when a sinus has formed (322).

Patients with active tuberculosis infection of the spine often benefit from surgical treatment (310). Indications for surgery include neurologic involvement, spinal instability, and failure of medical treatment (324). Although patients with neurologic involvement can recover with medical management, they seem to do so faster with surgical management (325). Surgical treatment of the kyphosis produces a higher rate of union and less deformity than regimens without surgical stabilization (326, 327). Therefore, it appears that with contemporary surgical and anesthetic techniques, tuberculous kyphosis is best treated early with anterior surgery for debridement and strut grafting if indicated, as well as posterior instrumentation. The treatment of spinal instability, especially that spanning more than two disc spaces, is difficult and requires both anterior arthrodesis with strut grafting and posterior arthrodesis with instrumentation (328). Surgical treatment must be accompanied by antituberculous treatment for at least a year, as shorter treatment duration has been associated with recurrent disease (310).

Surgical treatment of chronic spine involvement is controversial and has shown inconsistent benefit over antituberculous treatment alone. Many cases do well with medical management only (325–327).

Although the effectiveness of ambulatory drug treatment has been demonstrated (326, 327), there is evidence of an increasing incidence of resistant strains, due most likely to inadequate treatment of the initial infection (317). This emphasizes both the need for constant surveillance for drug resistance and the importance of careful supervision of outpatient oral therapy to be certain that compliance is optimal.

Antimicrobial therapy should be of at least 9 months' duration, longer in children and immunocompromised hosts.

Initial antimicrobial agent selection depends on the likelihood of drug-resistant organisms, whereas long-term selection should be guided by susceptibility testing. In those who are not at high risk for drug-resistant organisms, various regimens of isoniazid, rifampin, and pyrazinamide are recommended (329). In children who come from areas where antibiotics are sold over the counter, where high rates of drug-resistant tuberculosis occur, and when incomplete treatment may have resulted in multidrug-resistant strains, ethambutol or streptomycin should be added to the standard three-drug regimen. Treatment of bone and joint tuberculosis in children should be continued for 1 year.

Subacute Osteomyelitis. Subacute osteomyelitis is characterized by insidious onset of pain, absence of systemic signs, and radiographic presence of a bone lesion at the time of presentation with no previous acute episode to suggest evolution of an acute osteomyelitis to a chronic form (330). Subacute osteomyelitis is becoming an increasingly prevalent form of musculoskeletal infection and often results in a diagnostic and treatment dilemma (11). Because symptoms are often insidious in onset and less severe than in acute osteomyelitis, diagnosis is often delayed (331).

The atypical nature of subacute osteomyelitis is presumed to result from an increased host resistance, decreased virulence of the causative organism, and possible antibiotic exposure, causing alteration in the host–pathogen relationship. As a result, children typically present without the typical features of osteomyelitis, having only a mild limp or an intermittent pain of at least 1- to 2-week duration. Systemic symptoms such as fever, malaise, and anorexia are absent. Supportive laboratory data are often inconsistent. The leukocyte count is usually normal or only slightly elevated. The ESR is usually elevated, although usually not as high as in AHO, and CRP is often normal (332). Blood cultures are usually negative (333), although curettings from the lesions are frequently culture positive, usually for *S. aureus*. Histology is compatible with acute and chronic inflammation.

Subacute osteomyelitis most frequently involves lower extremity long bones, but the upper extremity, axial skeleton, hand, or foot may be involved (241, 333–335). Technetium-99 bone scintigraphy is very sensitive for subacute osteomyelitis and can be helpful when the location of a suspected lesion is unclear.

Standard radiographs show an abnormality in most patients, but the lesions often appear similar to neoplasm or other diagnoses. The radiographic classification system initially proposed by Gledhill (336) and modified by Roberts et al. (335) (Fig. 12-15) facilitates establishing a diagnosis. The most common type of subacute osteomyelitis in the pediatric age group is the metaphyseal lesion (types IA and IB) (337). This represents a true Brodie abscess, a localized abscess of bone without previous acute illness. The lesion is located eccentrically in the metaphysis, with frequent visible extension into the epiphysis. The second most common type is the epiphyseal lesion (type V)

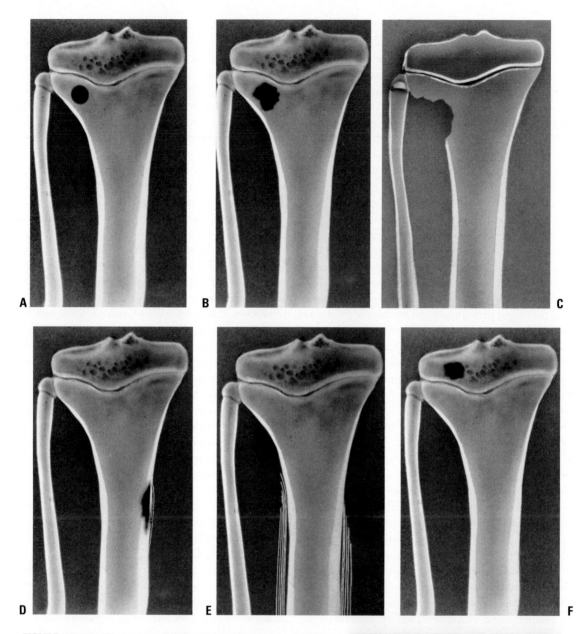

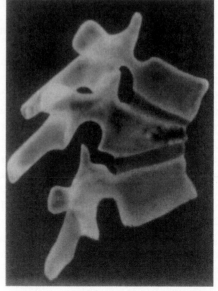

FIGURE 12-15.   The variety of presentations of subacute hematogenous osteomyelitis in the classification of Roberts et al. **A:** Type IA is a punched-out metaphyseal lesion resembling an eosinophilic granuloma. **B:** Type IB is similar to type IA, but has a sclerotic cortex. **C:** Type II lesions erode the metaphyseal bone, often including the cortex, and appear as aggressive lesions. **D:** Type III lesions are localized cortical and periosteal reactions, simulating osteoid osteoma. **E:** Type IV lesions produce onionskin-like periosteal reactions in the diaphysis and resemble Ewing sarcoma. **F:** Type V lesions are epiphyseal erosions. **G:** Type VI lesions involve the vertebral bodies. (From Roberts JM, Drummond DS, Breed AL, et al. Subacute hematogenous osteomyelitis in children: a retrospective study. *J Pediatr Orthop* 1982;2:249–254.)

(338–340). The radiographic appearance is similar to the lesion in the metaphysis, and it also may extend across the physis into the metaphysis. Despite crossing the physis, subacute osteomyelitis rarely causes permanent growth alteration (332).

The differential diagnosis for subacute osteomyelitis is dependent upon the radiographic appearance and the subtype of the lesion. The differential diagnoses for type I lesions include eosinophilic granuloma and, rarely, giant cell tumor. Type II metaphyseal lesions can mimic osteosarcoma, if aggressive, or metastatic neuroblastoma. Type III lesions cause cortical reaction and thickening and can be mistaken for an osteoid osteoma. The periosteal reaction seen in type IV lesions is a finding also seen with Ewing sarcoma. The differential diagnoses for type V lesions in the epiphysis include chondroblastoma, osteoid osteoma, eosinophilic granuloma, or enchondroma.

MRI and CT are helpful when characterizing an unknown lesion. CT has the advantage of being relatively inexpensive and more readily available, whereas MRI provides greater information about soft tissues, bone, and marrow edema. A characteristic "penumbra sign," which is reportedly helpful in differentiating subacute osteomyelitis from neoplasm, has been described on T1-weighted MR images (341).

Ross and Cole (309) divided the lesions into two categories: aggressive lesions and more benign-appearing cavities in the region of the metaphysis and epiphysis. All of the lesions in the aggressive group that were in the diaphysis or metaphysis demonstrated onionskin periosteal new bone. The other lesions were all in the metaphysis or epiphysis and had the typical radiologic features of type I and V lesions described in the preceding text. Benign-appearing epiphyseal and metaphyseal cavities were treated with 48 hours of intravenous semisynthetic penicillin or first-generation cephalosporin followed by 6 weeks of oral antibiotic. Eighty-seven percent of the children treated with antibiotics alone healed their lesion. Antibiotic treatment failure was associated with increased patient age. Hamdy reported similar successful results with antibiotic treatment alone for benign-appearing lesions (333). Aggressive lesions, where the diagnosis cannot be conclusively determined, should be biopsied and treated with curettage if osteomyelitis is confirmed (342).

Therefore, subacute osteomyelitis is distinctly different from acute or chronic osteomyelitis in that it responds predictably to antibiotic therapy, and surgical debridement is often unnecessary (11, 241, 309, 332, 333). Recommendations for route and duration of antibiotic treatment may vary, but the choice of antibiotic should cover *S. aureus* and typically consists of 2 to 7 days of parenteral antibiotics followed by oral antibiotics for a total treatment duration of 4 to 6 weeks. Surgery should be reserved for aggressive lesions and cases that do not respond to antibiotic therapy.

Myositis. Myositis is a spontaneous muscle infection prevalent in the developing world, accounting for up to 3% to 5% of hospital admissions (11, 343). Because pyomyositis is being reported with increased frequency in developed countries and

commonly affects the musculature about the hip, where it may confound the diagnosis of septic arthritis, all orthopaedists should be aware of the condition (344–348).

Because skeletal muscle inherently is resistant to bacterial infection, pyogenic muscle abscesses are infrequent. The development of pyomyositis, in the absence of penetrating trauma, presumably requires the coexistence of bacteremia and alterations in the microenvironment that facilitate the sequestration and proliferation of organisms. Many patients report a recent history of strenuous physical activity, which may in some way initiate the infectious process (217, 349). Once bacterial proliferation begins, pyomyositis may progress through three stages during which clinical findings parallel the progression from diffuse inflammation to focal suppuration. The initial, invasive stage involves the insidious onset of dull, cramping pain, with or without low-grade fevers that progresses over 10 to 21 days. An increase in the magnitude of symptoms, associated with systemic signs, heralds the suppurative phase of the disease. Most patients present during this stage, and physical findings are more focal. The late stage includes fluctuations and more profound systemic manifestations that require urgent treatment (350).

Although there does appear to be a propensity for involvement of muscles in the thigh and hip regions, other sites of involvement in children have included the chest wall, psoas, glutei, adductors, obturator internus and externus, quadriceps, hamstrings, gastrocsoleus, paraspinals, infraspinatus, subscapularis, biceps, triceps, and forearm muscles.

The differential diagnoses included with myositis typically include neoplasm, osteomyelitis, hematoma, and deep muscle contusion. The diagnosis is often delayed, and treatment mistakenly directed at incorrect diagnoses is common (109). Sedimentation rate is almost always elevated, and WBC count often is abnormal. Clinicians may have a strong sense of the presence of an infection but have difficulty localizing the source. Blood cultures are occasionally positive, and wound cultures frequently grow a causative organism, most often *S. aureus* (217, 351, 352). *Streptococcus pyomyositis* has been associated with varicella infection in children (353).

Ultrasonography and CT can identify fluid collections and provide guidance for placement of a drainage catheter. MRI provides excellent soft-tissue detail and can identify abscesses and coexisting regional pathology such as septic arthritis and osteomyelitis and therefore is the imaging modality most ideally suited for evaluation of myositis (217, 352, 354). MRI with gadolinium enhancement may be able to differentiate between the invasive and purulent stages of the disease. This distinction is important because nonsuppurative myositis can usually be treated with antibiotic therapy alone, while abscess formation is typically an indication for surgical or percutaneous drainage (109).

The treatment of pyomyositis depends on the stage in which it is diagnosed. Early stages of disease may be treated successfully with antibiotics. Later stages in which abscesses have formed require drainage. Although historically open surgical drainage has been used, recent reports have suggested that percutaneous drainage in conjunction with appropriate antibiotic therapy is efficacious (109). Empiric intravenous antibiotic therapy with good *Staphylococcus* coverage is recommended. Conversion to oral antibiotic is appropriate following clinical response to treatment. Because of the excellent healing potential of skeletal muscle, antibiotic therapy should not need to be continued for as long as it would be for osteomyelitis. Duration of antibiotics should range from 2 to 4 weeks. With appropriate drainage and antibiotic treatment, persistent or recurrent infection is uncommon.

Psoas Abscess. Psoas abscess is a bacterial infection that forms within or on the surface of the iliopsoas muscle. Psoas abscess may arise primary or secondary to associated conditions such as appendicitis, inflammatory bowel disease, discitis, or vertebral osteomyelitis. Differentiation of a psoas abscess from septic arthritis of the hip can be a diagnostic challenge made difficult by the wide variability in clinical presentation of children with psoas abscess and the uncommon occurrence of the condition.

Investigators in eastern Ontario reviewed 20 years of clinical data at 2 major pediatric hospitals and identified 11 children with an average age at presentation of 8 years who were treated for psoas abscess (355). All 11 patients had pseudoparalysis of the hip with apparent flexion contracture and pain with active or passive motion in all planes. Additional symptoms may include limp, groin pain and swelling, back pain, abdominal pain, genitourinary pain, and thigh pain (356).

The "psoas sign" has been described as being useful in differentiating septic arthritis from psoas abscess. It is performed by determining hip pain during ROM when the hip is in a flexed versus an extended position. When the hip is flexed, tension on the psoas is relaxed, and the patient with a psoas abscess may have minimal pain with hip internal and external rotation, whereas the patient with septic arthritis will have significant pain with the same motion. Extending the hip places the psoas muscle and the hip capsule under tension, resulting in severe pain with internal and external rotation in both patient groups. This sign is useful when present but is not very specific, with many patients ultimately diagnosed with psoas abscess having significant hip irritability in all positions, including flexion. Other patients may have no hip pain whatsoever. Atypical features such as femoral nerve neuropraxias or bladder irritability associated with hip pain are signs that may assist clinicians in differentiating between septic arthritis of the hip and psoas abscess.

Sedimentation rate and leukocyte count have been elevated in more than 98% of patients reported in the literature (355). Plain film radiography is rarely useful in establishing a diagnosis; CT, MRI, and ultrasound are most helpful. Frequently the hip is aspirated, and occasionally debridement is performed before the diagnosis of psoas abscess is made.

Once identified, a psoas abscess requires appropriate antibiotic treatment and, typically, drainage. The most common infecting organism is *S. aureus* (356). Traditionally, drainage has been performed surgically, but more recently CT or ultrasound-guided percutaneous drainage has achieved equally successful results (357). Duration of antibiotic therapy has varied from 3 weeks to 6 months depending on clinical response and normalization of sedimentation rate. Typically, most psoas abscesses can successfully be eradicated with adequate drainage and 3 to 6 weeks of appropriate antibiotic therapy.

Necrotizing Fasciitis. Necrotizing fasciitis is a rare but life-threatening infectious process that involves the deep dermis and the underlying fascia that must be treated emergently to avoid devastating consequences. Mortality associated with necortizing fasciitis in children has been reported in 5% to 20% of cases (358–361). Necrotizing fasciitis may occur without identifiable trauma, minor trauma, major trauma, or postoperatively. In 70% of cases, the lower extremity is involved (362), but upper extremity involvement has been described as well (363). Group A β-hemolytic *Streptococcus* is the most common bacteria but MRSA is becoming more common and up to 75% of infections may be polymicrobial (359). Varicella infection been identified as a predisposing risk factor in Streptococcal necrotizing fasciitis (358, 360). Group A Strep species containing the speC gene and ST-15/emm-3 genetic sequences have been associated with necrotizing fasciitis as well (364, 365). The use of nonsteroidal anti-inflammatory drugs (NSAIDs) has been questioned as a possible risk factor for developing necrotizing fasciitis and while an association has been established a causal relationship has not (366).

Initial clinical findings are often unimpressive, frequently consisting of merely a painful area of cellulitis. Necrotizing fasciitis, more fulminant cellulitis, skin bullae, ecchymoses, fever, tachycardia, and hemodynamic instability may follow (358, 361). It is the combination of rapidly progressive soft-tissue infection associated with hemodynamic instability that suggests the presence of necrotizing fasciitis. Ultrasound, CT, and MRI have been used to demonstrate fascial involvement, but definitive diagnosis is made by biopsy demonstrating involvement of skin, subcutaneous tissue, and underling fascia. Early diagnosis surgical treatment is imperative and should not be delayed by imaging studies. Emergent aggressive surgical debridement of all nonviable tissue is essential. Skin and subcutaneous tissue are often involved, muscle is typically spared, while the fascia is the primary focus of infection. "Dirty dishwater"-like fluid is usually encountered in fascial planes, which must be decompressed and irrigated. Open wound packing prevents reaccumulation of infected fluid, allows continued tissue decompression, and is followed by repeat irritation and debridement. Initial antibiotic treatment should include high-dose penicillin for Strep coverage as well as

Vancomycin for possible MRSA and then adjusted based on culture results.

Chronic Recurrent Multifocal Osteomyelitis.

Chronic recurrent multifocal osteomyelitis (CRMO) is an inflammatory bone disease of uncertain etiology characterized by an unpredictable and prolonged course with exacerbations and spontaneous remissions occurring over a period of at least 6 months. Some affected children do not have multiple lesions or a recurrent course and the term "chronic nonbacterial osteomyelitis" has been suggested (367). It is a nonpyogenic inflammatory process with a lack of demonstrable causative agent, occurring predominantly during childhood and adolescence (368). An increasing body of evidence is accumulating that suggests CRMO is an autoimmune process that may have a genetic basis. Reviewing 89 patients with CRMO, Jansson et al. (369) in Munich noted that 20% of all the patients demonstrated associ-

ated autoimmune disorders, particularly of the skin and the bowel, and 30% of patients had elevation in ANAs. The presence of autoimmune diseases in 40% of all the families and multiply affected family members led authors to suggest a genetic basis for CRMO.

At initial presentation, CRMO is often indistinguishable from bacterial osteomyelitis. The most common presenting symptom is local bone pain at one or more sites, often associated with fever. Girls are affected in approximately 70% of the cases (370). WBC is typically normal, but ESR and CRP are often elevated, and radiographs frequently show a lytic destructive lesion in a long bone metaphysis (368).

The characteristic metaphyseal lesions are usually well developed. These lesions consist of poorly delimited eccentric metaphyseal lucencies along the physeal border (Fig. 12-16). The lesions have been shown to cross into the epiphysis (371, 372). As healing occurs, sclerosis surrounds the lesion. When

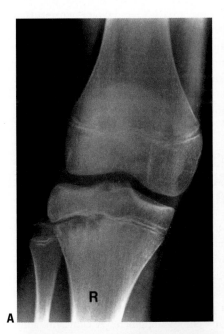
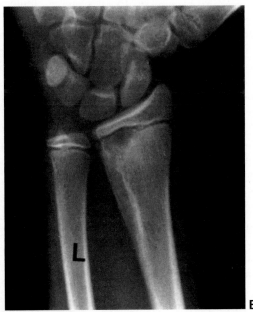
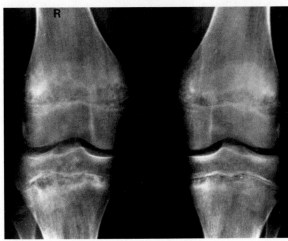

FIGURE 12-16. A: A 12-year-old girl presented with a recurrent limp over a period of 18 months. She complained of pain in the right knee. Examination demonstrated tenderness about the right knee, but no other signs of inflammation. Radiograph of the right knee showed metaphyseal irregularity of the proximal tibia. **B:** Skeletal survey demonstrated additional similar lesions in the opposite knee, distal tibia, and radius. These lesions were asymptomatic. **C:** Radiographs 1 year later show diffuse metaphyseal changes of the distal femur and proximal tibia of both legs. No antibiotics were administered, and the symptoms resolved over the next several months.

the lesion extends into the cortex, periosteal reaction may occur. This is more likely to be seen early in the course in the small tubular and flat bones. This picture can be confused with bony neoplasm, such as leukemia, Ewing sarcoma, or eosinophilic granuloma.

The most common sites for these lesions are the distal and proximal metaphyses of the tibia and femur, and there may be a tendency for symmetric involvement. Other affected sites are the distal radius and ulna, the distal fibula, and the metatarsals, as well as the medial aspect of bones in the anterior chest wall. When the clavicle is involved, it typically presents as a chronic sclerosing osteomyelitis originating at the medial end and may demonstrate both lucencies and an onionskin periosteal reaction (373). Multifocal involvement is present in over 90% of patients but is often not simultaneous (368). Frequently, patients may experience a single symptomatic lesion but have other asymptomatic lesions that are identifiable with bone scan, making technetium-99 bone scintigraphy very helpful at establishing multifocal involvement and the diagnosis of CRMO, sometime before lesions are visible on plain film radiographs. CRMO is associated with a variety of other curious disorders of bone and skin, including chronic sclerosing osteomyelitis of Garré, hyperostosis of the clavicle (374), sternocostoclavicular hyperostosis (375), and palmoplantar pustulosis (376–378). Because CRMO may be indistinguishable from bacterial osteomyelitis at initial presentation, bone culture and biopsy are often performed. Histopathologic features include chronic inflammation with a variety of cell types, occasional necrotic bone fragments, and fibrosis without the acute inflammation associated with bacterial osteomyelitis. Infiltration with fibrovascular tissue and inflammatory cells, followed by osteoblast proliferation and trabecular thickening, have been noted in later stages of the disease (261, 370, 377).

Response to anti-inflammatory drugs is predictable, with 90% of patients experiencing significant improvement in symptoms (368). Corticosteroids and interferon-γ have also been used on a limited basis with success (379). The mainstay of CRMO treatment is scheduled NSAID use during periods of exacerbations. A recent report suggests that Indomethacin may be especially effective (380). For those patients having inadequate response to NSAID therapy, the use of bisphosphonates is a promising new treatment (381–383).

The time from onset of illness to remission of symptoms is 3 to 5 years, by which time CRMO seems to burn itself out, but a minority of patients may experience a prolonged course despite intensive treatment (384). No association has been observed between the number of lesions and the response to treatment or outcome. Long-term sequelae are rare, but premature closure of a physis, bone deformity, kyphosis, chronic pain, and thoracic outlet syndrome have been reported (356, 385–387).

When associated with synovitis, acne, pustulosis, hyperostosis, and osteitis, the condition is called SAPHO syndrome (388). Like CRMO, SAPHO etiology has not been determined. There is speculation of a genetic predisposition, with immunologic response to an infective agent. *Propionibacterium acnes*, a skin saprophyte, has been detected in the cutaneous lesions of severe acne and in the articular and osseous lesions associated with pustulosis. However, most biopsies of involved areas are negative, demonstrating nonspecific inflammatory infiltrate. CRMO has also been associated with psoriasis and inflammatory bowel disease, lending further circumstantial evidence for an autoimmune-mediated cause (389, 390).

Almost certainly a variation in expression of the same disease, the SAPHO clinical course is similar to CRMO, characterized by recurrences and remissions; it is benign and self-limiting, with NSAID treatment usually effective at controlling symptoms. Chronic bone changes may persist, with the initial inflammatory changes being replaced by Paget-like features, including hypertrophic but inactive bone and fibrosis of the bone marrow (391).

Sclerosing osteomyelitis of Garré may be considered a unifocal form of CRMO and typically presents as an enlarged, painful segment of bone. The metaphysis of long bones and the mandible are the most commonly involved sites (11). Symptoms may fluctuate over time, resolving and then reappearing periodically over several years. Treatment typically consists of the symptomatic use of NSAIDs and bisphosphonates should be considered for refractory cases.

APPENDIX: A CLINICAL PRACTICE GUIDELINE FOR TREATMENT OF SEPTIC ARTHRITIS IN CHILDREN[1]

Clinical Practice Guidelines Disclaimer Statement: This Clinical Practice Guideline (Algorithm 12-1) is designed to provide clinicians an analytical framework for evaluation and treatment of a particular diagnosis or condition. It is not intended to establish a protocol or to identify all patients with a particular condition, nor is it intended to replace a clinician's clinical judgment. A clinician's adherence to this Clinical Practice Guideline is voluntary. It is understood that some patients will not fit into the clinical conditions contemplated by this Clinical Practice Guideline and that the recommendations contained in this Clinical Practice Guideline should not be considered inclusive of all proper methods or exclusive of other methods of care reasonably directed to obtaining the same results. Decisions to adopt any specific recommendation of this Clinical Practice Guideline must be made by the clinician in light of available resources and the individual circumstances presented by the patient.

---

[1]From Kocher MS, Mandiga R, Murphy JM, et al. A clinical practice guideline for treatment of septic arthritis in children: efficacy in improving process of care and effect on outcome of septic arthritis of the hip. *J Bone Joint Surg* 2003;85A:994–999, with permission.

Septic Arthritis CPG Algorithm

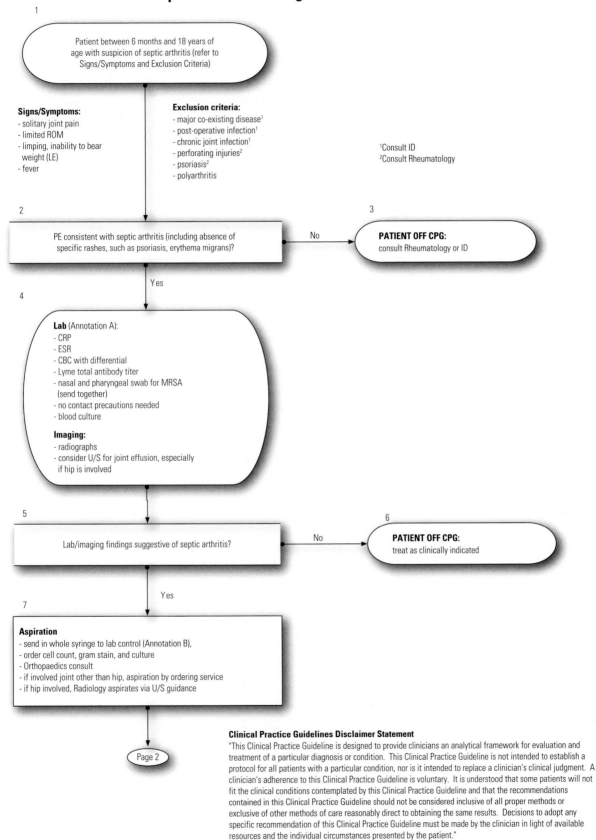

1

Patient between 6 months and 18 years of age with suspicion of septic arthritis (refer to Signs/Symptoms and Exclusion Criteria)

Signs/Symptoms:
- solitary joint pain
- limited ROM
- limping, inability to bear weight (LE)
- fever

Exclusion criteria:
- major co-existing disease[1]
- post-operative infection[1]
- chronic joint infection[1]
- perforating injuries[2]
- psoriasis[2]
- polyarthritis

[1]Consult ID
[2]Consult Rheumatology

2

PE consistent with septic arthritis (including absence of specific rashes, such as psoriasis, erythema migrans)?

No →

3

PATIENT OFF CPG:
consult Rheumatology or ID

Yes

4

Lab (Annotation A):
- CRP
- ESR
- CBC with differential
- Lyme total antibody titer
- nasal and pharyngeal swab for MRSA (send together)
- no contact precautions needed
- blood culture

Imaging:
- radiographs
- consider U/S for joint effusion, especially if hip is involved

5

Lab/imaging findings suggestive of septic arthritis?

No →

6

PATIENT OFF CPG:
treat as clinically indicated

Yes

7

Aspiration
- send in whole syringe to lab control (Annotation B),
- order cell count, gram stain, and culture
- Orthopaedics consult
- if involved joint other than hip, aspiration by ordering service
- if hip involved, Radiology aspirates via U/S guidance

Page 2

Clinical Practice Guidelines Disclaimer Statement
"This Clinical Practice Guideline is designed to provide clinicians an analytical framework for evaluation and treatment of a particular diagnosis or condition. This Clinical Practice Guideline is not intended to establish a protocol for all patients with a particular condition, nor is it intended to replace a clinician's clinical judgment. A clinician's adherence to this Clinical Practice Guideline is voluntary. It is understood that some patients will not fit the clinical conditions contemplated by this Clinical Practice Guideline and that the recommendations contained in this Clinical Practice Guideline should not be considered inclusive of all proper methods or exclusive of other methods of care reasonably direct to obtaining the same results. Decisions to adopt any specific recommendation of this Clinical Practice Guideline must be made by the clinician in light of available resources and the individual circumstances presented by the patient."

Septic Arthritis CPG Algorithm

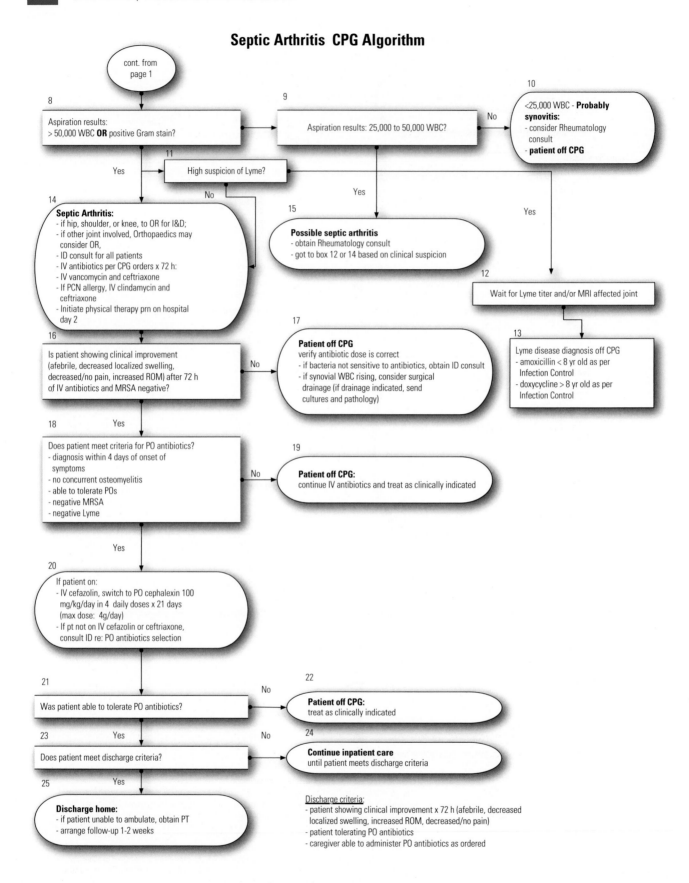

Septic Arthritis CPG Algorithm Annotations

Annotation A: Preliminary work-up laboratory information

Test	Blood Specimen Amount	Type of Tube Used with Patient Label	Form to Complete:	For:	Send Specimen To:	Results returned:
CRP C-Reaction Protein	Minimum 1 mL	Mint green top tube	Hematology/ Chemistry	Core Lab	Lab Control	3 d
Sed Rate (ESR) Erythrocyte Sedimentation Rate	2 mL	Lavender top tube	Hematology/ Chemistry	Hematology	Lab Control	< 4 h
CBC/Plt + Diff Complete Blood Count, Platelets and Differential	Minimum 1 mL ***Mix specimen by gentle inversion x10**	Lavender top tube	Hematology/ Chemistry	Hematology	Lab Control	Stat: 30 min Routine: 1 h
Lyme Titer	3 mL	Red top tube	Children's Hospital Misc. Form	ARUP laboratory	Lab Control	3 d
Blood Culture	5 mL: 1 mL minimum into Aerobic btl	Blood culture bottles	Bacteriology ***State clinical diagnosis**	Bacteriology	Lab Control	Prelim: 24 h and 48 h Final negative 6 d
Rapid Strep Throat Culture	N/A	Culturette Swab (two swabs)	1. Misc form 2. Bacteriology	Hematology Bacteriology	Lab Control	48 h
ASLO	1 mL	Red top tube	**Heme/Chem**	ARUP laboratory	Lab Control	2–5 d

Annotation B: Aspiration Laboratory Information

Aspirates	Blood Specimen Amount	Type of Tube Used with Patient Label	Form to Complete:	For:	Send Specimen To:	Results returned:
Cell count	1–2 mL	Sterile tube or send joint aspirate in its syringe	Hematology/Chemistry **Use Other Fluid column** ***Requisition must state specific site of specimen, age of patient and clinical diagnosis**	Hematology	Lab Control	Stat: 1 h Routine: 2 h
Gram stain	Minimum 2 drops or one swab ***If culture to be included, minimum two swabs and 0.5 mL**	Sterile specimen container, or sterile tub or appropriate tub for swab. Or send joint aspirate in its syringe	Bacteriology **Use wound, tissue, fluid, bone, bone marrow section C&S (gram)** ***Requisition must state specific site of specimen, age of patient and clinical diagnosis**	Bacteriology	Lab Control **asap**	**Stat: 1 h Routine: 8–12 h**

REFERENCES

1. Floyed RL, Steele RW. Culture negative osteomyelitis. *Pediatr Infect Dis J* 2003;22:731–736.
2. Morrey BF, Peterson HA. Hematogenous pyogenic osteomyelitis in children. *Orthop Clin North Am* 1975;6:935–951.
3. Peltola H, Vahvanen V. A comparative study of osteomyelitis and purulent arthritis with special reference to aetiology and recovery. *Infection* 1984;12:75–79.
4. Morrey BF, Bianco AJ Jr, Rhodes KH. Septic arthritis in children. *Orthop Clin North Am* 1975;6:923–934.
5. Sonnen GM, Henry NK. Pediatric bone and joint infections: diagnosis and antimicrobial management. *Pediatr Clin North Am* 1996;43:933–947.
6. Krogstad P, Smigh AL. Osteomyelitis and septic arthritis. In: Feigin RD, Cherry JD, eds. *Textbook of pediatric infectious diseases*. Philadelphia, PA: WB Saunders, 1998:683–704.
7. Gutierrez KM. Osteomyelitis. In: Long SS, Pickering LK, Prober CG, eds. *Principles and practice of pediatric infectious diseases*. New York, NY: Churchill Livingstone, 1997:528–536.
8. Riise OR, Kirkhus E, Handeland KS, et al. Childhood osteomyelitis-incidence and differentiation from other acute onset musculoskeletal features in a population-based study. *BMC Pediatr* 2008;8:45.
9. Gillespie WJ, Nade SML. *Musculoskeletal infections*. Melbourne, Australia: Blackwell Scientific, 1987.
10. Dormans J, Drummond DS. Pediatric hematogenous osteomyelitis: new trends in presentation, diagnosis, and treatment. *J Am Acad Orthop Surg* 1994:333–341.
11. Macnicol MF. Patterns of musculoskeletal infection in childhood. *J Bone Joint Surg* 2001;83B:1–2.
12. Blyth MJ, Kincaid R, Craigen MA, et al. The changing epidemiology of acute and subacute haematogenous osteomyelitis in children. *J Bone Joint Surg Br* 2001;83:99–102.
13. Karwowska A, Davies HD, Jadavji T. Epidemiology and outcome of osteomyelitis in the era of sequential intravenous-oral therapy. *Pediatr Infect Dis J* 1998;17:1021–1026.
14. Khachatourians AG, Patzakis MJ, Roidis N, et al. Laboratory monitoring in pediatric acute osteomyelitis and septic arthritis. *Clin Orthop* 2003;409:186–194.
15. Peltola H, Kallio MJ, Unkila-Kallio L. Reduced incidence of septic arthritis in children by *Haemophilus influenzae* type-b vaccination: implications for treatment. *J Bone Joint Surg Br* 1998;80:471–473.
16. Song KM, Sloboda JF. Acute hematogenous osteomyelitis in children. *J Am Acad Orthop Surg* 2001;9:166–175.
17. Wang CL, Wang SM, Yang YJ, et al. Septic arthritis in children: relationship of causative pathogens, complications and outcomes. *J Microbiol Immunol Infect* 2003;36:41–46.
18. Howard AW, Viskontas D, Sabbagh C. Reduction in osteomyelitis and septic arthritis related to *Haemophilus influenzae* type B vaccination. *J Pediatr Orthop* 1999;19:705–709.
19. Bowerman SG, Green NE, Mencio GA. Decline of bone and joint infections attributable to *Haemophilus influenzae* type B. *Clin Orthop* 1997;341:128–133.
20. Yagupsky P, Dagan R. *Kingella kingae*: an emerging cause of invasive infections in young children. *Clin Infect Dis* 1997;24:860–866.
21. Kiang KM, Ogunmodede F, Juni BA, et al. Outbreak of osteomyelitis/septic arthritis caused by *Kingella kingae* among child care center attendees. *Pediatrics* 2005;116(2):E206–E213.
22. Yagupsky P, Erlich Y, Ariela S, et al. Outbreak of *Kingella kingae* skeletal system infections in children in daycare. *Pediatr Infect Dis* 2006;25(6):526–532.
23. Dodman T, Robson J, Pincus D. *Kingella kingae* infections in children. *J Paediatr Child Health* 2000;36:87–90.
24. Lebel E, Rudensky B, Karasik M, et al. *Kingella kingae* infections in children. *J Pediatr Orthop B* 2006;15(4):289–292.
25. Moumile K, Merckx J, Glorion C, et al. Bacterial aetiology of acute osteo-articular infections in children. *Acta Paediatr* 2005;94(4):419–422.
26. Yagupsky P. *Kingella Kingae*: from medical rarity to an emerging paediatric pathogen. *Lancet Infect Dis* 2004;4(6):358–367.
27. Dubnov-Raz G, Scheuerman O, Chodick G, et al. Invasive *Kingella kingae* infections in children: clinical and laboratory characteristics. *Pediatrics* 2008;122(6):1305–1309.
28. Newton PO, Ballock RT, Bradley JS. Oral antibiotic therapy of bacterial arthritis. *Pediatr Infect Dis J* 1999;18:1102–1103.
29. Peltola H, Unkila-Kallio L, Kallio MJ. Simplified treatment of acute staphylococcal osteomyelitis of childhood. *Pediatrics* 1997;99:846–850.
30. Perlman MH, Patzakis MJ, Kumar PJ, et al. The incidence of joint involvement with adjacent osteomyelitis in pediatric patients. *J Pediatr Orthop* 2000;20:40–43.
31. Gafur OA, Copley LA, Hollmig ST, et al. The impact of the current epidemiology of pediatric musculoskeletal infection on evaluation and treatment guidelines. *J Ped Orthop* 2008;28(7):777–785.
32. Hobo T. Zur pathogenese de akuten haematogenen osteomyelitis, mit berucksichtigungder vitalfarbungs leher. *Acta Scolar Med Kioto* 1921;4:1–29.
33. Speers DJ, Nade SML. Ultrastructural studies of *Staphylococcus aureus* in experimental acute haematogenous osteomyelitis. *Infect Immun* 1985;49:443.
34. Cunningham R, Cockayne A, Humphreys H. Clinical and molecular aspects of the pathogenesis of *Staphylococcus aureus* bone and joint infections. *J Med Microbiol* 1996;44:157–164.
35. Dich VQ, Nelson JD, Haltalin KC. Osteomyelitis in infants and children. *Am J Dis Child* 1975;129:1273–1278.
36. Gilmour WN. Acute hematogenous osteomyelitis. *J Bone Joint Surg Br* 1962;44:842.
37. Manche E, Rombouts-Godin V, Rombouts JJ. Acute hematogenous osteomyelitis due to ordinary germs in children with closed injuries: study of a series of 44 cases. *Acta Orthop Belg* 1991;57:91–96.
38. Shandling B. Acute hematogenous osteomyelitis: a review of 300 cases treated during 1953–1959. *South Afr Med J* 1960;34:520.
39. Watson RJ, Burko H, Megas H, et al. The hand-foot syndrome in sickle cell disease in young children. *Pediatrics* 1963;31:975.
40. Morrissy RT, Haynes DW. Acute hematogenous osteomyelitis: a model with trauma as an etiology. *J Pediatr Orthop* 1989;9:447.
41. Whalen JL, Fitzgerald RH Jr, Morrissy RT. A histological study of acute hematogenous osteomyelitis following physeal injuries in rabbits. *J Bone Joint Surg Am* 1988;70:1383–1392.
42. Olney BW, Papasian CJ, Jacobs RR. Risk of iatrogenic septic arthritis in the presence of bacteremia: a rabbit study. *J Pediatr Orthop* 1987;7:524–526.
43. Schurman DJ, Mirra J, Ding A, et al. Experimental *E. coli* arthritis in the rabbit: a model of infectious and post-infectious inflammatory synovitis. *J Rheumatol* 1977;4:118–128.
44. Clark P, Davidson D, Letts M, et al. Necrotizing fasciitis secondary to chickenpox infection in children. *Can J Surg* 2003;46:9–14.
45. Mills WJ, Mosca VS, Nizet V. Orthopaedic manifestations of invasive group A streptococcal infections complicating primary varicella. *J Pediatr Orthop* 1996;16:522–528.
46. Schenk RK, Wiener J, Spiro D. Fine structural aspects of vascular invasion of the tibial epiphyseal plate of growing rats. *Acta Anat* 1968;69:1–17.
47. Tiku K, Tiku ML, Skosey JL. Interleukin-1 production by human polymorphonuclear neutrophils. *J Immunol* 1986;136:3677–3685.
48. Dinarello CA, Cannon JG, Mier W, et al. Multiple biological activities of human recombinant interleukin-1. *J Clin Invest* 1986;77:1734–1739.
49. Trueta J. The normal vascular anatomy of the human femoral head during growth. *J Bone Joint Surg Br* 1957;39:358.
50. Johnson AH, Campbell WG, Callahan BC. Infection of rabbit knee joints after intra-articular injection of *Staphylococcus aureus*. *Am J Pathol* 1970;60:165–202.
51. Gruber BF, Miller BS, Onnen J, et al. Antibacterial properties of synovial fluid in the knee. *J Knee Surg* 2008;21(3):180–185.
52. Arvidson S, Holme T, Lindholm B. The formation of extracellular proteolytic enzymes by *Staphylococcus aureus*. *Acta Pathol Microbiol Scand* 1972;80:835–844.
53. Dingle JT. The role of lysomal enzymes in skeletal tissue. *J Bone Joint Surg Br* 1973;55:87.

54. Harris ED, McCroskery PA. The influence of temperature and fibril stability on degradation of cartilage collagen by rheumatoid synovial collagenase. *N Engl J Med* 1974;290:1–6.

55. Harris EDJ, Parker HG, Radin EL, et al. Effects of proteolytic enzymes on structural and mechanical properties of cartilage. *Arthritis Rheum* 1972;15:497–503.

56. Oronsky A, Ignarro L, Perper R. Release of cartilage mucopolysaccharide-degrading neutral protease from human leukocytes. *J Exp Med* 1973;138:461–472.

57. Steinberg JJ, Sledge CB. Co-cultivation models of joint destruction. In: Dingle JT, Gordon JL, eds. *Cellular interactions.* Amsterdam, the Netherlands: Elsevier/North-Holland, 1981:263.

58. Smith L, Schurman DJ, Kajiyama G, et al. The effect of antibiotics on the destruction of cartilage in experimental infectious arthritis. *J Bone Joint Surg Am* 1987;69:1063–1068.

59. Curtiss PHJ, Klein L. Destruction of articular cartilage in septic arthritis. I. In vitro studies. *J Bone Joint Surg Am* 1963;45:797.

60. Curtiss PHJ, Klein L. Destruction of articular cartilage in septic arthritis. II. In vivo studies. *J Bone Joint Surg Am* 1965;47:1595–1604.

61. Daniel D, Akeson W, Amiel D, et al. Lavage of septic joints in rabbits: effects of chondrolysis. *J Bone Joint Surg Am* 1976;58:393–395.

62. Pessler F, Dai L, Diaz-Torne C, et al. Increased angiogenesis and cellular proliferation as hallmarks of the synovium in chronic septic arthritis. *Arthritis Rheum* 2008;59(8):1137–1146.

63. Faden H, Grossi M. Acute osteomyelitis in children: reassessment of etiologic agents and their clinical characteristics. *Am J Dis Child* 1991;145:65–69.

64. Scott RJ, Christofersen MR, Robertson WW Jr, et al. Acute osteomyelitis in children: a review of 116 cases. *J Pediatr Orthop* 1990;10:649–652.

65. Klein DM, Barbera C, Gray ST, et al. Sensitivity of objective parameters in the diagnosis of pediatric septic hips. *Clin Orthop* 1997;338:153–159.

66. Walsh S, Phillips F. Deep vein thrombosis associated with pediatric musculoskeletal sepsis. *J Pediatr Orthop* 2002;22:329–332.

67. Jackson MA, Nelson JD. Etiology and medical management of acute suppurative bone and joint infections in pediatric patients. *J Pediatr Orthop* 1982;2:313–323.

68. Peltola H, Vahvanen V, Aalto K. Fever, C-reactive protein, and erythrocyte sedimentation rate in monitoring recovery from septic arthritis: a preliminary study. *J Pediatr Orthop* 1984;4:170–174.

69. Pepys MB. C-reactive protein fifty years on. *Lancet* 1981;1:653–657.

70. Unkila-Kallio L, Kallio MJT, Eskola J, et al. Serum C-reactive protein, erythrocyte sedimentation rate, and white blood cell count in acute hematogenous osteomyelitis of children. *Pediatrics* 1994;93:59–62.

71. Roine I, Faingezich I, Arguedas A, et al. Serial serum C-reactive protein to monitor recovery from acute hematogenous osteomyelitis in children. *Pediatr Infect Dis J* 1995;14:40–44.

72. Levine MJ, McGuire KJ, McGowan KL, et al. Assessment of the test characteristics of C-reactive protein for septic arthritis in children. *J Pediatr Orthop* 2003;23:373–377.

73. Tejani N, Chonmaitree T, Rassin DK, et al. Use of C-reactive protein in differentiation between acute bacterial and viral otitis media. *Pediatrics* 1995;95:664–669.

74. Hoeffel DP, Hinrichs SH, Garvin KL. Molecular diagnostics for the detection of musculoskeletal infection. *Clin Orthop* 1999;360:37–46.

75. Mariani BD, Martin DS, Levine MJ, et al. Polymerase chain reaction detection of bacterial infection in total knee arthroplasty. *Clin Orthop* 1996;331:11–22.

76. Cherkaoui A, Ceroni D, Emonet S, et al. Molecular diagnosis of *Kingella kingae* osteoarticular infections by specific real-time PCR assay. *J Med Microbiol* 2009;58 (pt 1):65–68.

77. Chometon S, Benito Y, Chaker M, et al. Specific real-time polymerase chain reaction places *Kingella kingae* as the most common cause of osteoarticular infections in young children. *Pediatr Infect Dis J* 2007;26(5):377–381.

78. Verdier I, Gayet-Ageron A, Ploton C, et al. Contribution of a broad range polymerase chain reaction to the diagnosis of osteoarticular infections caused by *Kingella kingae*: description of twenty-four recent pediatric diagnoses. *Pediatr Infect Dis J* 2005;24(8):692–696.

79. Pineda C, Vargas A, Rodriguez AV. Imaging of osteomyelitis: current concepts. *Infect Dis Clin North Am* 2006;20(4):789–825.

80. Boutin RD, Brossmann J, Sartoris DJ, et al. Update on imaging of orthopedic infection. *Orthop Clin North Am* 1998;29:41–66.

81. Capitanio MA, Kirkpatrick JA. Early roentgen observations in acute osteomyelitis. *AJR Am J Roentgenol Radium Ther Nucl Med* 1970; 108:488–496.

82. Volberg FM, Sumner TE, Abramson JS, et al. Unreliability of radiographic diagnosis of septic hip in children. *Pediatrics* 1984;74: 118–120.

83. Cabanela ME, Sim FH, Beabout JW, et al. Osteomyelitis appearing as neoplasms: a diagnostic problem. *Arch Surg* 1974;109:68–72.

84. Lindenbaum S, Alexander H. Infections simulating bone tumors. *Clin Orthop* 1984;184:193–203.

85. Willis RB, Rozencwaig R. Pediatric osteomyelitis masquerading as skeletal neoplasia. *Orthop Clin North Am* 1996;27:625–634.

86. Howie DW, Savage JP, Wilson TG, et al. The technetium phosphate bone scan in the diagnosis of osteomyelitis in childhood. *J Bone Joint Surg Am* 1983;65:431–437.

87. Francis MD, Fogelman I. ^{99m}Tc diphosphonate uptake mechanism on bone. In: Fogelman I, ed. *Bone scanning in clinical practice*. London, UK: Springer-Verlag, 1987:7.

88. Mandell GA. Imaging in the diagnosis of musculoskeletal infections in children. *Curr Probl Pediatr* 1996;26:218–237.

89. Kothari NA, Pelchovitz DJ, Meyer JS. Imaging of musculoskeletal infections. *Radiol Clin N Am* 2001;39:653–671.

90. Canale ST, Harkness RM, Thomas PA, et al. Does aspiration of bones and joints affect results of later bone scanning? *J Pediatr Orthop* 1985;5: 23–26.

91. Tuson CE, Hoffman EB, Mann MD. Isotope bone scanning for acute osteomyelitis and septic arthritis in children. *J Bone Joint Surg Br* 1994;76:306–310.

92. Hod N, Home T. "Cold" and "hot" osteomyelitis on bone scintigraphy. *Clin Nucl Med* 2003;28(11):927–928.

93. Pennington WT, Mott MP, Thometz JG, et al. Photopenic bone scan osteomyelitis: a clinical perspective. *J Pediatr Orthop* 1999;19: 695–698.

94. Sundberg SB, Savage JP, Foster BK. Technetium phosphate bone scan in the diagnosis of septic arthritis in childhood. *J Pediatr Orthop* 1989;9:579–585.

95. Wong M, Isaacs D, Howman-Giles R, et al. Clinical and diagnostic features of osteomyelitis occurring in the first three months of life. *Pediatr Infect Dis J* 1995;14:1047–1053.

96. McCoy JR, Morrissy RT, Seibert J. Clinical experience with the technetium-99 scan in children. *Clin Orthop* 1981;154:175–180.

97. Kaiser S, Jacobsson H, Hirsch G. Specific or superfluous? Doubtful clinical value of granulocyte scintigraphy in osteomyelitis in children. *J Pediatr Orthop* 2001;10B:109–112.

98. Jaramillo D, Trevers ST, Kasser JR, et al. Osteomyelitis and septic arthritis in children: appropriate use of imaging to guide treatment. *AJR Am J Roentgenol* 1995;165:399–403.

99. Mazur JM, Ross G, Cummings RJ, et al. Usefulness of magnetic resonance imaging for the diagnosis of acute musculoskeletal infections in children. *J Pediatr Orthop* 1995;15:144–147.

100. Modic MT, Feiglin DH, Piraino DW, et al. Vertebral osteomyelitis: assessment using MR. *Radiology* 1985;157:157–166.

101. Shimose S, Sugita T, Kubo T, et al. Differential diagnosis between osteomyelitis and bone tumors. *Acta Radiol* 2008;49(8):928–933.

102. Umans H, Harameti N, Flusser G. The diagnostic role of gadolinium enhanced MRI in distinguishing between acute medullary bone infarct and osteomyelitis. *Magn Reson Imaging* 2000;18:255–262.

103. Browne LP, Mason EO, Kaplan SL, et al. Optimal imaging strategy for community-acquired *Staphylococcus aureus* musculoskeletal infections in children. *Pediatr Radiol* 2008;38(8):841–847.

104. Yang WJ, Im SA, Lim GY, et al. MR imaging of transient synovitis: differentiation from septic arthritis. *Pediatr Radiol* 2006;36(11): 1154–1158.

105. Karmazyn B, Loder RT, Kleiman MB, et al. The role of pelvic magnetic resonance in evaluating nonhip sources of infection in children with acute nontraumatic hip pain. *J Pediatr Orthop* 2007;27(2):158–164.

106. McPhee E, Eskander JP, Eskander MS, et al. Imaging in pelvic osteomyelitis: support for early magnetic resonance imaging. *J Pediatr Orthop* 2007;27(8):903–909.

107. Darge K, Jaramillo D, Siegel MJ. Whole-body MRI in children: current status and future applications. *Eur J Radiol* 2008;68(2):289–298.

108. Kan JH, Hilmes MA, Martus JE, et al. Value of MRI after recent diagnostic or surgical intervention in children with suspected osteomyelitis. *AJR Am J Roentgenol* 2008;191(5):1595–1600.

109. Spiegel DA, Meyer JS, Dormans JP, et al. Pyomyositis in children and adolescents: report of 12 cases and review of the literature. *J Pediatr Orthop* 1999;19(2):143–150.

110. Gordon JE, Huang M, Dobbs M, et al. Causes of false-negative ultrasound scans in the diagnosis of septic arthritis of the hip in children. *J Pediatr Orthop* 2002;22:312–316.

111. Dorr U, Zieger M, Hauke H. Ultrasonography of the painful hip: prospective studies in 204 patients. *Pediatr Radiol* 1988;19:36–40.

112. Royle SG. Investigation of the irritable hip. *J Pediatr Orthop* 1992; 12:396.

113. Azam Q, Ahmad I, Abbas M, et al. Ultrasound and colour Doppler sonography in acute osteomyelitis in children. *Acta Orthop Belg* 2005;71(5):590–596.

114. Sadat-Ali M, al-Umran K, al-Habdan I, et al. Ultrasonography: can it differentiate between vasoocclusive crisis and acute osteomyelitis in sickle cell disease? *J Pediatr Orthop* 1998;18:552–554.

115. Epperly TD. The value of needle aspiration in the management of cellulitis. *J Fam Pract* 1986;23:337–340.

116. Fink CW, Nelson JD. Septic arthritis and osteomyelitis in children. *Clin Rheum Dis* 1986;12:423–435.

117. Shmerling RH, Delbanco TL, Tosteson AN, et al. Synovial fluid tests: what should be ordered? *J Am Med Assoc* 1990;264:1009–1014.

118. Morrissy RT, Shore S. Septic arthritis in children. In: Gustilo RB, Gruninger RP, Tsukayama DT, eds. *Orthopaedic infection: diagnosis and treatment*. Philadelphia, PA: WB Saunders, 1989:261–270.

119. Press J, Peled N, Buskila D, et al. Leukocyte count in the synovial fluid of children with culture-proven brucellar arthritis. *Clin Rheumatol* 2002;21:191–193.

120. Wilson NI, DiPaola M. Acute septic arthritis in infancy and childhood: 10 years' experience. *J Bone Joint Surg Br* 1986;68:584–587.

121. Vaughan PA, Newman NM, Rosman MA. Acute hematogenous osteomyelitis in children. *J Pediatr Orthop* 1987;7:652–655.

122. Green NE, Edwards K. Bone and joint infections in children. *Orthop Clin North Am* 1987;18:555–576.

123. Lyon RM, Evanich JD. Culture negative septic arthritis in children. *J Pediatr Orthop* 1999;19:655–659.

124. Hann IM, Gupta S, Palmer MK, et al. The prognostic significance of radiological and symptomatic bone involvement in childhood acute lymphoblastic leukemia. *Med Pediatr Oncol* 1979;6:51–55.

125. Rogalsky RJ, Black GB, Reed MH. Orthopaedic manifestations of leukemia in children. *J Bone Joint Surg Am* 1986;68:494–501.

126. Clausen N, Gotze H, Pedersen A, et al. Skeletal scintigraphy and radiography at onset of acute lymphocytic leukemia in children. *Med Pediatr Oncol* 1983;11:291–296.

127. Kocher MS, Zurakowski D, Kasser JR. Differentiating between septic arthritis and transient synovitis of the hip in children: an evidence-based clinical prediction algorithm. *J Bone Joint Surg Am* 1999;81:1662–1670.

128. Kocher MS, Mandiga R, Zurakowski D, et al. Validation of a clinical prediction rule for the differentiation between septic arthritis and transient synovitis of the hip in children. *J Bone Joint Surg Am* 2004;86(8):1629–1635.

129. Luhmann SJ, Jones A, Schootman M, et al. Differentiation between septic arthritis and transient synovitis of the hip in children with clinical prediction algorithms. *J Bone Joint Surg Am* 2004;86A(5):956–962.

130. Caird MS, Flynn JM, Leung YL, et al. Factors distinguishing septic arthritis from transient synovitis of the hip in children. A prospective study. *J Bone Joint Surg Am* 2006;88(6):1251–1257.

131. Baldassare AR, Chang F, Zuckner J. Markedly raised synovial fluid leukocyte counts not associated with infectious arthritis in children. *Ann Rheum Dis* 1978;37:404–409.

132. Birdi N, Allen U, D'Astous J. Post-streptococcal reactive arthritis mimicking acute septic arthritis: a hospital-based study. *J Pediatr Orthop* 1995;15:661–665.

133. Bont L, Brus F, Dijkman-Neerinex RH, et al. The clinical spectrum of post-streptococcal syndromes with arthritis in children. *Clin Exp Rheumatol* 1998;16:750–752.

134. Giladi M, Maman E, Paran D, et al. Cat-scratch disease-associated arthropathy. *Arthritis Rheum* 2005;52(11):3611–3617.

135. Reinehr T, Burk G, Michel E, et al. Chronic osteomyelitis in childhood: is surgery always indicated? *Infection* 2000;28:282–286.

136. Ibia EO, Imoisili M, Pikis A. Group A beta-hemolytic streptococcal osteomyelitis in children. *Pediatrics* 2003;112(1 pt 1):e22–e26.

137. de Kort JG, Robben SG, Schrander JJ, et al. Multifocal osteomyelitis in a child: a rare manifestation of cat scratch disease: a case report and systematic review of the literature. *J Pediatr Orthop B* 2006;15(4):285–288.

138. Hajjaji N, Hocqueloux L, Kerdaon R, et al. Bone infection in cat-scratch disease: a review of the literature. *J Infect Dis* 2007;54(5):417–421.

139. Ridder-Schroter R, Marx A, Beer M, et al. Abscess-forming lymphadenopathy and osteomyelitis in children with Bartonella henselae infection. *J Med Microbiol* 2008;57 (pt 4):519–524.

140. Rozmanic V, Banac S, Miletic D, et al. Role of magnetic resonance imaging and scintigraphy in the diagnosis and follow-up of osteomyelitis in cat-scratch disease. *J Paediatr Child Health* 2007;43(7–8):568–570.

141. Nelson JD, Bucholz RW, Kusmiesz H, et al. Benefits and risks of sequential parenteral-oral cephalosporin therapy for suppurative bone and joint infections. *J Pediatr Orthop* 1982;2:255–262.

142. Bachur R, Pagon Z. Success of short-course parenteral antibiotic therapy for acute osteomyelitis of childhood. *Clin Pediatrics* 2007; 46(1):30–35.

143. Zaoutis T, Localio AR, Leckerman K, et al. Prolonged intravenous therapy versus early transition to oral antimicrobial therapy for acute osteomyelitis in children. *Pediatrics* 2009;123(2):636–642.

144. Daoud A, Saighi-Bouaouina A. Treatment of sequestra, pseudoarthroses and defects in the long bones of children who have chronic hematogenous osteomyelitis. *J Bone Joint Surg Am* 1989;71:1448–1468.

145. Kucukkaya M, Kabukcouglu Y, Tezer M, et al. Management of childhood chronic tibial osteomyelitis with the Ilizarov method. *J Pediatr Orthop* 2002;22:632–637.

146. Onuminya JE, Onuminya DS. Results of open wound technique in the treatment of post-sequestrectomy dead space. *S Afr J Surg* 2008; 46(1):26–27.

147. Nelson JD, Howard JB, Shelton S. Oral antibiotic therapy for skeletal infections of children. I. Antibiotic concentrations in suppurative synovial joint. *J Pediatr* 1978;92:131–134.

148. Gomez MM, Maraqa NF, Alvarez A, et al. Complications of outpatient parenteral antibiotic therapy in childhood. *Pediatr Infect Dis J* 2001;20:541–543.

149. Maraqa NF, Gomez MM, Rathore MH. Outpatient parenteral antimicrobial therapy in osteoarticular infections in children. *J Pediatr Orthop* 2002;22:506–510.

150. Jaberi FM, Shahcheraghi GH, Ahadzadeh M. Short-term intravenous antibiotic treatment of acute hematogenous bone and joint infection in children: a prospective randomized trial. *J Pediatr Orthop* 2002;22:317–320.

151. Kim HK, Alman B, Cole WG. A shortened course of parenteral antibiotic therapy in the management of acute septic arthritis. *J Pediatr Orthop* 2000;20:44–47.

152. Vinod MB, Matussek J, Curtis N, et al. Duration of antibiotics in children with osteomyelitis and septic arthritis. *J Pediatr Child Health* 2002;38:363–367.

153. Kocher MS, Mandiga R, Murphy JM, et al. A clinical practice guideline for treatment of septic arthritis in children: efficacy in improving process of care and effect on outcome of septic arthritis of the hip. *J Bone Joint Surg Am* 2003;85:994–999.

154. Gwynne-Jones DP, Stott NS. Community-acquired methicillin-resistant *Staphylococcus aureus*: a cause of musculoskeletal sepsis in children. *J Pediatr Orthop* 1999;19:413–416.

155. Martinez-Aguilar G, Hammerman WA, Mason EO Jr, et al. Clindamycin treatment of invasive infections caused by community-acquired, methicillin-resistant and methicillin-susceptible *Staphylococcus aureus* in children. *Pediatr Infect Dis J* 2003;22:593–598.

156. Perl TM. The threat of vancomycin resistance. *Am J Med* 1999;106:26s–37s.

157. Chen CJ, Chiu CH, Lin TY, et al. Experience with linezolid therapy in children with osteoarticular infections. *Pediatr Infect Dis J* 2007;26(11):985–988.

158. Harwood PJ, Glannoudis PV. The safety and efficacy of linezolid in orthopaedic practice for the treatment of infection due to antibiotic-resistant organisms. *Expert Opin Drug Saf* 2004;3(5):405–414.

159. Bryan LE, Van den Elzen HM. Streptomycin accumulation in susceptible and resistant strains of Escherichia coli and *Pseudomonas aeruginosa*. *Antimicrob Agents Chemother* 1976;9:928–938.

160. Bryant RE, Hammond D. Interaction of purulent material with antibiotics used to treat *Pseudomonas* infection. *Antimicrob Agents Chemother* 1974;6:700–707.

161. Donowitz GR, Mandell GL. Beta-lactam antibiotics. *N Engl J Med* 1988;318:419–426.

162. Farrar WE Jr, O'Dell NM. Comparative f3-lactamase resistance and antistaphylococcal activities of parenterally and orally administered cephalosporins. *J Infect Dis* 1978;137:490–493.

163. Sabath LD, Garner C, Wilcox C, et al. Effect of inoculum and of beta-lactamase on the anti-staphylococcal activity of thirteen penicillins and cephalosporins. *Antimicrob Agents Chemother* 1975;8:344–349.

164. Braude AI, Jones JL, Douglas HI. The behavior of *Escherichia coli* endotoxin (somatic antigen) during infectious arthritis. *J Immunol* 1963;90:297.

165. Ginsburg I, Sela MN. The role of leukocytes and their hydrolases in the persistence, degradation, and transport of bacterial constituents in tissues: relation to chronic inflammatory processes in staphylococcal, streptococcal, and mycobacterial infections and in chronic periodontal disease. *CRC Crit Rev Microbiol* 1976;4:249–322.

166. Ginsburg J, Goultchin A, Stabholtz N, et al. Streptococcal and staphylococcal arthritis: can chronic arthritis in the human be caused by highly chemotactic degradation products generated from bacteria by leukocyte enzymes and by the deactivation of leukocytes by inflammatory exudates, polyelectrolytes, leukocyte hydrolases and by cell sensitizing agents derived from bacteria? *Agents Actions* 1980;7:260–270.

167. Goldstein WM, Gleason TF, Barmada R. A comparison between arthrotomy and irrigation and multiple aspirations in the treatment of pyogenic arthritis. *Orthopaedics* 1983;6:1309.

168. Gordon JE, Wolff A, Luhmann SJ, et al. Primary and delayed closure after open irrigation and debridement of septic arthritis in children. *J Pediatr Orthop B* 2005;14(2):101–104.

169. Kim SJ, Choi NH, Ko SH, et al. Arthroscopic treatment of septic arthritis of the hip. *Clin Orthop* 2003;407:211–214.

170. Forward DP, Hunter JB. Arthroscopic washout of the shoulder for septic arthritis in infants. A new technique. *J Bone Joint Surg Br* 2002;84(8):1173–1175.

171. Nusem I, Jabur MK, Playford EG. Arthroscopic treatment of septic arthritis of the hip. *Arthroscopy* 2006;22(8):902.e1–902.e3.

172. Peltola H, Paakkonen M, Kallio P, et al. Prospective, randomized trial of 10 days versus 30 days of antimicrobial treatment, including a short-term course on parenteral therapy, for childhood septic arthritis. *Clin Infect Dis* 2009;48(9):1201–1210.

173. Ceroni D, Regusci M, Pazos JM, et al. Risks and complications of prolonged parenteral antibiotic treatment in children with acute osteoarticular infections. *Acta Orthop Belg* 2003;69(5):400–404.

174. Ruebner R, Keren R, Coffin S, et al. Complications of central venous catheters used for the treatment of acute hematogenous osteomyelitis. *Pediatrics* 2006;117(4):1210–1215.

175. Javaheri M, Khurana RN, O'heam TM, et al. Linezolid-induced optic neuropathy: a mitochondrial disorder? *Br J Ophthalmol* 2007;91(1):111–115.

176. van den Boom J, Kristiansen JB, Voss LM, et al. Flucloxacillin associated neutropenia in children treated for bone and joint infections. *J Paediatr Child Health* 2005;41(1–2):48–51.

177. Crary SE, Buchanan GR, Drake CE, et al. Venous thrombosis and thromboembolism in children with osteomyelitis. *J Pediatr Child Health* 2006;149(4):537–541.

178. Gonzalez BE, Martinez-Aguilar G, Hulten KG, et al. Severe Staphylococcal sepsis in adolescents in the era of community-acquired methicillin-resistant *Staphylococcus aureus*. *Pediatrics* 2005;115(3):642–648.

179. Gonzalez BE, Teruya J, Mahoney DH Jr, et al. Venous thrombosis associated with staphylococcal osteomyelitis in children. *Pediatrics* 2006;117:1673–1679.

180. Hollmig ST, Copley LA, Browne RH, et al. Deep venous thrombosis associated with osteomyelitis in children. *J Bone Joint Surg Am* 2007;89(7):1517–1523.

181. Saavedra-Lozano J, Mejias A, Ahmad N, et al. Changing trends in acute osteomyelitis in children: impact of methicillin-resistant *Staphylococcus aureus* infections. *J Pediatr Orthop* 2008;28(5):569–575.

182. Arnold SR, Elias D, Buckingham SC, et al. Changing patterns of acute hematogenous osteomyelitis and septic arthritis: emergency of community-associated methicillin-resistant *Staphylococcus aureus*. *J Pediatr Orthop* 2006;26(6):703–708.

183. Fergie JE, Purcell K. Community-acquired methicillin-resistant *Staphylococcus aureus* infections in South Texas children. *Pediatr Infect Dis* 2001;20(9):860–863.

184. Gillet Y, Dohin B, Dumitrescu O, et al. Osteoarticular infections with *Staphylococcus aureus* secreting Panton-Valentine leucocidin. *Arch Pediatr* 2007;14 (Suppl 2):S102–S107.

185. Hsu LY, Koh TH, Tan TY, et al. Emergence of community-associated methicillin-resistant *Staphylococcus aureus* in Singapore: a further six cases. *Singapore Med J* 2006;47(1):20–26.

186. Ghebremedhin B, Olugbosi MO, Raji AM, et al. Emergence of a community-associated methicillin-resistant *Staphylococcus aureus* strain with a unique resistance profile in Southwest Nigeria. *J Clin Microbiol* 2009;47(9):2975–2980.

187. Nimmo GR, Coombs GW. Community-associated methicillin-resistant *Staphylococcus aureus* (MRSA) in Australia. *Int J Antimicrob Agents* 2008;31(5):401–410.

188. Paganini H, Della Latta MP, B MO, et al. Community-acquired methicillin-resistant *Staphylococcus aureus* infections in children: multicenter trial. *Arch Argent Pediatr* 2008;106(5):397–403.

189. Manoura A, Korakaki E, Hatzidaki E, et al. Use of recombinant erythropoietin for the management of severe hemolytic disease of the newborn of a K0 phenotype mother. *Pediatr Hematol Oncol* 2007;24(1):69–73.

190. Crawford SE, Daum RS. Epidemic community-associated methicillin-resistant *Staphylococcus aureus*: modern times for an ancient pathogen. *Pediatr Infect Dis J* 2005;24(5):459–460.

191. Nourse C, Starr M, Munckhof W. Community-acquired methicillin-resistant *Staphylococcus aureus* causes severe disseminated infection and deep venous thrombosis in children: literature review and recommendations for management. *J Paediatr Child Health* 2007;43(10):656–661.

192. McCaskill ML, Mason EO Jr, Kaplan SL, et al. Increase of the USA300 clone among community-acquired methicillin-susceptible *Staphylococcus aureus* causing invasive infections. *Pediatr infect Dis J* 2007;26(12):1122–1127.

193. Sdougkos G, Chini V, Papanastasious DA, et al. Methicillin-resistant *Staphylococcus aureus* producing Panton-Valentine leukocidin as a cause of acute osteomyelitis in children. *Clin Microbiol Infect* 2007;13(6):651–654.

194. Kaplan SL. Community-acquired methicillin-resistant *Staphylococcus aureus* infections in children. *Semin Pediatr Infect Dis* 2006;17(3):113–119.

195. Copley LA. Pediatric musculoskeletal infection: trends and antibiotic recommendations. *J Am Acad Orthop Surg* 2009;17(10):618–626.

196. Hammond PJ, Macnicol MF. Osteomyelitis of the pelvis and proximal femur: diagnostic difficulties. *J Pediatr Orthop* 2001;10B:113–119.
197. Glazer PA, Hu SS. Pediatric spinal infections. *Orthop Clin North Am* 1996;27:111–123.
198. Bremner AE, Neligan GA. Benign form of acute osteitis of the spine in young children. *Br Med J* 1953;1:856.
199. Ghormley RK, Bickel WH, Dickson DD. A study of acute infectious lesions of the intervertebral disks. *South Med J* 1940;33:347.
200. Ring D, Johnston CE, Wenger KR. Pyogenic infectious spondylitis in children: the convergence of discitis and vertebral osteomyelitis. *J Pediatr Orthop* 1995;15:652–660.
201. Song KS, Ogden JA, Ganey T, et al. Contiguous discitis and osteomyelitis in children. *J Pediatr Orthop* 1997;17:470–477.
202. Coventry MB, Ghormley RK, Kernohan JW. The intervertebral discitis microscopic anatomy and pathology. Part I. Anatomy, development and physiology. *J Bone Joint Surg Am* 1945;27:105.
203. Crock HV, Yoshizawa H. *The blood supply of the vertebral column and spinal cord in man.* New York, NY: Springer-Verlag, 1977.
204. Hassler O. The human intervertebral disc: a microangiographical study on its vascular supply at various ages. *Acta Orthop Scand* 1969;40:765.
205. Wiley AM, Trueta J. The vascular anatomy of the spine and its relationship to pyogenic vertebral osteomyelitis. *J Bone Joint Surg Br* 1959;41:796.
206. Fernandez M, Carrol CL, Baker CJ. Discitis and vertebral osteomyelitis in children: an 18-year review. *Pediatrics* 2000;105:1299–1304.
207. Rocco HD, Erying EJ. Intervertebral disk infections in children. *Am J Dis Child* 1972;123:448–451.
208. Boston HC, Bianco AJ, Rhodes KH. Disk space infections in children. *Orthop Clin North Am* 1975;6:953–964.
209. Spiegel PG, Kengla KW, Isaacson AS, et al. Intervertebral disc space inflammation in children. *J Bone Joint Surg Am* 1972;54:284–296.
210. Wenger DR, Bobechko WP, Gilday DL. The spectrum of intervertebral disc-space infection in children. *J Bone Joint Surg Am* 1978;60:100–108.
211. Jensen AG, Espersen F, Skinhoj, et al. Increasing frequency of vertebral osteomyelitis following *Staphylococcus aureus* bacteraemia in Denmark 1980–1990. *J Infection* 1997;34:113–118.
212. Klein JD, Leach KA. Pediatric pelvic osteomyelitis. *Clin Pediatrics* 2007;46(9):787–790.
213. Song KS, Lee SM. Peripelvic infections mimicking septic arthritis of the hip in children: treatment with needle aspiration. *J Pediatr Orthop B* 2003;12(5):354–356.
214. Schaad UB, McCracken GH, Nelson JD. Pyogenic arthritis of the sacroiliac joint in pediatric patients. *Pediatrics* 1980;66:375–379.
215. Weber-Chrysochoou C, Corti N, Goetschel P, et al. Pelvic osteomyelitis: a diagnostic challenge in children. *J Pediatr Surg* 2007;42(3):553–557.
216. Connolly SA, Connolly LP, Drubach LA, et al. MRI for detection of abscess in acute osteomyelitis of the pelvis in children. *AJR Am J Roentgenol* 2007;189(4):867–872.
217. Karmazyn B, Kleiman MB, Buckwalter KA, et al. Acute pyomyositis of the pelvis: the spectrum of clinical presentations and MR findings. *Pediatr Radiol* 2006;36(4):338–343.
218. Edwards MS, Baker CJ, Granberry WM, et al. Pelvic osteomyelitis in children. *Pediatrics* 1978;61:62.
219. Jarvis J, McIntyre W, Udjus K, et al. Osteomyelitis of the ischiopubic synchondrosis. *J Pediatr Orthop* 1985;5:163.
220. Kloiber R, Udjus K, McIntyre W, et al. The scintigraphic and radiographic appearance of the ischiopubic synchondroses in normal children and in osteomyelitis. *Pediatr Radiol* 1988;18:57.
221. Ailsby RL, Staheli LT. Pyogenic infections of the sacroiliac joint in children. Radioisotope bone scanning as a diagnostic tool. *Clin Orthop* 1974;100:96.
222. Farley T, Conway J, Shulman ST. Hematogenous pelvic osteomyelitis in children. *Am J Dis Child* 1985;139:946–949.
223. Reilly JP, Gross RH, Emans JB, et al. Disorders of the sacroiliac joint in children. *J Bone Joint Surg* 1988;70A:31–40.
224. Sucato DJ, Gillespie R. Salmonella pelvic osteomyelitis in normal children: report of two cases and a review of the literature. *J Pediatr Orthop* 1997;17:463–466.
225. Beaupre A, Carroll N. The three syndromes of iliac osteomyelitis in children. *J Bone Joint Surg Am* 1979;61:1087–1092.
226. Coy JT III, Wolf CR, Brower TD, et al. Pyogenic arthritis of the sacroiliac joint: long-term follow-up. *J Bone Joint Surg Am* 1976;58:845–849.
227. Davidson D, Letts M, Khoshhal K. Pelvic osteomyelitis in children: a comparison of decades from 1980–1989 with 1990–2001. *J Pediatr Orthop* 2003;23:514–521.
228. Gervais DA, Brown SD, Connolly SA, et al. Percutaneous imaging-guided abdominal and pelvic abscess drainage in children. *Radiographics* 2004;24(3):737–754.
229. Johanson PH. Pseudomonas infections of the foot following puncture wounds. *JAMA* 1968;204:170.
230. Fisher MC, Goldsmith JF, Gilligan PH. Sneakers as a source of *Pseudomonas aeruginosa* in children with osteomyelitis following puncture wounds. *Pediatrics* 1985;106:607–609.
231. Weber CA, Wertheimer SJ, Ognjan A. *Aeromonas hydrophilia*—its implications in freshwater injuries. *J Foot Ankle Surg* 1995;34:442–446.
232. Fitzgerald RH, Cowan JDE. Puncture wounds of the foot. *Orthop Clin North Am* 1975;6:965–972.
233. Eidelman M, Bialik V, Miller Y, et al. Plantar puncture wounds in children: analysis of 80 hospitalized patients and late sequelae. *Isr Med Assoc J* 2003;5(4):268–271.
234. Lau LS, Bin G, Jaovisidua S, et al. Cost effectiveness of magnetic resonance imaging in diagnosing *Pseudomonas aeruginosa* infection after puncture wound. *J Foot Ankle Surg* 1997;36:36–43.
235. Jacobs RF, Adelman L, Sack CM, et al. Management of *Pseudomonas osteochondritis* complicating puncture wounds of the foot. *Pediatrics* 1982;69:432–435.
236. Jacobs RF, McCarthy RE, Elser JM. *Pseudomonas osteochondritis* complicating puncture wounds of the foot in children: a 10-year evaluation. *J Infect Dis* 1989;160:657–661.
237. Puffinbarger WR, Gruel CR, Herndon WA, et al. Osteomyelitis of the calcaneus in children. *J Pediatr Orthop* 1996;16:224–230.
238. Jaakkola J, Kehl DK. Hematogenous calcaneal osteomyelitis in children. *J Pediatr Orthop* 1999;19:699–704.
239. Rasool MN. Hematogenous osteomyelitis of the calcaneus in children. *J Pediatr Orthop* 2001;21:738–743.
240. Rasool MN. Osseous manifestations of tuberculosis in children. *J Pediatr Orthop* 2001;21:749–755.
241. Rasool MN. Primary subacute haematogenous osteomyelitis in children. *J Bone Joint Surg* 2001;83B:93–98.
242. Lim MO, Gresham EL, Franken EA Jr, et al. Osteomyelitis as a complication of umbilical artery catheterization. *Am J Dis Child* 1977;131:142–144.
243. Bergdahl S, Ekengren K, Eriksson M. Neonatal hematogenous osteomyelitis: risk factors for long-term sequelae. *J Pediatr Orthop* 1985;5:564–568.
244. Fox L, Sprunt K. Neonatal osteomyelitis. *Pediatrics* 1978;62:535–542.
245. Edwards MS, Baker CJ, Wagner ML, et al. An etiologic shift in infantile osteomyelitis: the emergence of the group B streptococcus. *J Pediatr* 1978;93:578–583.
246. Hoffman JA, Mason EO, Schutze GE, et al. *Streptococcus pneumoniae* infections in the neonate. *Pediatrics* 2003;112(5):1095–1102.
247. Aigner RM, Fueger GF, Ritter G. Results of three-phase bone scintigraphy and radiography in 20 cases of neonatal osteomyelitis. *Nucl Med Commun* 1996;17:20–28.
248. Trueta J. The three types of acute haematogenous osteomyelitis: a clinical and vascular study. *J Bone Joint Surg Br* 1959;41:671.
249. Ash JM, Gilday DL. The futility of bone scanning in neonatal osteomyelitis: concise communication. *J Nucl Med* 1980;21:417–420.
250. Ingram DL. *Neisseria gonorrhoeae* in children. *Pediatr Annals* 1994;23:341–345.
251. Israel KS, Rissing KB, Brooks GF. Neonatal and childhood gonococcal infections. *Clin Obstet Gynec* 1975;18:143–151.
252. Holmes KK, Counts GW, Beaty HN. Disseminated gonococcal infection. *Ann Intern Med* 1971;74:979–993.
253. Rimsza ME, Niggemann EH. Medical evaluation of sexually abused children: a review of 311 cases. *Pediatrics* 1982;69:8–14.

254. White ST, Loda FA, Ingram DL, et al. Sexually transmitted diseases in sexually abused children. *Pediatrics* 1983;72:16–21.

255. Masi AT, Eisenstein BI. Disseminated gonococcal infection (DGI) and gonococcal arthritis (GCA): II. Clinical manifestations, diagnosis, complications, treatment and prevention. *Sem Arth Rheum* 1981;10:173–197.

256. Cooperman MB. Gonococcus arthritis in infancy: a clinical study of forty-four cases. *Am J Dis Child* 1927;33:932.

257. Cooperman MB. End results of gonorrheal arthritis: a review of seventy cases. *Am J Surg* 1928;5:241.

258. Spink WW, Keefer CS. Gonococcic arthritis: pathogenesis, mechanism of recovery and treatment. *JAMA* 1938;109:1448.

259. Wehrbein HL. Gonococcus arthritis—a study of six hundred cases. *Surg Gyn Obstet* 1929;49:105.

260. Wise CM, Morris CR, Wasilauskas BL, et al. Gonococcal arthritis in an era of increasing penicillin resistance: presentations and outcomes in 41 recent cases (1985–1991). *Arch Intern Med* 1994;154:2690–2695.

261. Manson D, Wilmot DM, King S, et al. Physeal involvement in chronic recurrent multifocal osteomyelitis [see comments]. *Pediatr Radiol* 1989;20:76.

262. Bardin T. Gonococcal arthritis. *Best Pract Res Clin Rheumatol* 2003;17:201–208.

263. Martinez-Rojano H, Juarez Hernandez E, Ladron de Guevara G, et al. Rheumatologic manifestations of pediatric HIV infection. *AIDS Patient Care STDs* 2001;15:519–526.

264. Chinniah K, Mody GM, Bhimma R, et al. Arthritis in association with human immunodeficiency virus infection in Black African children: causal or coincidental? *Rheumatology (Oxford)* 2005;44(7):915–920.

265. Weinstein A, Britchkov M. Lyme arthritis and post-Lyme disease syndrome. *Curr Opin Rheumatol* 2002;14:383–387.

266. Thompson A, Mannix R, Bachur R. Acute pediatric monoarticular arthritis: distinguishing lyme arthritis from other etiologies. *Pediatrics* 2009;123(3):959–965.

267. Ecklund K, Vargas S, Zurakowski D, et al. MRI features of Lyme arthritis in children. *AJR Am J Roentgenol* 2005;184(6):1904–1909.

268. Bradley J, Nelson J. *Nelson's pocket handbook of pediatric antimicrobial therapy.* Philadelphia, PA: Lippincott Williams & Wilkins, 2002.

269. Willis AA, Widmann RF, Flynn JM, et al. Lyme arthritis presenting as acute septic arthritis in children. *J Pediatr Orthop* 2003;23:114–118.

270. Aebi C, Ahmed A, Ramilo O. Bacterial complications of primary varicella in children. *Clin Infect Dis* 1996;23:698–705.

271. Quach C, Weiss K, Moore D, et al. Clinical aspects and cost of invasive *Streptococcus pneumoniae* infections in children: resistant vs. susceptible strains. *Int J Antimicrob Agents* 2002;20(2):113–118.

272. Schreck P, Schreck P, Bradley JS, et al. Musculoskeletal complications of varicella. *J Bone Joint Surg Am* 1996;78:1713–1719.

273. Tyrrell GJ, Lovgren M, Kress B, et al. Varicella-associated invasive group A streptococcal disease in Alberta, Canada—2000–2002. *Clin Infect Dis* 2005;40(7):1055–1057.

274. Griebel M, Nahlen B, Jacobs RF, et al. Group A streptococcal postvaricella osteomyelitis. *J Pediatr Orthop* 1985;5:101.

275. Barrett-Connor E. Bacterial infection and sickle cell anemia. *Medicine* 1971;50:97–112.

276. Chambers JB, Forsythe DA, Bertrand SL, et al. Retrospective review of osteoarticular infections in a pediatric sickle cell age group. *J Pediatr Orthop* 2000;20:682–685.

277. Sadat-Ali M. The status of acute osteomyelitis in sickle cell disease: a 15 year review. *Int Surg* 1998;83:84–87.

278. Ware RE. *Salmonella* infection in sickle cell disease: a clear and present danger. *J Pediatr* 1997;130:350–351.

279. Zarkowsky HS, Gallagher D, Gill FM, et al. Bacteremia in sickle hemoglobinopathies. *J Pediatr* 1986;109:579–585.

280. Wright J, Thomas P, Sargeant GR. Septicemia caused by *Salmonella* infection: an overlooked complication of sickle cell disease. *J Pediatr* 1997;130:394–399.

281. Specht EE. Hemoglobinopathic *Salmonella* osteomyelitis. *Clin Orthop* 1971;79:110–118.

282. Engh CA, Hughes JL, Abrams RC, et al. Osteomyelitis in the patient with sickle-cell disease. *J Bone Joint Surg Am* 1971;53:1–14.

283. Keely K, Buchanan GR. Acute infarction of long bones in children with sickle cell anemia. *J Pediatr* 1982;101:170–175.

284. Akar NA, Adekile A. Ten-year review of hospital admissions among children with sickle cell disease in Kuwait. *Med Princ Pract* 2008;17(5):404–408.

285. Bouden AK, Kais C, Abdallah NB, et al. MRI contribution in diagnosis of acute bone infarcts in children with sickle cell disease. *Tunis Med* 2005;83(6):344–348.

286. Ejindu VC, Hine AL, Mashayekhi MS, et al. Musculoskeletal manifestations of sickle cell disease. *Radiographics* 2007;27(4):1005–1021.

287. Frush DP, Heyneman LE, Ware RE, et al. MR features of soft tissue abnormalities due to acute marrow infarction in five children with sickle cell disease. *AJR Am J Roentgenol* 1999;173:989–993.

288. Booz MM, Hariharan V, Aradi AJ, et al. The value of ultrasound and aspiration in differentiating vaso-occlusive crisis and osteomyelitis in sickle cell disease patients. *Clin Radiol* 1999;54:636–639.

289. Worrel VT, Butera V. Sickle-cell dactylitis. *J Bone Joint Surg* 1976;58A:1161–1163.

290. Greene WB, McMillan CW. *Salmonella* osteomyelitis and hand-foot syndrome in a child with sickle cell anemia. *J Pediatr Orthop* 1987;7:716–718.

291. Noonan WJ. *Salmonella* osteomyelitis presenting as "hand-foot syndrome" in sickle-cell disease. *Br Med J* 1982;284:1464–1465.

292. Sankaran-Kutty M, Sadat-Ali M, Kutty MK. Septic arthritis in sickle cell disease. *Int Orthop* 1988;12:255–257.

293. Adeyokunnu AA, Hendrickse RG. *Salmonella* osteomyelitis in childhood. *Arch Dis Child* 1980;55:175–184.

294. Mallouh A, Talab Y. Bone and joint infection in patients with sickle cell disease. *J Pediatr Orthop* 1985;5:158–162.

295. Syrogiannopoulos GA, McCracken GHJ, Nelson JD. Osteoarticular infections in children with sickle cell disease. *Pediatrics* 1986;78:1090–1096.

296. Adu-Gyamfi Y, Sankarankutty M, Marwa S. Use of a tourniquet in patients with sickle-cell disease. *Can J Anesth* 1993;40:24–27.

297. Stein RE, Urbaniak J. Use of the tourniquet during surgery in patients with sickle cell hemoglobinopathies. *Clin Orthop* 1980;151:231–233.

298. Riddington C, Williamson L. Preoperative blood transfusions for sickle cell disease. *Cochrane Database Syst Rev* 2001;3:CD003149.

299. Burnett MW, Bass JW, Cook BA. Etiology of osteomyelitis complicating sickle cell disease. *Pediatrics* 1998;10:296–297.

300. Henderson RC, Rosenstein BD. *Salmonella* septic and aseptic arthritis in sickle-cell disease: a case report. *Clin Orthop* 1989;248:261.

301. Espinoza LR, Spilberg I, Osterland CK. Joint manifestations of sickle-cell disease. *Medicine* 1974;53:295–305.

302. Orozoco-Alcala J, Baum J. Arthritis during sickle cell crisis. *N Engl J Med* 1973;288:420.

303. Ebong WW. Septic arthritis in patients with sickle-cell disease. *Br J Rheumatol* 1987;26:99–102.

304. Malaviya AN, Kotwal PP. Arthritis associated with tuberculosis. *Best Pract Res Clin Rheumatol* 2003;17:319–343.

305. Smith MJD, Stack KR, Marquis JR. Tuberculosis and opportunistic mycobacterial infections. In: Fegin RO, Cherry JD, eds. *Pediatric infectious diseases.* Philadelphia, PA: WB Saunders, 1992:1327.

306. Vohra R, Kang HS, Dogra S, et al. Tuberculous osteomyelitis. *J Bone Joint Surg Am* 1997;79:562–566.

307. Wang MN, Chen WM, Lee KS, et al. Tuberculous osteomyelitis in young children. *J Pediatr Orthop* 1999;19:151–155.

308. Engin G, Acunas B, Acunas G, et al. Imaging of extrapulmonary tuberculosis. *Radiographics* 2000;20:471–488.

309. Ross ERS, Cole WG. Treatment of subacute osteomyelitis in childhood. *J Bone Joint Surg Am* 1985;67:443–448.

310. Nussbaum ES, Rockswold GL, Bergman TA, et al. Spinal tuberculosis: a diagnostic and management challenge. *J Neurosurg* 1995;83:243–247.

311. Negusse W. Bone and joint tuberculosis in childhood in a children's hospital, Addis Abeba. *Ethiopian Med J* 1993;31:51–61.

312. Phemister DB, Hatcher CH. Correlation of pathological and roentgenological findings in the diagnosis of tuberculous arthritis. *AJR Am J Roentgenol* 1933;29:736.

313. Ruggieri M, Pavone V, Polizzi A, et al. Tuberculosis of the ankle in childhood: clinical, roentgenographic and computed tomography findings. *Clin Pediatrics* 1997;36:529–534.

314. Sawlani V, Chandra T, Mishra RN, et al. MRI features of tuberculosis of peripheral joints. *Clin Radiol* 2003;58:755–762.

315. Hardy JB, Hartmenn JR. Tuberculous dactylitis in childhood. *J Pediatr* 1947;30:146.

316. Shannon BF, Moore M, Houkom JA, et al. Multifocal cystic tuberculosis of bone. *J Bone Joint Surg Am* 1990;72:1089.

317. Jereb JA, Cauthen GM, Kelly GD, et al. The epidemiology of tuberculosis. In: Friedman LN, ed. *Tuberculosis: current concepts and treatment.* Boca Raton, FL: CRC, 1994:17.

318. Berk RH, Yazici M, Atabey N, et al. Detection of *Mycobacterium tuberculosis* in formaldehyde solution-fixed, paraffin-embedded tissue by polymerase chain reaction in Pott's disease. *Spine* 1996;21(17):1991–1995.

319. Brisson-Noel A, Gicquel B, Lecossier D, et al. Rapid diagnosis of tuberculosis by amplification of mycobacterial DNA in clinical samples. *Lancet* 1989;2(8671):1069–1971.

320. Pao CC, Yen TS, You JB, et al. Detection and identification of *Mycobacterium tuberculosis* by DNA amplification. *J Clin Microbiol* 1990;28(9):1877–1880.

321. Versfeld GA, Solomon A. A diagnostic approach to tuberculosis of bones and joints. *J Bone Joint Surg Br* 1982;64:446–469.

322. Martini M, Adjrad A, Boudjemaa A. Tuberculous osteomyelitis. A review of 125 cases. *Int Orthop* 1986;10:201–207.

323. Hoffman EB, Allin J, Campbell JA, et al. Tuberculosis of the knee. *Clin Orthop* 2002;398:100–106.

324. O'Brien JP. Kyphosis secondary to infectious disease. *Clin Orthop* 1977;128:56–64.

325. Lifeso RM, Weaver P, Harder EH. Tuberculous spondylitis in adults. *J Bone Joint Surg* 1985;67A:1405–1413.

326. A five-year assessment of controlled trials of in-patient and out-patient treatment and of plaster-of-Paris jackets for tuberculosis of the spine in children on standard chemotherapy. Studies in Masan and Pusan, Korea. Fifth report of the Medical Research Council Working Party on Tuberculosis of the Spine. *J Bone Joint Surg Br* 1976;58(4):399–411.

327. A five-year assessment of controlled trials of ambulatory treatment, debridement and anterior spinal fusion in the management of tuberculosis of the spine: studies in Bulawayo (Rhodesia) and in Hong Kong. *J Bone Joint Surg Br* 1978;60:163–177.

328. Rajasekaran S, Soundarapandian S. Progression of kyphosis in tuberculosis of the spine treated by anterior arthrodesis. *J Bone Joint Surg Am* 1989;71:1314–1323.

329. Pediatrics AAO. Tuberculosis. In: Peter G, ed. *Report of the Committee on Infectious Diseases*, 23rd ed. Elk Grove Village, IL: American Academy of Pediatrics, 1994:488.

330. King DM, Mayo KM. Subacute haematogenous osteomyelitis. *J Bone Joint Surg Br* 1969;51:458–463.

331. Gonzelez-Lopez JL, Soleto-Martin FJ, Cubillo-Martin A, et al. Subacute osteomyelitis in children. *J Pediatr Orthop* 2001;10B:101–104.

332. Ezra E, Cohen N, Segev E, et al. Primary subacute epiphyseal osteomyelitis: role of conservative treatment. *J Pediatr Orthop* 2002;22:333–337.

333. Hamdy RC, Lawton L, Carey T, et al. Subacute hematogenous osteomyelitis: are biopsy and surgery always indicated? *J Pediatr Orthop* 1996;16:220–223.

334. Ezra E, Wientroub S. Primary subacute haematogenous osteomyelitis of the tarsal bones in children. *J Bone Joint Surg Br* 1997;79:983–986.

335. Roberts JM, Drummond DS, Breed AL, et al. Subacute hematogenous osteomyelitis in children: a retrospective study. *J Pediatr Orthop* 1982;2:249–254.

336. Gledhill RB. Subacute osteomyelitis in children. *Clin Orthop* 1973;96:57–69.

337. Bogoch E, Thompson G, Salter RB. Foci of chronic circumscribed osteomyelitis (Brodie's abscess) that traverse the epiphyseal plate. *J Pediatr Orthop* 1984;4:162–169.

338. Azouz EM, Greenspan A, Marton D. CT evaluation of primary epiphyseal bone abscesses. *Skel Radiol* 1993;22:17–23.

339. Green NE, Beauchamp RD, Griffin PP. Primary subacute epiphyseal osteomyelitis. *J Bone Joint Surg Am* 1981;63:107–114.

340. Sorensen TS, Hedeboe J, Christensen ER. Primary epiphyseal osteomyelitis in children: report of three cases and review of the literature. *J Bone Joint Surg Br* 1988;70B:818–820.

341. Grey AC, Davies AM, Mangham DC, et al. The "penumbra sign" on T1-weighted MR imaging in subacute osteomyelitis: frequency, cause and significance. *Clin Radiol* 1998;53:587–592.

342. Cottias P, Tomeno B, Anract P, et al. Subacute osteomyelitis presenting as a bone tumour: a review of 21 cases. *Int Orthop* 1997;21:243–248.

343. Spiegel DA, Myer JS, Dormans JP, et al. Pyomyositis in children and adolescents: report of 12 cases and review of the literature. *J Pediatr Orthop* 1999;19:143–150.

344. Chen W-S, Wan Y-L. Iliacus pyomyositis mimicking septic arthritis of the hip joint. *Arch Orthop Trauma Surg* 1996;115(3–4):233–235.

345. Liew KL, Choong CS, Liu PN, et al. Pyomyositis in childhood: a case report. *Zhonghua Yi Xue Za Zhi (Taipei)* 1998;61(8):488–491.

346. Peckett WR, Butler-Manuel A, Apthorp LA. Pyomyositis of the iliacus muscle in a child. *J Bone Joint Surg Br* 2001;83(1):103–105.

347. Secmeer G, Toyran M, Kara A, et al. Primary haemophilus influenzae pyomyositis in an infant: a case report. *Turk J Pediatr* 2003;45(2):158–160.

348. Thomas S, Tytherleight-Strong G, Dodds R. Adductor myositis as a cause of childhood hip pain. *J Pediatr Orthop B* 2002;11(2):117–120.

349. Block AA, Marshall C, Ratcliffe A, et al. Staphylococcal pyomyositis in a temperate region: epidemiology and modern management. *Med J Aust* 2008;189(6):323–235.

350. Martinez-de Jesus FR, Mendiola-Segura I. Clinical stage, age and treatment in tropical pyomyositis: a retrospective study including forty cases. *Arch Med Res* 1996;27(2):165–170.

351. Lee SS, Chao EK, Chen CY, et al. Staphylococcal pyomyositis. *Changgeng Yi Xue Za Zhi* 1996;19(3):241–246.

352. Meena AK, Rajasekar S, Reddy JJ, et al. Pyomyositis: clinical and MRI characteristics report of three cases. *Neurol India* 1999;47(4):324–326.

353. Vugia D, Peterson CL, Meyers HB, et al. Invasive group A streptococcal infections in children with varicella in Southern California. *Pediatr Infect Dis J* 1996;15(2):146–150.

354. Glylys-Morin VM. MR imaging of pediatric musculoskeletal inflammatory and infectious disorders. *Magn Reson Imaging Clin N Am* 1998;6(3):537–559.

355. Song J, Letts M, Monson R. Differentiation of psoas muscle abscess from septic arthritis of the hip in children. *Clin Orthop* 2001;391:258–265.

356. Bresee JS, Edwards MS. Psoas abscess in children. *Pediatr Infect Dis* 1990;9:201–206.

357. Tong CW, Griffith JF, Lam TP, et al. The conservative management of acute pyogenic psoas abscess in children. *J Bone Joint Surg Br* 1998;80:83–85.

358. Bingol-Kologlu M, Yildiz RV, Alper B, et al. Necrotizing fasciitis in children: diagnostic and therapeutic aspects. *J Pediatr Surg* 2007;42(11):1892–1897.

359. Brook I. Aerobic and anaerobic microbiology of necrotizing fasciitis in children. *Pediatr Dermatol* 1996;13(4):281–284.

360. Eneli I, Davies HD. Epidemiology and outcome of necrotizing fasciitis in children: an active surveillance study of the Canadian Paediatric Surveillance Program. *J Pediatr* 2007;151(1):79–84.

361. Tang JS, Gold RH, Bassett LW, et al. Musculoskeletal infection of the extremities: evaluation with MR imaging. *Radiology* 1988;166:205.

362. McCarthy JJ, Dormans JP, Kozin SH, et al. Musculoskeletal infections in children: basic treatment principles and recent advancements. *Instr Course Lect* 2005;54:515–528.

363. Hankins CL, Southern S. Factors that affect the clinical course of group A beta-haemolytic streptococcal infections of the hand and upper extremity: a retrospective study. *Scand J Plast Reconstr Surg Hand Surg* 2008;42(3):153–157.

364. Meisal R, Hoiby EA, Aaberge IS, et al. Sequence type and emm type diversity in Streptococcus pyogenes isolates causing invasive disease in Norway between 1988 and 2003. *J Clin Microbiol* 2008;46(6):2102–2105.

365. Minodier P, Bidet P, Rallu F, et al. Clinical and microbiologic characteristics of group A streptococcal necrotizing fasciitis in children. *Pediatr Infect Dis* 2009;28(6):541–543.

366. Zerr DM, Rubens CE. NSAIDS and necrotizing fasciitis. *Pediatr Infect Dis J* 1999;18(8):724–725.

367. Girschick HJ, Raab P, Surbaum S, et al. Chronic non-bacterial osteomyelitis in children. *Ann Rheum Dis* 2005;64(2):279–285.

368. Schultz C, Holterhus PM, Seidel A, et al. Chronic recurrent multifocal osteomyelitis in children. *Pediatr Infect Dis* 1999;18:1008–1013.

369. Jansson A, Renner ED, Ramser J, et al. Classification of non-bacterial osteitis. *Rheumatology* 2007;46:154–160.

370. Jurik AG, Helmig O, Ternowitz T, et al. Chronic recurrent multifocal osteomyelitis: a follow-up study. *J Pediatr Orthop* 1988;8:49–58.

371. Manson D, Wilmot DM, King S, et al. Physeal involvement in chronic recurrent multifocal osteomyelitis. *Pediatr Radiol* 1989;20:76–79.

372. Carr AJ, Cole WG, Roberton DM, et al. Chronic multifocal osteomyelitis. *J Bone Joint Surg Br* 1993;75:582–591.

373. Jurik AG, Moller BN. Chronic sclerosing osteomyelitis of the clavicle: a manifestation of chronic recurrent multifocal osteomyelitis. *Arch Orthop Trauma Surg* 1987;104:144–151.

374. Keipert JA, Campbell PE. Recurrent hyperostosis of clavicles: an undiagnosed syndrome. *Aust Paediatr J* 1970;6:97–104.

375. Azouz EM, Jurik AG, Bernard C. Sternoclavicular hyperostosis in children: a report of eight cases. *AJR Am J Roentgenol* 1998;171:461–466.

376. Bjorksten B, Gustavson KH, Eriksson B, et al. Chronic recurrent multifocal osteomyelitis. *J Pediatr* 1978;93:227–231.

377. Kawai K, Doita M, Tateishi H, et al. Bone and joint lesions associated with pustulosis palmaris et plantaris: a clinical and histological study. *J Bone Joint Surg Br* 1988;70:117–122.

378. Bergdahl K, Bjorksten B, Gustavson KH, et al. Pustulosis palmoplantaris and its relation to chronic recurrent multifocal osteomyelitis. *Dermatologica* 1979;159(1):37–45.

379. Gallagher KT, Roberts RL, MacFarlane JA, et al. Treatment of chronic recurrent multifocal osteomyelitis with interferon gamma. *J Pediatr* 1997;131:470–472.

380. Abril JC, Ramirez A. Successful treatment of chronic recurrent multifocal osteomyelitis with indomethacin: a preliminary report of five cases. *J Pediatr Orthop* 2007;27(5):587–591.

381. Compeyrot-Lacassagne S, Rosenberg A, Babyn P, et al. Pamidronate treatment of chronic noninfectious inflammatory lesions of the mandible in children. *J Rheumatol* 2007;34(7):1585–1589.

382. Gleeson H, Wiltshire E, Briody J, et al. Childhood chronic recurrent multifocal osteomyelitis: pamidronate therapy decreases pain and improves vertebral shape. *J Rheumatol* 2008;35(4):707–712.

383. Yamazaki Y, Satoh C, Ishikawa M, et al. Remarkable response of juvenile diffuse sclerosing osteomyelitis of mandible to pamidronate. *Oral Surg Oral Med Oral Pathol Oral Radiol Endod* 2007;104(1):67–71.

384. Catalano-Pons C, Comte A, Wipff J, et al. Clinical outcome in children with chronic recurrent multifocal osteomyelitis. *Rheumatology (Oxford)* 2008;47(9):1397–1399.

385. Huber AM, Lam PY, Duffy CM, et al. Chronic recurrent multifocal osteomyelitis: clinical outcomes after more than five years of follow-up. *J Pediatr Orthop* 2002;141:198–203.

386. Piddo C, Reed MH, Black GB. Premature epiphyseal fusion and degenerative arthritis in chronic recurrent multifocal osteomyelitis. *Skel Radiol* 2000;29:94–96.

387. Duffy CM, Lam PY, Ditchfield M, et al. Chronic recurrent multifocal osteomyelitis: review of orthopaedic complications at maturity. *J Pediatr Orthop* 2002;22(4):501–505.

388. Letts M, Davidson D, Birdi N, et al. The SAPHO syndrome in children A rare cause of hyperostosis and osteitis. *J Pediatr Orthop* 1999;19(3):397–300.

389. Bousvaros A, Marcon M, Treem W, et al. Chronic recurrent multifocal osteomyelitis associated with chronic inflammatory bowel disease in children. *Dig Dis Sci* 1999;44:2500–2507.

390. Laxer RM, Shore SD, Manson D, et al. Chronic recurrent multifocal osteomyelitis and psoriasis: a report of a new association and review of related disorders. *Sem Arth Rheum* 1988;17:260–270.

391. Suei Y, Taguchi A, Tanimoto K. Diagnostic points and possible origin of osteomyelitis in synovitis, acne, pustulosis, hyperostosis, and osteitis (SAPHO) syndrome: a radiographic study of 77 mandibular osteomyelitis cases. *Rheumatology* 2003;42:1398–1403.

CHAPTER 13

Alexandre Arkader
Mark C. Gebhardt
John P. Dormans

Bone and Soft-Tissue Tumors

Pediatric bone and soft-tissue tumors are rare. Although uncommon, these tumors may impact significantly in the child's life, in terms of both survival and quality of life. Most musculoskeletal tumors seen in pediatric group are benign; however, malignancies do occur. The musculoskeletal primary malignancies that occur predominately in children are two bone sarcomas, namely osteosarcoma and Ewing sarcoma (EWS), and one soft-tissue sarcoma (STS), rhabdomyosarcoma (RMS). In addition, there are non-RMSs, such as congenital and infantile fibrosarcoma in young children and synovial sarcoma in adolescents. The orthopaedist must remain alert, because the malignant tumor is an unexpected event, and its infrequency can result in improper or delayed initial management. The orthopaedist who sees pediatric patients but is not prepared to manage a malignant or an aggressive benign musculoskeletal tumor needs to be comfortable with evaluating patients with these kinds of tumors and deciding which of them should be referred to an orthopaedic oncologist.

This chapter reviews the common bone and soft-tissue tumors of childhood; it discusses how the patients present, what physical findings to expect, and what the plain radiographs may show, and it suggests additional diagnostic and staging evaluations and treatment. This chapter is not intended to be a definitive text on musculoskeletal pathology, and tumor management, and includes only the most common tumors of childhood.

MOLECULAR BIOLOGY OF TUMORS

In the last 30 years, the use of adjuvant chemotherapy has led to dramatic improvement in the survival of children with previously lethal sarcomas. While 30 years ago, 80% of children with a primary bone sarcoma died, now at least that same number will survive (1, 2). One of the intriguing aspects of childhood sarcomas is that, despite similar histologies, stages, and prognostic factors, some patients respond well to treatment, whereas others seem to be resistant to chemotherapy. To date, patients with good prognoses cannot be distinguished from those with poor prognoses except by crude clinical characteristics, such as the presence of metastatic disease at diagnosis or the histologic response to preoperative chemotherapy (3). Recent molecular findings in sarcomas may shed light on their biologic behavior and their response to chemotherapy.

One method of looking for genetic alterations in tumors is to examine the chromosomes by karyotype analysis. The identification of recurrent chromosomal abnormalities provides clues regarding sites of potential gene mutations. Normally, there are 23 pairs of chromosomes in the nucleus of the human cell. Osteosarcomas in general have multiple, bizarre karyotypic abnormalities: some chromosomes are missing, some are duplicated, and some are grossly altered. To date, all studies of high-grade osteosarcomas have shown complex karyotypes and nonclonal chromosome aberrations superimposed on complex clonal events (4, 5). Low-grade juxtacortical osteosarcoma, on the other hand, is characterized by the presence of a ring chromosome accompanied by few other abnormalities or none at all (6). Although it is usually possible to distinguish high-grade from low-grade osteosarcoma by standard histology, the karyotype information may be diagnostically useful in the case of other tumors. In addition to possibly providing prognostic information, the specific chromosomal aberrations provide clues that assist molecular biologists who are looking for gene mutations (6).

In contrast to osteosarcoma, Ewing sarcoma (EWS)/peripheral neuroectodermal tumors (PNETs) and alveolar RMSs have single chromosomal translocations characteristic of their respective histologies. In these tumors, part of one chromosome is transposed to part of another chromosome through a breakpoint. A novel gene and gene protein product are created that presumably give the cell a growth advantage. The most common translocations for these tumors are listed in Table 13-1 (7, 8).

TABLE 13-1	Cytogenetic Findings in Pediatric Soft-Tissue Neoplasms	
Tumor	**Translocation**	**Genes**
EWS/PNET	t(11;22)(q24;q12)	EWS-FLI1
	t(21;22)(q21;q12)	EWS-ERG
Clear cell sarcoma	t(12;22)(q13;q12)	EWS-ATF1
Synovial sarcoma	t(X;18)(p11;q11)	SYT-SSX1
		SYT-SSX2
Desmoid tumor, fibromatosis	Trisomy 20	
Congenital fibrosarcoma	t(12;15)(p13;q25)	ETV6-NTRK3 (Tel-TrkC)
Dermatofibrosarcoma protuberans	t(17;22)(q22;q13)	COLIA1-PDGFβ
Lipoblastoma	8q rearrangement (8q11-q13)	
Alveolar RMS	t(2;13)(q35;q14)	PAX3-FHKR
	t(1;13)(p36;q14)	PAX7-FHKR
Alveolar soft parts sarcoma	t(X;17)(p11.2;q25)	ASPL-TFE3

EWS/PNET, Ewing sarcoma/peripheral (primitive) neuroectodermal tumor.

The demonstration of translocations has been useful in the differential diagnosis of round cell tumors. Under the light microscope, there is little to distinguish one of these tumor types from another, and although immunohistochemistry helps to a certain extent, it is at times difficult to be sure of the diagnosis. Demonstration of these characteristic karyotypic findings makes pathologists more secure in their diagnosis and has helped with the classification of these tumors. To perform a karyotype analysis, short-term cultures and metaphase spreads are necessary, but these are labor- intensive and require fresh tissue (7). Fluorescent *in situ* hybridization and reverse transcriptase–polymerase chain reaction (RT-PCR) allow rapid analysis for the presence of translocations; these techniques can be performed on frozen tissue and sometimes even on paraffin-embedded tissue (8–10). Therefore, it is important to give the pathologist appropriate fresh tissue to be snap frozen to preserve messenger ribonucleic acid (mRNA) and allow these studies to be performed (11).

These translocations have significance beyond merely establishing the diagnosis. These rearrangements lead to novel proteins that give the tumor cell a growth advantage. In EWS/PNET, for instance, a fragment of the EWS gene contains DNA-binding domains of the FLY1 gene. The protein acts by disrupting pathways that regulate DNA transcription (12). For several years, it was difficult to make the distinction between EWS and PNET, and clinicians were not sure whether to treat them differently. The observation that both EWS, a poorly differentiated mesenchymal tumor of uncertain cell lineage, and PNET, a tumor believed to be of neural crest origin, shared the same chromosomal translocation led pathologists to believe that both were related neuroectodermal tumors (13). As noted in Table 13-1, further studies revealed other translocations in

several of these tumors, each such translocation specifying a different novel protein. There is debate regarding whether one or the other of these is associated with a better prognosis, but the treatment strategies used today are the same for both tumors. While some authors suggest that tumors with the type 1 transcript (EWS-FLY1) are associated with a better prognosis than those with other transcripts, others have disputed this (14, 15).

More recently, these markers have been used in staging and follow-up of high-risk patients (16). Using RT-PCR technology, one can detect small numbers of tumor cells in a bone marrow or a peripheral blood cell population (17). This makes the interpretation of bone marrow aspirates more precise and may provide a method for the earlier detection of relapses after treatment. It is hoped that the gene products of these translocations can also be used in treatment strategies. Because the novel genes formed from the translocation make a novel protein that normal cells do not make, antibodies or targeted T cells can be generated to specifically kill tumor cells. This is being tried in early-phase trials of relapsed patients with RMS and EWS/PNET, and if it works, it may be a way of treating patients who fail standard drug therapy.

Genetic alterations in the DNA of sarcomas have been well demonstrated. Mutations in genes, called *oncogenes*, give some evidence about the pathogenesis of these tumors and may have some prognostic and therapeutic import (4, 18, 19). Oncogenes are normal cellular genes (*protooncogenes*) that are necessary for the normal development and functioning of the organism (20). When they are mutated, they may produce a protein that is capable of inducing the neoplastic state. Oncogenes act through a variety of mechanisms to deregulate cell growth. This is obviously a very complex process and may involve more than one genetic event.

There are two categories of oncogenes: *dominant oncogenes* and *tumor-suppressor genes* (20). The cumulative effect alters proteins that function as growth factors and their receptors, kinase inhibitors, signal transducers, and transcription factors (12). The dominant oncogenes encode proteins that are involved in signal transduction, that is, in transmitting an external stimulus from outside the cell to the machinery that controls replication in the cell nucleus. Mutant cellular signal transduction genes keep the cell permanently "turned on." The protein products of oncogenes also function as aberrant growth factors, growth factor receptors, or nuclear transcription factors. These types of genes seem to have less of a role in osteosarcomas. One exception is amplification of the *HER-2/NEU/ERBB-2* protooncogene in patients with breast cancer, which confers a poorer prognosis. Patients with this amplification are treated with a monoclonal antibody to this protooncogene [MAb45D5, trastuzumab (Herceptin)]. Overexpression of *HER2-NEU* in osteosarcoma has been reported and is associated with advanced disease and poorer prognosis (21, 22). Although this has been disputed by some studies (23, 24), it provides the potential for treatment strategies in patients with osteosarcoma who have amplification of HER2-NEU.

A second class of genes are the tumor-suppressor genes, which encode proteins whose normal role is to restrict cell proliferation (25, 26). They act as brakes rather than as accelerators of growth. Their normal role is to regulate the cell cycle and keep it in check. The retinoblastoma gene (*RB*) was the first gene recognized in this class (27). Osteosarcomas are very frequent in patients with hereditary retinoblastoma (1000× increased chance), both in the orbit and in the extremities, and are unrelated to irradiation. It was subsequently learned that osteosarcoma in these patients, as well as spontaneously occurring osteosarcomas, carries mutations or deletions of the *RB* gene. It was one of the first clues to the finding that osteosarcomas have a genetic cause. It is estimated that approximately 60% to 75% of sporadic osteosarcomas either have an abnormality of the *RB* gene or do not express a functional RB product (19). The *RB* gene is located on the long arm of chromosome 13 (13q14) and is 200 kb in length. Its product is a 105- to 110-kDa nuclear phosphoprotein (pRB) that appears to have a cell cycle regulatory role. The retinoblastoma protein acts as a signal protein, or a gatekeeper, to regulate the cell cycle through the transcription of genes that mediate the cell cycle. Deactivation of the *RB* gene or absence of pRB allows cells to enter the cell cycle in an unregulated fashion, a condition that imparts a growth advantage to the affected cell. It should be noted that one copy of the gene is sufficient for a normal phenotype. A child born with a normal allele and a mutant or an absent allele will not manifest retinoblastoma until some event occurs in retinoblasts to alter the normal allele. If both copies become deranged, the normal check on the cell cycle disappears, and the conditions for the neoplastic state are met. There are several other mechanisms by which the function of the RB protein can be altered; for instance, viral proteins may bind to the RB protein and inactivate it (5).

The second tumor-suppressor gene to be identified was the *p53* gene (28–30). Located on the short arm of chromosome 17 (17p), its product is a nuclear phosphoprotein that has a cell cycle–regulatory role similar to that of the RB protein. As in the case of *RB*, inactivation of p53 gives the cell a growth advantage, probably because of loss of cell cycle regulation. The p53 phosphoprotein may be inactivated by a variety of mutations, including a single base change (point mutation) that increases the half-life of the protein, allelic loss, rearrangements, and deletions of the *p53* gene. Each of these mechanisms can result in tumor formation by loss of growth control. The p53 protein functions as an extremely important cell cycle checkpoint that blocks cells with DNA damage until they can be repaired or directs damaged cells into apoptosis (programmed cell death) if they cannot be repaired. Cells lacking this checkpoint can accumulate successive genetic abnormalities and possibly become malignant. It is estimated that approximately 25% of osteosarcomas have detectable mutations of the *p53* gene (31).

The p53 protein is a transcription factor, meaning that it binds to regions of other genes (DNA) and controls the expression of genes responsible for cell cycle control (cell growth), apoptosis (programmed cell death), and other metabolic functions, such as control and repair of DNA damage. In concert with RB and a variety of other proteins, p53 acts to regulate the cell cycle through a complex cascade of enzymes, in which RB probably plays the central role. Apoptosis has recently become recognized as an important mechanism by which chemotherapy and radiotherapy kill cancer cells. p53 is involved in this process and appears to arrest cell division after sublethal damage (e.g., by radiation), to give the cell time to repair DNA defects before the next division (32–34). If repair does not take place, the cell undergoes apoptosis and dies. If p53 is not functional, the cell may survive and accumulate genetic defects, leading to malignant transformation. Osteosarcomas have been shown to have a variety of mutations of the *p53* gene (35–37). Preliminary evidence suggests that overexpression of mutant p53 protein (detected by immunohistochemistry) or loss of heterozygosity of the *p53* gene is related to human osteosarcoma (38, 39).

In sarcomas, genetic defects other than p53 and RB have also been detected. One example is a gene called *mdm-2*, which is a zinc finger protein that is amplified in some sarcomas (28, 40, 41). It inactivates p53 protein by binding to it, preventing its transcription factor activity. Cordon-Cardo et al. (42) studied 211 adult STSs by immunohistochemistry, using monoclonal antibodies to mdm-2 and p53, and demonstrated a correlation between overexpression of mdm-2/p53 and poor survival rates. Patients without mutations in either gene (mdm-2/p53–) had the best survival rates, those with one mutation (either mdm-2+/p53– or mdm-2–/p53+) had intermediate rates of survival, and those with mutations in both genes (mdm-2+/p53+) had the lowest survival rates. Another mechanism in which p53 protein can be inactivated is by viral proteins that bind and inactivate both RB and p53 protein (43).

Not only are genetic mutations found in the tumors of patients with sarcomas, but mutations may also be present in all somatic cells (*germ-line mutations*) in patients with heritable cancer (44–46). Although such defects do not appear to be common in the general population, germ-line p53 mutations are present in patients who are part of a familial cancer syndrome. These families have a variety of cancers, often at an early age, and osteosarcomas and STSs are a fairly common occurrence in these kindred. Identification of patients with p53 germ-line mutations can be useful in determining which patients in an affected family are at risk for developing cancers, but much more work is needed in the area of genetic counseling to determine how best to use this information. One study showed that germ-line mutations were present in approximately 3% to 4% of children with osteosarcoma, and that the detection of these mutations was more accurate than family history in predicting the family's susceptibility to cancer (47).

How is this information useful for treatment? One possibility is that the p53 mutations may be potential biologic markers of prognosis and response to treatment (chemotherapy). There is some preliminary evidence that p53 mutations in the tumor may portend a worse prognosis in osteosarcoma. More recently, the association of p53 with apoptosis has suggested possible strategies for chemotherapy, on the basis of the status of the p53 pathway (33, 34). Gene therapy (replacing the missing or mutated gene by transfection with viral carriers) is often discussed, but there are major technical hurdles to overcome before this technology can be used for treating cancers in humans. However, it might be possible to make tumor cells more antigenic, or to make them more sensitive to antineoplastic drugs, by gene transfer. Another strategy would be to alter normal cells to make them less sensitive to damage by chemotherapeutic agents. Currently, these techniques pose technical challenges, but they offer realistic promise for the near future.

Another exciting area of research in the molecular biology of sarcomas is multidrug resistance (MDR). MDR probably explains why some patients respond to chemotherapy and others do not. Drug resistance may be intrinsic (present at diagnosis) or acquired (appearing after treatment of a tumor) (48, 49). At least four basic mechanisms of drug resistance are now recognized under the category of the MDR phenotype. They are (a) changes in glutathione metabolism, (b) alterations in topoisomerase II, (c) non-P-glycoprotein (P-gp)–mediated mechanisms, and (d) P-gp–mediated mechanisms (6, 7, 48–50). Recent evidence has suggested that P-gp may be of particular relevance to osteosarcoma. P-gp is a glycoprotein encoded by the *MDR-1* gene on the long arm of chromosome 7 in humans (48, 49). *MDR-1* is one member of the aneurysmal bone cyst (ABC) superfamily of genes that encode membrane transport proteins; these proteins function as unidirectional membrane pumps using adenosine triphosphate hydrolysis to work against a concentration gradient. P-gp is a 170-kDa protein that is located in the cell membrane and functions as an energy (adenosine triphosphate)–requiring pump that excludes certain classes (amphipathic compounds) of drugs from the cell. This physiologic mechanism is believed to be important in certain organ systems, such as the blood–brain barrier, placenta, liver, kidney, and colon, for ridding the cell of unwanted toxins, but it is also responsible for actively excluding chemotherapeutic agents, such as *Vinca* alkaloids, anthracyclines, colchicine, etoposides, and taxol (many of which are active in osteosarcoma protocols) from the cancer cell. Another feature of the P-gp mechanism that may have some relevance to therapeutic strategies is that some classes of drugs can reverse the MDR phenotype by blocking the action of the pump. These drugs include verapamil, cyclosporin A, tamoxifen, and others.

Several studies have demonstrated that some sarcomas (25% to 69%) display the MDR phenotype at diagnosis, and that relapsed sarcomas show higher incidence and intensity of MDR expression (48, 49, 51, 52). Because of the small numbers of patients in these studies, and the variety of the methods by which MDR expression was tested, comparisons of the studies and an accurate determination of the incidence of MDR expression are difficult to accomplish. In addition, the age of the patient and the type of sarcoma appear to be related to the incidence of detectable P-gp at diagnosis. One study showed that osteosarcomas have a higher incidence of MDR than other types of adult sarcomas (51). Serra et al. (53) demonstrated that overexpression of P-gp protein was evident in 23% of primary and 50% of metastatic osteosarcomas.

Baldini et al. (54) reported on 92 patients with nonmetastatic osteosarcoma of an extremity who had been treated with chemotherapy and surgery. The study demonstrated that an immunohistochemically determined expression of P-gp

predicted a decreased probability of the patient having an event-free survival, and was more accurate in prediction than histologic response to preoperative chemotherapy. Another study failed to find a relation between MDR-1 mRNA expression and outcome in patients treated for osteosarcoma (55).

Findings such as these are important in planning future protocols in human osteosarcoma. The drug-resistant tumor is becoming better identified as one that has a poor histologic response to preoperative chemotherapy and that expresses P-gp. Undoubtedly, it is more complex than this, and other mechanisms will pertain. Several caveats exist. One is the complexity of defining the resistant tumor. Preoperative chemotherapy requires 10 to 12 weeks to provide an estimate of histologic necrosis, unless ways can be found to accurately predict percentage of necrosis by positron emission tomographic (PET) scans, thallium scans, and/or gadolinium-enhanced magnetic resonance imaging (MRI). Detection of P-gp at diagnosis is difficult, and no one method has proven superior. It is probably not sufficient to demonstrate the presence of P-gp; also important is whether the pump is functioning to exclude cytotoxic agents from the tumor cell. Ideally, one would like to reverse the action of the P-gp mechanism but, just as there are no new agents to rescue patients who show poor histologic response, the agents currently available to reverse MDR are of limited benefit. They are potentially problematic in that they make normal cells less tolerant of chemotherapy, and thereby increase toxicity; and in other tumors they have not proven to be effective. The future probably lies in developing more effective reversing agents and in defining other drug-resistant mechanisms.

EVALUATION

A thorough evaluation is necessary for any child presenting with a bone or soft-tissue mass. Although infection and trauma are much more common than a neoplastic process, the consequences of the mismanagement of a patient with a musculoskeletal tumor can be grave (Fig. 13-1).

Medical History. Most children have no significant past medical history, but inquiries should be made. Has the child had a previous fracture? Has the child had other illnesses? Have radiographs been taken previously? Do not assume that the patient or the family will volunteer significant past medical history. Questions that should be asked include: How long has the mass been present? The longer the mass has been present, the more likelihood of a benign process. Especially worrisome are new masses that arise and grow over a short period of time. Is the mass getting bigger or is it stable in size? Masses that are rapidly growing indicate an active process that could be aggressive. Depending on the location, however, such as axial skeleton, some masses may not be noticed until they reach substantial size. Among younger patients, a parent usually notices the mass first, and although the parent will usually think that the mass has appeared overnight, this is rarely the

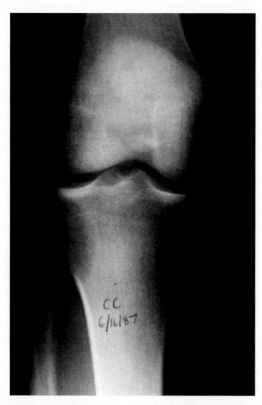

FIGURE 13-1. Anteroposterior radiograph of the knee of a young man who complained of it "giving way." The orthopaedist who saw the patient suspected a derangement, and the patient eventually had arthroscopic surgery. A radiolucent lesion can easily be seen in the lateral aspect of the proximal tibial metaphysis and epiphysis. This giant cell tumor of bone was missed because the physician did not consider this diagnosis when he was examining the patient or the radiograph.

case. Teenagers may report the presence of a mass, but often only after a few weeks or months of waiting for it to resolve spontaneously. Is the mass associated with pain? Pain at the lesional site is a frequent complaint (see below). Active and aggressive tumors will usually present with pain. Painful soft-tissue masses are most often abscesses. Most soft-tissue tumors do not produce significant symptoms until they are large. Although most of the soft-tissue masses seen in children prove to be benign, all soft-tissue masses, even those in children, should be considered to be malignant tumors until proven otherwise. The consequences of mistaking a malignant soft-tissue tumor for a benign tumor can be devastating, whereas the consequences of approaching a benign tumor as if it were a malignancy are minimal. Is there a history of cancer? Depending on the age and the type of tumor, metastatic disease may be the main differential diagnosis.

Chief Complaint. Generally, bone and soft-tissue tumors present in one of four ways:

1. Pain
2. Mass
3. Incidental finding on x-ray
4. Pathologic fracture

Pain is the most common presenting complaint of a child with a musculoskeletal tumor. The characteristics of the pain can help determine the diagnosis. Ask the patient: Where is the pain? How did it begin? Is it sharp, dull, radiating, or constant? Is it associated with activity? Is there a particular activity that makes the pain worse? What makes the pain better? Does it awaken you at night? Is the intensity of the pain increasing, staying the same, or diminishing?

Patients who have active or aggressive benign tumors (e.g., ABC, chondroblastoma, and osteoblastoma) usually have a mild, dull, slowly progressive pain that is worse at night and aggravated by activity. Patients with malignant musculoskeletal tumors complain of a more rapidly progressive symptom complex, not specifically related to activity, which often awakens them at night. Occasionally, the pain pattern is diagnostic. The classic example is the pain of an osteoid osteoma, which is a constant, intense pain that is worse at night, and is almost always relieved by aspirin or nonsteroidal anti-inflammatory drugs (NSAIDs). The pain caused by a Brodie abscess (subacute osteomyelitis) is similar to that of an osteoid osteoma, but is rarely relieved by aspirin.

Most children and parents date the onset of symptoms to a traumatic event. The specific nature of the trauma and the relation of the trauma to the current symptoms must be evaluated thoroughly. Trauma without a definitive fracture may be the explanation for an abnormal radiograph, but it should not be assumed to be the explanation, even for a periosteal reaction, unless the history is perfectly consistent. With the increased level of organized sports for children, there has been an increase in the incidence of fatigue or stress fractures, and these can sometimes be confused with neoplasias. Still, one should be cautious about ascribing a lesion to trauma.

The child presenting with a fracture should be questioned about the specifics of the injury that produced the fracture. Most lesions that lead to a pathologic fracture are easily recognized on a plain radiograph, but occasionally they may not be obvious. When the traumatic event seems insignificant, a pathologic fracture should be suspected. Patients should be asked about symptoms, no matter how minimal, that they experienced before the fracture. Most aggressive benign tumors and malignant tumors produce pain before the bone is weakened enough to fracture. Latent benign tumors such as unicameral bone cyst (UBC) and nonossifying fibroma (NOF) are often diagnosed following a trauma, as an incidental finding or a pathologic fracture.

A complete review of systems is mandatory. Ask specifically about fever, decreased appetite, irritability, and decreased activity. Most patients with musculoskeletal tumors do not have systemic symptoms at presentation, and their presence should alert the physician to the possibility of an underlying generalized disorder or osteomyelitis. Rarely, children with a malignant neoplasm, such as EWS, may present with fever, weight loss, and malaise, favoring an infectious etiology. Even children with large primary malignant musculoskeletal tumors usually appear healthy.

Physical Examination.

All patients with musculoskeletal complaints, especially those in the pediatric age group, should have a complete physical examination. Not only can important information be gained about the specific disorder being evaluated, but also other significant abnormalities may be found. For example, café au lait lesions of the skin are a clue that the patient has fibrous dysplasia or neurofibromatosis (Fig. 13-2); numerous hard, nontender, fixed masses near the ends of long bones are suggestive of multiple hereditary exostosis (MHE).

The affected extremity should be examined carefully. The mass should be measured; larger tumors are usually more active and worrisome. Although there isn't a specific number, soft-tissue masses over 5 cm and bone tumors over 8 cm have a higher likelihood of being malignant. The location is an important characteristic. STSs are usually located deep to the deep fascia, while bone sarcomas are usually located around the fastest growth areas (e.g., knee and shoulder). STSs are usually "fixed" to superficial or deep structures (no mobility) and firm to touch; soft, movable, nontender masses, especially those in the subcutaneous tissues, are usually benign. Transilluminate the mass, if light is transmitted more easily through the mass than through the surrounding tissue, the mass is a fluid-filled cyst. The gait pattern should be recorded; muscular atrophy measured, and the range of motion of the adjacent joint should be measured. The presence of erythema, tenderness, or increased temperature should be noted.

Neurovascular exam is essential. Often vascular malformations will be in the differential of soft-tissue tumors; check

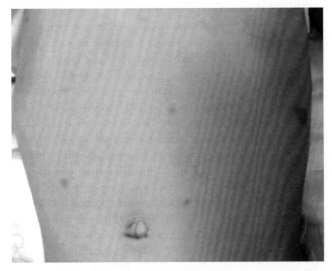

FIGURE 13-2. Appearance of the abdomen of a 4-year-old girl who presented with several café au lait spots and angular deformity of the tibia. Based on physical examination, the diagnosis of neurofibromatosis could be made. (Reproduced with permission from The Children's Orthopaedic Center, Los Angeles, CA.)

for pulsations or bruit. Detailed peripheral nerve check will assist in evaluating the proximity to these structures. Check for satellite lesions, the easiest lesion to miss is the second lesion. Examine the abdomen for hepatomegaly, splenomegaly, etc. Examine regional lymph nodes; although most musculoskeletal malignancies metastasize via hematogenous, some will do it via lymphatic. The most common ones are epithelioid sarcoma (16%), synovial sarcoma (15%), RMS (13%), and angiosarcoma (13%) (56).

Plain Radiograph Examination.

Plain radiographs are the single most useful image modality to assess a musculoskeletal tumor; all patients should have at least anteroposterior and lateral plain radiographs of the affected area. Often bone tumors are incidentally found after radiographs are taken for other reason. Pathologic fracture is also a common presentation, especially among some benign tumors such as UBC.

The entire lesion must be observed. The radiograph should be reviewed systematically. Look at the bone, all of it, and every bone on the radiograph. Ask yourself these questions: Is there an area of increased or decreased density? Is there endosteal or periosteal reaction, and if there is, what are the characteristics of the reaction? Is there cortical destruction? Is it localized or are there multiple defects? Is the margin in the tumor well defined or poorly defined? Is there a reactive rim of bone surrounding the lesion? Are there densities within a radiolucent lesion? Is the bone of normal, increased, or decreased overall density? Is the joint normal? Is there loss of articular cartilage? Is the subchondral bone normal, thick, or thin? Are there abnormalities in the bone on both sides of the joint? Are there intra-articular densities? Is there a soft-tissue mass? Are there calcifications or ossifications in the soft tissue? If one looks specifically for abnormalities, it is unlikely that an abnormality will be missed.

The pelvis and the scapula are exceptions to this rule. Large tumors involving the pelvis or the scapula, even those with marked destruction of bone, can be extremely difficult or impossible to see on a plain radiograph. If there is a suggestion that the patient has a pelvic or a scapular tumor, computerized axial tomography (CT) scan or magnetic resonance (MRI) is recommended.

Enneking (57) proposes that four sets of questions should be asked when looking at plain radiographs of a possible bone tumor.

1. Where is the tumor? This refers to the lesion's anatomic location: long bone or flat bone; epiphyseal, metaphyseal, or diaphyseal; and medullary canal, intracortical, or surface. Based on the tumor location and the patient's age, one can already formulate a differential list.
2. What is the tumor doing to the bone? Is there erosion of the bone, and if so, what is the pattern? This will determine the lesion aggressiveness.
3. What is the bone doing to the tumor? Is there periosteal or endosteal reaction? Is it continuous? Is it sharply defined? The periosteal reaction will reflect the efforts of the host bone to contain the lesion.

TABLE 13-2	Most Common Pediatric Bone Tumors by Location
Tumor Location	**Most Common Tumors**
Epiphysis	Chondroblastoma (growth plate open)
	Giant cell tumor (growth plate closed)
	Brodie abscess (subacute osteomyelitis)
	Langerhans cell histiocytosis
Metaphysis	Anything!
	Most benign and malignant bone tumors
Diaphysis	Fibrous dysplasia
	Osteofibrous dysplasia
	Adamantinoma
	Langerhans cell histiocytosis
	Osteoid osteoma
	Bone cyst
	Ewing sarcoma
	Leukemia/lymphoma
	Osteomyelitis
Anterior spine elements	Langerhans cell histiocytosis
	Hemangioma
	Infection
	Giant cell tumor
	Chordoma
	Leukemia
Posterior spine elements	Aneurysmal bone cyst
	Osteoblastoma
	Osteoid osteoma
	Osteochondroma

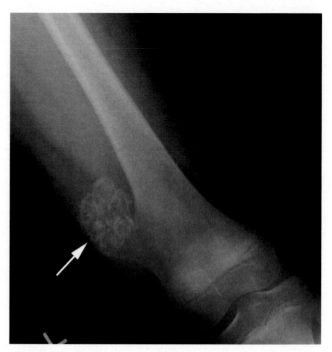

FIGURE 13-3. Anteroposterior radiograph of the distal femur of a 12-year-old boy with a hard, fixed mass that has been present for several years. Note the continuity of the cortex and the outline of the mass, as well as continuity of the intramedullary cavity and the interior of the mass. Also present are calcifications within the mass. The appearance is typical for a pedunculated osteochondroma. (Reproduced with permission from The Children's Orthopaedic Center, Los Angeles, CA.)

4. Are there any intrinsic characteristics within the tumor that indicate its histology? Is there bone formation by the tumor? Is there calcification? Is the lesion completely radiolucent?

In addition to this list approach, always consider patient's age and specific location of the tumor within the bone, as these characteristics will limit the differential diagnosis (Table 13-2). Most bone tumors can be diagnosed correctly after obtaining the history, performing a physical examination, and examining the plain radiograph. When the specific diagnosis is made from these examinations, additional studies are requested only if they are necessary for treatment. Often, specific treatment can be planned from only the history, physical examination, and plain radiographs. For example, a 12-year-old boy with a hard, fixed mass in the distal femur that has been present for several years and has not increased in size for more than 1 year complains of pain after direct trauma to this mass. Plain radiographs confirm the clinically suspected diagnosis of osteochondroma (Fig. 13-3). Further evaluation to make the diagnosis is not necessary.

When the specific diagnosis cannot be made, it should be possible to limit the differential to three or four diagnoses, and appropriate additional evaluations can be requested. CT, MRI, and nuclear bone scanning (technetium, gallium, thallium, or indium) may reveal findings that are diagnostic, or that provide the information required for planning a subsequent biopsy.

Additional Diagnostic Studies

Laboratory Examinations. For the most part, serum and urine laboratory values are usually normal in musculoskeletal neoplasia. Nonetheless, a few musculoskeletal tumors are associated with abnormal laboratory values. The erythrocyte sedimentation rate (ESR) is nonspecific but sensitive. Patients with infections or malignant tumors usually have an elevated ESR, but patients with benign disease should have a normal value. A normal ESR value can increase the physician's confidence that a suspected benign, inactive lesion is just that. Patients with active benign or malignant musculoskeletal tumors, particularly those with EWS, often have an elevated ESR, but it is rarely >80 mm/hour. A markedly elevated value (>180 mm/hour) favors a diagnosis of infection and may be just what is needed to justify an early aspiration of a bone or soft-tissue lesion. C-reactive protein (CRP) is another useful serum value that indicates systemic inflammation. Because it increases and returns to normal more quickly than ESR, CRP has been used as the main serum value to follow-up infection.

Serum alkaline phosphatase is present in most tissues in the body, but the bones and the hepatobiliary system are the predominant sources. In the pediatric age group, conventional high-grade osteosarcoma is associated with elevated levels of serum alkaline phosphatase (58). Not all patients with osteosarcoma have elevated levels of serum alkaline phosphatase, and therefore a normal level does not exclude osteosarcoma from the diagnosis. A minimal elevation can be observed with numerous processes, even a healing fracture. Adults with elevated levels of serum alkaline phosphatase secondary to bone disease are most likely to have Paget disease of bone or diffuse metastatic carcinoma. Patients with a primary liver disorder have elevated levels of serum alkaline phosphatase as well, but they also have elevated levels of serum 5-nucleotidase and leucine aminopeptidase, and glutamyl transpeptidase deficiency. The levels of 5-nucleotidase and leucine aminopeptidase are not elevated in primary bone tumors. Two- to threefold increase in the alkaline phosphatase levels has been associated with worse prognosis in patients with osteosarcoma (58).

Serum and urine calcium and phosphorus levels should be measured, especially if a metabolic bone disorder is suspected. Serum lactate dehydrogenase (LDH) level is elevated in some patients with osteosarcoma. Patients with EWS or osteosarcoma with elevated LDH have a worse prognosis (15, 59, 60). Elevated LDH levels may also indicate relapse in a patient who has been treated for these tumors (59). Patients entering chemotherapy treatment protocols will need to have LDH levels determined in order to stratify them on the protocol. Other laboratory determinations are not helpful and are not recommended.

Radionuclide Scans.   Technetium bone scanning is readily available, safe, and an excellent method for evaluating the activity of the primary lesion. In addition, bone scanning is the most practical method of surveying the entire skeleton (Fig. 13-4). Technetium-99 attached to a polyphosphate is injected intravenously, and, after a delay of 2 to 4 hours, the polyphosphate, with its attached technetium, concentrates in the skeleton proportional to the production of new bone. A disorder that is associated with an increase in bone production increases the local concentration of technetium-99 and produces a "hot spot" on the scan. The technetium bone scan can be used to evaluate the activity of a primary lesion, to search for other bone lesions, and to indicate extension of a lesion beyond what is seen on the plain radiograph. The polyphosphate–technetium-99 compound also concentrates in areas of increased blood flow, and soft-tissue tumors usually have increased activity compared with normal soft tissues. The technetium-99 bone scan can be used to evaluate blood flow if images are obtained during the early phases immediately after injection of the technetium-99. The polyphosphate–technetium-99 is cleared and excreted by the kidneys, so the kidneys and the bladder have more activity than other organs. The technetium-99 scan is sensitive but nonspecific, whereas infectious processes will usually present with "hot scans." The principal value of a radionuclide scan is as a means of surveying the entire skeleton for clinically unsuspected lesions. There are exceptions and false negative may occur, in approximately 25% of cases of Langerhans cell histiocytosis (LCH), the bone

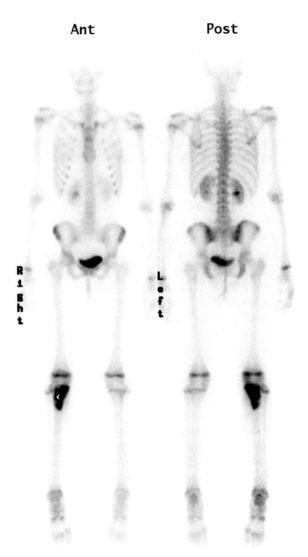

Ant   **Post**

FIGURE 13-4.   An anterior and posterior view of a whole-body technetium-99 bone scan. This was a 14-year-old girl with a right proximal tibia osteogenic sarcoma and there is increased activity in the lesional area. There were no other sites of disease based on the bone scan. Technetium-99 bone scanning is an efficient means of evaluating the entire skeleton of a patient with a bone lesion. It is important to have the entire skeleton scanned, rather than limit the scan to a small part of the skeleton. (Reproduced with permission from The Children's Orthopaedic Center, Los Angeles, CA.)

scan is normal, or there is decreased activity at the site of the lesion (42, 61, 62).

PET is being used more frequently in the evaluation of musculoskeletal tumors (42, 63). Fluoro-2-deoxy-D-glucose (FDG) PET is the type of PET used most frequently for the musculoskeletal system. Because there is a differential uptake of FDG between neoplastic tissue and normal tissue (neoplastic tissue has greater uptake), it is possible to identify neoplastic tissue on a PET scan. The role of PET in the evaluation and monitoring of patients with musculoskeletal neoplasia is under investigation, especially among children. PET with fluorine-18-FDG has proved particularly useful in evaluating patients with lymphoma (64, 65).

Computerized Axial Tomography.

When introduced in the late 1970s, CT scan dramatically improved the evaluation of bone and soft-tissue tumors. The anatomic location and extent of the tumor could be determined accurately. The improved accuracy of anatomic localization means that less radical surgery can be performed safely.

The density of a bone or soft-tissue mass on a CT scan is called its "attenuation coefficient" and is measured in Hounsfield units (HU). The density of water is 0 HU; tissues more dense than water have a positive value, and tissues less dense than water have a negative value. The vascularity of a lesion can be evaluated by measuring the increase in the attenuation coefficient of a lesion after intravenous infusion of contrast, and comparing this increase to that in an adjacent muscle. Normal muscle has an attenuation coefficient of approximately 60 HU, and increases 5 to 10 HU with a bolus of intravenous contrast. Fat has an attenuation coefficient of approximately 60 HU, and cortical bone usually has a value of more than 1000 HU.

CT scan can be performed quickly and is less anxiety producing than closed MR, so sedation is less likely to be needed when compared with MRI. The main downside is the amount of radiation delivered in a CT scan, particularly among children (66). CT scan is most useful in the evaluation of small lesions in or immediately adjacent to the cortex (e.g., osteoid osteoma) and lesions with fine mineralization or calcifications (e.g., chondroblastoma). CT is still the gold standard for chest evaluation and to rule out lung nodules (Fig. 13-5). CT has also been used for percutaneous biopsies and treatment of several different lesions.

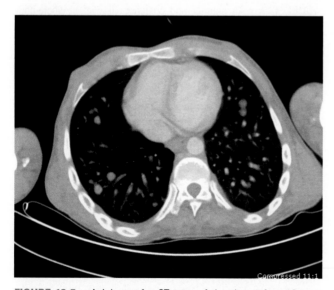

FIGURE 13-5. Axial cut of a CT scan of the chest of an 18-year-old male who had NF-1 and an MPNST of the shoulder girdle with metastatic involvement of the lung at presentation. (Reproduced with permission from The Children's Orthopaedic Center, Los Angeles, CA.)

Magnetic Resonance Imaging.

MRI does not expose the patient to radiation and has proved to be the most useful tool in the evaluation of soft-tissue lesions. MRI produces images of the body in all three planes (axial, sagittal, and coronal) as easily as in a single plane, and poses no known hazards to the patient.

The images are produced by a computer program that converts the reactions of tissue hydrogen ions in a strong magnetic field excited by radio waves. By adjusting excitation variables, images that are T1- and T2-weighted are obtained. A variety of techniques have been used to produce images of improved quality compared with routine T1- and T2-weighted images. The use of gadolinium as an intravascular contrast agent allows one to judge the vascularity of a lesion, thereby providing even more information about the tumor. Fat-suppression images with gadolinium enhancement are often especially useful in demonstrating a soft-tissue neoplasia. As with CT scan, it is important for the orthopaedist requesting MRI to discuss the case with the radiologist. The radiologist can then determine the optimal MRI settings required for visualizing the lesion.

MRI is the single most important diagnostic test after physical examination and plain radiography for evaluating a musculoskeletal lesion. The ability to view the lesion in three planes, determine its intraosseous extent, see the soft-tissue component clearly, and have an idea of the tissue type from one diagnostic test makes MRI a powerful tool. Unfortunately, variations in technique mean that it is important that the examination be planned carefully if the maximum information possible is to be obtained. T1-weighted (with and without gadolinium), T2-weighted, and fat-suppression techniques are the minimal images needed.

Staging.

Patients with neoplasia can be separated into groups on the basis of the extent of their tumor and its potential or presence for metastasis. These groups are called *stages*. Grouping patients by their stage helps the physician predict a patient's risk of local recurrence, metastasis, and outcome. This facilitates making treatment decisions about individual patients and helps in the comparison of treatment protocols. Staging systems are based on the histologic grade of the tumor, its size and location, and the presence of regional or distant metastases. The presence of a metastasis at the time of presentation is a bad prognostic sign and, regardless of other findings, puts the patient in the highest-risk stage. For patients without metastases at presentation, the histologic grade of the tumor is the principal prognostic predictor. Size is next in importance. Higher histologic grade and larger tumors are associated with the worse prognoses (67).

There are two common staging systems in use for musculoskeletal tumors. The task force on malignant bone tumors of the American Joint Commission on Cancer Staging and End Result Studies published a staging system for soft-tissue tumors in 1977, which was most recently revised in 2002 (68). This staging system is based on the histologic grade (G), local extent or size (T), whether the nodes are involved (N), and metastases (M). The tumors are separated into three histologic grades (G1, low grade; G2, medium grade; G3, high grade) and two sizes (T1 for <8 cm (for bone) or 5 cm (for soft tissue), T2 for equal to or greater than that). Patients with nodal involvement are designated N1, and those without nodal involvement are designated N0. Patients with metastatic disease are designated M1, and those without metastatic disease are designated M0. There are four stages, with subclasses in each stage. Tumors at stage I are associated with the best prognosis, and tumors at stage IV with the worst prognosis.

Enneking et al. (69) also proposed a musculoskeletal staging system. This system is used more often by orthopaedists involved in the management of patients with musculoskeletal tumors. It was designed to be simple, straightforward, and clinically practical. The tumors are separated into only two histologic grades (I, low grade; II, high grade) and two anatomic extents (A, intracompartmental; B, extracompartmental). Patients with metastatic disease in either a regional lymph node or a distant site are grouped together as stage III. Each bone is defined as its own separate anatomic compartment. The soft-tissue anatomic compartments are defined as muscle groups separated by fascial boundaries. There are five stages in this system (Table 13-3).

Enneking et al. (69) also introduced four terms to indicate the surgical margin of a tumor resection. These terms are in common use, and provide a means of describing the relation between the histologic extent of the tumor and the resection margin. The surgical margins are defined as *intralesional, marginal, wide,* and *radical*. An intralesional margin is the surgical margin achieved when a tumor's pseudocapsule is violated and gross tumor is removed from within the pseudocapsule. An incisional biopsy and curettage are two common examples of an intralesional margin. A marginal surgical margin is achieved when a tumor is removed by dissecting between the normal tissue and the tumor's pseudocapsule. This is a surgical margin obtained when a tumor is "shelled out." A wide surgical margin is achieved when the tumor is removed with a surrounding cuff of normal, uninvolved tissue. This is often referred to as *en bloc* resection and is the most common type of resection used for malignant tumors. A radical surgical margin is achieved when the tumor and the

entire compartment (or compartments) are removed together. This usually is accomplished only with an amputation proximal to the joint that is just proximal to the lesion (e.g., an above-knee amputation for a tibial tumor). As a rule, benign lesions can be managed with an intralesional or a marginal surgical margin, but malignant tumors require a wide surgical margin. Radical surgical margins are reserved for recurrent tumors and the most infiltrative malignancies.

Biopsy. Biopsy is an essential part of tumor staging and management decision making for children with a bone or a soft-tissue tumor. Sometimes, a biopsy can be avoided and diagnosis made on basis of history, physical examination, and imaging studies. When a biopsy is required, the prebiopsy evaluation improves the chance that adequate and representative tissue will be obtained, the least amount of normal tissue will be contaminated, and the pathologist will make an accurate diagnosis. It is recommended that the surgeon consult with the radiologist and the pathologist before performing the biopsy to get their suggestions for the best tissue to obtain; furthermore, discussing the case preoperatively with the pathologist will allow the pathologist to be better prepared to make a diagnosis from a frozen section.

The purpose of the biopsy is to confirm the diagnosis suspected by the physician after the evaluation, or to determine which diagnosis, from among a limited differential diagnosis, is correct. In addition to providing confirmation for a specific diagnosis, the tissue obtained must be sufficient for histologic grading. It must be representative of the tumor and, because many musculoskeletal tumors are heterogeneous, the specific site from which the tissue is taken is important. Biopsy is not a simple procedure; the musculoskeletal tumor society has shown that an unplanned or erroneous biopsy can impact negatively the outcome, with higher incidence of unneeded surgery, including amputation and worse outcome (70).

There are two forms of biopsies: percutaneous (needle biopsy) and open (incisional and excisional). Percutaneous biopsy can be done via fine needle aspirate or core. It has the advantage of having low morbidity and sometimes can be done in clinic (older patients). Some of the disadvantages include a small amount of tissue and a higher chance for sampling error that may limit the ability to perform special stains and cytogenetics. The reported accuracy of a needle biopsy is around 85% (71).

Open biopsy has the advantage of obtainment of a larger tumor sample that allows the pathologist to perform all necessary studies and decreases the chance of sampling error. The accuracy of open biopsy is close to 96% (71). Furthermore, most children will require general anesthesia for a biopsy and therefore is important to obtain adequate sampling. Open incisional biopsy is the most commonly used technique. It entails obtaining a sizeable fragment of the tumor without attempting excision of the whole mass. Ideally, the treating surgeon will be the one performing the biopsy. That should avoid several possible complications that could impact in the ability of performing limb salvage and adequate tumor resection. Some of

TABLE 13-3	Staging of Musculoskeletal Tumors	
Stage	**Grade**	**Site and Size**
IA	Low	Intracompartmental (T1)
IB	Low	Extracompartmental (T2)
IIA	High	Intracompartmental (T1)
IIB	High	Extracompartmental (T2)
III	Any grade; regional or distant metastasis	Any site or size

T1, tumor <5 cm; T2, tumor ≥5 cm.
From Enneking WF, Spanier SS, Goodman MA. A system for the surgical staging of musculoskeletal sarcoma. *Clin Orthop Relat Res* 1980;153:106, with permission.

the principles of open biopsy include drawing definitive limb salvage incision prior to start; avoiding transverse incisions on extremities; avoiding raising flaps or exposure of neurovascular structures; always performing an intraoperative frozen section to ensure acquisition of diagnostic tissue; if a drain is used, it should exit the skin in line with the incision; placing sutures within 5 mm of the incision; sending material for culture and sensitivity; achieving meticulous homeostasis (hematoma from the biopsy may contain tumor cells and will require resection if surgery is the treatment); and avoiding or judicious use of local anesthesia (72).

Occasionally an excisional biopsy, rather than an incisional biopsy, is indicated. Open excisional biopsy differs from incisional biopsy in that the entire tumor is excised and sent for analysis. An excisional biopsy is appropriate when the lesion is small and can be excised with a cuff of normal tissue. It is usually reserved for small (<3 cm) lesions that are likely benign. An excisional biopsy may be appropriate even when a major resection is required. If the preoperative evaluation strongly supports the diagnosis of a malignancy, particularly one for which a frozen section analysis will be difficult to do, an excisional biopsy should be considered. The advantages

include single surgical procedure; however, a significant disadvantage is the need for extensive tissue sacrifice if re-excision is necessary (malignant tumor) to obtain appropriate margins (i.e., unplanned excision) (Fig. 13-6). An added advantage of an excisional biopsy is that the pathologist is able to examine the entire lesion, thereby improving the accuracy of the pathologic examination. An incisional biopsy exposes uncontaminated tissues to the tumor, and if the tumor proves to be a malignancy, the definitive resection is more complicated. If the lesion can be treated with curettage or a marginal excision, the incisional biopsy leads to the least functional loss. The final decision is made for each patient on the basis of not only the tumor's characteristics but also the patient's preference. Some patients want to take the fewest chances, and are willing to accept the possibility of slight overtreatment, whereas others choose to take one step at a time. It is the surgeon's responsibility to explain the situation to the patient so that an informed decision can be made.

A final note of caution is offered with regard to the biopsy: osteomyelitis is more common than bone tumors, especially in children, and osteomyelitis often mimics neoplasia. The reverse is also true; therefore, when performing a biopsy, even

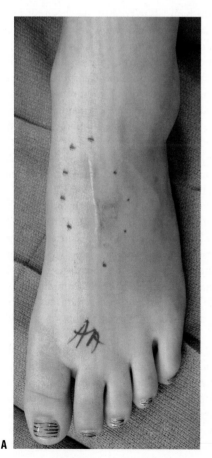
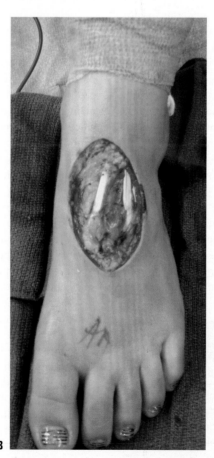
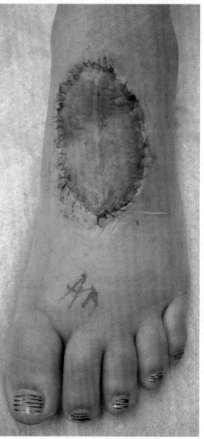

FIGURE 13-6. This 14-year-old girl had an unplanned excision of a "lipoma" of the dorsum of her foot, performed at an outside institution **(A)**. The definitive diagnosis was consistent with a fibrosarcoma. The patient needed re-excision of the lesion with oncologic margins **(B)** and the soft-tissue defect created needed skin grafting **(C)**. (Reproduced with permission from The Children's Orthopaedic Center, Los Angeles, CA.)

when the diagnosis seems obvious, culture every biopsy and biopsy every culture.

SPECIFIC BONE TUMORS

This chapter is not designed to be a definitive musculoskeletal pathology text, and only those tumors that are commonly seen in the pediatric orthopaedic practice are discussed. The authors have tried to confine the discussion to pertinent information regarding the tumors, their evaluation, and particularly their treatment.

BENIGN BONE TUMORS

Bone-Forming Tumors

Osteoid Osteoma.   Osteoid osteoma is a benign active bone tumor that accounts for 11% of the benign bone tumors in Dahlin series from the Mayo Clinic (73). Osteoid osteoma most commonly affects boys (3:1 girl) between 5 and 24 years of age (80% of all patients). McLeod (74) is credited with the initial description, distinguishing it from a Brodie abscess, and from Garre osteomyelitis.

The classic presentation is pain at lesional site. The pain is not related to activity. Prostaglandins produced by the tumor are suspected to cause the pain, which is sharp, piercing, worse at night, and readily alleviated by aspirin or NSAIDs. If a patient has the typical pain for an osteoid osteoma, but there is no relief by aspirin, the diagnosis should be doubted. Patients with osteoid osteoma show few abnormalities on physical examination, with the exception of scoliosis in patients with osteoid osteoma of the spine. The child may walk with a limp and have atrophy of the extremity involved. If the lesion is superficial, it may be tender on palpation.

Although osteoid osteomas may arise in any bone, around 50% are found in the femur and tibia. The usual radiographic appearance is one of dense reactive bone with new bone periosteal formation, the actual lesion (a.k.a. nidus) is small (<15 mm in diameter), radiolucent, and of difficult visualization especially in the axial skeleton. The nidus may be on the surface of the bone, within the cortex, or on the endosteal surface. Lesions on the endosteal surface have less reaction than lesions within or on the cortex (Fig. 13-7).

Spine is a common location for "occult" osteoid osteoma. Since osteoid osteoma of the spine does not elicit a significant bony reaction, and it is usually located in the posterior elements, it is very difficult to make the diagnosis based on plain radiographs (Fig. 13-8A). When a child presents with painful scoliosis, with or without atypical curve pattern, osteoid osteoma should be considered (75–77).

A technetium-99 bone scan is particularly useful to localize the lesion otherwise missed on the plain radiograph (78). CT is the best imaging modality for visualization of the nidus (79). The distance between the CT scan sections should be small (1 to 2 mm), so that the nidus is not missed (Fig. 13-8B). The window

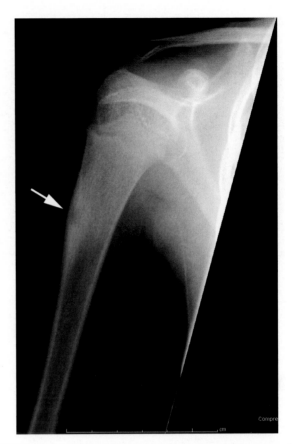

FIGURE 13-7.   Anterior–posterior radiograph of the humerus of a 5-year-old girl who presented with night pain that was readily relieved with NSAIDs. Note the intracortical lytic (nidus) lesion, surrounded by new bone formation, no periosteal reaction or soft-tissue mass (*arrow*). The nidus measured <1 cm and the lesion was consistent with an osteoid osteoma. (Reproduced with permission from The Children's Orthopaedic Center, Los Angeles, CA.)

settings of the CT scanner should be adjusted so that the dense reaction around the lesion does not obscure the small, low-density nidus. MRI can be misleading and demonstrate excessive soft-tissue reaction favoring an infectious or a more aggressive diagnosis (79). Serum and urine laboratory values are normal.

On gross inspection, the nidus of an osteoid osteoma is cherry-red and surrounded by dense white bone. The nidus is small, <5 to 10 mm in diameter. A lesion that is identical histologically to the nidus of an osteoid osteoma, but larger than 2 cm, is called an *osteoblastoma*. The nidus is composed of numerous vascular channels, osteoblasts, and thin, lacelike osteoid seams (Fig. 13-9). Multinucleated giant cells may be seen, but are not common (75).

Natural history shows that osteoid osteoma may heal spontaneously although that may take several years (75, 80). Occasionally, a patient may use aspirin or NSAIDs to control the symptoms until the pain disappears, but most often the intensity of pain, the time it takes for the lesion to heal spontaneously, and the amount of medication required are not tolerable, and surgery is indicated.

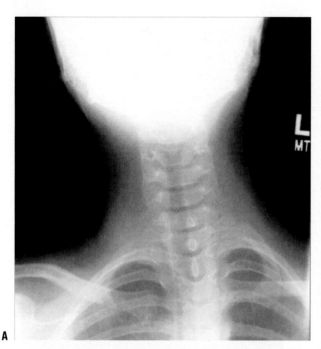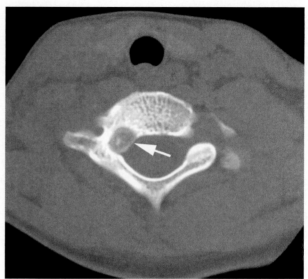

A   **B**

FIGURE 13-8.   This is a 13-year-old boy with lower neck pain, worse at night and torticollis; anterior–posterior **(A)** radiographs of the cervical spine is not diagnostic and only shows malalignment due to muscle spasm. Axial CT **(B)** shows the osteoid osteoma nidus located in the pedicle of C5 (*arrow*). (Reproduced with permission from The Children's Orthopaedic Center, Los Angeles, CA.)

Kneisl and Simon (80) treated 24 patients with osteoid osteoma. Thirteen were operated on immediately, and all had complete relief of pain. Nine others were treated with NSAIDs. Of these, three subsequently elected to have surgery, but the six others also eventually became free of pain (an average of 33 months). Complete removal of the nidus relieves the patient's pain. Partial removal may provide temporary relief,

but the pain usually returns (80). Only the nidus needs to be excised. The reactive bone around the nidus does not have to be removed.

Minimally invasive CT-guided techniques have become the preferred treatment for osteoid osteoma. The advantages include adequate visualization of the nidus, lower risk of recurrence, fast recovery, and its safety. Radiofrequency ablation is

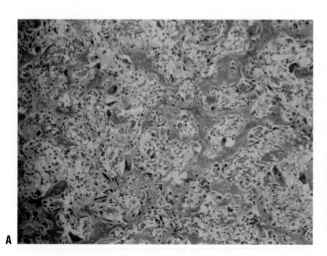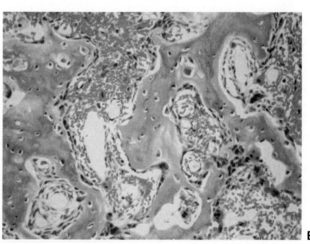

A   **B**

FIGURE 13-9.   **A:** Typical histologic appearance of an osteoid osteoma. There is immature (woven) bone lined with osteoblast. Between the woven bone is a vessel-rich fibrous stroma. There is no atypia, and the few mitotic figures are normal (10× magnification). **B:** Higher magnification (40×) of the histology of the osteoid osteoma shown in A. The woven bone lined with osteoblast is easily seen. The red blood cells indicate the intense vascularity that is typical of this lesion.

one of the most common methods used. The procedure is performed under as an outpatient with general anesthesia. A needle biopsy is performed under CT guidance that is followed by placing the radiofrequency electrode with an internal thermistor and ablating the nidus. The success rate is of up to 90% (81).

Sometimes surgery is indicated, especially for recurrent tumors and spine lesions. Once identified, the nidus is curetted. Although this technique usually does not weaken the bone significantly, sometimes bone grafting is required; for spinal lesions, instrumentation may be needed. Failure in removing the entire nidus will cause recurrence of pain (77, 81). Preoperative planning and careful localization of the nidus is the most important means of ensuring that the nidus can be found during the operation. The reactive bone does not need to be removed.

Osteoblastoma.   Osteoblastoma is a benign active or aggressive tumor. It is histologically identical to osteoid osteoma, but larger. Osteoblastoma is less common than osteoid osteoma, accounting for <1% of the primary bone tumors in Dahlin series (73). Unlike osteoid osteoma, osteoblastoma is not surrounded by dense reactive bone.

It is most commonly seen in boys in the second decade of life (50% of the patients are between 10 and 20 years of age, although the age range is from 5 to 35 years). Pain at lesional site is the classic presentation; most patients have an average delay of 6 months from start of symptoms and diagnosis (82). The pain of an osteoblastoma is not as severe as the pain of an osteoid osteoma, and aspirin or NSAIDs do not have such a dramatic effect. At least one-third of the lesions are located in the spine, in those cases, scoliosis is present in almost half of the patients (82). Lesions of the extremities are usually diaphyseal; the patient often has a limp and mild atrophy, and complains of pain directly over the lesion, especially on palpation.

The appearance of osteoblastoma on a radiograph is variable. It is usually a mixed radiolucent, radiodense lesion, more lucent than dense. There is usually reactive bone formation but less intense than with osteoid osteoma. When the nidus can be observed, it measures over 2 cm. Lesions in the spine may be difficult or impossible to see when initially examining the plain radiograph, but when located by other studies, the subtle abnormality on the plain radiograph can usually be appreciated. Clues to look for on the plain radiograph to indicate the location of an osteoblastoma are an irregular cortex, loss of pedicle definition, and enlargement of the spinous process (83, 84). As with osteoid osteoma, a technetium-99 bone scan is the best method of localization. On a radionuclide scan an osteoblastoma shows increased uptake, and technetium-99 bone scanning is an excellent method of initially screening a patient suspected of having an osteoblastoma. CT scans are the best method of determining the diagnosis and extent of the lesion (Fig. 13-10A–C). On the CT scan, the lesion usually "expands the bone" and has intralesional stippled ossifications and a high attenuation coefficient (100 HU or more). Laboratory examinations of blood and urine show normal results.

The histology of an osteoblastoma is identical to the nidus of an osteoid osteoma. There should not be abnormal mitoses, although mitotic activity may be observed. There are osteoblasts, multinucleated giant cells, seams of osteoid, and a rich vascular bed. Schajowicz and Lemos (85) suggested that a subset of osteoblastoma be termed *malignant osteoblastoma*. They believe that this subset has histologic features that are worse than those of the usual osteoblastoma, is more aggressive locally, and is more likely to recur after limited surgery. Rarely, an osteoblastoma metastasizes (<1%) but still meets the histologic definitions of a benign tumor, although in those cases it should probably be classified as low-grade osteosarcoma.

Biopsy for diagnostic confirmation is usually indicated. The definitive treatment is surgical, as these lesions will continue to enlarge and damage the bone and adjacent structures. A wide surgical resection is theoretically preferred when practical, to reduce chance of recurrence. A four-step approach (extended curettage, high-speed burring, electrocauterization of cavity wall, and phenol 5% solution) has been shown to be effective with recurrence rates around 5% (82) (Fig. 13-10E,F). Children younger than 6 years tend to recur more frequently (82).

Osteochondroma and Multiple Hereditary Exostoses. Also known as exostosis, osteochondroma is a benign latent or active cartilaginous tumor. Although the pathogenesis of this lesion is not known, an abnormality or injury to the periphery of the growth plate has been suggested as the cause (86). It has been shown in an experimental animal study that the periphery of the growth plate can be traumatized and a typical exostosis can be produced.

The patient with a solitary exostosis is usually brought in by a parent who has just noticed a mass adjacent to a joint. Often, the patient may have been aware of the mass for months or even years, and says that it has been slowly enlarging. Pain at presentation is unusual unless there is a trauma. Occasionally, there is loss of motion in the adjacent joint attributable to the size of the mass. Some patients have pain resulting from irritation of an overlying muscle, bursa formation, repeated trauma, pressure on an adjacent neurovascular bundle, or inflammation in an overlying bursa. Other symptoms may include "catching" or "popping" around the knee due to impingement to tendons and muscles.

On physical examination, the mass is nontender, hard, and fixed to the bone. The rest of the physical examination may show no abnormality. Complete neurovascular examination is important.

Osteochondromas can be diagnosed based on their radiographic appearance alone (Fig. 13-3). The mass is a combination of a radiolucent cartilaginous cap with varying amounts of ossification and calcification. The amount of calcification and bone formation increases with age. The base may be broad (sessile exostosis) or narrow (pedunculated exostosis). In both types, the cortex of the underlying bone opens to join the cortex of the exostosis, so that the medullary canal of the bone is in continuity. This can usually be appreciated on the plain radiograph itself, but if not, CT scan or MRI establishes this finding and confirms the diagnosis.

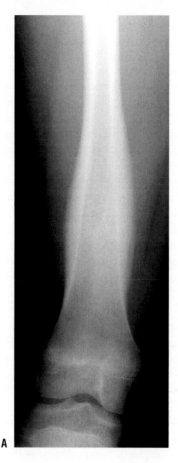

A

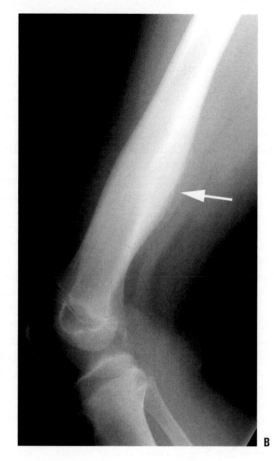

B

FIGURE 13-10. Osteoblastoma. Anteroposterior **(A)** and lateral **(B)** radiographs of a 13-year-old boy with a 3-month history of increasing thigh pain. There is abundant new bone formation and continuous periosteal reaction. A small lucency is seen in the posterior aspect of the femur (*arrow*). The bone scan **(C)** shows increased uptake in the lesional area, and CT axial cut

Ant   Post

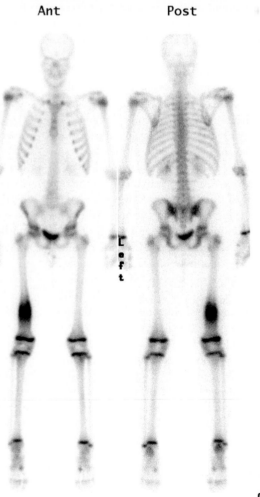

C

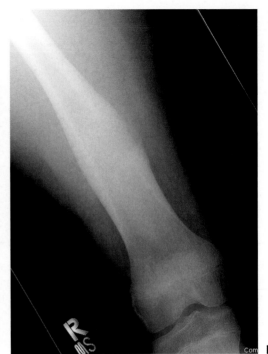

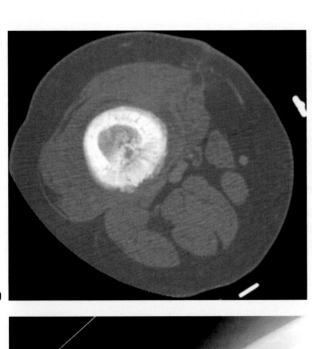

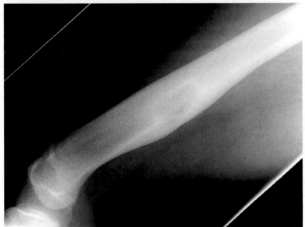

FIGURE 13-10. *(continued)* **(D)** demonstrates the well-defined nidus. Twelve months after a four-step approach **(E** and **F)**, the bone has remodeled; there is no signs of recurrence, and the patient is pain free. (Reproduced with permission from The Children's Orthopaedic Center, Los Angeles, CA.)

In the pediatric age group, osteochondromas should be expected to grow. This is not a sign of malignancy. After skeletal maturity, continued growth of an exostosis is usually an indication for removal (87). The growth rate is not steady, and occasionally a lesion grows more rapidly than expected. Removal of the lesion in a child is indicated only for those patients who have symptoms attributable to pressure on a neurovascular bundle or irritation of the overlying muscle. Removal of the lesion in a young child may result in damage to the growth plate and recurrence of the lesion. Degeneration of the lesion into a malignancy is extremely rare in children and uncommon in adults. The definition of malignant degeneration of a solitary exostosis is confusing. Clinically, an exostosis is considered to be malignant in a patient as old as 30 years or older if there is an enlarging cartilage cap and when the cap is more than approximately 2 cm thick. This so-called malignant degeneration is more common in lesions of the

scapula, the pelvis, and the proximal femur. The real incidence of malignant degeneration is not known. It is probably <2% (88).

Gross examination of an exostosis reveals a lesion that looks like a cauliflower. It has an irregular surface covered with cartilage. The cartilage is usually <1 cm thick, except in the young child, in which it may be 2 or 3 cm thick. Deep in the cartilaginous cap, there is a variable amount of calcification, enchondral ossification, and normal bone with a cortex and cancellous marrow cavity. Typically, the microscopic appearance of the cartilaginous cap is that of benign hyaline cartilage, which has the configuration of a slightly disordered growth plate (Fig. 13-11).

Some patients have multiple osteochondromas, a condition called multiple hereditary exostosis (MHE) (89–91). A patient may have 3 or 4 lesions, but more often there are 10 to 15. Usually, the patient has exostoses of all shapes and

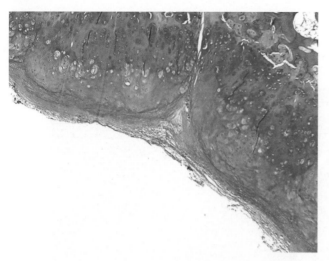

FIGURE 13-11. Low-power view of an osteochondroma cartilage cap, showing the very blend benign hyaline cartilage, low cellularity, no mitoses or pleomorphism. (Reproduced with permission from The Children's Orthopaedic Center, Los Angeles, CA.)

sizes. They are concentrated in the metaphysis of the long bones, but may be in the spine, the ribs, the pelvis, and the scapula. On physical examination, they are hard, fixed masses adjacent to joints. Patients with multiple exostoses are usually shorter than average but not shorter than the normal range. The affected joints show loss of range of motion, especially forearm rotation, elbow extension, hip abduction and adduction, and ankle inversion and eversion.

MHE is transmitted by an autosomal dominant gene with a variable penetrance, and there is an approximately 50% chance that a child of a parent with the heritable gene will show clinical manifestations of this condition (88, 89, 92, 93).

Up to half of the cases are spontaneous mutation (88). The disease may manifest with extensive involvement in the parent, but with minimal involvement in the child, or vice versa (88). In most patients with MHE, the radiographic appearance of the proximal femur or the knees is diagnostic (Fig. 13-12).

Occasionally, one or more of the exostoses need to be removed in order to relieve the pain related to repeated local trauma, or to improve the motion of the adjacent joint. Lesions in the pelvis and the spine should be observed closely because they have the greatest risk of undergoing malignant degeneration. We do not recommend that these lesions be removed simply because they are present. MHE patients often need surgery for correction of angular deformities. Secondary chondrosarcoma is rare in the pediatric age group (94, 95). After the third decade, patients with MHE are at increased risk of developing secondary chondrosarcoma (96, 97). Among large series on chondrosarcoma in children, around 25% of the cases are secondary to a benign cartilaginous lesion (96, 97). We advise patients with exostosis, in particular MHE, to be examined at least yearly. Patients are told to report symptoms or increasing size immediately.

Enchondroma. The origin of enchondroma is debatable; it may be the result of epiphyseal growth cartilage that does not remodel and persists in the metaphysis, or it may result from persistence of the original cartilaginous anlage of the bone (86). Both possibilities have been suggested as the cause of this common benign latent or active tumor. Most patients with a solitary enchondroma present with either a pathologic fracture through a lesion in the phalanx, which is the most common location (86, 98); or a history of the lesion having been an incidental finding on a radiograph taken for another reason (Fig. 13-13). Enchondromas are common lesions that account for 11% of benign bone tumors (99, 100), and they

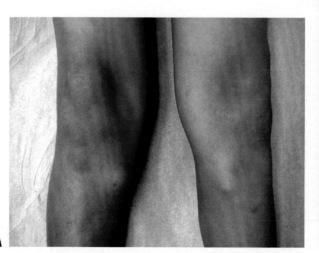

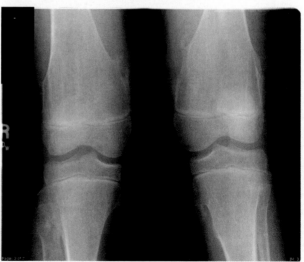

FIGURE 13-12. Clinical appearance **(A)** and anteroposterior radiograph **(B)** of a 12-year-old boy with MHE demonstrates several osteochondromas arising from distal femur and proximal tibia. (Reproduced with permission from The Children's Orthopaedic Center, Los Angeles, CA.)

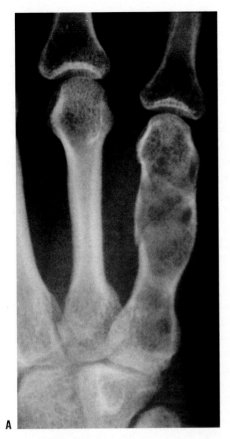

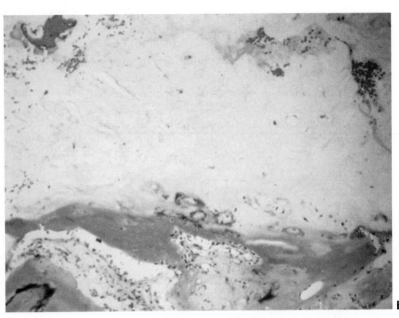

A   B

FIGURE 13-13.   **A:** This enchondroma of the fifth metacarpal is typical. The shaft is enlarged, and the lesion is radiolucent, with cortical thinning. This patient had been aware of this lesion since she was 10 years of age. She had sustained numerous pathologic fractures and decided to have it curetted. The curettage was done after the fracture had healed. **B:** Enchondroma can have varied histologic appearances with varying cellularity, but generally the cartilage, the amorphous material in the center of the image, has few chondrocytes. Typically, the cartilage is lined by a thin band of bone, and the adjacent marrow is normal. Often there is considerable calcification within the cartilage component of the lesion (10× magnification).

do not necessarily need to be removed. However, they may be difficult to diagnose. Usually, the diagnosis can be made from the clinical setting and the plain radiograph. Forty percent of enchondromas are found in the bones of the hands or feet, usually a phalanx. An enchondroma should not produce symptoms unless there is a pathologic fracture. There are no associated abnormalities of blood or urine. The femur and proximal humerus are the next most common sites.

Enchondromas are located in the metaphysis and are central lesions in the medullary canal. The bone may be wider than normal, but this is caused by the lack of remodeling in the metaphysis rather than by expansion of the bone by the tumor. The cortex may be either thin or normal; the lesion is radiolucent in the pediatric age group, but at later stages it shows intralesional calcifications (101). There is usually no periosteal reaction. The appearance of an enchondroma on MRI is typical. The cartilage matrix has intermediate signal intensity on the T1-weighted image and high signal intensity on the T2-weighted image (102, 103). It has a sharp margin with the adjacent bone, without peripheral edema (102, 103).

When the findings are typical of an enchondroma, no biopsy is necessary. Repeat plain radiography and physical examination should be performed in approximately 6 weeks, then every 3 to 6 months for 2 years. Although there are reports of solitary enchondromas differentiating into chondrosarcomas, usually late in adult life, this does not occur frequently enough to justify the removal of all enchondromas. The patient should be advised that after age 30 years, if the lesion becomes painful or enlarges, it should be considered a low-grade chondrosarcoma and be surgically resected. Bone scan is also used to evaluate the tumor activity level and to help determining preferred treatment (101–103).

Incisional biopsy is usually contraindicated. Pathologists have difficulty distinguishing between active enchondroma (most pediatric patients have active lesions) and low-grade chondrosarcoma. The clinical course is the best measure of the lesion's significance, and an incisional biopsy alters the status of the lesion and makes subsequent evaluation difficult. If the patient or the patient's parents insist on biopsy, it is best that the entire lesion be removed.

Patients with multiple enchondromatosis (Ollier disease) are far fewer than those with solitary enchondromas. Multiple enchondromatosis was originally described in the late 1800s by Ollier (104). Most patients with Ollier disease have bilateral involvement but with unilateral predominance. These patients have growth deformities, both angular and in length (Fig. 13-14). The deformities of the extremities should be managed surgically in order to maintain the function of the limbs, without specific regard to the enchondroma. Patients with Ollier disease have an increased risk of developing secondary chondrosarcoma later in life and should be so advised (105, 106). The incidence of secondary chondrosarcoma and other tumors in patients with Ollier disease is not known but may be as high as 25% (96, 107). The pelvis and the shoulder girdle are the most common locations of secondary chondrosarcoma.

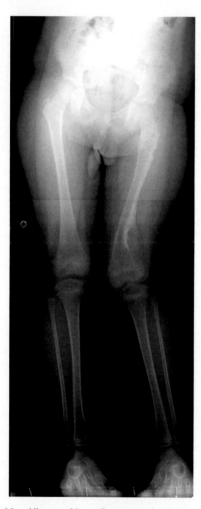

FIGURE 13-14. Hip-to-ankle radiographs of a 5-year-old boy that presented for evaluation of angular deformity. Note the well-defined, mostly radiolucent lesion in the proximal femur and in the distal femur, with cortical thinning, no periosteal reaction, no soft-tissue mass and resultant valgus deformity of the femur. Ollier disease often predominates in one side of the body. (Reproduced with permission from The Children's Orthopaedic Center, Los Angeles, CA.)

Maffucci disease consists of multiple enchondromatosis and soft-tissue hemangiomas (108). Patients with this disorder have an even greater risk of developing malignant tumors than do patients with Ollier disease; more importantly, beside the risk of malignant degeneration, they have a great risk of developing carcinoma of an internal organ (96, 107, 109).

Chondroblastoma. Chondroblastoma, or Codman tumor, is a benign active tumor. It was first described by Codman in 1931 as an "epiphyseal chondromatous giant cell tumor" (110); since Codman was particularly interested in the shoulder, he thought this lesion was found mostly in the proximal humerus (Fig. 13-15A). It has since become clear that chondroblastoma is found in many bones, but the proximal humerus is the most common site (approximately 20%) (99).

Chondroblastoma accounts for 1% of bone tumors (111, 112). The patient with a chondroblastoma is usually in the second decade of life, with an open growth plate, but the condition may occur in older patients as well. The initial symptom is pain in the joint adjacent to the lesion. The findings on physical examination also may suggest an intra-articular disorder because most patients have an effusion and diminished motion in the adjacent joint. Frequently, the patient is believed to have chronic synovitis; he or she does not have other symptoms or abnormal physical findings. The patient's laboratory data are normal.

The lesion arises in the secondary ossification center. In children, it is the most common neoplastic lesion of the secondary ossification center (74); in adults, only giant cell tumor of bone involves the secondary ossification center more often. In children, osteomyelitis is the most common condition that can produce a lesion in the secondary ossification center.

On the plain radiograph, the lesion is radiolucent, usually with small foci of calcification (99). The calcification is best seen on a CT scan (Fig. 13-15B). There is usually a reactive rim of bone surrounding the lesion and, sometimes, metaphyseal periosteal reaction. The edema associated with chondroblastoma can be appreciated on MRI (Fig. 13-16). There is increased uptake on a technetium-99 bone scan. Chest radiography or CT scan should be performed because chondroblastoma is one of the benign bone tumors that can have lung implants and still be considered benign (<2% incidence) (113).

Chondroblastoma and osteochondritis dissecans can have similar appearances on plain radiographs, but they should not be confused with each other. Osteochondritis dissecans produces an abnormality in the subchondral bone; in chondroblastoma, on the other hand, the subchondral bone is almost always normal. Patients with chondroblastoma have more of an effusion than patients with osteochondritis dissecans, and their pain is constant and not related to activity as it is in patients with osteochondritis dissecans.

Histologically, the appearance of chondroblastoma is typical and is rarely confused with other diagnoses. It consists of small cuboidal cells (chondroblasts) closely packed together to give the appearance of a cobblestone street (114). In addition,

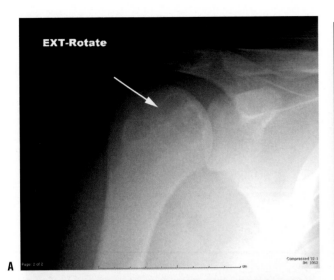

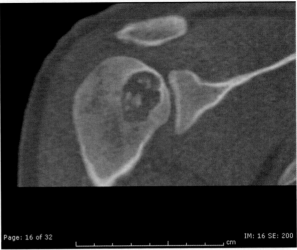

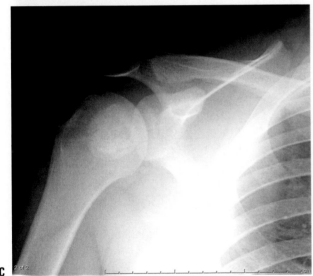

FIGURE 13-15. This is a 15-year-old boy with a chondroblastoma of the right proximal humerus epiphysis. Radiographs **(A)** at presentation shows a well-defined lytic lesion within the epiphysis and opened growth plate; coronal CT images **(B)** better define this lesion and demonstrate intralesional calcification; 12 months after a "four-step procedure" **(C)** the lesion is completely healed and the patient is pain free. (Reproduced with permission from The Children's Orthopaedic Center, Los Angeles, CA.)

there are areas with varying amounts of amorphous matrix that often contains streaks of calcification, and usually there are numerous multinucleated giant cells. Chondroblastoma is not as vascular as osteoblastoma; there are few, if any, mitoses, and no abnormal ones (Fig. 13-17).

Chondroblastomas progress and invade the joint. They should be treated when found (111). Following biopsy for diagnostic confirmation, curettage is the treatment of choice, but it should be a thorough curettage and should extend beyond the reactive rim (four-step approach described above) (Fig. 13-15C). The lesion should be seen adequately at the time of the curettage, which usually means that the joint should be opened. Iatrogenic seeding of a joint is not a significant risk, and intra-articular surgical exposure is recommended if this facilitates visualization. Most recurrences are cured with a second curettage, but a rare lesion can be locally aggressive and requires a wide resection (111). Chondroblastoma of the pelvis frequently behaves more aggressively than that in long bones, and an initial wide excision is recommended if it can be done with limited functional loss and morbidity. Most patients

are close to skeletal maturity when the diagnosis is made, and the risk of growth disturbance from the tumor or its treatment is usually minimal. When the patient is younger than 10 years old, care should be taken not to damage the growth plate. Intra-articular penetration and articular cartilage damage are real risks that should be avoided.

Chondromyxoid Fibroma. Chondromyxoid fibroma is a rare benign active, rarely aggressive tumor. The patient is usually of the male sex (men are more frequently affected than women, at a ratio of 2:1) in the second or third decade of life (99, 115). The patient complains of a dull, steady pain that is usually worse at night. The only positive physical finding is tenderness over the involved area, and occasionally a deep mass can be detected.

Approximately one-third of chondromyxoid fibromas occur in the tibia, usually proximally. It is a radiolucent lesion that involves the medullary canal but is eccentric and erodes the cortex (100, 116) (Fig. 13-18). It may be covered by only periosteum, and is often mistaken for the more common ABC.

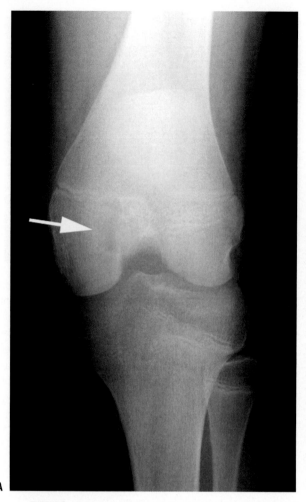

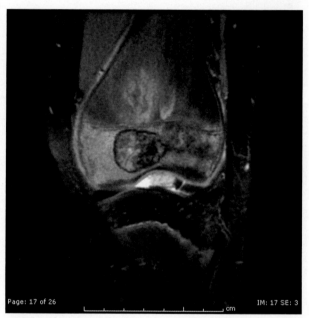

A

B

FIGURE 13-16. A 14-year-old boy with a diagnosis of a distal femur chondroblastoma. Plain radiographs **(A)** show a well-defined, lytic lesion within the distal femoral epiphysis; T2-weighted coronal MRI **(B)** demonstrates the lesion better, its relationship to the joint line and the growth plate. Note the abundant surrounding osseous edema. (Reproduced with permission from The Children's Orthopaedic Center, Los Angeles, CA.)

FIGURE 13-17. Histologic appearance of a chondroblastoma. The tumor consists of cuboidal cells (i.e., chondroblasts), varying amounts of amorphous matrix (some of which is calcified), and multinucleated giant cells. Calcification is seen (**left**). The cuboidal cells fit together in such a manner that they have the appearance of cobblestones (original magnification ×10).

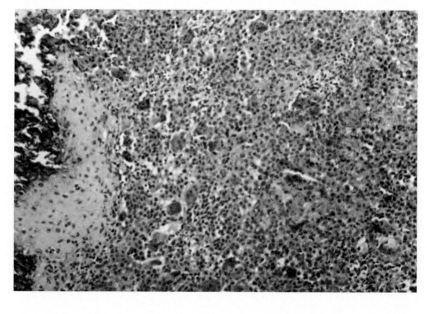

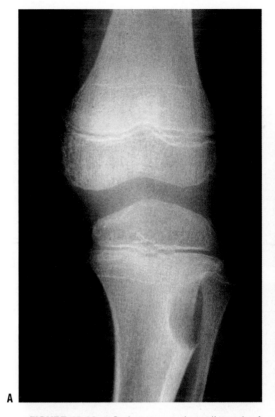
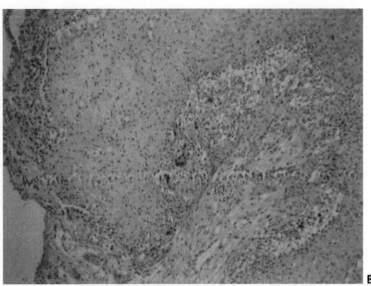

A   B

FIGURE 13-18. **A:** Anteroposterior radiograph of a chondromyxoid fibroma of the proximal lateral tibia. The lesion is typically an eccentric, radiolucent abnormality that usually destroys the cortex but is contained by the periosteum. As in this case, the radiographic appearance of chondromyxoid fibroma is often similar to that of an ABC. **B:** Chondromyxoid fibroma does not have typical hyaline cartilage. It is a cellular lesion with areas of chondroid matrix, myxoid matrix, and abundant fibrous tissue. It can be mistaken for a low-grade malignancy if the diagnosis of chondromyxoid fibroma is not considered (4× magnification).

The solid nature of chondromyxoid fibroma versus the cystic nature of an ABC, as seen on MRI, is a means of differentiating between these two lesions. The natural history is not known because the condition itself is infrequent and surgical treatment is nearly universal. Thorough curettage and bone grafting are recommended. Recurrence is a risk, and patients and parents should be so advised.

Juxtacortical Chondroma. This is an uncommon active or latent benign lesion that arises from the surface of the cortex, deep to the periosteum. The patient may present with pain at the site of the lesion or a painless "bump." More than half of such lesions are found in the proximal humerus, and the others are evenly dispersed through the long bones. The lesion can often be palpated. It is a nontender, hard mass that is fixed to the bone. On plain radiographs, it is a scalloped defect on the outer surface of the cortex, occasionally with intralesional calcifications and minimal periosteal reaction. Sometimes, MRI can be used to help in the diagnosis (Fig. 13-19). On microscopic examination, juxtacortical chondroma is a benign cartilage, but it appears more active than enchondroma. It has been mistaken for chondrosarcoma (117). Because local recurrence is a risk, a marginal or wide

excision, sometimes including the underlying cortex, is the treatment of choice (117, 118).

Lesions of Fibrous Origin
Nonossifying Fibroma and Fibrous Cortical Defect.
Also known as fibroma of bone, nonosteogenic fibroma, and metaphyseal fibrous defect, NOF and fibrous cortical defect are probably the most common lesions of bone (119–121). Fibrous cortical defects are subperiosteal and erode into the outer surface of the cortex, whereas NOFs are medullary lesions that thin the cortex from within. Up to 40% of children have this lesion, which is found most often between the ages of 4 and 8 years (122). Ninety percent of the lesions found are in the distal femur. These are asymptomatic lesions that are usually found when a radiograph is taken for another reason or when the patient has a pathologic fracture. The patient shows no abnormal physical findings, and the serum and urine chemistries are normal.

NOF and fibrous cortical defects should be recognized on the basis of the clinical presentation and plain radiographic findings (123). Biopsy is rarely necessary for diagnosis. Two radiographic appearances are possible. The one that most authors refer to as *fibrous cortical defect* is a

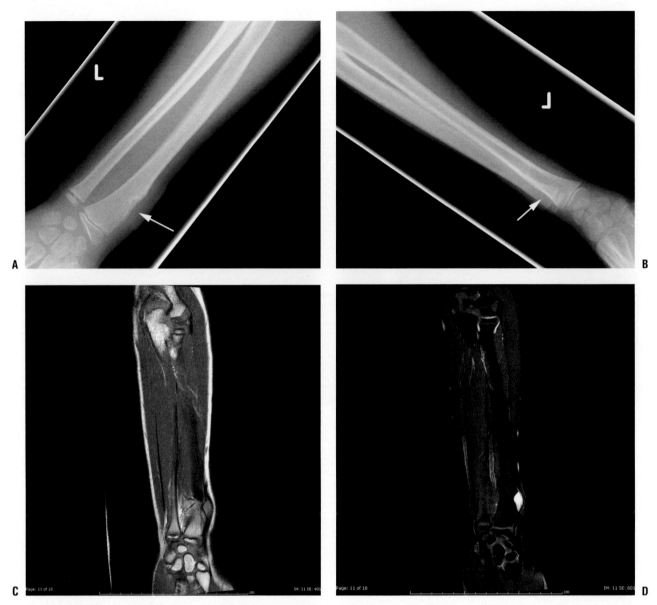

FIGURE 13-19. Juxtacortical chondroma. Plain radiographs of a 10-year-old boy with a history of painless hard mass in the wrist. There are secondary changes in the distal radius metaphysis (*arrow*), but the lesion can be poorly visualized in plain films (**A** and **B**). T1- (**C**) and T2-weighted (**D**) MRI better shows the cartilage lesion located next to the cortex. (Reproduced with permission from The Children's Orthopaedic Center, Los Angeles, CA.)

small (<0.5 cm) radiolucent lesion within the cortex, with a sharply defined border (99). There is little or no increased uptake on the technetium-99 bone scan. A NOF is a metaphyseal lesion eccentrically located (Fig. 13-20). This lesion grows into the medullary canal. It is surrounded by a well-defined, sharp rim of sclerotic reactive bone. There should be no acute periosteal reaction unless there has been a fracture. There may be slightly increased uptake on the technetium-99 bone scan. Multiple NOFs occur in approximately 20% of the patients.

Both lesions consist of benign, spindle, fibroblastic cells arranged in a storiform pattern (123, 124) (Fig. 13-21).

Multinucleated giant cells are common, and areas of large, lipid-laden macrophages can often be seen. Hemosiderin is often present within the fibroblastic stromal cells and multinucleated giant cells. There is no bone formation within the lesion, and mitoses are not seen.

The small cortical lesion (fibrous cortical defect) needs no treatment, but should be observed. Radiographs at 3- to 6-month intervals for 1 to 2 years are suggested. These lesions tend to heal spontaneously. NOF may need surgery. The indication for surgery is to reduce the risk of a pathologic fracture. It is however difficult to predict who is at risk of sustaining a pathologic fracture. The less active and

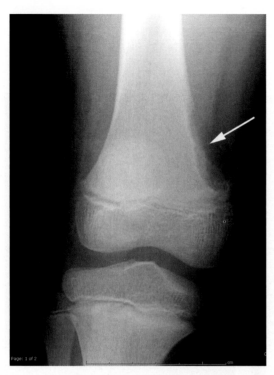

FIGURE 13-20. Anterior–posterior radiograph of the distal femur of a 11-year-old boy that had a minor trauma to the knee and obtained this x-ray. Note this is an eccentric, well-defined, mostly lytic lesion, without periosteal reaction or soft-tissue mass (*arrow*). This appearance is typical for NOF. (Reproduced with permission from The Children's Orthopaedic Center, Los Angeles, CA.)

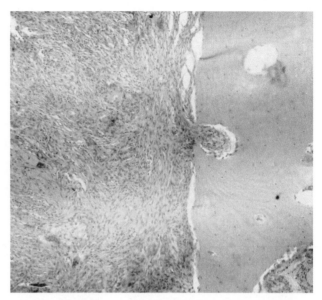

FIGURE 13-21. Low-power histologic view of a typical NOF. The fibroma is composed of benign fibrous tissue and multinucleated giant cells. Hemosiderin is often present. The NOF is invading cortical bone (**right**) (original magnification ×10).

the smaller the child, the less risk there is of the child sustaining a pathologic fracture. NOFs that are <50% of the diameter of the bone can be merely observed because they have little risk of fracture, but curettage and packing with bone graft should be considered if they enlarge (119–121). Patients who present with NOFs that are more than 50% of the diameter of the bone have a risk of fracture with even a minimal injury and should at least be considered for surgery, particularly for lesions in the weight-bearing bones. Recently, an approach using CT analysis and biomechanical modeling has been shown to be of value in more precisely predicting which lesions may be at risk for fracture (115). Many patients with these large NOFs elect not to have surgery and reduce their activity instead. This is an alternative treatment.

Patients who present with pathologic fractures should have the fractures treated nonoperatively if possible. The fracture should heal without difficulty in a normal length of time (Fig. 13-22). There is no evidence that the healing of the fracture increases the chances of spontaneous healing of an NOF. NOF usually heals spontaneously, and this may happen after the fracture; but usually the fracture callus obscures the radiolucent lesion, and the physician is fooled into thinking that the lesion is healing when it is not. When the callus has remodeled and the cortices become distinct on the

radiograph, the lesion can be seen again. Patients with pathologic fractures must be followed until the callus has remodeled sufficiently so that a final determination can be made about the status of the underlying NOF. If it persists after the fracture has healed, curettage and bone grafting may be considered.

Fibrous Dysplasia. Fibrous dysplasia may not be a true neoplasm but a developmental abnormality caused by a somatic mutation leading to a defect in the formation of bone. It is a common disorder that produces a variety of symptoms and physical findings. Most patients (approximately 85%) have a single skeletal lesion (monostotic fibrous dysplasia), whereas the remainder has numerous lesions (polyostotic fibrous dysplasia). The patients with polyostotic fibrous dysplasia may have only two or three small areas of involvement, or may have extensive skeletal abnormalities with grossly deformed bones.

The patient with monostotic fibrous dysplasia usually presents without symptoms, and the lesion is found when a radiograph is taken for unrelated reasons (125–127). Occasionally, the child presents with a pathologic fracture or an angular deformity (Fig. 13-23). The rib is the most common location of monostotic fibrous dysplasia, but any bone can be involved. There are no physical findings that are specifically associated with monostotic fibrous dysplasia, and the café au lait lesions and endocrine abnormalities sometimes found in patients with polyostotic fibrous dysplasia do not occur in patients with the monostotic variant. Serum and urine chemistries are normal in patients with fibrous dysplasia.

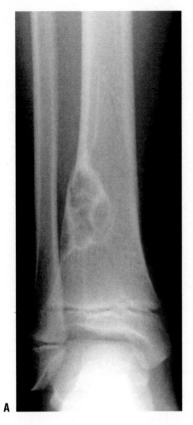

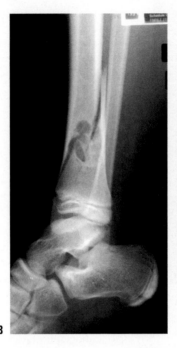

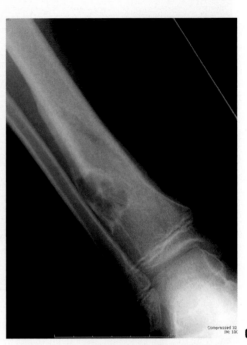

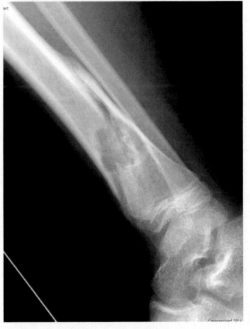

FIGURE 13-22. Anterior–posterior **(A)** and lateral **(B)** radiographs of the distal tibia and ankle of a 13-year-old boy that sustained a fall while riding his bicycle. There is a pathologic fracture true. An eccentric, large, well-defined, mixed, but mostly lytic lesion in the distal tibia metaphysis, consistent with a NOF. Six weeks after cast immobilization, the fracture is essential healed **(C** and **D)**, but the lesion has not changed its appearance. (Reproduced with permission from The Children's Orthopaedic Center, Los Angeles, CA.)

The plain radiograph is often diagnostic, although the radiographic appearance of fibrous dysplasia is variable (Fig. 13-24A). It is a medullary process that typically produces a ground-glass appearance on the radiograph. The lesion is usually diaphyseal. The diaphysis is larger than normal, and the ground-glass appearance of the medullary canal blends into the thinned cortex so that it is difficult to define the border between the medullary canal and the cortex. When typical-appearing lesions are seen in a single bone or in a single limb, the diagnosis is almost certain. There may be an angular deformity in the bone, especially when the lesion is large. The lesions may mature with age and become radiodense or cystic. Fibrous dysplasia may show excessive uptake on a technetium-99 bone scan, out of proportion to what one might predict from the plain radiographic appearance.

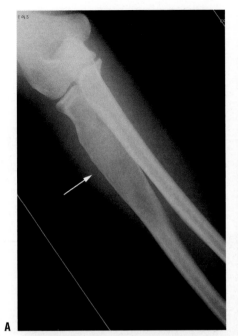

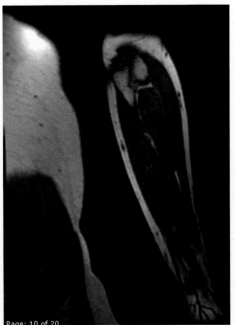

A

B

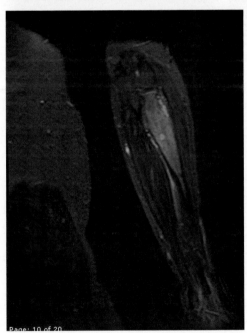

C

FIGURE 13-23. Fibrous dysplasia; this is a 15-year-old girl with history of left arm pain following a minor fall. The plain radiograph **(A)** demonstrates a well-defined, mostly lytic lesion, with cortical thinning, ground-glass appearance, mild expansion, and no periosteal reaction or soft-tissue mass (*arrow*). T1- **(B)** and T2-weighted MRI **(C)** better demonstrates the lesion, low and high intensity, respectively, and no soft-tissue mass. (Reproduced with permission from The Children's Orthopaedic Center, Los Angeles, CA.)

The patient with polyostotic fibrous dysplasia usually presents at about the age of 10 years with an angular deformity of a bone (127, 128). The most common deformity is varus of the proximal femur, or shepherd's crook deformity. The light brown skin lesions with irregular borders are called *coast of Maine* café au lait spots. The lesions that have smooth borders and are associated with neurofibromatosis are called *coast of California* café au lait spots.

Hyperthyroidism and diabetes mellitus have been reported as associated endocrinopathies, and vascular tumors have been seen in association with fibrous dysplasia. McCune-Albright syndrome is a triad of fibrous dysplasia, café au lait

spots, and precocious puberty (126). The lesions in polyostotic fibrous dysplasia tend to be unilateral rather than bilateral. The radiographic appearance of the lesion is the same as in patients with monostotic disease. The structural strength of bones with fibrous dysplasia is reduced because of the poorly organized trabecular pattern and the thinned cortex. The weakness of the bones leads to the deformities that are usually present.

On microscopic examination, fibrous dysplasia, both the monostotic and polyostotic forms, is composed of fibrous tissue with normal-appearing nuclei and irregularly shaped strands of osteoid and bone (Fig. 13-24B). There are few, if

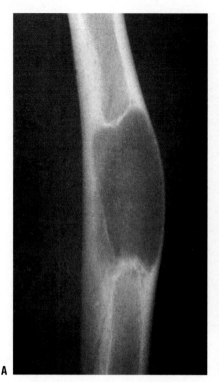
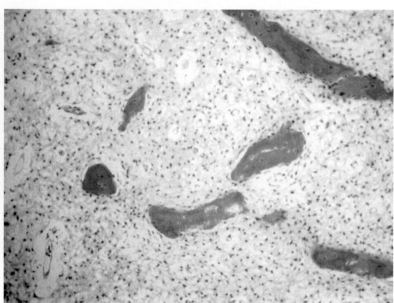

A   B

FIGURE 13-24. **A:** Radiograph of a fibrous dysplasia in the diaphysis of a long bone. The ground-glass appearance, the thin cortex, and the angular deformity of the bone are all typical features of fibrous dysplasia. **B:** The tumor is mostly fibrous tissue composed of collagen and fibroblast. Small bits of bone and osteoid, often having a "C" or an "O" shape, seem to have been sprinkled on the fibrous tissue. Osteoblasts are not seen, and the bone seems to be produced by the fibroblastic cells (40× magnification).

any, osteoblasts present, and the osteoid and bone seem to arise directly from the background fibrous stoma. The bone is irregularly organized, and often has a "C" or an "O" shape. Multinucleated giant cells are rare and there are few mitoses, none of which is abnormal. Nodules of cartilage may be present in typical fibrous dysplasia.

Monostotic fibrous dysplasia usually does not need surgical treatment (125, 126). Occasionally, a solitary lesion will be painful and curettage with grafting is required. Small lesions can be packed with cortical cancellous bone graft (autogenous or allogenic), whereas large lesions are probably better treated with cortical bone grafts, and a high incidence of recurrence and/or fibrous dysplasia transformation of the grafted bone is to be expected (129). A special circumstance is a lesion in the femoral neck. These lesions may be associated with a risk of fatigue fractures, and cortical strut bone grafting has been recommended (125, 126). Resorption of the bone graft with recurrence of fibrous dysplasia can occur, and the patient should be followed up for at least 5 years. Occasionally, surgical intervention is needed to prevent or treat fractures or deformity and relieve pain. Progressive bone deformity is unusual in patients with monostotic; however, in the poliostotic disease, bone deformity is frequent. The proximal femur is one of the most common areas of deformity; once a varus deformity develops, curettage and grafting are associated with

internal fixation. Recently, coral grafts have been shown to reduce the chance of recurrence. In terms of fixation, intramedullary devices are superior to plates and screws (130, 131). Bisphosphonates have been used with success in polyostotic fibrous dysplasia and McCune-Albright; they prevent fractures, deformities, and most importantly, they seem to decrease pain (132).

Osteofibrous Dysplasia. Osteofibrous dysplasia is a benign active, sometimes locally aggressive bone lesion. The most common presenting symptoms are swelling and painless bowing of the tibia. The lesion is almost always located within the anterior cortex of the tibia and is best seen on the lateral radiograph (Fig. 13-25). Radius and ulna may also be involved (133–135). Sometimes, the diagnosis is made at time of a pathologic fracture. There are often numerous radiolucent lesions with a rim of reactive bone. On the technetium-99 bone scan, there is increased uptake in the area of the lesion.

Osteofibrous dysplasia arises from the cortex and involves the medullary canal late in the disease process. It is usually associated with a bowed tibia and quickly recurs if curetted. There are not many data on patients with osteofibrous dysplasia who have been adequately followed up. The natural history is of gradual growth until around 15 years of age.

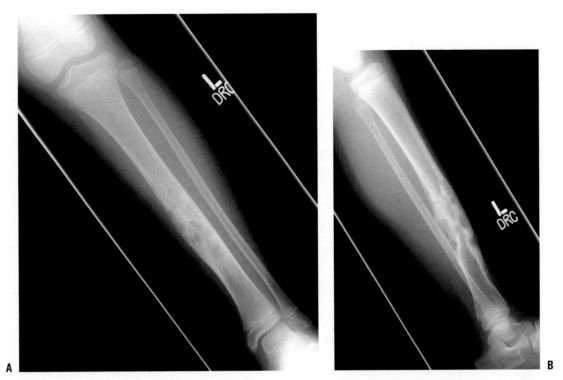

FIGURE 13-25. This is a 6-year-old girl with pain and swelling over the left tibia. Anterior-posterior **(A)** and lateral **(B)** x-rays demonstrate the classic appearance of osteofibrous dysplasia, this is a lytic, loculated lesion, involving the midshaft of the tibia, with mild expansion, angulation, and no soft-tissue mass or periosteal reaction (Reproduced with permission from The Children's Orthopaedic Center, Los Angeles, CA.)

We recommend observation of the lesion when it is found in a patient younger than 10 years of age. Incisional biopsy is not necessary in most cases because the clinical presentation is diagnostic. Also, the biopsy reveals only a small portion of the lesion and does not change the initial management. Bracing can be used to prevent pathologic fracture, pain, and progressive bowing. If the lesion progresses rapidly before closure of the growth plate, biopsy and resection are suggested. If the patient presents after closure of the growth plate, especially if the lesion is large (more than 3 or 4 cm in diameter) or has aggressive features on plain radiographs, a biopsy is suggested. If an adamantinoma is found, a wide resection is recommended. If the biopsy reveals osteofibrous dysplasia, it is best to excise the entire lesion for a complete histologic examination to rule out the possibility of there being a focus of adamantinoma. If the lesion is small (<3 cm) and the patient has no symptoms, continued observation is suggested.

Adamantinoma is a low-grade malignancy that has a clinical presentation similar to osteofibrous dysplasia. In adamantinoma, however, the patient is usually older (third decade of life), and the lesion appears more aggressive on the radiographs (e.g., soft-tissue extension, acute periosteal reaction, large size, involvement of the medullary canal). It has been suggested that there is a type of adamantinoma that looks very similar to osteofibrous dysplasia, even on histologic examination. Some hypothesize that osteofibrous dysplasia could be a precursor for adamantinoma (136, 137). One must be suspicious of the

diagnosis of osteofibrous dysplasia, especially in a progressive lesion in a patient older than 10 years of age (138). If a lesion suspected of being an osteofibrous dysplasia is going to be observed, the patient should undergo radiography at least every 6 months until the lesion stabilizes, heals, or is resected. Typical adamantinoma has a risk of metastasizing, but it is not known whether the adamantinoma that looks like osteofibrous dysplasia can metastasize (133). Nonetheless, osteofibrous dysplasia, osteofibrous dysplasia–like adamantinoma, and classic adamantinoma appear to show a progressive complexity of cytogenetic aberrations, perhaps indicative of a multistep neoplastic transformation (139–141).

Langerhans Cell Histiocytosis. LCH is a rare group of disorders, of unknown etiology, with a wide spectrum of clinical presentation. Solitary osseous lesions are referred as to eosinophilic granuloma; Hand-Schüller-Christian includes the triad of cranial lesions, diabetes insipidus, and exophthalmos; Letterer-Siwe disease is a malignant form of LCH, whereas most patients present before 3 years of age with skin, visceral, and brain lesions, with or without bone lesions, and high incidence of mortality (61, 141–143). This is a disorder of the Langerhans histiocytes, and although eosinophils are a common component of the lesion, they are not necessary for the diagnosis (Fig. 13-26). Theories behind LCH etiology range from an inflammatory process to viral infection (94, 144, 145).

FIGURE 13-26. Low-power view of an eosinophilic granuloma (Langerhans granuloma). The eosinophils are numerous, but it is the presence of histiocytes that defines this tumor. The histiocytes are large cells with a clear, folded nucleus and a prominent nucleolus (original magnification ×10).

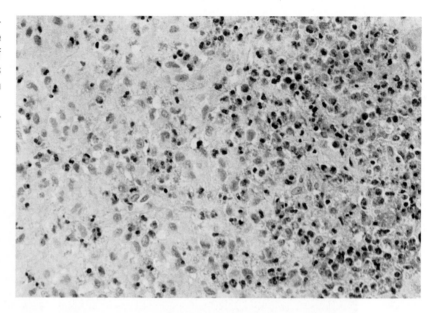

LCH is predominantly a disease of childhood, with more than 50% of cases diagnosed between the ages of 5 and 15 years (146). The skull is the most common site of bone involvement (61, 146, 147). Many of the skull lesions are probably not diagnosed because the only abnormality is a painless, small, spontaneously resolving lump in the scalp. The vertebral bodies and the ilium are the next most common sites of involvement (148, 149). When the lesions occur in the long bones, they may weaken the bone to such an extent that the patient presents with activity-related pain suggestive of a fatigue fracture, or with a pathologic fracture.

Due to the highly variable radiographic appearance, LCH has been referred as to the "great imitator." Most lesions are well defined, lytic, with or without sharp sclerotic rim, no periosteal reaction or soft-tissue mass (Fig. 13-27). Although LCH usually presents with increased uptake on a technetium bone scan, as many as 25% of the lesions will not be associated with abnormal bone scans (61), for that reason skeletal survey is often recommended to rule out other lesions (Fig. 13-27E). MRI is sometimes needed, especially for spine lesions, to rule out soft-tissue mass and intraspinal extension.

The clinical course of LCH is quite variable. Isolated osseous LCH is more frequent than the multisystem disease (61). The clinical manifestations depend on the location of the lesion; however, local "bone" pain is the initial symptom in 50% to 90% of the patients with osseous lesion (139, 143, 150, 151). Other reported symptoms in osseous LCH include night pain, soft-tissue swelling, tenderness, pathologic fractures, headaches (skull lesions), diminished hearing and otitis media (mastoid lesions), or loose teeth (mandible lesions) (152–156). Dull, aching neck or back pain is usually the presenting symptom of children with spinal LCH; vertebral collapse may also produce pain and spasm. Torticollis may be seen with cervical spine lesions, and kyphosis might be present with thoracic lesions (157–163).

Patients with eosinophilic granuloma do not progress to Hand-Schüller-Christian disease, but should be evaluated on presentation to exclude the presence of that syndrome. The easiest way to evaluate the patient for diabetes insipidus is to obtain a lateral skull film in order to observe the size of the sella turcica, and test a first voided urine specimen after overnight fluid restriction to determine whether the patient can concentrate his or her urine. Liver enzymes should be determined.

The treatment of LCH remains controversial. Some of the treatment options described include topical steroids, intralesional injections of steroids, NSAIDs, phototherapy, bone marrow allografting, surgical excision, stem cell transplantation, and chemotherapy. The decision should be made based on the severity of osseous involvement, location and size of the lesions, and presence or absence of systemic involvement (61). Biopsy is usually recommended. For isolated bone lesions, the treatment is mainly conservative and aims at controlling the symptoms, maximizing functional recovery, and limiting any long-term disability (141). The clinical course of these patients is generally benign; solitary bone lesions often heal without intervention or after biopsy with curettage of the lesion (61). Multiple bone lesions or systemic involvement is an indication for chemotherapy, and the pediatric oncologist should be consulted (164, 165).

Unicameral Bone Cysts. UBC or simple bone cyst is a common benign active or latent lesion that most often involves the metaphysis of long bones. Most of the lesions involve the proximal femur and proximal humerus (approximately 80% of the lesions) in children around the second decade (166). They are usually painless lesions and approximately 85% of UBCs are diagnosed at time of a pathologic fracture. Their radiographic appearance is so typical that most can be diagnosed without a biopsy (Fig. 13-28). UBCs are a well-defined, central, lytic lesion in the metaphysis. Cortical thinning may

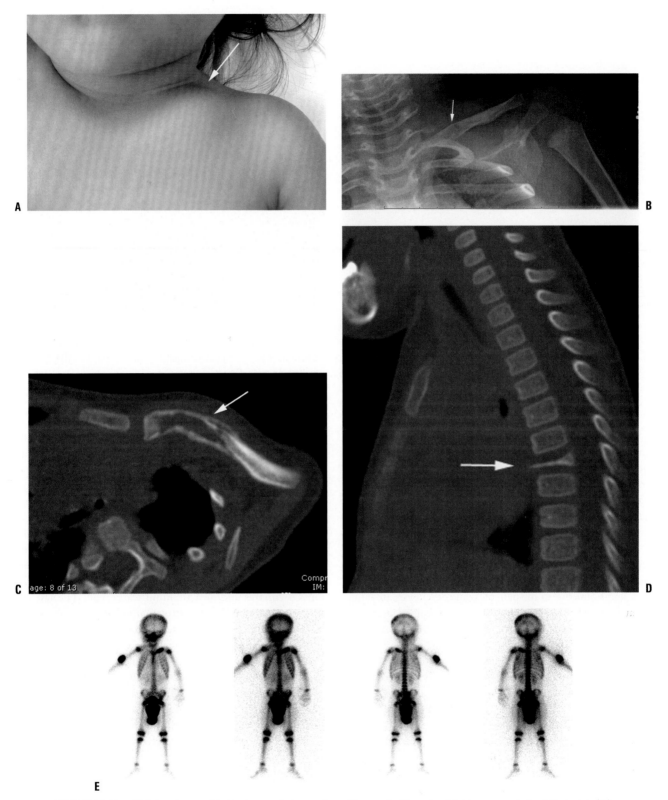

FIGURE 13-27.   This is a 4-year-old girl who was being evaluated for a palpable and painful bone mass in the left clavicle **(A)**. Radiograph **(B)** shows a poorly defined lytic lesion within the medial half of the clavicle. CT of the clavicle **(C)** better defines the lesion and shows periosteal reaction with new bone formation and no soft-tissue mass. During the CT of the clavicle, sagittal image of the t-spine **(D)** shows a vertebra plana of T6, favoring the latter confirmed diagnosis of LCH. Bone scan **(E)** didn't show any other bone lesion and failed to demonstrate the T6 lesion. (Reproduced with permission from The Children's Orthopaedic Center, Los Angeles, CA.)

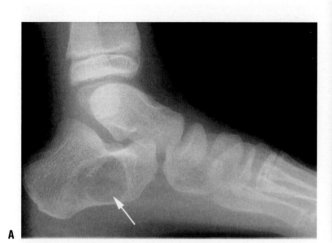
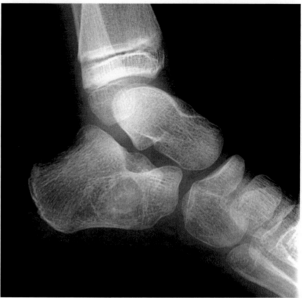

FIGURE 13-28. A 7-year-old boy presents with constant heel pain. Initial lateral radiograph of the calcaneus **(A)** demonstrates a well-defined, lytic lesion, without periosteal reaction or soft-tissue mass. This is a classic location and appearance of UBC. Postoperative image shows complete healing of the cyst, 3 months after a minimally invasive surgical procedure **(B)**. (Reproduced with permission from The Children's Orthopaedic Center, Los Angeles, CA.)

occur with larger cysts, but there is no periosteal reaction or soft-tissue mass (166, 167). The metaphyseal bone does not remodel and the metaphysis is broader than normal, but not broader than the width of the epiphyseal plate. When the cyst becomes mature (latent), usually after the patient reaches the age of 10 years, the epiphysis "grows away" from the lesion. The cyst may eventually heal spontaneously and fills in with bone.

The indications for treatment include large cysts in weight-bearing regions, high risk for pathologic fracture, and continued pain. Some UBCs remain small and do not present a significant risk to the patient, while other cysts are large, situated in high-stress anatomic sites (e.g., femoral neck), or persist after the patient has become a young adult, and in these cases treatment is also indicated (168).

For many years, steroid injection was the treatment of choice. The advantages are the low morbidity, low cost, and quick recovery, while the disadvantages include a very high persistence rate and the need to repeat the procedure several times before healing is obtained (169, 170). Before the use of corticosteroid injections became common, curettage and autogenous bone grafting had been the most common treatment. Operative treatment with curettage and autogenous bone grafting is now reserved for those lesions that do not respond to less invasive procedures. Injecting autogenous bone marrow is a technique advocated by some with better results than steroids (171, 172).

Several authors have more recently been advocating cyst decompression as the most efficient way to treat UBCs (173). We described a minimally invasive technique for the treatment of UBCs (174). The procedure is done under general anesthesia with fluoroscopic guidance. The cyst is penetrated with a Jamshidi needle and aspiration follows. Cystogram with Renografin diluted 50% is then performed to evaluate for loculations within the cyst. A 0.5-cm incision is made over the needle site, and the cortex is penetrated with a 6-mm trocar. If there is any question regarding the treatment, an incisional biopsy is done with a pituitary rongeur and specimen is sent for frozen section. The cyst is curetted under fluoroscopy, and any cyst lining or fibrous tissue (following fracture) is excised. The cyst is now decompressed using curved curettes and/or a titanium elastic nail. The last step of the procedure is bone grafting with medical-grade calcium sulfate pellets. In a recent review of intermediate-to-long-term results, the healing rates were around 80% after one procedure and over 90% after repeat procedure (*unpublished data*). Many other substances including demineralized bone matrix gel, bone marrow, allograft or autograft bone chips, and calcium phosphate materials have been proposed as "fillers." Some seem to be better than steroid injections alone, but none of these treatments has been definitively proven to be superior to another. When open excision is performed with intralesional curettage, autogenous bone or allograft cortical cancellous bone can be used for packing the cavity. Freeze-dried cortical cancellous allograft is particularly advantageous because it is associated with an excellent healing rate and little, if any, incidence of complications; also, a secondary incision is not required for obtaining the autogenous bone graft. Calcium sulfate tablets are an alternative material that can be used for filling the cavity. When the cyst is adjacent to the growth plate, care should be taken not to damage the epiphyseal cartilage during the procedure. If there is doubt about the integrity of the growth plate, it is wise to obtain an MRI to document whether or not it has been violated by the cyst prior to instituting treatment.

Aneurysmal Bone Cysts.

ABC is a benign active and sometimes aggressive lesion. ABCs often occur in association with a number of other tumors (e.g., giant cell tumor, chondroblastoma, osteoblastoma, and osteosarcoma). When it is a secondary lesion, the primary lesion is usually obvious, and the ABC component is limited to only a small portion of the tumor. Secondary ABCs are classified by their underlying diagnosis. The presence of a secondary ABC does not change the therapy or prognosis of the underlying primary tumor. The neoplastic basis of primary ABCs has been, at least in part, demonstrated by the chromosomal translocation t(16;17) (q22;p13) that places the ubiquitin protease USP6 gene under the regulatory influence of the highly active osteoblast cadherin 11 gene (CDH11), which is strongly expressed in bones (175, 176).

A primary ABC occurs most commonly in teenagers (80%). More than 50% of these cysts arise in large tubular bones, and almost 30% occur in the spine (175, 176). The patient usually complains of a mild, dull pain, and only rarely is there a clinically apparent pathologic fracture. The physical examination usually shows normal results, and there is no abnormal laboratory finding associated with ABC.

On the plain radiograph, an ABC is a radiolucent lesion arising eccentrically within the medullary canal of the metaphysis (Fig. 13-29). It resorbs the cortex and elevates the periosteum, generally making the bone wider than the epiphyseal plate (characteristic finding). Usually, there is a thin shell of reactive periosteal bone, but occasionally this bone cannot be seen. When ABC arises in a long bone, it is metaphyseal. When it arises in the spine, it originates in the posterior elements but it may extend into the body and, not uncommonly, will extend also to an adjacent vertebral body or rib. The radiograph of an ABC may appear identical to those of giant cell tumor of the bone and telangiectatic osteosarcoma. The periosteal reaction appears to be aggressive, and the lesion may be mistaken for an aggressive or a malignant tumor. ABCs may arise in the cortex and elevate the periosteum with or without involving the medullary canal.

A CT scan is helpful in making the diagnosis of ABC. The lesion should have a density of approximately 20 HU, and this does not increase with intravenous contrast injection. When the patient lies still for 20 to 30 minutes, the cells in the fluid within the cyst cavity settle, and a fluid/fluid level can be seen. Similar findings can be seen on MRI. Fluid/fluid level was originally described in ABC but has subsequently been seen in a number of other lesions, so it cannot be considered to be diagnostic of ABC. An ABC has an increased uptake of technetium on the bone scan, but often the scan has a central area of decreased uptake.

ABCs should undergo a biopsy to establish the diagnosis (175–177). The pathologist should be advised in advance,

and the possibility of a telangiectatic osteosarcoma should be discussed. It is uncommon for the histologic appearance of an ABC to be mistaken for that of a telangiectatic osteosarcoma, although the radiographic and the gross appearances can be identical. On gross inspection, an ABC is a cavitary lesion with a villous lining. Microscopic examination reveals the lining to be composed of hemosiderin-laden macrophages, multinucleated giant cells, a fibrous stroma, and usually small amounts of woven bone (Fig. 13-30). The microscopic appearance of the lining of the ABC is similar to that of a giant cell tumor of bone.

Most recommend treatment by curettage and packing of bone graft, but recurrence rates are high (up to 60%) (175–177). Embolization may be used in order to decrease blood loss during surgery and has been associated with fewer recurrences. Whether embolization is necessary or helpful is debatable. Cryosurgery has also been reportedly tried. Cryosurgery may produce complications, and it is not considered necessary in most cases. It may play a role in the treatment of recurrent lesions. Definitive resection (wide or en bloc resection) can be performed when the consequences of the resection are minimal, but it is absolutely necessary only when the lesion has a particularly aggressive clinical growth pattern. We recommend a four-step-approach including extended intralesional curettage, high-speed burring, adjuvant use (such as phenol), and electrocauterization. The recurrence rate in children with this technique is <20% (38).

An ABC of the spine (approximately 30% of cases) can present a particularly challenging problem. The lesion always involves the posterior elements, but can also involve the vertebral body. The patients initially complain of pain at the site of the lesion, but the ABC is often not found until the patient has nerve root or cord compression. Most cases heal with the four-step approach described anteriorly; caution should be taken if adjuvant is used, due to the proximity to the spinal cord and nerve roots (175). Usually the posterior elements are resected, and any involvement of the pedicles or the body is curetted. If complete laminectomy is performed, a short posterior fusion is advised using titanium instrumentation to allow for postoperative MRI or CT scan (178).

MALIGNANT BONE TUMORS

Guidelines for Surgical Treatment of Bone Tumors.

Some benign tumors may not need treatment and can be merely observed. Others are successfully treated with simple intralesional curettage. In general, when curettage is indicated it is best to visualize the cavity thoroughly and carefully remove the entire tumor under direct visualization. The use of a high-speed burr can help assure complete removal of all tumor cells and is especially advised for benign aggressive tumors (179). The use and effectiveness of a local adjuvant such as phenol, argon-beam, and cryosurgery is controversial but common (180–182).

In children, most malignant bone tumors, with the exception of lymphoma, should be surgically resected. The goal of

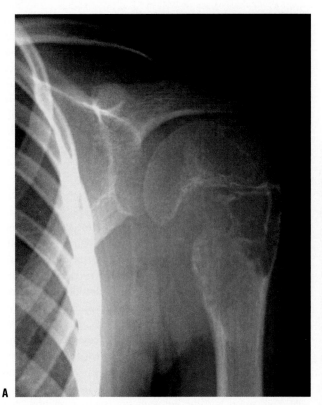

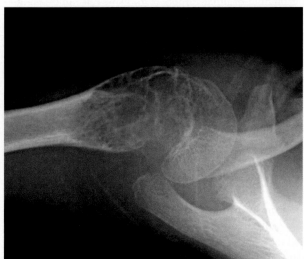

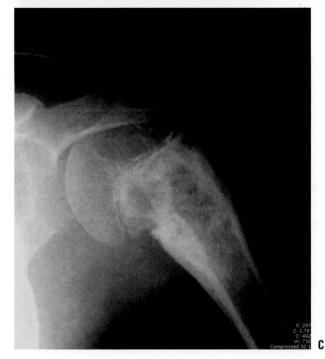

FIGURE 13-29. A 9-year-old boy presents with a several months history of shoulder pain and muscle wasting. Anterior–posterior **(A)** and axillary **(B)** radiographs of the left shoulder demonstrate a mixed, well-defined, loculated lesion in the proximal humerus metaphysis, with cortical thinning and bone expansion. There is no soft-tissue mass or periosteal reaction. This ABC was excised utilizing a four-step approach, and 3 months postoperatively, there was complete resolution of the lesion and bone remodeling **(C)**. (Reproduced with permission from The Children's Orthopaedic Center, Los Angeles, CA.)

surgical treatment of these malignant bone tumors is to resect the entire tumor. To accomplish this, some of the adjacent normal tissue must be removed because the tumor infiltrates these tissues. The exact extent of involvement of the normal tissue is impossible to determine preoperatively, although MRI is a reasonably accurate method of determining the extent of the tumor. The greater the amount of adjacent tissue removed, the less likely the patient is to have a local recurrence; therefore, as much adjacent tissue as is practical should be removed (182, 183). Although the goal of treatment is to eliminate local recurrence, it is not practical to try to guarantee that local recurrences never happen, because such an approach would lead to excessive surgery for most patients without a proven benefit in survival.

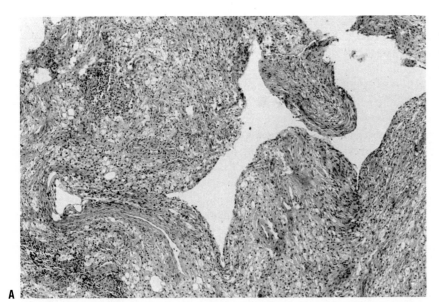

A

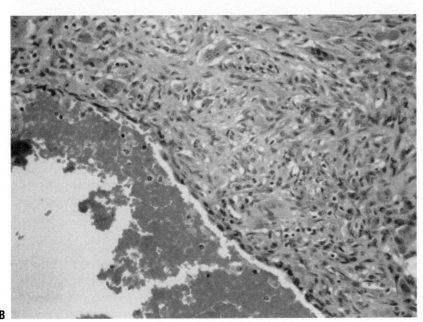

B

FIGURE 13-30.   **A:** Low-power view of the tissue lining an ABC. The lining is composed of fibrous tissue with multinucleated giant cells, foamy histiocytes, hemosiderin and, often, spicules of immature bone (not seen). The fronds and spaces are typical (original magnification × 10). **B:** Higher-power view (40 ×) of ABC. Benign spindle cells, vessels, hemosiderin, and multinucleated giant cells make up the solid component. There is a cystic component filled with blood.

In order to determine how much normal adjacent tissue should be removed, it is useful to first determine what is the minimal amount of tissue that must be removed in order to completely remove the tumor as shown on an MRI. Then add as much additional adjacent tissue to the resection as possible without changing the functional impact of the surgery. For example, if 15 cm of a distal femur must be removed, it is just as functional to replace 25 cm (i.e., a 10-cm bone margin), as it is to replace 17 cm (which would be only a 2-cm margin). If adjacent muscle has been invaded to the extent that what remains is not functional, all of the muscle should be removed. If no additional adjacent tissue can be removed without impacting on the patient's functioning, either an adjuvant is needed, or the patient should undergo the more functionally impacting resection.

Limb-salvage surgery is done for most sarcomas of the extremities, but the decision is often difficult because the surgical margin achieved with an amputation would almost always be much better than the one obtained with a limb-salvage resection (182, 183). In a limb-salvage operation, local recurrence may be higher than with amputation, but no adverse effect on disease outcome (survival) has been shown. The time to recovery is longer, the complexity of the surgery is greater, there are more local complications, the chance of needing additional surgery is increased, and the safe level of physical activity is lower as compared to an amputation, but the patient retains his or her own foot or hand. Since the introduction of adjuvant chemotherapy, especially preoperative (neoadjuvant) chemotherapy, and the availability of CT scanning and MRI, limb-salvage surgery has become more common. The materials used in reconstruction, and the surgeons' experience with these materials and techniques, have improved to such an extent that limb-salvage resections have become commonplace in most medical centers. Nowadays, a patient rarely needs to undergo an amputation for a sarcoma of the extremity (184).

An amputation may be necessary in those patients in whom surgical resection will remove so much tissue that the remaining limb will be less useful than a prosthesis (184, 185). To make this decision, the patients have to indicate how they want to use the extremity (184, 185). The more sedentary the patient, the greater the amount of tissue that can be removed in limb-salvage surgery without amputation becoming the better option, and vice versa (186). In general, bone, joints, arteries, veins, and muscles can be removed and still leave the extremity functional. Even the need to resect a major nerve is not in itself an indication for an amputation (60, 183, 187–189). It is when a combination of these tissues, including a major nerve, has to be resected that amputation should be seriously considered. Each patient's situation and preferences should be considered individually.

There is a fairly wide experience with limb salvage in adults. For children, however, the surgeon encounters problems including growth, small size, and (it is hoped) greater longevity, all of which make reconstruction more challenging (190, 191). The options for limb salvage include osteoarticular and intercalary allograft, metallic prostheses, and vascularized and nonvascularized autograft transplants. All of these are used at various times by the tumor surgeon. Rotationplasty is another option somewhere between limb salvage and amputation; it is occasionally useful in very young patients (187, 192).

In some locations, such as the fibula and clavicle, no bone reconstruction is necessary. Very young children with bone tumors of the foot and ankle are usually best treated by amputation of the ray, or Syme amputation, or below-knee amputation.

The unique issue regarding limb salvage in children is growth of the opposite extremity and the limb-length inequality that follows. For the child who is within 2 or 3 years of completion of growth, this is not a significant issue (187, 193, 194). Fortunately, most malignant bone tumors occur within this age group or in older children. In a patient who is between 10 and 13 years of age, there is sufficient growth potential (particularly in the distal femur, proximal tibia, and proximal humerus, the most common sites for malignant bone tumors) that if limb-salvage surgery is done, special attention is needed to achieve near-equal limb lengths at maturity. Equal or near-equal limb lengths can be achieved with traditional methods initially making the operated leg longer and, if needed, by epiphysiodesis. Usually, for patients whose limb-length inequality will be 2 cm or less, no surgical adjustment is necessary and the patient can use a lift if desired. For limb-length inequality between approximately 2 and 5 cm, an epiphysiodesis is usually the best means of achieving equal limb lengths. For limb-length differences >5 cm, some type of limb lengthening or rotationplasty is advised (195).

For lesions of the proximal humerus, intra-articular or extra-articular resection is performed. If the rotator cuff and part of the deltoid can be preserved, the expected functional outcome is reasonable (195, 196). Reconstruction options include osteoarticular allograft, allograft-prosthetic composite, or endoprosthesis. The advantage of the allograft is better attachment of the rotator cuff and soft tissues; endoprosthesis may prevent late collapse of the joint and fracture (195, 196). For extra-articular resections in which both the deltoid and the rotator cuff are sacrificed, arthrodesis, using allograft, vascularized fibula, or both, may be indicated and tends to be very functional (196). When a formal Tikhoff-Linberg resection including the scapula is necessary, the reconstruction is more difficult; options include custom prosthesis, allograft reconstruction of the scapula associated with humeral reconstruction, or at times flail upper extremity (197).

For tumors around the knee (most common area involved), the resection will almost certainly include an epiphyseal center. One option is to reconstruct with an osteoarticular allograft, and treat the limb-length discrepancy using standard methods of epiphysiodesis, closed femoral shortening, or limb lengthening (185). The results of allograft for limb salvage in osteosarcoma are reasonably good, but the patient should not expect normal limb function. It should be noted that there are no ideal measures of function after limb salvage (although several have been developed), and this remains an area of investigation (197–199). In general, if patients can return to normal walking activities without supports or braces, it is considered to be a good result. Seldom can they return to contact sports or activities involving running. Complications include infection, nonunion, fracture, and joint instability (176, 200). If the patient survives, he or she may need joint arthroplasty at some time in the future, but by then the patient should be old enough that growth is no longer a consideration. Growth equalization can be achieved by contralateral epiphysiodesis, limb shortening, or ipsilateral lengthening (189). The experience with limb lengthening in these patients is limited because limb length is seldom a major issue.

Another option is the use of a metallic prosthesis. Modular prostheses are available and allow the surgeon to construct an implant of suitable length in the operating room (187, 193, 194). Custom implants are seldom necessary. Some prostheses have the ability to be extended or grow as the child grows (201). There are many methods that can be used to lengthen endoprosthetic devices. Some require a major operative procedure, some can be done with limited surgery (Fig. 13-31), and a few endoprostheses can be lengthened without surgery (192–194, 202) (Fig. 13-32). The efficacy and longevity of these "growing" prostheses are the focus of several studies (194). Usually, it is possible to achieve at least 2 cm of length per procedure. In very young patients, this must be repeated every 6 months until maturity, at which point revision to an adult prosthesis may be necessary. There are few data on these prostheses, but at least one report shows that it is possible to gain 2 to 18 cm in length, and to have equal limb lengths at skeletal maturity (187, 192–194). The issues of prosthetic failure, loosening, wear of polyethylene, and infection remain unresolved. The choice between an implant and a reconstructive procedure has to be made by the surgeon and the patient's family. Prostheses are more functional initially, but their longevity is unknown. Extendible prostheses have a high failure rate (187). More than

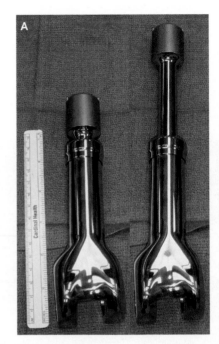
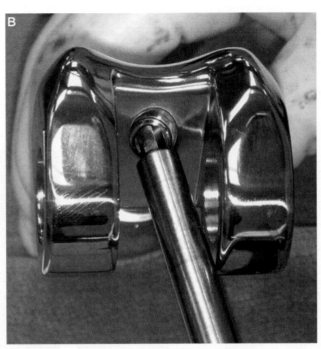

FIGURE 13-31. A,B: Example of a coaxial extendible prosthesis that can be lengthened with a minimally invasive procedure, utilizing a screw driver placed into the notch (Reproduced from Arkader A, et al. Coaxial extendible knee equalizes limb length in children with osteogenic sarcoma. *Clin Orthop Relat Res* 2007;459:60–65, with permission.)

80% require revision by 5 years, and the revision rate appears to be higher in uncemented prostheses (183, 189, 192, 194). Many of these patients will have knee stiffness, and the infection rate, especially in the tibia, may be as high as 38%, although this can be improved with the liberal use of gastrocnemius flaps. The modular prosthesis has been reported to have a 5-year revision-free and amputation-free survival rate of 75%, presumably because it is mechanically stronger and less complex (184, 185). Functioning appears to be better in children who are older than 8 years at the time of the reconstruction. Rehabilitation is more difficult with allograft, but they hold the promise of superior longevity. It is very important to tell the patient in either case that the function will not be normal and that neither method of reconstruction will return the patient to sports activities; amputations can still be more functional if the patient is willing to engage in high-level activity (203, 204). Distraction osteogenesis is another means of achieving equal limb length that can be done for patients who have had resections of malignant bone tumors. This should be done only after the patient has completed chemotherapy.

For diaphyseal lesions, an intercalary resection can be performed, sparing the adjacent joints and occasionally the epiphyseal plates. In these patients, reconstruction can be carried out with intercalary allografts and/or vascularized fibula (203, 204). A method of using an allograft to provide initial stability, augmented by a vascularized fibular graft to achieve quicker union and long-term healing potential (205). This technique is especially helpful when only a small segment of the epiphysis remains after the resection (206, 207).

For very young patients with tumors of the distal femur, or older patients who want to be athletically active, rotationplasty is a good option (207). In these patients, above-knee amputation would lead to a very short stump with a poor lever arm with high energy consumption during gait (206). Rotationplasty, by taking advantage of the tibia and foot, provides a longer lever arm and an active "knee" joint. It also avoids resection of the major nerves, so that phantom pain is not an issue. The physical appearance without the prosthesis is disturbing to some patients, but with prosthesis they look similar to other amputees with better function than above-knee amputees (Fig. 13-33). The technical details are well described elsewhere, and the technique has been described for lesions of the proximal tibia and the proximal femur (73). It is very important to have frank discussions with the patient and his or her family about the appearance and the expected outcome of this reconstruction. It can be very helpful to the patient to be able to meet another patient, who has undergone rotationplasty, or at least view a video and meet with an experienced physical therapist and prosthetist. Interestingly, young patients do not view this as an amputation, because the foot is still present, and the long-term psychological outcomes in these patients have been very good.

The more distal the tumor is in the lower extremity, the more likely it is that amputation will be the better treatment choice. A hip disarticulation has so much more functional consequence compared to an ankle disarticulation that limb-salvage surgery for a tumor in the proximal femur is always more valuable compared to limb-salvage surgery for a tumor in the calcaneus.

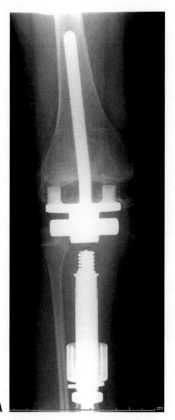
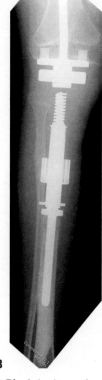
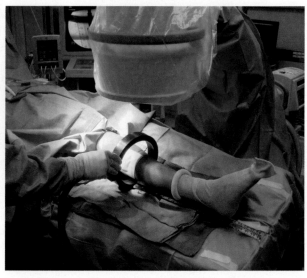

FIGURE 13-32. Radiographs **(A** and **B)** of the knee of a 12-year-old boy that underwent limb salvage surgery with a Repiphysis prosthesis for proximal tibia osteosarcoma. Note the spring-loaded system that expanded following lengthening. The procedure is done under sedation, and the lengthening is obtained by placing the extremity in an electromagnetic field **(C)**. (Reproduced with permission from The Children's Orthopaedic Center, Los Angeles, CA.)

Locally recurrent tumor is often indication for an amputation. These patients' tumors have proved that they are more aggressive or more extensive than had been appreciated at the time of their initial treatment and therefore need more aggressive surgery than usual. In these circumstances, limb salvage is less likely to be effective and should be done with caution.

Chemotherapy for Musculoskeletal Tumors. It was not until the 1970s that chemotherapy was believed to be effective in the treatment of malignant tumors of the musculoskeletal system. The extremely high incidence of metastatic disease in patients with osteosarcoma (more than 80%) and EWS (more than 85%), and some promising results in patients with metastatic sarcoma, prompted the use of adjuvant chemotherapy in patients who did not have documented disease but in whom the risk of having subclinical metastases was high. The early results were exciting, and even the use of what was considered minimal amounts of less-than-optimal drugs improved survival. These early studies led to the acceptance of adjuvant chemotherapy for primary bone sarcomas. In the 1980s, preoperative chemotherapy was introduced, and it is now standard for the initial chemotherapy for patients with EWS, osteosarcoma, and RMS. *Neoadjuvant chemotherapy* is a

term used to indicate that the patient receives chemotherapy before the definitive treatment of the primary lesion. This was initially used as a means of treating patients with osteosarcoma who were waiting for the production of a custom prosthesis. The effect of chemotherapy on the tumor was considerable and of prognostic significance, and this has led to the routine use of preoperative chemotherapy.

There are numerous chemotherapeutic protocols for the three main skeletal malignancies (EWS, osteosarcoma, and RMS) for which chemotherapy is used. All these protocols use more than one drug, usually three to five. Most protocols are between 9 and 12 months in duration. Approximately one-third of the chemotherapy is given preoperatively, and the remainder is given after surgery.

The drugs used for musculoskeletal tumors include

- Doxorubicin (Adriamycin), a cytotoxic anthracycline antibiotic that passively enters the cell to diffuse into the nucleus, where it binds nucleic acids and disrupts DNA synthesis. It is cardiotoxic, myelosuppressive, and produces alopecia. It is given intravenously in divided doses over 6 months, with $450 \ mg/m^2$ recommended as the maximum dose.
- Methotrexate is an antimetabolite that inhibits dihydrofolic acid reductase. This interferes with DNA synthesis and

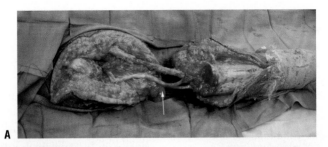

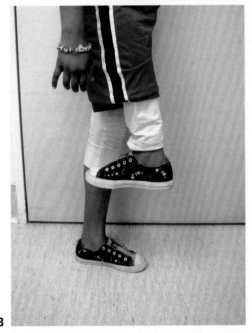

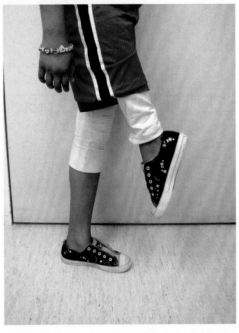

FIGURE 13-33. This 8-year-old girl had an extensive osteogenic sarcoma of the femur, complicated by a pathologic fracture and inappropriate ORIF performed at an outside institution; she underwent a Van Nes rotationplasty with extensive neurovascular dissection **(A)** (*arrow* points to sciatic nerve dividing into tibial and peroneal branches) and retained movement of her ankle (**B** and **C**), that will now be used as a knee. (Reproduced with permission from The Children's Orthopaedic Center, Los Angeles, CA.)

repair, and alters cellular replication. When administered in high doses (12 mg/m^2 intravenously), leucovorin or citrovorum factor is given to the patient to rescue the normal cells. Leucovorin is a chemically reduced derivative of folic acid and is used by the cells to complete normal cell functions without the need for dihydrofolic acid reductase. Tumor cells seem less able to use leucovorin than normal cells, and this difference allows methotrexate to be effective against malignant tumors. The primary side effects of methotrexate are gastrointestinal, including nausea, vomiting, and loss of appetite.

- Cisplatin is a heavy metal that is thought to cause intrastrand crosslinks in DNA, and thereby interfere with the DNA. It is given intravenously in doses of 75 to 100 mg/m^2 repeatedly over the course of the treatment. The principal side effect of cisplatin is nephrotoxicity.
- Cyclophosphamide (Cytoxan) is a synthetic drug chemically related to nitrogen mustard. It crosslinks DNA and interferes with DNA functions. It is given intravenously at

a dose of 40 to 50 mg/kg in divided doses over 4 to 5 days. The major side effects of cyclophosphamide are gastrointestinal disorders and myelosuppression.

- Ifosfamide is a synthetic analog of cyclophosphamide, with similar actions. It is given intravenously at 1.2 g/m^2/day for 5 days.
- Vincristine is an alkaloid from the periwinkle plant. It is thought to arrest dividing cells in the metaphase state by inhibiting microtubule formation in the mitotic spindle. It is given intravenously at weekly intervals at doses of 1.4 mg/m^2 in adults and 2.0 mg/m^2 in children. The major side effect of vincristine is peripheral neuropathy.
- Bleomycin is a cytotoxic glycopeptide antibiotic from a strain of *Streptomyces verticillus* that inhibits DNA synthesis. It also probably inhibits ribonucleic acid (RNA) and protein synthesis. It is given intravenously at 0.25 to 0.50 U/kg once or twice per week. The most serious side effect of bleomycin is a 10% incidence of severe pulmonary fibrosis.

- Actinomycin D (Dactinomycin) is one of a number of actinomycin antibiotics from *Streptomyces*. It binds to DNA by intercalation with the phenoxazone ring. This inhibits the DNA from being a template for RNA and synthesizing itself. It is given intravenously at 0.5 mg/day for 5 days. Dactinomycin produces nausea and vomiting and is myelosuppressive.

These drugs are given in various combinations and doses, depending on the specific diagnosis, the protocol, the response of the patient, and the aggressiveness of approach of the medical oncologist.

Osteosarcoma.

Osteogenic sarcoma or osteosarcoma is defined as a tumor in which malignant spindle cells produce bone. There are two major variants that have significantly different clinical presentations and prognoses. The more common osteosarcoma is called classic high grade, or conventional, and the other is juxtacortical (73). Less common variants of osteosarcoma (e.g., intracortical, soft tissue, radiation-induced, Paget disease) are not discussed in this text.

Conventional Osteosarcoma. The patient is usually a teenager (approximately 50% of the patients present during the second decade of life; more than 75% are between 8 and 25 years of age) with symptoms of pain and a mass around the knee (187, 200, 208). In approximately half of the patients, the lesions are located in the distal femur or the proximal tibia. The proximal humerus, proximal femur, and pelvis are the next most common sites. The pain precedes the appreciation of the mass by a few weeks to 2 or 3 months. Boys and girls are affected with equal frequency. The patient does not have systemic symptoms and usually feels well. The mass is slightly tender, firm to hard, and fixed to the bone but not inflamed. The adjacent joint may have mild restriction of motion.

The remainder of the physical examination is normal, except in the rare (<1%) patient who presents with bone metastases or multiple focal osteosarcoma. One-half of all patients have elevated serum alkaline phosphatase (extremely high serum alkaline phosphatase values indicate a worse prognosis), and approximately one-fourth of all patients have elevated serum LDH level (an elevated LDH level also is associated with a worse prognosis). The rest of the laboratory values for blood and urine are normal.

The plain radiograph of an osteosarcoma is usually diagnostic. The typical lesion is located in the metaphysis, involves the medullary canal, is both lytic (radiolucent) and blastic (radiodense), and has an extraosseous component and a periosteal reaction suggestive of a rapid growth (Codman triangle or sunburst pattern) (Fig. 13-34A). Most osteosarcomas have a soft-tissue component, of a fluffy density suggestive of neoplastic bone, adjacent to the more obvious bone lesion. Those osteosarcomas that consist primarily of cartilage or fibrous tissue are almost purely radiolucent. Telangiectatic osteosarcoma, a histologic variant of classic high-grade osteosarcoma, may be mistaken on a radiograph for an ABC or a giant cell tumor.

Usually, this will not be a clinical problem for the pathologist if the surgeon provides adequate clinical information.

MRI is the method of choice for evaluating suspected osteosarcoma. The extent of the lesion, especially the intraosseous component, is more clearly defined by MRI. The lesion can be seen in all three planes, and its soft-tissue extension is easily appreciated. It is critical that the entire bone be included on at least one plane (usually the coronal view). The tumor should be viewed with at least a T1-weighted (with and without gadolinium) image, a T2-weighted image, and a fat-suppressed image (Fig. 13-34B,C).

Osteosarcomas should be resected with at least a wide surgical margin, and the anatomic extent of the tumor is the principal determinant of what operation will be required (209). MRI is the best method of determining the anatomic extent of an osteosarcoma (Fig. 13-34D). The relation of osteosarcoma to the major neurovascular bundle should be determined. The muscles that have been invaded by the soft-tissue component should be identified. Involvement of the adjacent joint must be looked for, the intraosseous extent measured, and the presence of metastasis noted. Talking to the radiologist before MRI is performed helps to ensure that all this information is obtained.

Chest CT scan is performed because of the relatively high percentage (approximately 20%) of patients present with pulmonary metastasis (209). The lung is the most common site for metastatic involvement (osteosarcoma metastasize via hematogenous) (210, 211). The technetium-99 bone scan shows increased uptake in the area of the tumor. Occasionally it is useful in determining the intraosseous extent, although MRI is more accurate. More importantly, technetium-99 bone scanning is an excellent screen of the entire skeleton for occult bone lesions. This screening process is the most important reason for obtaining a bone scan. On rare occasions, a lung metastasis is seen on the bone scan, but usually a hot spot in the chest on the bone scan is secondary to involvement of a rib.

There are five major histologic types of conventional osteosarcoma, and each is graded for the degree of malignancy. The predominant tumor cell type determines the histologic subtype. It is debatable whether the different types have distinct prognoses (210, 211); some believe that if matched for size and histologic grade, all types have the same prognosis. Even telangiectatic osteosarcoma, which was originally described as having a particularly poor prognosis, is thought to have the same prognosis as the other classic high-grade osteosarcomas. The five types are osteoblastic, chondroblastic, fibroblastic, mixed, and telangiectatic (188, 200, 210, 212). These tumors are graded on a scale of either 1 to 3 or 1 to 4; by definition, the higher the grade is, the worse the prognosis. Most osteosarcomas are grade 3 or 4, and of the mixed type. The tumor is composed of a mixture of neoplastic cells, but must contain malignant spindle cells making osteoid. Atypical mitoses are common, and small areas of necrosis are usually seen (Fig. 13-35).

Treatment of classic high-grade osteosarcoma includes adjuvant chemotherapy and surgical resection. The standard protocol consists of chemotherapy (neoadjuvant; usually three

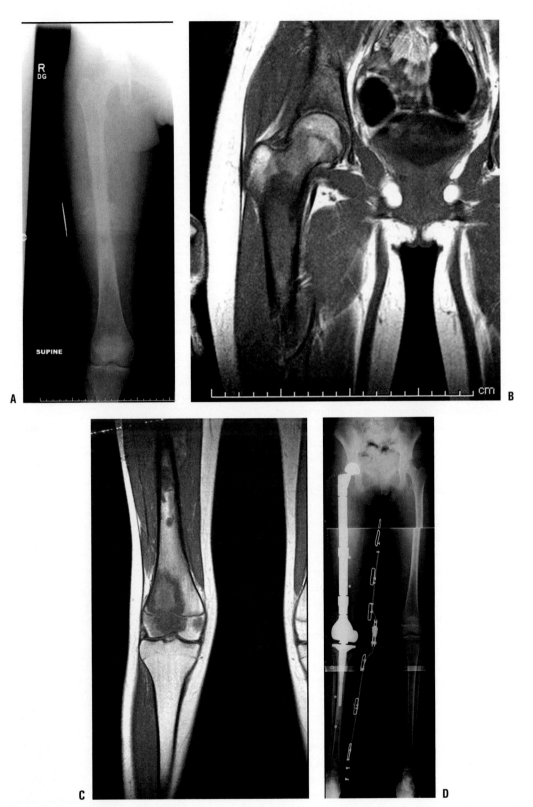

FIGURE 13-34.   Hip-to-ankle anterior–posterior radiograph **(A)** of a 14-year-old girl with recently diagnosed osteogenic sarcoma. The image shows an aggressive-looking, permeative, and ill-defined mixed lesion, disorganized periosteal reaction and sunburst appearance, and associated with a soft-tissue mass. Coronal T1-weighted MRI of the proximal femur **(B)** and distal femur **(C)** shows the extension of disease, involving the entire femur. The patient underwent wide resection of the femur with negative margins and reconstruction with a total femur endoprosthesis **(D)**. (Reproduced with permission from The Children's Orthopaedic Center, Los Angeles, CA.)

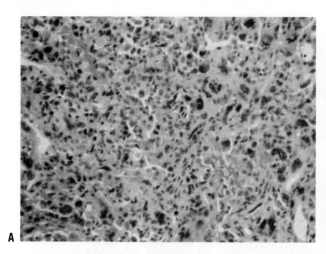
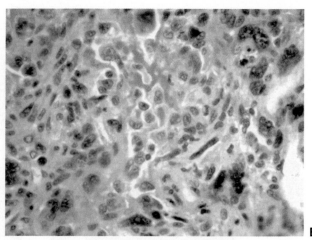

FIGURE 13-35. **A:** Typical histologic appearance of an osteoblastic osteosarcoma. There is immature bone being formed from cells that vary in size, shape, and amount of nuclear material. These findings are typical of malignant cells (10× magnification). **B:** Higher magnification (40×) of the osteosarcoma in (A). The nuclear detail is more clearly seen, and the bone seemingly coming directly from these bizarre cells makes the diagnosis of an osteosarcoma.

or four courses of a multidrug regimen), then surgical resection, and finally additional chemotherapy. The entire treatment takes almost 1 year (188, 200, 210, 212). The surgical resection can almost always be done without an amputation of the extremity, and less radical surgery is being performed now compared with only a few years ago. The use of neoadjuvant chemotherapy has not produced increased survival compared with postoperative adjuvant chemotherapy alone, but it does make surgery easier, and gives the pediatric oncologist a predictor of the patient's chance of survival (Fig. 13-36).

The three most important drugs used in the treatment of osteosarcoma are doxorubicin (Adriamycin), high-dose methotrexate, and cisplatin (188, 200, 208, 210, 212–214). Most chemotherapy protocols include these three drugs in various dosage schedules, in addition to one or more other drugs. The development of granulocyte-stimulating factor (GSF) to counteract bone marrow suppression has allowed intensification of the treatment with fewer complications; GSF is now used routinely. Overall survival has increased to more than 60%, with even better survival rates being reported for patients with >90% necrosis of the tumor after chemotherapy (182, 183).

Limb-salvage surgery is being performed for all but the largest of osteosarcomas. Amputation is done in fewer than 20% of all cases (183). The accepted incidence of local recurrence with limb-sparing procedure is between 5% and 10% (209, 215). Although the local recurrence does not seem to be directly related to worse survival, this is an area of concern, because it appears that most patients with local recurrence die of osteosarcoma (200, 215, 216). One explanation is that local recurrence is a sign of a more aggressive tumor, not solely the consequence of poor surgery. That being said, however, the insistence on wide (free) margins is paramount (50, 191, 217, 218).

There is currently some controversy about the best method of treatment for patients with pathologic fractures. There is an increased incidence of local recurrence if limb-salvage resection

is performed, but this increased incidence of local recurrence does not seem to increase the risk of death (50, 191, 217, 218). The usual treatment of a patient with a pathologic fracture and

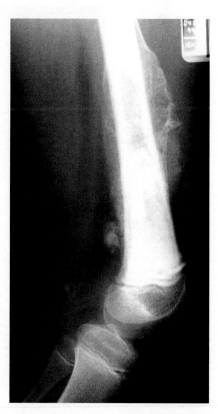

FIGURE 13-36. This plain radiograph is a lateral view of the distal femur of a patient who has had standard preoperative chemotherapy. The original lesion had a large extraosseous component that has been reduced in size, and there has been "maturing" of the periosteal reaction. The patient's pain diminished, and the range of motion in her knee returned to normal.

osteosarcoma is to treat the fracture closed (if amenable) or by minimally invasive technique (avoid further contamination), give neoadjuvant chemotherapy, and perform limb salvage if negative surgical margins can be obtained (73, 219).

Juxtacortical Osteosarcoma.   Osteosarcomas that arise from or are adjacent to the external surface of the bone behave differently from those that arise from within the medullary canal (73). They are usually less aggressive locally, have less potential for distant metastasis, and occur less commonly than conventional osteosarcoma. The "old" classification divides these lesions into parosteal and periosteal; neither is common, and how distinct they are from each other remains a topic of debate. Parosteal osteosarcoma is most commonly located in the posterior aspect of the distal femur, and is composed of bone and low-grade malignant fibrous tissue. Periosteal osteosarcoma is more often located in the diaphysis of the tibia, and is composed of bone and cartilage with malignant spindle cells (220). The current nomenclature includes both types under juxtacortical, low or high grade (220).

The patient's age at presentation varies over a greater range (10 to 45 years) than in classic high-grade osteosarcoma, and the median age at presentation tends to be slightly higher (73, 219, 220). The patient usually reports a painless mass that blocks motion in the adjacent joint. This is most often knee flexion because the posterior distal femur is the most common site of a juxtacortical osteosarcoma (73, 219). Occasionally the patient has a mild, dull ache in the area of the tumor, but the symptoms are minimal. The mass is fixed, hard, and nontender. The adjacent joint may have limited passive and active motion because of the mechanical block from the tumor. Inflammation is not observed. The laboratory values of the patient's blood and urine are normal.

The plain radiograph is almost always diagnostic, but the findings may be mistaken for a juxtacortical chondroma or an osteochondroma (Fig. 13-37). The lesion arises from the cortex, which may be normal or thickened. The juxtacortical osteosarcoma often wraps around the bone, with the periosteum between the tumor and the underlying cortex. This growth pattern (wrapping around the bone) produces the "string sign" on

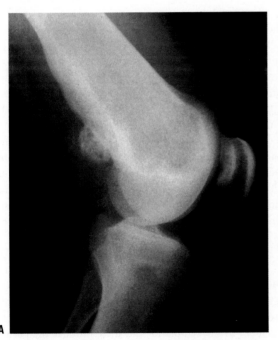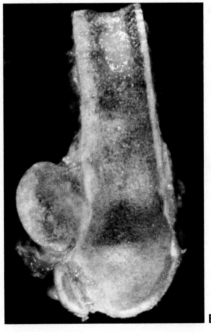

FIGURE 13-37.   A: Lateral radiograph of the distal femur and knee of a patient with a juxtacortical osteogenic sarcoma. The posterior distal femoral cortex is thickened and slightly irregular. The radiodensity adjacent to the posterior cortex is the central portion of the juxtacortical osteosarcoma. Surrounding this bony mass is a nonossified component of the tumor, composed primarily of fibrous tissue, but with some cartilage. This patient was treated with limb-salvage wide resection of the distal femur and underwent reconstruction with an osteoarticular allograft. No chemotherapy was used since this was a low-grade tumor, and the patient has remained free of disease for 5 years. **B:** The juxtacortical osteogenic sarcoma is larger than it appears on the plain radiograph. The cap of fibrous tissue and cartilage can be seen covering the bony center. The tumor is attached to the cortex, but does not extend through it. This gross relation is similar to that of an exostosis and may lead to a mistaken histologic diagnosis. The gross difference between an exostosis and a juxtacortical osteosarcoma is that the stalk of an exostosis is cortical bone that blends with the cortex of the host bone, and the medullary canal of the stalk and host bone are connected. The juxtacortical osteosarcoma, conversely, is attached to the cortex, but the cortex of host bone is intact, and the medullary canal does not communicate with the parosteal osteosarcoma.

the plain radiograph, with a thin radiolucent line between the lesion and the cortex of the bone. The lesion itself is dense, and has the pattern of bone. There is increased uptake on a technetium-99 bone scan. The appearance of the lesion on a CT scan is characteristic and distinguishes a juxtacortical osteosarcoma from an exostosis. Juxtacortical osteosarcoma is attached to the cortex growing out into the soft tissue and may invade the cortex, but the normal cortex is intact (219, 220). An exostosis arises from the cortex, and the cortex of the normal bone becomes the cortex of the exostosis, with the medullary canal of the bone communicating with the medullary canal of the exostosis. These relations, and also the intraosseous extension of the tumor, are better seen with MRI than with CT scan.

An incisional biopsy of a juxtacortical osteosarcoma can be difficult to interpret and, on the basis of histology alone, the lesion may be mistaken for an exostosis. This is particularly true when juxtacortical osteosarcoma is not suspected by the clinician, or when the pathologist does not examine the radiograph (219, 220). This lesion, more than most other lesions, is diagnosed by its clinical and radiographic presentation and is confirmed by histology. An excisional biopsy is sometimes recommended to avoid local contamination. Higher grade lesions, especially those with medullary involvement, have a greater risk of metastasizing (usually to the lung) than those of lower grade without medullary extension (101, 219, 220).

The cortical margin should be generous and the tumor pseudocapsule should not be disturbed. When a lesion from the posterior distal femur is resected, the neurovascular bundle can usually be freed from the lesion without dissecting the pseudocapsule, but the posterior capsule of the knee and the posterior aspect of the femoral condyle must usually be resected with the tumor. Those lesions that wrap around the bone and show gross invasion of the medullary canal may require a resection that includes the entire end of the bone. The initial resection is the best opportunity to control the lesion without an amputation. Most patients do not need adjuvant chemotherapy (unless the lesion is high grade) because the cure with surgery alone is approximately 80% (221, 222).

Ewing Sarcoma/Peripheral Neuroectodermal Tumor.

EWS and PNET are discussed together here because they are basically the same tumor, or are at least closely related. Both have the same chromosomal translocation between chromosomes 11 and 22, similar presentations, identical treatments, and almost identical histologic characteristics (223). PNET is also called Askin tumor and was originally identified from tumors classified as EWS. EWS/PNETs are thought to arise from the neural crest. At least 90% of them have a characteristic chromosomal translocation [t(11:22) (q24:q12)]. This translocation leads to a novel fusion protein called EWS-FLI1 (224).

Before the use of adjuvant chemotherapy, EWS/PNET was associated with a 5-year survival of approximately 15%, being considered the most lethal of all primary bone tumors (225). Before adjuvant chemotherapy came into use, most patients were treated with irradiation alone (224, 226, 227).

With improved survival associated with adjuvant chemotherapy the role of surgery has been reevaluated, and there is growing evidence that surgical resection combined with chemotherapy produces improved survival rates, compared with survival after irradiation and chemotherapy (59).

Patients with EWS/PNET initially experience pain. Some have generalized symptoms of fever, weight loss, and malaise, but this is not the usual presentation. Male patients outnumber female patients by a ratio of 3:2, and most patients are between the ages of 5 and 30 years. Any bone may be affected. The femur is the most common site of origin (20%); the pelvis and the humerus are also common sites. There is usually a soft-tissue mass associated with the bone lesion, and this mass can often be palpated during a physical examination. The mass is warm, firm, and tender, and it may be pulsatile. There are no specific abnormal laboratory values that are diagnostic of EWS/PNET, but the sedimentation rate is often increased. Elevated LDH level indicates a poor prognosis (60).

The typical plain radiograph of an EWS/PNET reveals diffuse destruction of the bone, extension of the tumor through the cortex, a soft-tissue component, and a periosteal reaction (Fig. 13-38A). The periosteal reaction may produce a Codman triangle, an "onionskin" appearance, or a sunburst appearance. These suggest an aggressive lesion that has rapidly penetrated the cortex and elevated the periosteum. The extraosseous soft-tissue mass and the medullary canal involvement can be seen on CT scans and MRI scans, and are usually more extensive than what might have been expected from the appearance of the plain radiograph. MRI has proved to be more accurate than CT scan in determining the intramedullary extent of EWS. The inflammation around the tumor is seen more easily with MRI than with other studies, and the extent of inflammation is often more than would be suggested from the findings of other tests. The technetium bone scan is most useful in finding occult bone metastasis. Approximately 20% of these patients present with metastatic disease (lung is the most common site) (60, 225, 226).

The histologic appearance of EWS/PNET is that of a small, round, cell tumor. The EWS/PNET cell has a distinct nucleus with minimal cytoplasm and an indistinct cytoplasmic border. The cells are similar and mitoses are uncommon. Necrotic areas are usually seen (Fig. 13-38B,C). There are glycogen granules in the cytoplasm, and these produce the positive periodic acid Schiff (PAS) stain on routine histologic examination. The intracellular glycogen granules are diastase positive (i.e., exposure to diastase will break the glycogen down, eliminating PAS staining). Under the electron microscope, the glycogen can be seen as dense cytoplasmic granules. Increasingly, genetic analysis is being done in EWS/PNET in order to identify the 11:22 translocation as a means of establish the diagnosis.

The treatment for EWS/PNET is a combination of chemotherapy and local control, either by surgery, radiation therapy, or a combination of both (60, 225, 226) (Fig. 13-39). The drugs commonly used include vincristine, doxorubicin, cyclophosphamide, ifosfamide, and etoposide. Actinomycin D, a drug used earlier, is currently used less often. Most

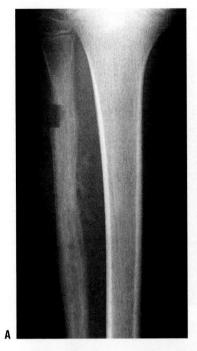
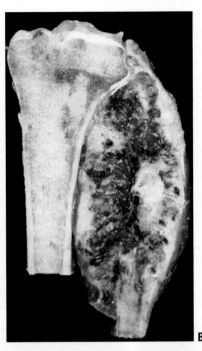
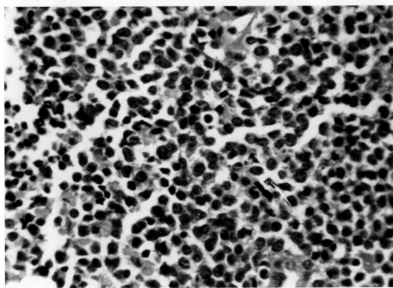

FIGURE 13-38. **A:** Anteroposterior radiograph of the proximal tibia and fibula of a patient with EWS involving the proximal fibula. The fibular cortical detail is lost, and erosion of the medial surface, soft-tissue mass, and periosteal reaction—all typical findings of EWS—are present. The combination of these findings is indicative of an aggressive process. Acute osteomyelitis may have this appearance, but the patient would usually have other signs of infection. The defect in the lateral aspect of the fibula is attributable to an incisional biopsy of the bone. A biopsy of the bone should not be performed if there is sufficient soft-tissue extension. This will lower the risk of pathologic fracture. In addition, the extraosseous tumor is usually easier to cut, and the histologic appearance is better. **B:** Gross specimen of EWS of the proximal fibula, similar to the case in A. The tumor has replaced the proximal fibula, and there is a large soft-tissue mass, with invasion of surrounding muscles and no involvement of the tibia. This patient chose to have an immediate amputation, although this is not standard treatment. **C:** Histologic appearance of EWS. The nuclei are easily seen, and there are nucleoli within each nucleus. The cells are small and round, with very little variation in appearance of the nuclei. Mitoses are rare. The cytoplasm is faint and difficult to see, and the cytoplasmic borders are poorly defined (original magnification × 10).

protocols begin with two to four courses of chemotherapy before a decision is made on how to manage the primary tumor. This usually results in a significant reduction in the size of the primary tumor. Surgical resection is recommended if the consequences of the resection (limitation or loss of function) are acceptable to the patient. If the margins are close and viable tumor is present in the resected specimen, postoperative irradiation is recommended (59, 224, 225, 227). If the primary tumor cannot be resected without undue morbidity, irradiation alone can be used (228). The total dosage should be kept as low as possible, usually around 50 Gy, and certainly <60 Gy, because dosages of more than 60 Gy are associated with an unacceptable incidence of irradiation-associated sarcomas at a later time, as well as other complications in this young age group (59, 224, 227). Current survival statistics for patients presenting without metastasis reveal a 5-year disease-free survival of >5%. Patients who present with metastasis have less chance of being cured, but should be treated aggressively because some will survive (229).

SOFT-TISSUE TUMORS

Soft-tissue tumors are a heterogeneous group of mesenchymal origin lesions that include lesions of different etiology such as congenital, traumatic, benign, and malignant neoplasms. Benign soft-tissue tumors are latent or active lesions and there are as many as 200 different types. Malignant soft-tissue

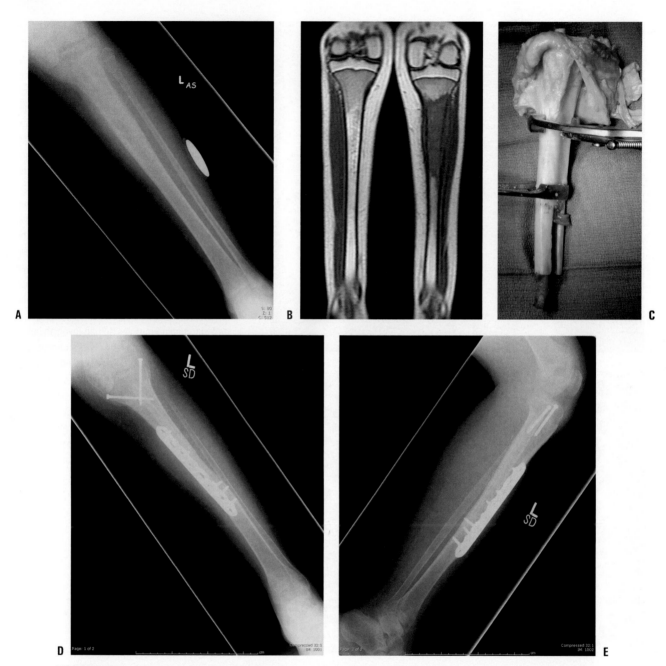

FIGURE 13-39. Ewing Sarcoma; this is the anterior–posterior radiograph **(A)** of the tibia of a 11-year-old girl who presented with a 4-month history of leg pain, demonstrating ill-defined, permeative lytic lesion with "onionskinning" periosteal reaction. After inductive chemotherapy, the tumor shrunk in size as shown in this MRI **(B),** and resection was carried out sparing the proximal tibia epiphysis. An intercalary allograft, combined with a vascularized fibula **(C),** was performed for reconstruction and the patient is disease free and back to full activity 24 months after surgery **(D,E).** (Reproduced with permission from The Children's Orthopaedic Center, Los Angeles, CA.)

tumors, in particular STSs, are aggressive tumors, capable of distant metastatic spread; there are over 70 types of STS. Most soft-tissue tumors in children are benign (230). Hemangioma, fibromatoses, and nerve tumors are probably the most common. Among malignancies, only RMS in the younger age group and synovial sarcoma in teenagers and older patients occur with any frequency, and still they are both rare tumors (231). In any instance, the physician must be aware of the

possibility of malignant soft-tissue tumor in the child and evaluate any lump carefully (232).

Benign Vascular Tumors. Benign vascular tumors are common and most frequently involve the skin. Controversies exist in regards to the tumor classification and the determination between benign vascular lesions, true neoplasms, and vascular malformations. Furthermore, clinicians, radiologists, and pathologists tend to classify these lesions differently, adding to the confusing differentiation. Understanding the differences and intricacies of vasculogenesis and angiogenesis helps understanding the differentiation between these lesions. A biologic classification, based on cellular kinetics and clinical behavior, has attempted to help resolve the confusion; there are two major categories of vascular anomalies: vascular tumors that arise from endothelial hyperplasia and vascular anomalies that arise from dysmorphogenesis (diffuse or localized errors of embryonic development) and have normal endothelial turnover (233).

Some congenital vascular malformations will not be diagnosed until later in life, suggesting a new appearing vascular tumor. Vascular anomalies can be divided into slow-flow and fast-slow lesions. They can also be divided according to their predominant vessel type (capillary, venous, lymphatic, arterial, or a combination). It is beyond the scope of this chapter to discuss vascular malformations in further detail.

Among true vascular tumors, hemangioma is the most common, particularly in infancy and childhood. Its origin is controversial. A true hemangioma is a benign lesion that often regresses spontaneously. Most are superficial lesions with predilection for the head and neck regions, but sometimes also found in internal organs, especially the liver.

Enzinger and Weiss (232) provide a classification of different forms of hemangioma that includes capillary, cavernous, pyogenic, venous, arteriovenous (racemose hemangioma), epithelioid (angiolymphoid hyperplasia, Kimura disease), diffuse or angiomatosis, and miscellaneous (synovial, intramuscular, neural). We only discuss the most common types in children.

- Capillary hemangioma (including juvenile type): Constitutes the largest group of benign vascular tumors. The juvenile hemangioma variant of capillary hemangioma occurs in 1 out of every 200 live births. They may be cutaneous or deep, and are usually seen within the first few weeks of life, often enlarging for the first 6 months but then regressing and becoming 75% to 95% involute by the age of 7 years. Capillary hemangiomas do not require treatment.
- Cavernous hemangioma: Less common than the capillary variant, but with similar age group and distribution. Cavernous hemangiomas do not spontaneously regress and may require treatment. They most commonly arise within muscle and invade tissue planes extensively. The patient often presents with complaints of swelling, tenderness, and inflammation secondary to thrombophlebitis within the hemangioma. This inflammation resolves within a few days, and can be treated with local heat and oral aspirin. The noninflamed hemangioma is soft and ill defined. The patient may have either no symptoms at all, or the sensation of heaviness or a tight feeling in the extremity. On the plain radiograph, there are often small, smooth, round calcifications called *phleboliths*. The appearance of hemangiomas on MRI is almost completely diagnostic because they are composed of smooth, regular blood vessels and normal fat.

Cavernous hemangiomas have an indirect communication with the major vascular tree and do not easily fill with contrast for angiography or venography; they are better visualized with MRI. Occasionally, a tourniquet proximal to the hemangioma permits filling of the tumor veins at the time of venography or angiography. If an intravenous injection does not demonstrate the hemangioma, the dye can be injected directly into the hemangioma. Biopsy may be performed to confirm the diagnosis, but often, the clinical presentation is sufficiently characteristic to render biopsy unnecessary. Resection is not necessary unless the patient has repeated bouts of inflammation or complaints of discomfort (usually a full or tight feeling), or the parents are anxious about the mass.

Surgical excision is usually not required. When surgery is performed, the hemangioma often recurs unless the entire muscle (or muscles) involved is resected. These lesions are probably best considered as congenital abnormalities that involve most of the veins in the extremity. When the grossly involved veins are resected, the surrounding vessels dilate, resulting in clinical recurrence. Hemangiomas do not undergo malignant degeneration, and although they can produce significant abnormalities in the extremity, surgical resection is rarely curative. However, resection may reduce the symptoms. Embolization and sclerotherapy have also been used in patients who have severe pain.

Hemangioma of bone, either solitary or diffuse, is a hamartoma, and not a true neoplasm. The solitary lesions are more frequent, especially in the vertebral bodies where they are most often found (Fig. 13-40). Solitary lesions may occur in any bone, but the skull is the second most common site. These lesions do not produce symptoms and are usually found

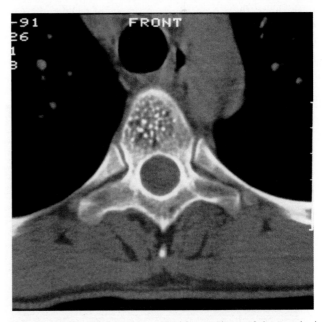

FIGURE 13-40. CT scan of a typical hemangioma of the vertebral body. The small foci of increased density are thickened trabeculae of bone, and the low-density areas are filled with the hemangiomatous tissue.

when a radiograph is taken for another reason. They are most often diagnosed in adults. The radiograph and the CT scan are diagnostic. The bone has a honeycomb appearance, with increased trabecular markings around radiolucencies.

Patients with multiple lesions are more likely to present during the first or the second decade of life, with either mild discomfort or pathologic fracture. The viscera and the skin of these patients may be involved. When multiple sites are involved, they are usually the long bones of the extremities and the short bones of the hands and feet. Treatment should be symptomatic, with curettage and bone grafting for lesions that weaken the bone. Lesions that do not produce symptoms or that are not associated with a risk for fracture should be merely observed. They usually resolve with time.

Fibromatoses.   Benign fibrous lesions in children are relatively common and rarely malignant. Extra-abdominal desmoid, or aggressive fibromatosis, is the most common benign fibrous lesion seen in children (234, 235). The less common lesions are not discussed in this text and can be found in detail elsewhere (232, 236).

The patient presents with mild pain and a slowly enlarging mass. The mass is deep, firm, and slightly tender but is not inflamed. The adjacent joint is normal. Approximately 60% of the lesions involve the extremities (234, 237, 238). A soft-tissue mass can be seen on a plain radiograph, but there are no distinguishing features. Calcifications are not expected to be present within the mass.

Technetium bone scan usually shows increased activity in the lesion, but some large masses will not display increased uptake. Often, even when the lesion is immediately adjacent to the bone, there is no increased uptake of technetium. On CT scan, the mass has a density similar to that of muscle, but it is usually more vascular and can be distinguished best from the surrounding tissue by performing the CT scan with an intravenous contrast. On MRI, the classic collagen bundles produce a relative signal void (dark on T1- and T2-weighted images) but, because the cellularity varies, fibromatoses may have an appearance similar to any soft-tissue neoplasia (Fig. 13-41) (235, 239).

Histologically, fibromatosis has the appearance of scar tissue (240). It is composed of dense bundles of collagen with evenly dispersed benign cells. The cell of origin is believed to be the myofibroblast. The histologic appearance and the cell of origin of fibromatosis are identical to those of plantar fibromatosis and Dupuytren contracture, but those lesions are not as clinically aggressive as fibromatosis. Although they too recur, they do not extend proximally from the feet or hands, as they do in aggressive fibromatosis.

Wide excision is the treatment of choice; however, since aggressive fibromatosis is an infiltrative lesion, often the pathologist finds a positive margin during examination under a microscope (236). Fortunately, the presence of a positive margin at the initial resection does not always lead to a local recurrence, and it is recommended that the patient be observed for a local recurrence (234). Approximately half of the patients will develop recurrent disease regardless of the histologic margin. When lesions recur, they must be widely excised if local control is to be achieved. Patients younger than 10 years have a greater risk of developing a local recurrence than older patients. When a wide surgical margin is ensured during the resection of the recurring lesion, local control is usually achieved. When the second surgical margin is also positive on microscopic examination, radiation therapy may be considered (240–243). Most lesions will be controlled with this combination. Chemotherapy is used sometimes, especially for aggressive, nonresectable lesions. There is still debate on whether chemotherapy is efficient (234, 235, 239, 244). Fibromatosis has a variable clinical course, and the treatment needs to be individualized for each patient.

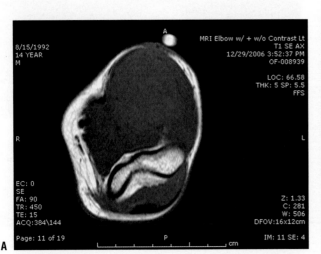
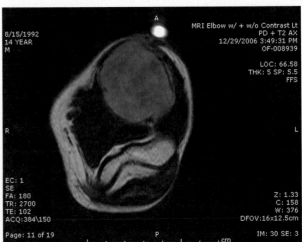

FIGURE 13-41.   A 14-year-old boy presented with a slow-growing, painful mass in the anterior aspect of the left elbow. T1- **(A)** and T2-weighted **(B)** axial images demonstrate this well-defined, soft-tissue mass consistent with desmoid tumor. (Reproduced with permission from The Children's Orthopaedic Center, Los Angeles, CA.)

Benign Tumors of Nerve Origin. There are two common benign tumors that arise from nerves: schwannomas and neurofibroma (244). Neurilemomas, or schwannomas (now the preferred term), arise from the nerve sheath. They occur most often in early adulthood, and are usually solitary and slow growing. The patient usually presents with a painless mass, and may have a Tinel sign when the mass is tapped. The mass may be from any nerve, but it is often in the superficial tissue arising from a small sensory nerve. When arising from a spinal nerve root, the foramen may be enlarged because of the pressure of the tumor on the bone. Nerve dysfunction is uncommon, and is seen only when the nerve is compressed between the tumor and an adjacent rigid structure. Patients with superficial nerve lesions usually present early with small tumors, but deep-seated lesions may be large before they are discovered (Fig. 13-42).

Schwannomas are nodular masses with a distinct capsule and are easily separated from the nerve of origin. Under the microscope, they appear as a combination of a cellular area (Antoni A) and a myxoid area (Antoni B). The Antoni A area is composed of benign spindle cells that tend to have their nuclei stacked with intervening cytoplasm (Fig. 13-43). This nuclear stacking produces a *palisaded appearance*, and the arrangement of alternating nuclei and cytoplasm is called a *Verocay body*. The Antoni B area is composed of myxomatous tissue that has less cellularity than does the Antoni A area. Schwannomas are

treated by observation, or marginal excision without sacrificing the affected nerve (244). Schwannomas do not usually recur.

Neurofibroma may arise as a solitary lesion or as multiple lesions. Approximately 90% are solitary and are not characteristic of von Recklinghausen disease, although most patients with neurofibromatosis will have multiple neurofibromas. They may arise in the skin or be associated with a recognizable peripheral nerve. Like schwannomas, they usually present as a painless mass with a Tinel sign. Unlike schwannomas, however, they tend to be intimately associated with the nerve fibers (244). Fortunately, most arise from small cutaneous nerves and can be removed without loss of nerve function. Histologically, neurofibromas are not encapsulated, and they invade the nerve fibers and, rarely, the adjacent soft tissue. The cells are elongated and wavy, and have dark-staining nuclei. There is a collagen matrix composed of stringy-looking fibers. Neurites are usually seen within the lesion. Surgical resection is recommended for those lesions that are solitary and not associated with a major nerve. Lesions arising from a major nerve can be resected, but the nerve fascicles should be split and the neurofibroma should be removed from between them. Careful resection is important as there is an inherited risk for nerve damage and worsening of symptoms following resection (235). Neither solitary schwannoma nor neurofibroma is associated with a significant incidence of malignant degeneration, but patients with neurofibromatosis have a higher risk of developing neurofibrosarcoma.

Benign Synovial Tumors

Synovial Chondromatosis. Synovial chondromatosis is a disorder of the synovial tissues (245). It occurs most often in the knee, but can arise in any joint, tendon sheath, or bursa. Its cause is unknown, and it has no recognized familial pattern of occurrence. Although some authors believe that this is a reactive rather than a neoplastic process, it is mostly a benign metaplastic disease that has malignant potential (245, 246). The subliminal lining of the joint produces small nodules of hyaline-like cartilage that are extruded from the synovial lining to become loose bodies within the joint. If they become large, the cartilage may become necrotic; if they have blood supply, they may undergo enchondral ossification.

The disease is rare in children and presents most commonly between the ages of 20 and 50 years, slightly more common in males (245). The most common joint involved is the knee (approximately 70%), followed by hip and elbow (247). The patient usually presents with mild discomfort, minimal loss of motion, and an effusion in a joint. There may be a history of locking and previous trauma. The knee may appear normal on examination, but usually there is a moderate-to-large effusion, limited motion, and a boggy synovium.

The plain radiographs may be normal, or show only small intra-articular calcified bodies. The arthrogram is usually diagnostic, showing an irregular synovial surface and normal-to-thinned synovial fluid. MRI is most useful imaging for diagnosis of synovial chondromatosis. There are three distinct MR

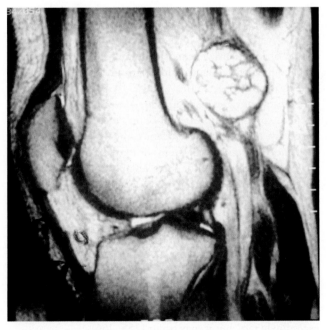

FIGURE 13-42. This is a sagittal view of a T1-weighted magnetic resonance image. The round, well-circumscribed mass posterior to the femur is within the peroneal nerve. It proved to be a schwannoma. Schwannomas have a typical appearance on magnetic resonance images. If they arise from a major nerve, as is the case in this patient, the nerve can usually be traced into the lesion. The schwannoma is smooth, slightly oblong, and has both bright and intermediate signals.

FIGURE 13-43. Histologic appearance of schwannoma (Antoni A area). The nuclei are stacked, giving the lesion a palisaded appearance (original magnification × 10).

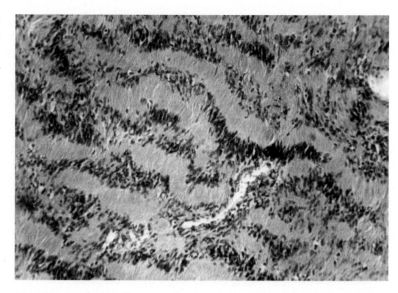

patterns: lobulated homogeneous intra-articular signal isointense to slightly hyperintense to muscle on T1-weighted images and hyperintense on T2-weighted images; the previous pattern plus foci of signal void on all pulse sequences (corresponding to areas of calcification); and features of both patterns plus foci of peripheral low signal surrounding central fat-like signal (corresponding to areas of ossification) (245, 248).

Most patients have sufficient symptoms to require removal of the loose bodies. Usually synovectomy is performed, but recurrence is high (approximately 15%) as the synovial lining is regenerated (245). The process seems to have a limited natural course, and the production of new loose bodies ceases after 1 or 2 years. In cases with large amount of lesional tissue, resection is also recommended to avoid secondary joint destruction with degenerative arthritis; the risk of malignant degeneration (approximately <5%) is a relative indication for resection (249–251).

Pigmented Villonodular Synovitis.   Pigmented villonodular synovitis (PVNS) is a rare disorder of the synovial tissues, characterized by destructive proliferation of synovial-like mononuclear cells. The synovial lining becomes proliferative and hypertrophic. It can involve a joint (most commonly the knee) or a tendon sheath (referred as to giant-cell tumor of tendon sheath). Most involvement is intra-articular, but extra-articular disease also occurs. When tendon sheaths are involved, PVNS usually occurs in the hand or the foot. Most patients with PVNS are between 20 and 40 years of age (250). The patient presents with a swollen joint that is usually painless. The synovial tissue is boggy on examination. Locking and giving-away sensation may be reported, and symptoms that mimic meniscal tear are common (252). There is a diffuse form of disease that presents with slow clinical course of insidious onset of pain, swelling, and stiffness in the involved joint, often being misdiagnosed as early osteoarthritis, rheumatoid arthritis, meniscal tear, or other ligamentous injury.

The plain radiograph is usually normal except for the soft-tissue swelling, but occasionally, the proliferative synovial tissues invade the bones adjacent to the joint. This happens most frequently when the hip joint is involved. The fluid in the joint has old, dark blood in it, and it is common for the diagnosis to be suspected first when the joint is aspirated just before the injection of contrast material for arthrography. The arthrogram or the MRI scan is diagnostic, with a thickened shaggy lining and demonstration of dark pigment signal on MRI; the high hemosiderin content causes the mass to appear as low signal on T1- and T2-weighted images. (249) (Fig. 13-44). MRI is the best radiographic method to evaluate the extent of the lesion. Bone invasion can be appreciated, as can the extent of enlargement of the synovial cavity. Gradient-echo imaging together with enhanced imaging is the most useful sequence for pediatric patients. The most common areas of involvement are the suprapatellar pouch, Hoffa fat pad, and behind the cruciate ligaments (251, 253).

Treatment varies from surgical synovectomy (arthroscopic, open, or combined) to external-beam radiation. Synovectomy is usually the treatment of choice, but there is a variable incidence of recurrence (from 8 to 50% in some series) (250, 251, 253). Anterior knee lesions, especially for localized disease are best treated with an arthroscopic synovectomy. Posterior knee lesions are difficult to approach via arthroscopic and a combined anterior synovectomy via scope combined with formal open posterior synovectomy is recommended (251). Recurrence may not warrant re-excision (decision is made upon location, size, and symptoms). Some patients have minimal symptoms and will accept the chronic swelling. As long as the bones remain uninvolved, there is no absolute indication for surgical removal (254). Malignant degeneration is exceedingly rare, but it may occur (255, 256).

Rhabdomyosarcoma.   RMS is a malignant tumor of skeletal muscle. RMS is the most common STS in children with an approximate annual incidence of approximately 350 new cases in the United States (257–259). RMS is slightly more common in men and in Caucasians. The majority is sporadic; however, some will occur in association with neurofibromatosis,

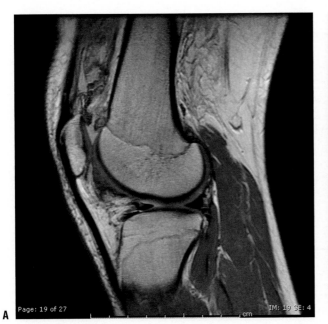
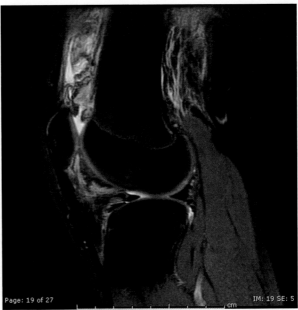

FIGURE 13-44. A 14-year-old boy presenting with knee pain and swelling. Sagittal T1- **(A)** and T2-weighted **(B)** MRI demonstrate the classic appearance of PVNS with dark/ dark intensity. (Reproduced with permission from The Children's Orthopaedic Center, Los Angeles, CA.)

Beckwith-Wiedemann syndrome, Li-Fraumeni disease, Costello syndrome, and others. There are four histologic patterns: embryonal, botryoid type, alveolar, and pleomorphic (260, 261).

Embryonal RMS is the most common type, and usually arises in the head, neck, genitourinary tract, and retroperitoneum. It is rare in the extremities. Botryoid-type RMS is histologically identical to the embryonal pattern, but is considered as a separate entity because of its appearance on gross examination. A botryoid RMS is an embryonal cell type that involves a hollow viscus. Botryoid RMS tends to occur in the first decade of life. The histologic appearance of embryonal RMS can vary (262). This lesion consists of poorly differentiated rhabdomyoblasts with limited collagen matrix. The rhabdomyoblasts are small, round-to-oval cells with dark-staining nuclei and limited amounts of eosinophilic cytoplasm. Cross-striations are not seen regularly.

Alveolar RMS is more common in the extremities than in the trunk, and is seen in older children and young adults, usually between 10 and 25 years of age (263). Characteristic chromosomal abnormalities [t(2;13)(q35;q14) and t(1;13)(p36-q14)] have been identified. Approximately 70% of the tumors will have a translocation between chromosomes 13 and 2, whereas another 30% will have the translocation between chromosomes 13 and 1. This occurs with equal frequency in the upper and lower extremities. Alveolar RMS is composed of small, round-to-oval tumor cells loosely arranged together in groups by dense collagen bundles. This arrangement of cells in groups produces an alveolar appearance; hence the name. The patient presents with a rapidly growing deep mass within the muscle (Fig. 13-45).

Pleomorphic RMS is the histologic type seen in adults, and it is the least common. It represents <20% of all cases. It is of difficult differentiation from EWS, neuroblastoma, and melanoma. Pleomorphic RMS has the worst prognosis.

The current treatment is a combination of chemotherapy, surgery, and, if the malignancy is not totally excised, irradiation (235, 254). When chemotherapy is given preoperatively, the surgery required is less radical, and adequate surgical margins are more easily achieved. If the lesion is small, it should be totally resected initially. If an RMS lesion occurs in an extremity, preoperative chemotherapy should be considered. A wide surgical margin is recommended (264). Regional lymph is sometimes indicated. Preoperative irradiation is reserved for lesions that would require an amputation in order to obtain a wide margin. Postoperative irradiation is used when the surgical margins are positive for tumor (265, 266).

The Intergroup Rhabdomyosarcoma Committee, with representation from both the Pediatric Oncology Group and the Children's Cancer Study Group, has been the dominant group treating RMS in the United States. Their coordinated efforts have resulted in major advances in the management of this malignancy (235, 266). Their staging system for patients with RMS is currently in use (267, 268). Prognostic variables include histologic subtype, size of the tumor, site of the tumor, and age of the patient (235, 263, 265, 267). Alveolar subtype, larger tumors, patients older than 10 years, and extremity tumors are associated with a poor prognosis (263, 265, 267, 268). Therefore, the patients that the orthopaedist treats tend to do worse than those treated by the urologist and the otolaryngologist. Better prognosis and improved 5-year overall survival (OS) is seen with younger age (ages 1 to 4 years: ~80% OS) at diagnosis, localized disease (approximately 80% OS),

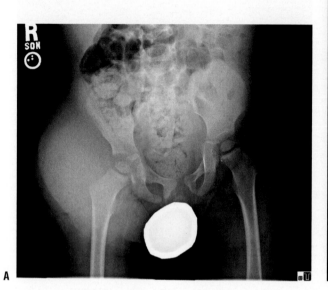
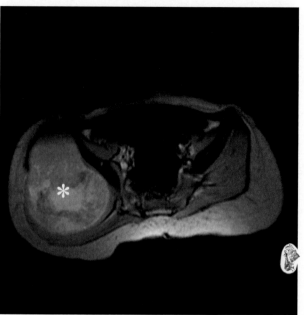

FIGURE 13-45.   This is a 5-year-old boy with a large alveolar RMS of the right buttock. Plain radiograph **(A)** shows the soft-tissue shadow, and axial cut MRI **(B)** clearly demonstrates the large, infiltrative mass, located deep within the gluteus musculature (*).

embryonal histology (approximately 70% OS), orbital (approximately 85% OS) and genitourinary (approximately 80% OS) tumors (86, 98, 268–270).

Synovial Sarcoma. Synovial sarcoma is a malignant soft-tissue tumor of cell of unknown origin. It is not related to the synovium, and the term synovial *cell* sarcoma should be avoided. It is the most common non-RMS STS in young adults, it accounts for 10% of all STSs. It has a typical chromosomal translocation, t(x;18)(p11.2;q11.2). Most patients are between 15 and 35 years of age, with male patients being slightly predominant in number. Approximately 75% occur in the extremities with a tendency to develop near large joints (most commonly the knee) (Fig. 13-46). Less than 10% are intra-articular and it is the most common sarcoma of the foot.

Patients often experience pain before they have palpable masses, and many patients give a history of having pain for 2 to 4 years before the lesion was found. Other patients have a palpable mass that has not grown in many years, and suddenly it starts increasing in size. The usual physical finding is a firm, slightly tender mass. Up to 25% of these patients have metastasis to regional lymph nodes, and the lymph nodes should therefore be examined carefully. The patient's blood and urine laboratory values are usually normal.

The lesion may occur in any part of the body. The head, neck, and trunk account for approximately 15% of the lesions, whereas the upper and lower extremities account for more than 50%. Almost 10% of the lesions occur in the hands or feet.

Synovial sarcomas may have calcifications or ossifications within the tumor, and these are often seen on plain radiographs.

Neurofibrosarcoma and fibrosarcoma also may have intralesional calcification, but synovial sarcoma is the most common tumor with intralesional densities. The radiodensities are usually very low. Small, irregular calcific foci, or irregular ossification within a soft-tissue tumor, should suggest the diagnosis of synovial cell sarcoma. The CT scan demonstrates a soft-tissue mass, with calcified densities deep within the tumor. Although the small foci of calcification or mineralization are not seen as well with MRI as with CT scan, MRI is preferred to CT scan as the staging test.

The characteristic translocation t(X;18;p11;q11) creates a gene fusion SYT-SSX1 or SSX2. Patients with SSX2 seem to have a better prognosis at least in a small series of patients. At a histologic level, synovial sarcoma can be monophasic with epithelial or spindled cells (more often SSX2); or biphasic with epithelial and glandular-like differentiation (predominately SSX1) (100). Usually, the spindle cell component predominates (Fig. 13-47). Synovial sarcoma is almost always a high-grade STS.

Surgical resection has been and continues to be the principal treatment for synovial sarcoma. Adjuvant chemotherapy is used, but the data regarding its efficacy in synovial sarcoma are equivocal at best. In adults and older children with synovial sarcoma, as in those with other STSs, radiotherapy is considered in conjunction with nonradical surgery in an attempt to salvage the extremities. It used to be thought that the scarring from irradiation precluded its use in the feet and hands but, but with modern techniques, adjuvant irradiation and marginal resection can be performed in most sarcomas of the feet or hands, with preservation of the functioning of the extremity. Radiation may improve local control, but the impact in overall survival is questionable (86, 270, 271).

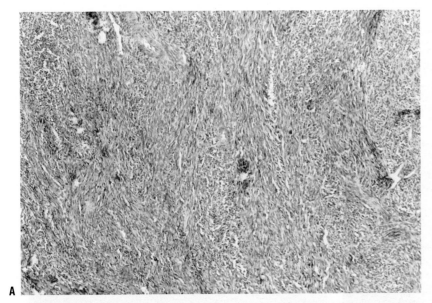

A

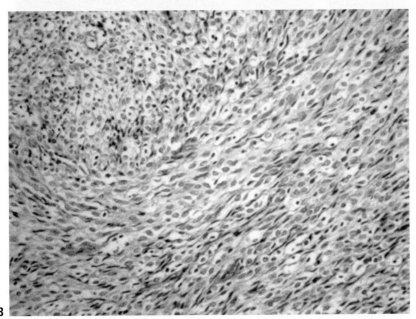

B

FIGURE 13-46. A: Low-power view of the spindle component of a synovial sarcoma. This lesion is composed of malignant spindle cells with a minimal amount of matrix. At a higher power, mitotic figures are seen. Other areas of this tumor have a glandular appearance, which is why synovial sarcoma is a biphasic tumor (original magnification ×10). **B:** Synovial sarcoma does not arise from within joints. It may be monophasic to biphasic. This is a monophasic synovial sarcoma. It is composed of fibrous stroma cells with minimal matrix formation. As can be seen in this image, the direction of the fibers is often at right angles, so that there are areas where the fibers run horizontally (**center**) and other areas where the fibers run vertically (**lower right**) (original magnification ×40).

In a large study including only young patients, the overall survival among 219 patients at 5 years was 80% ± 3% and disease free-survival 72% ± 3%; the incidence of local recurrence 14% at an average 1.3 years, and 42% developed distant recurrence. Among the identified prognostic factors were invasiveness, Intergroup Rhabdomyosarcoma Study (IRS) group, age, metastasis at presentation, margins, and size (272, 273).

Infantile Fibrosarcoma. Congenital or infantile fibrosarcoma (IFS) is the most common STS in children below 1 year of age. It is different than the adult countertype (fibrosarcoma) in that it has a more benign course and very low metastatic potential (approximately 10%) (272–274).

Although wide resection is preferred, due to the relative low risk of metastatic dissemination and the usual young age at presentation, IFS may be treated by a "conservative" surgical

management and positive margins may be accepted (95). Late recurrence does not seem to affect survival and there are few reports of spontaneous regression of incompletely excised IFS (95, 272, 273). It is still unclear how effective chemotherapy is; however, it is usually used for large and unresectable lesions (275).

Malignant Peripheral Nerve Sheath Tumor. Malignant peripheral nerve sheath tumor (MPNST) is a malignant nerve tumor that may arise *de novo* or from a neurofibroma; they do not arise from schwannomas. MPNSTs have previously been called neurofibrosarcoma. They represent approximately 5% to 10% of all NRSTS in children, and may occur sporadically (50% to 80%), or in association to neurofibromatosis type 1 (NF-1) (20% to 50%). Interestingly, only 2% to 13% of children with NF-1 will develop MPNST (104).

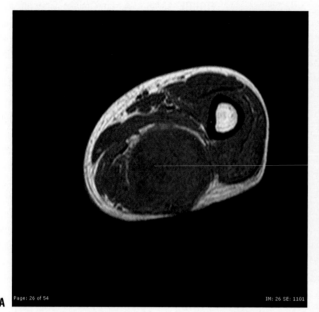
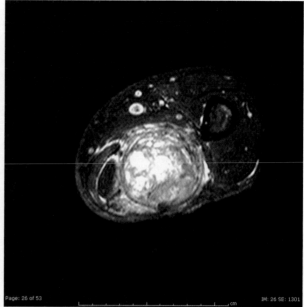

FIGURE 13-47. MPNST; An 18-year-old male with NF-1 and a rapidly growing mass. T1- **(A)** and T2-weighted **(B)** MRI shows the large mass within the sciatic nerve. The gross specimen is shown **(C)**. (Reproduced with permission from The Children's Orthopaedic Center, Los Angeles, CA.)

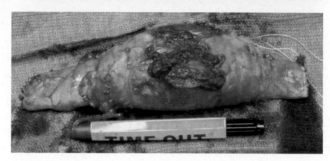

MPNSTs may also develop at the site of prior radiation. The clinical presentation is one of a slow-growing mass, initially painless but that usually becomes painful as it grows. The tumor usually arises from small peripheral nerves, but at times major nerves can be involved (Fig. 13-47).

Local control of MPNST is best achieved by surgery; chemotherapy is often used for systemic control and radiation can be used both pre- and postoperatively, especially for positive margins. A large study including 167 patients with MPNST showed that NF-1 was present in 17%, there was a good response to chemotherapy in 45%, radiation decreased local recurrence and IRS staging correlated with survival, 82% and 26% at 5 years for IRS I and IRS V, respectively (104, 275, 276). Among the poor prognostic factors are early age at diagnosis, NF-1 positive, large and high-grade tumors.

REFERENCES

1. Rosen G, et al. Chemotherapy, en bloc resection, and prosthetic bone replacement in the treatment of osteogenic sarcoma. *Cancer* 1976; 37(1):1–11.
2. Ferrari S, Palmerini E. Adjuvant and neoadjuvant combination chemotherapy for osteogenic sarcoma. *Curr Opin Oncol* 2007;19(4):341–346.
3. Rosen G, et al. Primary osteogenic sarcoma: the rationale for preoperative chemotherapy and delayed surgery. *Cancer* 1979;43(6):2163–2177.
4. Krishnan B, Khanna G, Clohisy D. Gene translocations in musculoskeletal neoplasms. *Clin Orthop Relat Res* 2008;466(9):2131–2146.
5. Tang, N, et al. Osteosarcoma development and stem cell differentiation. *Clin Orthop Relat Res* 2008;466(9):2114–2130.
6. Bridge JA, et al. Cytogenetic findings in 73 osteosarcoma specimens and a review of the literature. *Cancer Genet Cytogenet* 1997;95(1):74–87.
7. Fletcher J, Kozakewich H, Hoffer F. Diagnostic relevance of clonal cytogenetic aberrations in malignant soft-tissue tumors. *N Engl J Med* 1991;324:436.
8. Triche TJ. Molecular biological aspects of soft tissue tumors. *Curr Top Pathol* 1995;89:47–72.
9. Berkova A, et al. A comparison of RT-PCR and FISH techniques in molecular diagnosis of Ewing's sarcoma in paraffin-embedded tissue. *Cesk Patol* 2008;44(3):67–70.
10. Barr FG, et al. Molecular assays for chromosomal translocations in the diagnosis of pediatric soft tissue sarcomas. *JAMA* 1995;273(7):553–557.
11. Trische T, Sorensen P. Molecular pathology of pediatric malignancies. In: Pizzo PA, Poplack DG, eds. *Principles and practice of pediatric oncology.* Philadelphia, PA: Lippincott Williams & Wilkins, 2002:161–204.
12. Look A, Kirsch I. Molecular basis for childhood cancer. In: Pizzo PA, Poplack DG, eds. *Principles and practice of pediatric oncology.* Philadelphia, PA: Lippincott Williams & Wilkins, 2002:45–88.
13. Navarro S, et al. Comparison of Ewing's sarcoma of bone and peripheral neuroepithelioma. An immunocytochemical and ultrastructural analysis of two primitive neuroectodermal neoplasms. *Arch Pathol Lab Med* 1994;118(6):608–615.

14. de Alava E, et al. EWS-FLI1 fusion transcript structure is an independent determinant of prognosis in Ewing's sarcoma. *J Clin Oncol* 1998; 16(4):1248–1255.

15. Riley RD, et al. A systematic review of molecular and biological markers in tumours of the Ewing's sarcoma family. *Eur J Cancer* 2003;39(1): 19–30.

16. West D, Grier H, Swallow M. Detection of circulating tumor cells in patients with Ewing's sarcoma and peripheral primitive neuroectodermal tumor. *J Clin Oncol* 1997;15:583.

17. Avigad S. The predictive potential of molecular detection in the nonmetastatic Ewing family of tumors. *Cancer* 2004;100(5):1053–1058.

18. Gebhardt M. Molecular biology of sarcomas. *Orthop Clin N Am* 1996; 27:421.

19. Hansen M. Molecular genetic considerations in osteosarcoma. *Clin Orthop* 1991;270:237.

20. Varmus J, Weinberg R. *Genes and the biology of cancer*. New York, NY: Scientific American Library, 1993:67.

21. Gorlick, R, Huvos A, Heller G. Expression of HER2/erbB-2 correlates with survival in osteosarcoma. *J Clin Oncol* 1999;17(9):2781–2788.

22. Scotlandi K, et al. Prognostic and therapeutic relevance of HER2 expression in osteosarcoma and Ewing's sarcoma. *Eur J Cancer* 2005;41(9): 1349–1361.

23. Thomas DG, et al. Absence of HER2/neu gene expression in osteosarcoma and skeletal Ewing's sarcoma. *Clin Cancer Res* 2002;8(3):788–793.

24. Tsai JY, et al. HER-2/neu and p53 in osteosarcoma: an immunohistochemical and fluorescence in situ hybridization analysis. *Cancer Invest* 2004;22(1):16–24.

25. Weinberg RA. Tumor suppressor genes. *Science* 1991;254(5035):1138–1146.

26. Hinds PW, Weinberg RA. Tumor suppressor genes. *Curr Opin Genet Dev* 1994;4(1):135–141.

27. Friend S, Bernards R, Rogelj S. A human DNA segment with properties of the gene that predisposes to retinoblastoma and osteosarcoma. *Nature* 1986;323:643.

28. Hung J, Anderson R. p53: functions, mutations and sarcomas. *Acta Orthop Scand Suppl* 1997;273:68.

29. Lane D. Cancer: p53, guardian of the genome. *Nature* 1992;358:15.

30. Miller C, Koeffler H. p53 mutations in human cancer. *Leukemia* 1993; 7:S18.

31. Link M, Eilber F, Osteosarcoma. In: Pizzo P, Poplack DG, eds. *Principles and practice of pediatric oncology*. Philadelphia, PA: Lippincott Williams & Wilkins, 2002:1051.

32. Ding H, Fisher D. Mechanisms of p53-mediated apoptosis. *Crit Rev Oncol* 1998;9:83.

33. Fisher D. Apoptosis in cancer therapy: crossing the threshold. *Cell* 1994; 78:539.

34. Lowe S, Bodis S, Bardeesy N. Apoptosis and the prognostic significance of p53 mutation. *Cold Spring Harb Symp Quant Biol* 1994;59:419.

35. Ueda Y, et al. Analysis of mutant P53 protein in osteosarcomas and other malignant and benign lesions of bone. *J Cancer Res Clin Oncol* 1993;119(3):172–178.

36. Wadayama B, et al. p53 expression and its relationship to DNA alterations in bone and soft tissue sarcomas. *Br J Cancer* 1993;68(6):1134–1139.

37. Lonardo F, et al. p53 and MDM2 alterations in osteosarcomas: correlation with clinicopathologic features and proliferative rate. *Cancer* 1997;79(8):1541–1547.

38. Abudu A, Mangham D, Reynolds G. Overexpression of p53 protein in primary Ewing's sarcoma of bone: relationship to tumour stage, response and prognosis. *Br J Cancer* 1999;79:1185.

39. Yamaguchi T, Toguchida J, Yamamuro T. Allelotype analysis in osteosarcomas: frequent allele loss on 3q, 13q, 17p, and 18q. *Cancer Res* 1992;52:2419.

40. Chan H, Grogan T, DeBoer G. Diagnosis and reversal of multidrug resistance in paediatric cancers. *Eur J Cancer* 1996;32A:1051.

41. Chan H, Grogan T, Haddad G. P-glycoprotein expression: critical determinant in the response to osteosarcoma chemotherapy. *J Natl Cancer Inst* 1997;89:1706.

42. Cordon-Cardo C, Latres E, Drobnjak M, et al. Molecular abnormalities 8 mdm2 and p53 genes in adult soft tissue sarcomas. *Cancer Res* 1994;54(3):794–799.

43. Carbone M, Rizzo P, Procopio A. SV40-like sequences in human bone tumors. *Oncogene* 1996;13(3):527–535.

44. Li FP, Fraumeni JF Jr. Prospective study of a family cancer syndrome. *JAMA* 1982;247(19):2692–2694.

45. Malkin D, et al. Germ line p53 mutations in a familial syndrome of breast cancer, sarcomas, and other neoplasms. *Science* 1990;250(4985):1233–1238.

46. Diller L, et al. Germline p53 mutations are frequently detected in young children with rhabdomyosarcoma. *J Clin Invest* 1995;95(4):1606–1611.

47. McIntyre J, Smith-Sorensen B, Friend S. Germline mutations of the p53 tumor suppressor gene in children with osteosarcoma. *J Clin Oncol* 1994;12:925.

48. Kuttesch JF Jr. Multidrug resistance in pediatric oncology. *Invest New Drugs* 1996;14(1):55–67.

49. Chan HS, et al. Multidrug drug resistance in pediatric sarcomas. *Hematol Oncol Clin North Am* 1995;9(4):889–908.

50. Abudu A, et al. The surgical treatment and outcome of pathological fractures in localised osteosarcoma. *J Bone Joint Surg Br* 1996;78(5):694–698.

51. Stein U, Wunderlich V, Haensch W. Expression of the mdr1 gene in bone and soft tissue sarcomas of adult patients. *Eur J Cancer* 1993;29A:1979.

52. Scotlandi K, et al. Multidrug resistance and malignancy in human osteosarcoma. *Cancer Res* 1996;56(10):2434–2439.

53. Serra M, Scotlandi K, Manara M. Analysis of P-glycoprotein expression in osteosarcoma. *Eur J Cancer* 1995;31A:1998.

54. Baldini N, Scotlandi K, Barbanti-Brodano G. Expression of P-glycoprotein in high-grade osteosarcomas in relation to clinical outcome. *N Engl J Med* 1995;333:1380.

55. Wunder J. MDR1 gene expression and outcome in osteosarcoma: a prospective, multicenter study. *J Clin Oncol* 2000;18(14):2685–2694.

56. Fong Y, et al. Lymph node metastasis from soft tissue sarcoma in adults. Analysis of data from a prospective database of 1772 sarcoma patients. *Ann Surg* 1993;217(1):72–77.

57. Enneking W. *Musculoskeletal tumor surgery*. New York, NY: Churchill Livingstone, 1983.

58. Bacci G, Dallari D, Battistini A. The prognostic value of serum alkaline phosphatase in osteosarcoma of the limbs. *Chir Organi Mov* 1992;77:171.

59. Leavey PJ, et al. Prognostic factors for patients with Ewing sarcoma (EWS) at first recurrence following multi-modality therapy: a report from the Children's Oncology Group. *Pediatr Blood Cancer* 2008;51(3):334–338.

60. Bacci G, et al. Prognostic factors in non-metastatic Ewing's sarcoma tumor of bone: an analysis of 579 patients treated at a single institution with adjuvant or neoadjuvant chemotherapy between 1972 and 1998. *Acta Oncol* 2006;45(4):469–475.

61. Arkader A, et al. Primary musculoskeletal Langerhans cell histiocytosis in children: an analysis for a 3-decade period. *J Pediatr Orthop* 2009;29(2):201–207.

62. Goo HW, et al. Whole-body MRI of Langerhans cell histiocytosis: comparison with radiography and bone scintigraphy. *Pediatr Radiol* 2006;36(10):1019–1031.

63. Leskinen S, Lapela M, Lindholm P. Metabolic imaging by positron emission tomography in oncology. *Ann Med* 1997;29:271.

64. Becherer A, Jaeger U, Szabo M. Prognostic value of FDG-PET in malignant lymphoma. *Q J Nucl Med* 2003;47:14–21.

65. Friedberg S, Chengazi V. Pet scans in the staging of lymphoma: current status. *Oncologist* 2003;8:438–447.

66. Frush DP, Donnelly LF, Rosen NS. Computed tomography and radiation risks: what pediatric health care providers should know. *Pediatrics* 2003;112(4):951–957.

67. Wunder JS, et al. A comparison of staging systems for localized extremity soft tissue sarcoma. *Cancer* 2000;88(12):2721–2730.

68. AJCC. *AJCC cancer staging manual*, 6th ed. New York, NY: Springer, 2002.

69. Enneking WF, Spanier SS, Goodman MA. A system for the surgical staging of musculoskeletal sarcoma. *Clin Orthop Relat Res* 1980;153:106–120.

70. Mankin HJ, Mankin CJ, Simon MA. The hazards of the biopsy, revisited. Members of the Musculoskeletal Tumor Society. *J Bone Joint Surg Am* 1996;78(5):656–663.
71. Heslin MJ, et al. Core needle biopsy for diagnosis of extremity soft tissue sarcoma. *Ann Surg Oncol* 1997;4(5):425–431.
72. Bickels J, et al. Biopsy of musculoskeletal tumors. Current concepts. *Clin Orthop Relat Res* 1999;368:212–219.
73. Unni K. *Dahlin's bone tumors: general aspects and data on 11,087 cases.* Philadelphia, PA: Lippincott-Raven, 1996:143.
74. McLeod R, Beabout J. The roentgenographic features of chondroblastoma. *AJR Am J Roentgenol* 1973;118:464.
75. Frassica FJ, et al. Clinicopathologic features and treatment of osteoid osteoma and osteoblastoma in children and adolescents. *Orthop Clin North Am* 1996;27(3):559–574.
76. Keim H, Reina E. Osteoid-osteoma as a cause of scoliosis. *J Bone Joint Surg Am* 1975;57:159.
77. Pettine KA, Klassen RA. Osteoid-osteoma and osteoblastoma of the spine. *J Bone Joint Surg Am* 1986;68(3):354–361.
78. Smith F, Gilday D. Scintigraphic appearances of osteoid osteoma. *Radiology* 1980;137:191.
79. Hosalkar HS, et al. The diagnostic accuracy of MRI versus CT imaging for osteoid osteoma in children. *Clin Orthop Relat Res* 2005;433:171–177.
80. Kneisl J, Simon M. Medical management compared with operative treatment for osteoid-osteoma. *J Bone Joint Surg Am* 1992;74:179.
81. Donkol RH, Al-Nammi A, Moghazi K. Efficacy of percutaneous radiofrequency ablation of osteoid osteoma in children. *Pediatr Radiol* 2008;38(2):180–185.
82. Arkader A, Dormans JP. Osteoblastoma in the skeletally immature. *J Pediatr Orthop* 2008;28(5):555–560.
83. Kroon HM, Schurmans J. Osteoblastoma: clinical and radiologic findings in 98 new cases. *Radiology* 1990;175(3):783–790.
84. Lucas DR, et al. Osteoblastoma: clinicopathologic study of 306 cases. *Hum Pathol* 1994;25(2):117–134.
85. Schajowicz F, Lemos C. Malignant osteoblastoma. *J Bone Joint Surg Br* 1976;58(2):202–211.
86. Lewis JJ, et al. Synovial sarcoma: a multivariate analysis of prognostic factors in 112 patients with primary localized tumors of the extremity. *J Clin Oncol* 2000;18(10):2087–2094.
87. Hudson T. *Radiographic pathologic correlation of musculoskeletal lesions.* Baltimore, MD: Williams & Wilkins, 1987.
88. Schmale GA, Conrad EU III, Raskind WH. The natural history of hereditary multiple exostoses. *J Bone Joint Surg Am* 1994;76(7):986–992.
89. Solomon L. Hereditary multiple exostosis. *J Bone Joint Surg Am* 1963;45:292.
90. Jaffe H. Hereditary multiple exostosis. *Arch Pathol* 1943;36:335.
91. Shapiro F, Simon S, Glimcher M. Hereditary multiple exostoses: anthropometric, roentgenographic, and clinical aspects. *J Bone Joint Surg Am* 1979;61:815.
92. Schmale G, Conrad E, Raskind W. The natural history of hereditary multiple exostoses. *J Bone Joint Surg Am* 1994;76:986.
93. Peterson H. Multiple hereditary osteochondromata. *Clin Orthop* 1989;239:222.
94. Glotzbecker MP, et al. Langerhans cell histiocytosis and human herpes virus 6 (HHV-6), an analysis by real-time polymerase chain reaction. *J Orthop Res* 2006;24(3):313–320.
95. Loh ML, et al. Treatment of infantile fibrosarcoma with chemotherapy and surgery: results from the Dana-Farber Cancer Institute and Children's Hospital, Boston. *J Pediatr Hematol Oncol* 2002;24(9):722–726.
96. Huvos AG, Marcove RC. Chondrosarcoma in the young. A clinicopathologic analysis of 79 patients younger than 21 years of age. *Am J Surg Pathol* 1987;11(12):930–942.
97. Young CL, et al. Chondrosarcoma of bone in children. *Cancer* 1990;66(7):1641–1648.
98. Ladanyi M, et al. Impact of SYT-SSX fusion type on the clinical behavior of synovial sarcoma: a multi-institutional retrospective study of 243 patients. *Cancer Res* 2002;62(1):135–140.
99. Green P, Whittaker R. Benign chondroblastoma: case report with pulmonary metastasis. *J Bone Joint Surg Am* 1975;57:418.
100. Wolden SL. Radiation therapy for non-rhabdomyosarcoma soft tissue sarcomas in adolescents and young adults. *J Pediatr Hematol Oncol* 2005;27(4):212–214.
101. Geirnaerdt MJ, et al. Usefulness of radiography in differentiating enchondroma from central grade 1 chondrosarcoma. *AJR Am J Roentgenol* 1997;169(4):1097–1104.
102. Geirnaerdt MJ, et al. Cartilaginous tumors: correlation of gadolinium-enhanced MR imaging and histopathologic findings. *Radiology* 1993;186(3):813–817.
103. Geirnaerdt MJ, et al. Cartilaginous tumors: fast contrast-enhanced MR imaging. *Radiology* 2000;214(2):539–546.
104. Carli M, et al. Pediatric malignant peripheral nerve sheath tumor: the Italian and German soft tissue sarcoma cooperative group. *J Clin Oncol* 2005;23(33):8422–8430.
105. Schwartz H, Zimmerman N, Simon M. The malignant potential of enchondromatosis. *J Bone Joint Surg Am* 1987;69:269.
106. Cannon S, Sweetnam D. Multiple chondrosarcomas in dyschondroplasia (Ollier's disease). *Cancer* 1985;55:836.
107. Schwartz HS, et al. The malignant potential of enchondromatosis. *J Bone Joint Surg Am* 1987;69(2):269–274.
108. Bean W. Dyschondroplasia and hemangiomata (Maffucci's syndrome). *Arch Intern Med* 1955;95:767.
109. Lewis R, Ketcham A. Maffucci's syndrome: functional and neoplastic significance. Case report and review of the literature. *J Bone Joint Surg Am* 1973;55:1465.
110. Codman E. Epiphyseal chondromatous giant cell tumor of the upper end of the humerus. *Surg Gynecol Obstet* 1931;52:543.
111. Lin PP, et al. Treatment and prognosis of chondroblastoma. *Clin Orthop Relat Res* 2005;438:103–109.
112. Gardner D, Azouz E. Solitary lucent epiphyseal lesions in children. *Skeletal Radiol* 1988;17:497.
113. Springfield D, Capanna R, Gherlinzoni F. Chondrobla-stoma: a review of seventy cases. *J Bone Joint Surg Am* 1985;67:748.
114. Huvos A, Marcove R. Chondroblastoma of bone: a critical review. *Clin Orthop* 1973;95:300.
115. Snyder BD, et al. Predicting fracture through benign skeletal lesions with quantitative computed tomography. *J Bone Joint Surg Am* 2006;88(1):55–70.
116. Bertoni F, Bacchini P. Classification of bone tumors. *Eur J Radiol* 1998;27:S74.
117. Bauer TW, Dorfman HD, Latham JT Jr. Periosteal chondroma. A clinicopathologic study of 23 cases. *Am J Surg Pathol* 1982;6(7):631–637.
118. Boriani S, Bacchini P, Bertoni F. Periosteal chondroma: a review of twenty cases. *J Bone Joint Surg Am* 1983;65:205.
119. Easley M, Kneisl J. Pathologic fractures through nonossifying fibromas: is prophylactic treatment warranted? *J Pediatr Orthop* 1997;17:808.
120. Peterson H, Fitzgerald E. Fractures through nonossifying fibromata in children. *Minn Med* 1980;63:139.
121. Arata M, Peterson H, Dahlin D. Pathological fractures through nonossifying fibromas: review of the Mayo Clinic experience. *J Bone Joint Surg Am* 1981;63:980.
122. Caffey J. On fibrous defects in cortical walls of growing tubular bones. In: Levine S, ed. *Advances in pediatrics.* Vol. 7, Chicago, IL: Year Book, 1955:13.
123. Friedland J, Reinus W, Fisher A. Quantitative analysis of the plain radiographic appearance of nonossifying fibroma. *Invest Radiol* 1995;30:474.
124. Bullough P, Walley J. Fibrous cortical defect and non-ossifying fibroma. *Postgrad Med J* 1965;41:672.
125. DiCaprio MR, Enneking WF. Fibrous dysplasia. Pathophysiology, evaluation, and treatment. *J Bone Joint Surg Am* 2005;87(8):1848–1864.
126. Ippolito E, et al. Natural history and treatment of fibrous dysplasia of bone: a multicenter clinicopathologic study promoted by the European Pediatric Orthopaedic Society. *J Pediatr Orthop B* 2003;12(3):155–177.
127. Lee PA, Van Dop C, Migeon CJ. McCune-Albright syndrome. Long-term follow-up. *JAMA* 1986;256(21):2980–2984.

128. Albright F, Butler A, Hampton A. Syndrome characterized by osteitis fibrosa disseminata, area of pigmentation and endocrine dysfunction, with precocious puberty in females. *N Engl J Med* 1937;216:727.

129. Enneking W, Gearen P. Fibrous dysplasia of the femoral neck: treatment by cortical bone-grafting. *J Bone Joint Surg Am* 1986;68:1415.

130. Lala R, et al. Bisphosphonate treatment of bone fibrous dysplasia in McCune-Albright syndrome. *J Pediatr Endocrinol Metab* 2006;19(Suppl 2): 583–593.

131. Plotkin H, et al. Effect of pamidronate treatment in children with polyostotic fibrous dysplasia of bone. *J Clin Endocrinol Metab* 2003; 88(10):4569–4575.

132. Kamineni S, et al. Osteofibrous dysplasia of the ulna. *J Bone Joint Surg Br* 2001;83(8):1178–1180.

133. Gleason BC, et al. Osteofibrous dysplasia and adamantinoma in children and adolescents: a clinicopathologic reappraisal. *Am J Surg Pathol* 2008;32(3):363–376.

134. Maki M, Athanasou N. Osteofibrous dysplasia and adamantinoma: correlation of proto-oncogene product and matrix protein expression. *Hum Pathol* 2004;35(1):69–74.

135. Springfield DS, et al. Relationship between osteofibrous dysplasia and adamantinoma. *Clin Orthop Relat Res* 1994;309:234–244.

136. Schajowicz F, Santini-Araujo E. Adamantinoma of the tibia masked by fibrous dysplasia: report of three cases. *Clin Orthop* 1989;238:294.

137. Hazelbag H, Taminiau A, Fleuren G. Adamantinoma of the long bones: a clinicopathological study of thirty-two patients with emphasis on histological subtype, precursor lesion, and biological behavior. *J Bone Joint Surg Am* 1994;76:1482.

138. Springfield D, Rosenberg A, Mankin H. Relationship between osteofibrous dysplasia and adamantinoma. *Clin Orthop* 1994;309:234.

139. Meyer JS, et al. Langerhans cell histiocytosis: presentation and evolution of radiologic findings with clinical correlation. *Radiographics* 1995;15(5):1135–1146.

140. Howarth DM, et al. Langerhans cell histiocytosis: diagnosis, natural history, management, and outcome. *Cancer* 1999;85(10):2278–2290.

141. Ghanem I, et al. Langerhans cell histiocytosis of bone in children and adolescents. *J Pediatr Orthop* 2003;23(1):124–130.

142. Bhatia S, et al. Epidemiologic study of Langerhans cell histiocytosis in children. *J Pediatr* 1997;130(5):774–784.

143. Braier J, et al. Langerhans cell histiocytosis: retrospective evaluation of 123 patients at a single institution. *Pediatr Hematol Oncol* 1999;16(5):377–385.

144. Bank MI, et al. p53 expression in biopsies from children with Langerhans cell histiocytosis. *J Pediatr Hematol Oncol* 2002;24(9):733–736.

145. Glotzbecker MP, Carpentieri DF, Dormans JP. Langerhans cell histiocytosis: a primary viral infection of bone? Human herpes virus 6 latent protein detected in lymphocytes from tissue of children. *J Pediatr Orthop* 2004;24(1):123–129.

146. Kilpatrick S, Wenger D, Gilchrist G. Langerhans' cell histiocytosis (histiocytosis X) of bone: a clinicopathologic analysis of 263 pediatric and adult cases. *Cancer* 1995;76:2471.

147. Sessa S, Sommelet D, Lascombes P. Treatment of Langerhans-cell histiocytosis in children: experience at the Children's Hospital of Nancy. *J Bone Joint Surg Am* 1994;76:1513.

148. Oppenheim W, Galleno H. Operative treatment versus steroid injection in the management of unicameral bone cysts. *J Pediatr Orthop* 1984;4:1.

149. Scaglietti O, Marchetti P, Bartolozzi P. Final results obtained in the treatment of bone cysts with methylprednisolone acetate (Depo-Medrol) and a discussion of results achieved in other bone lesions. *Clin Orthop* 1982;165:33.

150. Kilpatrick SE, et al. Langerhans' cell histiocytosis (histiocytosis X) of bone. A clinicopathologic analysis of 263 pediatric and adult cases. *Cancer* 1995;76(12):2471–2484.

151. Garg S, Mehta S, Dormans JP. Langerhans cell histiocytosis of the spine in children. Long-term follow-up. *J Bone Joint Surg Am* 2004;86-A(8):1740–1750.

152. Levine SE, et al. Langerhans' cell histiocytosis of the spine in children. *Clin Orthop* 1996;323:288–293.

153. Floman Y, et al. Eosinophilic granuloma of the spine. *J Pediatr Orthop B* 1997;6(4):260–265.

154. Raab P, et al. Vertebral remodeling in eosinophilic granuloma of the spine. A long-term follow-up. *Spine* 1998;23(12):1351–1354.

155. Ippolito E, Farsetti P, Tudisco C. Vertebra plana. Long-term follow-up in five patients. *J Bone Joint Surg Am* 1984;66(9):1364–1368.

156. Kamimura M, et al. Eosinophilic granuloma of the spine: early spontaneous disappearance of tumor detected on magnetic resonance imaging. Case report. *J Neurosurg Spine* 2000;93(2):312–316.

157. Kilborn TN, The J, Goodman TR. Paediatric manifestations of Langerhans cell histiocytosis: a review of the clinical and radiological findings. *Clin Radiol* 2003;58(4):269–278.

158. Leonidas JC, Guelfguat M, Valderrama E. Langerhans' cell histiocytosis. *Lancet* 2003;361(9365):1293–1295.

159. Broadbent V, Gadner H. Current therapy for Langerhans cell histiocytosis. *Hematol Oncol Clin North Am* 1998;12(2):327–338.

160. Gadner H, et al. A randomized trial of treatment for multisystem Langerhans' cell histiocytosis. *J Pediatr* 2001;138(5):728–734.

161. Greenberger JS, et al. Results of treatment of 127 patients with systemic histiocytosis. *Medicine (Baltimore)* 1981;60(5):311–338.

162. Greis PE, Hankin FM. Eosinophilic granuloma. The management of solitary lesions of bone. *Clin Orthop* 1990;257:204–211.

163. Minkov M, Whitlock J. *The Importance of Clinical Trials in the Fight Against Histiocytosis.* Pitman, NJ: Histiocytosis Association of America, 2004.

164. Altermatt S, Schwobel M, Pochon J. Operative treatment of solitary bone cysts with tricalcium phosphate ceramic: a 1 to 7 year follow-up. *Ear J Pediatr Surg* 1992;2:180.

165. Peltier L, Jones R. Treatment of unicameral bone cysts by curettage and packing with plaster-of-Paris pellets. *J Bone Joint Surg Am* 1978;60:820.

166. Martinez V, Sissons H. Aneurysmal bone cyst: a review of 123 cases including primary lesions and those secondary to other bone pathology. *Cancer* 1988;61:2291.

167. Hecht A, Gebhardt M. Diagnosis and treatment of unicameral and aneurysmal bone cysts in children. *Curr Opin Pediatr* 1998;10:87.

168. Capanna R, Campanacci D, Manfrini M. Unicameral and aneurysmal bone cysts. *Orthop Clin North Am* 1996;27:605.

169. Chang CH, Stanton RP, Glutting J. Unicameral bone cysts treated by injection of bone marrow or methylprednisolone. *J Bone Joint Surg Br* 2002;84(3):407–412.

170. Cho HS, et al. Unicameral bone cysts: a comparison of injection of steroid and grafting with autologous bone marrow. *J Bone Joint Surg Br* 2007;89(2):222–226.

171. de Sanctis N, Andreacchio A. Elastic stable intramedullary nailing is the best treatment of unicameral bone cysts of the long bones in children? Prospective long-term follow-up study. *J Pediatr Orthop* 2006; 26(4):520–525.

172. Roposch A, Saraph V, Linhart WE. Flexible intramedullary nailing for the treatment of unicameral bone cysts in long bones. *J Bone Joint Surg Am* 2000;82-A(10):1447–1453.

173. Dormans JP, et al. Percutaneous intramedullary decompression, curettage, and grafting with medical-grade calcium sulfate pellets for unicameral bone cysts in children: a new minimally invasive technique. *J Pediatr Orthop* 2005;25(6):804–811.

174. Oliveira AM, et al. USP6 and CDH11 oncogenes identify the neoplastic cell in primary aneurysmal bone cysts and are absent in so-called secondary aneurysmal bone cysts. *Am J Pathol* 2004;165(5):1773–1780.

175. Garg S, Mehta S, Dormans JP. Modern surgical treatment of primary aneurysmal bone cyst of the spine in children and adolescents. *J Pediatr Orthop* 2005;25(3):387–392.

176. Mankin HJ, et al. Aneurysmal bone cyst: a review of 150 patients. *J Clin Oncol* 2005;23(27):6756–6762.

177. Dormans JP, et al. Surgical treatment and recurrence rate of aneurysmal bone cysts in children. *Clin Orthop Relat Res* 2004;421:205–211.

178. Torpey BM, Dormans JP, Drummond DS. The use of MRI-compatible titanium segmental spinal instrumentation in pediatric patients with intraspinal tumor. *J Spinal Disord* 1995;8(1):76–81.

179. Meller I, et al. Fifteen years of bone tumor cryosurgery: a single-center experience of 440 procedures and long-term follow-up. *Eur J Surg Oncol* 2008;34(8):921–927.

180. Blakely ML, et al. The impact of margin of resection on outcome in pediatric nonrhabdomyosarcoma soft tissue sarcoma. *J Pediatr Surg* 1999;34(5):672–675.

181. Futani H, et al. Long-term follow-up after limb salvage in skeletally immature children with a primary malignant tumor of the distal end of the femur. *J Bone Joint Surg Am* 2006;88(3):595–603.

182. Gherlinzoni F, et al. Limb sparing versus amputation in osteosarcoma. Correlation between local control, surgical margins and tumor necrosis: Istituto Rizzoli experience. *Ann Oncol* 1992;3(Suppl 2):S23–S27.

183. Springfield DS, et al. Surgical treatment for osteosarcoma. *J Bone Joint Surg Am* 1988;70(8):1124–1130.

184. Kawai A, et al. Interrelationships of clinical outcome, length of resection, and energy cost of walking after prosthetic knee replacement following resection of a malignant tumor of the distal aspect of the femur. *J Bone Joint Surg Am* 1998;80(6):822–831.

185. Frances JM, et al. What is quality of life in children with bone sarcoma? *Clin Orthop Relat Res* 2007;459:34–39.

186. Brooks AD, et al. Resection of the sciatic, peroneal, or tibial nerves: assessment of functional status. *Ann Surg Oncol* 2002;9(1):41–47.

187. Arkader A, et al. Coaxial extendible knee equalizes limb length in children with osteogenic sarcoma. *Clin Orthop Relat Res* 2007;459:60–65.

188. Bacci G, et al. Prognostic factors for osteosarcoma of the extremity treated with neoadjuvant chemotherapy: 15-year experience in 789 patients treated at a single institution. *Cancer* 2006;106(5):1154–1161.

189. Kawai A, et al. A rotating-hinge knee replacement for malignant tumors of the femur and tibia. *J Arthroplasty* 1999;14(2):187–196.

190. Jacobs P. Limb salvage and rotationplasty for osteosarcoma in children. *Clin Orthop* 1984;188:217.

191. Bacci G, et al. Nonmetastatic osteosarcoma of the extremity with pathologic fracture at presentation: local and systemic control by amputation or limb salvage after preoperative chemotherapy. *Acta Orthop Scand* 2003;74(4):449–454.

192. Unwin PS, Walker PS. Extendible endoprostheses for the skeletally immature. *Clin Orthop Relat Res* 1996;322:179–193.

193. Baumgart R, et al. The bioexpandable prosthesis: a new perspective after resection of malignant bone tumors in children. *J Pediatr Hematol Oncol* 2005;27(8):452–455.

194. Eckardt JJ, et al. Expandable endoprosthesis reconstruction in skeletally immature patients with tumors. *Clin Orthop Relat Res* 2000;373:51–61.

195. Cannon CP, Paraliticci GU, Lin PP, et al. Functional outcome following endoprosthetic reconstruction of the proximal humerus. *J Shoulder Elbow Surg* 2009;18:705–710.

196. Potter BK, et al. Proximal humerus reconstructions for tumors. *Clin Orthop Relat Res* 2009;467(4):1035–1041.

197. Alman BA, De Bari A, Krajbich JI. Massive allografts in the treatment of osteosarcoma and Ewing sarcoma in children and adolescents. *J Bone Joint Surg Am* 1995;77(1):54–64.

198. Mankin HJ, et al. Long-term results of allograft replacement in the management of bone tumors. *Clin Orthop Relat Res* 1996;324:86–97.

199. Mankin HJ, Hornicek FJ, Raskin KA. Infection in massive bone allografts. *Clin Orthop Relat Res* 2005;432:210–216.

200. Meyers PA, et al. Chemotherapy for nonmetastatic osteogenic sarcoma: the Memorial Sloan-Kettering experience. *J Clin Oncol* 1992;10(1):5–15.

201. Neel MD, et al. Early multicenter experience with a noninvasive expandable prosthesis. *Clin Orthop Relat Res* 2003;415:72–81.

202. Tillman RM, et al. Growing endoprostheses for primary malignant bone tumors. *Semin Surg Oncol* 1997;13(1):41–48.

203. Muscolo DL, MA Ayerza, Aponte-Tinao LA. Massive allograft use in orthopedic oncology. *Orthop Clin North Am* 2006;37(1):65–74.

204. Muscolo DL, et al. Intercalary femur and tibia segmental allografts provide an acceptable alternative in reconstructing tumor resections. *Clin Orthop Relat Res* 2004;426:97–102.

205. Muscolo DL, et al. Partial epiphyseal preservation and intercalary allograft reconstruction in high-grade metaphyseal osteosarcoma of the knee. *J Bone Joint Surg Am* 2005;87(Suppl 1, pt 2):226–236.

206. Gottsauner-Wolf F, et al. Rotationplasty for limb salvage in the treatment of malignant tumors at the knee. A follow-up study of seventy patients. *J Bone Joint Surg Am* 1991;73(9):1365–1375.

207. McClenaghan BA, et al. Comparative assessment of gait after limb-salvage procedures. *J Bone Joint Surg Am* 1989;71(8):1178–1182.

208. Picci P, Sangiorgi L, Rougraff B. Relationship of chemotherapy-induced necrosis and surgical margins to local recurrence in osteosarcoma. *J Clin Oncol* 1994;12:2699.

209. Meyers PA, et al. Osteogenic sarcoma with clinically detectable metastasis at initial presentation. *J Clin Oncol* 1993;11(3):449–453.

210. Bacci G, et al. Neoadjuvant chemotherapy for high-grade central osteosarcoma of the extremity. Histologic response to preoperative chemotherapy correlates with histologic subtype of the tumor. *Cancer* 2003;97(12):3068–3075.

211. Hauben EI, et al. Does the histological subtype of high-grade central osteosarcoma influence the response to treatment with chemotherapy and does it affect overall survival? A study on 570 patients of two consecutive trials of the European Osteosarcoma Intergroup. *Eur J Cancer* 2002;38(9):1218–1225.

212. Meyers PA, et al. Osteosarcoma: a randomized, prospective trial of the addition of ifosfamide and/or muramyl tripeptide to cisplatin, doxorubicin, and high-dose methotrexate. *J Clin Oncol* 2005;23(9):2004–2011.

213. Link MP, et al. The effect of adjuvant chemotherapy on relapse-free survival in patients with osteosarcoma of the extremity. *N Engl J Med* 1986;314(25):1600–1606.

214. Rosen G, et al. Preoperative chemotherapy for osteogenic sarcoma: selection of postoperative adjuvant chemotherapy based on the response of the primary tumor to preoperative chemotherapy. *Cancer* 1982;49(6):1221–1230.

215. Ferrari S, et al. Late relapse in osteosarcoma. *J Pediatr Hematol Oncol* 2006;28(7):418–422.

216. Winkler K, et al. Local control and survival from the Cooperative Osteosarcoma Study Group studies of the German Society of Pediatric Oncology and the Vienna Bone Tumor Registry. *Clin Orthop Relat Res* 1991;270:79–86.

217. Bramer JA, et al. Do pathological fractures influence survival and local recurrence rate in bony sarcomas? *Eur J Cancer* 2007;43(13):1944–1951.

218. Scully SP, et al. Pathologic fracture in osteosarcoma: prognostic importance and treatment implications. *J Bone Joint Surg Am* 2002;84-A(1):49–57.

219. Kaste SC, et al. Pediatric surface osteosarcoma: clinical, pathologic, and radiologic features. *Pediatr Blood Cancer* 2006;47(2):152–162.

220. Schwab JH, et al. A comparison of intramedullary and juxtacortical low-grade osteogenic sarcoma. *Clin Orthop Relat Res* 2008;466(6):1318–1322.

221. Delattre O, Zucman J, Melot T. The Ewing family of tumors: a subgroup of small-round-cell tumors defined by specific chimeric transcripts. *N Engl J Med* 1994;331:294.

222. Grier H. The Ewing family of tumors: Ewing's sarcoma and primitive neuroectodermal tumors. *Pediatr Clin North Am* 1997;44:991.

223. Meier V, Kuhne T, Jundt G. Molecular diagnosis of Ewing tumors: improved detection of EWS-FLI-1 and EWS-ERG chimeric transcripts and rapid determination of exon combinations. *Diagn Mol Pathol* 1998;7:29.

224. Pritchard D, Dahlin D, Dauphine R. Ewing's sarcoma: a clinicopathological and statistical analysis of patients surviving five years or longer. *J Bone Joint Surg Am* 1975;57:10.

225. Paulino AC, Nguyen TX, Mai WY. An analysis of primary site control and late effects according to local control modality in non-metastatic Ewing sarcoma. *Pediatr Blood Cancer* 2007;48(4):423–429.

226. Bacci G, et al. Role of surgery in local treatment of Ewing's sarcoma of the extremities in patients undergoing adjuvant and neoadjuvant chemotherapy. *Oncol Rep* 2004;11(1):111–120.

227. Dunst J, Jurgens H, Sauer R. Radiation therapy in Ewing's sarcoma: an update of the CESS 86 trial. *Int J Radiat Oncol Biol Phys* 1995;32:919.

228. Paulino AC. Late effects of radiotherapy for pediatric extremity sarcomas. *Int J Radiat Oncol Biol Phys* 2004;60(1):265–274.

229. Smith J, Yandow S. Benign soft-tissue lesions in children. *Orthop Clin North Am* 1996;27:645.

230. Pappo A, Pratt C. Soft tissue sarcomas in children. *Cancer Treat Res* 1997;91:205.

231. Meyer J, Dormans J. Differential diagnosis of pediatric musculoskeletal masses. *Magn Reson Imaging Clin N Am* 1998;6:561.

232. Weiss S, Goldblum J. *Enzinger and Weiss's Soft tissue tumors*, 5th ed. New York, NY: Mosby Elsevier, 2008.

233. Mulliken JB, Fishman SJ, Burrows PE. Vascular anomalies. *Curr Probl Surg* 2000;37(8):517–584.

234. Spiegel DA, et al. Aggressive fibromatosis from infancy to adolescence. *J Pediatr Orthop* 1999;19(6):776–784.

235. Enzinger F, Weiss S. *Soft tissue tumors*. New York, NY: CV Mosby, 1993.

236. Faulkner L, Hajdu S, Kher U. Pediatric desmoid tumor: retrospective analysis of 63 cases. *J Clin Oncol* 1995;13:2813.

237. Eich G, Hoeffel J, Tschappeler H. Fibrous tumours in children: imaging features of a heterogeneous group of disorders. *Pediatr Radiol* 1998;28:500.

238. Sundaram M, McGuire M, Herbold D. Magnetic resonance imaging of soft tissue masses: an evaluation of fifty-three histologically proven tumors. *Magn Reson Imaging* 1988;6:237.

239. Hajdu S. *Pathology of soft tissue tumors*. Philadelphia, PA: Lea & Febiger, 1979.

240. Buitendijk S, et al. Pediatric aggressive fibromatosis: a retrospective analysis of 13 patients and review of literature. *Cancer* 2005;104(5):1090–1099.

241. Skapek SX, et al. Vinblastine and methotrexate for desmoid fibromatosis in children: results of a Pediatric Oncology Group Phase II Trial. *J Clin Oncol* 2007;25(5):501–506.

242. Raney R. Chemotherapy for children with aggressive fibromatosis and Langerhans' cell histiocytosis. *Clin Orthop* 1991;262:58.

243. Weiss A, Lackman R. Low-dose chemotherapy of desmoid tumors. *Cancer* 1989;64:1192.

244. Kehoe NJ, Reid RP, Semple JC. Solitary benign peripheral-nerve tumours. Review of 32 years' experience. *J Bone Joint Surg Br* 1995;77(3):497–500.

245. Davis RI, Hamilton A, Biggart JD. Primary synovial chondromatosis: a clinicopathologic review and assessment of malignant potential. *Hum Pathol* 1998;29(7):683–688.

246. Tiedjen K, et al. Synovial osteochondromatosis in a 9-year-old girl: clinical and histopathological appearance. *Knee Surg Sports Traumatol Arthrosc* 2006;14(5):460–464.

247. Kramer J, et al. MR appearance of idiopathic synovial osteochondromatosis. *J Comput Assist Tomogr* 1993;17(5):772–776.

248. Shpitzer T, Ganel A, Engelberg S. Surgery for synovial chondromatosis: 26 cases followed up for 6 years. *Acta Orthop Scand* 1990;61:567.

249. Eckhardt BP, Hernandez RJ. Pigmented villonodular synovitis: MR imaging in pediatric patients. *Pediatr Radiol* 2004;34(12):943–947.

250. Dines JS, et al. Long-term follow-up of surgically treated localized pigmented villonodular synovitis of the knee. *Arthroscopy* 2007;23(9):930–937.

251. Chin KR, et al. Treatment of advanced primary and recurrent diffuse pigmented villonodular synovitis of the knee. *J Bone Joint Surg Am* 2002;84-A(12):2192–2202.

252. Steinbach L, Neumann C, Stoller D. MRI of the knee in diffuse pigmented villonodular synovitis. *Clin Imaging* 1989;13:305.

253. Flandry FC, et al. Surgical treatment of diffuse pigmented villonodular synovitis of the knee. *Clin Orthop Relat Res* 1994;300:183–192.

254. Layfield LJ, et al. Malignant giant cell tumor of synovium (malignant pigmented villonodular synovitis). *Arch Pathol Lab Med* 2000;124(11):1636–1641.

255. Kransdorf MJ. Malignant soft-tissue tumors in a large referral population: distribution of diagnoses by age, sex, and location. *AJR Am J Roentgenol* 1995;164(1):129–134.

256. Gurney JG, Young JL, Roffers SD. Soft tissue sarcomas. In: *Cancer Incidence and Survival Among Children and Adolescents: United States SEER Program, 1975–1995*. Bethesda, MD: N.C.I.S. Program. NIH No. 99-4649, 1999:111–123.

257. Pappo A. Rhabdomyosarcoma and other soft tissue sarcomas of childhood. *Curr Opin Oncol* 1995;7:361.

258. Pappo A, Shapiro D, Crist W. Biology and therapy of pediatric rhabdomyosarcoma. *J Clin Oncol* 1995;13:2123.

259. Pappo A, Shapiro D, Crist W. Rhabdomyosarcoma: biology and treatment. *Pediatr Clin North Am* 1997;44:953.

260. Dodd S, Malone M, McCulloch W. Rhabdomyosarcoma in children: a histological and immunohistochemical study of 59 cases. *J Pathol* 1989;158:13.

261. Newton W, Soule E, Hamoudi A. Histopathology of childhood sarcomas: Intergroup Rhabdomyosarcoma Studies I and II. Clinicopathologic correlation. *J Clin Oncol* 1988;6:67.

262. Newton WA Jr, et al. Early history of pathology studies by the Intergroup Rhabdomyosarcoma Study Group. *Pediatr Dev Pathol* 1999;2(3):275–285.

263. Ruymann FB, Grovas AC. Progress in the diagnosis and treatment of rhabdomyosarcoma and related soft tissue sarcomas. *Cancer Invest* 2000;18(3):223–241.

264. Gross E, Rao B, Bowman L. Outcome of treatment for pediatric sarcoma of the foot: a retrospective review over a 20-year period. *J Pediatr Surg* 1997;32:1181.

265. Andrassy RJ, et al. Extremity sarcomas: an analysis of prognostic factors from the Intergroup Rhabdomyosarcoma Study III. *J Pediatr Surg* 1996;31(1):191–196.

266. Newton WA Jr, et al. Classification of rhabdomyosarcomas and related sarcomas. Pathologic aspects and proposal for a new classification—an Intergroup Rhabdomyosarcoma Study. *Cancer* 1995;76(6):1073–1085.

267. Punyko JA, et al. Long-term survival probabilities for childhood rhabdomyosarcoma. A population-based evaluation. *Cancer* 2005;103(7):1475–1483.

268. Spunt SL, et al. Prognostic factors for children and adolescents with surgically resected nonrhabdomyosarcoma soft tissue sarcoma: an analysis of 121 patients treated at St. Jude Children's Research Hospital. *J Clin Oncol* 1999;17(12):3697–3705.

269. Raney RB. Synovial sarcoma in young people: background, prognostic factors, and therapeutic questions. *J Pediatr Hematol Oncol* 2005;27(4):207–211.

270. Deshmukh R, Mankin HJ, Singer S. Synovial sarcoma: the importance of size and location for survival. *Clin Orthop Relat Res* 2004;419:155–161.

271. Okcu MF, et al. Synovial sarcoma of childhood and adolescence: a multicenter, multivariate analysis of outcome. *J Clin Oncol* 2003;21(8):1602–1611.

272. Cecchetto G, et al. Fibrosarcoma in pediatric patients: results of the Italian Cooperative Group studies(1979–1995). *J Surg Oncol* 2001;78(4):225–231.

273. Kurkchubasche AG, et al. The role of preoperative chemotherapy in the treatment of infantile fibrosarcoma. *J Pediatr Surg* 2000;35(6):880–883.

274. Madden NP, et al. Spontaneous regression of neonatal fibrosarcoma. *Br J Cancer Suppl* 1992;18:S72–S75.

275. Ferrari A, et al. Soft-tissue sarcomas in children and adolescents with neurofibromatosis type 1. *Cancer* 2007;109(7):1406–1412.

276. Casanova M, et al. Malignant peripheral nerve sheath tumors in children: a single-institution twenty-year experience. *J Pediatr Hematol Oncol* 1999;21(6):509–513.

CHAPTER 14

H. Kerr Graham
Pam Thomason
Tom F. Novacheck

Cerebral Palsy

INTRODUCTION

Cerebral palsy (CP) is the most common cause of physical disability affecting children in developed countries. The prevalence is about 2 per 1000 live births and is not decreasing. Children with CP have complex needs and are usually managed by a multidisciplinary team. The medical literature dealing with CP is extensive and varies from level I (Randomized Clinical Trials [RCTs]), to cohort studies and case reports (levels IV and V). In this chapter, the most recent and the highest level of evidence will be cited, where possible. However, randomized trials in CP are difficult to perform and relatively few have been published, especially on the orthopaedic aspects of CP. When RCTs are not available, cohort studies, with long-term follow up and objective outcome measures, will be referenced.

CEREBRAL PALSY: DEFINITION

Cerebral palsy was described in 1861 by the English Physician William Little, who recognized a link between difficult births and the development of deformities (1). For many years, CP was known as "Little's Disease." Little popularized tenotomy to correct deformity in CP and was the first to bridge the gap between neurology and orthopaedics. Although his understanding of the *link* between brain injury and deformity has stood the test of time, his views on the *causation* of CP have been superseded. It is now accepted that only 10% to 20% of CP is related to perinatal events. The influence of "difficult births" may have been much greater in Little's era, when maternal health was poor, maternal and infant mortality was high, and obstetric services were primitive.

The term cerebral palsy was also used by Sir William Osler in 1889 in a book titled "The Cerebral Palsies of Children" (2). Freud considered CP to be caused not just at parturition but also earlier in pregnancy because of "deeper effects that influenced the development of the foetus" (3). Many other definitions have been proposed and debated since then (4).

THE 2007 REVISED DEFINITION AND CLASSIFICATION OF CEREBRAL PALSY

The revised definition of CP, published in 2007, is as follows:

Cerebral palsy (CP) describes a group of permanent disorders of the development of movement and posture, causing activity limitation, that are attributed to nonprogressive disturbances that occurred in the developing fetal or infant brain. The motor disorders of cerebral palsy are often accompanied by disturbances of sensation, perception, cognition, communication, and behavior, by epilepsy, and by secondary musculoskeletal problems (5).

The new definition has been widely accepted and is recommended as the most useful current operational definition of CP. However, it should be remembered that there is no test, genetic, metabolic, immunologic or otherwise, that demonstrates the existence or absence of CP. There is no specified cause such as cerebral pathology or even type of motor impairment, only that motor impairment exists resulting from nonprogressive cerebral pathology, acquired early in life (6).

BRAIN DEVELOPMENT AND GROSS MOTOR FUNCTION

During the first trimester of pregnancy, the growth of the brain is rapid and the brain differentiates into a recognizable cerebrum, cerebellum, brain stem, and spinal cord at a very early age of fetal development. During this time of explosive growth, the developing brain is highly susceptible to genetic influences, exogenous toxins, nutritional deficiencies and other insults, some of which can be characterized by meconium analysis (7). Neuronal development peaks in the second trimester. Neurons differentiate from neural stem cells around the periventricular regions and migrate centrifugally toward the surface of the cerebral cortex. This results in functional activity in neurons by 7 weeks of differentiation with reflex movements detectable in the fetus by the 15th week of gestation (8). By the end of the second trimester, the majority of neurons have been formed. Loss of neurons can be accommodated by neuronal plasticity but not by the generation of new neurons. The third trimester is characterized by extensive synaptogenesis and remodeling with glialization commencing in the second trimester and continuing at least until the age of 2 years. Myelination of neurons begins late in the third trimester, reaches a peak in the early years of childhood, and continues into adolescence, following a well-defined pattern (9). The myelination of complex pathways results in the progressive elimination of primitive reflexes, during the first 6 months of neonatal life as normal postural reflexes appear and the acquisition of gross motor skills occurs. In the typically developing infant, head control is achieved by age 3 months, independent sitting by 6 months, crawling by 8 months (usually accompanied by pulling to stand) and independent walking by the age of 12 months. However, even typically developing infants may take 3 to 6 months longer than these mean figures and still be considered to have typical development (10).

MOTOR CURVES AND CEREBRAL PALSY

The development of gross motor function in children with CP can be described by a series of curves that were derived from longitudinal measurements of gross motor function, using the Gross Motor Function Measure (GMFM) (11, 12) (Fig. 14-1). The curves show rapid acquisition of gross motor function in infants with a progressive separation of the curves especially between the ages of 2 and 4 years. The curves plateau between the ages of 3 and 6 years. The five gross motor curves constitute the five levels of the Gross Motor Function Classification System (GMFCS) (11–15).

Understanding the position of a child's development in relation to their gross motor curve provides a rational basis for the understanding of management strategies, goal setting, and long-term gross motor function. For example, a 2-year-old child GMFCS level II with signs of spastic diplegia is treated with a physical therapy program, ankle-foot orthoses (AFOs), and injections of Botulinum toxin A (BoNT-A) to the gastrocsoleus and hamstring muscles. Within 3 months, the child is noted to have progressed from standing with support to independent walking. While the intervention may well have contributed to these gains in gross motor function, the child is at the stage of rapid acquisition of gross motor function with or without intervention (12). This underlines the need for intervention studies in the first 6 years of life to be controlled. The popularity of many forms of intervention in early childhood in children with CP is the mistaken attribution of improvements in gross motor function to the intervention, when natural history has an undoubtedly much greater effect. Association is not causation.

In the majority of children aged 6 to 12 years, gross motor function has reached a plateau (Fig. 14-1). At the same time, gait parameters are noted to show deterioration as contractures and bony deformities increase (16–19). Changes in gross

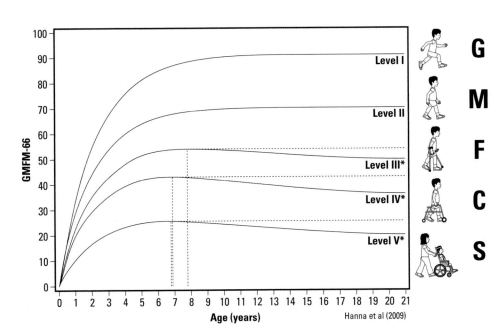

FIGURE 14-1. Gross motor curves in children with CP. The curves are based on longitudinal measurements of gross motor function, using the Gross Motor Function Measure (GMFM). Note the rapid acquisition of gross motor function between birth and age 2 years in all groups. Between the age of 2 and 6 years, the curves reach a plateau and level out into the five levels of the Gross Motor Function Classification System (GMFCS). (From Gallagher C, Sheedy M, Graham HK. Integrated management with botulinum neurotoxin A. In: Panteliadis CP, ed. *Cerebral palsy. A multidisciplinary approach.* Munchen, Germany: Dustri-Verlag; 2011:213–236, with permission.)

motor function and in gait during this plateau can be more realistically attributed to intervention, and longitudinal cohort studies are less liable to misinterpretation than in the birth to 6 years age group.

PREVALENCE OF CEREBRAL PALSY AND CAUSAL PATHWAYS

The incidence of CP varies from 1 to 7 children per 1000 live births, according to maternal health, prenatal and perinatal maternal, and child health care services (6, 20). Prevalence rates are accurately reported in countries with well-developed health care services and are most reliable in countries with national CP registers including some European countries and Australia. In these countries, prevalence rates are comparable at around 2 per 1000 live births (20, 21). In most countries, prevalence rates are either static or increasing.

There is a paradoxical relationship between prevalence rates and the provision of neonatal intensive care. Sophisticated neonatal intensive care for premature and low birth weight infants may reduce the risk of brain injury in some and eliminate brain injury in other high-risk neonates. However, the lives of very premature and very low birth weight neonates with a severity of health problems, which would previously have resulted in premature mortality, are saved. These infants may survive with an increased risk of moderate and severe CP (6, 20).

Males are at higher risk of CP, perhaps due to gender-specific neuronal vulnerabilities (22). The risk of CP increases with decreasing gestational age. However, because births before 32 weeks contribute <2% of neonatal survivors, they contribute a minority (20% to 25%) of all CP in developed countries (6, 20, 23). The majority of CP cases are born at term.

The risk of CP increases 4-fold in twins and 18-fold in triplets (24–27). The widespread use of *in vitro* fertilization has greatly increased the rate of multiple births, which has resulted in an increase in CP rates (6, 28). The high CP rates in multiple births are in part explained by shorter gestation and low birth weight, but these are not the only factors. Any factor causing preterm birth may lie on a causal pathway to CP (6).

The introduction of statewide and national registers is extremely important in monitoring the prevalence of CP and detecting changes. In this way, causative factors and causal pathways may be identified that in turn may lead to primary and secondary preventive strategies (6, 21, 24).

CENTRAL NERVOUS SYSTEM PATHOLOGY AND ETIOLOGY

CP is the most common cause of the upper motor neuron (UMN) syndrome in childhood, a syndrome characterized by positive features (spasticity, hyperreflexia, and co-contraction)

and negative features (weakness, loss of selective motor control, sensory deficits, and poor balance) (Fig. 14-2). Clinicians have traditionally focused more on the positive features because it is possible to treat spasticity. However, it is the negative features, which determine the locomotor prognosis. Weakness and loss of selective motor control determine when or if a child will walk. Balance deficits may dictate long-term dependence on a walking aid (13, 15).

The brain lesion, which results in CP, is a "static encephalopathy." In other words, the brain lesion is not progressive and is unchanging. This is in contrast to musculoskeletal pathology in the limbs, which is progressive and constantly changing during growth and development (6, 29, 30).

At least 70% of cases have antecedents during pregnancy and only 10% to 20% have any relation to the child's delivery (6, 20, 31). The mechanism of causal pathways suggests that in any one case of established CP a number of factors may have contributed to the brain lesion resulting in the specific clinical phenotype. There are a number of genetic predispositions to CP that may require an addition of an environmental trigger such as a maternal infection to be expressed as a brain lesion and CP. The genotype may load the gun and the environment pulls the trigger. A large number of major brain malformations have a genetic basis, and subtle genetic polymorphisms may also play a role (31, 32).

About 10% of infants with CP weigh <1500 g at birth. In this low birth weight group, the risk of CP is 90 per 1000, compared to 3 per 1000 in infants born at term and weighing more than 2500 g. Maternal risk factors include viral infections, urinary tract infections in late pregnancy, dietary deficiency, some prescription drugs, drug or alcohol abuse, maternal epilepsy, mental retardation, hypothyroidism, preeclamptic toxemia, cervical incompetence, and third-trimester bleeding. Obstetric risk factors include multiple births, placental abruption, premature rupture of membranes, chorioamnionitis, and prolonged labor. Other obstetric factors include the administration of oxytocin, cord prolapse, and breech presentation, when accompanied by low Apgar scores (6, 28). Neither routine use of fetal monitoring during labor nor increasing rate of Cesarean section has resulted in a decrease in the prevalence of CP (6).

The older the child at the time of the acquired brain lesion, the more the clinical syndrome is likely to differ from classical CP. Age 2 to 3 years is an important watershed (5).

CP was formerly a clinical diagnosis with occasional confirmation by central nervous system (CNS) imaging. With the availability of MRI and safer anesthesia for children, the majority of children suspected of having a CP will have brain imaging (31). A recent practice parameter from the American Neurological Association recommended that the diagnosis of CP be confirmed by imaging (33). In a large recently published multicenter study, the brain lesions identified by MRI are given in Table 14.1.

On the basis of their MRI scans, only 20% of cases of CP were considered as *possibly* being secondary to some type

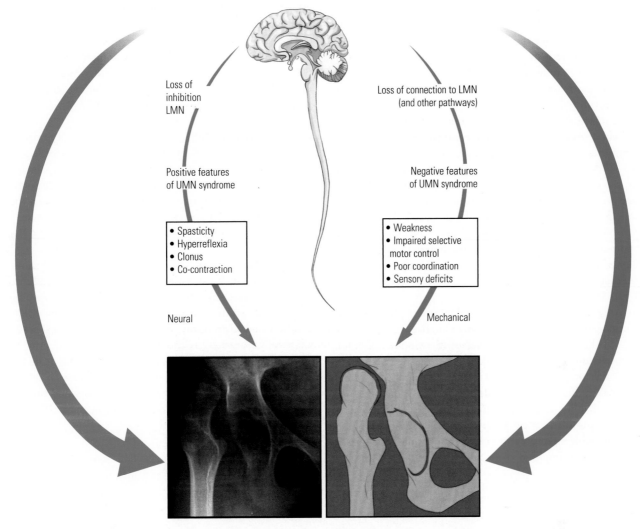

Loss of
inhibition
LMN

Loss of connection to LMN
(and other pathways)

Positive features
of UMN syndrome

Negative features
of UMN syndrome

- Spasticity
- Hyperreflexia
- Clonus
- Co-contraction

- Weakness
- Impaired selective
  motor control
- Poor coordination
- Sensory deficits

Neural

Mechanical

FIGURE 14-2. CP is a neuromusculoskeletal disorder. The CNS lesion has profound effects on the growing skeleton leading to deformities in both the upper and the lower limbs. Note the effects of both the positive and the negative features of the Upper Motor Neuron (UMN) syndrome.

of obstetric mishap. Twelve percent of cases, with a clinical diagnosis of CP, had a normal MRI scan (31).

PROGRESSIVE MUSCULOSKELETAL PATHOLOGY: CP IS A NEUROMUSCULOSKELETAL DISORDER

By definition CP is a static encephalopathy, but the musculoskeletal pathology is progressive (6, 30). Chronic neurologic impairment affects the development of bones and muscles (Fig. 14-3). In spastic hemiplegia, the affected side demonstrates muscle atrophy and limb shortening, compared to the unaffected side. Thus, CP is a neuromusculoskeletal disorder (29, 30).

The key feature of the musculoskeletal pathology in CP is failure of longitudinal growth of skeletal muscle. An apt synonym for CP is "short muscle disease." The conditions

for normal muscle growth are regular stretching of relaxed muscle, under physiologic loading conditions and normal levels of activity (29). In children with CP, skeletal muscle does not relax during activity because of spasticity and the

TABLE 14.1	Frequency of Brain Pathology by MRI
1. White matter damage of prematurity: 43%	
2. Basal ganglia damage: 13%	
3. Cortical/subcortical damage: 9%	
4. Brain malformations: 9%	
5. Focal infarcts: 7%	
6. Miscellaneous lesions: 7%	
7. Normal MRI: 12%	

Bax M, Tydeman C, Flodmark O. Clinical and MRI correlates of cerebral palsy: the European Cerebral Palsy Study. *JAMA* 2006;296:1602–1608.

children have greatly reduced levels of activity because of weakness and poor balance (30). In animal models of CP, such as the hereditary spastic mouse, there is failure of longitudinal muscle growth, in relation to bone growth. Affected mice develop equinus deformities because of a failure of longitudinal gastrocsoleus muscle growth when compared to tibial growth (34). However, muscle growth can be enhanced by the injection of BoNT-A soon after birth (35). The newborn child with CP does not have contractures or lower limb deformities, and most do not show signs of spasticity (29, 30). With time, spasticity develops, activity levels remain low, the growth of muscle-tendon units (MTUs) lags behind bone growth and contractures develop. Although the MTU is short in CP, muscle fibers may not be short (36, 37). Because of disordered growth and abnormal biomechanics, torsional abnormalities persist or develop in the long bones and instability of joints including the hip and subtalar joint develop. Eventually, premature degenerative arthritis may develop (6, 30, 38–41).

An important therapeutic window exists for spasticity management before the development of fixed contractures (38, 39) (Fig. 14-3). A second therapeutic window exists for the correction of fixed musculoskeletal deformities, before the onset of decompensation (39). There are three important longitudinal studies of gait in children with spastic diplegia that confirm that the musculoskeletal pathology and the attendant gait disorder are progressive during childhood. These studies provide an important insight into natural history and a framework to interpret the results of surgical intervention (16–18).

CLASSIFYING CEREBRAL PALSY

CP may be classified by the cause (when known) and the brain lesion as determined by MRI. Classification by movement disorder, topographical distribution, and gross motor function may be relevant to management, including orthopaedic surgery (13, 31, 42, 43) (Figs. 14-4 and 14-5A,B).

Movement Disorder. The most common approach to classification by movement disorder divides the disorders into pyramidal (spastic) and extrapyramidal (dystonic, athetoid) types (44). The majority of children with CP show features of both pyramidal and extrapyramidal involvement. When there is involvement of both pyramidal and extrapyramidal systems, spasticity and dystonia may coexist to varying degrees (43).

Spasticity. Spastic CP is by far the most common subtype and in most series comprises between 60% and 85% of all cases (21, 29, 43–46) (Fig. 14-4). A large population-based study of children with CP found that 85% of children had a primarily spastic movement disorder (21). Classically, spasticity is the result of a lesion affecting the pyramidal system and results in velocity-dependent increase in muscle tone with increased spastic tonic stretch reflexes. Spasticity is often associated with prematurity and the characteristic lesion of periventricular leucomalacia (PVL) on MRI (31).

Dystonia. Dystonia is the second most common form of movement disorder in CP and may not develop until late

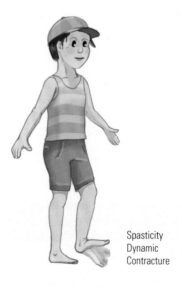

Spasticity
Dynamic
Contracture

• Physical Therapy
• Orthotics
• Botulinum Neurotoxin A

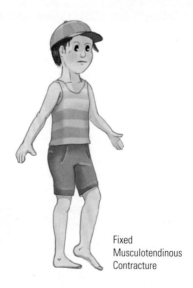

Fixed
Musculotendinous
Contracture

• Tendon Lengthening

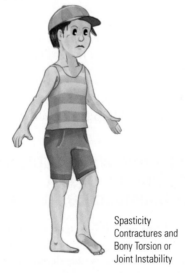

Spasticity
Contractures and
Bony Torsion or
Joint Instability

• Tendon Lengthening
• Rotational Osteotomies
• Arthrodeses

FIGURE 14-3. Musculoskeletal pathology in children with CP is progressive. At Stage 1, children have spasticity but no fixed contractures and can be managed nonoperatively. At Stage 2, there are fixed contractures and at Stage 3 contractures and bony deformities that may require corrective orthopaedic surgery. (Modified after Dr. Mercer Rang.)

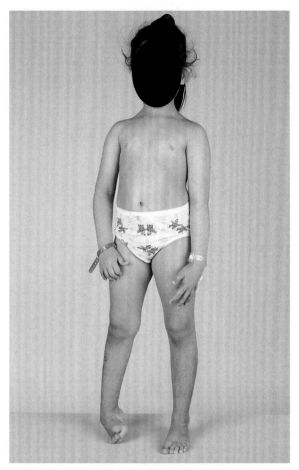

FIGURE 14-4. This girl has a right spastic hemiplegia. Her upper limb involvement is "dynamic." She has spasticity in her elbow flexors and this becomes apparent when she walks and even more pronounced when she runs. She has a severe varus deformity affecting her right foot because of spasticity in both tibialis anterior and tibialis posterior. The varus posture is consistent and does not change from day to day. Spastic CP tends to be predictable and amenable to corrective orthopaedic surgery.

childhood. Dystonia is often underreported in CP registers and population-based reviews (21, 45). Dystonia is diagnosed by observing abnormal twisting postures and writhing movements that vary in intensity. Dystonia may be triggered or worsened by attention, distraction, startling, overuse, fatigue, touch, or pain (43). Resting tone is variable and postures in both the upper and lower limbs vary with time. The brain lesion resulting in dystonia is usually in the basal ganglia and is more likely to be associated with a child who has had a term birth and widespread white matter lesions (31, 46). Uncontrolled movements seen in response to stimulation of the nervous system (e.g., volitional movements, loud noises, pain, etc.) are considered dystonic, while similar uncontrolled movements seen at rest are athetoid (43). Oral medications such as L-dopa and Artane may be beneficial in some children with dystonia. Severe dystonia can be managed by intrathecal baclofen (ITB) pump (38, 46) (Fig. 14-5A,B).

Mixed Movement Disorder. Many children with CP born at term have extensive brain lesions on MRI and have a mixture of pyramidal and extrapyramidal movement disorders. Defining the major movement disorder and the secondary and associated disorders can be challenging (43, 46). Dystonia and spasticity may occur in the same limb segments and distinction requires separation of the velocity-dependent from the action-induced and posture-responsive components of the hypertonia. Spasticity is evaluated by passively moving limb segments and joints at variable speeds. Dystonia is more easily confirmed by observation than palpation (39).

Ataxia. Ataxia may be part of a genetically determined syndrome and is uncommon as a pure movement disorder in CP (21, 45). Ataxia is disturbance of coordination and therefore most easily observed during walking. There may be associated signs of cerebellar dysfunction, including tremor. Because the resting tone is normal, and the majority of children have quite good walking ability, contractures are uncommon, and children with pure ataxia do not develop hip dysplasia or scoliosis (30).

Hypotonia. Many children who develop hypertonic CP are initially hypotonic, and this phase may last for several years. Hypertonia may not be expressed until myelination reaches a certain stage of completion (9) Many children with intellectual disabilities and certain other syndromes exhibit hypotonia, joint laxity, and developmental delay. Unless there is, in addition to the hypotonia, a defined static brain lesion, these children are not classified as having CP (6, 30).

Topographical Distribution
Unilateral Bilateral

1. *Unilateral*
   Monoplegia, hemiplegia
2. *Bilateral*
   Diplegia, quadraplegia

Topographical distribution is a classification of CP according to which limb segments are affected. As with classification by movement disorder, there is considerable variability in the terminology used, especially between different countries. The emphasis in Europe is the subdivision of CP into unilateral and bilateral types (44). The unilateral types can be subdivided into monoplegia (affecting only one limb) and hemiplegia (affecting one side of the body. The majority of children who seem to have a lower limb monoplegia with spastic equinus and toe walking, when asked to run, will show some abnormal upper limb posturing (21).

The common forms of bilateral CP are diplegia and quadriplegia (21, 45). Children with diplegia have bilateral lower limb involvement that may be symmetric or asymmetric. The involvement of the upper limbs is restricted to deficits in fine motor function, and overall upper limb function

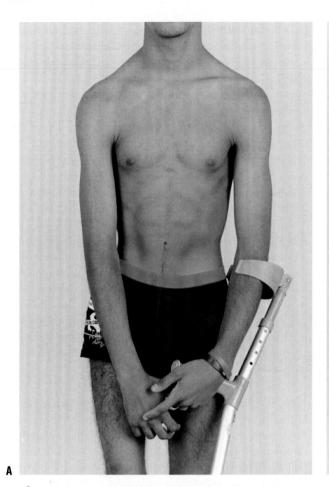
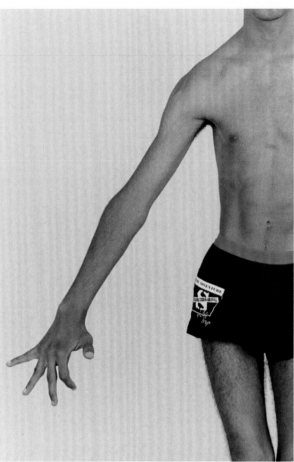

A

B

FIGURE 14-5. **A and B:** This teenage boy also has a right hemiplegia but his movement disorder is dystonic. He is using his uninvolved left hand to restrain his right hand. When the restraint is removed, his right arm undergoes variable dystonic posturing, with abduction at the shoulder, extension at the elbow, and abduction of the fingers. His dystonia is so severe that he requires a crutch and functions at GMFCS level III. Dystonic posturing can rarely be improved by orthopaedic surgery but may respond to medications including ITB.

is good. Spastic diplegia is most commonly associated with prematurity and PVL (31). The affected children usually have normal intelligence and a good prognosis for independent walking although many have visual deficits and learning difficulties. Quadriplegia refers to involvement of the upper and the lower limbs, and such children are usually born at term and have extensive brain involvement (46). They usually have a mixed movement disorder with spastic and dystonic features. The severity of involvement varies between the upper and the lower limbs and between the two sides. Because of the greater degree of brain involvement, quadriplegia is far more likely to be associated with comorbidities such as seizure disorder, learning challenges, and impairments of speech or cognition (5).

A small number of children appear to have a "triplegia" or three-limb involvement. This usually is a combination of hemiplegic involvement with both lower limbs involved to an asymmetric degree. One upper limb seems to be largely spared. This is an uncommon type of CP and is sometimes

grouped with spastic quadriplegia (42, 45). Classification by topographical distribution is not a strictly functional classification, but there are functional implications. Almost all children with hemiplegia walk independently in the community, about 80% of children with diplegia walk either independently or with assistive devices, but only 20% of children with quadriplegia walk and then only with assistance (21). The separation of children into diplegia and quadriplegia is arbitrary and unsatisfactory, hence the need for a classification based on a valid and reliable measure of gross motor function (13, 42, 44).

Classification by Gross Motor Function. The development of the GMFCS has for the first time given a common language to communicate about CP (13). The GMFCS is a five-level ordinal grading system in which a series of descriptors, supplemented by illustrations, can be used in five different age groups to classify gross motor function in CP (Figs. 14-6 and 14-7). The GMFCS has established validity

GMFCS E & R between 6th and 12th birthday: Descriptors and illustrations

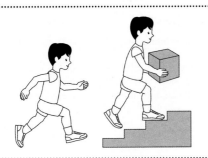

GMFCS Level I

Children walk at home, school, outdoors and in the community. They can climb stairs without the use of a railing. Children perform gross motor skills such as running and jumping, but speed, balance and coordination are limited

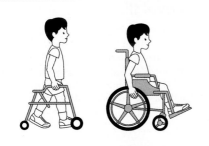

GMFCS Level II

Children walk in most settings and climb stairs holding onto a railing. They may experience difficulty walking long distances and balancing on uneven terrain, inclines, in crowded areas or confined spaces. Children may walk with physical assistance, a hand-held mobility device or used wheeled mobility over long distances. Children have only minimal ability to perform gross motor skills such as running and jumping.

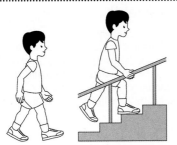

GMFCS Level III

Children walk using a hand-held mobility device in most indoor settings. They may climb stairs holding onto a railing with supervision or assistance. Children use wheeled mobility when traveling long distances and may self-propel for shorter distances.

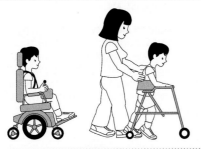

GMFCS Level IV

Children use methods of mobility that require physical assistance or powered mobility in most settings. They may walk for short distances at home with physical assistance or use powered mobility or a body support walker when positioned. At school, outdoors and in the community children are transported in a manual wheelchair or use powered mobility.

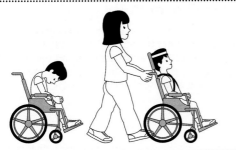

GMFCS Level V

Children are transported in a manual wheelchair in all settings. Children are limited in their ability to maintain antigravity head and trunk postures and control leg and arm movements.

GMFCS descriptors: Palisano et al. (1997) Dev Med Child Neurol 39:214-23
CanChild: www.canchild.ca

Illustrations copyright © Kerr Graham, Bill Reid and Adrienne Harvey,
The Royal Children's Hospital, Melbourne

FIGURE 14-6. GMFCS E & R (Expanded and Revised) between 6th and 12th birthday: Descriptors and illustrations.

GMFCS E & R between 12th and 18th birthday: Descriptors and illustrations

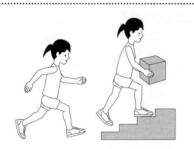

GMFCS Level I

Youth walk at home, school, outdoors and in the community. Youth are able to climb curbs and stairs without physical assistance or a railing. They perform gross motor skills such as running and jumping but speed, balance and coordination are limited.

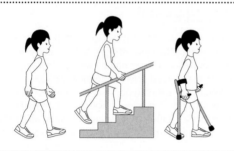

GMFCS Level II

Youth walk in most settings but environmental factors and personal choice influence mobility choices. At school or work they may require a hand held mobility device for safety and climb stairs holding onto a railing. Outdoors and in the community youth may use wheeled mobility when traveling long distances.

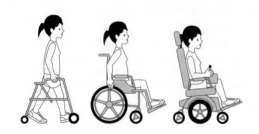

GMFCS Level III

Youth are capable of walking using a hand-held mobility device. Youth may climb stairs holding onto a railing with supervision or assistance. At school they may self-propel a manual wheelchair or use powered mobility. Outdoors and in the community youth are transported in a wheelchair or use powered mobility.

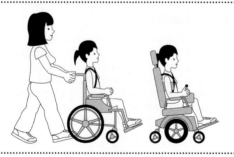

GMFCS Level IV

Youth use wheeled mobility in most settings. Physical assistance of 1-2 people is required for transfers. Indoors, youth may walk short distances with physical assistance, use wheeled mobility or a body support walker when positioned. They may operate a powered chair, otherwise are transported in a manual wheelchair.

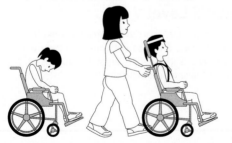

GMFCS Level V

Youth are transported in a manual wheelchair in all settings. Youth are limited in their ability to maintain antigravity head and trunk postures and control leg and arm movements. Self-mobility is severely limited, even with the use of assistive technology.

GMFCS descriptors: Palisano et al. (1997) Dev Med Child Neurol 39:214-23
CanChild: www.canchild.ca

Illustrations copyright © Kerr Graham, Bill Reid and Adrienne Harvey,
The Royal Children's Hospital, Melbourne

FIGURE 14-7. GMFCS E & R (Expanded and Revised) between 12th and 18th birthday: Descriptors and illustrations.

(based on the GMFM), reliability, and stability. There is good agreement between clinicians and also between clinicians and parents (47). Given that the GMFCS is a grading system and not an outcome measure, it is the major prognostic information which must be considered in all children with CP. Knowing a child's long-term gross motor prognosis has management implications. For example, a child between the ages of 6 and 12 years at GMFCS level IV may perform some stepping with a heavily adapted walker, under the supervision of a therapist or a parent (13). However, following the pubertal growth spurt, useful walking is not sustained (15). It would be inappropriate to offer such children invasive treatments to improve or prolong walking because these will not be successful in the long term. Appropriate goal setting would be maintaining standing transfers (15).

The prevalence and severity of medical comorbidities shows good correlation with GMFCS (48). Severe respiratory disease, nutritional deficiencies, and premature mortality are largely seen at GMFCS levels IV and V. Children who are at GMFCS levels I and II do not have severe medical comorbidities (apart from epilepsy) nor do they show significant excess mortality.

Certain musculoskeletal features and deformities are also closely related to GMFCS level. The shape of the proximal femur shows a strong correlation with GMFCS level. Femoral neck anteversion (FNA) increases from GMFCS level I to level III and then plateaus at a mean of 40 degrees at GMFCS levels III, IV, and V. Mean neck shaft angle (NSA) increases stepwise from GMFCS levels I through to V (49). The incidence and severity of hip displacement is directly predicted by GMFCS level. In one study, children at GMFCS level I showed no hip displacement and those at GMFCS level V had a 90% incidence of having a migration percentage in excess of 30% (50). The relationship between GMFCS and hip displacement has direct implication for screening and management protocols.

CEREBRAL PALSY: COMORBIDITIES

The spinal cord is not involved in CP and the most common neurologic impairment is epilepsy, affecting about 30% of children. Epilepsy is most commonly seen in hemiplegia, especially when it is acquired postnatally and in children with quadriplegia (48, 51). Intellectual disability is variable and more severe in children at GMFCS levels IV and V. However, many children at GMFCS levels I to III exhibit learning difficulties, autism spectrum disorders, and behavioral and emotional difficulties. Impairments of hearing, speech, and vision are also common and may adversely impact schooling and learning. The prevalence of visual problems is so high (about 50%) that routine screening is advised (52).

Respiratory Disorders. Children with CP have excess mortality at GMFCS levels IV and V, the levels previously described as spastic quadriplegia. The commonest cause of death is from respiratory disease especially aspiration pneumonia (48, 53). A major risk factor for respiratory disease is "pseudobulbar palsy" in which there are varying combinations of impaired swallowing, esophageal reflux, aspiration, and chest infection. Nocturnal coughing and asthma are also very common. The management of chronic respiratory disease involves careful assessment of swallowing and may necessitate investigation of the upper gastrointestinal tract. Fundoplication and the use of feeding tubes are often beneficial in the management of severe respiratory disease, when aspiration has been confirmed to be a major contributory factor (54).

Gastrointestinal System. The most severe problems are in GMFCS levels IV and V (48). Pseudobulbar palsy leads to impaired swallowing, vomiting, esophageal reflux, and aspiration. Oral feeding can be slow and inefficient leading to chronic malnutrition, impaired growth, and poor nutritional reserves (55). Malnourished children are at greatly increased risk of postoperative complications after hip reconstruction and scoliosis surgery. Assessment of nutritional status includes a careful dietary history and a radiologic assessment of swallowing in those with suspected gastroesophageal reflux. Nutritional status can be assessed by measurement of serum albumin, iron, and transferrin levels and examination for iron deficiency anemia. Correction of malnutrition may require the introduction of improved oral feeding. In many children, a percutaneous enterogastrostomy or a jejunostomy may transform the child's nutritional status and general health. Gastroesophageal reflux may respond to medical management but often requires a fundoplication (55, 56).

Of all problems affecting the gastrointestinal system, slow transit and chronic constipation is by far the most common (56). The excessively loaded colon is often noted as an incidental finding during hip surveillance radiographs. Chronic constipation assumes even more importance in the perioperative period when fecal impaction, vomiting, and the inability to achieve satisfactory intake of food and fluids postoperatively causes severe distress and results in prolonged hospitalization. Strategies to ensure that children at GMFCS levels IV and V have a satisfactory bowel management program prior to admission for orthopaedic surgery are advised.

DIAGNOSIS AND ASSESSMENT: THE DIAGNOSTIC MATRIX

In the majority of children who are referred to an orthopaedic surgeon, the diagnosis of CP has already been established by a pediatrician or a pediatric neurologist. The exception is a small number of children with mild hemiplegia and monoplegia who present after walking age with toe walking or some other subtle disturbance of gait. The postural abnormalities associated with monoplegia and hemiplegia are best observed by asking the child to walk and then run in a sufficiently long, well-lit corridor (Fig. 14-8).

History. The "neonate at risk" and the majority of children with mild CP are diagnosed because they are observed to have

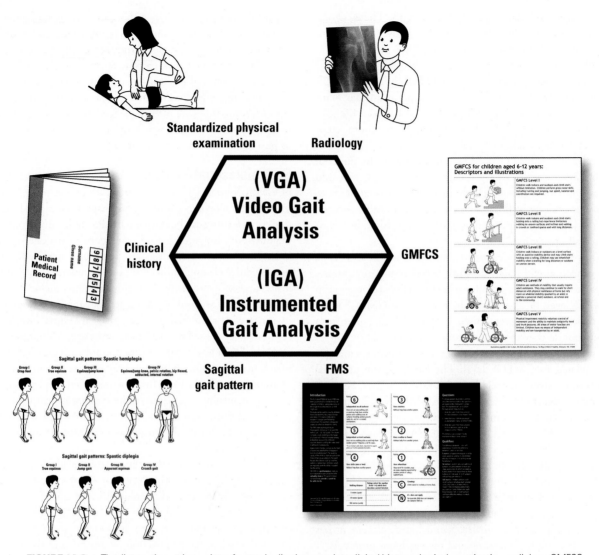

FIGURE 14-8. The diagnostic matrix consists of a standardized approach to clinical history, physical examination, radiology, GMFCS, functional scales (FMS and FAQ), and sagittal gait pattern identification. These components can be used in conjunction with either video gait analysis (VGA) or instrumented gait analysis (IGA). (Illustration copyright © Kerr Graham, Bill Reid and Adrienne Harvey.)

a delay in reaching gross motor milestones. A knowledge of the normal age (and range) of achieving these milestones is important. In typically developing infants, head control is acquired at age 3 months, sitting at 6 months, crawling and pulling to stand at 8 to 9 months, and independent walking at 12 months (10).

Recognition of abnormal muscle tone is also important (43). This may include hypotonia in the infant and hypertonia in the child. The mothers of children with CP, who have previously had a typically developing child, often sense that "something is wrong" at a very early stage. It is clearly wise to take the concerns of an experienced parent seriously. Details of the history of the pregnancy, the birth, and early development are very important in establishing the diagnosis of CP. The family history is important to detect such conditions as hereditary spastic paraplegia (HSP) and congenital ataxias (57).

Physical Examination. Physical examination is important in both preliminary examinations to establish the diagnosis of CP and in subsequent assessments in which the child's tone, gross motor function, and secondary musculoskeletal pathology are evaluated:

1. Observation of posture, movement and gait
2. Assessment of gross motor function: GMFCS, FMS, and FAQ
3. Evaluation of muscle tone by a combination of observation, palpation, and testing of reflexes.
4. Assessment of soft-tissue contracture by evaluation of passive joint range of motion and muscle length measurement.
5. Assessment of torsional abnormalities in the long bones: FNA; tibial torsion; deformities of the spine, hands, and feet.
6. Sensory evaluation: especially the hemiplegic upper limb.

Assessment of Gross Motor Function: GMFCS.
Knowing the child's GMFCS level is fundamental in establishing gross motor prognosis and monitoring changes. The GMFCS can be easily and reliably determined by age 4 years and all orthopaedic surgeons should be competent in assigning a grade after the age of 6 years. Changes in GMFCS levels should be carefully documented. The most common reason for a change in GMFCS is an error in the previous or current examination (58). Given that the GMFCS is a categorical grading system, true changes in GMFCS level sometimes occur and these may occur in both directions, that is improvement or deterioration. After major intervention such as selective dorsal rhizotomy (SDR) or multilevel surgery, a small number of children move up a level, but this is uncommon and should not be expected in more than about 5% to 10% of a study population. Deterioration in GMFCS level is more common. Lengthening of the Achilles tendons in children at GMFCS level II can result in progressive crouch gait and the need for assistive devices. Such children may deteriorate from GMFCS level II to III (59).

The GMFCS is a classification system and not an outcome measure. It is expected to be stable throughout a child's growth and development but is often misused as a proxy outcome measure in intervention studies. Simple scales of gross motor function that can be used as outcome measures

are the Functional Mobility Scale (FMS) and the Functional Assessment Questionnaire (FAQ) (60, 61).

The World Health Organization's International Classification of Functioning (ICF) describes health conditions in several domains, including body structure and function, activities, and participation (62) (Fig. 14-9). These domains are modified by environmental factors and personal factors. Various tools exist to measure parameters relevant to CP in the ICF domains and new measurement tools are being developed. Fortunately, there are now valid and reliable tools to classify and measure gross motor function in both the upper and lower limbs.

Functional Mobility Scale. The Functional Mobility Scale describes the level of assistance a child requires to mobilize in three different environments, the home (distances of up to 5 m), school (distances of up to 50 m), and the community (distances of 500 m) (60). Hence, three numbers are assigned depending on the level of assistance required in each of these settings. For example, a child at GMFCS level III is frequently capable of independent walking in a sheltered familiar environment such as the home. The same child may require the use of Canadian crutches to move around in the school environment but may be too slow to keep up with the rest of the

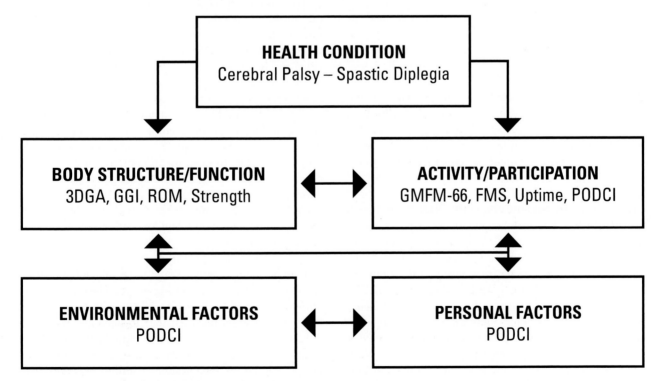

FIGURE 14-9. The World Health Organization International Classification of Functioning (WHO-ICF) as applied to spastic diplegia. Suggested assessment tools are indicated in each domain. (3DGA, three-dimensional gait analysis; GGI, Gillette Gait Index; PODCI, Pediatric Outcomes Data Collection Instrument.)

family during trips to the shopping mall, when a wheelchair may be preferred. The FMS grading for such a child is 5, 3, 1. Unlike the GMFCS, the FMS was designed as an outcome measure and is sensitive to change (59, 63). For example, children at GMFCS level III often require a posterior walker to ambulate prior to multilevel surgery. After optimum biomechanical realignment and correction of spastic contractures, these children can often progress to lesser levels of support. Some will be able to walk increasing distances independently; others will require crutches or sticks when previously they were dependent on a posterior walker. These important changes can be monitored and reported using the FMS (63).

Functional Assessment Questionnaire. The Gillette FAQ is a 10-level, parent report walking scale that describes a range of walking abilities across the spectrum of CP, from nonambulatory to independent ambulation at a high level. In addition to the 10-level walking scale, there is an additional list of 22 items describing a variety of higher-level functional activities requiring varying degrees of walking ability, balance, strength, and coordination. The scale has been shown to be reliable and validity has been established by comparison with other scales used in neuromuscular diseases. It has also been shown to have sensitivity to change with improvements seen in children with CP after such interventions as SDR and single-event multilevel surgery (SEMLS). It is a simple scale, which can be quickly completed by parents or caregivers and provides an excellent longitudinal view of the child's gross motor and walking abilities.

The FMS and FAQ are complementary scales and are both gaining acceptance in assessing children with CP as baseline measures and as outcome measures after intervention (59–61, 63).

Additional Diagnostic Tests. Between 10% and 20% of children with a clinical syndrome typical of CP will have a normal MRI of the brain and spinal cord (31). In these children additional investigation for causes such as HSP, genetic, dysmorphic, metabolic and muscular diseases and syndromes is important (57).

Longitudinal Assessments with Radiology: Hip Surveillance. The early stage of hip displacement is silent and formal screening by radiographs of the hips with careful positioning is advised (64, 65). The frequency of such radiographs should be directly related to the risk of hip displacement which is in turn related to the child's GMFCS level. At GMFCS level I, there is little risk of hip displacement and radiographs are only required if there are findings on clinical examination. More regular radiographs are required at GMFCS levels II and III. Radiographs every 6 to 12 months may be required at GMFCS levels IV and V to monitor progressive hip displacement (66).

Deformities of the feet are very common in all GMFCS levels. Standing weight-bearing radiographs of the feet are extremely useful in the longitudinal assessment of progressive foot deformity. Recently, a series of radiologic indices have been published in typically developing children that are an excellent baseline with which the results in CP can be compared (67).

Instrumented Gait Analysis. Evaluation of gait and functioning in children with CP can be considered in the format of a diagnostic matrix (68). The role of instrumented gait analysis (IGA) is crucial to the evaluation of gait dysfunction, especially in relation to planning and assessing the outcome of major interventions such as SDR and SEMLS (69). Historically, problems with reliability undermined the utility of IGA and the confidence in using such information for planning interventions (70–72). Recent work from several centers has reestablished confidence in the reliability of gait kinematics (73, 74). Only about half of the orthopaedic surgeons in North America who care for children with CP have access to IGA (75). There are children with symmetric gait deviations that through the eyes of experienced examiners are relatively easy to recognize. Even for those with experience, there are many children with complex movement disorders, asymmetric gait patterns, and complexities that require IGA for understanding and planning (40, 69). As gait analysis becomes more reliable, cheaper, and more accessible, the quality of assessments and outcomes should continue to improve.

Video Gait Analysis. Even in centers with access to IGA, video gait analysis (VGA) is a central part of the diagnostic matrix (38). A visual record of a child's gait and functioning on digital video is of much greater value than observational gait analysis and a written report (39). Digital video can be archived in a permanent fashion, is objective, and can be shared by multiple observers over time. It allows observation and recording of gait from multiple viewpoints, can be replayed in slow motion, and can be reviewed repeatedly, including late in the evening prior to an operating list, when real-time observation of a child's gait is not feasible (40). In an effort to quantify and objectify the outcome of observational gait analysis, a number of gait scores have been developed of varying degrees of complexity, sophistication, and reliability. These include the Physician Rating Scale, the Observational Gait Scale, and the Edinburgh Visual Gait Score (76–78).

VGA has wider application than IGA. IGA requires a child to be about a meter tall and to be able to follow simple commands over a 2-hour testing period. There is much useful information to be gained in children with hemiplegia and diplegia from when they first start to stand and walk which cannot be obtained from IGA. Longitudinal assessment of children following interventions such as injection of BoNT-A, the prescription or modification of orthoses, is also conveniently achieved using serial VGA (39, 79). Gait deviations for children at GMFCS IV may be so severe that the extra cost and effort of IGA may not be necessary (15). VGA and physical exam may be all that is needed.

PHYSIOTHERAPY AND OCCUPATIONAL THERAPY IN CP

Physiotherapy is the most popular and widely used management strategy in children with CP (80–83). Some have access to therapy services integrated within the school program and others outside of the school program. The frequency of such programs may be related to the severity of the individual child's involvement but rarely reflect the family and the child's real needs. This type of background physical therapy support is valued by the parents of children with CP. These programs provide education and emotional support to the parents coping with the diagnosis of CP and starting the journey through the uncharted waters of raising a child with a lifelong physical disability. Roles that may be assumed by therapists may include education, counseling, coordination of access to other services including physical medicine and rehabilitation, orthotics, and orthopaedic surgery. The parents will often seek the view of the child's therapist on recommendations for spasticity management, the type of orthosis, and the timing and type of surgical intervention (80). The need for clear communication and teamwork within the multidisciplinary team is obvious. These "background" programs of physical therapy are rarely adequate to ensure an optimum rehabilitation from major interventions such as SDR or SEMLS. Therapy around such episodes needs to be carefully planned and is often best as a team approach involving the child's community therapist as well as providing the additional therapy in the tertiary hospital or rehabilitation center.

The physical therapy management of children with CP has been based on a variety of theoretical perspectives. The theoretical frameworks most commonly applied can be broadly categorized into biomechanical (splints, orthoses, stretching, and strength training), neurodevelopmental, cognitive (including conductive education [CE] and motor learning), and constraint-induced movement therapy (CIMT) (80–83). These approaches are not mutually exclusive. They can have shared components and most therapists use a combination of approaches. Given that the surgical management of CP has a biomechanical basis, surgeons find it easier to communicate with therapists who share this approach (80).

Biomechanical Approach.

The biomechanical approaches (80) aim to maintain range of motion and muscle length. Techniques used include manual passive ranging of joints, stretching of muscles, and splinting and casting. Serial casting can be combined with Botox injections, for dynamic contractures (84). The introduction of a suitable ankle foot orthosis is often a critical step in providing an improved base of support and achieving progress in a child progressing to standing and walking (38). Muscle weakness is a significant functional and biomechanical problem in children with CP. In children with hemiplegia, muscle weakness is also often compounded by nonuse of the affected limb (39). Progressive resistance strength training may be used to increase muscle strength and endurance (85).

Neurodevelopmental Therapy: The Bobath Approach.

Neurodevelopmental therapy (NDT) (81) is a widely used approach in children with CP. It aims to inhibit abnormal, primitive postural patterns and facilitate developmentally more mature movement patterns with improved function. NDT therapists use specific physical handling, including facilitation, to provide sensorimotor input and to guide motor output. Inhibitive casting is sometimes used with NDT to help achieve a reduction in tone and increased range of motion.

Cognitive Approach.

Cognitive or learning approaches (82) focus on learning control of movement for function rather than emphasizing quality of movement. Motor learning or training programs use task analysis to breakdown functional tasks into basic motor components or patterns. These components are then practiced and learned as a motor skill for functional use. Conductive Education (CE) or the Peto method is a cognitive approach that utilizes rhythm, music, and counting to initiate and moderate movements. CE is used extensively by therapists to develop skills necessary for the performance of daily activities such as dressing and self-feeding.

Constraint-Induced Movement Therapy.

CIMT (83) is used for learned nonuse of the affected upper limb, which is common in hemiplegia (39). It involves the forced use of the most affected upper limb by restricting use of the less involved hand in a cast, splint, or glove for periods of activity during the day.

The approach used by occupational therapists and physical therapists to manage children with CP is influenced by many factors. Intervention requires sensitivity to the child's age, cognitive, sensory, and perceptual factors as well as type and severity of CP. The child's environment, including family and culture, is important. Interventions will be less effective if they are not carried over into the child's management at home. The treatment setting, whether based in a hospital, at school or home, and the focus of these services are also factors. The setting and the frequency of treatments are often influenced by the financial resources available.

Despite widespread use, evidence on the efficacy of physiotherapy to improve function in children with CP is equivocal. In randomized, controlled trials, treatment effects have generally been small.

MOVEMENT DISORDER MANAGEMENT AND THE SPASTICITY COMPASS

The "spasticity compass" can be used to classify and compare interventions for spasticity management, as focal or generalized in their effect and as temporary or permanent (84). Each intervention can then be located in the appropriate quadrant. For example, oral medications are general (all nerves or all muscles in all body areas) but temporary in effect (86). SDR is a neurosurgical procedure in which 30% to 50% of the dorsal rootlets between L1 and S1 are transected for the permanent relief of spasticity in a highly selected group of children with

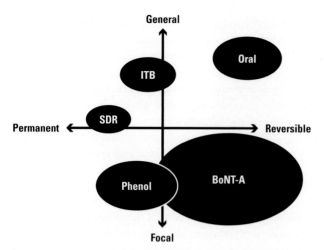

FIGURE 14-10. The spasticity compass as a guide to movement disorder management in CP. Interventions are classified on the north–south axis according to whether they are "general" or "focal" in their action. They are also classified on the east–west axis as to whether they are "permanent" or "reversible." (From Gallagher C, Sheedy M, Graham HK. Integrated management with botulinum neurotoxin A. In: Panteliadis CP, ed. *Cerebral palsy. A multidisciplinary approach.* Munchen, Germany: Dustri-Verlag; 2011:213–236, with permission.)

spastic diplegia. The principal effects are on the lower limbs although there may be minor effects on the upper limbs. The position on the grid is therefore permanent and half way between general and focal (87, 88) (Fig. 14-10).

Oral medications used for the management of spasticity in children with CP include diazepam, baclofen, dantrolene sodium, and tizanidine. Artane and L-dopa are used in dystonia. All are limited in usefulness by a combination of limited benefits and side effects. They have been extensively reviewed in several recent publications (84, 89).

The limited lipid solubility of baclofen when administered orally can be overcome by intrathecal administration using a programmable, battery-operated implantable pump connected to a catheter and delivery system to the intrathecal space (86). This is an invasive procedure with associated morbidity and

mortality (38, 39, 88). However, it is the most effective current method available for the management of severe spasticity, dystonia, and mixed movement disorders in CP and a number of other conditions including spasticity of spinal origin and acquired brain injury. The role of ITB has been reviewed extensively in several recent publications (86, 88).

Chemodenervation is useful in the management of focal spasticity and dystonia. Phenol neurolysis was much more widely utilized before the introduction of Botulinum neurotoxin A (BoNT-A). The principal limitation on its use is pain at the site of injection and post injection dysesthesia. Phenol is not selective and has the same effect on sensory nerve fibers as motor fibers. The principal indications are neurolysis of the musculocutaneous nerve for elbow flexor spasticity and the obturator nerve for adductor spasticity. These nerves have limited sensory distribution (84, 90).

BOTULINUM NEUROTOXIN A IN CEREBRAL PALSY

Injection of skeletal muscle with BoNT-A results in a dose-dependent, reversible chemodenervation, by blocking presynaptic release of acetylcholine at the neuromuscular junctions (84). Because of the toxin's rapid and high-affinity binding to receptors at the neuromuscular junctions of the target muscle, little systemic spread occurs. Neurotransmission is restored first by sprouting of new nerve endings, followed by the original nerve endings regaining their ability to release acetylcholine (91, 92). BoNT-A may be useful in children with CP to manage dynamic gait problems and to delay the need for orthopaedic surgery until the child is older (Fig. 14-11).

Spastic Equinus. The most common and most important indication for BoNT-A therapy in children with CP is the injection of the gastrocsoleus for spastic equinus (93, 94). Before widespread use of BoNT-A for spastic equinus, the majority of children with CP who walked on their toes had a lengthening of their Achilles' tendons by age 4 to 6 years (95). This resulted in crouch gait that was much more disabling than the original equinus gait.

FIGURE 14-11. The CP musculoskeletal management algorithm. Neurolytic blocks, botulinum toxin A, and phenol are used in younger children with spasticity. Under the age of 6 years, the only surgery required is preventive hip surgery. Surgery for contracture and bony torsion is most often required between the ages of 6 and 12 years by which stage the role of Botulinum toxin is very limited. (From Gallagher C, Sheedy M, Graham HK. Integrated management with botulinum neurotoxin A. In: Panteliadis CP, ed. *Cerebral palsy. A multidisciplinary approach.* Munchen, Germany: Dustri-Verlag; 2011:213–236, with permission.)

CP: Musculoskeletal Management Algorithm

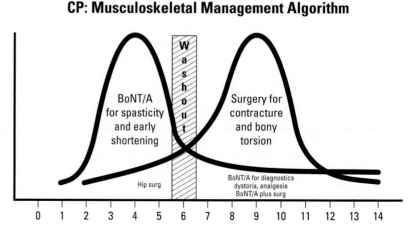

Now children with spastic equinus usually commence BoNT-A therapy aged between 1 and 3 years, in conjunction with physical therapy and the use of appropriate AFOs. They receive injections every 6 to 12 months for several years until gross motor function plateaus, at 4 to 6 years of age. Residual contractures and bony torsion can then be dealt with as SEMLS (96). A program of care utilizing BoNT-A should be viewed as complementary to surgical reconstruction and not as an alternative (96, 97) (Fig. 14-11). Information about dosing, dilution, muscle targeting, and safety has been published elsewhere (98–102).

Injection of BoNT-A for spastic equinus increases the dynamic length of the gastrocsoleus with improvements in ankle dorsiflexion during gait, as determined by the Physician Rating Scale (93, 103). Improvements have been reported in studies using IGA, including kinematics, kinetics, and electromyography (94, 104). This may lead to small but important gains in gross motor function (105–107). The evidence base supporting the use of BoNT-A in CP is quite good as confirmed in several randomized controlled trials and systematic reviews (108, 109). However, the treatment effect is small and short lived. The drug is expensive limiting access and is not approved by the FDA in the management of children with CP in the United States. All current use in the United States is therefore "off label."

Spastic Equinovarus and Equinovalgus.
Spastic equinovarus is the result of spasticity in the gastrocsoleus, tibialis posterior and/or tibialis anterior (110). In spastic equinovarus, the most effective strategy is to inject the gastrocsoleus and the tibialis posterior (94). Equinovalgus is not usually the result of muscle imbalance but altered biomechanics. It is best managed by injection of the gastrocsoleus and provision of an appropriate AFO (109).

Injection of the Hamstrings and the Adductor Muscles in Cerebral Palsy.
Spasticity in the hamstring and adductor muscles is prevalent in the severely involved child and may result in scissoring postures and spastic hip displacement (38). Injection of the adductor and hamstring muscles with BoNT-A every 6 months combined with an abduction brace had no appreciable effect on the prevention of hip displacement, in a large RCT (111). The majority of the children required surgical stabilization of their hips either during the study or soon after the study concluded (111).

Multilevel Injections of Botulinum Neurotoxin A in Cerebral Palsy.
Techniques have been developed for injecting the iliopsoas as part of a multilevel injection protocol for children with spastic diplegia. Multiple target muscles are injected under mask anesthesia and followed by supplemental casting, orthoses, and intensive rehabilitation. Temporary improvements in gait and function have been reported (112, 113). Phenol neurolysis for adductor spasticity can be combined with BoNT-A chemodenervation of the hamstring and calf muscles (90). The principal indication is the younger child with spastic hip displacement and walking difficulties (39, 84).

Botulinum Neurotoxin A in the Upper Limb in Cerebral Palsy.
In typical hemiplegic posturing the most common target muscles are biceps, brachialis, pronator teres, flexor carpi ulnaris, flexor carpi radialis, and adductor pollicis. The long finger flexors should usually be avoided to prevent weakening grip strength, except when the aim is improved palmar hygiene (92, 114, 115). Precise targeting with electrical stimulation, electromyography, or ultrasound is mandatory (101, 102). Palpation is inaccurate. Upper limb dose guides have been published elsewhere (92, 98, 99, 115). Botox injections in the upper limb results in a reduction in muscle tone but robust evidence for improvements in function is limited, in studies that employed valid and reliable functional outcome measures (116–121).

ADVERSE EVENTS AND BOTULINUM NEUROTOXIN THERAPY IN CEREBRAL PALSY

BoNT-A is generally safe in children with CP (93, 94, 98, 99). Most adverse events are localized, minor, and self-limiting. Systemic side effects including temporary incontinence and dysphagia have been reported (100). Dysphagia, aspiration, and chest infection are the most serious complications after injection of BoNT-A and if unrecognized or inadequately treated could lead to death from asphyxia (100, 122).

BOTULINUM NEUROTOXIN A AS AN ANALGESIC AGENT IN CEREBRAL PALSY

BoNT-A can be used to treat muscle spasm following operative procedures, such as adductor-release surgery (123). Injection of BoNT-A can be useful for short-term relief of pain associated with hip displacement (124). Target muscles include the hip adductors, medial hamstrings, and hip flexors. Pain relief is associated with a decrease in spastic adduction and scissoring postures (123, 124). It is not clear if short-term pain relief can be sustained by repeat injections and the need for salvage surgery avoided. Some children with neglected hip displacement have limited life expectancy and may not survive salvage surgery. BoNT-A may provide useful palliation in such circumstances (124). Better still is to prevent painful hip displacement.

SAGITTAL GAIT PATTERNS: SPASTIC HEMIPLEGIA—WINTERS, GAGE, AND HICKS

In 1987, a four-group classification of sagittal gait patterns in spastic hemiplegia was developed by Winters et al. (125). Their four-group classification has been extensively used by

Sagittal gait patterns: Spastic hemiplegia

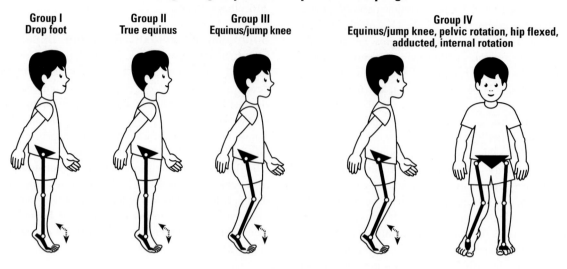

| Group I Drop foot | Group II True equinus | Group III Equinus/jump knee | Group IV Equinus/jump knee, pelvic rotation, hip flexed, adducted, internal rotation |

Sagittal gait patterns: Spastic diplegia

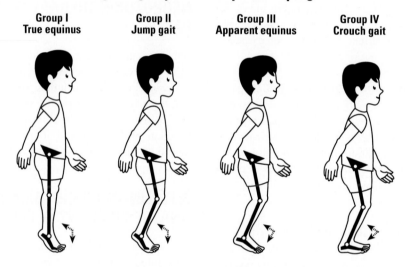

| Group I True equinus | Group II Jump gait | Group III Apparent equinus | Group IV Crouch gait |

Sagittal gait patterns

FIGURE 14-12. Sagittal gait patterns in spastic hemiplegia (based on the classification by Winters, Gage, and Hicks (127)). Sagittal gait patterns in spastic diplegia (based on Rodda and Graham (97)).

clinicians as a template for clinical management including prescription of orthoses, spasticity management by injection of BoNT-A, and musculoskeletal surgery (Fig. 14-12).

Type I Hemiplegia.
In type I hemiplegia, there is a drop foot in the swing phase of gait due to loss of selective motor control in tibialis anterior. There is no contracture of the gastrocsoleus and second rocker is relatively normal. Neither spasticity management nor musculoskeletal surgery is necessary.

Gait and function can be improved by the use of an AFO, usually a leaf spring AFO or a hinged AFO.

Type II Hemiplegia.
In type II hemiplegia, there is spasticity in the gastrocsoleus that gradually becomes fixed resulting in a contracture and equinus gait. First and second rockers at the ankle are disrupted and there may be proximal deviations related to the excessive plantar flexion at the ankle, but these are not primary gait deviations. Management of type II hemiplegia

requires correction of fixed contracture in the gastrocsoleus (to correct second rocker) and provision of an AFO (to provide heel strike and first rocker in stance as well as swing phase clearance and appropriate prepositioning of the foot during preswing).

Type III Hemiplegia.

In type III hemiplegia, there is a contracture of the gastrocsoleus at the ankle and knee involvement with co-contraction of the hamstrings and rectus femoris. Children in this transitional group may benefit from lengthening of the medial hamstrings and rectus femoris transfer (see Figs. 14-29 to 14-33), in addition to gastrocsoleus lengthening.

Type IV Hemiplegia.

In type IV hemiplegia, pathology is present at all three joints of the lower extremity. In the sagittal plane, in addition to ankle equinus and knee stiffness, there is incomplete hip extension. In the coronal plane at the hip, there is excessive adduction and in the transverse plane, excessive internal rotation. Hip dysplasia is common and often presents late. In addition to the treatments outlined above for type III, correction of type IV hemiplegic gait includes lengthening of both the adductor longus and the psoas over the brim (POTB) of the pelvis as well as a proximal femoral derotation osteotomy.

Not all children with hemiplegia fit neatly into one of the four groups described (126). Nonetheless, this is an entirely logical and very useful way of classifying hemiplegic gait with direct relevance to clinical management (127).

SAGITTAL GAIT PATTERNS—SPASTIC DIPLEGIA

Knee patterns in spastic diplegia have been classified as recurvatum knee, jump knee, stiff knee, and crouch (128). The knee classification has been extended to the sagittal plane as true equinus, jump gait, apparent equinus, and crouch gait (97) (Fig. 14-12).

True Equinus.

True equinus is characterized by walking on tip toe with extended hips and knees, as is commonly seen in younger children with spastic diplegia when they first learn to walk. The plantarflexion-knee extension couple is overactive and the ground reaction force (GRF) is in front of the knee throughout stance phase. True equinus can be managed in the younger child by injections of BoNT-A to the gastrocsoleus and the provision of hinged AFOs. By the time children develop fixed contractures and require surgery, true equinus is rare. When it persists, there are usually occult contractures of the hamstrings and iliopsoas. Single-level surgery (gastrocsoleus lengthening) is almost never the correct strategy, no matter how tempting it may appear on observational gait analysis.

Jump Gait.

Jump gait is characterized by equinus at the ankle associated with incomplete extension at the knee and hip. In the original description by Sutherland and Davids, the jump knee pattern is characterized by excessive flexion at initial contact with rapid extension in later stance to near-normal

range (128). In the pattern described by Rodda and Graham, jump gait encompasses this pattern as well as patterns in which knee extension is more severely compromised and in which there is incomplete extension at the hip (97, 127). This is the most common pattern in the preadolescent with spastic diplegia. Many children benefit from SEMLS.

Apparent Equinus.

Many children with spastic diplegia who walk on their toes, never achieving heel contact, have an ankle range of motion within the normal range. Such children are at risk of inappropriate management with injections of BoNT-A to the gastrocsoleus or even worse, lengthening of the gastrocsoleus. The important contractures are proximal at the level of the knee and hip. The recognition of "apparent equinus" in contradistinction to "true equinus" is very important to avoid inappropriate lengthening and weakening of the gastrocsoleus with further deterioration in gait and functioning. IGA is very helpful in differentiating "apparent equinus" from "true" equinus. Apparent equinus pattern is often transitional. With further growth and progression of lever arm deformities, the majority of children will eventually develop "crouch gait."

Crouch Gait.

Crouch gait is characterized by excessive knee flexion in stance, incomplete extension at the hip, and excessive ankle dorsiflexion. Knee stiffness in swing is common. The soleus is excessively long and usually weak. This is a very common gait pattern in adolescence and is often the result of natural history, accelerated by lengthening of the gastrocsoleus, especially percutaneous lengthening of the Achilles tendons. In recent reviews of crouch gait, the majority of children had lengthening of the Achilles tendons in childhood (59). A key feature of crouch gait is that the majority of MTUs are excessively long. This is by definition true for all of the one joint muscles such as soleus, quadriceps, and gluteus maximus and often for the two joint hamstrings. The only consistent contractures are of the iliopsoas. In crouch gait, the hamstrings are short only in patients with a posterior pelvic tilt. When the pelvis is in the neural range, the hamstrings are of normal length and when the pelvis is anteriorly tilted, the hamstrings are excessively long. Without the use of IGA and the plotting of muscle lengths, it is very difficult to appreciate these findings. Consequently, the majority of children with crouch gait are managed by excessive hamstring lengthening to improve knee extension when in fact the hamstrings are of normal length or excessively long. Such surgery results in increased anterior pelvic tilt that in the long term may bring its own set of problems with low back pain and increased risks of spondylolisthesis and spondylolysis (59).

BIOMECHANICAL STUDIES RELEVANT TO ORTHOPAEDIC SURGERY IN SPASTIC DIPLEGIA

In a study of muscle excursion and cross-sectional area, it was demonstrated that the gastrocsoleus and ankle dorsiflexors have such different physical characteristics that they cannot be considered to be "in balance," in either normal subjects or in children with CP (129). The plantarflexors are six times as strong as the dorsiflexors. The plantarflexors of the ankle must be balanced against the GRF not the dorsiflexors. Lifting the foot and ankle during swing phase (dorsiflexor function) requires a very small muscle moment. Push-off in terminal stance (plantarflexor function) requires a large muscle moment. The concept of muscle balance should be redefined as a requirement for balance between the three anatomical levels, hip, knee and ankle, in the sagittal plane, not at a single level (129).

Lower limb muscles have different sensitivities to surgical lengthening, related to their gross anatomy and morphology. The soleus is exquisitely sensitive to lengthening, but the iliopsoas and semitendinosus are relatively resistant. A 1-cm lengthening of the soleus reduces its moment-generating ability by 30% and a 2-cm lengthening reduces its moment by 85% (130). A small error in terms of overlengthening the soleus may be disastrous. A 4-cm lengthening of the psoas is required to reduce its moment by 50% (130). The surgical implications are to lengthen the gastrocnemius only, when there is no contracture of the soleus. When the soleus requires lengthening, a precise and stable technique should be used, with careful control of the position postoperatively in a cast. By contrast, it is difficult to overlengthen the psoas. Intramuscular lengthening at the pelvic brim without immobilization postoperatively is safe and effective.

Many children who walk with flexed knee gait have hamstrings that are of normal length. It is the psoas that is shortened and requires lengthening, not the hamstrings. It is easy to do too much hamstring lengthening and not enough psoas lengthening (59, 131, 132).

MUSCULOSKELETAL MANAGEMENT IN CEREBRAL PALSY BY GMFCS LEVEL: INTRODUCTION

The GMFCS gives an accurate summary of a child's current gross motor function and long-term prognosis (13, 15). It is difficult to frame a logical discussion of musculoskeletal management outside of the context of the GMFCS. Most disagreements in the literature are apparent rather than real because those taking opposing views are often considering a child in a different GMFCS level. The terms mild, moderate, and severe diplegia along with mild, moderate, and severe quadriplegia are not meaningful or useful. Age-appropriate GMFCS descriptors are valid, reliable, stable, and clinically meaningful (47, 49, 50). Recommendations for both gait correction surgery and surgery for hip displacement are much more easily understood when the child's GMFCS level is known. In the following sections, musculoskeletal management will be discussed by GMFCS level, in conjunction with both topographical classification and sagittal gait patterns. Gait correction surgery is an option for many children with CP at GMFCS levels I to III but with differences at each level. SEMLS will be discussed primarily in the GMFCS level II section. Preventive

hip surgery will be discussed in the GMFCS level III section, reconstructive hip surgery in the GMFCS level IV section, and salvage surgery in the GMFCS level V section. Obviously, reconstructive surgery may be appropriate at GMFCS levels III to V and salvage surgery is sometimes needed at both GMFCS IV and V but is best avoided.

GMFCS I

1. **Between 6th and 12th birthday**
   Children walk at home, school, outdoors, and in the community. They can climb stairs without the use of a railing. Children perform gross motor skills such as running and jumping, but speed, balance, and coordination are limited (13).
2. **Between 12th and 18th birthday**
   Youth walk at home, school, outdoors, and in the community. They are able to climb curbs and stairs without physical assistance or a railing. They perform gross motor skills such as running and jumping, but speed, balance, and coordination are limited (15).
3. **Risk of hip displacement:** Developmental dislocation of the hip occurs at the same rate as in the normally developing population. Spastic hip displacement is not seen (49, 50).
4. **Mean femoral neck anteversion (FNA):** 30 degrees
5. **Mean neck shaft angle (NSA):** 136 degrees
   Children at GMFCS level I participate in physical recreational activities, have a normal life expectancy, few medical comorbidities apart from epilepsy, and good levels of intellectual functioning.

Movement Disorder. Children at GMFCS level I usually have mild spasticity that is often distal with little proximal involvement. Some have mild dystonia. The movement disorder is mild and easily managed by injections of BoNT-A. Neither SDR nor ITB are appropriate choices (38, 39, 84).

Topographical Distribution. Children at GMFCS level I have either spastic hemiplegia or mild spastic diplegia. In terms of sagittal gait patterns, those with hemiplegia are usually type I or II. Those with diplegia usually have true equinus or mild jump gait.

Musculoskeletal Impairments. Hip disease and scoliosis are rare and occur with a similar prevalence as would be expected in typically developing children. If hip displacement is detected, it is usually a developmental dysplasia. If a spinal curvature develops, it will be an adolescent idiopathic-type curve.

Musculoskeletal Management GMFCS Level I: Spastic Hemiplegia
Lower Limb Surgery. Children with type I hemiplegia have a drop foot in the swing phase of gait. They may benefit from a leaf spring or a hinged AFO. Orthopaedic surgery is not required (125).

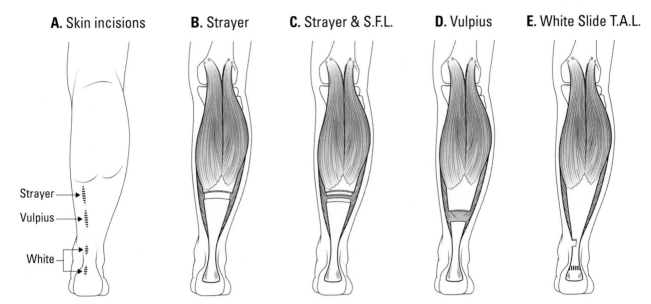

A. Skin incisions   **B.** Strayer   **C.** Strayer & S.F.L.   **D.** Vulpius   **E.** White Slide T.A.L.

Strayer

Vulpius

White

FIGURE 14-13.   Surgery for equinus deformity in cerebral palsy. **A:** The location of the skin incisions is usually posteromedial and with accurate identification of the level can be kept small, typically 2 to 3 cm for the Strayer and Vulpius procedures. The White slide TAL may be performed percutaneously, but our preference is for two small posteromedial incisions each 1.5 cm long. We prefer to see the tendon and avoid accidental complete tenotomy. **B:** The Strayer procedure is a distal gastrocnemius recession and lengthens only the gastrocnemius portion of the gastrocsoleus. It is the most useful procedure in children with diplegia and "gastrocnemius equinus." **C:** The Strayer procedure can be combined with soleal fascial lengthening (SFL). This results in a lengthening of both gastrocnemius and soleus but by different amounts, a 2:1 ratio, that is, twice as much lengthening of the gastrocnemius as for the soleus. This is the most useful procedure in children with spastic diplegia who have a moderate contracture of the gastrocnemius and a less severe contracture of the soleus. **D:** The Vulpius procedure is a Zone 2 recession of the gastrocsoleus. The shape of the cut can be the familiar inverted V. However, a simple transverse cut requires a smaller skin incision and is just as effective. This is a useful procedure in children with hemiplegia who have a moderate degree of fixed contracture affecting both the gastrocnemius and the soleus. **E:** Slide lengthening of the Achilles tendon may be performed by double hemisection as described by White. This is the most useful procedure in children with hemiplegia who have a severe contracture affecting the gastrocnemius and the soleus. For further discussion please see reference 133.

Children with type II hemiplegia develop equinus contractures and may benefit from lengthening of the gastrocsoleus. Surgery can usually be deferred until age 4 to 6 years by the use of an AFO combined with injections of BoNT-A and physical therapy. The choice of lengthening procedure is based on a careful Silverskiold test to determine the amount of contracture in the gastrocnemius and soleus, respectively (133). There are four main options as illustrated in Figure 14-13 (see Figs. 14-14 and 14-15).

Upper Limb Surgery in Spastic Hemiplegia.   Many children with hemiplegia are not candidates for upper limb surgery. Occupational therapy and physiotherapy have small treatment effects alone but are essential adjuncts to surgical management. As with lower limb surgery, there is a move toward detailed preoperative analysis, the identification of component deformities and muscle imbalances, and the development of a detailed single-event, multilevel surgical plan which is followed by casting, splinting, and rehabilitation (134, 135) (Figs. 14-16 to 14-18).

The typical upper limb deformities in CP include adduction and internal rotation of the shoulder, pronation of the forearm, wrist flexion and ulnar deviation, finger flexion, and thumb in palm (134).

Functional Impairment.   Functional deficits include problems with reaching, grasping, releasing, and manipulation and should be carefully evaluated in each child. The appearance of the limb is also a concern to children and caregivers. Gross motor function in the upper limbs in children with CP is classified using the Manual Ability Classification System (MACS), the upper limb equivalent of the GMFCS (136).

Principles of Management.   Children with spastic hemiplegia function at a high level and may require interventions aimed at developing sophisticated fine motor control for bimanual hand activities. Improving cosmesis by reducing flexion posturing of the elbow during running and flexion of the wrist with grasping activities are important goals. Simpler hand activities such as grasping and releasing assistive walking devices are the main objectives of treatment in children with more severe involvement. In those still more severely involved, ease of dressing and hygiene are the primary reasons for correcting upper limb deformities (134).

Assessment of the Upper Limb in CP.   Detailed history, standardized physical examination, and radiographs are the

Text continued on page 508

The Strayer Distal Gastrocnemius Recession (Fig. 14-14)

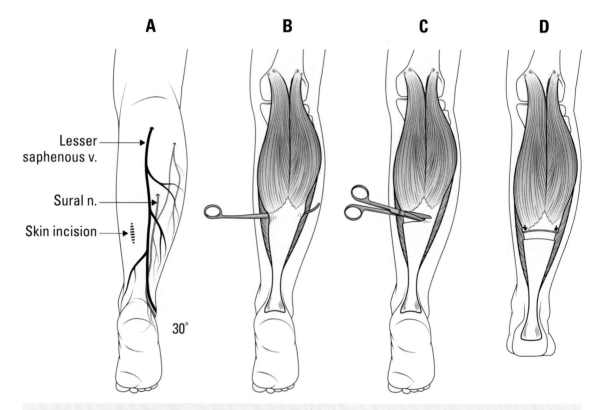

A   B   C   D

Lesser saphenous v.

Sural n.

Skin incision

30°

FIGURE 14-14. **The Strayer Distal Gastrocnemius Recession. A:** For all methods of gastrocsoleus lengthening, the superficial structures at risk of injury include the sural nerve and the lesser saphenous vein. **B:** The Strayer distal gastrocnemius recession is sometimes criticized because of the length of the skin incision required and subsequent scarring. However, with accurate identification of the interval between the gastrocnemius aponeurosis and the soleal fascia, the incision can be kept very small, typically 2 to 3 cm long. The termination of the distal medial belly of the gastrocnemius can be determined by palpation and the skin incision should be centered on this point. For those who are less experienced, this interval can be determined accurately by preoperative ultrasound and marking the skin with a surgical pen. The interval between the bellies of the gastrocnemius and the underlying soleal fascia can be developed by a combination of blunt dissection with the surgeon's finger and the use of a blunt dissector. A blunt dissector can be passed from medial to lateral through this interval and the lesser saphenous vein and sural nerve protected by retraction. **C:** Following mobilization of the gastrocnemius aponeurosis from the underlying soleal fascia, the aponeurosis is divided transversely from medial to lateral, using dissecting scissors. **D:** Following dorsiflexion of the foot, a gap opens up in the aponeurosis (without lengthening of the underlying soleus). With the knee in extension and the foot plantargrade, the gastrocnemius aponeurosis can be sutured to the underlying soleal fascia by two sutures to prevent excessive proximal retraction. We are unsure about the need for this step. We usually omit the suture in the interest of a shorter incision. Dorsiflexion of the foot to five degrees is sufficient for the majority of children with spastic diplegia because "a little equinus is better than calcaneus."

Strayer Distal Gastrocnemius Recession Combined with Soleal Fascial Lengthening (Fig. 14-15)

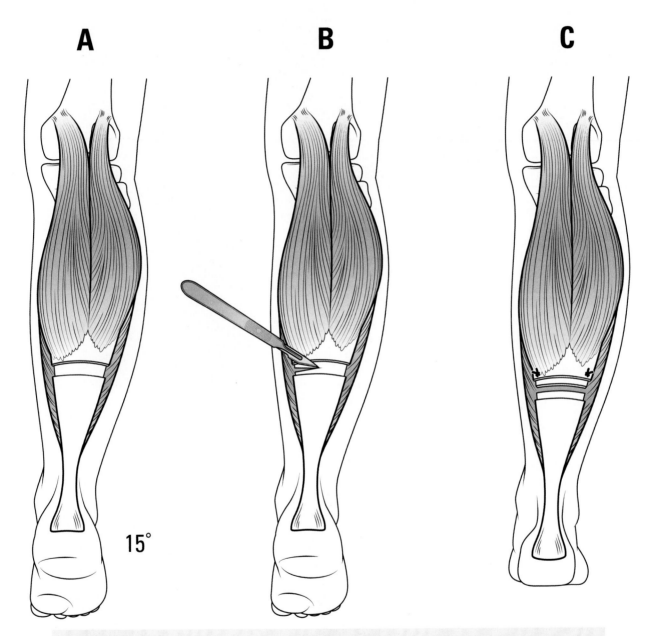

FIGURE 14-15. Strayer Distal Gastrocnemius Recession Combined with Soleal Fascial Lengthening. A: In some children, the Strayer procedure is insufficient to gain a plantargrade position of the foot. This can be confirmed by an intraoperative Silfverskiold test. When this is the case, lengthening of the soleal fascia should be considered. **B:** Following division of the gastrocnemius aponeurosis as previously described, the underlying soleal fascia can be divided transversely by sharp dissection using a scalpel. The midline raphé should also be identified and divided in the midline of the underlying soleal muscle. **C:** Following further dorsiflexion of the foot, the gastrocnemius can be sutured to the underlying soleal fascia as indicated.

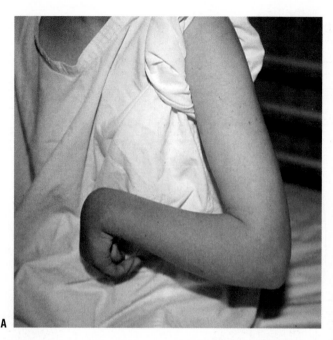

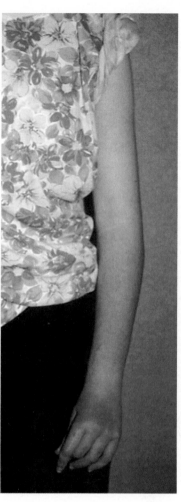

FIGURE 14-16. SEMLS for the upper extremity in spastic hemiplegia. Note the flexed elbow, flexed wrist, finger flexion, and thumb adduction following elbow flexor release. Green transfer, pronator teres rerouting fractional lengthening of the finger flexors and correction of thumb in palm, the resting posture of the limb is improved with improved function including reaching, grasp, and release. The whole view of the forearm and hand before and after is illustrated in Figure 14-16A,B. (From Chin TYP, Duncan JA, Johnstone BR, et al. Management of the upper limb in cerebral palsy. *J Pediatr Orthop B* 2005;14(6):398, with permission.)

FIGURE 14-17. The Green transfer is the single most useful tendon transfer in the hemiplegic upper limb to improve function. The flexor carpi ulnarus (FCU) is the strongest wrist flexor and ulnar deviator of the wrist. When transferred around the subcutaneous border of the ulna to the extensor carpi radialis brevis (ECRB), wrist extension is strengthened and the tendency to ulnar deviation corrected. The line of the transfer also strengthens supination. An alternative site for the transfer is to the extensor digitorum communis (EDC).

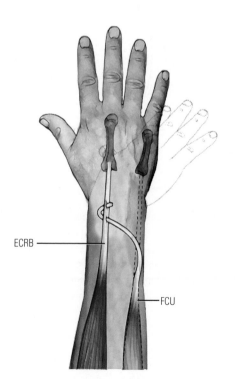

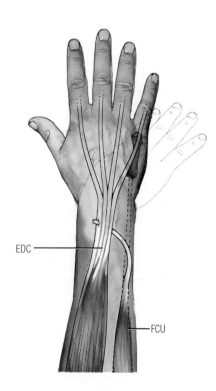

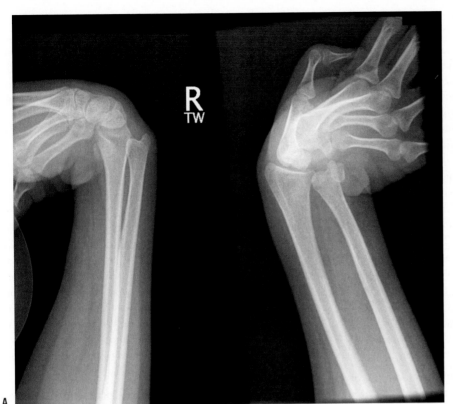

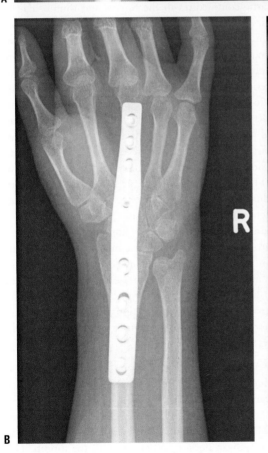

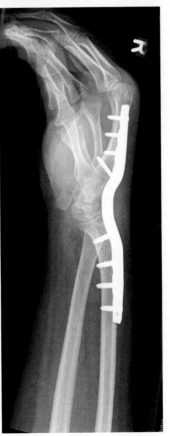

FIGURE 14-18. **A–C:** Severe wrist flexion and ulnar deviation in an adolescent with spastic hemiplegia before and after wrist fusion using a custom, contoured fixation plate. Fusion was combined with superficialis-to-profundus transfer of the finger flexors, and plication of the extensor tendons. Improvements in comfort and cosmesis were obtained with no change in function.

cornerstones of upper limb assessment. The active and passive range of motion, presence of spasticity, dystonia, contractures, selective motor control, muscle strength, and sensory deficits should be recorded (134). The child's functional use of the affected hand may be quantified according to the House Classification of Upper Extremity Functional Use (136). This nine-level classification is useful to establish baseline function, communicate functional levels and goals to parents and other clinicians, and monitor progress of treatment.

Objective evaluation of upper limb function using standardized, validated instruments such as the Melbourne Unilateral Upper Limb Assessment (Melbourne Assessment) or Quality of Upper Extremity Skills Test (QUEST) is strongly recommended to document baseline function and also assess changes following treatment (119, 120). Both scales have established reliability and validity. Video recordings of postural and functional assessments are very useful, especially when combined with an objective scoring system such as Shriner's Hospital for Children Upper Extremity Evaluation (SHUEE) (137). Kinematic analysis is developing rapidly but is not yet standardized or widely available.

Principles of Surgical Management. Almost any fixed contracture may benefit from lengthening but which procedures to use and when, requires experience and judgment (135, 138). Tendon transfers can be utilized to improve hand or wrist function. BoNT-A may also be used together with surgery as a spasticity-reducing measure or to aid with perioperative pain relief (139). Surgical results are most predictable in spastic movement disorders and are unpredictable in dystonia. Realistic expectations are vital because surgery cannot restore normal hand function or appearance (134, 135).

Elbow. Dynamic flexion contracture of the elbow is frequently seen in hemiplegic CP and is particularly marked as an associated movement during running. A transverse incision across the elbow crease can provide adequate access to perform Z lengthening of the biceps tendon, as well as a fractional lengthening of the brachialis (138) (Fig. 14-16)

Forearm Pronation. The pronator teres is the first MTU to develop a contracture in the hemiplegic upper limb. A fibrotic pronator teres can be simply released but if it has a reasonable excursion, it can be rerouted to act as a supinator (140). The forearm is immobilized in maximum passive supination with the elbow flexed to 90 degrees. Forearm pronation can also be improved by transferring flexor carpi ulnarus (FCU) to extensor carpi radialis brevis (ECRB) (Green transfer). By virtue of the dorsoulnar course of the transferred tendon, FCU becomes a secondary supinator in addition to its new role as a wrist extensor (138).

Wrist. The majority of children with hemiplegic CP have wrist flexion deformities. The two most useful procedures for wrist flexion deformities are the Green transfer and arthrodesis but for different indications. Children who have a functional hand with constant flexed wrist posturing, secondary to out-of-phase

activity in FCU, may be candidates for the Green transfer (Fig. 14-17) (135, 138). Activation of FCU can be assessed by palpating the FCU tendon as patients open and close their fingers and confirmed using dynamic electromyography. Some children have poor finger extension and an FCU working in phase with finger extensors. These children may benefit from transfer of the FCU to the extensor digitorum communis (EDC). Contractures of FCR, Palmaris longus, and the long finger flexors must be addressed at the same time (134, 135, 138).

Adolescents with severe wrist flexion contractures and limited function may appreciate the cosmetic gains and improvements in palmar hygiene from arthrodesis of the wrist, combined with soft-tissue releases (Fig. 14-18). A dorsal wrist fusion plate provides stable fixation, permits early mobilization, and has good outcomes in terms of fusion rates and deformity correction (141). The soft tissues should be rebalanced by an extensive release of all contracted MTUs and plication of the redundant wrist and finger extensors. Improvements in cosmesis are substantial because the atrophic limb appears to be longer following correction of the severe wrist flexion deformity as well as partial correction of the digital contractures. There may be minor improvements in "helper hand" functions. In appropriately selected cases, satisfaction with the procedure is very high (134, 141).

Fingers. When wrist flexion is corrected, as described above, occult spastic contractures in the fingers and thumb may be unmasked. There are three main options. Mild spastic contractures in the long flexors may respond to Botox, combined with casting (139). Fractional lengthening at the musculotendinous junctions of FDS and FDP, especially when combined with injections of BoNT-A and splinting, is effective and preserves function (138). In severe contractures, when functional goals are more limited, FDS to FDP transfer may be performed (134). The FDS tendons are divided distally, close to the wrist. The FDP tendons are exposed and are divided more proximally toward the musculotendinous junction. The proximal FDS MTUs are then repaired en masse to the distal FDP tendons to provide a degree of tension. This works well in conjunction with wrist arthrodesis.

Release of the finger flexors may unmask swan neck deformities, particularly when the intrinsic muscles of the hand are spastic. An uncorrected wrist flexion posture has a tenodesis effect on the extensors, which is expressed by deformities at the PIP joint. In addition to rebalancing the flexor and extensor tension across the PIP joints, correction of unstable swan neck deformities is performed where there is incompetence of the volar plates (142, 143).

Thumb in Palm. The "thumb-in-palm" deformity is variable and may include adduction of the first metacarpal, flexion at the metacarpophalangeal (MCP) joint, and either flexion or extension at the IP joint (143). Many children have hyperextendable MCP joints and, with adduction of the metacarpal, this leads to a swan neck–type deformity of the thumb. This is managed with a release of adductor pollicis, and the flexor pollicis brevis from the flexor retinaculum. Release of the first dorsal interosseous and the overlying fascia is also frequently required. A contracted first web space may be corrected by Z-plasty or "square flap" (143). Instability of the thumb MCP joint can be corrected by arthrodesis of the radial sesamoid of the thumb to the underlying metacarpal (143). Rerouting the EPL to the volar side of the wrist makes it an abductor, rather than an adductor of the thumb. EPL function can be augmented by transferring palmaris longus. An opponensplasty using the FDS to the ring or middle fingers can provide functional correction of a thumb-in-palm deformity.

Surgical Results. Several large retrospective studies have reported improvements in House scale, grasp and release, self-care, grip strength, and dexterity (132, 135, 144, 145). Satisfaction with both functional and cosmetic outcomes by both children and care givers is generally high (146).

Spastic Diplegia—GMFCS Level I.

Children with spastic diplegia at GMFCS level I usually have a true equinus gait pattern with mild spasticity in the gastrocsoleus and little proximal involvement. The spasticity is typically too mild and too focal to require SDR. It responds well to injections of BoNT-A and the provision of an AFO. Some children develop a mild contracture, usually involving only the gastrocnemius and not the soleus. This can be managed by distal gastrocnemius recession as described by Strayer. Careful assessment by IGA is essential to identify proximal involvement that require simultaneous correction. Isolated, single-level surgery for equinus is rarely indicated and is associated with a 40% risk of severe crouch gait, in long-term follow-up (95). The correction of proximal gait deviations will be discussed in the section on children at GMFCS level II.

GMFCS II

1. **Between 6th and 12th birthday**
   Children walk in most settings and climb stairs holding onto a railing. They may experience difficulty walking long distances and balancing on uneven terrain, inclines, in crowded areas, or confined spaces. Children may walk with physical assistance, a handheld mobility device or use wheeled mobility over long distances. Children have only minimal ability to perform gross motor skills such as running and jumping (13).
2. **Between 12th and 18th birthday**
   Youth walk in most settings but environmental factors and personal choice influence mobility choices. At school or work, they may require a handheld mobility device for safety and climb stairs holding onto a railing. Outdoors and in the community youth may use wheeled mobility when traveling long distances (15).
3. **Risk of hip displacement (MP > 30%):** 15%
4. **Mean femoral Neck Anteversion (FNA):** 36 degrees
5. **Mean Neck Shaft Angle (NSA):** 141 degrees (49, 50)
   The majority of children at GMFCS level II have either a type IV hemiplegia or a mild spastic diplegia.

Type IV Hemiplegia. In type IV hemiplegia, there is involvement of the entire lower limb. The usual pattern is equinus (equinovarus or equinovalgus) at the ankle; a stiff flexed knee; a hip that is internally rotated, adducted, and flexed; and a pelvis that is retracted (125, 147, 148). The lower limb is usually but not always spastic. The upper limb often has mixed spasticity and dystonia. In addition to increased FNA, there may be external tibial torsion (ETT) resulting in "malignant malalignment." The foot progression angle may be normal, but there is internal rotation of the femur and external rotation of the tibia. Complete correction will usually require an external rotation osteotomy of the femur and an internal rotation osteotomy at the supramalleolar level of the tibia and the fibula. Long-term reliance on the contralateral "sound" leg for push off may result in excessive ETT. It is difficult to evaluate "sound side" ETT without IGA, but it rarely requires correction.

Unilateral multilevel surgery is usually required between the ages of 6 and 10 years (147–150). It is important to note that type IV hemiplegia is associated with progressive hip displacement in a significant number of children. In the initial phases, this is clinically silent, so the hips should always have radiologic evaluation. Progressive subluxation of the hip is an indication to proceed with unilateral multilevel surgery in which stabilization of the hip and correction of the limb deformities is combined. IGA is essential in type IV hemiplegia because of the number of gait deviations and the need to differentiate between primary deviations, secondary compensations, and tertiary coping mechanisms. Shortening of both the leg and the shank is often significant (148). Clinical and CT measurement of limb segment lengths is strongly advised as well as periodic assessment of bone age. A number of children with hemiplegia benefit from contralateral epiphysiodesis to reduce limb-length discrepancy. In these children, bone age is often well ahead of chronologic age. Unilateral SEMLS in type IV hemiplegia can result in correction of hip displacement, improvements in lower limb alignment, correction of gait dysfunction, and significant improvements in both the efficiency and cosmesis of gait (147). Because of unilateral surgery and the intact lower limb, these children rehabilitate quickly and relatively easily.

Spastic Equinovarus at GMFCS II: Differences between Diplegia and Hemiplegia.

Spastic equinovarus is much more common in hemiplegia than in diplegia. Symptoms may include pain, tripping, brace intolerance, and callosities over the lateral border of the foot (110, 133). In diplegia, varus may be more apparent than real because of excessive FNA and "rollover varus." In diplegia varus is usually mild, flexible, and more prone to overcorrection into valgus than in hemiplegia. In hemiplegia, varus is often more severe, more stiff, and more likely to progress or relapse than in children with diplegia.

Evaluation should include IGA including dynamic EMG, pedobarography, and standardized radiographs in the weight-bearing position (67, 110).

There are many options for the management of spastic equinovarus in CP (133). There are few comparative studies and no clinical trials with high levels of evidence have been

CLINICAL PRESENTATION	SUGGESTED MANAGEMENT (Fig. 14-19)
Mild, dynamic varus in the younger child	Inject GS and TP with BoNT-A + AFO (84)
Mild to moderate flexible varus: diplegia	IMT TP + GR + AFO + SEMLS (151)
Moderate, flexible varus: hemiplegia	IMT TP or SPOTT + GSR+ AFO (151–153)
Moderate to severe flexible varus hemiplegia	IMT TP + SPLATT + GSR + AFO (151,154,155)
Moderate fixed varus	Soft Tissue Balancing + cal. osteotomy/shorten lateral column (133)
Severe fixed varus	Soft tissue balancing + triple arthrodesis (133, 156)

IMT, intramuscular tenotomy; GR, gastrocnemius recession; GSR, gastrocsoleus recession; SPOTT, split posterior tibialis tendon transfer; SPLATT, split anterior tibialis tendon transfer.

published. As with many management issues in CP, the stage of musculoskeletal pathology is important to determine and some appreciation of surgical "dose" is helpful.

In diplegia, intramuscular tenotomy of tibialis posterior, combined with correction of FNA, as part of SEMLS gives good results (157). In hemiplegia, equinovarus deformities are more variable in severity and more resistant to surgical correction. In younger children with documented overactivity in tibialis posterior, both intramuscular recession and SPOTT transfer are good options (110, 133, 150–152). Ideally this should be undertaken before deformities become fixed, avoiding the need for bony surgery. In children with documented overactivity in both tibialis anterior and tibialis posterior, a combination of SPLATT transfer and intramuscular tenotomy of tibialis posterior gives good long-term results (110, 133). It is easy to overestimate and overtreat the equinus component

of the equinovarus deformity. An Achilles tendon lengthening combined with a tibialis posterior lengthening may result in excessive weakening of plantarflexion, overcorrection, and poor push off. A careful examination under anesthesia will confirm that a gastrocnemius or gastrocsoleus recession is all that is required for equinus correction, in most equinovarus feet.

In children with diplegia, overcorrection to valgus is common. In children with hemiplegia, relapse to recurrent equinovarus is common (133). Postoperative bracing with an AFO may be helpful. Bony surgery may be required for fixed deformities and for some recurrent deformities but must always be combined with soft-tissue balancing. A lateral closing wedge osteotomy of the calcaneum or heel shift is useful for fixed heel varus. Calcaneocuboid shortening/fusion is useful to correct adductus and supination. Triple arthrodesis should be avoided because it is unsatisfactory end-stage, salvage

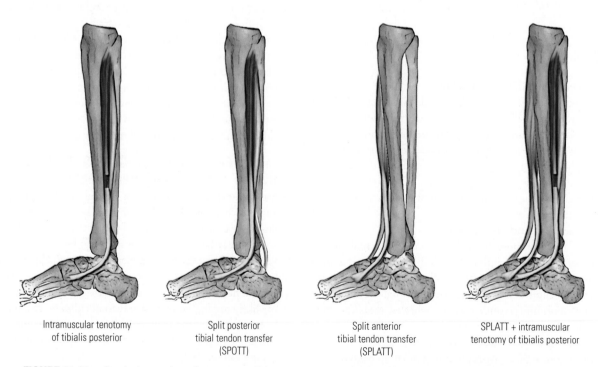

| Intramuscular tenotomy of tibialis posterior | Split posterior tibial tendon transfer (SPOTT) | Split anterior tibial tendon transfer (SPLATT) | SPLATT + intramuscular tenotomy of tibialis posterior |

FIGURE 14-19. Surgical procedures for pes varus. (Modified from Graham HK. Cerebral palsy. In: McCarthy JJ, Drennan JC. *Drennan's the child's foot & ankle*, 2nd ed. Philadelphia, PA: Lippincott Williams & Wilkins; 2010:188–218, Chapter 13.)

Birthday Syndrome: Mercer Rang

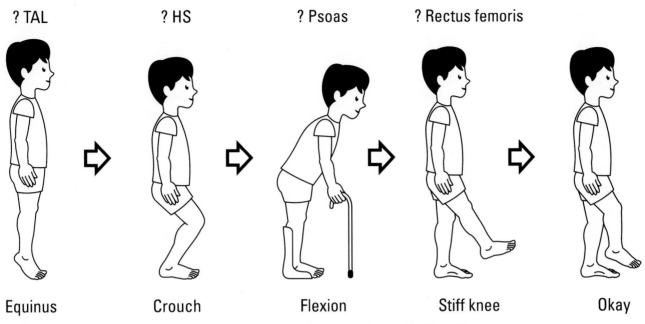

FIGURE 14-20.   The Birthday Syndrome as described by Mercer Rang.

surgery (156). It will not be necessary if soft-tissue balancing is performed at the appropriate age and stage (133).

GMFCS II—Moderate Spastic Diplegia

Movement Disorder Management.   The movement disorder is usually spastic, especially in those born prematurely. If the spasticity is mild and mainly distal, it can be managed by multilevel injections of BoNT-A repeated at 6- to 12-month intervals. SDR may be a better option when the spasticity is severe, generalized, and adversely affecting gait and function (38, 88).

Hip Displacement GMFCS II.   In spastic diplegia, GMFCS level II, the shape of the proximal femur is abnormal with a mean FNA of 36 degrees and a 15% risk of hip displacement (49, 50). The hip displacement is generally mild and progresses slowly. Preventive surgery consisting of lengthening of the hip adductors is usually effective (148). Lengthening of the psoas at the pelvic brim may be required (157, 158). Hip displacement and gait dysfunction can be successfully managed by intertrochanteric proximal femoral osteotomy with derotation and a very small amount of varus. The hip abductors are frequently weak and correction of the NSA should therefore be to normal values. Excessive varus weakens the hip abductors and causes a Trendelenburg gait.

Musculoskeletal Pathology.   Musculoskeletal pathology in spastic diplegia GMFCS level II includes increased FNA and contractures of the two joint muscles, the psoas, hamstrings, and gastrocnemius (29, 30). There is usually pes valgus and in

adolescents hallux valgus. There is sometimes excessive ETT resulting in lower limb malalignment. In asymmetric diplegia, pelvic retraction may make clinical estimation of rotational alignment during gait very difficult, without IGA (Fig. 14-20).

The Birthday Syndrome and SEMLS.   The natural history of *deformities* in the lower limbs at GMFCS level II is for gradual progression during childhood with more rapid deterioration during the adolescent growth spurt (29). The natural history of *gait* is progressive deterioration including increasing stiffness throughout the lower limb joints and increasing tendency to flexed knee gait and ultimately crouch gait (16–18). The transition from equinus gait to crouch gait is often accelerated by procedures that weaken the gastrocsoleus, especially lengthening of the Achilles tendons (95) (Fig. 14-21).

Surgery for children with spastic diplegia used to start at the ankles with TALs for equinus gait. This achieved foot-flat but at the expense of rapidly increasing hip and knee flexion (95). The second stage of surgery was then to lengthen the hamstrings in order to improve knee extension. This resulted in increased hip flexion and anterior pelvic tilt, so eventually the hip flexors were lengthened. Finally, transfer of the rectus femoris was considered for knee stiffness. This approach was caricatured by Mercer Rang as the "Birthday Syndrome" (148). Children spent most of their birthdays in hospital, in casts, or in rehabilitation.

The current concept for the management of musculoskeletal deformities is SEMLS (40, 148). In this approach, the gait pattern is identified and evaluated by IGA as part of

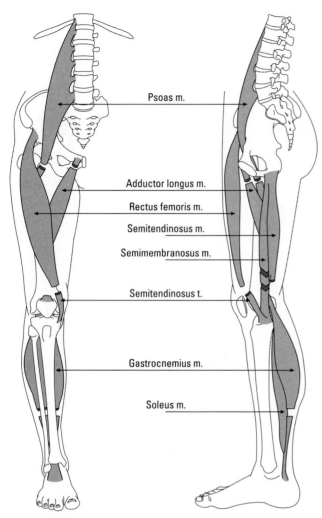

FIGURE 14-21. The most commonly used soft-tissue procedures in Single Event Multilevel Surgery. (From Bache CE, Selber P, Graham HK. Mini-Symposium: cerebral palsy: the management of spastic diplegia. *Curr Orthopaed* 2003;17:88–104, with permission.)

6. Close monitoring of functional recovery (63)
7. Follow-up gait analysis at 12 to 24 months after the index surgery (159)
8. Removal of fixation plates and other implants (159)
9. Follow-up until skeletal maturity, for new or recurrent deformities (63).

The surgical team should consist of two experienced surgeons and two assistants. None of the surgical procedures are particularly complex, but a single surgeon is unable to perform 8 to 16 consecutive procedures without fatigue and diminished performance (159). Expert anesthesia and pain management is essential. Epidural analgesia is required to make SEMLS acceptable on social and humanitarian grounds (157). Postoperative nursing care must be vigilant. The use of epidural analgesia carries risks of masking the signs of compartment syndromes, nerve stretch palsies, and decubitus ulceration. The surgery is a series of steps that correct deformity. However, for 6 to 9 months after surgery, children are more dependent and less functional than they were prior to surgery. A child who walks into hospital with a typical diplegic gait pattern, leaves hospital in a wheelchair with straighter legs but may be unable to walk independently for weeks or even months. Only a carefully tailored and carefully monitored rehabilitation program can ensure that the child will reach a higher level of function (63, 157).

Weight bearing should commence within a few days if there has been no bony surgery, or a femoral osteotomy with stable internal fixation. The maximum acceptable delay to full weight bearing is 2 weeks, if there has been extensive reconstructive surgery at the foot-ankle level (157). Casts are only required after foot and ankle surgery. Removable extension splints may be used at the knee level after hamstring-rectus surgery. The goal is to achieve full extension of the knee, combined with regaining full flexion, so that the transferred rectus femoris does not become scarred and adherent in its new site. New AFOs must be prepared for immediate fitting after cast removal, usually 6 weeks after surgery. The initial postoperative brace is either a Ground Reaction or Saltiel AFO (GRAFO) or a solid AFO. The orthotic prescription must be carefully monitored throughout the first year after surgery (63, 157). A less supportive AFO, such as a hinged or a posterior leaf spring, may be introduced when the sagittal plane balance has been restored and the plantar-flexion, knee-extension couple is competent. Functional recovery and orthotic prescription can be monitored by a gait laboratory visit every 3 months for the first year after surgery and yearly thereafter.

the diagnostic matrix (40, 68). A comprehensive plan is then developed for the correction of all muscle tendon contractures, torsional malalignments, and joint instabilities in one operative session (157, 159). Rehabilitation requires at least 1 year and improvements continue into the 2nd and 3rd years, postoperatively. The GMFCS descriptors for children at level II, aged 12 to 18, include the need for assistive devices for longer distances (15). Children who have optimal biomechanical alignment of their lower limbs by multilevel surgery continue to function independently throughout the second and third decades of life.

The principal components of a successful SEMLS program are:

1. Planning based on the diagnostic matrix, including gait analysis (68)
2. Preparation and education of the child and family (157)
3. Optimal perioperative care, including epidural analgesia (157)
4. Carefully planned and supervised rehabilitation (159)
5. Appropriate orthotic prescription (157)

Soft-Tissue Surgery: Lengthening of Contracted Muscle-tendon Units (The Two Joint Muscles)

1. Lengthening of the psoas "over the brim" (POTB) (158, 160)
2. Percutaneous or open lengthening of adductor longus (157) (see Figs. 14-35 to 14-40)
3. Medial hamstring lengthening (MHS) (161)
4. Distal gastrocnemius recession (Strayer) (162) (Fig. 14-22) (see Figs. 14-14 and 14-15)

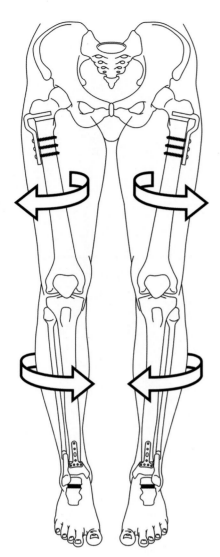

FIGURE 14-22. The most commonly used bony procedures in single event multilevel surgery; femoral derotation, supramalleolar osteotomy of the tibia, and stabilization of the midfoot. (From Bache CE, Selber P, Graham HK. Mini-Symposium: cerebral palsy: the management of spastic diplegia. *Curr Orthopaed* 2003;17:88–104, with permission.)

Soft-Tissue Surgery: Tendon Transfers

1. Transfer of rectus femoris to the semitendinosus or gracilis (163, 164)
2. Transfer of the semitendinosus to the adductor tubercle.
3. SPLATT for the varus foot (154, 155)

Bony Surgery: Rotational Osteotomies

1. External rotation osteotomy of the femur (165, 166)
2. Internal rotation osteotomy of the tibia (167–169) (Fig. 14-22)

Bony Surgery: Joint Stabilization

1. Hip: varus derotation osteotomy (VDRO) (150, 169).
2. Os calcis lengthening (170).
3. Talo-navicular fusion.
4. Subtalar fusion (171).

Occasional Procedures

1. Pelvic osteotomy (172)
2. Fusion first MTP joint for hallux valgus (173)
3. Epiphysiodesis for LLD (157)
4. "Guided Growth": Staples or "8" plates for knee flexion deformity (174, 175)

Principles of Surgical Treatment: Dynamic Ankle Function. Contractures of the gastrocnemius and soleus can be measured by comparing the range of ankle dorsiflexion with the knee flexed (soleus) and extended (gastrocnemius). The Silverskiold test should be performed both before surgery and during surgery for equinus in order to select the correct surgical "dose" (133). Hindfoot valgus in weight bearing is often associated with breaching of the midfoot, lateral subluxation of the navicular on the talus, abduction of the forefoot, and an increasingly external foot progression angle. This reduces stance phase stability and the GRF is also maldirected out of the plane of progression, resulting in abnormal stresses on proximal joints (176).

Standardized weight-bearing radiographs of the foot and ankle mortise are required in all children (67). Excessive ETT is frequently found with the valgus/abducted foot, and careful clinical and radiologic assessment is required to determine how much of each deformity is present (133). Accurate measurement of tibial torsion by physical examination is difficult. Three techniques have been described: the thigh-foot-angle, the bimalleolar axis, and the "second toe test" (176, 177).

Foot and Ankle: Soft-Tissue Surgery. The gastrocnemius is always more contracted than the soleus in spastic diplegia, and selective lengthening of the gastrocnemius is best for the majority of children (162). Even when a contracture of the soleus is present, differential lengthening of the gastrocnemius and soleus by a combination of the Strayer procedure combined with soleal fascial lengthening (SFL) is biomechanically more appropriate and safer than other procedures. Only very severe and neglected equinus deformity requires lengthening of the Achilles tendons. The White slide technique, performed under direct vision, is a much more controlled and satisfactory procedure than the triple hemisection technique, performed percutaneously (133, 178).

The main complication is gradual failure of the plantar-flexion, knee extension couple, leading to calcaneus gait, which is more disabling and difficult to treat than the original equinus gait. In diplegia, "a little equinus is better than calcaneus" (148). Isolated lengthening of the gastrocsoleus will result in the crouch gait in up to 40% of children with spastic diplegia (95). The "overlengthening" is mediated by biomechanical changes and growth, not surgical imprecision. When the GRF falls behind the knee, the soleus responds to the continual stretch by adding more sarcomeres in series. In time, the soleus becomes functionally too long, biomechanically incompetent and calcaneus-crouch progresses rapidly (59). Deferring the surgery until age 6 to 8 years reduces the risks of

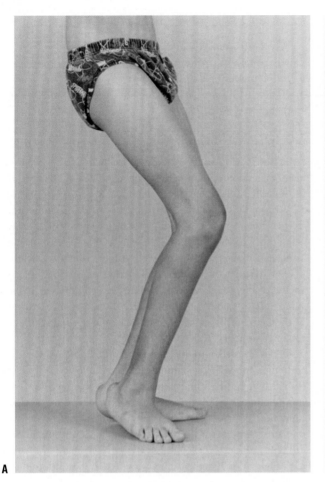
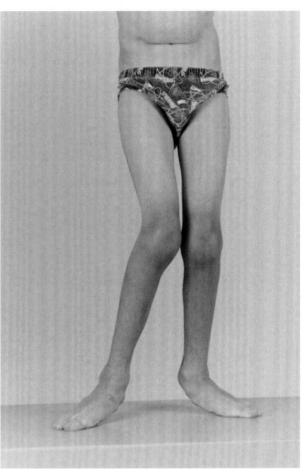

A

B

FIGURE 14-23. **A and B:** Sagittal and coronal views of a 10-year-old boy with spastic diplegia showing the characteristic musculoskeletal pathology. The sagittal view shows jump alignment with mild equinus at the ankle and significant flexion deformities at the hip and knee. In the coronal plane, there is internal rotation of both femora, external rotation deformities in both tibiae resulting in "malignant malalignment" that is asymmetric. The external foot progression angle is a combination of external tibial torsion and pes valgus.

both recurrence and overcorrection (95). The more proximal operations on the gastrocsoleus are the most stable and safest in terms of avoiding calcaneus (162, 179–181) (Fig. 14-23).

Surgical Technique (Strayer). With the patient in the prone position, a posteromedial incision, 2 to 3 cm long, is made, centered over the musculotendinous junction of the gastrocnemius. The deep fascia is divided longitudinally, and the sural nerve and lesser saphenous vein are identified and protected. The plane between the gastrocnemius and the soleus is identified from the medial side and developed by blunt dissection. Once the two layers have been separated, the aponeurosis of gastrocnemius is divided transversely, the muscle bellies are allowed to recess proximally and are then sutured in the appropriate position (ankle in neutral, knee in extension). If the range of dorsiflexion is still limited to less than plantigrade, with the knee in extension, the fascia overlying the muscle belly of soleus can be divided transversely. After wound

closure, a below knee cast is applied, with the ankle at neutral. This remains in place for 6 weeks and is then replaced by an ankle foot orthosis. This surgery is inherently stable and immediate weight bearing is encouraged (133, 151, 162, 182, 183) (Fig. 14-24A,B).

Foot and Ankle: Bony Surgery. Equinus leads to excessive loading of the forefoot and with time may cause breaching of the midfoot. A series of complex segmental malalignments of the midfoot, hindfoot, and forefoot develops referred to as pes equinoplanovalgus, pes planoabductovalgus, or simply "pes valgus." The component parts are valgus of the heel, pronation of the midfoot with flattening of the medial longitudinal arch, pronation and abduction of the forefoot with hallux valgus (Figs. 14-25 and 14-26A,B). Symptoms may include pain and callosities over the collapsed medial arch, particularly the head of the talus. This leads to pain, inability to wear AFOs, and discomfort in shoes. Evaluation includes the usual

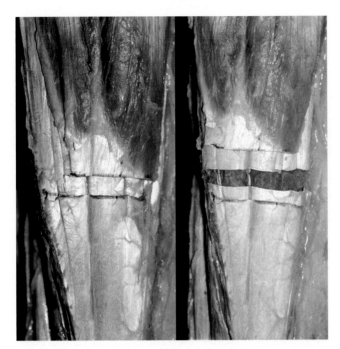

FIGURE 14-24. Cadaver dissection to demonstrate the distal gastrocnemius recession described by Strayer. The broad gastrocnemius aponeurosis has been divided transversely, at the distal extent of the medial gastrocnemius belly. This results in isolated lengthening of the gastrocnemius and is the safest procedure for equinus in diplegia because it avoids the risk of weakening of the soleus. In some children, lengthening of the soleus maybe required and this is illustrated on the right where the soleus fascia has been divided transversely exposing the soleus muscle fibers in the intervening gap. Note that when the Strayer procedure is combined with soleal fascial lengthening, the gastrocnemius is lengthened by more than the soleus that is biomechanically appropriate for the majority of children with spastic diplegia. (From Firth GB, McMullan M, Chin T, et al. Lengthening of the gastrocnemius-soleus complex. An anatomical and biomechanical study in human cadavers. *J Bone Joint Surg* 2013;95-A:1489–1496, with permission.)

components of the diagnostic matrix with special emphasis on weight-bearing radiographs of the feet and ankles, rather than motion analysis (68). A useful guide to the radiographic functional anatomy of the foot, with normal values for a series

of radiographic parameters, has been published (67). Factors affecting the choice of operative procedure include the age of the patient and the clinical and radiographic severity of the deformity (133). The flexibility of the deformity is crucial because the commonly used surgical techniques depend on ligamentotaxis for the correction of all component parts of the deformity. The corrigibility of the deformity should be checked by placing the foot in an equinovarus position, while palpating the medial arch with special attention to the talonavicular joint. As the foot moves into equinovarus, the medial arch should be restored and the navicular should cover the head of the talus.

The midfoot can be stabilized and deformity corrected by lengthening of the lateral column of the foot (os calcis lengthening) or extra-articular fusion of the subtalar joint (170, 171, 184–186). Os calcis lengthening corrects subtalar joint eversion and midfoot breaching by elongating the lateral column of the foot, driving the heel out of valgus, into relative varus and raising the medial arch. This procedure has the advantage of preserving subtalar motion. The indication for os calcis lengthening is a flexible valgus deformity of the heel in association with an abductus deformity of the forefoot, in a patient who walks independently, GMFCS I or II (133, 186). Arthrodesis of the subtalar joint is a reliable means of correcting hindfoot valgus and with secondary correction of the midfoot. It is useful for more severe deformities in patients who require assistive devices and long-term orthotic support, GMFCS III and IV (133, 185). A modified Fulford technique is best, with a cannulated screw passed through the talar neck, across the sinus tarsi into the calcaneum, combined with iliac crest autograft or allograft (171). A third option for the correction of pes valgus in CP is calcaneo-cuboid-cuneiform (triple C) osteotomy (187). A fourth option which is gaining in popularity is isolated fusion of the talo-navicular joint.

Hallux valgus is commonly associated with deformities in the hindfoot, midfoot, and proximal gait deviations, such as stiff-knee gait, which causes toe scuffing. The most reliable procedure is fusion of the first MCP joint, either in conjunction with, or after correction of the proximal deformities. A cup-and-cone reamer technique with dorsal plate and screw fixation is effective and reliable (133, 173).

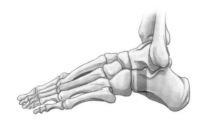 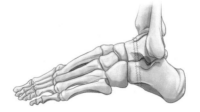 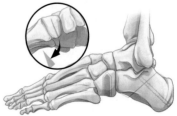

A Lateral column lengthening   **B** Extra-articular subtalar fusion   Calcaneo-cuboid-cuneiform osteotomy   **C**

FIGURE 14-25. The three principal procedures for the correction of flexible pes valgus in CP. **A:** Lateral column lengthening. **B:** Extra-articular subtalar fusion (Dennyson and Fulford technique). **C:** The triple C osteotomy, closing lateral wedge of the cuboid, heel shift to the calcaneum, and opening medial wedge in the medial cuneiform. (Modified from Graham HK. Cerebral palsy. In: McCarthy JJ, Drennan JC. *Drennan's the child's foot & ankle,* 2nd ed. Philadelphia, PA: Lippincott Williams & Wilkins; 2010:188–218, Chapter 13.)

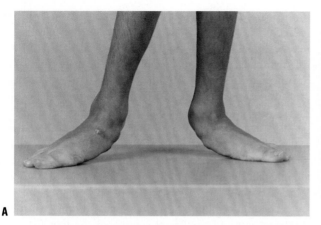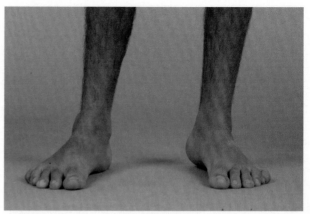

FIGURE 14-26. **A and B:** Severe pes valgus, and ETT in a 10-year-old boy with severe spastic diplegia before and after surgical correction that included Strayer gastrocnemius recessions, internal supramalleolar osteotomy of the tibia, and bilateral midfoot stabilization. Foot pain was relieved and he was able to resume wearing AFOs.

Surgical Technique: Os Calcis Lengthening. There are four principal steps, correct the equinus deformity, lengthen the lateral column, assess the medial column, and assess the ankle and tibia. Gastrocnemius recession to permit 5 degrees of dorsiflexion in subtalar neural is usually required (133) (Fig. 14-25).

An Ollier incision or a longitudinal incision can be used to approach the lateral aspect of the Os calcis. The aim of the surgery is to perform an osteotomy parallel to and approximately 1 cm proximal to the calcaneocuboid joint. The osteotomy should be between the middle and anterior facets of the subtalar joint. The osteotomy site is distracted with special distraction forceps, and a trapezoid of autologous or allograft corticocancellous bone is inserted. Some surgeons use a longitudinal K wire to transfix the osteotomy, the graft, and the calcaneocuboid joint. Calcaneocuboid subluxation is a risk that must be avoided. We prefer a stable, "press-fit" tricortical iliac crest allograft, without internal fixation, in the majority of children. After insertion of the graft, the alignment of the first ray and forefoot should be checked to determine if a plantarflexion osteotomy of the medial cuneiform is required to correct supination of the forefoot, unmasked by correction of the midfoot. The need for this procedure is not well defined and differences in practice in the literature may relate to the age of the patient and the stage of the deformity (133). Additional deformities that may need correction include ETT (SMO) and ankle valgus (SMO, guided growth).

Postoperatively, non–weight bearing in a below knee cast is advised for 2 weeks, followed by 4 weeks of weight bearing, protected in a cast, to a total of 6 weeks. At 6 weeks after surgery, graft incorporation is usually adequate to permit cast removal and fitting of an AFO. Short-term results are very good but failure may occur with time, particularly in more involved children, GMFCS III and IV (133, 170).

Foot and Ankle: Supramalleolar Osteotomy of the Tibia. ETT may occur in isolation or in conjunction with medial femoral torsion. In isolation, ETT results in an external foot progression angle and "lever arm disease" because the foot lever is effectively shortened and maldirected, in relation to the line of progression. Derotational osteotomy of the tibia is an effective means of addressing this problem (150). A very distal, supramalleolar osteotomy of the tibia is preferred 1-2 cm proximal to the distal tibial physis, which increases the cross-sectional area of contact between the two osteotomy surfaces. This increases stability, facilitates early weight bearing, minimizes the risk of secondary deformities, and is associated with reliable and rapid union. In order to gain the desired degree of rotation (which can be determined using transverse plane kinematic data), the fibula may sometimes need to be divided at the same level as the tibia. The osteotomy of the tibia may be stabilized using a straight DC plate, crossed Kirschner wires or the AO/ASIF small fragment, contoured T plate (150, 161, 163, 164). External foot progression angle is usually the result of combined pes valgus and ETT. The decision to perform os calcis lengthening, SMO, or a combination requires a very careful assessment using all components of the diagnostic matrix (68, 133). Finally, ETT may be disguised by increased FNA (malignant malalignment). The torsional deformities in both the femur and tibia should be corrected (Fig. 14-27).

Knee. The principal gait dysfunctions are stiffness and excessive flexion. Recurvatum is sometimes seen after excessive hamstring lengthening with an equinus contracture. Hamstring spasticity and contracture are often evaluated by measuring the popliteal angle. Unfortunately, the popliteal angle has little correlation with knee flexion during gait. Hamstring function is better assessed dynamically, based on muscle elongation rates and muscle lengths in the second half of swing (149). Improvements in knee extension during late swing occur when decisions regarding hamstring lengthening are made consistent with muscle length and velocity data. When hamstrings are lengthened in cases of normal hamstring function (normal muscle length and velocity in swing), excessive anterior pelvic tilt and pelvic range of motion may develop (Fig. 14-28).

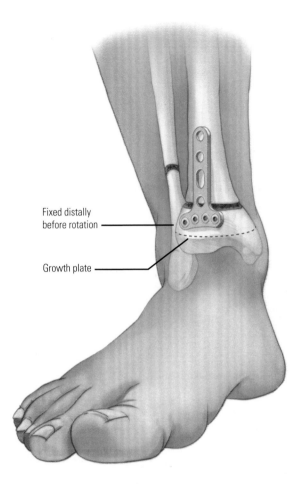
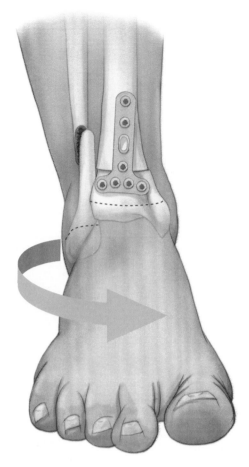

Fixed distally
before rotation

Growth plate

FIGURE 14-27.   The technique of supramalleolar osteotomy of the distal tibia and fibula, with "T" plate fixation. The "T" plate is fixed to the distal tibia, 1 cm above the physis, prior to osteotomy of the tibia and fibula. The plate is then removed, the osteotomy is performed, the external rotation deformity is corrected, and the plate reapplied to fix the distal tibia, in the corrected position. (Modified from Selber P, Filho ER, Dallalana R, et al. Supramalleolar derotation osteotomy of the tibia, with T plate fixation: technique and results in patients with neuromuscular disease. *J Bone Joint Surg* 2004;86-B:1170–1175.)

Knee: Soft-Tissue Surgery.   Fractional lengthening of the medial hamstrings can be accomplished through a midline posterior incision just above the knee. Gracilis and semitendinosus are lengthened in continuity by intramuscular tenotomy and the semimembranosus, by performing one or two stripes through its broad aponeurosis (157, 161). The semitendinosus or gracilis may be harvested at the time of medial hamstring lengthening, for subsequent transfer of the rectus femoris. The rectus can be detached distally from the patella and "tubed" around the harvested semitendinosus or gracilis tendon. Early mobilization is required to prevent adhesion formation (157) (Fig. 14-28).

There are two major problems with distal hamstring lengthening. Firstly, it frequently fails to achieve adequate knee extension during gait suggesting that other factors are causative. Secondly, it may cause or exacerbate anterior pelvic tilt (59). If an anterior pelvic tilt is present preoperatively, hamstring lengthening should either not be done or should be done cautiously and in conjunction with other efforts to treat the anterior pelvic tilt. Distal hamstring lengthening works best for mild dynamic deformities, in children at GMFCS levels I and

II without any fixed flexion contracture at the knee. Distal hamstring lengthening is ineffective when knee flexion contracture exceeds about 5 to 10 degrees. When knee flexion deformity exceeds 5 degrees, in GMFCS III and IV, we prefer distal hamstring lengthening combined with transfer of the semitendinosus to the adductor tubercle (188) (see Figs. 14-29 to 14-33).

Hip.   Hip flexion contractures are common and should be managed by lengthening of the psoas tendon at the brim of the pelvis (157, 158). Tenotomy at the lesser trochanter may result in excessive weakness of hip flexion and is reserved for the nonambulant patient. In the Sutherland technique, the femoral nerve is first identified and protected, before the psoas tendon is sectioned. It is inherently safer than the alternative technique, a modification of the approach to the psoas tendon described by Salter for innominate osteotomy of the pelvis. In this approach, the psoas is identified by palpation, lying between the iliacus muscle and the periosteum of the ilium, but the femoral nerve is not visualized (158). Both techniques are effective in the correction of hip flexion contracture and the associated gait

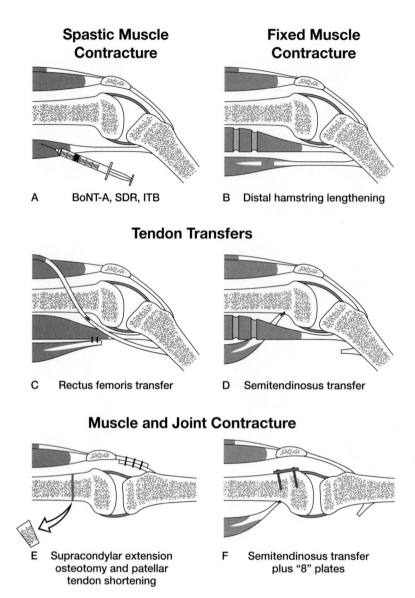

FIGURE 14-28. Management options for flexed knee gait in CP. (From Young JL, Rodda J, Selber P, et al. Management of the knee in spastic diplegia: what is the dose? *Orthoped Clin North Am* 2010;41:561–577, with permission.)

disturbance. The principal risk is injury to the femoral nerve because it is mistaken for the psoas tendon. Bilateral femoral nerve injuries have occurred but have not been reported by experienced surgeons. The Sutherland technique may be safer for less experienced surgeons (158). This is a stable lengthening and does not require immobilization. Prone positioning is required postoperatively to encourage hip extension.

Hip: Bony Surgery. Proximal femoral osteotomy is usually performed with the patient in the prone position, when the rotational arcs of both hips can be easily checked before and during surgery. A 90- or 100-degree AO/ASIF blade plate is used to achieve stable fixation. Anteversion is corrected to about 10 degrees, leaving only 10 to 20 degrees of internal rotation at the hip. The proximal osteotomy effectively lengthens the psoas and is the preferred technique (159) (see Figs. 14-35 to 14-40).

SEMLS is an exercise in correcting anatomical deformities based on clinical and radiologic examination and a biomechanical analysis of gait deviations. However, children with spastic diplegia have psychological and physiologic dimensions, which make successful surgical outcomes unpredictable. Weakness is a fundamental issue that is easily overlooked and may have a greater impact on energy cost of walking and function in the community than multiple musculoskeletal deformities (151). Careful preoperative assessment and goal setting helps to ensure that parent and surgeon goals are consistent. The majority of children have a satisfactory correction of gait but remain in their preoperative GMFCS level.

A recent systematic review of SEMLS found evidence for large improvements in gait dysfunction and moderate improvements in health-related quality of life. Changes in gross motor function were generally small and inconsistent (189).

Text continued on page 520

Distal Medial Hamstring Lengthening Combined with Transfer of the Rectus Femoris to Semitendinosus (Figs. 14-29 to 14-33)

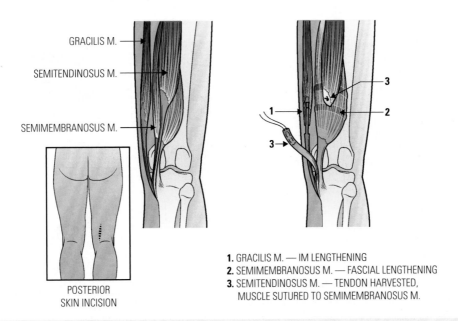

GRACILIS M.

SEMITENDINOSUS M.

SEMIMEMBRANOSUS M.

POSTERIOR
SKIN INCISION

3
1
2
3

1. GRACILIS M. — IM LENGTHENING
2. SEMIMEMBRANOSUS M. — FASCIAL LENGTHENING
3. SEMITENDINOSUS M. — TENDON HARVESTED,
   MUSCLE SUTURED TO SEMIMEMBRANOSUS M.

FIGURE 14-29. **Distal Medial Hamstring Lengthening Combined with Transfer of the Rectus Femoris to Semitendinosus.** In the majority of children, lengthening of the medial hamstrings is performed first, with the patient in the prone position. The position of the skin incision is indicated and with experience and good retraction, can be restricted to between 4 and 6 cm long on the posteromedial aspect of the distal thigh, terminating just above the popliteal crease. The gracilis is lengthened by an intramuscular technique. The semimembranosus muscle is lengthened by one or two transverse divisions of the fascial coat. The semitendinosus muscle is sutured to the underlying semimembranosus to prevent retraction and loss of important hip extensor function. The semitendinosus is then divided at the musculotendinous junction, secured with a whip stitch and mobilized distally to its insertion on the posteromedial aspect of the proximal tibia. The harvested semitendinosus tendon is placed in a subcutaneous position on the medial aspect of the distal thigh. A subcutaneous pocket is developed by blunt finger dissection. The incision is then closed in layers, a sterile dressing is applied. The patient is then turned into the supine position and the lower limbs prepared and redraped.

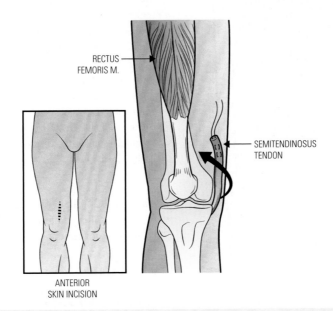

RECTUS
FEMORIS M.

SEMITENDINOSUS
TENDON

ANTERIOR
SKIN INCISION

FIGURE 14-30. With the patient in the supine position a second incision is made on the anteromedial aspect of the thigh starting at the proximal medial pole of the patella and extending 4 to 6 cm proximally. The interval between the rectus femoris tendon and the underlying vastus intermedius is identified and mobilized by blunt dissection.

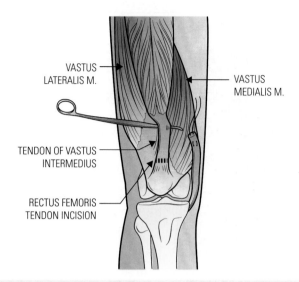

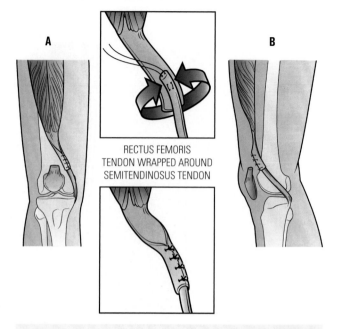

FIGURE 14-31. The rectus femoris tendon needs to be fully mobilized from the underlying tendon of the vastus intermedius distally. Proximally it needs to be separated from the overlapping bellies of the vastus medialis and lateralis. In the interests of cosmesis, it is important to use a small skin incision and to accomplish the proximal dissection by visualization using well placed retractors. Once the tendon of the rectus femoris has been fully mobilized from the underlying vastus intermedius, it is divided transversely just above its insertion on the patella.

FIGURE 14-33. The relatively flat tendon of the rectus femoris is then transferred medially to meet the previously harvested tendon of the semitendinosus. The flat rectus femoris tendon is wrapped around the semitendinosus to form a tube and secured by a combination of the previous whip stitch in the semitendinosus combined with interrupted sutures to the rectus femoris. To permit a stable repair and early mobilization it is recommended that a nonabsorbable suture such as Ethibond is utilized. It is vitally important that the trajectory of the rectus femoris be smooth and unencumbered by adhesions or subcutaneous fascia as shown in both **A** and **B** from the anterior and medial aspects. Postoperative rehabilitation is crucial. Active and passive range of motion exercises are commenced on the first postoperative day. We recommend regaining 30 degrees of knee flexion by the end of the first postoperative week, 60 degrees of knee flexion by the end of the second postoperative week, and 90 degrees at the end of the third postoperative week. During this time, full knee extension is maintained by the use of a removable knee immobilizer. Cast immobilization cannot be used because adhesions will form and the transferred tendon will not regain gliding motion. If there are any concerns about the patient's ability to comply with early active and passive range of motion exercises then continuous passive motion (CPM) is a useful alternative.

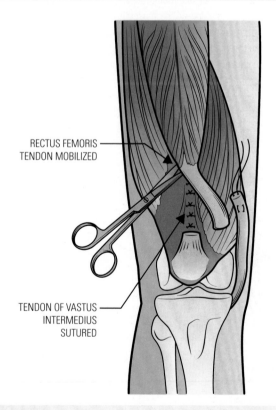

FIGURE 14-32. Any defects in the vastus intermedius and the capsule of the knee joint are carefully repaired. It is also helpful to approximate the vastus medialis to the lateralis underneath the rectus femoris to minimize dead space and prevent adhesions.

The first RCT of SEMLS reported a 50% improvement in gait function (Gillette Gait Index, GGI) and a 4.9% improvement in gross motor function (GMFM-66) (159).

GMFCS III

1. **Between 6th and 12th birthday**
   Children walk using a handheld mobility device in most outdoor settings. They may climb stairs holding onto a railing with supervision or assistance. Children use wheeled mobility when traveling long distances and may self-propel for shorter distances (13).

2. **Between 12th and 18th birthday**

   Youth are capable of walking using a handheld mobility device. They may climb stairs holding onto a railing with supervision or assistance. At school, they may self-propel a manual wheelchair or use powered mobility. Outdoors and in the community youth are transported in a wheelchair or use powered mobility (15).

3. **Risk of hip displacement:** 41%
4. **Mean femoral neck anteversion (FNA):** 40 degrees
5. **Mean neck shaft angle (NSA):** 149 degrees (49, 50)

At GMFCS level III, children and adults ambulate in the community using an assistive device. The predominant movement disorder at GMFCS level III is spasticity, but some children have dystonia or a mixed movement disorder. Weakness of the major lower limb muscles, particularly those contributing to body support, is a major feature. Flexed knee gait patterns predominate and weakness is usually the primary determinant of long-term gait and community function rather than spasticity (79, 97). It is important to differentiate between those individuals who are "being pulled down" by spasticity and those who are "falling down" because of weakness (85). The strength and selective motor control of the muscle groups that contribute to the body support moment, the gastrocsoleus, quadriceps, and hip extensors is crucial (85).

The musculoskeletal pathology at GMFCS level III is similar to that at GMFCS level II, but the contractures of the MTUs are usually more severe and the deformities in the bony levers (femur and tibia) and joint instability (hip and foot) are more pronounced. Severe "lever arm deformities" are common

at GMFCS level III with increased FNA, marked ETT, and pes valgus (30, 41).

Hip Displacement at GMFCS III: Hip Surveillance and Preventive Hip Surgery. Mercer Rang suggested many years ago that all children with CP should have regular hip examinations and radiographs (148). The goal was to prevent dislocation by early detection and early preventive (adductor release) surgery. He famously stated that no child with CP was actually helped by having a dislocated hip. Several centers in Europe and Australia have developed these concepts into formal "Hip Surveillance Programs." Children with a confirmed diagnosis of CP are offered regular clinical and radiographic examination of their hips and access to both preventive and reconstructive surgery. In both Southern Sweden and Victoria, Australia, the prevalence of late dislocation has decreased and the need for salvage surgery has been reduced (65, 190) (Fig. 14-34) (see Figs. 14-35 to 14-40).

Hip displacement in children with CP is different to DDH in typically developing children. The hip is normal at birth and then displaces because of limitations in activity, accompanied by contractures and bony deformities. Factors that may contribute to hip displacement include increased magnitude of muscle forces across the hip, which have been modeled to be increased sixfold (191). The shape of the proximal femur is also important and is predicted by GMFCS level, in terms of torsion (femoral neck anteversion, FNA) and NSA (49).

Hip displacement in children with CP can be reliably measured from AP hip radiographs, taken in the supine

Prevention

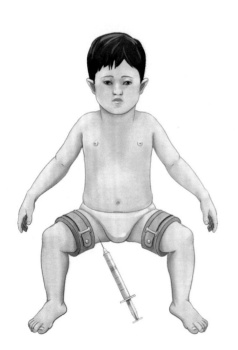

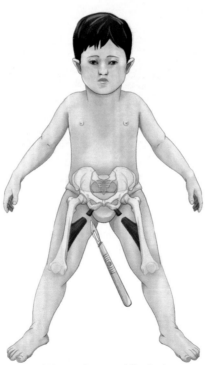

Botox + bracing: not effective

Adductor release: partially effective

FIGURE 14-34. Prevention of hip displacement in younger children with CP is difficult. Repeated injection of Botulinum toxin to the hip adductors combined with an abduction brace is not effective. Adductor release surgery is partially effective. Success rate is high at GMFCS level II and lower at GMFCS level III. The failure rate in nonambulators, GMFCS IV and V, is very high.

Text continued on page 525

Adductor and Iliopsoas Release (Figs. 14-35 to 14-40)

FIGURE 14-35.   **Adductor and Iliopsoas Release.** The patient is placed supine, near the end of the operating table and the perineum is isolated with a waterproof dressing. Both legs are draped free so that the range of abduction in both flexion and extension can be checked. A transverse incision 2 to 3 cm long is made 1 cm distal to the groin crease, parallel to the groin crease, and centred over the adductor longus. The incision is opened down to the deep fascia with careful hemostasis.

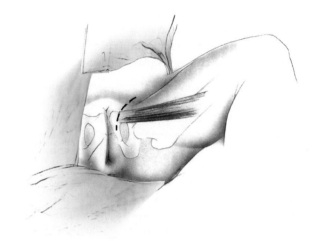

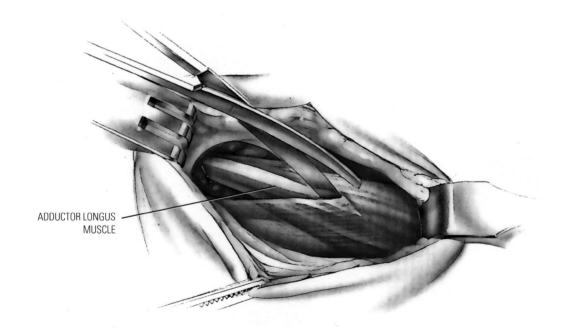

ADDUCTOR LONGUS
MUSCLE

FIGURE 14-36.   The adductor longus tendon and the interval between the adductor longus and brevis are carefully identified by blunt dissection. The fascia overlying the adductor longus is opened longitudinally, that is, at right angles to the skin incision and parallel with the axis of the adductor longus tendon.

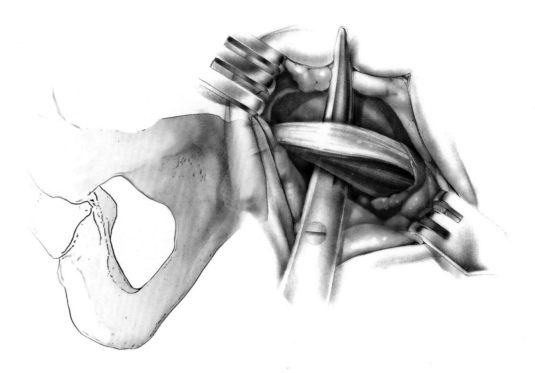

FIGURE 14-37. The tendon of the adductor longus is mobilized and divided close to its attachment to the pelvis, because this minimizes bleeding and dead space. The anterior branches of the obturator nerve can be identified in the interval between the adductor longus and brevis and should either be protected (in ambulators) or consideration given to phenol neurolysis in nonambulant patients with severe spasticity.

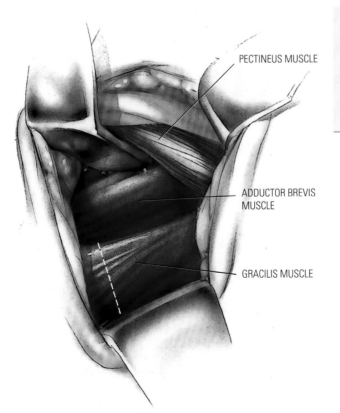

PECTINEUS MUSCLE

ADDUCTOR BREVIS MUSCLE

GRACILIS MUSCLE

FIGURE 14-38. At this point the range of abduction in flexion should be checked carefully and the underlying adductor brevis can usually be manually stretched to provide sufficient abduction.

Next the origin of the gracilis is identified and mobilized. This can be facilitated by having the assistant extend the knee while abducting the hips. The gracilis is divided close to its origin from the pubis using electrocautery with attention to hemostasis.

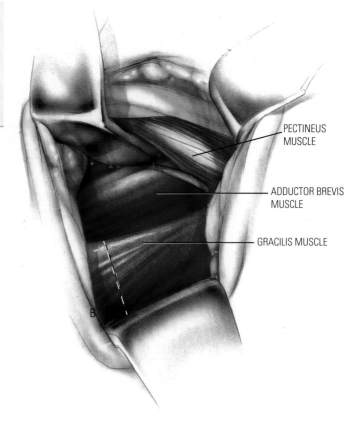

FIGURE 14-39. The adductor brevis rarely requires division, it is better to manually stretch this muscle. In severe or neglected cases partial division may be required. Complete division should not be undertaken lightly because the posterior branch of the obturator nerve will be at risk. Excessive muscle division and/or injury to the posterior branch of the obturator nerve may lead to a fixed abduction deformity.

PECTINEUS MUSCLE

ADDUCTOR BREVIS MUSCLE

GRACILIS MUSCLE

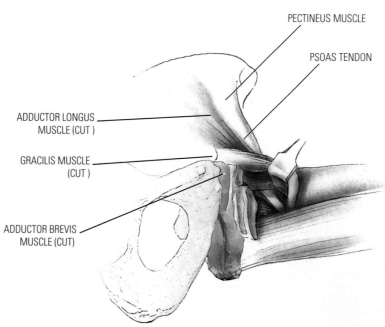

PECTINEUS MUSCLE

PSOAS TENDON

ADDUCTOR LONGUS MUSCLE (CUT)

GRACILIS MUSCLE (CUT)

ADDUCTOR BREVIS MUSCLE (CUT)

A

FIGURE 14-40. **A:** The decision whether to lengthen the iliopsoas at the lesser trochanter is based on the presence of a hip flexion deformity and the ambulatory status of the patient. If the hip flexion contracture is less than 5 degrees and the patient is an ambulator, lengthening at the lesser trochanter is not desirable. In nonambulators with a flexion contracture of more than 5 to 10 degrees, lengthening of the iliopsoas at the lesser trochanter is usually recommended. It is important to identify the correct intramuscular interval. This is best done by finger dissection along the posterior border of the divided adductor longus. The hip is held in abduction and flexion, with the surgeon's index finger palpating the proximal femur. The underlying femur can be identified by gently rotating the hip internally and externally followed by feeling the "bump" of the lesser trochanter. Then appropriate retractors can be inserted above and below the femur taking care to retract the neurovascular bundle anteriorly. It is important to place the retractors carefully and ensure a good view of the lesser trochanter with the psoas tendon running obliquely from the proximal thigh and inserting on the lesser trochanter. There is often a small amount of overlying fat which needs to be bluntly removed. A right angle clamp can be placed underneath the tendon of the iliopsoas which can then be divided completely under direct vision.

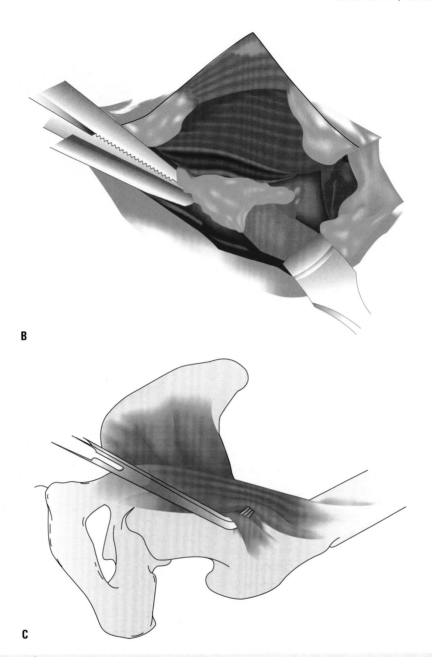

B

C

FIGURE 14-40. (*continued*) **B and C:** Following division of the iliopsoas tendon close to the lesser trochanter, a second inspection is advised to ensure that the division has been complete and that the tendon has been seen to retract proximally. It is important to inspect the incision carefully for bleeding and to secure hemostasis. The most frequent cause of a wound infection in this vulnerable groin area is a deep hematoma. If there is any doubt about the quality of hemostasis, a suction drain is advisable. The dead space should be reduced by closing the deep fascia. The skin is closed with a subcuticular absorbable suture. It is very important to carefully apply a waterproof dressing. The majority of children who require this surgery are incontinent and a further cause of deep wound infection is contamination of the incision.

position, with good positioning, and a standardized technique (192). The most useful radiographic index is the migration percentage (MP) of Reimers. This is the percentage of the femoral head that lies outside the acetabulum. The measurement error should be <10% and serial measurement of MP is the most useful means to study hip displacement in children with CP. It is the key index for making decisions regarding surgical management and to monitor hip displacement both

before and after operative intervention (50, 64). In children with CP, the MP increases by 2% to 5% per year until the MP reaches about 50%. At this point, the displacement may increase rapidly and is associated with progressive deformities in the femoral head and acetabulum, loss of articular cartilage, and degenerative arthritis (189, 193).

Nonoperative measures including physical therapy, abduction bracing, and injections of BoNT-A do not prevent progressive hip displacement in children with CP (111). Hip surgery for children with CP can be classified as preventive, reconstructive, and salvage (191). Surgery to prevent hip displacement refers to soft-tissue releases of the hip adductors and flexors to prevent or reverse early hip displacement in younger children (194). Because the outcome of preventive surgery depends on the age of the child (younger children have better results) and the initial migration percentage (MP <40%), early and regular hip surveillance is recommended (64, 65, 195). The majority of children will require open lengthening of the adductor longus and gracilis with lengthening of the psoas over the brim of the pelvis (POTB). The results in children at GMFCS III, who are walking with external support, are very good. Several studies have reported that the outcome of preventive surgery is much better in ambulators than in nonambulators (194–196). The effectiveness of adductor surgery is predicted by GMFCS level (197).

Surgical Correction of Crouch Gait in Spastic Diplegia.

Crouch gait may occur at GMFCS level I but is usually mild because children at GMFCS level I have good strength and good selective motor control. Severe crouch gait may occur at GMFCS level IV, but given that sustained ambulation is not feasible in adult life, correction by invasive surgery is not appropriate. Severe crouch gait is the major functional issue at GMFCS levels II and III. It can be part of the natural history of gait in spastic diplegia but in most recent series, the majority of affected individuals had prior lengthening of the Achilles tendons (59, 189).

There is usually a delay between lengthening of the gastrocsoleus and the development of crouch gait (95). The Achilles tendons are often lengthened in children with spastic diplegia between the ages of 3 and 6 years. It may take another 3 to 6 years before crouch gait becomes a significant functional problem, and it is often not until the adolescent growth spurt when the maximum deterioration in gait and functioning occurs (29, 95, 189). Instead of "growing up" the adolescent with progressive crouch gait "sinks down," with an inability to maintain an extension posture at the hip and knee during the stance phase of gait. Contributing factors seem to be a mismatch between the strength of the one-joint muscles contributing to the body support moment (gluteals, quadriceps, and soleus) and the increased demand because of rapid increases in height and weight at the pubertal growth spurt. This typically occurs in conjunction with progressive bony deformities known as lever arm disease. Around the time of the pubertal growth spurt, increasing patella alta (sometimes with fractures of the patella or avulsions of the inferior pole) increasing ETT and breakdown of the midfoot with severe pes valgus, all contribute to increasing crouch, fatigue and decreasing ability to walk (30, 41, 95) (Figs. 14-41 and 14-42). Understanding the biomechanics of severe crouch gait has led to improved surgical management in recent years with the development of more effective techniques to achieve lasting correction. This can be summarized by classifying surgical techniques as first-generation techniques, second-generation techniques, and hybrid techniques.

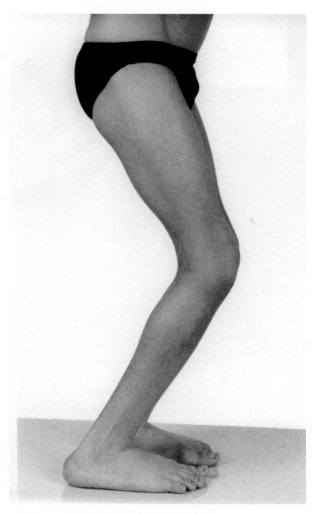

FIGURE 14-41. Sagittal alignment in crouch gait includes excessive dorsiflexion at the ankle, following previous TALs, with flexion deformities at the hips and knees.

First-Generation Techniques

Principles: Lengthening of proximal contractures (psoas, hamstrings) and correction of lever arm deformities. External support using ground reaction AFOs (GRAFOs) is required until adaptive shortening of the quadriceps occurs. This mechanism is more effective in growing children (59) (Fig. 14-43).

Advantages: Familiar techniques with acceptable morbidity.

Disadvantages: Incomplete correction in many patients leads to early relapse and recurrence. This is often related to the inefficiency of distal hamstring lengthening to achieve full and lasting correction of knee flexion contractures of >5 to 10 degrees.

Current Role. First-generation techniques are most effective in younger children with crouch gait caused by Achilles tendon lengthening with good proximal strength and selective motor control, knee flexion contractures of <5 to 10 degrees, good cooperation with a rehabilitation program, and compliance with the use of ground reaction AFOs.

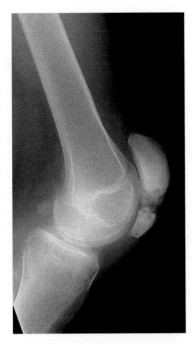

FIGURE 14-42. In crouch gait, there is frequently chronic overload of the extensor mechanism. In this 15-year-old boy, severe crouch gait was associated with bilateral fatigue fractures of the patellae.

Satisfactory correction of crouch gait using these techniques was reported with results maintained at 5 years (59). Increased knee extension was reported with healing of patellar fractures and resolution of knee pain. An important finding was that the soleus gradually shortened with a reduction in excessive dorsiflexion in the stance phase of gait, improved power generation at the ankle and the ability to ambulate without AFOs (59). Disadvantages include the slow recovery and reliance on ground reaction AFOs for at least 2 years after the surgery (59). Patella alta remains, even after the quadriceps has retensioned.

Second-Generation Techniques. First-generation techniques do not correct patella alta and distal hamstring lengthening is an inefficient method for the correction of knee flexion deformity of >10 degrees. More direct surgical approaches to the knee extensor mechanism insufficiency and the knee flexion deformity have been developed including distal femoral extension osteotomy (DFEO) with stable internal fixation, combined with shortening or advancement of the patellar tendon (198, 199) (Fig. 14-44).

Principles: Acute surgical shortening of the excessively long knee extensor mechanism combined with correction of knee flexion deformity by DFEO. Correction of all lever arm deformities is also required.

Advantages: Direct correction of the knee flexion contracture using extension osteotomy avoids weakening of MTUs (hamstrings) with more effective and predictable results. Direct correction of the patella alta and correction of quadriceps insufficiency by advancement or shortening of the extensor mechanism.

Disadvantages: These techniques are less familiar to many surgeons and are more invasive than first-generation techniques. They have a significant "learning curve," during which even experienced surgeons may report significant morbidity including neurovascular injury, loss of fixation, and incomplete correction.

Current role: DFEO combined with advancement or shortening of the extensor mechanism are powerful tools for the correction of severe crouch gait. Long-term studies are awaited to determine if the results will be durable (198, 199).

Crouch Gait: 1ˢᵗ Generation Techniques

FIGURE 14-43. First-generation techniques for the management of crouch gait.

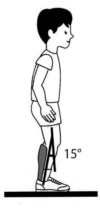

15°

1. **Lengthening psoas over the brim**
2. **Distal hamstring lengthening**
3. **Fix distal levers**
4. **Ground Reaction AFO**

Knee flexion deformity:
- **difficult to brace**
- **leads to relapse**
- **Ground Reaction AFO**

FIGURE 14-44. Second-generation techniques for the management of crouch gait.

Crouch Gait: 2nd Generation Techniques

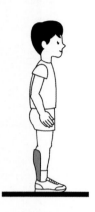

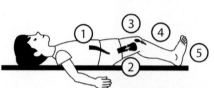

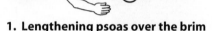

1. **Lengthening psoas over the brim**
2. **Distal femoral extension osteotomy**
3. **Patella tendon shortening**
4. **Fix distal levers**
5. **Solid AFO**

Full knee extension
Solid AFO

Hybrid Methods. Some children develop severe crouch gait before skeletal maturity. In these children, a hybrid approach to surgical correction, consisting of a combination of hamstring surgery and distal femoral growth plate surgery, is showing promising results (168, 169, 176).

Principles: Distal hamstring lengthening/semitendinosus transfer deals with the spastic hamstring contracture (186). Guided growth deals with residual knee flexion deformity (174, 175).

Advantages: Semitendinosus transfer and guided growth are variations on familiar, existing techniques.

Disadvantages: Correction depends on growth and is gradual. Indications and outcomes not yet established in the literature.

Current Role: Preliminary reports have been published. Further reports and comparative studies are necessary.

Fractional lengthening of the semimembranosus, intramuscular tenotomy of the gracilis and transfer of the semitendinosus to the adductor tubercle can deliver improved knee extension, without weakening hip extension and without causing increased anterior pelvic tilt (188) (Figs. 14-45 and 14-46). Hamstring lengthening often reduces a knee flexion contracture but frequently fails to abolish it. In a typical case, a knee flexion deformity of 15 to 20 degrees will reduce to 5 to 10 degrees. The residual knee flexion deformity is enough to prevent correction of crouch gait and to impair the effectiveness of a ground reaction AFO (Fig. 14-45). Correction of

FIGURE 14-45. Hybrid techniques for the management of crouch gait.

Crouch Gait: Hybrid Techniques

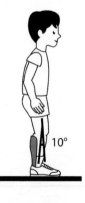

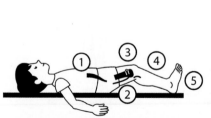

10°

1. **Lengthening psoas over the brim**
2. **Semitendinosus transfer to adductor tubercle**
3. **"8" plates to distal femur**
4. **Fix distal levers**
5. **Solid AFO**

Prerequisites:
1. **Must be pre-pubertal**
2. **Must know bone age (wrist & elbow)**
3. **Must be monitored carefully**

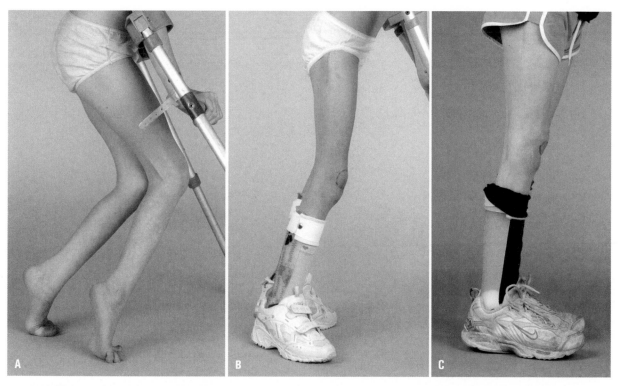

FIGURE 14-46. Severe jump gait alignment prior to SEMLS **(A)**. Improved alignment following SEMLS that included bilateral semitendinosus transfers and Strayer gastrocnemius recessions. Note the residual knee flexion deformities and external foot progression **(B)**. Full knee extension was achieved by a combination of guided growth, with staples to the anterior part of the distal femoral physis, and bilateral rotation supramalleolar osteotomies **(C)**. (From Young JL, Rodda J, Selber P, et al. Management of the knee in spastic diplegia: what is the dose? *Orthoped Clin North Am* 2010;41:561–577, with permission.)

the residual knee flexion deformity using growth plate surgery can be effective. This may be performed using staples or "8" plates placed in the anterior aspect of the distal femoral growth plate (175, 176) (Fig. 14-47). It is important to know both the chronologic age and the bone age of the patient. At least 2 years of remaining growth is necessary for clinically significant improvements in knee flexion contracture to occur.

Growth plate surgeries are consistent with early and full weight bearing and a rapid return of knee motion in most children (174, 175). However, some children can develop bursitis

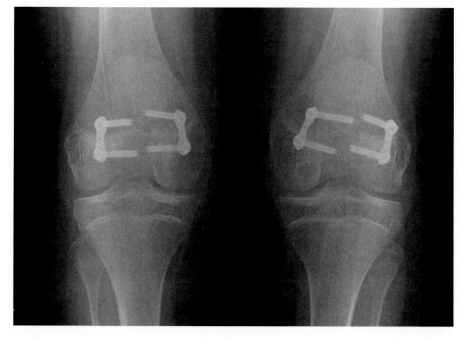

FIGURE 14-47. "8" plates for guided growth to correct residual flexion deformity at both knees. These are more prominent than staples and may cause bursitis and pain in some children.

Text continued on page 533

Subtalar Fusion (Figs. 14-48 to 14-55)

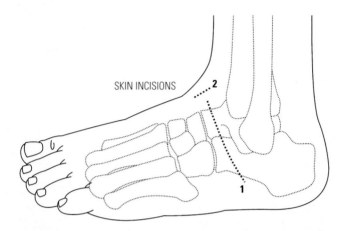

SKIN INCISIONS

FIGURE 14-48. **Subtalar Fusion.** The skin incisions for subtalar fusion are as shown. They include a modified Ollier skin crease incision, which is ideal for exposing the subtalar joint, and a second small dorsal incision for the insertion of the cannulated screw. The operation is facilitated by having the patient in the supine position and using a pneumatic thigh tourniquet. The lower limb is prepared and draped free in the usual way. The flexibility and reducibility of the pes valgus is confirmed, and the margins of the sinus tarsi, the talonavicular joint, and calcaneocuboid joint are carefully palpated. The Ollier incision is made in a skin crease, extending across the midpoint of the sinus tarsi to give good access to the sinus as shown. At the inferior margin of the incision, the sural nerve and peroneal tendons need to be identified and protected. The dorsal incision for insertion of the screw is made by palpation of the anterior part of the talus and making a 1 cm incision in the midline of the talus. Blunt dissection is carried down to the anterior part of the talus avoiding injury to the extensor tendons and the neurovascular structures. (From Shore BJ, Smith KR, Riazi A, et al. Subtalar fusion for pes valgus in cerebral palsy: Results of a modified technique in the setting of single event multilevel surgery. *J Pediatr Orthop* 2013;33: 431–438, with permission.)

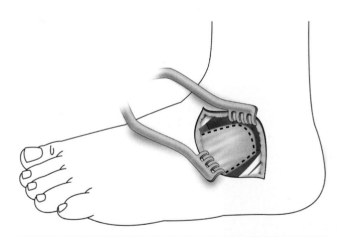

FIGURE 14-49. The skin incision extends down to the deep fascia overlying the extensor digitorum brevis (EDB) (which is often atrophic in neuromuscular patients) and a self retaining retractor is gently inserted. A distally based U-shape flap is outlined in the fascia and extensor brevis. This is carefully elevated with a combination of diathermy, cutting, and sharp dissection. (From Shore BJ, Smith KR, Riazi A, et al. Subtalar fusion for pes valgus in cerebral palsy: Results of a modified technique in the setting of single event multilevel surgery. *J Pediatr Orthop* 2013;33:431–438, with permission.)

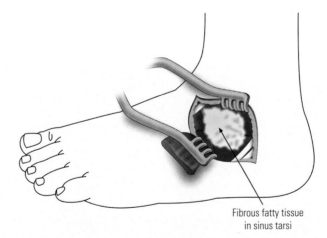

Fibrous fatty tissue in sinus tarsi

FIGURE 14-50. The elevated EDB is retracted from the sinus, and the fibrous fatty contents of the sinus are fully removed using a combination of sharp dissection, rongeurs, and best of all a hemispherical Coughlin reamer. (From Shore BJ, Smith KR, Riazi A, et al. Subtalar fusion for pes valgus in cerebral palsy: Results of a modified technique in the setting of single event multilevel surgery. *J Pediatr Orthop* 2013;33:431–438, with permission.)

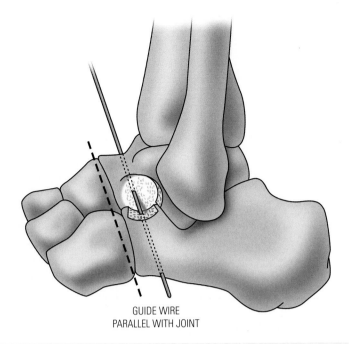

GUIDE WIRE
PARALLEL WITH JOINT

FIGURE 14-51. Once the sinus tarsi has been exposed and the contents cleared, the dorsal lateral peritalar subluxation (DLPTS) is manually reduced and a guide wire is inserted through the dorsal incision, across the depths of the sinus tarsi and into the anterior process of the os calcis, approximately parallel to both the talonavicular and calcaneocuboid joints. (From Shore BJ, Smith KR, Riazi A, et al. Subtalar fusion for pes valgus in cerebral palsy: Results of a modified technique in the setting of single event multilevel surgery. *J Pediatr Orthop* 2013;33:431–438, with permission.)

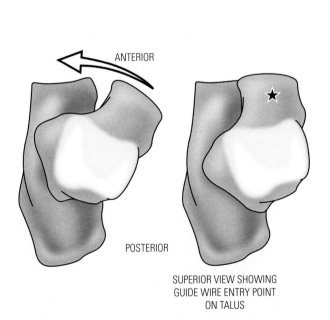

ANTERIOR

POSTERIOR

SUPERIOR VIEW SHOWING
GUIDE WIRE ENTRY POINT
ON TALUS

FIGURE 14-52. The reduction of the AP talocalcaneal subluxation is seen in Figure 14-53. The reduction needs to be checked both clinically and radiologically to ensure that full correction, but not over correction has been achieved. A useful guide is the navicular covering the head of the talus and the restoration of the medial arch of the foot. (From Shore BJ, Smith KR, Riazi A, et al. Subtalar fusion for pes valgus in cerebral palsy: Results of a modified technique in the setting of single event multilevel surgery. *J Pediatr Orthop* 2013;33:431–438, with permission.)

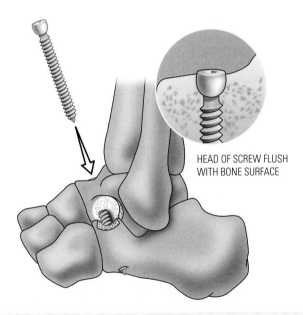

HEAD OF SCREW FLUSH
WITH BONE SURFACE

FIGURE 14-53. A fully threaded cannulated screw of appropriate length is now inserted across the guide wire to stabilize the reduction of the subtalar joint. It is very important to pay attention to the screw length. It should be fully counter sunk within the superior surface of the talus (to avoid impingement during ankle dorsiflexion). However, it must not protrude into the sole of the foot where it would cause pain and require early removal. (From Shore BJ, Smith KR, Riazi A, et al. Subtalar fusion for pes valgus in cerebral palsy: Results of a modified technique in the setting of single event multilevel surgery. *J Pediatr Orthop* 2013;33:431–438, with permission.)

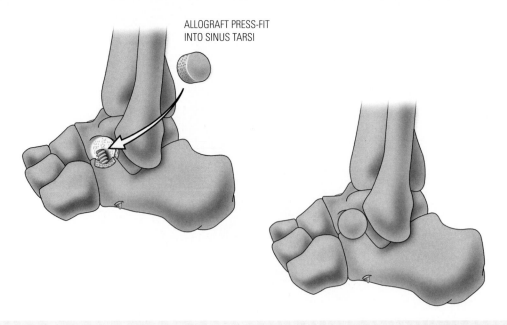

ALLOGRAFT PRESS-FIT
INTO SINUS TARSI

FIGURE 14-54. Following stabilization of the subtalar joint, the sinus tarsi is then grafted. The best options are a circular autograft (harvested from the patient's iliac crest) or a pre-cut circular allograft. Given the benefits of avoiding an additional incision to harvest an autograft, and the need for at least two grafts, our preference is a pre-cut circular cortico-cancellous allograft cut from an iliac crest. By using the Coughlin reamers to harvest this graft, it will be a secure press fit within the sinus tarsi. Given the circumferential contact between the cancellous bone of the allograft and the denuded margins of the sinus tarsi, rapid healing and incorporation is to be expected. In addition, the cortical surface of the iliac crest graft confers additional structural stability. Following irrigation, the incisions are closed in layers with interrupted nylon sutures to the skin. Following irrigation, the U-shaped flap of EDB is sutured back across the grafts covering the sinus tarsi. The incision is then closed in layers with fine interrupted nylon sutures to the skin. Using absorbable sutures risks wound separation and exposure of the allograft, which is in the relatively superficial position. We avoid this by using nylon sutures and leaving them in place for 3 weeks. The position of the graft and the fixation screw is checked on fluoroscopy prior to the application of a well padded below knee plaster cast. If a pneumatic tourniquet has been used or surgery has been prolonged it is wise to split the cast. We recommend non–weight-bearing for approximately 1 week until swelling has settled and then allow full weight bearing as tolerated. The combination of the press fit graft and the cannulated screw is stable for full weight bearing. After 2 to 3 weeks the first cast is removed, healing of the incisions is assessed, sutures are removed, and casting for a new solid AFO is done at this stage, if required. A second cast is applied for a further 4 to 6 weeks. It is often 6 to 9 months before complete healing and integration of the graft is noted on follow-up radiographs. However, bridging trabeculae can often be seen around the circular margins of the graft from as early as 3 months postoperatively. (From Shore BJ, Smith KR, Riazi A, et al. Subtalar fusion for pes valgus in cerebral palsy: Results of a modified technique in the setting of single event multilevel surgery. *J Pediatr Orthop* 2013;33:431–438, with permission.)

FIGURE 14-55. The position of the screw and the graft is seen intraoperatively, and a clinical example of foot stabilization by this method is shown in Figure 14-26A, B. (From Shore BJ, Smith KR, Riazi A, et al. Subtalar fusion for pes valgus in cerebral palsy: Results of a modified technique in the setting of single event multilevel surgery. *J Pediatr Orthop* 2013;33:431–438, with permission.)

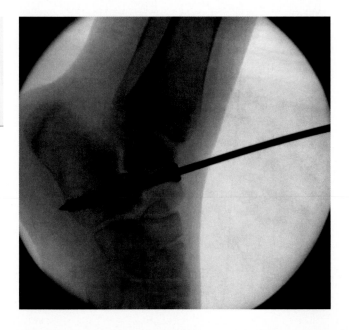

over the prominent "8" plates especially if they have a dystonic or a mixed movement disorder. Rehabilitation may be very slow in these children and in some, persistent pain and bursitis necessitate early removal of the hardware. The combination of correction of spastic hamstring contracture by semitendinosus transfer with fractional lengthening of the remaining medial hamstrings and dealing with the residual knee flexion contracture by growth plate surgery have not yet been reported in the literature. The place of these techniques in the correction of crouch gait is not yet established.

GMFCS IV

1. **Between 6th and 12th birthday**
   Children use methods of mobility that require physical assistance or powered mobility in most settings. They may walk for short distances at home with physical assistance or use powered mobility or a body support walker when positioned. At school, outdoors, and in the community, children are transported in a manual wheelchair or use powered mobility (13).
2. **Between 12th and 18th birthday**
   Youth use wheeled mobility in most settings. Physical assistance of one to two people is required for transfers. Indoors, youth may walk short distances with physical assistance, use wheeled mobility or a body support walker when positioned. They may operate a powered chair, otherwise are transported in a manual wheelchair (15).
3. **Risk of hip displacement:** 69%
4. **Mean femoral neck anteversion (FNA):** 40 degrees
5. **Mean neck shaft angle (NSA):** 155 degrees (49, 50)

Movement Disorder. The majority of children at GMFCS level IV have mixed tone, or "spastic-dystonia." In children and adolescents with severe generalized hypertonia, ITB by implanted pump offers the most reliable method of sustained tone reduction (86, 88). The position of the catheter in the intrathecal space can be adjusted to titrate the effects of the Baclofen in the upper limbs versus the lower limbs. Weakness of the trunk and paraspinal muscles may contribute to a postural kyphosis, and the incidence of scoliosis is high (30, 46).

Management goals, based on a realistic appraisal of long-term motor prognosis, include standing and assisted walking in early childhood. In later childhood, maintenance of comfortable sitting by detecting and treating early hip displacement and managing tone when necessary with ITB is important. Later, monitoring of spinal deformity with appropriate treatment and provision of custom seating are the most important issues.

Preventive Hip Surgery GMFCS Level IV. Lengthening of the hip adductors to achieve >50 degrees abduction in both hips, with the hips and knees extended, is an appropriate goal. This requires lengthening of the adductor longus and gracilis and sometimes a partial lengthening of the adductor brevis, depending on the age of the child and the degree of fixed contracture. Tenotomy of the iliopsoas at the lesser trochanter is helpful for hip flexion contracture. Lengthening at this level is more effective than lengthening at

the pelvic brim. Weakness of hip flexion is of less consequence for a child at GMFCS IV. Phenol neurolysis of the anterior branch of the obturator nerve is safe and effective at the time of adductor release (90). Most reports of adductor releases with long-term follow-up report a high failure rate after adductor surgery in nonambulators (GMFCS IV and V) (196, 197).

Reconstructive Hip Surgery GMFCS Level IV. The most common indication for reconstructive surgery is a persistently high MP after adductor releases. If the MP remains >40%, at >12 months after adequate adductor releases and the child is >4 years, reconstructive surgery is indicated (191, 195). Reconstructive surgery is also advised as the index surgery in children >8 years presenting with MP >40% (191, 193) (Fig. 14-56).

Reconstructive hip surgery poses a major challenge to children with CP and general health should be optimized before embarking on bilateral hip surgery. Nutrition and respiratory status should be optimized before surgery (193). Potential sites for infection, including feeding tubes, chest, and bladder, should be screened. Many children have low-grade, iron deficiency anemia and may benefit from iron supplements. The single most common complication after reconstructive hip surgery is the exacerbation of chronic constipation that can be detected and corrected prior to hip surgery (56).

Reconstructive surgery consists of three main components: **Adductor Releases:** Lengthening of the soft tissues to ensure an adequate range of passive hip abduction (>50 degrees) is the first step in reconstructive surgery. For those children who have recurrent displacement after previous adductor releases, a revision adductor release at the time of bony reconstruction is always required (189, 190, 192). Revision adductor releases have a higher complication rate than first-time surgery. Meticulous hemostasis, suction drainage, and sealed waterproof dressings may reduce the rate of hematoma formation and deep infection. **Femoral Osteotomy:** Correction of the abnormal femur is achieved by varus derotation, shortening osteotomy of the proximal femur. Given that these children never ambulate independently and most are walkers for a relatively short period, correction of the NSA to about 100 degrees is an appropriate goal with reduction of anteversion to about 10 degrees (166, 169). The osteotomy should be performed at the intertrochanteric level. Most children at GMFCS IV have true coxa valga and will need excision of a 1 to 3 cm medially based wedge or trapezoid from the femur (49). The wedge includes the lesser trochanter and the psoas insertion. Shortening of the proximal femur is an effective way to reduce soft-tissue tension and restore range of motion and symmetry about the hips. In windswept deformities, symmetry can be achieved by a combination of soft-tissue releases and adjusting the amount of rotation in each osteotomy (191).

Stable internal fixation with the AO-ASIF 90- or 100-degree blade plate is the preferred fixation device (166). Older, two part fixation devices are not reliable but the newer proximal femoral locking plates are a good option, particularly in osteopenic bone. Hip spicas should be avoided, but poor bone quality may necessitate short-term use in a minority of children (191).

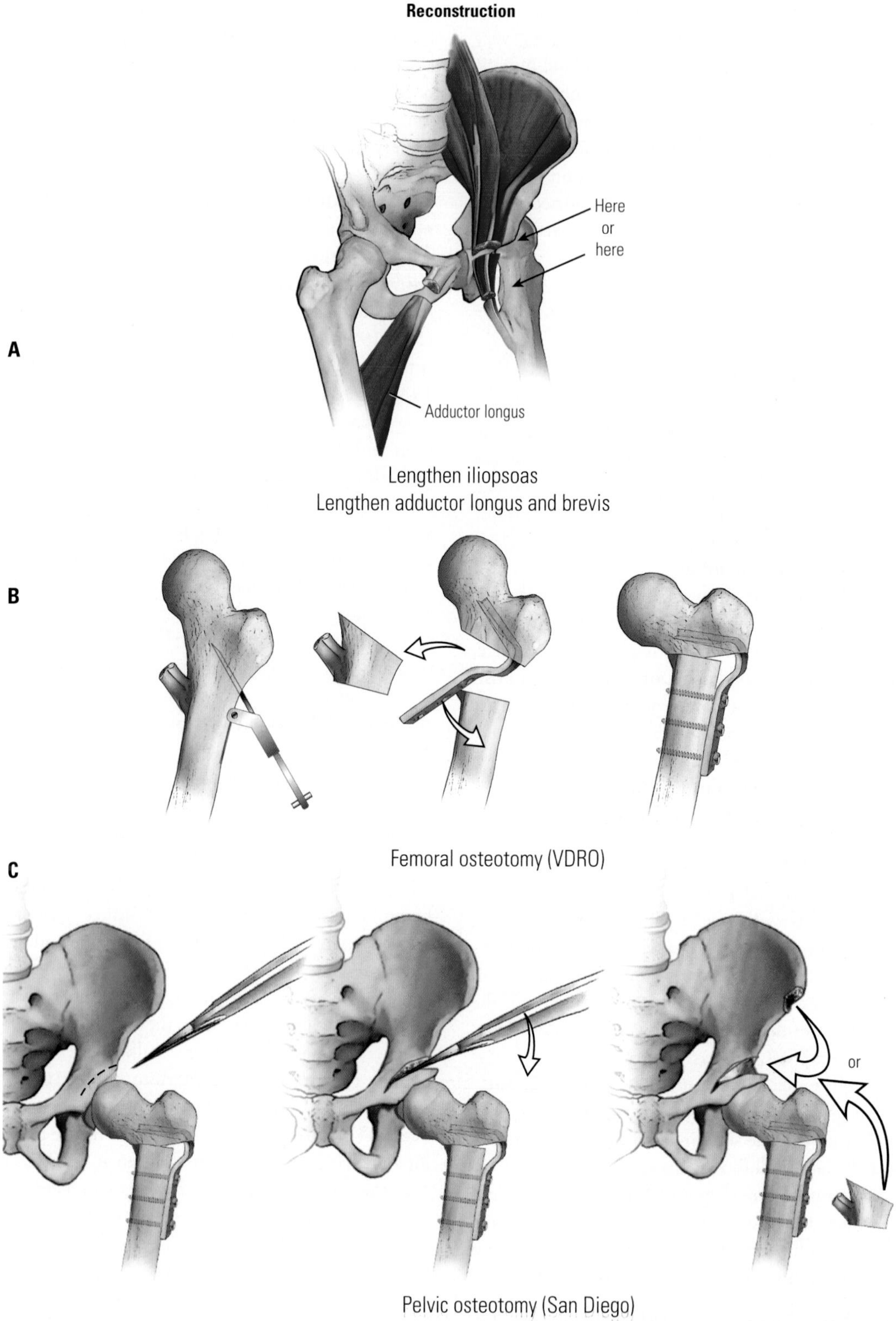

Reconstruction

Here
or
here

Adductor longus

A

Lengthen iliopsoas
Lengthen adductor longus and brevis

B

Femoral osteotomy (VDRO)

C

or

Pelvic osteotomy (San Diego)

FIGURE 14-56. The essential three components of reconstructive hip surgery include the following: **A:** Primary or revision adductor and psoas lengthening. **B:** Femoral varus derotation osteotomy with appropriate shortening, internal fixation with a fixed angle blade plate or a proximal femoral locking plate and providing additional graft for **C:** Pelvic osteotomy of the San Diego type.

Pelvic Osteotomy: Significant acetabular dysplasia should be corrected by a pelvic osteotomy at the time of bony reconstruction. Innominate osteotomy is contraindicated in CP, and salvage procedures such as the Chiari or shelf procedures are not good options. A curved osteotomy, close to the acetabular margin as popularized by the San Diego and Du Pont groups, is by far the best option for the majority of younger children (172, 200, 201). The San Diego and Du Pont surgeons have refined the direction of the cut, the opening of the osteotomy site, and the stabilization with "press fit" bony wedges to make the procedure effective and reliable in CP. Older children and teenagers may benefit from a triple pelvic osteotomy or a periacetabular osteotomy (202, 203).

Postoperative Care. At the end of the reconstruction, the hip and the fixation should be stable and a hip spica should not be required (200). More preventable morbidity comes from hip spica immobilization than from the surgery. Expert pain management, nutritional and respiratory support should continue well into the postoperative period. General complications include respiratory infections, exacerbation of constipation, emesis, and weight loss. Surgical complications of reconstructive hip surgery include avascular necrosis, infection, nerve palsy, loss of fixation, periprosthetic fracture, and recurrent hip displacement. Windswept deformity, leg-length inequality, and heterotopic ossification are also seen.

Outcomes: One-stage correction of hip displacement, as described above, is a very effective and reliable method of stabilizing the severely subluxated or dislocated hip in CP as reported in several large series (172, 200, 201). The radiologic status of most hips remains satisfactory in the short and longer terms. Pain is prevented or relieved and sitting tolerance is usually improved (193). Prominent hardware (blade plates) are usually removed about 12 months after surgery. Radiologic monitoring of hip development should continue until skeletal maturity, at least. The biggest threat to hip status after successful hip reconstruction is progression of scoliosis and pelvic obliquity. It is very difficult to maintain hip stability on the high side of an oblique pelvis (191).

Special Circumstances. Anterior dislocations are rare and present clinically with extension posturing, restricted hip flexion, and inability to sit comfortably. Improved anterior cover, using a Pemberton osteotomy, is required as part of the reconstruction (191). Windblown hips require a very careful analysis of movement disorder, soft-tissue contractures, and a tailored asymmetric surgical prescription. In children with severe dystonic posturing, an ITB pump may be required before the hip reconstruction. The abducted hip may need an abductor release and a VDRO. The adducted hip may require an adductor release, a VDRO, and San Diego pelvic osteotomy (191).

Lower Limb Surgery at GMFCS Level IV. Flexion deformities at the hip and knee are very common as well as deformities at the foot and ankle, especially ETT and pes valgus. Hallux valgus and dorsal bunions are also quite common. In early childhood, if the child is enjoying assisted ambulation, it may be appropriate to employ some of the procedures described for children at GMFCS levels II and III, to help the child stand and achieve the goal of limited walking. However, parents, carers, and therapists should recognize that sustained ambulation into adult life is not achievable (15). Therefore, extraordinary measures to maintain ambulation are not indicated. Despite cospastic stiffness at the knee, transfer of the rectus femoris is contraindicated at this GMFCS level because it does not work and may weaken knee extension, which is needed for transfers. More invasive measures such as DFEO and patellar tendon shortening for crouch gait are also contraindicated because with or without these measures, ambulation will eventually be lost (15).

Managing deformity of the foot and ankle is important to allow bracing, the wearing of normal shoes, and for the feet to be able to rest on the foot rest of a wheelchair. Calcaneus is very common after gastrocsoleus lengthening and it is best to manage spastic equinus in these children by injections of BoNT-A or by a modest gastrocnemius recession (95). Correction of severe ETT by supramalleolar osteotomy of the tibia may be necessary for positioning on the wheelchair footrest. Stabilization of the foot for pes valgus is more reliably achieved by a subtalar fusion than by os calcis lengthening (133). Correction of hallux valgus and dorsal bunion by soft-tissue balancing and fusion of the first MTP joint is effective for deformity correction, pain relief, and comfortable shoe wear (133).

Spinal Deformities at GMFCS Level IV

Kyphosis. Postural kyphosis is very common at GMFCS level IV due to paraspinal muscle weakness and impairments of posture and balance. Dorsal kyphosis remains flexible and corrects in prone lying in early childhood. It is best managed by appropriate seating and occasionally by the use of thoracolumbosacral orthosis (TLSO). With advancing age, the thoracic kyphosis and the secondary cervical lordosis may become more fixed. Cervical pain in adults with CP is common. Spinal reconstructive surgery may be indicated to improve alignment, minimize pain, and promote comfort in sitting.

Scoliosis. Progressive scoliosis is common at GMFCS level IV but differs from that seen at GMFCS level V (30). It tends to start a little later, is not so rapidly progressive, and the outcomes of surgery are better because medical comorbidities are fewer and less severe. Pelvic obliquity and hip disease are less severe. Management of scoliosis will be considered in more detail in the section on GMFCS level V. The question of orthotic management of scoliosis at GMFCS level IV is frequently raised because parents, caregivers, and therapists may wish to avoid the risks of spinal fusion surgery. Studies have suggested that bracing rarely prevents progression of spinal deformity at GMFCS level IV although it may slow down progression (204). Previous studies have not subdivided children according to GMFCS level. From the point of view of parents, it is important to provide information about the limited benefit of bracing. Even when surgery is likely to be required in the near future, it may be helpful for parents to feel that they have tried nonoperative measures. Curve progression should be monitored because it can be very rapid.

GMFCS V

1. **Between 6th and 12th birthday**
   Children are transported in a manual wheelchair in all settings. Children are limited in their ability to maintain antigravity head and trunk postures and control leg and arm movements (13).

2. **Between 12th and 18th birthday**
   Youth are transported in a manual wheelchair in all settings. They are limited in their ability to maintain antigravity head and trunk postures and control leg and arm movements. Self-mobility is severely limited, even with the use of assistive technology (15).

3. **Risk of hip displacement:** 90%
4. **Mean femoral neck anteversion (FNA):** 40 degrees
5. **Mean neck shaft angle (NSA):** 163 degrees (49, 50)

Seating Requirements GMFCS Levels IV and V.

Comfortable sitting requires a straight spine, over a level pelvis, with flexible hips that are in joint. Hip flexion should be >90 degrees and extension to within 30 degrees of full extension, with 20 to 40 degrees of abduction at each hip and no fixed abduction or "windswept" deformity. Flexible knees with little fixed flexion and no extension deformity and plantargrade feet that will rest comfortably on the foot plates

of wheelchairs are also important. At GMFCS level IV, the wheelchair is a "total body orthosis" requiring prescription, fitting, and maintenance by an expert team (205). The ability to transfer independently in and out of specialized seating is crucial for the option of young adults to be able to live in a group home setting (Fig. 14-57).

The Chair Back.   The back should support the patient's trunk from the shoulders to the pelvis and be wide enough to accommodate trunk and lateral supports that are often needed. The chair back should be firm enough to provide support and soft enough for comfort throughout the day. The chair back requires the ability to recline as this provides additional spinal support. A reclined position may inhibit extensor thrust as well as remove some of the demands on the paraspinal muscles to maintain the upright position (205) (Fig. 14-57A,B).

The Seat.   The feet should reach the foot rests and the seat should be wide enough to accommodate a central pommel and lateral supports for the control of "windswept" hips. The seat should support the thigh segments that may be unequal in the windswept deformity. The seat should be firm enough to provide support and soft enough for comfort. Customized contouring for windswept deformity can be very helpful. The use

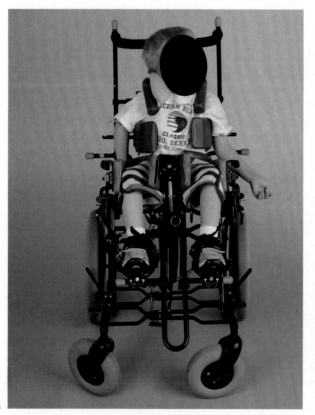
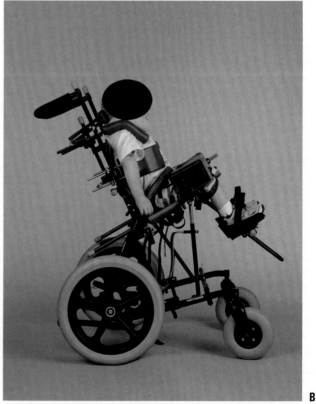

A   B

FIGURE 14-57.   A and B: Modular, adjustable seating for a 5-year-old child with severe CP, GMFCS level V, who lacks head control and sitting balance. Note the ability to provide supports for the neck, shoulders, trunk, and legs. The chair is partially reclined to reduce extensor thrust and the feet are well supported by the foot plates. Maintenance of comfortable sitting at GMFCS level V frequently requires management of hypertonia, reconstructive hip surgery, and spinal fusion surgery.

of pressure mapping to define areas of high contact pressures can be helpful in problem children (205).

The Foot Rest.

The foot rest should support the entire foot in a plantargrade position and be designed to swing out of the way during sitting and during transfers in and out of the chair. Given the high incidence of spastic dystonia, foot restraints, supplemented by straps at the knee level, may be helpful to avoid one or both lower limbs escaping from the chair and risking injury during transport. Additional supports or restraints may be helpful at the level of the head and neck, trunk, pelvis, knees, foot, and ankle (205).

Functional Mobility.

The ability to move the chair easily in and out of an adapted vehicle is an important consideration for many families. Independent control by the patient using hand controls may add significantly to the patient's self-esteem, quality of life, and independence.

Preventive and Reconstructive Hip Surgery: GMFCS V.

Preventive surgery has a high failure rate and should be considered to be a temporizing measure for most children at GMFCS V. Reconstructive surgery is technically easier and probably more successful in older children. Scoliosis and pelvic obliquity are so prevalent that hip and spine management should be considered together (193). Windswept deformities are more common and more severe at GMFCS V. If the hips are windswept, a more extensive release on the adducted side is required sometimes combined with phenolization of the anterior branch of the obturator nerve or a neurectomy. If there is fixed abduction contracture, this should be addressed by release of the hip abductors. Bilateral femoral VDRO should be performed with shortening and appropriate derotation, taking into consideration the patient's posture while awake and any torsional deformities identified clinically or confirmed by CT.

Salvage Surgery GMFCS Level V.

The degree of femoral head deformity and acetabular deformity should be carefully evaluated in the context of the child's health, functioning, and life expectancy. The principal symptoms from neglected hip displacement are pain, which is reported to occur in between 10% and 90% of cases (191, 193). Fixed deformity, especially the windswept deformity, is also a major impediment to comfortable sitting and care. None of the salvage options that are available are reliable and predictable. The need for salvage surgery is best avoided by early hip surveillance and appropriately timed preventive and reconstructive surgery. Before considering salvage surgery, consultation with the multidisciplinary team to optimize the patient's general health is very important. Referral to an appropriate pain management service is important as a number of teenagers can be managed nonoperatively, in the short term. Reflex spasms of the hip adductors and flexors are almost always part of the pain problem in dislocated hips. Short-term symptomatic relief can often be achieved by injecting the hip joint with bupivicaine and corticosteroid and injecting the hip adductors and flexors with BoNT-A (123, 124). Open releases of the contracted hip adductors

and phenolization of the obturator nerve may also help. These interventions have been reported to give short-term pain relief, but no long-term studies have been reported (123, 124).

It is also important to optimize tone management prior to salvage surgery. If an ITB pump is an appropriate choice for the child and accepted by the parents, this should be done before hip surgery (86). The marked reduction in tone around the hips may reduce pain and postural deformities to a degree that salvage surgery is not required. If salvage surgery is still necessary, it is much more easily performed in the context of global tone reduction afforded by the ITB pump (88). During salvage surgery, the pump can be reprogrammed to increase the amount of Baclofen available to the child in the immediate postoperative period resulting in reduced postoperative pain and a reduction in the need for narcotic analgesia. During surgery, the pump should be protected from hematogenous infection by perioperative antibiotics.

There is no single, reliable salvage surgery for the painful dislocated hip at GMFCS level V. The Castle procedure is an extraperiosteal resection of the entire proximal femur, below the lesser trochanter, with vastus lateralis and rectus femoris sewn over the end of the femur and as much hip capsule and gluteal muscle as possible interposed between the femoral stump and acetabulum (206). Postoperative care has included skin traction, skeletal traction, external fixators, hip distracters, hip spica casts, and bracing. Postoperative complications include pneumonia, decubitus ulceration, deep infection, wound breakdown, and death. Pain relief is usually delayed and unpredictable. After the Castle procedure, adolescents may take a year to show improvement in pain and there are high rates of heterotopic ossification, proximal migration, inadequate pain relief, and the need for revision surgery (207, 208). The family and caregivers must know that the hip will be unusually "floppy" and that weight bearing will no longer be possible.

The McHale combination of femoral head resection combined with valgus osteotomy is more stable, has a reduced risk of heterotopic ossification and less proximal migration than the Castle subtrochanteric resection (209, 210). However, impingement may occur between the lesser trochanter and the acetabulum or pelvic wall. Valgus osteotomy, without femoral head resection, has been reported in a recent study to have good pain relief in 24 patients followed for a mean of 44 months (211).

Interposition arthroplasty with a variety of devices has been reported in several small series with relatively short follow-up (212). Prophylaxis of heterotopic ossification with preoperative radiation or the administration of nonsteroidal anti-inflammatory drugs should be considered. Radiation may increase discomfort and affect healing. Nonsteroidal anti-inflammatory drugs are risky in this population but so is the development of severe heterotopic ossification.

Arthrodesis is very effective in terms of pain relief but is indicated only in unilateral hip disease in patients with dystonia in a hemiplegic distribution (213). Conventional total hip arthroplasty (THA) is very effective but is only indicated in a small subset of ambulant patients with well-controlled movement disorders (213). Metal on metal, resurfacing arthroplasty combined with proximal femoral derotation and shortening has a wider range of indications because the risk of dislocation is lower than with conventional THA. Resurfacing arthroplasty can give good pain relief and improve function (214) (Figs. 14-58 to 14-60).

Lower Limb Surgery GMFCS Level V.

Maintaining the ability to wear normal shoes and place the feet on a foot plate of a wheelchair is a basic but important goal. Deformities around the foot and ankle are often severe. Lengthening of the gastrocsoleus is contraindicated because it almost invariably leads to the subsequent development of a fixed calcaneus deformity. In the younger child, neurolytic blocks and AFOs are appropriate to maintain the feet in a plantargrade alignment. In the older child, soft-tissue surgery combined with bony stabilization for severe deformities may be appropriate. Triple arthrodesis may be necessary to manage problematic equinovarus or equinovalgus foot deformities. Occasionally, a severe calcaneovalgus deformity can be managed by a tibiotalocalcaneal fusion, eliminating all ankle motion and motion of the hindfoot, but resulting in a plantargrade foot that is easily accommodated within a normal shoe and on the wheelchair foot rest (215).

Dorsal bunion in severely involved children is common and often becomes symptomatic in the teenage years. Management requires soft-tissue rebalancing and a fusion of

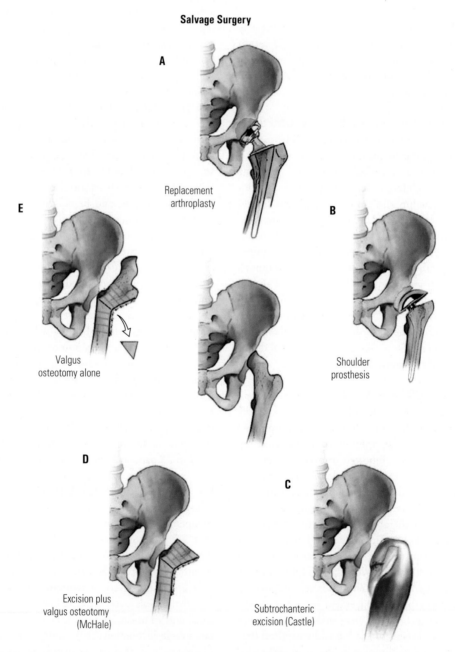

Salvage Surgery

A
Replacement arthroplasty

B
Shoulder prosthesis

C
Subtrochanteric excision (Castle)

D
Excision plus valgus osteotomy (McHale)

E
Valgus osteotomy alone

FIGURE 14-58. Options in salvage surgery for the hip in CP include the following: **A:** Replacement arthroplasty. **B:** Interposition arthroplasty with a shoulder prosthesis. **C:** Subtrochanteric excision of the proximal femur as described by Castle. **D:** Limited excision of the proximal femur along the intertrochanteric line combined with a valgus osteotomy as described by McHale. **E:** Valgus osteotomy without resection of the femoral head.

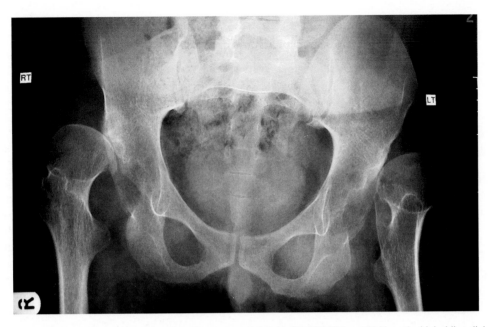

FIGURE 14-59. Bilateral painful hip dislocations in a young adult with CP, GMFCS level IV. Note the high riding dislocations, contact between the femoral head and pelvis, and severe acetabular dysplasia.

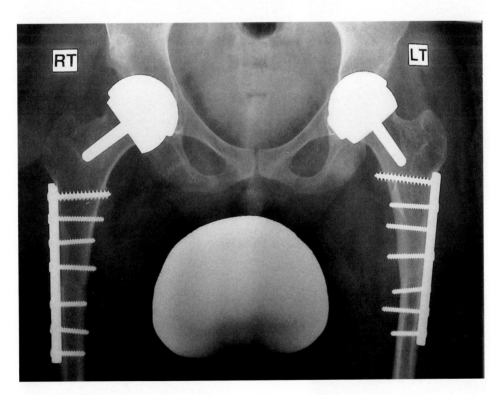

FIGURE 14-60. Post bilateral reconstruction including:
   1. Bilateral femoral shortening with derotation and DCP fixation
   2. Metal on metal resurfacing (Mr John O'Hara, Birmingham, England).

This type of reconstruction combines extensive soft-tissue lengthening, by virtue of the femoral shortening and the stability of large diameter metal on metal resurfacing. It effectively extends the range of joint arthroplasty to one of the most difficult patient populations (214).

the first MTP joint. One cm should be excised from the tibialis anterior, the remaining dorsiflexors should be lengthened, and the first MTP joint fused and fixed with a dorsal plate. The FDB and FHL will then act as a depressor of the first ray, as they act across a rigid first MTP joint (133).

SPINAL DEFORMITY AND SCOLIOSIS SURGERY GMFCS LEVEL V

Natural History. Spinal deformity affects approximately two-thirds of children at GMFCS level V but is variable in its onset, severity, progression, and effects (216). Dorsal kyphosis is very common in younger children with weak paraspinal muscles and is best managed by having the wheelchair seat slightly reclined, the use of chest straps and occasionally a TLSO (204, 205). Kyphosis in the lumbar spine is less common and may be caused by tight hamstrings. Proximal hamstring recession at the time of adduc-

tor releases may be beneficial. Lumbar lordosis is much more common and is frequently related to hip flexion contractures. Lengthening of the hip flexors before the lordosis becomes fixed may help. An ITB pump may be helpful in the management of muscle imbalances about the hip that are contributing to lumbar lordosis or kyphosis (86, 88) (Figs. 14-61 and 14-62).

Scoliosis. Scoliosis in children with CP is particularly prevalent in nonambulant children, GMFCS levels IV and V. Curves in ambulant patients are uncommon, are more likely to be idiopathic in type, and are managed accordingly. The cause of scoliosis in CP remains speculative, but spasticity, dystonia, muscle imbalance, weakness, postural impairment, and immobility have been suggested as contributing factors. SDR may be associated with kyphosis, lumbar lordosis, spondylolysis, and spondylolisthesis (217). The high rate of scoliosis in CP and the lack of controls make the interpretation of this association difficult. As with hip displacement, there is growing evidence

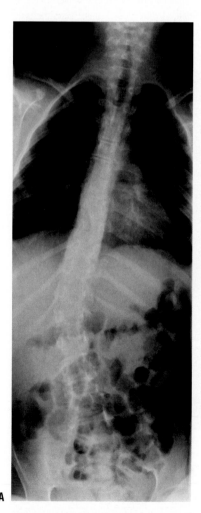
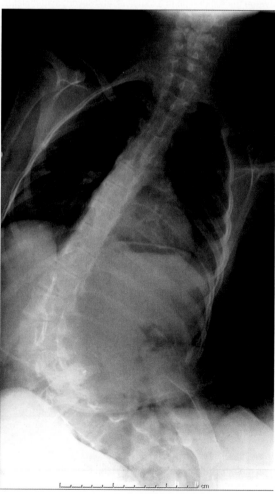

FIGURE 14-61. **A and B:** Scoliosis may progress very rapidly during the pubertal growth spurt in children with CP, especially at GMFCS level V. These two radiographs were taken only 14 months apart, at age 13 and just over age 14 years. Note the severity of the curve, and its extension into the sacrum and pelvis with marked pelvic obliquity.

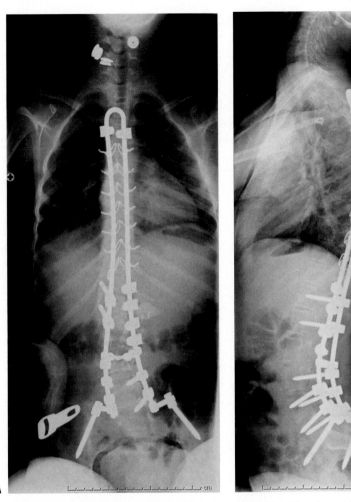

FIGURE 14-62. **A and B:** Long posterior instrumented fusion from T3 to the pelvis using a unit rod construct, and a combination of segmental fixation techniques, combined with iliac screw fixation to the pelvis in a manner similar to the Galveston technique.

that GMFCS level is the single strongest predictor of spinal deformity in children with CP (50).

Natural History of Scoliosis in Cerebral Palsy.

The long "C"-shaped CP curves present earlier in childhood than idiopathic curves, are more likely to be progressive, progress more rapidly, and may continue to progress after skeletal maturity if the curve is more than 40 degrees (218–220). The curves may be convex to the left, which is rarely seen in idiopathic scoliosis. Scoliosis may present as early as age 6 to 8 years (and occasionally even younger). In the initial stages, curves are flexible. They progress faster than idiopathic curves. The rate of progression accelerates when the curve reaches 40 to 50 degrees and especially as the child enters the pubertal growth (Fig. 14-61A,B). The speed of progression may catch parents, pediatricians, and physical therapists unawares. Some adolescents present with acute loss of sitting ability, especially when there is pelvic obliquity and windswept hips. In the space of 1 to 2 years, it is possible for a curve to progress from a moderate flexible curve, easily correctible in single-stage posterior surgery with moderate risks, to a severe rigid curve requiring

anterior and posterior surgery, with substantially increased risks of morbidity and mortality.

Neurologic deterioration, related to shunt malfunction, is also associated with rapid curve progression (216). Recent longitudinal studies of gross motor function in CP confirm that deterioration during the second decade is common, at GMFCS levels IV and V (19). Scoliosis may progress very rapidly, coincident with the deterioration in gross motor function. Curves progressed by 4.4 degrees per annum in a group of patients with a decline in function, as compared to 3.0 degrees per annum in a group with stable function (219). Larger curves progress more rapidly, including after skeletal maturity. In skeletally mature individuals, with curves <50 degrees, the progression was 0.8 degrees per annum and 1.4 degrees per annum for curves >50 degrees (219).

Nonoperative Management.

Physical therapy, injections of BoNT-A, and electrical stimulation have been tried and are not effective (216). Customized seating with molded inserts improves sitting balance and comfort but does not slow curve progression. Bracing of scoliosis in CP is poorly

Text continued on page 548

Galveston Pelvic Instrumentation (Figs. 14-63 to 14-73)

FIGURE 14-63. **Galveston Pelvic Instrumentation.** In the Galveston technique, the segment of the rod that is in the pelvis passes between the two tables of cortical bone in the thickest portion of the ilium, the transverse portion just cephalad to the sciatic notch.

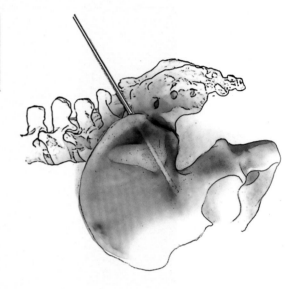

FIGURE 14-64. From the midline incision, both iliac crests are exposed. Unlike the exposure for obtaining a bone graft from a midline incision, this entire dissection is best carried out deep to the paravertebral muscles so that the rod can lie in contact with the bone and be covered with the muscle. Some surgeons prefer to split this muscle transversely for ease and speed of execution. Elevation of the muscle is aided by a transverse cut at the caudal extent of the muscle. The periosteum over the posterior crest is incised, and the posterior crest and the outer table of the ilium are exposed. The sciatic notch should be visible because it serves as a guide to the pelvic segment of the rod. The bone graft can be obtained from the more cephalad portion of the ilium, where it will not interfere with the purchase of the rod. In most cases in which this technique is used, however (e.g., paralytic scoliosis), the ilium is very thin, and what little bone is harvested does not make it worthwhile. After the area is exposed, a drill of correct size for the rod is used to drill the path for the rod.

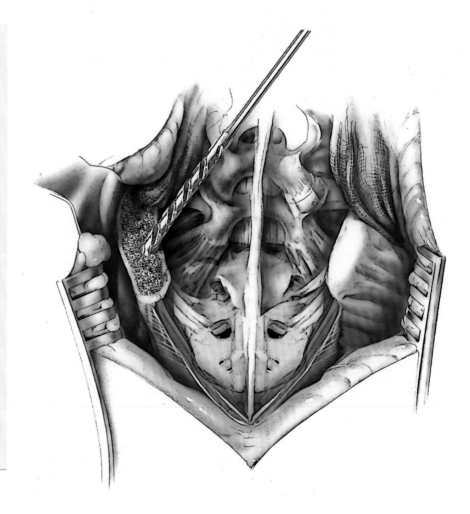

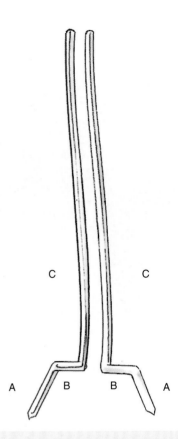

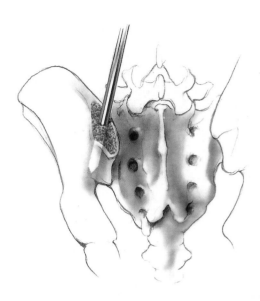

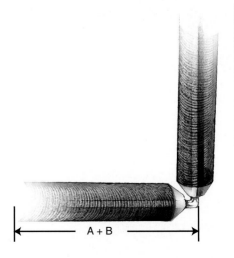

FIGURE 14-65. It will take two bends and one twist to produce the finished rod that consists of three segments. The first segment (*A*) is that which lies between the two cortical tables of the ilium and is called the *iliac segment*. The second part of the rod (*B*) runs from the ilium transversely to the area adjacent to the sacral spinous process and is called the *sacral segment*. The last segment (*C*) is that fixed to the spinal vertebrae and is called the *spinal segment*.

FIGURE 14-66. The hole for the iliac segment is made with a drill. The hole is started slightly cephalad to the posteroinferior iliac spine, and the drill is directed between the two tables of the ilium to pass just cephalad to the sciatic notch. The depth of the hole varies between 6 and 9 cm, depending on the size of the child. If desired, a guide pin can be inserted in this hole to be used with a special jig to aid in bending the correct contours into the rod (see Fig. 14-71). After a little experience, however, it is easier simply to bend the rods and make minor adjustments with the rod in place.

FIGURE 14-67. The depth of the hole should be noted; it is usually 7 to 8 cm. This is the length of the iliac segment of the rod (*A*). In addition, the distance from the hole to a point adjacent to the sacral spinous process should be noted. This is usually 2 to 2.5 cm (*B*) and represents the sacral segment of the rod. *C*: The spinal segment of the rod. The rod is now bent with two tube rod benders to place a 60-degree to 80-degree bend in the rod at a distance from the end of the rod that is equal to the length of both the iliac and the sacral segments of the rod. On the concave side of the curve, the rod fits better if the bend is less (i.e., approximately 60 degrees). On the convex side, 80 degrees is usually correct.

FIGURE 14-68. The next step is to place the bend that separates the iliac segment from the sacral segment. With a tube bender on the iliac section and a rod clamp on the sacral segment, a bend is placed that allows the rod to reach the sacral lamina when the iliac segment is inserted. In calculating the measurement with the bend, it should be remembered that the bend in the rod itself accounts for at least 0.5 cm. In addition, although the technique for bending the opposite rods is identical, the rods will be mirror images of each other.

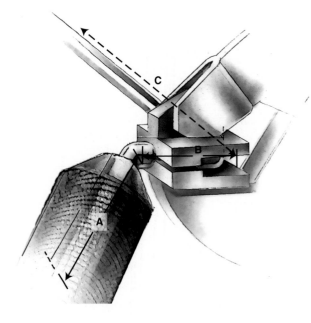

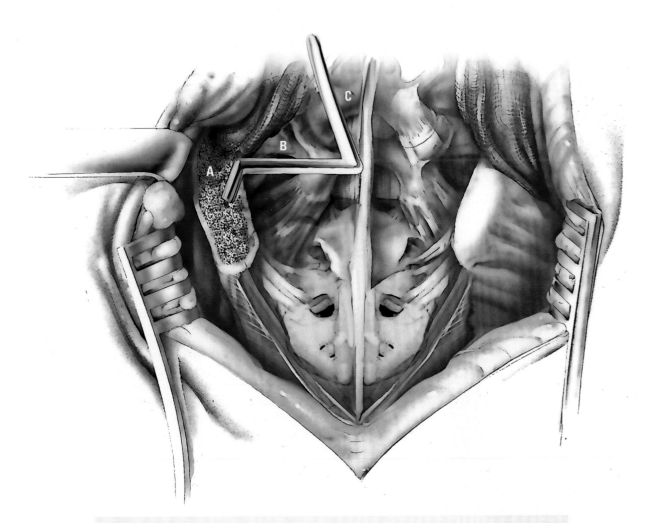

FIGURE 14-69. The three sections of the rod are now formed. At this point the rod cannot be placed.

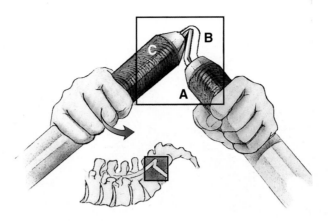

FIGURE 14-70. The last step (*B*) is to place a twist in the rod in the sacral segment. This allows the rod to conform to the sacral inclination. Although this can be done to some extent by bending lordosis into the rod, it is usually difficult to incorporate sufficient lordosis close enough to the junction of the sacral and spinal sections to have the rod lie on the sacral lamina. This twist is created by placing a tube rod bender on the spinal (*C*) and iliac (*A*) segments. The benders are brought toward each other. This produces a more ventrally directed spinal section, which conforms better to the sacrum. The amount of twist to be placed must be estimated because the rod cannot be placed at this point.

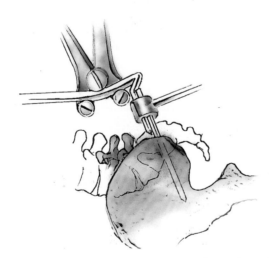

FIGURE 14-71. Finally, the desired spinal contours are bent into the rod. It is best to start with lordosis because it will not be possible to place the rod in the iliac hole and next to the spine until this is done. Although a rod guide can be used with a pelvic guide pin in the iliac hole and the double-rod guide, this technique usually results in a less than perfect fit and, after a short learning curve, is easily omitted.

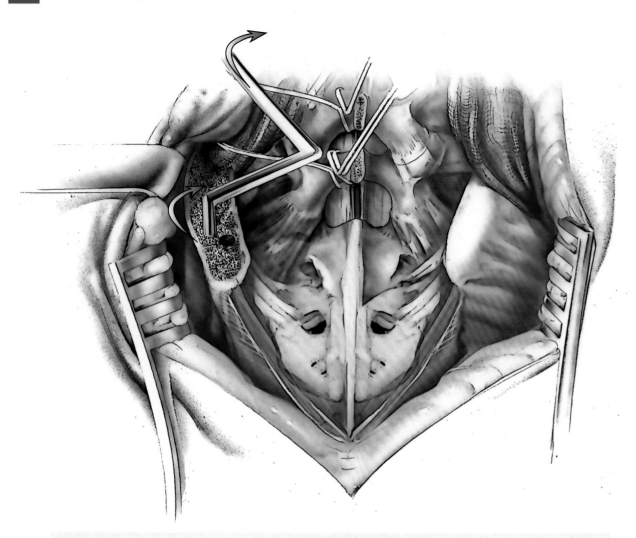

FIGURE 14-72. After the rod is contoured and the proper fit of both rods is ensured, the facet excision, any desired decortication, and passage of the sublaminar wires is completed. The rod can be inserted and wired into place.

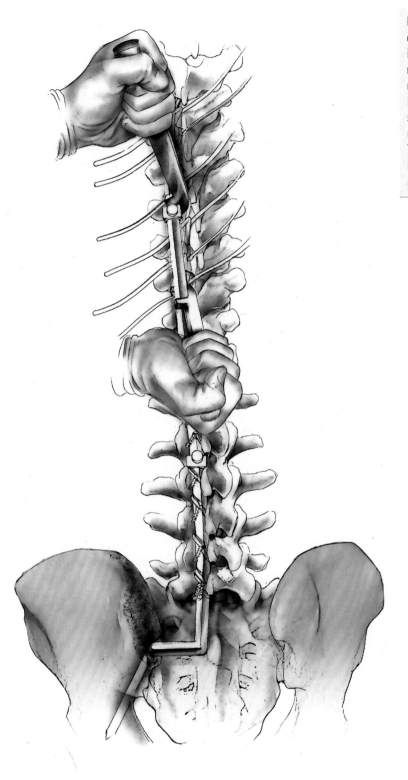

FIGURE 14-73. After the rods are in place, and even after some of the wires have been tightened, it is possible to make adjustments in the spinal segment with a pair of in situ rod benders. After the first rod is in place, consideration should be given to placing the second rod. It is likely that after tightening some of the wires on the spinal segment of the first rod, the contour of the spine would have changed. The contour of the spinal segment of the second rod may need to be adjusted. After all the adjustments are made, the cross-links are secured.

tolerated and is ineffective in avoiding progression in the long term (204). Nevertheless, in an effort to maximize spinal growth and to demonstrate that all reasonable steps have been taken prior to surgery, it is sometimes appropriate to offer bracing or seating modifications with close clinical and radiographic monitoring. This gives the parents and caregivers the opportunity to learn about the natural history of the curve in their child and come to terms with the need for major spinal surgery. In one study, bracing was helpful in curves <40 degrees in ambulant patients, but these are not the typical GMFCS V patients (204). Bracing in GMFCS V children may, at best, slow curve progression in immature patients with small curves and good compliance. Surgery may be postponed but will still be required for the vast majority of patients (216).

Preoperative Assessment. Poor nutritional status is associated with increased morbidity and mortality. Optimizing nutritional status requires adequate time for assessment and correction. Serum albumin <35 g/L and a lymphocyte count of <1.5 g/L were associated with increased rate of deep infection, prolonged intubation, and delayed discharge from hospital in one study (221). Nutritional supplementation is more effective and safer by the enteral route than by the parenteral route. Supplementation of gastrostomy feeds can be very effective in children with a feeding tube in place. Otherwise, supplementary feeding via a fine nasogastric tube may be offered for 3 to 6 weeks, prior to surgery. The period of preoperative preparation should be closely supervised and monitored by a gastroenterologist and dietician. Low serum iron and transferrin levels are common and may result in iron deficiency anemia. Gastroesophageal reflux is common and must be treated medically or by fundoplication, prior to major surgery. Perioperative conversion of the gastrostomy tube to a gastrojejunal feeding tube allows effective enteral nutrition early in the postoperative period when the risk of gastroparesis and gastroesophageal reflux is highest due to narcotic analgesics.

Good respiratory function is vital. Children with known respiratory disease require evaluation and preoperative chest management including physical therapy. Those with seasonal asthma should be offered surgery at the optimum time of year from the respiratory point of view.

Some seizure medications such as valproate are associated with both an anti–vitamin D effect (resulting in osteopenia and increased fracture risk) as well as increased bleeding (increased transfusion requirements) (216, 222). It may be prudent to wean valproate and convert to other antiepileptics as needed to control seizures if possible. Because the primary effect is on platelet function, routine screening parameters fail to detect the problem. The platelet function assay is the necessary test. Seizure management should be optimized and closely supervised throughout the perioperative period.

Comfortable sitting, for prolonged periods of time, is essential for participation in family life, schooling, and community activities. The functional goal of scoliosis surgery in CP is to improve sitting balance and ease the burden of care. The biomechanical goal is to achieve a stiff, well-balanced spine over a level pelvis with flexible, pain-free hips. The surgical goal is a long posterior spinal fusion with the fusion limits from high in the dorsal spine to the pelvis in the majority of children (223). If the fusion does not extend to high in the thoracic spine, there is a risk of a junctional kyphosis that may interfere with the patient's ability to see above the horizontal, make eye contact, and interact with their family and environment (see Figs. 14-63 to 14-73).

Technical Issues (Figs. 14-14, 14-15, and 14-62 to 14-73). Multisegmental fixation using sublaminar wires or combinations of hooks and pedicle screws to strong double rods are necessary to distribute the corrective forces throughout the length of the fusion. The unit rod has excellent results and costs a fraction of other systems (223, 224). Fusion should include the pelvis when pelvic obliquity exceeds 10 to 15 degrees, on an anteroposterior radiograph of the pelvis with the patient in the sitting position (216, 223). Without fusion to the pelvis, pelvic obliquity may continue to progress, resulting in impaired seating, recurrent hip displacement, and failure to reach the goals of the operation (225). Many surgeons recommend fusion to the pelvis in all GMFCS V patients regardless of preoperative pelvic obliquity. Fixation to the pelvis may include hooks, rods, and screws with the best documented and most reliable results reported using the Galveston technique (224, 225) (Fig. 14-62A,B) (see Figs. 14-14 and 14-15). To improve sitting, spinal balance in both the coronal and the sagittal planes is essential. Maintenance of this desired alignment is feasible with a solid fusion throughout the length of the spine. A strong fusion mass will necessitate large quantities of allograft, autograft, bone substitutes, and/or the addition of growth factors (223).

With regular monitoring and surgery at an appropriate age and stage of curve progression, anterior spinal surgery and anterior spinal fusion is not required. However, some children develop rigid curves and an anterior spinal release may be necessary as part of a one- or two-stage correction before instrumented posterior fusion. Specific indications for anterior spinal surgery may include the need to correct severe pelvic obliquity, to achieve balance in large rigid curves that do not correct to <50 degrees during lateral bending or traction radiographs. The release of severe rigid curves may be achieved by resection of the anterior longitudinal ligament, excision of the annulus, and removal of disc material and end-plate cartilage back to the posterior annulus and posterior longitudinal ligament. This may be done via an open or thoracoscopic approach (226). The role of anterior instrumentation is not established and may not be necessary when a rigid posterior instrumentation is performed. Anterior fusion may be indicated in immature children with growth potential to avoid the crankshaft phenomenon.

Spinal surgery in severe CP carries a significant risk of mortality and severe morbidity. Hence prior consultation with the multidisciplinary team, optimization of nutrition, respiratory function, and tone management are essential. If an ITB pump is present, this can be adjusted postoperatively to reduce tone and the need for analgesia. However, the skin over the pump needs to be protected during surgery from injury on the spine frame, hematogenous infection of the pump must be avoided by all means, and the catheter needs to be protected or resited through the fusion mass. Postoperative fluid management is critical in these compromised patients. Intraoperative blood loss should be minimized by surgical technique and sometimes the use of additional agents such as Aprotinin (227). Both hypovolemia and coagulopathy must be avoided. The use of the cell saver intraoperatively may also be beneficial. The role of intraoperative monitoring of neurologic function remains controversial in nonambulant children with CP. There are problems with both somatosensory spinal evoked potentials and cooperation and communication during a wake-up test (216).

Postoperative bracing is not usually required. A brace may be helpful when osteopenia is identified intraoperatively and fixation is deemed to be tenuous. Parents and caregivers need clear instructions in regard to activity limitations and precautions in the immediate postoperative period.

Outcomes of Spinal Surgery in Cerebral Palsy.
Spinal surgery in CP has been shown to effectively correct the deformity, with curve correction varying from 45% to 75% accompanied by good correction of pelvic obliquity. Curve progression after successful fusion is usually <10 degrees although this may be greater in immature individuals with growth potential (223–225, 228, 229). Surgical complications are common, often severe, and sometimes life threatening. Complications include fixation failure, respiratory failure, wound infection, decubitus ulceration, neurologic injury, intestinal obstruction, pancreatitis, and death. Major complication rates vary from 40% to 80% and mortality rates from 5% to 7% (230). Pseudarthrosis may be asymptomatic but may result in progression of deformity, implant failure, and the need for revision surgery. Deep wound infections are relatively common, compared to idiopathic scoliois but may be reduced by using allograft impregnated with antibiotics (231). Deep infection requires surgical debridement, antibiotics, nutritional and respiratory support. Vacuum-assisted closure may be very helpful in managing some wound complications.

Spinal fusion in children with CP improves sitting position and appears to improve upper limb function, eating, and respiratory function (216, 232). It may also prolong life (232). What is not yet clearly established is the effect of spinal surgery on the patient's quality of life and in reducing the burden of care (232, 233). It is very likely that quality of life and reduced burden of care can be achieved, but we have until recently lacked appropriate tools to measure these outcomes. Such tools are now being developed and will allow the effects of spinal surgery to be assessed in the domains of most importance to the patient and their families (234).

ACKNOWLEDGMENTS

We acknowledge the support and help of the staff of the Educational Resource Centre, The Royal Children's Hospital in Melbourne, who provided the clinical photographs. Our sincere thanks to Medical Illustrator, Bill Reid, who drew all of the original illustrations.

REFERENCES

1. Little WJ. On the incidence of abnormal parturition, difficult labour, premature birth and asphyxia neonatorum on the mental and physical condition of the child, especially in relation to deformities. In: Transactions of the Obstetrical Society of London. London, UK: Obstetrical Society of London, 1862:293–344.
2. Osler W. *The cerebral palsies of children. A clinical study for the infirmary for nervous diseases.* Philadelphia, PA: Blakiston, 1889.
3. Freud S. Die infantile Cerebrallahmung. In: Northnagel H, ed. *Specielle Pathologie und Therapie*, Bd IX, Teil III. Vienna, Austria: Holder, 1897:1–327.
4. Mac Keith RC, MacKenzie ICK, Polani PE, eds. The Little Club Memorandum on terminology and classification of 'cerebral palsy'. *Cerebral Palsy Bull* 1959;1:27–35.
5. Rosenbaum P, Paneth N, Leviton A. et al. A report: the definition and classification of cerebral palsy April 2006. *Dev Med Child Neurol* 2007;49(Suppl 109):8–14.
6. Blair E. Epidemiology of the cerebral palsies. *Orthop Clin North Am* 2010;41:441–455.
7. Ostrea EM, Morales V, Ngoumgna E, et al. Prevalence of fetal exposure to environmental toxins as determined by meconium analysis. *Neurotoxicology* 2002;23:329–339.
8. Johnson MA, Weick JP, Pearce RA, et al. Functional neural development from human embryonic stem cells: accelerated synaptic activity via astrocyte coculture. *J Neurosci* 2007;27:3069–3077.
9. Gogtay N, Giedd JN, Lusk L, et al. Dynamic mapping of human cortical development during childhood through early childhood. *Proc Natl Acad Sci U S A* 2004;101:8174–8179.
10. WHO Multicentre Growth Reference Study Group. WHO Motor Development Study: windows of achievement for six gross motor development milestones. *Acta Paediatr* 2006;450(Suppl):86–95.
11. ©CanChild Centre for Childhood Disability Research. Ontario Motor Growth (OMG) Study Project Report, 2002.
12. Rosenbaum PL, Walter SD, Hanna SE, et al. Prognosis for gross motor function in cerebral palsy: creation of motor development curves. *JAMA* 2002;288:1357–1363.
13. Palisano R, Rosenbaum P, Walter S, et al. Development and reliability of a system to classify gross motor function in children with cerebral palsy. *Dev Med Child Neurol* 1997;39:214–223.
14. Russell DJ, Rosenbaum PL, Cadman DT, et al. The gross motor function measure: a means to evaluate the effects of physical therapy. *Dev Med Child Neurol* 1989;31:341–352.
15. Palisano RJ, Rosenbaum P, Bartlett P. Content validity of the expanded and revised Gross Motor Function Classification System. *Dev Med Child Neurol* 2008;50:744–750.
16. Johnson DC, Damiano DL, Abel MF. The evolution of gait in childhood and adolescent cerebral palsy. *J Pediatr Orthop* 1997;17:392–396.
17. Bell KJ, Ounpuu S, DeLuca P, et al. Natural progression of gait in children with cerebral palsy. *J Pediatr Orthop* 2002;22:677–682.
18. Gough M, Eve LC, Robinson RO. Short-term outcome of multilevel surgical intervention in spastic diplegic cerebral palsy compared with the natural history. *Dev Med Child Neurol* 2004;96:91–97.
19. Hanna SE, Rosenbaum PL, Bartlett DJ, et al. Stability and decline in gross motor function among children and youth with cerebral palsy aged 2 to 21 years. *Dev Med Child Neurol* 2009;51:295–302.
20. Stanley F, Blair E, Alberman E. *"What are the cerebral palsies?" Cerebral Palsies: epidemiology and causal pathways*, Chapter 2. London, UK: Mac Keith Press, 2000:8–13.
21. Howard J, Soo B, Graham HK, et al. Cerebral palsy in Victoria: motor types, topography and gross motor function. *J Paediatr Child Health* 2005;41:479–483.
22. Johnston M, Hagberg H. Sex and the pathogenesis of cerebral palsy. *Dev Med Child Neurol* 2007;49:74–78.
23. McManus V, Guillem P, Surman G, et al. SCPE work, standardization and definition—an overview of the activities of SCPE: a collaboration of European CP registers. *Zhongguo Dang Dai Er Ke Za Zhi* 2006;8:261–265.

24. Watson L, Blair E, Stanley FJ. Report of the Western Australian Cerebral Palsy Register to birth year 1999. Perth Telethon Institute for Child Health Research, 2006. Available at http://www.ichr.uwa.edu.au/files/user1/WACR_Report_a4.pdf

25. Stanley F, Blair E, Alberman E. *'The special case of multiple pregnancy'. Cerebral palsies: epidemiology and causal pathways*, Chapter 10. London, UK: Mac Keith Press, 2000:109–137.

26. Sher A, Petterson B, Blair E, et al. The risk of mortality or cerebral palsy in twins: a collaborative population-based study. *Pediatr Res* 2002;52:671–681.

27. Topp M, Huusom L, Langhoff-Roos J, et al. Multiple birth and cerebral palsy in Europe: a multicenter study. *Acta Obstet Gynecol Scand* 2004;83:548–553.

28. Panteliadis CP, Hausler M. Aetiological factors. In: *Cerebral palsy. A multidisciplinary approach*. Munchen: Dustri-Verlag, 2011:P55–P67.

29. Graham HK, Selber P. Musculoskeletal aspects of cerebral palsy. *J Bone Joint Surg Br* 2003;85-B:157–166.

30. Graham HK. Mechanisms of deformity. In: Scrutton D, Damiano D, Mayston M, eds. *Management of the motor disorders of children with cerebral palsy*, Chapter 8, 2nd ed. Clinics Dev Med No 161. London, UK: Mac Keith Press, 2004:105–129.

31. Bax M, Tydeman C, Flodmark O. Clinical and MRI correlates of cerebral palsy: the European Cerebral Palsy Study. *JAMA* 2006;296:1602–1608.

32. Gibson CS, MacLennan AH, Dekker GA. Genetic polymorphisms and spontaneous preterm birth. *Obstet Gynecol* 2007;109:384–391.

33. Ashwai S, Russman BS, Blasco PA, et al. Practice parameter: diagnostic assessment of the child with cerebral palsy. *Neurology* 2004;62:851–863.

34. Ziv I, Blackburn N, Rang M, et al. Muscle growth in the normal and spastic mouse. *Dev Med Child Neurol* 1984;26:94–99.

35. Cosgrove AP, Graham HK. Botulinum toxin A prevents the development of contractures in the hereditary spastic mouse. *Dev Med Child Neurol* 1994;36:379–385.

36. Lieber RL, Friden J. Spasticity causes a fundamental rearrangement of muscle-joint interaction. *Muscle Nerve* 2002;25:265–270.

37. Shortland AP, Harris CA, Gough M, et al. Architecture of the medial gastrocnemius in children with spastic diplegia. *Dev Med Child Neurol* 2002;44:158–163.

38. Hutchinson R, Graham HK. Management of spasticity in children. In: Barnes MP, Johnson GR, eds. *Upper motor neurone syndrome and spasticity. Clinical management and neurophysiology*, 2nd ed., Chapter 12. Cambridge, UK: Cambridge University Press, 2008:214–239.

39. M.E.N.T.O.R.S. (Methodologies for Experts in Neurotoxin Therapy: Outreach, Resources and Support). Focus on Cerebral Palsy. Monograph: A continuing Medical Education DVD Activity. New York, NY: The Institute for Medical Studies, 2004.

40. Gage JR. *Gait analysis in cerebral palsy*. London, UK: Mac Keith Press, 1991.

41. Paley D. Dynamic deformities and lever arm considerations. In: Herzenberg JE, ed. *Principles of deformity correction*, Chapter 22. Berlin, Germany: Springer-Verlag, 2002:761–775.

42. Graham HK. Classifying cerebral palsy (on the other hand). *J Pediatr Orthop* 2005;25:127–128.

43. Sanger TD, Delgado MR, Gaebler-Spira D, et al. Task force on childhood motor disorders. Classification and definition of disorders causing hypertonia in childhood. *Pediatrics* 2003;111:e89–e97.

44. SCPE. Surveillance of cerebral palsy in Europe: a collaboration of cerebral palsy surveys and registers. *Dev Med Child Neurol* 2000;42:816–824.

45. Rice J, Russo R, Halbert J, et al. Motor function in 5-year-old children with cerebral palsy in the South Australian population. *Dev Med Child Neurol* 2009;51:551–556.

46. Albright L. Basal ganglia injury and resulting movement disorders. In: Gage JR, Schwartz MH, Koop SE, et al., eds. The identification and treatment of gait problems in cerebral palsy, Chapter 2.3. Clin Dev Med No 180–181. London, UK: Mac Keith Press, 2009.

47. McDowell BC, Kerr C, Parkes J. Interobserver agreement of the Gross Motor Function Classification System in an ambulant population of children with cerebral palsy. *Dev Med Child Neurol* 2007;49:528–533.

48. Shevell MI, Dagenais L, Hall N. Comorbidities in cerebral palsy and their relationship to neurologic subtype and GMFCS level. *Neurology* 2009;72:2090–2096.

49. Robin J, Graham HK, Selber P, et al. Proximal femoral geometry in cerebral palsy. A population-based cross-sectional study. *J Bone Joint Surg Br* 2008;90-B:1372–1379.

50. Soo B, Howard J, Boyd RN, et al. Hip displacement in cerebral palsy: a population based study of incidence in relation to motor type, topographical distribution and gross motor function. *J Bone Joint Surgery Am* 2006;88-A:121–129.

51. Wallace SJ. Epilepsy in cerebral palsy. *Dev Med Child Neurol* 2001;43:713–717.

52. Schenk-Rootlieb AJ, van Niewenhuizen O, van der Graaf Y, et al. The prevalence of cerebral visual disturbance in children with cerebral palsy. *Dev Med Child Neurol* 1992;34:473–480.

53. Seddon PC, Khan Y. Respiratory problems in children with neurological impairment. *Arch Dis Child* 2003;88:75–78.

54. Okuyama H, Kubota A, Kawahara A, et al. The efficacy and long-term outcome of laparoscopic Nissen Fundoplication in neurologically impaired children. *Pediatr Endosurg Innov Tech* 2004;8:5–11.

55. Samson-Fang LJ, Stevenson RD. Identification of malnutrition in children with cerebral palsy: poor performance of weight-for-height centiles. *Dev Med Child Neurol* 2000;42:162–168.

56. Sullivan B. Gastrointestinal disorders in children with neurodevelopmental disabilities. *Dev Disabil Res Rev* 2008;14:128–136.

57. Tallaksen CME, Durr A, Brice A. Recent advances in hereditary spastic paraplegia. *Curr Opin Neurol* 2001;14:457–463.

58. Harvey A, Rosenbaum P, Graham HK, et al. Current and future uses of the Gross Motor Function Classification System. Letter to the Editor. *Dev Med Child Neurol* 2009;51:328–329.

59. Rodda JM, Graham HK, Galea MP. Correction of severe crouch gait in spastic diplegia by multilevel orthopaedic surgery: outcome at one and five years. *J Bone Joint Surg Am* 2006;88-A:2653–2664.

60. Graham HK, Harvey A, Rodda J, et al. The functional mobility scale. *J Pediatr Orthop* 2004;24:514–520.

61. Novacheck TF, Stout JL, Tervo R. Reliability and validity of the Gillette Functional Assessment Questionnaire as an outcome measure in children with walking disabilities. *J Pediatr Orthop* 2000;20:75–81.

62. World Health Organization. International Classification of Functioning, Disability and Health (ICF) 2001. Geneva, Switzerland: World Health Organization.

63. Harvey A, Graham HK, Morris ME, et al. The Functional Mobility Scale: ability to detect change following single event multilevel surgery. *Dev Med Child Neurol* 2007;49:603–607.

64. Scrutton D, Baird G, Smeeton N. Hip dysplasia in bilateral cerebral palsy: incidence and natural history in children aged 18 months to 5 years. *Dev Med Child Neurol* 2001;43:586–600.

65. Dobson F, Boyd RN, Parrott J, et al. Hip surveillance in children with cerebral palsy: impact on the surgical management of spastic hip disease. *J Bone Joint Surg Br* 2002;84-B:720–726.

66. Wynter M, Gibson N, Kentish M, et al. Consensus Statement on Hip Surveillance for Children with Cerebral Palsy. Australian Standards of Care. www.cpaustralia.com.au/ausacpdm

67. Davids JR, Gibson TW, Pugh LI. Quantitative segmental analysis of weight-bearing radiographs of the foot and ankle for children: normal alignment. *J Pediatr Orthop* 2005;25:769–776.

68. Davids JR, Ounpuu S, DeLuca PA, et al. Optimization of walking ability of children with cerebral palsy. *J Bone Joint Surg Am* 2003;85-A:2224–2234.

69. Gage JR. Con: interobserver variability of gait analysis. Editorial. *J Pediatr Orthop* 2003;23:290–291.

70. Wright JG. Pro: interobserver variability of gait analysis. Editorial. *J Pediatr Orthop* 2003;23:288–289.

71. Gorton GE, Hebert DA, Gannotti ME. Assessment of the kinematic variability among 12 motion analysis laboratories. *Gait Posture* 2009;29:398–402.

72. Noonan KJ, Halliday S, Browne R, et al. Interobserver variability of gait analysis in patients with cerebral palsy. *J Pediatr Orthop* 2003;23:279–287.

73. Schwartz MH, Trost JP, Wervey RA. Measurement and management of errors in quantitative gait data. *Gait Posture* 2004;20:196–203.

74. Baker R. An engineering approach to reducing measurement error in clinical gait analysis. *J Biomech* 2007;40(Suppl 2):26.

75. Narayanan UG. The role of gait analysis in the orthopaedic management of ambulatory cerebral palsy. *Curr Opin Pediatr* 2007;19:38–43.

76. Koman LA, Mooney JF, Smith B, et al. Management of cerebral palsy with botulinum-A toxin: preliminary investigation. *J Pediatr Orthop* 1993;4:489–495.

77. Mackey AH, Lobb GL, Walt SE, et al. Reliability and validity of the Observational Gait Scale in children with spastic diplegia. *Dev Med Child Neurol* 2003;45:4–11.

78. Read HS, Hazlewood ME, Hillman SJ, et al. Edinburgh visual gait score for use in cerebral palsy. *J Pediatr Orthop* 2003;23:296–301.

79. Graham HK. Botulinum toxin type A management of spasticity in the context of orthopaedic surgery for children with spastic cerebral palsy. *Eur J Neurol* 2001;8(Suppl 5):S30–S39.

80. Boyd RN, Graham HK. Objective measurement of clinical findings in the use of botulinum toxin type A for the management of children with cerebral palsy. *Eur J Neurol* 1999;6(Suppl 4):S23–S35.

81. Butler C, Darrah J. Effects of neurodevelopmental treatment (NDT) for cerebral palsy: an AACPDM evidence report. *Dev Med Child Neurol* 2001;43:778–790.

82. Darrah J, Watkins B, Chen L, et al. Conductive education intervention for children with cerebral palsy: an AACPDM evidence report. *Dev Med Child Neurol* 2004;46:187–203.

83. Facchin P, Rosa-Rizzotto M, Turconi A, et al. Multisite trial on efficacy of constraint-induced movement therapy in children with hemiplegia: study design and methodology. *Am J Phys Med Rehab* 2009;88:216–230.

84. Leonard J, Graham HK. Treatment of motor disorders in cerebral palsy with Botulinum neurotoxin. In: Jankovic J, ed. *Botulinum toxin: therapeutic clinical practice and science*, Chapter 14. Philadelphia, PA: Saunders Elsevier Inc, 2009:172–191.

85. Dodd KJ, Taylor NF, Graham HK. A randomized clinical trial of strength training in young people with cerebral palsy. *Dev Med Child Neurol* 2003;45:652–657.

86. Butler C, Campbell S. Evidence of the effects of intrathecal Baclofen for spastic and dystonic cerebral palsy. *Dev Med Child Neurol* 2000;42:634–645.

87. McLaughlin J, Bjornson K, Temkin N, et al. Selective dorsal rhizotomy: meta-analysis of three randomized controlled trials. *Dev Med Child Neurol* 2002;44:17–25.

88. Albright AL. Neurosurgical options in cerebral palsy. *Paediatr Child Health* 2008;18:414–418.

89. Ward M. Pharmacologic treatment with oral medications. In: Gage JR, Schwartz MH, Koop SE, et al., eds. *The identification and treatment of gait problems in cerebral palsy*, Chapter 4.3. Clin Dev Med No 180–181. London, UK: Mac Keith Press, 2009.

90. Khot A, Sloan S, Desai S, et al. Adductor release and chemodenervation in children with cerebral palsy: a pilot study in 16 children. *J Child Orthop* 2008;2:293–299.

91. De Paiva A, Meunier FA, Molgo J, et al. Functional repair of motor endplates after botulinum neurotoxin type A poisoning: biphasic switch of synaptic activity between nerve sprouts and their parent terminals. *Proc Natl Acad Sci U S A* 1999;96:3200–3205.

92. Corry IS, Cosgrove AP, Walsh EG, et al. Botulinum toxin A in the hemiplegic upper limb: a double-blind trial. *Dev Med Child Neurol* 1997;39:185–193.

93. Koman AL, Mooney JF, Smith BP, et al. Management of spasticity in cerebral palsy with botulinum toxin A: preliminary investigation. *J Pediatr Orthop* 1993;13:489–495.

94. Cosgrove AP, Corry IS, Graham HK. Botulinum toxin in the management of the lower limb in cerebral palsy. *Dev Med Child Neurol* 1994;36:386–396.

95. Borton DC, Walker K, Pirpiris M, et al. Isolated calf lengthening in cerebral palsy. Outcome analysis of risk factors. *J Bone Joint Surg Br* 2001;83-B:364–370.

96. Boyd RN, Graham HK. Botulinum toxin A in the management of children with cerebral palsy: indications and outcome. *Eur J Neurol* 1997;4(Suppl 2):S15–S22.

97. Rodda JM, Graham HK, Carson L, et al. Sagittal gait patterns in spastic diplegia. *J Bone Joint Surg Br* 2004;86-B:251–258.

98. Graham HK, Aoki KR, Autti-Ramo I, et al. Recommendations for the use of botulinum toxin type A in the management of cerebral palsy. *Gait Posture* 2000;11:67–79.

99. Heinen F, Molenaers G, Fairhurst C, et al. European consensus table 2006 on botulinum toxin for children with cerebral palsy. *Eur J Paediatr Neurol* 2006;10:215–225.

100. Naidu K, Smith K, Sheedy M, et al. Systemic adverse events following Botulinum toxin A therapy in children with cerebral palsy. *Dev Med Child Neurol* 2010;52:139–144.

101. Chin TYP, Nattrass GR, Selber P, et al. Accuracy of intramuscular injection of botulinum toxin A in juvenile cerebral palsy. *J Pediatr Orthop* 2005;25:286–291.

102. Berweck S, Schroeder AS, Fietzek UM, et al. Sonography-guided injection of botulinum toxin in children with cerebral palsy. *Lancet* 2004;363:249–250.

103. Eames N, Baker R, Hill N, et al. The effect of botulinum toxin A on gastrocnemius length: magnitude and duration of response. *Dev Med Child Neurol* 1999;41:226–232.

104. Sutherland DH, Kaufman KR, Wyatt MP, et al. Double-blind study of botulinum toxin injections into the gastrocnemius muscle in patients with cerebral palsy. *Gait Posture* 1999;10:1–9.

105. Scholtes VA, Dallmeijer AJ, Knol DL, et al. The combined effect of lower-limb multilevel botulinum toxin type A and comprehensive rehabilitation on mobility in children with cerebral palsy: a randomized clinical trial. *Arch Phys Med Rehabil* 2006;87:1551–1558.

106. Bjornson K, Hays R, Graubert C, et al. Botulinum toxin for spasticity in children with cerebral palsy: a comprehensive evaluation. *Pediatrics* 2007;120:49–58.

107. Desloovere K, Molenaers G, Jonkers I, et al. A randomized study of combined botulinum toxin type A and casting in the ambulant child with cerebral palsy using objective outcome measures. *Eur J Neurol* 2001;8(Suppl 5):75–87.

108. Simpson DM, Gracies J-M, Graham HK, et al. Assessment: botulinum neurotoxin for the treatment of spasticity (an evidence-based review): report of the Therapeutics and Technology Assessment Subcommittee of the American Academy of Neurology. *Neurology* 2008;70:1691–1698.

109. Love SC, Novak I, Kentish M, et al. Botulinum toxin assessment, intervention and after-care for lower limb spasticity in children with cerebral palsy: international consensus statement. *Eur J Neurol* 2010;17(Suppl 2):9–37.

110. Michlitsch MG, Rethlefsen SA, Kay RM. The contributions of anterior and posterior tibialis dysfunction to varus foot deformity in patients with cerebral palsy. *J Bone Joint Surg Am* 2006;88-A:1764–1768.

111. Graham HK, Boyd R, Carlin JB, et al. Does botulinum toxin A combined with hip bracing prevent hip displacement in children with cerebral palsy and "hips-at-risk"? A randomized controlled trial. *J Bone Joint Surgery Am* 2008;90-A:23–33.

112. Molenaers G, Desloovere K, Fabry G, et al. The effects of quantitative gait assessment and botulinum toxin A on musculoskeletal surgery in children with cerebral palsy. *J Bone Joint Surg Am* 2006;88-A:161–170.

113. Molenaers G, Desloovere K, De Cat J, et al. Single event multilevel botulinum toxin type A treatment and surgery: similarities and differences. *Eur J Neurol* 2001;8(Suppl 5):S88–S97.

114. Gibson N, Graham HK, Love S. Botulinum toxin in the management of focal muscle over activity in children with cerebral palsy. *Disabil Rehabil* 2007;29(23):1813–1822.

115. Fehlings D, Rang M, Glazier J, et al. An evaluation of botulinum-A toxin injections to improve upper extremity function in children with hemiplegic cerebral palsy. *J Pediatr* 2000;137:331–337.

116. Wallen M, O'Flaherty SJ, Waugh M-CA. Functional outcomes of intramuscular botulinum toxin type A and occupational therapy in the upper limbs of children with cerebral palsy: a randomized controlled trial. *Arch Phys Med Rehabil* 2007;88:1–10.

117. Russo RN, Crotty M, Miller MD, et al. Upper-limb botulinum toxin A injection and occupational therapy in children with hemiplegic cerebral palsy identified from a population register: a single-blind, randomized, controlled trial. *Pediatrics* 2007;119:e1149–e1158.

118. Lowe K, Novak I, Cusick A. Repeat injection of botulinum toxin A is safe and effective for upper limb movement and function in children with cerebral palsy. *Dev Med Child Neurol* 2007;49:823–829.

119. DeMatteo C, Law M, Russell D, et al. *QUEST: Quality of Upper Extremity Skills Test manual*. Hamilton, ON: Neurodevelopmental Research Unit, Chedoke Campus, Chedoke-McMasters Hospital, 2000.

120. Randall MJ, Carlin J, Reddihough DS, et al. Reliability of the Melbourne Assessment of unilateral upper limb function—a quantitative test of quality of movement in children with neurological impairment. *Dev Med Child Neurol* 2001;43:761–767.

121. Krumlinde-Sundholm L, Holmefur M, Kottorp A, et al. The Assisting Hand Assessment: current evidence of validity, reliability, and responsiveness to change. *Dev Med Child Neurol* 2007;49:259–264.

122. Howell K, Selber P, Graham HK, et al. Botulinum neurotoxin A: an unusual systemic effect. *J Paediatr Child Health* 2007;43:499–501.

123. Barwood S, Baillieu C, Boyd RN, et al. Analgesic effects of botulinum toxin A: a randomized placebo-controlled clinical trial. *Dev Med Child Neurol* 2000;42:116–121.

124. Lundy CT, Doherty GM, Fairhurst CB. Botulinum toxin type A injections can be effective treatment for pain with hip spasms and cerebral palsy. *Dev Med Child Neurol* 2009;51:705–710.

125. Winters T, Gage J, Hicks R. Gait patterns in spastic hemiplegia in children and adults. *J Bone Joint Surg Am* 1987;69-A:437–441.

126. Riad J, Haglund-Akerlind Y, Miller F. Classification of spastic hemiplegic cerebral palsy in children. *J Pediatr Orthop* 2007;27:758–764.

127. Rodda J, Graham HK. Classification of gait patterns in spastic hemiplegia and spastic diplegia: a basis for a management algorithm. *Eur J Neurol* 2001;8(Supp 5): S98–S108.

128. Sutherland DH, Davids JR. Common gait abnormalities of the knee in cerebral palsy. *Clin Orthop Relat Res* 1993;288:139–147.

129. Silver RL, de la Garza J, Rang M. The myth of muscle balance. A study of relative strengths and excursions of normal muscles about the foot and ankle. *J Bone Joint Surg Br* 1985;67-B:432–437.

130. Delp SL, Zajac FE. Force- and moment-generating capacity of lower extremity muscles before and after tendon lengthening. *Clin Orthop Relat Res* 1992;284:247–259.

131. Delp SL, Arnold AS, Speirs RA, et al. Hamstrings and psoas lengths during normal and crouch gait implications for muscle-tendon surgery. *J Orthop Res* 1996;14:144–151.

132. Hoffinger SA, Rab GT, Abou-Ghaida H. Hamstrings in crouch gait. *J Pediatr Orthop* 1993;13:722–726.

133. Graham HK. Cerebral palsy. In: McCarthy JJ, Drennan JC, eds. *Drennan's the child's foot and ankle*, 2nd ed., Chapter 13. Philadelphia, PA: Lippincott, Williams & Wilkins, 2010:188–218.

134. Chin TYP, Duncan JA, Johnstone BR, et al. Management of the upper limb in cerebral palsy. *J Pediatr Orthop B* 2005;14:389–404.

135. Smitherman JA, Davids JR, Tanner S, et al. Functional outcomes following single-event multilevel surgery of the upper extremity for children with hemiplegic cerebral palsy. *J Bone Joint Surg* 2011;93:655–661.

136. Eliasson A-C, Krumlinde-Sundholm L, Rosblad B, et al. The Manual Ability Classification System (MACS) for children with cerebral palsy: scale development and evidence of validity and reliability. *Dev Med Child Neurol* 2006;48:549–554.

137. Davids JR, Peace LC, Wagner LV, et al. Validation of the Shriners Hospital for Children Upper extremity Evaluation (SHUEE) for children with hemiplegic cerebral palsy. *J Bone Joint Surg Am* 2006;88-A:326–333.

138. Van Heest AE, House JH, Cariello C. Upper extremity surgical treatment of cerebral palsy. *J Hand Surg* 1999;24-A:323–330.

139. Chin TYP, Graham HK. Botulinum toxin in the management of upper limb spasticity in cerebral palsy. *Hand Clin* 2003;19:591–600.

140. Bunata RE. Pronator teres rerouting in children with cerebral palsy. *J Hand Surg* 2006;31-A:474–482.

141. Sodl JF, Kozin SH, Kaulmann RA. Development and use of a wrist fusion plate for children and adolescents. *J Pediatr Orthop* 2002;2:146–149.

142. Carlson MG, Gallagher K, Spirtos M. Surgical treatment of swan-neck deformity in hemiplegic cerebral palsy. *J Hand Surg* 2007;32-A: 1418–1422.

143. Koman LA, Sarlikiotis T, Smith BP. Surgery of the upper extremity in cerebral palsy. *Orthop Clin North Am* 2010;41:519–529.

144. Dahlin LB, Komoto-Tufvesson Y, Salgeback S. Surgery of the spastic hand in cerebral palsy. *J Hand Surg* 1998;23-B:334–339.

145. Eliasson A-C, Ekholm C, Carstedt T. Hand function in children with cerebral palsy after upper limb tendon transfer and muscle release. *Dev Med Child Neurol* 1998;40:612–621.

146. Johnstone BR, Richardson PWF, Coombs CJ, et al. Functional and cosmetic outcome of surgery for cerebral palsy in the upper limb. *Hand Clin* 2003;19:679–686.

147. Dobson F, Graham HK, Baker R, et al. Multilevel orthopaedic surgery in group IV spastic hemiplegia. *J Bone Joint Surg Br* 2005;87-B:548–555.

148. Rang M. Cerebral palsy. In: Morrissey RT, ed. *Lovell and Winter's paediatric orthopaedics*, 3rd ed. Vol. 1. Philadelphia, PA: JB Lippincott, 1990:465–506.

149. Novacheck TF. Orthopaedic treatment of muscle contractures. In: Gage JR, Schwartz MH, Koop SE, et al., eds. *The identification and treatment of gait problems in cerebral palsy*, Chapter 5.5. Clin Dev Med No 180–181. London, UK: Mac Keith Press, 2009.

150. Gage JR. Orthopaedic treatment of long bone torsions. In: Gage JR, Schwartz MH, Koop SE, et al., eds. *The identification and treatment of gait problems in cerebral palsy*. Clin Dev Med No 180–181. London, UK: Mac Keith Press, 2009:473–491.

151. Ruda R, Frost HM. Cerebral palsy: spastic varus and forefoot adductus treated by intramuscular posterior tibialis tendon lengthening. *Clin Orthop* 1971;79:61–70.

152. Green NE, Griffin PP, Shiavi R. Split posterior tibial-tendon transfer in spastic cerebral palsy. *J Bone Joint Surg Am* 1983;65-A:748–754.

153. Kling TF, Kaufer H, Hensinger RN. Split posterior tibial-tendon transfers in children with cerebral spastic paralysis and equinovarus deformity. *J Bone Joint Surg* 1985;67:186–194.

154. Hoffer MM, Reiswig JA, Garrett AM, et al. The split anterior tibial tendon transfer in the treatment of spastic varus hindfoot of childhood. *Orthop Clin North Am* 1974;5:31–37.

155. Hoffer MM, Barakat G, Koffman M. 10-Year follow-up of split anterior tibial tendon transfer in cerebral palsied patients with spastic equinovarus deformity. *J Pediatr Orthop* 1985;5:432–434.

156. Ireland ML, Hoffer M. Triple arthrodesis for children with spastic cerebral palsy. *Dev Med Child Neurol* 1985;27:623–627.

157. Bache CE, Selber P, Graham HK. Mini-symposium: cerebral palsy: the management of spastic diplegia. *Curr Orthop* 2003;17:88–104.

158. Novacheck TF, Trost JP, Schwartz MH. Intramuscular psoas lengthening improves dynamic hip function in children with cerebral palsy. *J Pediatr Orthop* 2002;22:158–164.

159. Thomason P, Baker R, Dodd K, et al. Single event multilevel surgery in children with spastic diplegia: a pilot randomized controlled trial. *J Bone Joint Surg Am* 2011;93-A:451–460.

160. Sutherland DH, Zilberfarb JL, Kaufman KR, et al. Psoas release at the pelvic brim in ambulatory patients with cerebral palsy: operative technique and functional outcome. *J Pediatr Orthop* 1997;17:563–570.

161. Baumann JU, Ruetsch H, Schurmann K. Distal hamstring lengthening in cerebral palsy. An evaluation by gait analysis. *Int Orthop* 1980;3: 305–309.

162. Strayer LM. Recession of the gastrocnemius. An operation to relieve spastic contracture of the calf muscles. *J Bone Joint Surg Am* 1950; 32-A:671–676.

163. Chambers H, Lauer AL, Kaufman K, et al. Prediction of outcome after rectus femoris surgery in cerebral palsy: the role of cocontraction of the rectus femoris and vastus lateralis. *J Pediatr Orthop* 1998;18:703–711.

164. Muthusamy K, Seidl AJ, Friesen RM, et al. Rectus femoris transfer in children with cerebral palsy. Evaluation of transfer site and preoperative indicators. *J Pediatr Orthop* 2008;28:674–678.

165. Pirpiris M, Trivett A, Baker R, et al. Femoral derotation osteotomy in spastic diplegia. *J Bone Joint Surg Br* 2003;85-B:265–272.

166. Beauchesne R, Miller F, Moseley C. Proximal femoral osteotomy using the AO fixed-angle blade plate. *J Pediatr Orthop* 1992;12:735–740.

167. Selber P, Filho ER, Dallalana R, et al. Supramalleolar derotation osteotomy of the tibia, with T plate fixation: technique and results. *J Bone Joint Surg Br* 2004;86-B:1170–1175.

168. Inan M, Ferri-de Baros F, Chan G, et al. Correction of rotational deformity of the tibia in cerebral palsy by percutaneous supramalleolar osteotomy. *J Bone Joint Surg Br* 2005;87-B:1411–1415.

169. Hau R, Dickens DRV, Nattrass GR, et al. Which implant for proximal femoral osteotomy in children? A comparison of the AO (ASIF) 90° fixed-angle blade plate and the Richards intermediate hip screw. *J Pediatr Orthop* 2000;20:336–343.

170. Mosca VS. Calcaneal lengthening for valgus deformity of the hindfoot. Results in children who had severe, symptomatic flatfoot and skewfoot. *J Bone Joint Surg Am* 1995;77-A:500–512.

171. Dennyson WG, Fulford GE. Subtalar arthrodesis by cancellous grafts and metallic internal fixation. *J Bone Joint Surg Br* 1976;58-B: 507–510.

172. McNerney NP, Mubarak SJ, Wenger DR. One-stage correction of the dysplastic hip in cerebral palsy with the San Diego acetabuloplasty: results and complications in 104 hips. *J Pediatr Orthop* 2000;20:93–103.

173. Davids JR, Mason TA, Danko A, et al. Surgical management of hallux valgus deformity in children with cerebral palsy. *J Pediatr Orthop* 2001;21:89–94.

174. Kramer A, Stevens PM. Anterior femoral stapling. *J Pediatr Orthop* 2001;21:804–807.

175. Stevens PM. Guided growth for angular correction. A preliminary series using a tension band plate. *J Pediatr Orthop* 2007;27:253–259.

176. Sohrweide S. Foot biomechanics and pathology. In: Gage JR, Schwartz MH, Koop SE, et al., eds. *The identification and treatment of gait problems in cerebral palsy*, Chapter 3.2. Clin Dev Med No 180–181. London, UK: Mac Keith Press, 2009.

177. Trost JP. Clinical assessment. In: Gage JR, Schwartz MH, Koop SE, et al., eds. *The identification and treatment of gait problems in cerebral palsy*, Chapter 3.1. Clin Dev Med No 180–181. London, UK: Mac Keith Press, 2009.

178. White JW. Torsion of the Achilles tendon: its surgical significance. *Arch Surg* 1943;46:748–787.

179. Baker LD. Triceps surae syndrome in cerebral palsy. *Arch Surg* 1954;63:216–221.

180. Vulpius O, Stoffel A. Tenotomie der end schen der mm. Gastrocnemius el soleus mittels rutschenlassens nach Vulpius. In: *Orthopaedische Operationslehre*. Ferdinand Enke, 1920:29–31.

181. Hoke M. An operation for the correction of extremely relaxed flat feet. *J Bone Joint Surg Am* 1931;13-A:773–783.

182. Firth GB, Passmore E, Sangeux M, et al. Surgery for equinus in children with spastic diplegia: medium term follow-up with gait analysis. *J Bone Joint Surg* 2013;95-A(10):931–938.

183. Firth GB, McMullan M, Chin T, et al. Lengthening of the gastrocnemius-soleus complex. An anatomical and biomechanical study in human cadavers. *J Bone Joint Surg* 2013;95-A:1489–1496.

184. Davids JR. Orthopaedic treatment of foot deformities. In: Gage JR, Schwartz MH, Koop SE, eds. *The identification and treatment of gait problems in cerebral palsy*, Chapter 5.8. Clin Dev Med No 180–181. London, UK: Mac Keith Press, 2009.

185. Dogan A, Zorer G, Mumcuoglu EI, et al. A comparison of two different techniques in the surgical treatment of flexible pes planovalgus: calcaneal lengthening and extra-articular subtalar arthrodesis. *J Pediatr Orthop B* 2009;18:167–175.

186. Davids JR. The foot and ankle in cerebral palsy. In: Orthopaedic Management of Cerebral Palsy. *Orthop Clin North Am* 2010;41:579–593.

187. Rathjen KE, Mubarak SJ. Calcaneal-cuboid-cuneiform osteotomy for the correction of valgus foot deformities in children. *J Pediatr Orthop* 1998;18:775–782.

188. Ma FYP, Selber P, Nattrass GR, et al. Lengthening and transfer of hamstrings for a flexion deformity of the knee in children with bilateral cerebral palsy: technique and preliminary results. *J Bone Joint Surg Br* 2006;88-B:248–254.

189. McGinley JL, Dobson F, Ganeshalingam R, et al. Single event multilevel surgery for children with cerebral palsy: a systematic review. *Dev Med Child Neurol* 2012;54:117–128.

190. Hagglund G, Andersson S, Duppe H, et al. Prevention of dislocation of the hip in children with cerebral palsy. *J Bone Joint Surg Br* 2005; 87-B:95–101.

191. Miller F, Dabney KW, Rang M. Complications in cerebral palsy treatment. In: Epps CH, Bowen JR, eds. *Complications in pediatric orthopaedic surgery*. Philadelphia, PA: JB Lippincott Company, 1995:477–544.

192. Parrott J, Boyd RN, Dobson F, et al. Hip displacement in spastic cerebral palsy: repeatability of radiologic measurement. *J Pediatr Orthop* 2002;22:660–667.

193. Flynn JF, Miller F. Management of hip disorders in patients with cerebral palsy. *J Am Acad Orthop Surg* 2002;10:198–209.

194. Silver RL, Rang M, Chan J, et al. Adductor release in nonambulant children with cerebral palsy. *J Pediatr Orthop* 1985;5:672–677.

195. Presedo A, Oh C-W, Dabney KW, et al. Soft-tissue releases to treat spastic hip subluxation in children with cerebral palsy. *J Bone Joint Surg Am* 2005;87-A:832–841.

196. Stott NS, Piedrahita L. Effects of surgical adductor releases for hip subluxation in cerebral palsy: an AACPDM evidence report. *Dev Med Child Neurol* 2004;46:628–645.

197. Shore BJ, Yu X, Desai S, et al. Adductor surgery to prevent hip dislocation in children with cerebral palsy: the predictive role of the Gross Motor Function Classification System. *J Bone Joint Surg Am* 2012;94:326–334.

198. Ferraretto I, Machado PO, Filho ELR, et al. Preliminary results of patellar tendon shortening, as a salvage procedure for crouch gait in cerebral palsy. POSNA 2000 Annual Meeting, Vancouver, Canada, 1–4 May, 2000.

199. Stout JL, Gage JR, Schwartz MH, et al. Distal femoral extension osteotomy and patellar tendon advancement to treat persistent crouch gait in cerebral palsy. *J Bone Joint Surg Am* 2008;90-A:2470–2484.

200. Miller F, Girardi HJ, Lipton GE, et al. Reconstruction of the dysplastic hip with per-ilial pelvic and femoral osteotomy followed by immediate immobilization. *J Pediatr Orthop* 1997;17:592–602.

201. Mubarak SJ, Valencia FG, Wenger DR. One-stage correction of the spastic dislocated hip. Use of pericapsular acetabuloplasty to improve coverage. *J Bone Joint Surg Am* 1992;74-A:1347–1357.

202. Nagoya S, Nagao M, Takada J, et al. Long-term results of rotational acetabular osteotomy for dysplasia of the hip in adult ambulatory patients with cerebral palsy. *J Bone Joint Surg Br* 2005;87-B:1627–1630.

203. Clohisy JC, Barrett SE, Gordon JE, et al. Periacetabular osteotomy in the treatment of severe acetabular dysplasia. *J Bone Joint Surg Am* 2006;88-A(Suppl 1):65–83.

204. Olafsson Y, Saraste H, Soderlund V, et al. Boston brace in the treatment of idiopathic scoliosis. *J Pediatr Orthop* 1995;15:524–527.

205. Rang M, Douglas G, Bennet GC, et al. Seating for children with cerebral palsy. *J Pediatr Orthop* 1981;1:279–287.

206. Castle MF, Schneider C. Proximal femoral resection-interposition arthroplasty. *J Bone Joint Surg Am* 1978;60-A:1051–1054.

207. Widmann RF, Do TT, Doyle SM, et al. Resection arthroplasty of the hip for patients with cerebral palsy: an outcome study. *J Pediatr Orthop* 1999;19:805–810.

208. Abu-Rajab RB, Bennet GC. Proximal femoral resection-interposition arthroplasty in cerebral palsy. *J Pediatr Orthop B* 2007;16:181–184.

209. McHale KA, Bagg M, Nason SS. Treatment of the chronically dislocated hip in adolescents with cerebral palsy with femoral head resection and subtrochanteric valgus osteotomy. *J Pediatr Orthop* 1990;10:504–509.

210. Van Riet A, Moens P. The McHale procedure in the treatment of the painful chronically dislocated hip in adolescents and adults with cerebral palsy. *Acta Orthop Belg* 2009;75:181–188.

211. Hogan KA, Blake M, Gross RH. Subtrochanteric valgus osteotomy for chronically dislocated, painful spastic hips. *J Bone Joint Surg Am* 2006;88-A:2624–2631.

212. Gabos PG, Miller F, Galban MA, et al. Prosthetic interposition arthroplasty for the palliative treatment of end-stage spastic hip disease in nonambulatory patients with cerebral palsy. *J Pediatr Orthop* 1999;19: 796–804.

213. Root L, Goss JR, Mendes J. The treatment of the painful hip in cerebral palsy by total hip replacement or hip arthrodesis. *J Bone Joint Surg Am* 1986;68-A:590–598.

214. Prosser GH, Shears E, O'Hara JN. Hip resurfacing with femoral osteotomy for painful subluxed or dislocated hip sin patients with cerebral palsy. *J Bone Joint Surg* 2012;94-B:483–487.

215. Muir D, Angliss RD, Nattrass GR, et al. Tibiotalocalcaneal arthrodesis for severe calcaneovalgus deformity in cerebral palsy. *J Pediatr Orthop* 2005;25:651–656.

216. Miller F. Spinal deformity secondary to impaired neurologic control. *J Bone Joint Surg Am* 2007;89-A(Suppl 1):143–147.

217. Spiegel DA, Loder RT, Alley KA, et al. Spinal deformity following selective dorsal rhizotomy. *J Pediatr Orthop* 2004;24:30–36.

218. Kalen V, Conklin MM, Sherman FC. Untreated scoliosis in severe cerebral palsy. *J Pediatr Orthop* 1992;12:337–340.

219. Majd ME, Muldowny DS, Holt RT. Natural history of scoliosis in the institutionalized adult cerebral palsy population. *Spine* 1997;22: 1461–1466.

220. Thometz JG, Simon SR. Progression of scoliosis after skeletal maturity in institutionalized adults who have cerebral palsy. *J Bone Joint Surg Am* 1988;70-A:1290–1296.

221. Jevsevar DS, Karlin LI. The relationship between preoperative nutritional status and complications after an operation for scoliosis in patients who have cerebral palsy. *J Bone Joint Surg Am* 1993;75-A:880–884.

222. Heth R. Bone health in pediatric epilepsy. *Epilepsy Behav* 2004;5(Suppl 2): S30–S35.

223. Tsirikos AI, Lipton G, Chang W-N, et al. Surgical correction of scoliosis in pediatric patients with cerebral palsy using the Unit rod. *Spine* 2008;33:1133–1140.

224. Bulman WA, Dormans JP, Ecker ML, et al. Posterior spinal fusion for scoliosis in patients with cerebral palsy: a comparison of Luque rod and unit rod instrumentation. *J Pediatr Orthop* 1996;16:314–323.

225. Yaziei M, Asher MA, Hardacker JW. The safety and efficacy of Isola-Galveston instrumentation and arthrodesis in the treatment of neuromuscular spinal deformities. *J Bone Joint Surg Am* 2000;82-A:524–543.

226. Arlet V. Anterior thoracoscopic spine release in deformity surgery: a meta-analysis and review. *Eur Spine J* 2000;9(Suppl 1):S17–S23.

227. Cole J, Murray D, Snider RJ, et al. Aprotinin reduces blood loss during spinal surgery in children. *Spine* 2003;28:2482–2485.

228. Sussman MD, Little D, Alley RM, et al. Posterior instrumentation and fusion of the thoracolumbar spine for treatment of neuromuscular scoliosis. *J Pediatr Orthop* 1996;16:304–313.

229. Dias RC, Miller F, Dabney K, et al. Surgical correction of spinal deformity using a unit rod in children with cerebral palsy. *J Pediatr Orthop* 1996;16:734–740.

230. Lipton GE, Miller F, Dabney KW, et al. Factors predicting postoperative complications following spinal fusions in children with cerebral palsy. *J Spinal Disord* 1999;12:197–205.

231. Borkhuu B, Borowski A, Shah S, et al. Antibiotic-loaded allograft decreases the rate of acute deep wound infection after spinal fusion in cerebral palsy. *Spine* 2008;33:2300–2304.

232. Mercado E, Alman B, Wright JG. Does spinal fusion influence quality of life in neuromuscular scoliosis? *Spine* 2007;32(Suppl 19):S120–S125.

233. Tsirikos AI, Chang W-N, Dabney KW, et al. Comparison of parents' and caregivers' satisfaction after spinal fusion in children with cerebral palsy. *J Pediatr Orthop* 2004;24:54–58.

234. Narayanan UG, Fehlings D, Weir S, et al. Initial development and validation of the Caregiver Priorities and Child Health Index of Life with Disabilities (CPCHILD). *Dev Med Child Neurol* 2006;48: 804–812.

FURTHER READING

Hortsmann HM, Bleck EE. *Orthopaedic management in cerebral palsy. Clinics in Developmental Medicine No 173-174.* London, UK: Mac Keith Press, 2007.

Miller F. *Cerebral palsy.* New York, NY: Springer, 2005.

The Identification and Treatment of Gait Problems in Cerebral Palsy. In: Gage JR, Schwartz MH, Koop SE, et al., eds. Clin Dev Med No 180–181. London, UK: Mac Keith Press, 2009.

Thomason P, Graham HK. Consequences of interventions. In: Gage JR, Schwartz MH, Koop SE, et al., eds. *The identification and treatment of gait problems in cerebral palsy,* Chapter 6.1. Clin Dev Med No 180–181. London, UK: Mac Keith Press, 2009.

Young JL, Rodda J, Selber P, et al. Management of the knee in spastic diplegia: what is the dose? In: Guest CH, ed. *Orthopaedic management of cerebral palsy. Orthop Clin N Am* 2010;41:561–577. Philadelphia, PA: WB Saunders.

Myelomeningocele

Neural tube defects result from failure of the neural tube to close during embryogenesis. Although the incidence of neural tube defects has declined in recent decades, it remains the cause of chronic disability of between 70,000 and 100,000 individuals in the United States (1). Myelomeningocele, also referred to as spina bifida, is the most common neural tube defect and is the most severely disabling birth defect compatible with survival (1).

Myelomeningocele is a fluid filled cystic swelling, formed by dura and arachnoid. Myelodysplasia of the neural elements manifests in the vertebrae as a defect in the posterior elements. The sac protrudes through this defect and contains spinal nerve roots. Dysplasia of the spinal cord and nerve roots leads to bowel, bladder, motor, and sensory paralysis below the level of the lesion (2). Patients with myelomeningocele can also have concomitant lesions of the spinal cord, such as diastematomyelia or hydromyelia, or structural abnormalities of the brain, such as hydrocephalus or Arnold-Chiari malformation, which can also compromise neurologic function.

The survival rate for patients with myelomeningocele in the 1950s was only about 10%. Due to advances in the management of several important complications, a recent series reported at least 75% of children born with an open myelomeningocele defect can be expected to reach their early adult years (3). However, comprehensive treatment requires optimal care to prevent, monitor, and treat a variety of potential complications that can affect function, quality of life, and survival. This is best accomplished by a multidisciplinary team approach including specialists in orthopaedic surgery, neurosurgery, urology, rehabilitation, physical and occupational therapy, and orthotics. Access to nutritionists, social workers, wound specialists, and psychologists is also helpful.

As a result of the increased survival into adulthood, many patients with myelomeningocele now live long enough to eventually require transition to adult medical providers. This presents a great challenge since adult providers may lack the expertise necessary to manage these patients. Additionally, adults with myelomeningocele who failed to develop the skills they require to live independently remain dependent on aging family members who may be unable to care for them.

INCIDENCE

The incidence of infants born with neural tube defects shows regional and racial variations but is decreasing overall. The birth prevalence rate of myelomeningocele from 1983 to 1990 in the United States was 4.6 per 10,000 (4). Since that time, there has been a decrease in the number of new cases of myelomeningocele. This decrease can be attributed to two main factors: prenatal screening with elective termination of affected pregnancies and increased awareness of the importance of administration of folate to women before and during pregnancy. The United States Public Health Service recommends that all women of childbearing age who are capable of becoming pregnant should consume 400 μg of folic acid per day for the purpose of reducing their risk of having a pregnancy affected with myelomeningocele or other neural tube defects (5). Total folate consumption should be <1 mg per day because the effects of higher intakes are not well known (5).

An estimated 50% to 70% of neural tube defects can be prevented through the daily consumption of 400 μg of folic acid (5). The U.S. Food and Drug Administration mandated adding folic acid to all enriched cereal grain products by January 1998 (6). From October 1998 to December 1999, the birth prevalence rate of myelomeningocele in the United States decreased 22.9% compared with 1995–1996 (6). Notably, the prevalence of myelomeningocele remained higher among Hispanic women than among women in other racial/ethnic populations (6). This finding may be attributable to differences in folic acid consumption, eating habits, or genetic factors. In addition, religious and cultural preferences may play a role in the persistently higher prevalence of myelomeningocele in Hispanic women who may be less likely to terminate an affected pregnancy.

Overall the trend of decreasing incidence of myelomeningocele in the United States has continued after the folic acid mandate. From the early postfortification period of 1999–2000 to the recent postfortification period of 2003–2005, the birth prevalence of myelomeningocele among infants born to mothers of all racial/ethnic populations decreased 6.9%, from 2.04 to 1.90 cases per 10,000 live births (6).

A similar trend of decreased incidence of myelomeningocele related to folic acid consumption has been reported in Europe. Two of the first European countries to develop a periconceptional folic acid supplementation policy were the United Kingdom (1992) and Ireland (1993) (7). In a population-based study examining the effect of folic acid supplementation on the prevalence of neural tube defects in 16 European countries, a 32% decrease was found when comparing the periods 1989–1991 and 1999–2001 in the United Kingdom and Ireland (7). A 17% reduction in prevalence of neural tube defects was found in countries with folic acid supplementation introduced by 1999. In contrast, a decrease of 9% was seen in countries with no supplementation policy by 1999.

ETIOLOGY

Myelomeningocele is believed to result from failure of fusion of the neural folds during neurulation, which occurs at 26 to 28 days of gestation. Conditions that result from abnormalities during the phase of closure of the neural tube, such as myelomeningocele and anencephaly, are referred to as neurulation defects. In contrast, conditions such as meningocele, lipomeningocele, and diastematomyelia arise from abnormalities that occur during the canalization phase from 28 to 48 days of gestation and are referred to as postneurulation defects.

The cause of this embryonic failure is not known but is suspected to be multifactorial in origin, involving both genetic and environmental factors. Folate deficiency is an important contributor to the cause of neural tube defects as evidenced by the decrease in incidence observed after folate supplementation. Other environmental factors have also been examined for a potential role in neural tube defects, including temperature; drug exposure; substance abuse; maternal infection; and other nutritional factors, such as vitamin B_{12} and zinc (8).

Genetic factors seem to play an important role in the development of myelomeningocele. Animal studies have shown as many as 100 mutant genes that affect neurulation, and almost all have homologs in humans (8). Studies have suggested a higher incidence of neural tube defects in siblings of affected children than in the general population. A positive family history has been reported in 6% to 14% of cases (9, 10). Overall, for a couple with a child with myelomeningocele,

the chance that a subsequent sibling would be affected by a major malformation of the central nervous system is approximately 1 in 14 (11). Although association with single gene defects, increased recurrence risk among siblings, and a higher frequency in twins than in singletons indicate a genetic contribution to the etiology, the low frequency of families with a significant number of neural tube defect cases makes research into genetic causation difficult (8).

DIAGNOSIS

Prenatal screening for myelomeningocele and other neural tube defects involves biochemical testing of maternal blood for alpha-fetoprotein or the use of ultrasound evaluation. Maternal serum alpha-fetoprotein, a glycoprotein secreted by the fetal yolk sac and liver, has been used as a screening test for open neural tube defects for over 30 years. The detection rate for anencephaly is >95% and for open neural tube defects between 65% and 80% (12). Since closed neural tube defects do not increase alpha-fetoprotein, biochemical screening is not effective. Additionally, an increased serum alpha-fetoprotein is not diagnostic for open neural tube defects since it can also be associated with other abnormalities including gastroschisis, omphalocele, congenital nephrosis, and fetal demise.

With improvement in ultrasonographic techniques, prenatal diagnosis using ultrasound can be quite accurate. A recent report on prenatal screening in Europe found 88% of 725 cases of neural tube defects were detected prenatally using ultrasound at a median gestation of 17 weeks (13). The technique of three-dimensional ultrasound using multiplanar views can achieve diagnostic accuracy within one vertebral body in around 80% of patients (12).

When a diagnosis of myelomeningocele is suspected on ultrasound, careful evaluation of the entire spine and a search for other abnormalities is warranted as associated malformations are found in around 23% of patients (14).

ASSOCIATED CONDITIONS

Hydrocephalus. After repair and closure of the myelomeningocele defect, which is done in the first 48 hours of life, many infants will develop some degree of hydrocephalus. Using new protocols aimed at reducing shunt placement rates in patients with myelomeningocele, approximately 60% of infants with require a shunt (15). The incidence of hydrocephalus with need for cerebrospinal fluid diversion has been reported to correlate with functional level of the myelomeningocele lesion. Between 97% and 100% of patients with a thoracic level lesion require shunt placement compared to 87% of lumbar-level patients and 37% of sacral-level patients (15, 16).

Patients who do not require shunting may have a better prognosis in terms of upper extremity function and trunk balance as compared to patients who require shunting (17). One study comparing a group of 98 patients with myelomeningocele and a shunt with a group of 63 patients with no shunt found that patients without a shunt were more independent in their ambulation at medium and longer distances (18). In addition, the authors noted patients with no shunt tend to walk at a significantly greater velocity and stride length as compared with those with a shunt (18).

Infection and obstruction of cerebrospinal fluid shunts are serious complications that have the potential to affect a patient's motor and intellectual development. In one study following a group of 61 patients with myelomeningocele and a cerebrospinal fluid shunt, 95% patients underwent at least one shunt revision (3). Data not yet published by the senior author of this chapter also show that patients with an incidence of shunt infection have a decrease in functional mobility in the school and in the community compared to patients who have not experienced an infection (Dias L., personal communication). Awareness of this information will allow caregivers to effectively counsel patients with myelomeningocele and a ventriculoperitoneal shunt regarding functional ambulatory expectations.

Chiari II Malformation. The Chiari II malformation is present in almost all patients with myelomeningocele (1). It is characterized by caudal displacement of the posterior lobe of the developing fetal cerebellum and medulla into the spinal canal. If the brainstem or spinal cord is compressed within the spinal canal, progressive dysfunction may result, manifesting as weakness or paralysis of the vocal cords, or difficulty feeding, crying, or breathing (1). However, these symptoms are nonspecific and may also result from a shunt malfunction, which should be excluded prior to surgical decompression for the Chiari II malformation.

Tethered Spinal Cord. Tethered cord syndrome is a stretch-induced functional disorder of the spinal cord with its caudal part anchored by an inelastic structure such as scar tissue (19). Magnetic resonance imaging of the spine will show signs of tethering in most patients with myelomeningocele; however, the clinical signs are present in only about 30% (17). The most common clinical symptom of tethered cord is progressive scoliosis (44%) (3). Especially concerning is scoliosis that develops before 6 years of age in the absence of congenital vertebral anomalies. Also, since scoliosis is not as common in myelomeningocele patients with low lumbar- and sacral-level involvement, when seen in this population, it may signify tethered cord syndrome. Other common symptoms are gait changes associated with loss of muscle strength (35%) and spasticity (26%) (3) especially in the medial hamstrings and ankle dorsiflexors and evertors. Additional common symptoms associated with tethered cord are loss of motor function, back pain at the site of the repaired spina bifida defect (20), or changes in urologic function. As with hydromyelia, a shunt malfunction must be ruled out first when tethered cord is suspected. When a diagnosis of tethered cord syndrome is made, surgical treatment by a skilled neurosurgeon with experience with this procedure is indicated to prevent further deterioration. Often, symptoms will stabilize or improve with surgical untethering (1).

Hydromyelia. Hydromyelia is an accumulation of cerebrospinal fluid in the enlarged central canal of the spinal cord. In patients with myelomeningocele, hydromyelia develops due to shunt malfunction or untreated hydrocephalus. Magnetic resonance imaging of the spine in a group of 231 patients with myelomeningocele revealed hydromyelia in 49% (21). However, not all patients develop symptoms that require treatment of the hydromyelia. Those who are symptomatic may present with progressive scoliosis, urologic problems, pain, and motor or sensory defects (1). Decreased grip strength and thenar atrophy are also reliable signs of hydromyelia (17).

Urinary Tract. Most patients with myelomeningocele have neurogenic bladder dysfunction and may go on to develop progressive deterioration of the upper urinary tract and chronic renal disease. Treatment to reduce bladder pressure and minimize urine stasis is important to prevent these complications. In addition, regular monitoring of urinary tract function is necessary in order to detect changes in bladder function that may indicate shunt malfunction or tethered cord syndrome (1). Management includes clean intermittent catheterization of the bladder, which is necessary in approximately 85% patients with myelomeningocele (3). In addition, antibiotic prophylaxis and anticholinergic medication to reduce vesicoureteral reflux may be beneficial. A variety of surgical options exist for those patients that fail medical treatment or in order to facilitate self-management. These include vesicostomy, a diversion of the bladder to the lower abdominal wall to facilitate catheterization, and bladder augmentation in which a segment of the ileum is added to the bladder to increase capacity and reduce bladder pressure.

Bowel Management. Innervation of the bowel and anus is affected in most patients with myelomeningocele leading to dysmotility, poor sphincter control, and often fecal incontinence. Decreased bowel motility can cause constipation and fecal impaction, which in turn may cause increased intra-abdominal pressure leading to ventriculoperitoneal shunt malfunction (1). The goal of bowel management is to achieve continence and avoid fecal impaction by prompting regular elimination of stool using oral laxatives, suppositories, and/or enemas. If these measures are not successful, the Malone antegrade continence enema (MACE) procedure is an option. The MACE is a surgical procedure in which the appendix and the cecum are used to create a catheterizable stoma through which the patient irrigates the colon. In one study evaluating the results of the MACE procedure in 108 patients with myelomeningocele, approximately 85% achieved continence (22).

GENERAL HEALTH ISSUES

Patients with myelomeningocele have a high incidence of latex allergic reactions since they are exposed to latex products as a consequence of repeated surgical procedures, implantation of latex-containing materials, and catheterization (23). Latex allergy occurs in 18% to 40% of patients with myelomeningocele (3, 23, 24). The reaction may be a severe, life-threatening anaphylaxis in up to 26% (3). For this reason, it is imperative to avoid exposure to latex in myelomeningocele patients both in and out of the hospital environment. All surgical procedures performed on myelomeningocele patients should be done in a strictly latex-free setting.

Nutrition is an important issue in patients with myelomeningocele and appropriate counseling should begin at an early age. Childhood and adolescent obesity is common in patients with myelomeningocele and likely results from a variety of factors including energy intake and motor impairment. One study of 100 children and adolescents with myelomeningocele found 40% were markedly overweight, defined as Body Mass Index above the 95th percentile (25).

The psychosocial impact of myelomeningocele on the patient and the family should not be overlooked. Parents of children with myelomeningocele report more psychosocial stresses compared to parents of able-bodied children. One study found parents of myelomeningocele patients reported less parental satisfaction, less perceived parental competence, more social isolation, and less adaptability to change in comparison to a matched group of parents of able-bodied children (26). Another study looked at depressive symptoms in patients from 9 to 18 years of age with myelomeningocele compared to matched able-bodied patients. The authors found greater risk of depressive mood, low self-worth, and suicidal ideation in the myelomeningocele patients (27). The multidisciplinary care team should be aware of the potential for psychosocial issues and be prepared to refer or treat any concerns appropriately.

COMPLICATIONS

Skin Breakdown. The risk of skin breakdown and development of pressure sores is a significant problem in patients with myelomeningocele who lack protective sensation. Reported incidence of pressure sores varies in the literature from 17% to 82% of patients (28–32). The most common locations are over the sacrum, ischial tuberosity, greater trochanter, or on the feet (31). One study followed a group of 75 patients with myelomeningocele treated for pressure sores and determined that over the 13-year study period more than two million dollars were spent on their treatment (33). Another group reported 415 admissions at their institution between 1988 and 2005 for the treatment of pressure ulcers (31).

Care must be taken to aggressively prevent the development of pressure sores. All patients should be instructed from a young age to avoid walking without adequate foot protection, especially on rough or hot surfaces. Orthotic devices should be inspected on a regular basis, at least annually, to ensure proper fit and no pressure points or sharp edges. When casting, ample padding must be used and applied in a smooth fashion. Self-adhering foam pads can be used to supplement padding over pressure points such as the anterior knee, heel, or ankle malleoli. In addition, surgical arthrodesis within the foot should be strictly avoided since the resulting inflexibility in an insensate foot has been shown to be related to the development of neuropathic skin changes (30).

Fractures. Long bone fractures occur in up to 20% of patients with myelomeningocele and may involve the physis, metaphysis, or diaphysis (34, 35). The increased risk for fracture is thought to be related to a variety of factors including disuse osteoporosis, joint contractures, and postsurgical immobilization, especially spica casting. In addition, the level of neurologic involvement has been found to correspond to prevalence of fracture, with the higher the level of involvement, the higher the prevalence of fracture (34). This is thought to be attributable to osteopenia related to relative lack of mobility.

In myelomeningocele patients, fractures may result from minor trauma or physical therapy, and caregivers must have a high index of suspicion. In addition, caregivers need to be aware of the typical presentation of a metaphyseal or diaphyseal fracture in myelomeningocele patients who may not have pain due to lack of normal sensation. In this population, fracture should be suspected when a patient presents with a warm, swollen extremity (35). Other signs of fracture include erythema, temperature elevation >100°F, white blood cell count >10,000/mm^3, elevated erythrocyte sedimentation rate, general malaise, or nausea and vomiting (34–36). If not aware of this presentation for fracture, a mistaken diagnosis of cellulitis or osteomyelitis may be made and delay proper treatment. When a diagnosis of metaphyseal or diaphyseal fracture is made, healing often proceeds quickly. Most fractures can be treated nonsurgically, and immobilization is usually required for only 2 to 4 weeks (34, 35).

In contrast to metaphyseal and diaphyseal fractures, physeal fractures often have a different cause and clinical presentation. Physeal fractures are most common in ambulatory patients with low lumbar level of involvement (34, 35). Patients may complain of mild pain and often have warmth and swelling but may have only minimal increase in temperature, erythrocyte sedimentation rate, and white blood cell count (35). Radiographs may show a widened growth plate with an irregular and slightly widened metaphysis (34). These fractures heal at a slower rate and often require immobilization for up to 8 weeks.

Infection. Patients with myelomeningocele have an increased risk of postoperative infection that is likely multifactorial in origin. Contributing factors are lack of protective sensation, bladder paralysis, and poor soft-tissue envelope. With regard to spine surgery in particular, wound infection may occur in up to 50% of patients (4). Bacterial colonization of the urinary tract may occur due to bladder paralysis and its management. Infection rates in spinal surgery have been found to be higher in the presence of concurrent urinary tract infection; hence, some recommend obtaining preoperative urinary cultures (4).

PROGNOSIS FOR AMBULATION

Within the orthopaedic community, there is debate over whether or not working to achieve the goal of early ambulation in patients with myelomeningocele is worthwhile. Some attest early ambulation can provide physiologic and psychological benefits to a child with myelomeningocele even if that child will later become a sitter, while others dispute these benefits. One study compared a group of 36 high-level myelomeningocele patients who participated in a walking program with 36 matched patients who were prescribed a wheelchair early in life (37). At final follow-up, only 12 patients in the walking group retained the ability for effective ambulation. Despite this, patients who had walked early had fewer fractures and pressure sores, were more independent, and were better able to transfer compared to the wheelchair group (37).

Many factors influence the potential for ambulation in an individual patient with myelomeningocele. One of the most important is the motor level of involvement. Other contributing factors include sitting balance, upper extremity spasticity, obesity, age, and availability of appropriate orthotic support. Musculoskeletal deformity of the spine, pelvis, knees, and feet has also been shown to significantly influence ability to walk (38).

Neurologic level of involvement and the resulting muscle group strength plays a crucial role in achieving and maintaining ambulation. Asher and Olson studied the ambulatory status of 98 patients with myelomeningocele and found a notable difference in the ability to walk between patients with fourth lumbar level of involvement and third lumbar level. Most of the patients with fourth lumbar level involvement were functional household or community ambulators compared to the third lumbar level patients, who were mostly nonfunctional ambulators (38). In the same study, 20 of 21 patients with fifth lumbar or sacral level of involvement were community ambulators.

Maintenance of walking ability as an adult also correlates with the functional level of involvement. A review of 29 adult myelomeningocele patients aged 20 to 43 years found 95% of patients with third lumbar level of involvement or lower remained ambulatory (39). In contrast, only 22% of patients with second lumbar level of involvement or higher remained ambulatory. The difficulty with maintaining the ability to walk as an adult relates to the high energy cost required to walk. Also, in patients with high level of involvement, there is a high incidence of spinal deformity requiring surgical treatment. Hip and knee flexion contractures are also common and prone to recurrence as an adult despite aggressive treatment during childhood (17).

Correlating with functional level of involvement, one of the most important physical factors for maintaining ambulation is the strength of the quadriceps and the hamstrings muscles (38, 40). Seitzberg et al. (40) looked at a group of 32 patients with myelomeningocele and found a significantly better chance for maintaining ambulation as an adult if quadriceps strength was at least grade 4 during childhood.

They also found that overall patients with grade 3 or higher hamstring function during childhood had a significantly better chance for adult ambulation. However, they noted that hamstring function was not relevant in patients with normal quadriceps strength (40). Another study of 109 patients also found a correlation between quadriceps strength and ambulatory ability (41). In this group, 82% of patients with grade 4 or higher quadriceps power were community ambulators, whereas 88% of patients with grade 2 or less were not functional ambulators.

The strength of the iliopsoas muscle has also been shown to be important for ambulation. McDonald et al. (42) looked at a group of 291 patients with an average age of 14.5 years and found that 100% of the patients with symmetrical grade 4 or 5 iliopsoas strength were ambulatory. In contrast, 89% of the patients with iliopsoas strength grade 3 or less were non-ambulatory.

Sitting balance is a factor that can be assessed at a young age and has also been shown to be predictive of ambulatory potential in patients with higher levels of involvement. The ability to sit without hand support indicates nearly normal functioning of the central nervous system. When hand support is needed for sitting, use of an orthosis and external support for ambulation is likely to be severely impaired (17). A study of 206 patients with myelomeningocele confirmed that sitting balance was an independent predictor of community ambulation (43). In this study, lumbar and sacral level patients with no sitting-balance deficit and sacral level patients with a mild sitting-balance deficit were likely to be independent ambulators.

FUNCTIONAL CLASSIFICATION

The best known and most widely used classification of myelomeningocele is based on the neurologic level of the lesion (43, 44). Four main groups are identified based on the level of the lesion and associated functional and ambulatory capability (Table 15-1).

Thoracic/High-Lumbar Level of Involvement. The first group includes the thoracic and high-lumbar level patients, which represents approximately 30% of patients with myelomeningocele. This group is defined by the lack of functional quadriceps activity and has a neurologic level of L3 or above (43). To achieve ambulation during childhood, patients in this group require bracing to the level of the pelvis with either a reciprocating gait orthosis (RGO) (Fig. 15-1) or a hip–knee–ankle–foot orthosis (HKAFO) (Fig. 15-2). The majority of patients in this group, between 70% and 99%, require a wheelchair for mobility as an adult (17, 45). The inability to maintain community ambulation in adulthood relates to the high energy cost required to achieve ambulation with either an RGO or an HKAFO.

Low-Lumbar Level of Involvement. The next group, approximately 30% of patients with myelomeningocele, has

TABLE 15-1	Functional Classification of Myelomeningocele				
Group	**Neurologic Level of Lesion**	**Prevalence**	**Functional Capacity**	**Ambulatory Capability**	**FMS**
Thoracic/high lumbar	L3 or above	30%	No functional quadriceps (≤ grade 2)	During childhood, require bracing to level of pelvis for ambulation (RGO, HKAFO) 70%–99% require wheelchair for mobility in adulthood	1,1,1
Low lumbar	L3–L5	30%	Quadriceps, medial hamstring ≥ grade 3. No functional activity (≤ grade 2) of gluteus medius and maximus, gastrocsoleus.	Require AFOs and crutches for ambulation 80%–95% maintain community ambulation in adulthood	3,3,1
High sacral	S1–S3	30%	Quadriceps, gluteus medius ≥ grade 3 No functional activity (≤ grade 2) of gastrocsoleus	Require AFOs for ambulation 94%–100% maintain community ambulation in adulthood	6,6,6
Low sacral	S3–S5	5%–10%	Quadriceps, gluteus medius, gastrocsoleus ≥ grade 3	Ambulate without braces or support 94%–100% maintain community ambulation in adulthood	6,6,6

low-lumbar level of involvement. Functionally patients in this group have purposeful (grade 3 or higher) quadriceps and medial hamstring activity but lack purposeful activity (below grade 2) of the gluteus medius, gluteus maximus, and gastrocsoleus muscles. Hence, these patients require braces to control the position of the foot and ankle as well as crutches or a walker in order to ambulate. Between 80% and 95% of patients in this group maintain community ambulation in adulthood, but

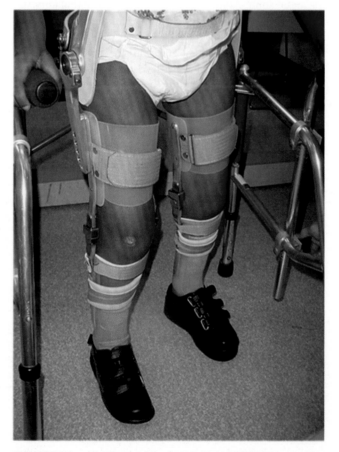

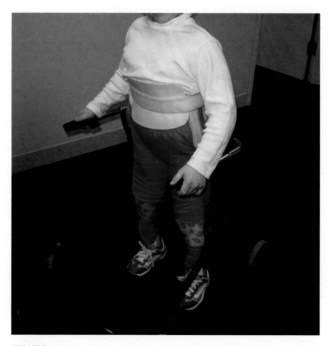

FIGURE 15-1. Reciprocating gait orthosis (RGO) with a reverse walker.

FIGURE 15-2. Hip–knee–ankle–foot orthosis (HKAFO).

most will use a wheelchair for long-distance mobility (43, 45). This group includes patients from L3 to L5 level of involvement, although patients with L3 level of involvement represent a transitional population and are included in this group only if they have evidence of strong quadriceps and medial hamstring function (43). Since medial hamstring function is needed for community ambulation, there is a significant difference in the ability to walk between children with L3 and L4 level of involvement (38). Because of this, children with L4 level of involvement have the most potential benefit from proper orthopaedic care of musculoskeletal deformities. Aggressive treatment of hip contractures; rotational malalignment of the tibia; and deformities of the knee, ankle, and foot are essential to maintain functional ambulation.

High-Sacral Level of Involvement.
Patients with high-sacral level of involvement represent approximately 30% of patients with myelomeningocele. Patients in this group have functional activity in the quadriceps and gluteus medius (grade 2 or higher) but lack functional activity in the gastrocnemius-soleus. Patients with high-sacral level walk without assistive devices but do require an ankle–foot orthosis (AFO) (Fig. 15-3). These children have a characteristic gluteus lurch with excessive pelvic obliquity and rotation during gait.

Low-Sacral Level of Involvement.
The last group of patients, approximately 5% to 10% of patients with myelomeningocele, has low-sacral level of involvement. These patients also have both quadriceps and gluteus medius function, but are distinguished from the high-sacral level patients based on the presence of gastrocnemius-soleus functional activity. Patients with low-sacral level of involvement walk without braces or assistive devices and have a gait pattern that is close to normal gait because they have normal gluteus medius and maximus function.

Between 94% and 100% of patients with sacral level involvement maintain community ambulation as adults (38, 45, 46). In this group, aggressive treatment of tethered cord syndrome; avoidance of arthrodesis in the foot; and treatment of deformities of the knee, ankle, and foot are important to promote functional ambulation.

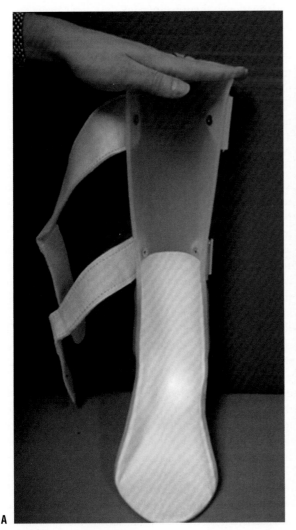
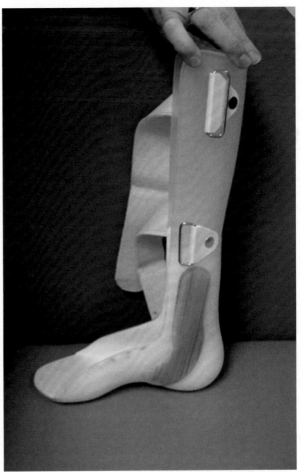

A   B

FIGURE 15-3.   Ankle–foot orthosis (AFO), front view **(A)** and side view **(B)**.

FUNCTIONAL MOBILITY SCALE

Many instruments specific to the pediatric population exist to assess quality of life, health status, physical function, and mobility in patients with physical disabilities. However, many of these instruments, such as the Pediatric Outcome Data Collection Instrument and the Child Health Questionnaire, are time consuming to administer and analyze. Because of this, the Functional Mobility Scale (FMS) was described in 2004 as a useful, simple tool to describe the more focused issue of functional mobility in children with disabilities and to aid communication between orthopaedic surgeons and health professionals (47).

The FMS was initially devised to describe functional mobility in children with cerebral palsy, but the authors reported they had also successfully used it to assess children with myelomeningocele (47). Recently, the FMS was used in a study by Battibugli et al. (18) to compare function in groups of patients with myelomeningocele. The FMS is unique because it allows quick, practical scoring of mobility over three distinct distances representing mobility in the home (5 m), at school (50 m), and in the community (500 m). In this way, it is effective for distinguishing between groups of children with varying levels of disabilities and provides a means for standardized communication between health professionals (47). The FMS has also been found to be sensitive to detect change after operative intervention (47).

To apply the FMS, a child is given a score from one to six based on their walking ability for each of the three distances assessed (Table 15-2). A score of one is used when a child uses a wheelchair, two for a walker, three for the use of two crutches, four for the use of one crutch or two walking sticks, five for a child who is independent on level surfaces, and six for a child who is independent on all surfaces. Two additional possible ratings are C for a child who crawls for mobility in the home and N for a child who does not complete the given distance. For example, a child who ambulates with crutches at home and at school and uses a wheelchair for long distances but would be an FMS 3,3,1.

Use of the FMS allows for an accurate clinical picture of a given patient's functional status at a distinct point in time. Often parents or the patient may have difficulty choosing a single response to a question regarding function and will default to the highest level of function. This can impact interpretation of outcome studies if parents choose different responses at different time intervals when there has been little actual change in function (47). A major advantage of the FMS is its ability to account separately for distances representing home, school, and the community hence addressing the complexities of functional mobility in the real world.

GAIT ANALYSIS

Gait analysis is defined as the systematic measurement, description, and assessment of quantities that characterize human locomotion (48). Clinical gait analysis has received a great deal of attention in regard to its application to the treatment of children with cerebral palsy. Increasingly gait analysis is also being recognized as a valuable component of the comprehensive orthopaedic evaluation of patients with myelomeningocele. Its use has been reported in the literature for assessing various manifestations of myelomeningocele including hip subluxation/dislocation, lower extremity contracture, and rotational abnormalities (49–53). Two main groups of patients with myelomeningocele can especially benefit from gait analysis: (a) patients with a low-lumbar lesion who walk with external support and a below-knee orthosis and (b) patients with sacral-level lesions who walk with no external support and AFOs (17). Studies have shown the average walking velocity for a patient with low lumbar-level involvement is 60% of normal (50). The average walking velocity for a patient with high sacral-level involvement is approximately 70% of normal (52).

The components of gait analysis may include kinematics, kinetics, electromyographic data, measurement of videotape recordings, energy expenditures, clinical observation, and foot pressure readings (48). The data obtained from these areas are presented as graphic and numerical data (for kinematics, kinetics, and ground-reaction forces), as electromyographic activity, and as videotape recordings. All of these data are then analyzed by a clinician with training in the interpretation of gait studies and a report of the gait analysis is generated. Several high-quality, commercial gait analysis systems are now available. The more comprehensive of these systems provide the clinician with three-dimensional kinematics and kinetics as well as dynamic electromyography (48). Three-dimensional gait analysis is especially useful for analyzing transverse plane deformities such as rotational problems. However, when a three-dimensional study is not available, the data obtained from a two-dimensional study have useful applications in the documentation of coronal and sagittal plane deformities such as crouch gait and foot deformities.

Kinematics describe the spatial movement of a body without consideration of the forces that cause the movement. These movements are linear and angular displacements, velocities, and accelerations. Kinematic data answer the question of what is happening at the level of each of the major lower extremity joints but not why it is happening (54). Kinematics are useful

TABLE 15-2	Functional Mobility Scale
Rating	**Function**
1	Uses a wheelchair
2	Uses a walker independently
3	Uses crutches independently
4	Uses one or two sticks independently
5	Independent on level surfaces
6	Independent on all surfaces
C	Crawls for the given distance
N	Does not complete the given distance

in determining treatment outcome through the comparison of preoperative and postoperative gait analysis data.

Kinetics on the other hand describe the mechanisms that cause movement around a joint. Hence, kinetics answer the question of why a particular movement or gait deviation occurs (54). Kinetic data include ground-reaction forces, joint moments, and joint powers. In order to calculate kinetic data, simultaneous acquisition of joint motion and force-plate data is necessary (48). The study of kinetics leads to improved understanding and knowledge of the pathogenesis of gait patterns (54).

Gait analysis is useful in preoperative planning for ambulatory myelomeningocele patients because it allows accurate dynamic assessment of an individual patient's gait problems. Postoperatively gait analysis is used to obtain a much more accurate, objective, and quantitative assessment of outcome than was previously possible (54). Often a patient's true functional status differs from what would be expected based on information obtained during the static clinical examination. Moen et al. demonstrated this in a study examining crouch gait in myelomeningocele patients. They found significantly greater dynamic knee flexion during ambulation using gait analysis than what was measured on clinical examination. Gait analysis is a useful component of the comprehensive evaluation of ambulatory myelomeningocele patients, especially when surgical treatment is being considered.

With specific regard to patients with myelomeningocele, gait analysis is useful to assess the abnormal movements that occur as compensation for muscle weakness. For example, due to weakness of the gluteus medius and maximus muscles, compensatory movements at the pelvis and hip such as increased active pelvic rotation and stance phase hip abduction develop to facilitate forward progression of the limb and maintain independent ambulation. All children with low lumbar-level involvement show increased anterior pelvic tilt, but compensatory movements become less pronounced with lower levels of motor involvement (17).

Gait analysis is helpful in determining the course of treatment for patients with hip flexion-adduction contracture and low lumbar or sacral-level patients with unilateral hip subluxation or dislocation (50). Gait analysis has also proved useful in increasing the appreciation of the effects of rotational malalignment of the lower extremity. Specifically, it has helped with understanding the relationship between external tibial torsion and a significantly increased valgus stress at the knee joint (49). In addition, the information gained from gait analysis in regard to the coronal and transverse plane kinematics at the pelvis and hip and the coronal plane kinetics at the hip and knee is important in the prescription of effective orthotics and walking aids (53).

OVERVIEW OF ORTHOPAEDIC CARE

Over the past 30 years, the overall care of children with myelomeningocele has changed substantially in regard to all specialties including neurosurgery, urology, rehabilitation, orthotics,

and orthopaedics. Specifically relating to orthopaedics, the advent of gait analysis in the late 1980s contributed to a better understanding of the underlying deformities and their effect on function. This has led to a shift in the focus of orthopaedic treatment from the goal of radiographic changes to functional improvement (55).

The main goal of orthopaedic care of a patient with myelomeningocele is to make the musculoskeletal system as functional as possible. As discussed earlier, walking ability is highly dependent on the neuromuscular level of the lesion. Whether or not ambulation should be the goal for every child with myelomeningocele is controversial. The role of the orthopaedic surgeon is to assist the patient and the family in developing realistic individualized goals and to provide the necessary care to meet these goals. Additionally, providers must help families to avoid neglecting the child's total development while focusing on the use of the lower extremities. Emphasizing intellectual and personality development utilizing wheelchair mobility, wheelchair sports programs beginning in preschool, and educational mainstreaming can lead to dramatically increased independence (17).

Both congenital and acquired orthopaedic deformities are seen in patients with myelomeningocele. Congenital deformities are present at birth and include kyphosis, hemivertebrae, teratologic hip dislocation, clubfoot, and vertical talus. Acquired developmental deformities are related to the level of involvement (4) and are caused by paralysis, decreased sensation in the lower extremities, and muscle imbalance (34). For example, calcaneus foot and hip dislocation are two acquired orthopaedic deformities caused in part by muscle imbalance. Orthopaedic deformities may also be result from iatrogenic injury such as postoperative tethered cord syndrome. Accordingly, the orthopaedic surgeon must monitor spinal balance and deformity and assist with monitoring the neurologic status of each patient.

The newborn examination of a patient with myelomeningocele should include identification of the level of paralysis for each extremity. Any associated conditions such as clubfoot or hip or knee contractures should be recognized and treated appropriately. In addition, a manual muscle test should be performed by a skilled physical therapist to evaluate the neurologic level of function. This should be done before closure of the spinal defect, again 10 to 14 days after closure, and then on an annual basis. Since a given patient's motor level should remain the same throughout their lifetime, a change in muscle strength may be a sign of tethered spinal cord.

After the initial newborn examination, orthopaedic follow-up should occur regularly every 3 to 4 months during the 1st year of life. After that, patients are seen every 6 months until the age of 11 or 12 years after which time patients are followed annually. The follow-up periodic orthopaedic examination should include assessment and monitoring of motor and sensory function, spinal alignment, and skin integrity. Orthoses should be inspected on a regular basis to ensure appropriate fit with no areas of irritation or pressure points on the skin. Patients with myelomeningocele have multiple medical comorbidities that must be considered as part of any orthopaedic treatment. Because of this, orthopaedic care should ideally be administered as part of a multidisciplinary team including neurosurgery, urology, and physiatry.

ORTHOPAEDIC MANAGEMENT

Spine. Spinal deformities such as scoliosis and kyphosis have a high prevalence in patients with myelomeningocele. Spinal deformity may present as a developmental deformity that is acquired and related to the level of paralysis, as a congenital deformity resulting from malformations such as hemivertebrae or unsegmented bars, or as a combination of both (4). The frequency of spinal deformity correlates with level of neurologic involvement. Hence, patients with a high-level lesion should have radiographs of the spine at least annually to evaluate any deformity. Patients with low-lumbar or sacral level of involvement have a low incidence of scoliosis; hence, any abnormal curvature in these patients should alert the caregiver to the possibility of an underlying tethered cord.

Scoliosis. Developmental scoliosis typically presents with a long, sweeping, C-shaped curve with the convexity often on the opposite side of the elevated pelvis (4). Overall, the prevalence of scoliosis in patients with myelomeningocele is reported to be between 62% and 90% (56–59). Many factors have been identified in patients with myelomeningocele that correlates to the development of scoliosis. One important factor is the functional level of involvement (4, 56, 59, 60). Trivedi et al. applied rigid criteria to a population of 141 patients in order to define incidence of developmental scoliosis defined as a Cobb angle >20 degrees. They found the prevalence of scoliosis to be 93% in patients with thoracic functional level, 72% in upper lumbar, 43% in lower lumbar, and <1% in sacral level patients (59). Other important factors in predicting development of scoliosis are ambulatory status (4, 56, 61) and the level of the last intact laminar arch (57, 59, 62). Less important predictive factors are hip dislocation/subluxation and lower extremity spasticity (4).

Scoliosis typically develops gradually in patients <10 years of age and then increases rapidly with the adolescent growth spurt. When a curve develops in a child younger than 6 years of age, it may be related to an underlying hydromyelia or a tethered cord syndrome. Muller et al. (61) found that curve progression was related to size of the curve with curves <20 degrees progressing slowly. In contrast, curves >40 degrees progressed severely and quickly at almost 13 degrees per year.

For a patient with curve magnitude <20 degrees, the recommended treatment is observation with follow-up radiographs every 4 to 6 months (4). When curve magnitude exceeds 20 degrees, brace treatment can be considered but has been controversial in patients with myelomeningocele. There is general consensus that brace treatment does not halt curve progression. However, the goal of using a brace in this population is not to correct the deformity but rather to support the

trunk in a functional position and control the curve during growth hence possibly delaying the need for surgical stabilization (63). Bracing typically consists of a custom-molded thoracolumbosacral orthosis used during the day. Ideally, the brace should assist with sitting balance and free the hands for functional usage but not interfere with pulmonary function, lower extremity bracing, self-catheterization, or sitting (4). When an orthosis is prescribed for a patient with myelomeningocele, it is imperative to ensure proper fitting and counsel patients to have their skin assessed daily to prevent skin complications.

Indications for operative treatment of scoliosis in patients with myelomeningocele have not been strictly defined. Most agree that progressive curves with magnitude >50 degrees that interfere with sitting balance warrant surgical treatment. Given the high risk of complications in patients with myelomeningocele, such as infection and pseudoarthrosis, surgical treatment should be considered on an individual basis. The functional consequences of spinal surgery on ambulation, motor skills, and activities of daily living should be reviewed. Some studies specifically evaluating the effect of spinal fusion on ambulatory ability have suggested ambulation may be more difficult following surgery (64–66). Furthermore, multiple studies have also shown no significant difference in the ability to perform activities of daily living after surgical intervention (64–66). However, with newer instrumentation and changes in postoperative management, considerable improvement in final outcome is possible (55).

The goal of surgical treatment of spinal curvature in patients with myelomeningocele is to prevent further deformity and create a stable, balanced spine while avoiding complications (31). Multiple studies have established that combined anterior and posterior instrumented arthrodesis is the treatment of choice in most patients to achieve fusion and provide the best long-term correction (31, 67–71). In combination with the posterior approach, the anterior approach allows for diskectomy to improve curve flexibility and anterior interbody fusion to increase strength of the fusion mass (4). Use of the posterior approach alone for instrumented arthrodesis has shown high failure rates with hardware complications and subsequent loss of correction (71, 31). Anterior arthrodesis and instrumentation alone may be considered for a select group of patients with a thoracolumbar curve <75 degrees, compensatory curve <40 degrees, no increased kyphosis, and no syrinx (72).

When planning for correction, the fusion should include all curves and should extend from the upper thoracic vertebrae to the sacrum in nonambulators (4, 31).

DUNN-MCCARTHY PELVIC FIXATION An alternative to the Galveston type of pelvic fixation is that described by McCarthy et al. (73). In this technique, the ends of the Luque rods are prebent to fit over the sacral ala in the manner of large alar hooks (Figs. 15-4 to 15-6). This technique may be indicated particularly when the pelvis is very thin or small. It is mechanically at its best in the correction of kyphosis and is contraindicated in lordosis.

The end of the rod that is to fit over the sacral ala must be bent before the operation. The tight bends necessitate that the

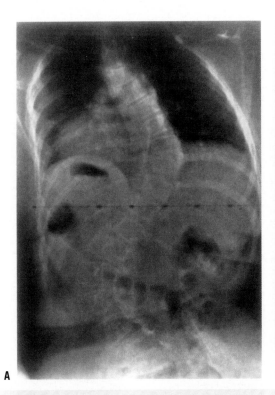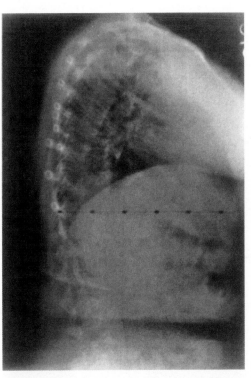

A   **B**

FIGURE 15-4.   Dunn McCarthy Pelvic Fixation. Measurement from the preoperative radiographs aids in achieving the correct dimensions of the bends. The first consideration is that the midportion of the sacral ala is lateral to the midportion of the lamina. This amount of lateral offset in the rod **(A)** can be estimated by measuring the distance from the midportion of the L5 lamina to the midportion of the sacral ala. In the typical patient, this is about 1 to 1.5 cm. The width of the segment that is to go over the sacral ala **(B)** is measured from the lateral radiograph of the pelvis. This width is usually between 1 and 1.5 cm. When this procedure is used in the bifid myelodysplastic spine, careful preoperative planning is necessary to be sure that the rod lies in the desired position. At surgery, the sacral ala is cleaned as it would be for lumbosacral arthrodesis. It is important that the hook portion of the rod passes anterior to the alae, thus necessitating the dissection be carried out slightly more anterior than usual. Before seating the rod, it should be possible to pass a finger around the front of the alae.

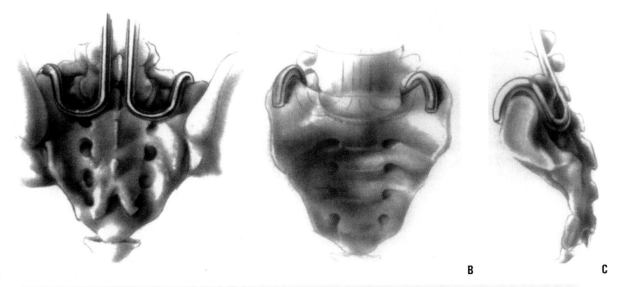

A   **B**   **C**

FIGURE 15-5.   A-C: The prebent portion of the rod is hooked on the ala like a giant sacral hook. It does not penetrate the cortex. It is possible to make minor adjustments to the rods during surgery, but it is not possible to bend all of the necessary curves into the rod on the operating room. Contouring lordosis into the sacral segment of the rod positions it more firmly against the sacral alae. Use of the Texas Scottish Rite crosslinks on the spinal segment of the rods prevents movement of one rod in relation to another and provides a rigid construct. The rod is held in place over the sacral alae by the sublaminar wires.

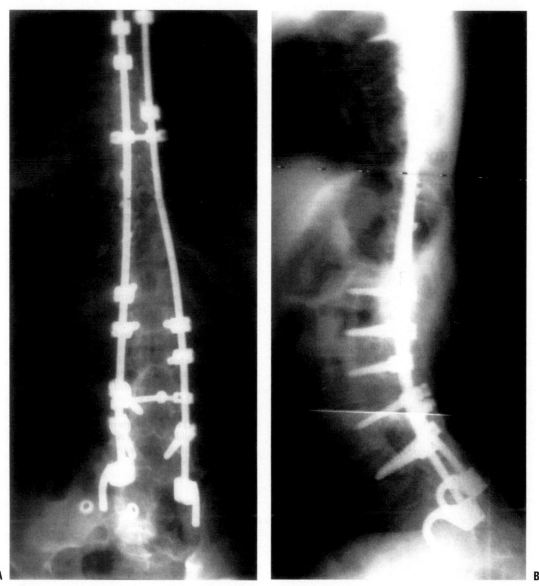

FIGURE 15-6. Anteroposterior **(A)** and lateral **(B)** radiographs after posterior arthrodesis and instrumentation with the Dunn-McCarthy technique in a child with myelomeningocele. Note the sacral alar hooks that connect independently to the rods. (Courtesy of Richard McCarthy, MD, Little Rock, AR.)

rods be heated over a flame to soften the metal before bending. Bends of two different dimensions can be made, one at each end of a long Luque rod. The end that fits less well can be cut off at surgery and discarded. It is necessary that the rods be bent so that they are mirror images of each other . These rods are available prebent.

A new variation of this method is now available using a special sacral hook that is made of titanium and designed to be used with a titanium rod. This allows for ease of use since contouring of the rod can be done independently of the sacral portion. It is necessary to use this hook in conjunction with a pedicle screw above (usually at least one screw at L4) so that distraction firmly seats the sacral hook in place. This

technique can be used in a variety of neuromuscular spinal deformities in which fixation to the sacrum is required.

In ambulatory patients, preserving pelvic motion is important for function; hence, whenever possible, lumbosacral fusion should be avoided. Pedicle screw instrumentation offers some advantages in patients with myelomeningocele in terms of correcting scoliosis while preserving lumbar lordosis and lumbar motion in ambulatory patients (74). However, difficulties with pedicle screw instrumentation may be encountered in patients with small, tightly packed vertebrae in lordotic segments or with small, dysplastic, and rotated pedicles. In these cases, familiarity with other instrumentation constructs such as multihook systems or sublaminar wires is necessary.

An important consideration for patients with myelomeningocele and scoliosis is the increased risk of complications associated with spine surgery in this population. Complications encountered with frequency include hardware problems such as implant failure, dislocation, and pseudoarthrosis, infections, postoperative lower extremity fractures, and neurologic complications. Hardware problems have been reported in approximately 30% of patients and often lead to loss of correction (31, 75). Pseudoarthrosis rates have been reported as high as 76% and are dependent on the approach and instrumentation utilized, with the highest rates associated with isolated posterior fusion (37, 66, 67, 69, 71). Wound infection and incisional necrosis are common and correlate with the incision used. The triradiate incision has been associated with a 40% rate of skin necrosis and should be avoided (69). The risk of wound infection is increased by the presence of a concurrent urinary tract infection, common in this population. For this reason, preoperative urinary cultures should be obtained. Lower extremity fractures due to disuse osteoporosis have been reported in up to 29% of patients in the first 6 months after surgery (66). Neurologic deficit occurs with a low frequency but can be permanent (66, 69).

Kyphosis. In patients with myelomeningocele, an associated kyphotic deformity is present in 8% to 21% of patients and occurs most commonly in the upper lumbar or thoracolumbar region (76–80). Patients may present with a large, rigid curve at the time of birth, often exceeding 80 degrees (31, 78). Progression of the curve has been related to the level of the neurologic lesion (75) and ranges from 4 to 12 degrees each year (31, 77–79). The natural history of rigid congenital kyphosis is rapid progression, especially after the 1st year of life when the child begins to sit (4). The apex of the curve is usually located in the upper lumbar spine (78). Rigid curves may be associated with vertebral anomalies, a sharp apical angulation, and the potential for skin breakdown over the prominence of the deformity (81). Development of trunk control and sitting balance can lead to the development of compensatory thoracic lordosis in older patients (80).

Treatment of rigid kyphosis is indicated to prevent progression of deformity, correct abnormal sitting posture, and prevent skin breakdown over the apex of the deformity (4). Conservative treatment using bracing and/or modified wheelchair seating systems has been largely ineffective (82). Surgery has been recommended as the treatment of choice; however, absolute criteria have not yet been well defined in the literature for indications and timing of surgical treatment, extent of resection and fusion, or type of instrumentation. Kyphectomy with osteotomy and resection of the vertebral bodies and spinal fusion has been the standard surgical treatment (83). Kyphectomy has been one of the most challenging procedures for spine surgeons and has been associated with high complication and mortality rates (78, 31, 82, 55) (Fig. 15-7). Improvements in final outcome have been seen using newer techniques, such as early intervention, longer fusion, and the decancellation described by Lindseth and Stelzer (78). With

this technique, the authors reported persistent correction with the potential for continued growth of the remaining lumbar vertebrae increasing the capacity of the abdominal cavity (78).

HIP

Deformity about the hip is very common in patients with myelomeningocele and may consist of hip joint contractures, subluxation, or dislocation. The development of hip deformity is related to the patient's neurologic level of involvement. For each type of hip deformity, treatment depends on the level of neurologic involvement, the type of deformity present, and the functional capacity of the patient (31).

Hip Contractures. Several factors contribute to the development of hip contractures in patients with myelomeningocele including muscle imbalance, positioning, and spasticity (31, 84). Muscle imbalance plays a major role, as seen in a patient with low-lumbar level of involvement who lacks normal strength in the gluteal muscles. In this case, the relatively greater strength in the hip flexors and adductors leads to deformity about the hip. The type and severity of contracture depends in part on the degree of muscle imbalance present (84). Positioning is a contributing factor especially in patients with high levels of involvement who rely on wheelchairs for mobility (31). Spasticity of the hip musculature may be seen in patients with tethered cord syndrome.

Hip contractures and the resultant loss of motion can affect a patient's function more than hip subluxation or dislocation. If not treated properly, pelvic obliquity and compensatory spinal deformity may result (34). In ambulatory patients, hip flexion contracture causes the patient to stand with increased lordosis leaning forward to use the arms for support resulting in greater energy cost (85). The effect of hip contractures on gait has been documented with gait analysis. Gabrieli et al. found that patients with unilateral hip flexion and/or adduction contractures had increased pelvic obliquity leading to asymmetric gait and compensatory scoliosis. The authors concluded that a symmetric gait pattern was related to absence of hip contracture or bilateral symmetric hip contractures but had no relation to hip dislocation. Current treatment goals based on studies of functional results focus on maintaining hip range of motion with contracture release, especially unilateral hip adduction and flexion contractures (50, 85–87).

The routine clinical examination of a patient with myelomeningocele should include the Thomas test to assess for hip flexion contracture. Because hip flexion deformity tends to decrease in the first 2 years of life, except in patients with high levels of involvement, treatment is rarely indicated in this age group. Specific treatment recommendations are based on a patient's functional level of involvement. In patients with thoracic or high-lumbar levels of involvement, flexion contracture of up to 30 to 40 degrees may be tolerated as long as it does not interfere with orthotic use and ambulation. In a high level patient attempting to walk with a RGO, more

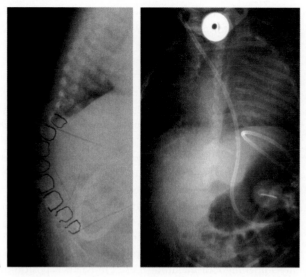

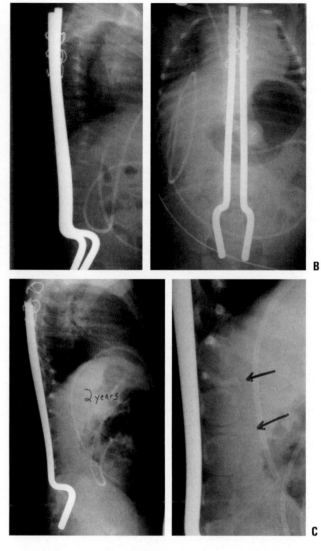

FIGURE 15-7. **A:** Anteroposterior and lateral radiographs of an 8-month-old infant with thoracic level of paralysis and C-shaped kyphosis. **B:** Anteroposterior and lateral bodies above and below the apex with posterior instrumentation. Rods are placed into the S1 foramen and fixed proximally with sublaminar wires in an extraperiosteal fashion. The rods are left long to allow for continued spine growth. **C:** Follow-up radiographs at 2 years demonstrate reduction of kyphosis and growth of the spine away from the rods proximally. Consolidation of the egg-shelled vertebrae are noted (*arrows*).

severe hip flexion contractures may cause a very short stride length and increased lumbar lordosis. Treatment is indicated to provide sufficient range of motion to allow the patient to sit comfortably in a wheelchair, lie supine in bed, and use an orthosis for standing and walking (31). Soft-tissue release is performed through an anterior approach and usually includes the sartorius, rectus femoris, iliopsoas, and tensor fascia latae. If needed, the anterior hip capsule can be divided as well. To prevent recurrence of contracture, physical therapy is necessary to maintain range of motion and a total body splint (TBS) can be used at night-time. In very severe cases with deformity >60 degrees, proximal femur extension osteotomy can be used, especially if pressure sores result from the hip deformity (31, 85).

For patients with low-lumbar level of involvement, lesser hip flexion contractures can result in major functional impairment. In such a patient who walks with AFOs and crutches, a hip flexion contracture of >20 degrees can lead to significant anterior pelvic tilt causing decreased walking velocity and increased demand on the upper extremities (50, 52). When surgical treatment is indicated in this group, care must be taken

to preserve hip flexor power. For contractures >20 degrees that interfere with function, the tensor fascia latae and the rectus femoris are released. The sartorius is detached from the anterosuperior iliac spine and reattached to the anterioinferior iliac spine. If iliopsoas lengthening is necessary, it is done so in an intramuscular fashion above the pelvic brim.

When adduction contracture is present and interferes with function, treatment includes myotomy of the adductor longus and gracilis. The adductor brevis is included if necessary. A subtrochanteric valgus osteotomy of the proximal femur may be necessary in severe cases in order to achieve sufficient abduction to improve pelvic obliquity. Abduction contractures usually respond well to the Ober-Yount procedure (88, 89). Cast immobilization after release of hip contractures is unnecessary. A TBS is used full time for the initial 10 days followed by early mobilization and night-time usage of the splint.

Hip Subluxation/Dislocation. Hip instability affects up to one-half of patients with myelomeningocele during the first 10 years of life with either hip dislocation or subluxation

(17, 31). Treatment of this common and complicated problem remains a controversial issue. In the 1960s and 1970s, an aggressive treatment approach was advised, and the procedure of choice was transfer of the iliopsoas tendon (90, 91). Other approaches used included the external oblique transfer and varus osteotomy of the femur. The goal of treatment was anatomic reduction of the hip. Then, in 1978, Feiwell et al. (88) described the importance of a level pelvis and adequate range of motion of the hips rather than anatomic reduction of the joint. Since then, the focus has shifted from obtaining radiographic reduction of the hip to achieving maximal functional results (85, 86). Data from gait analysis support this approach (50). Modern treatment of hip instability is based on the patient's functional level of involvement and consists largely of maintaining hip range of motion with contracture release only.

With the earlier treatment approach for hip instability, reconstruction was offered to both ambulatory and nonambulatory patients. Reported rates of success or failure were often based solely on anatomic and radiographic results with little regard given to the functional consequences of surgical treatment. Subsequently, concerns developed over whether radiographically successful hip reduction led to decreased range of motion and pathologic fractures compromising functional results (92). Feiwell et al. (88) compared functional results in patients who had undergone hip reduction to those who had not and found no improvement in range of motion or ability to ambulate in those who had undergone surgery. In addition, they found surgery did not lead to decrease in pain or need for bracing.

Rather, multiple studies have demonstrated a high complication rate leading to decreased ambulatory function in patients who have undergone surgical reduction of hip dislocation. Sherk et al. (93) compared a series of patients who had undergone surgical treatment of dislocation to those who had not and found 36% in the surgically treated group had worsened ambulatory capacity as a result of surgical complications. Worsening neurologic deficit has also been reported after surgical treatment of hip dislocation (92). Another series reported a high complication rate in surgically treated patients with 29% incidence of loss of motion and 17% with pathologic fractures (87).

There is general agreement in the literature that ambulatory ability does not depend on the status of the hip, but instead the most important factor in determining ambulation is the level of functional involvement (39, 85, 87, 94, 93). Preserving muscle strength of the iliopsoas and quadriceps is more relevant to potential for continued ambulation in adulthood than the status of the hip joint.

For patients with thoracic and high-lumbar levels of involvement, the stability of the hip joint has little clinical effect on function (85, 87, 93). Treatment should be limited to contracture release to allow for proper sitting posture, perineal care, and facilitate use of orthoses for ambulation. Convincing evidence does not exist to support hip reduction in this group of patients.

There is a high incidence of hip instability in patients with low-lumbar levels of involvement because of underlying muscle imbalance. Using gait analysis, it has been shown that hip instability in this group of patients has minimal effect on gait symmetry (50). In addition, the walking speed of patients with a unilateral hip dislocation was 60% of normal, which corresponds to that of patients without hip dislocations in previous studies from the same center (50). Hence surgical relocation of the unilaterally unstable hip in patients with low-lumbar level of involvement is not recommended. As discussed above, unilateral soft-tissue contractures should be treated to maintain a level pelvis and flexible hips (50, 85).

Hip instability in patients with sacral level of involvement is relatively rare but presents a challenging treatment dilemma. Hip dislocation in a patient who walks with no support can lead to level arm dysfunction (50, 55). Patients may develop an increased lurch due to the loss of a fulcrum from the dislocated hip (95). Patients in this group place high demand on the hip and have functional hip abductor strength that can be compromised with hip instability (50). Careful consideration should be given to surgical reduction in this group as a concentric reduction may help to maintain independent ambulation into adulthood, prevent asymmetry in gait, and preserve the integrity of the hip joint (50). When surgical treatment is being considered, a computerized tomography scan of the hips with three-dimensional reconstructions may be useful for preoperative planning to better assess acetabular deficiency and select the most appropriate type of pelvic osteotomy. Capsular plication is indicated when laxity is present, and rotational malalignment of the femur should be corrected at the same time. Excessive varus should be avoided to preserve hip abductor function for stability during stance and foot clearance during swing. Further studies are necessary to better assess the results of surgical treatment of hip instability in this select group of patients.

Hip Stiffness. Severe stiffness of the hip joint in patients who have undergone attempted surgical treatment presents a major problem (85). One option for treatment is the Castle procedure that entails resection of the proximal femur past the level of the lesser trochanter (96). A capsular flap is then closed across the acetabulum, and the quadriceps muscle is sutured around the resected end of the femur. The goal of the procedure is to allow patients improved range of motion for function, but disadvantages include the need for postoperative traction and high risk of postoperative heterotopic ossification.

The McHale et al. (97) procedure is another option for treatment of this serious complication. This procedure consists of femoral head resection with a valgus subtrochanteric osteotomy of the femur. In the author's experience in patients with cerebral palsy, this allows good range of motion in flexion, extension, abduction, and adduction leading to improved sitting ability and ease of perineal care. Postoperatively, we use the TBS (Fig. 15-8) instead of cast immobilization to allow early range of motion and easier care of the patient.

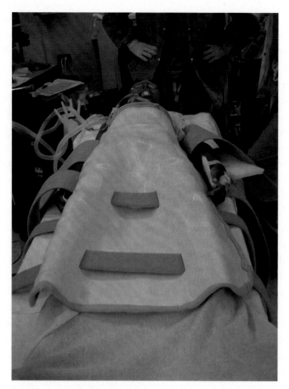

FIGURE 15-8. Total body splint.

KNEE DEFORMITIES

The two most common deformities about the knee in patients with myelomeningocele are knee flexion contracture and knee extension contracture. Other less commonly seen deformities are knee valgus deformity, knee varus deformity, or late knee instability with pain. Contractures occur most commonly in patients with thoracic and high lumbar level of involvement, and less often in patients with low lumbar level involvement (34). Deformity at the knee joint may occur as a result of many contributing factors, including static forces of positioning, fibrosis of surrounding muscles, muscle imbalance around the knee joint, and fracture malunion (95).

Knee Flexion Contracture. At birth, flexion contracture of the knee is a common finding in healthy newborns that often resolves during the first 6 months of life (98). This is in contrast to the fixed knee flexion contracture that can occur in both ambulatory and nonambulatory patients with myelomeningocele. Generally, more severe contractures are present in patients with thoracic level of involvement compared to those with lumbar level involvement (98–101). Early splinting can help to prevent knee flexion contracture in patients with high-level lesions.

The etiology of knee flexion contracture is multifactorial and may result in part from the typical supine positioning of patients with the hips abducted, flexed, and externally rotated and the knees flexed. Another factor relates to underly-

ing quadriceps weakness combined with prolonged time spent in a sitting position that leads to a gradual contracture of the hamstrings and biceps femoris and eventually contracture of the posterior knee capsule. Spasticity and contracture of the hamstrings may also result from tethered cord syndrome. In ambulatory patients, quadriceps weakness combined with paralysis of the gastrocnemius-soleus and gluteus muscles leads to flexion at the knee. Finally, flexion deformity at the knee may be exacerbated by fracture malunion (102).

In most nonambulatory patients, knee flexion contracture does not have a major impact on mobility or ability to transfer. However, in ambulatory patients, knee flexion contracture causes crouch gait, which has a high energy cost. Increased knee flexion during ambulation leads to increased oxygen cost and less efficient ambulation (51). Flexion deformity of >20 degrees has been shown to interfere with orthotic fitting, which can prevent the patient from being upright and ambulating (99). Gait analysis is useful in quantifying the amount of knee flexion during ambulation, which can differ from that seen on a static clinical examination. Using computerized gait analysis, one study found the degree of actual knee flexion during gait was significantly greater than the degree of clinical contracture (51). This information is useful in evaluating patients and planning proper treatment.

Because of the increased energy cost of a crouched gait, surgical treatment of knee flexion contracture is indicated when contracture exceeds 20 degrees in a patient with ambulatory potential (51, 99). Contracture release may also be indicated in nonambulatory patients if the fixed flexion position interferes with sitting balance, standing to transfer, or transfer from chair to bed (100). Treatment consists of radical knee flexor release including the hamstrings, gastrocnemius, and posterior capsule. It is also important to correct any hip flexion contracture at the same time, if present.

The knee release is done using a transverse incision located approximately 1 cm above the posterior flexor crease extending from medial to lateral. In a patient with thoracic or high-lumbar involvement, all of the medial and lateral hamstrings tendons are divided and resected. Lengthening of the tendons can be done in patients with lower level of involvement to preserve some flexor power. After this, the origin of the gastrocnemius tendon is released from the medial and lateral femoral condyles allowing exposure of the posterior knee articular capsule. An extensive capsulectomy is then performed leaving the posterior cruciate ligament intact. After closure of the wound with nonabsorbable suture, a long leg cast is placed with the knee in extension taking care to pad the patella to prevent pressure. If full extension is achieved at the time of surgery, the cast is left in place for 3 weeks. If complete extension is not achieved, a cast change may be performed 1 week later in order to achieve further correction. After 3 weeks, a knee immobilizer is used at night-time to maintain correction.

In rare instances, a supracondylar extension osteotomy of the femur may be necessary to achieve full extension of the knee if radical knee flexor release is not successful. This is primarily used for older patients who maintain the ability for community ambulation but are limited by a fixed knee flexion contracture.

In most cases, radical knee flexor release is successful in correcting the knee flexion deformity. Dias (99) reported a series of 23 knees undergoing radical flexor release. At final follow-up of 38 months, 21 of 23 knees maintained correction with flexion contracture of <10 degrees. In another study, a prospective review of 45 knees treated with radical flexor release found the mean knee flexion contracture decreased from 39 to 5 degrees after surgical release (100). The final average knee flexion contracture at follow-up of 13 years was 13 degrees (100). The authors noted a higher rate of recurrence of knee flexion contracture in patients with thoracic level of involvement compared to those with lumbar or lumbosacral. They also noted functional improvement in terms of walking ability in patients with L3/4 and L5/S1 levels of involvement.

Knee Extension Contracture.
Knee extension contracture is much less common than a flexion deformity. In most cases, knee extension contracture occurs bilaterally and is present at birth (99). Knee extension is frequently associated with other congenital anomalies such as dislocation of the ipsilateral hip, external rotation contracture of the hip, and equinovarus deformity of the foot (99, 103) (Fig. 15-9). Other causes of fixed extension contractures are unopposed quadriceps function with weak hamstrings, extensive bracing in extension, malunion after supracondylar fracture of the femur, and iatrogenic after surgical treatment of flexion contracture (34, 101).

Initial treatment entails a serial casting program with the goal of achieving at least 90 degrees of knee flexion. In most young patients, casting followed by physical therapy is successful. Surgical treatment is indicated when persistent extension contracture interferes with gait, sitting, using a wheelchair,

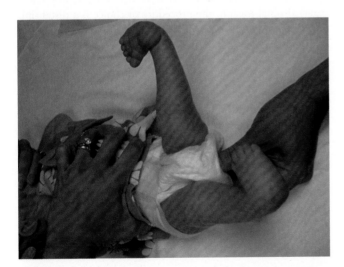

FIGURE 15-9. Newborn patient with myelomeningocele and knee extension contracture with ipsilateral hip dislocation and equinovarus deformity of the foot.

or performing transfers (101, 104). The preferred procedure is V–Y quadriceps lengthening with anterior capsulotomy as needed to obtain 90 degrees of flexion at the time of surgery (99, 101, 104). This is done using an anterior oblique incision beginning superomedially below the lesser trochanter and extending distally and laterally (99, 103). The extensor mechanism is divided superior to the patella with an inverted V incision. If needed, the anterior capsule is divided transversely to the medial and lateral collateral ligaments. The quadriceps is then sutured with the knee held in 45 degrees of flexion. The knee is then immobilized in a long leg cast with 45 degrees of knee flexion for 2 to 3 weeks. Physical therapy with active and passive motion starts after 2 to 3 weeks. Results with quadriceps plasty have been positive in terms of improving gait and sitting. Parsch and Manner (101) reported very good results after quadriceps plasty in 9 out of 10 patients. Dias (99) reported 13 of 15 patients treated with quadriceps plasty maintained at least 90 degrees of flexion at 43 months follow-up.

In nonambulatory patients without normal quadriceps function, another treatment option for knee extension contracture is tenotomy of the patellar tendon (104, 105). Sandhu et al. (105) reported a successful result in five out of eight patients with no further surgery required at 4 years follow-up. The authors achieved 50 to 70 degrees of knee flexion with tenotomy of the patellar tendon and 90 degrees or more of flexion with division of the medial and lateral retinacula as well. However, the authors stress that patellar tenotomy is recommended only for patients without normal quadriceps function and would otherwise recommend a formal quadricepsplasty.

Knee Valgus Deformity and Late Instability.
Valgus deformity of the knee, seen especially in patients with low-lumbar and sacral level of involvement, leads to instability, pain, and arthritis in adulthood. A specific gait pattern has been identified in symptomatic patients who have weakness of the hip abductors and gastrocsoleus muscles. The characteristic gait, described by Williams et al. (106), is an abductor lurch with the knee deforming into valgus and flexion during stance, followed by a swivel push-off on a fixed pronated foot. This gait pattern leads to increased stress on the knee ligaments and articular surfaces. Williams et al. (106) reported a series of 72 community ambulators over the age of 23 years and found 17 (24%) had significant knee symptoms.

The use of gait analysis has contributed to the understanding of abnormal valgus stress at the knee by allowing the identification of multiple factors leading to this stress. This includes rotational malalignment of the femur, femoral anteversion in association with excessive external tibial torsion, excessive trunk and pelvic movement, and knee flexion contracture (46, 55, 107, 108). Surgical treatment of excessive rotational deformities can decrease valgus stress at the knee and is indicated in patients over 6 years of age (55). Correction of rotational deformities leads to a significant improvement in knee stress and pain and may prevent the onset of late degenerative changes (49, 108). In addition, if knee valgus is associated with knee flexion contracture or hindfoot valgus, these deformities must be addressed at the same surgical setting (95). Patients found to have valgus stress at the knee should be encouraged to use an AFO and forearm crutches to decrease pelvic obliquity and rotation and hence increase stance-phase stability and decrease stress at the knee joint (46, 107).

ROTATIONAL DEFORMITY

Rotational deformities of the lower extremities develop commonly in both ambulatory and nonambulatory patients with myelomeningocele. The femur may be involved with an external rotation deformity of the hip that occurs due to contracture of the posterior hip capsule and short external rotator muscles. In addition, with the abnormal gait and activity levels in children with myelomeningocele, the normal newborn femoral torsion does not reliably decrease with growth (34). Even more common in patients with myelomeningocele are torsional deformities involving the tibia. Internal tibial torsion is a congenital deformity and is frequently associated with clubfoot. External tibial torsion, often associated with a shortened fibula and valgus deformity of the ankle, is an acquired deformity resulting from muscle imbalance. In certain ambulatory patients, the persistent proximal swivel motion of the pelvis and hip over the planted stance foot induces external tibial torsion (17).

In nonambulatory patients, rotational deformities are mainly a cosmetic problem. Treatment is indicated in ambulatory patients whose gait is impacted by the deformity, such as with internal tibial torsion, which can cause significant intoeing causing patients to trip and fall. Initially, treatment should be conservative utilizing twister cables attached to an AFO brace. In patients older than 5 to 6 years of age with severe femoral or tibial rotational deformity, surgical treatment indications include labored gait, difficulty with orthotic fitting resulting in skin ulceration, and pain (49). A detailed assessment of the patient's gait pattern utilizing three-dimensional gait analysis when available should be done to determine the extent of deformity correction necessary. The goal of treatment is to minimize bracing requirements while achieving as normal a gait pattern as possible (109).

Femoral Torsion.   In ambulatory patients with myelomeningocele, both excessive hip external and internal rotation can occur and impact gait. An internal rotation deformity of the hip can cause severe valgus stress at the knee when associated with external tibial torsion. External rotation at the hip joint can contribute to severe out-toeing when associated with external tibial torsion. Careful physical examination, including three-dimensional gait analysis if available, is necessary to ensure all the components of rotational deformity affecting gait are identified. As mentioned above, the initial treatment is with a twister cable attached to an AFO brace. If the deformity and resulting gait problem persist past the age of 5 to 6 years,

femoral osteotomy is indicated. In this case, the osteotomy is performed at the subtrochanteric level, and the distal segment is rotated to bring the foot into a position of neutral rotation (109). An AO dynamic compression plate, either 5 hole or 6 hole, is used for fixation. Postoperatively either a TBS or abduction wedge is used for 4 to 6 weeks until sufficient healing is present to allow mobilization and weight bearing.

Internal Tibial Torsion.   Internal tibial torsion requires surgical treatment when the resulting intoeing causes significant gait disturbance with frequent tripping. At the time of surgery, it is important to recognize any associated muscle imbalance. For instance, a spastic anterior tibialis muscle may require tenotomy with tendon excision at the same time as correction of the rotational deformity.

External Tibial Torsion.   Excessive external tibial torsion can also affect gait, cosmesis, and cause difficulty with orthotic fit. External rotation of the tibia places the medial malleolus more anteriorly leading to rubbing against the AFO and may cause a pressure sore on the medial aspect of the ankle (109). Improving external tibial torsion will not only alleviate skin issues, but also improve the effectiveness of the AFO brace in achieving knee extension. Even in the absence of a fixed knee flexion contracture, external tibial torsion >20 degrees can lead to a crouch gait pattern because the AFO is unable to improve the extension of the knee during stance phase (110). Hence, internal rotation osteotomy should be considered when the amount of external torsion exceeds 20 degrees in order to improve knee extension during stance phase (110). When planning for surgical correction, the patient's entire lower extremity should be carefully examined with particular attention to the hindfoot as hindfoot valgus may occur in association with external tibial torsion. In this case, both deformities require treatment in order to achieve a successful result (95).

When surgical treatment is indicated for either internal or external tibial torsion, the procedure of choice is a distal tibia and fibula derotation osteotomy (111). However, in patients with myelomeningocele, rotational osteotomies of the tibia are known to have a high rate of complications, such as delayed union and wound infection (112), so careful attention must be paid to the technical details of the procedure. The osteotomy should be performed just above the distal tibial physis, and the distal fibula osteotomy should be performed through a separate incision. The osteotomy should be created using multiple drill holes and a corticotomy in an attempt to decrease the thermal insult to the bone and preserve healing potential. An AO dynamic compression plate, usually a 5-hole plate, is used to provide stable fixation. The wound is then closed over a drain with interrupted, nonabsorbable sutures, and a short leg cast is placed. For the first 3 weeks, no weight bearing is allowed. After that time, a cast change is performed and the sutures are removed. The patient is allowed to weight bear in a walking cast for an additional 3 weeks or until sufficient healing is present. Utilizing this approach in a series of 10 osteotomies, there were no incidences of nonunion (49).

Using lower extremity osteotomies to treat rotational deformities has resulted in successful outcomes in terms of gait parameters and range of motion in 80% to 90% patients (109, 112). With regard to excessive external tibial torsion, derotation osteotomy will improve knee extension during stance phase. Corrective osteotomy may also delay or prevent the onset of late degenerative changes about the knee (49). Dunteman et al. used three-dimensional gait analysis to examine eight patients with external tibial torsion. They found increased valgus knee stress in 100% of the patients. After derotational tibial osteotomy, a significant improvement in the abnormal knee moment was seen along with improvement of knee extension during stance phase (49). In order to avoid the increased risk of complications such as delayed union and wound infection in patients with myelomeningocele, meticulous attention to technical details is important.

FOOT/ANKLE DEFORMITY

Foot deformity is present in almost all patients with myelomeningocele (34, 113). The spectrum of foot deformities seen includes calcaneus, equinus, varus, valgus, clubfoot, and vertical talus. Foot deformities can preclude effective bracing to allow ambulation, cause difficulty with shoe wear, create cosmetic problems, or lead to pressure sores. The common goal of treatment is a plantigrade, braceable foot with maximally preserved range of motion. Serial manual muscle testing is important for the detection of subtle muscle imbalance, which can lead to more significant deformities. Early intervention with casting, bracing, or surgical treatment may prevent fixed bony deformities. Surgical principles include the use of tendon excisions that are more reliable than tendon transfer or lengthenings. For bony deformities, osteotomies provide correction while preserving joint motion. Surgical arthrodesis

should be strictly avoided because the stiffness that results combined with an insensate foot has been shown to result in the development of neuropathic skin changes (30, 114). After surgical treatment, an AFO brace should be used to maintain correction and prevent recurrence.

Clubfoot. Clubfoot is the most common foot deformity in patients with myelomeningocele and has been reported in 30% to 50% of patients (31, 34, 115). Incidence of clubfoot varies with neurologic level of involvement. It occurs in approximately 90% of patients with thoracic or lumbar levels of involvement and 50% of patients with sacral level involvement (31). The clubfoot deformity in patients with myelomeningocele is quite different from the idiopathic clubfoot. In myelomeningocele, the clubfoot is often severely rigid (Fig. 15-10), similar to that seen in patients with arthrogryposis. Many patients also have severe internal tibial torsion.

Traditional teaching has been that nonsurgical management is rarely successful, and extensive soft-tissue release surgery is necessary for correction. However, two recent studies have reported promising early results using the Ponseti method of serial manipulation and casting in clubfeet associated with myelomeningocele (116, 117). Gerlach et al. (116) reported that initial correction was achieved in 27 of 28 clubfeet. Relapses occurred in 68% of the clubfeet but were treated successfully without extensive soft-tissue release surgery in all but 4 ft. Similarly, Janicki et al. reported initial correction with the Ponseti method in 9 out of 9 clubfeet. Five feet had recurrences and three of these required extensive soft-tissue release. They did note skin breakdown in 2 of the clubfeet. The Ponseti method can be useful in decreasing the need for extensive soft-tissue surgery, but families should be counseled about the high risk of recurrence, potential for need for further treatment, and risk of skin breakdown and fractures.

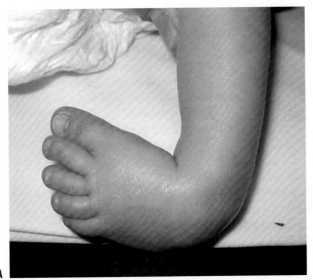
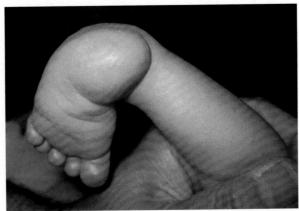

FIGURE 15-10. Rigid clubfoot in infant with myelomeningocele, anterior (**A**) and posterior (**B**) views.

When soft-tissue release surgery is indicated, the optimum time for treatment is at approximately 10 to 12 months of age. The surgical treatment consists of a radical posteromedial–lateral release using a Cincinnati incision (see Chapter 29). All tendons are excised rather than lengthened, including the anterior tibialis tendon. The subtalar, calcaneocuboid, and talonavicular joints are completely released. A separate plantar release may be needed through a plantar incision. Improved results have been shown with the use of a temporary Kirschner wire (K-wire) to derotate the talus in the ankle mortise (Fig. 15-11).

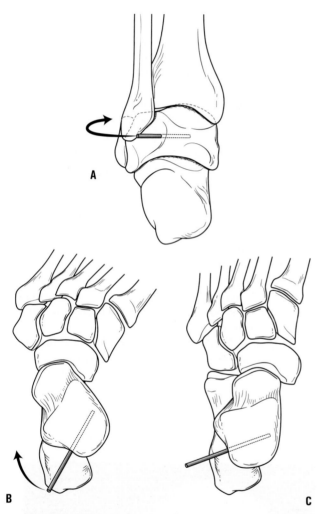

FIGURE 15-11. Temporary K-wire inserted into the posterolateral aspect of the talus to derotate the talus medially in the ankle mortise. **A:** Posterior view of the ankle and talus. The K-wire is inserted in the posterolateral surface of the talus. Note the external rotation of the talus in the ankle mortise. **B:** The abnormal rotation of the talus is seen. The K-wire is used to derotate the talus to its normal position. **C:** With the talus in a normal alignment and the talonavicular joint reduced, a second K-wire is then used to maintain this correction. (Reprinted from de Carvalho Neto J, Dias LS, Gabrieli AP. Congenital talipes equinovarus in spina bifida: treatment and results. *J Pediatr Orthop* 1996;16:782–5, with permission.)

(115). The K-wire is placed into the posterolateral aspect of the talus to rotate the talus medially, and the navicular is reduced on the talar head. A second K-wire is driven through the body of the talus into the navicular to hold the reduction and the temporary K-wire is then removed. Another K-wire is used to maintain the proper alignment of the talocalcaneal joint. Postoperatively, a long leg posterior mold splint is used with the foot in slight equinus to decrease tension on the interrupted sutures used for skin closure. After 2 weeks, the patient is changed to a long leg cast with the foot held in the corrected position. This remains in place for 6 weeks. After casting day and nighttime AFOs are used to maintain correction.

Good results after surgical release have been reported in 61% to 83% of patients (31, 115, 118). Outcome varies with motor level of involvement. de Carvalho Neto et al. (115) reported 50% poor results in patients with thoracic and high-lumbar level of involvement compared to only 11% poor results in patients with low-lumbar and sacral levels of involvement. The recurrence rate after surgical treatment is higher than in patients with idiopathic clubfoot and may be due in part to the lack of normal muscles around the ankle joint and lack of weight bearing (115). For this reason, it is important that at the time of cast removal, a standing A-frame is prescribed as well as the AFO.

Partial or complete recurrence occurs in 20% to 50% of patients after primary surgical correction (31). Patients with partial recurrence often develop adduction deformity, which may result from growth imbalance between an elongated lateral column and a shortened medial column. If bracing is not successful, surgical correction consists of a combination of lateral column shortening and medial column lengthening (see Chapter 29). This is done with the "double osteotomy," which consists of a closing wedge osteotomy of the cuboid with an opening wedge osteotomy of the medial cuneiform (Fig. 15-12) (119). Good results have been shown using this technique in children older than 4 years of age (119).

When complete recurrence occurs, the best procedure for achieving a plantigrade foot is talectomy (Fig. 15-13) (92, 120). Using an Ollier incision, an attempt is made to remove the talus as one piece. The tibiotalar, subtalar, and talonavicular joints are identified and opened widely. If contracture and scar make dissection difficult, needles can be used with intraoperative imaging to confirm location of the joints. To avoid recurrence, it is important not to leave any fragments of the talus remaining. Once the talus is removed, the calcaneus is thrust posteriorly in the ankle mortise and held in position with a K-wire. A short leg cast is then applied for at least 6 weeks. Dias and Stern (120) reported good results in 82% of feet treated with talectomy. The authors noted that severe forefoot deformities are not corrected by the talectomy; hence, any residual adduction deformity must be treated separately with concomitant closing wedge osteotomy of the cuboid.

Equinus. Equinus deformity occurs more commonly in patients with thoracic and high-lumbar levels of involvement but has been reported in patients with all levels of involvement

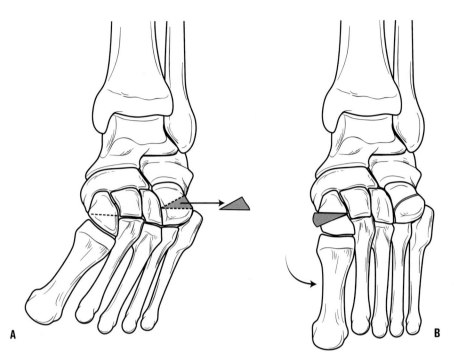

FIGURE 15-12. "Double osteotomy" to correct forefoot adduction. **A:** closing wedge osteotomy of the cuboid. **B:** opening wedge osteotomy of the medial cuneiform. (Reprinted from Lourenco AF, Dias LS, Zoellick DM, et al. Treatment of residual adduction deformity in clubfoot: the double osteotomy. *J Pediatr Orthop* 2001;21:713–8, with permission.)

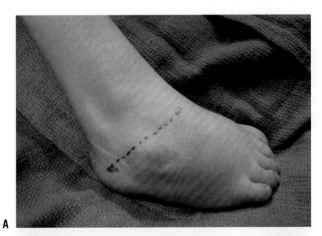

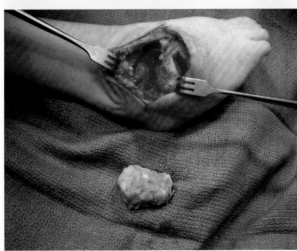

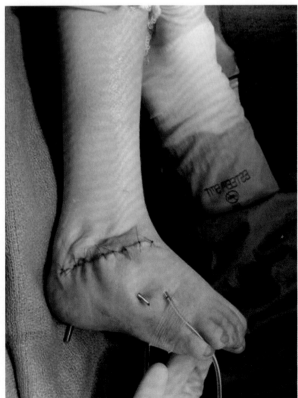

FIGURE 15-13. Talectomy for recurrent clubfoot. **A:** Photograph of foot showing deformity and location of incision. **B:** Intraoperative photograph showing talus removed en bloc. **C:** Postoperative photograph showing correction obtained.

(121). An AFO may be used to attempt to prevent equinus. Surgical treatment is indicated to achieve a plantigrade, braceable foot. The type of surgical procedure selected depends on the severity of deformity. Mild deformities respond to simple Achilles tendon excision. More severe contractures require a radical posterior release including the posterior tibiotalar and talocalcaneal joints. The authors prefer to use a limited Cincinnati incision and excise all tendons. The calcaneofibular ligament must be divided to achieve full correction. A K-wire may be used in the talocalcaneal joint to maintain neutral hindfoot alignment. A short leg cast is used for at least 6 weeks postoperatively followed by an AFO during the day and night.

Vertical Talus. Vertical talus deformity occurs in approximately 10% of patients with myelomeningocele (34) and is characterized by a rigid rocker-bottom flatfoot deformity with malalignment of the hindfoot and midfoot. The talus is nearly vertical and the calcaneus is in equinus and valgus. The navicular is dislocated dorsally and laterally on the talus. Vertical talus occurs in two forms in patients with myelomeningocele, either congenital that is more common, or developmental. The goal of treatment is to restore the normal relationship between the talus, navicular, and calcaneus and provide a plantigrade weight-bearing surface (122). Traditional treatment has been

with complete posteromedial–lateral and dorsal release when the patient is between 10 and 12 months of age. However, a new technique of serial manipulation and cast immobilization followed by open talonavicular pin fixation and percutaneous tenotomy of the Achilles tendon has been reported in idiopathic congenital vertical talus with excellent short-term results (123). The authors have begun using this method for initial correction of vertical talus in newborns with myelomeningocele with good initial success (Fig. 15-14).

When extensive soft-tissue release is necessary, good results have been reported with single-stage surgical correction addressing both the hindfoot and the forefoot (122). Using a Cincinnati incision, the Achilles tendon is z-lengthened, and the posterior capsules of the tibiotalar and subtalar joints are opened. The posterior and anterior tibial tendons are detached from their insertions and tagged for later repair. After this, the medial and dorsal aspects of the talonavicular joint, and the medial and lateral aspects of the subtalar joint are released. If necessary, the calcaneocuboid joint is released as well. Next a small K-wire is placed into the posterolateral aspect of the talus and used as a joystick to elevate the talus into a reduced position while plantarflexing the navicular and the forefoot (Fig. 15-15). Both the talonavicular and subtalar joints are then pinned in a reduced position, and if needed the extensor and peroneal tendons can be lengthened.

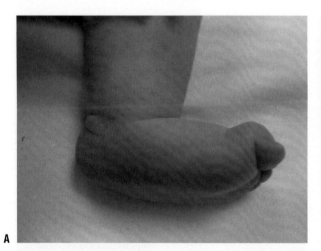

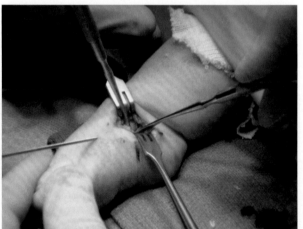

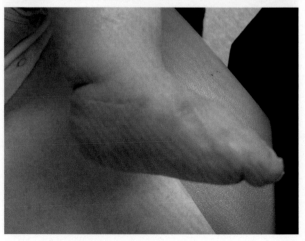

FIGURE 15-14. Vertical talus deformity in infant with myelomeningocele. **A:** Pretreatment photograph demonstrating foot deformity. **B:** After serial casting, patient underwent open talonavicular pin fixation and percutaneous tenotomy of the Achilles tendon. **C:** Postoperative photograph demonstrating deformity correction

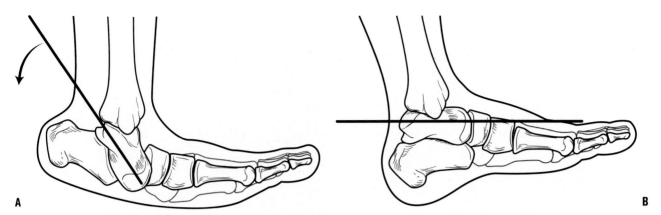

FIGURE 15-15. **A,B:** K-wire placed into posterolateral aspect of talus and used as joystick to elevate talus into reduced position while plantarflexing the navicular and forefoot. (Reprinted from Kodros SA, Dias LS. Single-stage surgical correction of congenital vertical talus. *J Pediatr Orthop* 1999;19:42–8, with permission.)

Calcaneus and Calcaneovalgus. Calcaneus deformity occurs in approximately 30% of patients with myelomeningocele. It is most common in patients with L4 or L5 level of involvement due to strength or spasticity of the ankle dorsiflexors combined with weakness of plantar flexion (31, 34, 124). Calcaneovalgus results from imbalance between the ankle evertors and the invertors. If the deformity is not rigid, an AFO may be useful to maintain the foot in neutral position. When the deformity is rigid, it can be very difficult to treat conservatively or surgically.

If left untreated, calcaneus deformity causes loss of normal toe-off and a crouch gait (31, 124). Persistent weight bearing on a calcaneus deformity leads to a bulbous heel prone to pressure sores and secondary osteomyelitis (31). External tibia torsion frequently develops in association with calcaneovalgus but can be avoided by early correction of the muscle imbalance (17). Surgical treatment with anterolateral release including tenotomy of all ankle dorsiflexors and the peroneus brevis and longus can achieve a plantigrade, braceable foot. Rodrigues and Dias (125) reported a series of 76 patients treated with anterolateral release and achieved a good result in 82%. The poor results were due to either recurrence requiring a second release or equinus deformity requiring release of the Achilles tendon. The authors have found the anterolateral release to be a simpler procedure than the anterior tibial tendon transfer to the os calcis with similar results. However, Park et al. (124) recently reported a series of 31 calcaneus feet treated with anterior tibialis tendon transfer with concomitant osseous surgeries in 12 ft. They noted no recurrence or worsening of the deformity in any patient and no other type of foot deformity developed after the surgery.

In older patients who have developed significant bony deformity, surgical correction requires not only release of all the extensor tendons and peroneals if needed, but also bony correction. A closing wedge osteotomy of the calcaneus with a plantar release can improve hindfoot alignment. If calcaneal valgus is present, a lateral opening wedge osteotomy of the cuboid may be necessary to achieve complete correction.

Ankle and Hindfoot Valgus. Valgus deformities of the hindfoot and ankle are common in ambulatory patients with myelomeningocele. Successful treatment depends on identifying the precise anatomical location of the deformity that can arise from the distal tibia, hindfoot, or both. Valgus deformities tend to become more pronounced as a child matures, begins ambulation, and gains weight (114). Valgus deformity (Fig. 15-16) is common in patients with low lumbar levels of involvement due to muscle imbalance, weight bearing, and the effects of gravity. When flexible, these deformities are initially managed with a rigid AFO to provide stability. Often as the hindfoot progresses into more valgus, skin irritation and breakdown over the medial malleolus and talar head result from excessive pressure against the brace. Surgery is indicated for severe, rigid deformities causing pain, difficulty with brace wear, or ulceration (114). Treatment options include distal tibia osteotomy, hemiepiphyseodesis of the distal tibia, or medial displacement osteotomy of the calcaneus.

For ankle valgus due to deformity in the distal tibia (Fig. 15-17), surgical treatment depends on the severity of the deformity and the amount of growth remaining. Hemiepiphysiodesis is indicated for mild deformities with sufficient growth remaining. Temporary growth arrest of the medial physis with continued growth of the lateral physis allows gradual correction of the valgus tilt. Use of a single cannulated screw has been reported in a series of 50 ft with satisfactory improvement of ankle valgus, low morbidity, and no incidence of permanent physeal closure (126). To avoid permanent closure of the physis, the screw should be removed within 2 years of its insertion. For more severe ankle valgus or in an older child with little growth remaining, a distal tibia osteotomy is indicated. Osteotomies of the distal tibia are associated with a high incidence of complications such as delayed union, nonunion, wound infection, and loss of correction. However, the authors have had good success with the transphyseal osteotomy described by Lubicky and Altiok (127). Care should be taken to create the osteotomy with multiple drill holes connected by an osteotome rather than with power instruments. If concomitant

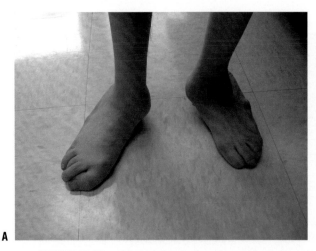
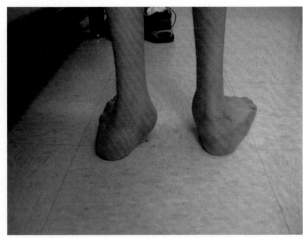

A

B

FIGURE 15-16. Valgus deformity in patient with myelomeningocele. **A:** Anterior view demonstrating bursa formation due to irritation over medial malleolus from brace. **B:** Posterior view demonstrating hindfoot valgus.

external tibial torsion is present as is often the case, internal rotation of the distal fragment should be done at the same time.

Surgical treatment for valgus deformity of the hindfoot consists of medial sliding osteotomy of the calcaneus in an effort to preserve subtalar motion while correcting the deformity. This procedure was initially described as a treatment for idiopathic flatfoot by Koutsogiannis (128) but has been also been reported in a series of patients with myelomeningocele (114). Using a lateral L-shaped incision to provide adequate exposure, full-thickness flaps are elevated to allow extraperiosteal

dissection of the calcaneus. An oblique osteotomy is made, and the amount of displacement of the distal fragment required for correction is usually 50% of the width of the fragment (114). A threaded K-wire should be used for internal fixation that is left in place for 3 weeks. After 3 weeks, the K-wire is removed and the patient is allowed to begin weight bearing in a short-leg walking cast. Using this procedure in 38 ft in patients with myelomeningocele, good results were obtained in 82% (114). In this series, three of the poor results were due to unrecognized concomitant distal tibia valgus deformity.

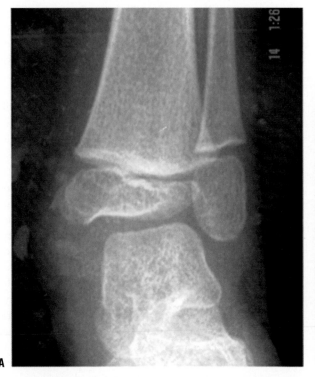
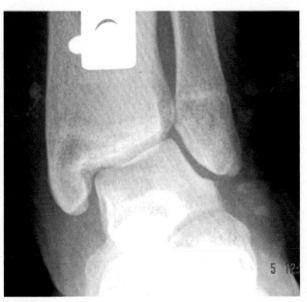

A

B

FIGURE 15-17. Distal tibia valgus deformity. **A:** Mild valgus in a skeletally immature patient. **B:** Severe valgus in a skeletally mature patient.

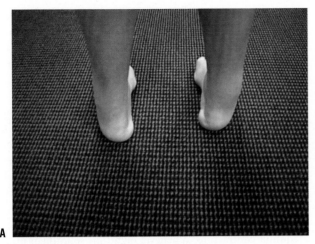
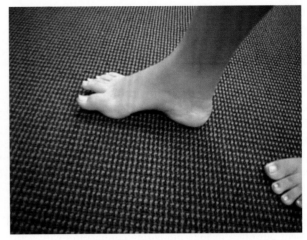

FIGURE 15-18. Cavovarus deformity in patient with myelomeningocele. **A:** Posterior view demonstrating hindfoot varus. **B:** Side view demonstrating cavus.

Cavus, Varus, and Cavovarus. Cavovarus deformity (Fig. 15-18) occurs in patients with sacral level myelomeningocele and in patients with lipomeningocele. The primary deformity is cavus and varus is caused by the muscle imbalance between the posterior tibialis and the peroneal muscles as well as intrinsic muscle weakness. Treatment is based on the flexibility of the deformity. The Coleman block test can be used to determine whether the hindfoot deformity is flexible or fixed (129). When the hindfoot varus is flexible, treatment is limited to the forefoot and consists of a radical plantar release. If the hindfoot varus is rigid, correction involves both the forefoot and the hindfoot (130). Muscle imbalance must be corrected at the same time. Mubarak and Van Valin (131) have described the use of selective, joint-sparing osteotomies to address deformity correction. They recommend a closing wedge osteotomy of the first metatarsal, opening plantar wedge osteotomy of the medial cuneiform, closing wedge osteotomy of the cuboid and if necessary a sliding osteotomy of the calcaneus and osteotomies of the second and third metatarsals. They also performed plantar release and peroneus longus-to-brevis tendon transfer when needed. In a series of 20 ft in patients with varying underlying etiologies, 95% had good or very good outcomes with this protocol (131). Triple arthrodesis should be avoided in this patient population with impaired sensation (130).

POSTOPERATIVE CARE

Patients with myelomeningocele are at a higher risk for certain postoperative complications compared to the general population. Care must be taken to prevent these complications, including skin breakdown, nonunion, and fractures. With regard to choice of immobilization, whenever possible a total body spica cast should be strictly avoided. A removable custom-molded TBS is a useful alternative to spica casting

(Figs. 15-7 and 15-19). It provides adequate immobilization even for patients who have undergone bony surgical procedures while allowing for easier care and comfort of the patient. In addition, the TBS can be removed for gentle range of motion once adequate healing is present to avoid stiffness and contracture. Another benefit of the TBS is that it can be used at nighttime after the initial postoperative immobilization period to provide additional stretch in order to augment the effects of surgery and prevent recurrence of deformity. While immobilized after surgery, it is important to educate the patient's family and caregivers to avoid pressure on the posterior aspect of the patient's heels. We instruct them to use a small towel rolled up under the distal calf to keep the heel floating freely in order to avoid creating a pressure sore.

The use of rigid internal fixation with plate and screw fixation of osteotomy sites instead of K-wire fixation has many advantages. Rigid fixation allows a shorter period of immobilization

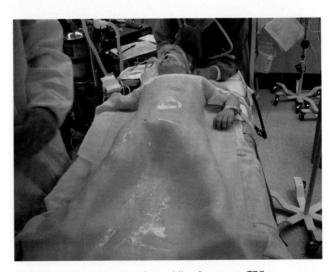

FIGURE 15-19. Intraoperative molding for custom TBS.

with earlier range of motion and weight bearing. In addition, rigid fixation helps to decrease the risk of nonunion.

The surgeon must properly educate the patient and family on how to avoid certain postoperative complications. Especially important is to strictly forbid crawling for at least 3 to 4 weeks after immobilization is discontinued. Crawling places a large amount of stress at the supracondylar region of the femur, which is a common location for postimmobilization fracture. The family is more likely to adhere to postoperative instructions if educated on the reason behind the recommendation.

Postoperative therapy should begin early—as soon as surgical wounds are stable and adequate healing is present. Goals of physical therapy should be tailored to the individual patient but often include preventing contractures with active and passive range of motion, strengthening program, early weight bearing, and gait training.

ORTHOSES

Almost all children with myelomeningocele will require orthotic support to achieve ambulation. The exception to this is some patients with low-sacral level of involvement. With regard to ambulation, the goal of orthotic treatment is to facilitate independent mobility while minimizing restrictions. The type of brace required depends on the motor deficit present and trunk balance. There are many other indications for the use of orthoses in patients with myelomeningocele aside from ambulation. These include maintenance of proper alignment and prevention of deformity, correction of flexible deformity, and protection of the insensate limb (95).

Nighttime bracing may be indicated to prevent orthopaedic deformities. As an example, a patient with thoracic level involvement may benefit from a nighttime TBS to prevent hip flexion and external rotation contractures, knee flexion contractures, and equinus. For this usage, the TBS is molded with the hips in fifteen degrees of abduction, knee extension, and the ankle in neutral (17). For patients with lower levels of involvement, an AFO can be used at night to prevent equinus contracture. Whenever nighttime splinting is utilized, the patient and the family should be carefully educated on skin care and proper fit in order to prevent areas of pressure irritation.

In patients with thoracic and high-lumbar level involvement, orthoses are needed for upright weight bearing and mobility. A standing frame (Fig. 15-20), which is a prefabricated trunk–hip lower extremity brace, allows the child to stand without hand support. This is usually prescribed for children aged 12 to 18 months or once the child demonstrates adequate head and neck control. It should be used up to 3 hours a day, divided into periods of 20 to 30 minutes.

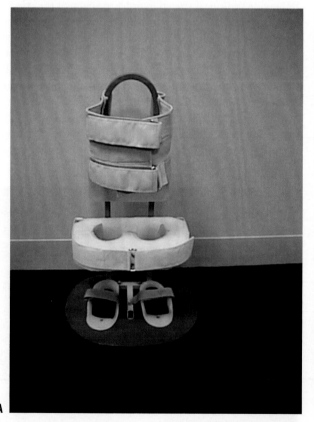

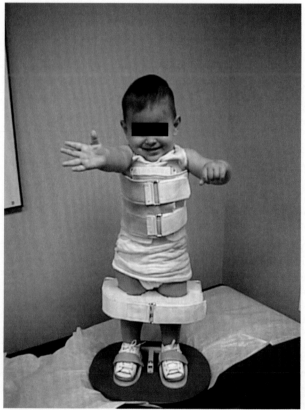

A

B

FIGURE 15-20. Standing frame, **(A)** alone and **(B)** with patient.

To achieve mobility, patients with thoracic and high-lumbar level involvement will require an orthosis that crosses the hip in order to control the trunk over the pelvis and lower limbs (95). Examples of this are the RGO (Fig. 15-1) and HKAFO (Fig. 15-2). The RGO, often used with a walker, is indicated for a child around 24 months of age with good sitting balance without hand support and good upper extremity function. An RGO is contraindicated in patients with severe scoliosis, hip flexion contracture >30 to 40 degrees, or severe visual deficit. As an alternative to the RGO, a parapodium (Fig. 15-21) is indicated for a child with poor trunk balance or upper extremity spasticity.

The HKAFO can be used for a patient with high-lumbar level involvement who has achieved swing-through ambulation with crutches. It is important however for providers to understand that most patients with higher levels of involvement will eventually opt to use a wheelchair for mobility. The wheelchair allows an energy-efficient means to achieve independent mobility. Several factors should be considered in the design of the wheelchair. In regard to the seat, special cushions may be needed to offload pressure areas and prevent decubitus ulcers over the ischium or the sacrum. Trunk supports should be added to the back rest as needed, and detachable arm rests allow for easier transfer in and out of the chair.

Patients with sacral or low-lumbar level of involvement will require a solid AFO (Fig. 15-3) to compensate for muscle weakness below the knee (52). The AFO acts as a substitute for weak or absent ankle plantar flexors and dorsiflexors. The AFO should be designed to be rigid enough to provide ankle and foot stability while maintaining the shank-ankle angle at 90 degrees to prevent excessive dorsiflexion leading to crouch at the knee. Carbon reinforcement is often needed in the older child. In addition, special padding may be necessary over pressure points such as the medial malleolus and head of talus to prevent pressure sores. Certain patients with a tendency for crouch gait will benefit from use of a ground reaction AFO (Fig. 15-22) to assist with knee extension during stance.

Occasionally, a patient with low lumbar level of involvement will benefit from a knee–ankle–foot orthosis (KAFO) to prevent excessive valgus stress at the knee if the patient is too young for derotation osteotomy. Whether using KAFOs or AFOs, patients with low lumbar or high sacral level of involvement who have weakness of the hip extensors and abductors may benefit from the use of crutches to improve pelvic and hip kinematics. In this instance, crutches allow the upper extremities to share in weight bearing decreasing the stress on the lower extremity musculature and allowing a more functional gait pattern (52). Patients who are introduced to crutches at a young age are more receptive to their use compared to adolescent and young adult patients.

Rotational malalignment is common in patients with low lumbar and high sacral level of involvement. AFOs with twister cables are useful to correct either intoeing or out-toeing gait until an appropriate age for surgical correction is reached. These may be introduced as early as 2 years of age.

ADULT CARE

As overall care for patients with myelomeningocele improves and more and more patients are surviving into adulthood, increased attention is required to the issues unique to adult patients with myelomeningocele. It can be difficult for adult patients to find appropriate providers as few adult physicians have experience with the detailed care of patients with myelomeningocele. Ideally, adult care should be provided in a multidisciplinary setting similar to that for the pediatric patient.

Orthopaedic issues in adult patients tend to correspond to the patient's functional level of involvement. Thoracic level patients usually have an FMS of 1,1,1 or 2,2,1 and very occasionally 3,3,1. They have a high incidence of spinal deformity requiring surgical treatment and hip and knee flexion contractures. Even despite aggressive treatment during childhood, some amount of recurrence of contracture as an adult is common. Patients with low lumbar lesions are likely to maintain the ability to ambulate as adults (39) and often have an FMS of 3,3,1. To assist patients with maintenance of

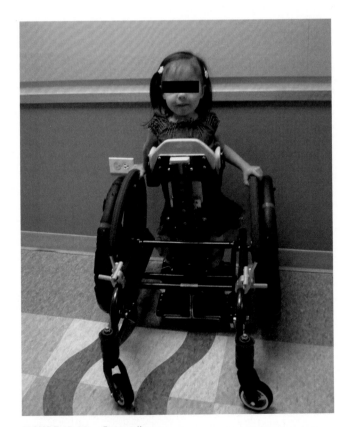

FIGURE 15-21. Parapodium.

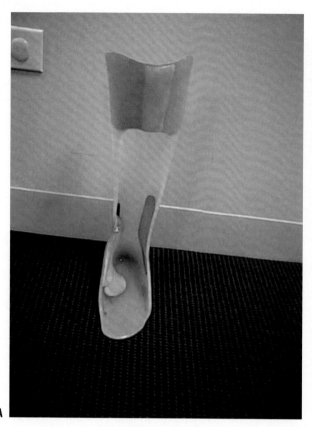
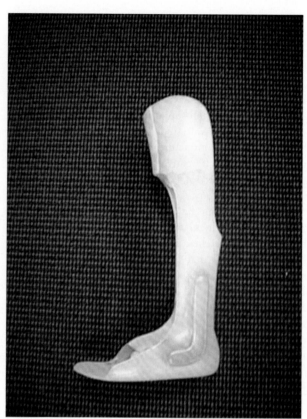

FIGURE 15-22. Ground reaction ankle foot orthosis (GRAFO). **A:** Front view. **B:** Side view.

ambulation, hip contractures should be treated aggressively as should any deformity of the knee, ankle, foot or rotational malalignment. The majority of patients with sacral level of involvement will maintain community ambulation as adults (38, 46) with an FMS of 6,6,3. As with low lumbar level patients, any rotational malalignment or deformity of the knee, ankle, or foot should be corrected. In addition, tethered cord syndrome should be treated aggressively and arthrodesis at the level of the foot should be avoided (46, 30).

Pressure sores are a major problem in adult myelomeningocele patients. In one study of 87 adult patients, 82% had experienced a pressure sore within the past 5 years (32). In this study, the sores were mainly located on the feet in areas of impaired sensation. The authors identified a significantly higher risk for pressure sores in patients with memory deficit, Arnold-Chiari malformation, and a history of previous sores. Patients with these conditions should be monitored closely and educated on a program of personal skin inspection and care.

In addition, we have observed a number of adult patients with thoracic or high-lumbar level of involvement who have developed severe lower extremity lymphedema. This causes problems with brace fitting and pressure sores leading to a functional decline. Prevention and treatment is with carefully fitted elastic compression stockings. If available, referral to occupational therapy or a lymphedema treatment clinic is beneficial.

The long-term outcome of adult patients with sacral level involvement has been evaluated in the literature (46,Brinker). Brinker et al. looked at a group of 36 patients ranging in age from 19 to 51 years followed for an average of 10 years. Although 97% patients were initially community ambulators, only 69% remained so at final follow-up. The authors also found a decrease in plantar sensation in 42% patients with skin breakdown in 75% patients. In addition, 64% patients had developed soft-tissue infections on the plantar surface of the metatarsal heads and heel. Forty-two percent of patients developed osteomyelitis necessitating a total of 14 amputations at various levels. In all 33 patients had undergone a total of 371 orthopaedic procedures.

Selber and Dias evaluated a group of 46 adult patients ranging in age from 18 to 38 years. In all 39 patients underwent 217 orthopaedic procedures. However, in contrast to Brinker et al, they found 89% patients maintained community ambulation at final follow-up, of whom 70% required no external support. In addition, only two amputations were performed. Selber and Dias attributed these results to aggressive treatment of tethered cord syndrome, surgical correction of musculoskeletal deformities, and avoidance of arthrodesis at the foot.

INTRASPINAL LIPOMA

Lipoma associated with the spinal cord, occurring in 1 in 4000 births, is the most common type of occult spinal dysraphism (132). Lipomeningocele is a subcutaneous lipoma connected to the conus medullaris by a vertebral and dural defect that can result in a tethered spinal cord and is the most common type. Other possibilities are intradural lipomas or lipoma of the filum (fatty filum terminale). In all, lipomas of the lumbosacral spine account for 25% to 35% of the cases of tethered cord syndrome (132).

Intraspinal lipoma is a separate entity from myelomeningocele with different embryogenesis, clinical presentation, and prognosis. Unlike with myelomeningocele, folate supplementation has not been shown to have an effect on reducing the incidence of intraspinal lipomas (133). Patients with intraspinal lipoma do not develop hydrocephalus or Chiari malformation and have normal intelligence (134). Also, the neurologic deficits resulting from tethered cord are asymmetric and can skip adjacent dermatomes (132).

Although most patients with intraspinal lipomas have normal neurologic function at birth, neurologic deterioration can occur at any age into adulthood. When not detected and treated appropriately, this can cause severe lower extremity dysfunction. With proper treatment and care, most patients with intraspinal lipomas maintain an FMS of 6,6,6. Rarely some patients have an FMS of 3,3,3.

Since the defect in patients with intraspinal lipomas is closed, the two main findings that prompt evaluation are cutaneous markers and neurologic deficits (133). The cutaneous manifestations of spinal lipoma include sacral dimples, masses, dermal sinuses, hemangiomas, and hairy patches in the lumbosacral area (132, 133). Neurologic deficits result from spinal cord tethering or compression of the cord and often occur during periods of rapid height or weight gain. Muscle imbalance caused by tethering of the cord leads to orthopaedic deformities, especially of the foot, which often require surgical correction.

Once tethering of the spinal cord causes muscle imbalance, surgical excision of the lipoma with cord untethering often does not lead to complete recovery (17). Hence, early aggressive neurosurgical treatment is indicated. In addition, since retethering occurs in approximately 30% patients (132), lifetime follow-up with manual muscle strength testing is recommended to facilitate early detection and intervention.

A recent review of 151 patients found acquired foot deformity was the most common orthopaedic manifestation occurring in 75% feet in patients with lipomeningocele (132). Of these, the most common deformity was cavovarus, followed by cavus with or without claw toes. Surgical correction (see "Cavus, Varus, and Cavovarus") was required in approximately 30% patients with lipomeningocele. Congenital foot deformities were also noted including clubfoot, vertical talus, and hypoplastic foot. Other common orthopaedic manifestations included scoliosis, which occurred in 20% of patients, none of whom required surgical treatment. Limb-length discrepancy

was present in 11% patients. The shorter side was the side with weakness or deformity.

REFERENCES

1. McClone DG, Bowman RM: Overview of the management of myelomeningocele UpToDate, 2009. Available at http://www.uptodate.com/contents/overview-of-the-management-of-myelomeningocele-spina-bifida
2. Herring JA. Neuromuscular disorders. In: Herring JA, ed. *Tachdjian's pediatric orthopaedics*. Philadelphia, PA: Saunders Elsevier, 2008:1405–1453.
3. Bowman RM, McLone DG, Grant JA, et al. Spina bifida outcome: a 25-year retrospective. *Pediatr Neurosurg* 2001;34:114.
4. Guille JT, Sarwark JF, Sherk HH, et al. Congenital and developmental deformities of the spine in children with myelomeningocele. *J Am Acad Orthop Surg* 2006;14:294–302.
5. Centers for Disease Control and Prevention (CDC). Recommendations for the use of folic acid to reduce the number of cases of spina bifida and other neural tube defects. *MMWR Recomm Rep* 1992;41 (RR-14):1–7.
6. Centers for Disease Control and Prevention (CDC). Racial/ethnic differences in the birth prevalence of spina bifida—United States, 1995–2005. *MMWR Morb Mortal Wkly Rep* 2009;57(53):1409–1413.
7. Busby A, Abramsky L, Dolk H, et al.; Eurocat Folic Acid Working Group. Preventing neural tube defects in Europe: population based study. *BMJ* 2005;330:574–575.
8. Padmanabhan R. Etiology, pathogenesis and prevention of neural tube defects. *Congenit Anom (Kyoto)* 2006;46:55–67.
9. Doran PA, Guthkelch AN. Studies in spina bifida cystica. I. General survey and reassessment of the problem. *J Neurol Neurosurg Psychiatry* 1961;24:331.
10. Ingraham FD, Swam H. Spina bifida and cranium bifida. I. A survey of five hundred forty six cases. *N Engl J Med* 1943;228:559.
11. Lorber J. Incidence and epidemiology of myelomeningocele. *Clin Orthop Relat Res* 1966;45:81.
12. Cameron M, Moran P. Prenatal screening and diagnosis of neural tube defects. *Prenat Diagn* 2009;29:402–411.
13. Boyd PA, Devigan C, Khoshnood B, et al.; EUROCAT Working Group. Survey of prenatal screening policies in Europe for structural malformations and chromosome anomalies, and their impact on detection and termination rates for neural tube defects and Down's syndrome. *BJOG* 2008;115(6):689–696.
14. Stoll C, Alembik Y, Dott B. Associated malformations in cases with neural tube defects. *Genet Couns* 2007;18(2):209–215.
15. Chakraborty A, Crimmins D, Hayward R, et al. Toward reducing shunt placement rates in patients with myelomeningocele. *J Neurosurg Pediatrics* 2008;1:361.
16. Rintoul NE, Sutton LN, Hubbard AM, et al. A new look at myelomeningoceles: functional level, vertebral level, shunting and the implications for fetal intervention. *Pediatrics* 2002;109:409–413.
17. Dias L. Myelomeningocele and intraspinal lipoma. In: Sponseller PD, ed. *Orthopaedic knowledge update: pediatrics*, 2nd ed. Rosemont, IL: American Academy of Orthopaedic Surgeons, 2002:249–259.
18. Battibugli S, Gryfakis N, Dias L, et al. Functional gait comparison between children with myelomeningocele: shunt versus no shunt. *Dev Med Child Neurol* 2007;49(10):764–769.
19. Yamada S, Won DJ, Siddiqi J, et al. Tethered cord syndrome: overview of diagnosis and treatment. *Neurol Res* 2004;26(7):719–721.
20. Sarwark JF, Weber DT, Gabrieli AP, et al. Tethered cord syndrome in low motor level children with myelomeningocele. *Pediatr Neurosurg* 1996;25(6):295–301.
21. La Marca F, Herman M, Grant JA, et al. Presentation and management of hydromyelia in children with Chiari type-II malformation. *Pediatr Neurosurg* 1997;26:57.

22. Curry JI, Osborne A, Malone PS. The MACE procedure: experience in the United Kingdom. *J Pediatr Surg* 1999;34:338.

23. Rendeli C, Nucera E, Ausili E, et al. Latex sensitization and allergy in children with myelomeningocele. *Childs Nerv Syst* 2006;22:28.

24. Emans JB. Current concepts review: allergy to latex in patients who have myelodysplasia. *J Bone Joint Surg Am* 1992;74:1103–1109.

25. Fiore P, Picco P, Castagnola E, et al. Nutritional survey of children and adolescents with myelomeningocele (MMC): overweight associated with reduced energy intake. *Eur J Pediatr Surg* 1998;8(Suppl 1):34–36.

26. Holmbeck GN, Gorey-Ferguson L, Hudson T, et al. Maternal, paternal, and marital functioning in families of preadolescents with spina bifida. *J Pediatr Psychol* 1997;22:167.

27. Appleton PL, Ellis NC, Minchom PE, et al. Depressive symptoms and self-concept in young people with spina bifida. *J Pediatr Psychol* 1997;22:707.

28. Bartonek A, Saraste H, Samuelsson L, et al. Ambulation in patients with myelomeningocele: a 12-year follow-up. *J Pediatr Orthop* 1999; 19(2):202–206.

30. Maynard MJ, Weiner LS, Burke SW. Neuropathic foot ulceration in patients with myelodysplasia. *J Pediatr Orthop* 1992;12:786.

31. Akbar M, Bresch B, Seyler TM, et al. Management of orthopaedic sequelae of congenital spinal disorders. *J Bone Joint Surg Am* 2009;91:87–100.

32. Plaum PE, Riemer G, Frøslie KF. Risk factors for pressure sores in adult patients with myelomeningocele—a questionnaire-based study. *Cerebrospinal Fluid Res* 2006;3:14.

33. Díaz Llopis I, Bea Muñoz M, Martinez Agulló E, et al. Ambulation in patients with myelomeningocele: a study of 1500 patients. *Paraplegia* 1993;31(1):28–32.

34. Westcott MA, Dynes MC, Remer EM, et al. Congenital and acquired orthopedic abnormalities in patients with myelomeningocele. *Radiographics* 1992;12:1155–1173.

35. Kumar SJ, Cowell HR, Townsend P. Physeal, metaphyseal and diaphyseal injuries of the lower extremities in children with myelomeningocele. *J Pediatr Onthop* 1984;4:25–27.

36. Anschuetz RH, Freehafer AA, Shaffer JW, et al. Severe fracture complications in myelodysplasia. *J Pediatr Orthop* 1984;4:22–24.

37. Mazur JM, Shurtleff D, Menelaus M, et al. Orthopaedic management of high-level spina bifida. Early walking compared with early use of a wheelchair. *J Bone Joint Surg Am* 1989;71:56–61.

38. Asher M, Olson J. Factors affecting the ambulatory status of patients with spina bifida cystica. *J Bone Joint Surg Am* 1983;65:350–356.

39. Barden GA, Meyer LC, Stelling FH III. Myelodysplastics—fate of those followed for twenty years or more. *J Bone Joint Surg Am* 1975;57: 643–647.

40. Seitzberg A, Lind M, Biering-Sørensen F. Ambulation in adults with myelomeningocele. Is it possible to predict the level of ambulation in early life? *Childs Nerv Syst* 2008;24:231–237.

41. Schopler SA, Menelaus MB. Significance of the strength of the quadriceps muscles in children with myelomeningocele. *J Pediatr Orthop* 1987;7:507–512.

42. McDonald CM, Jaffe KM, Mosca VS, et al. Ambulatory outcome of children with myelomeningocele: effect of lower-extremity muscle strength. *Dev Med Child Neurol* 1991;33:482–490.

43. Swank M, Dias LS. Walking ability in spina bifida patients: a model for predicting future ambulatory status based on sitting balance and motor level. *J Pediatr Orthop* 1994;14:715–718.

44. Sharrard WJ. The orthopaedic surgery of spina bifida. *Clin Orthop Relat Res* 1973;92:195–213.

45. Stillwell A, Menelaus MB. Walking ability in mature patients with spina bifida. *J Pediatr Orthop* 1983;3:184–190.

46. Selber P, Dias L. Sacral-level myelomeningocele: long-term outcome in adults. *J Pediatr Orthop* 1998;18:423–427.

47. Graham HK, Harvey A, Rodda J, et al. The Functional Mobility Scale (FMS). *J Pediatr Orthop* 2004;24(5):514–520.

48. Gage JR, DeLuca PA, Renshaw TS. Gait analysis: principles and applications; emphasis on its use in cerebral palsy. *J Bone Joint Surg* 1995;77:1607–1623.

49. Dunteman RC, Vankoski SJ, Dias LS. Internal derotation osteotomy of the tibia: pre- and postoperative gait analysis in persons with high sacral myelomeningocele. *J Pediatr Orthop* 2000;20:623–628.

50. Gabrieli APT, Vankoski SJ, Dias LS, et al. Gait analysis in low lumbar myelomeningocele patients with unilateral hip dislocation or subluxation. *J Pediatr Orthop* 2003;23:330–334.

51. Moen T, Gryfakis N, Dias L, et al. Crouched gait in myelomeningocele: a comparison between the degree of knee flexion contracture in the clinical examination and during gait. *J Pediatr Orthop* 2005;25(5):657–666.

52. Vankoski SJ, Sarwark JF, Moore C, et al. Characteristic pelvic, hip and knee kinematic patterns in children with lumbosacral myelomeningocele. *Gait Posture* 1995;3:51–57.

53. Duffy CM, Hill AE, Cosgrove AP, et al. Three-dimensional gait analysis in spina bifida. *J Pediatr Orthop* 1996;16:786–791.

54. Gage JR, Novacheck TF. An update on the treatment of gait problems in cerebral palsy. *J Pediatr Orthop B* 2001;10:265–274.

55. Dias L. Orthopaedic care in spina bifida: past, present, and future. *Dev Med Child Neurol* 2004;46:579.

56. Muller EB, Nordwall A, von Wendt L. Influence of surgical treatment of scoliosis in children with spina bifida on ambulation and motoric skills. *Acta Paediatr* 1992;81:173–176.

57. Piggott H. The natural history of scoliosis in myelodysplasia. *J Bone Joint Surg Br* 1980;62:54–58.

58. Samuelsson L, Eklof O. Scoliosis in myelomeningocele. *Acta Orthop Scand* 1988;59:122–127.

59. Trivedi J, Thomson JD, Slakey JB, et al. Clinical and radiographic predictors of scoliosis in patients with myelomeningocele. *J Bone Joint Surg Am* 2002;84:1389–1394.

60. Glard Y, Launay F, Viehweger E, et al. Neurological classification in myelomeningocele as a spine deformity predictor. *J Pediatr Orthop B* 2007;16:287–292.

61. Muller EB, Nordwall A, Oden A. Progression of scoliosis in children with myelomeningocele. *Spine* 1994;19:147–150.

62. Shurtleff DB, Goiney R, Gordon LH, et al. Myelodysplasia: The natural history of kyphosis and scoliosis. A preliminary report. *Dev Med Child Neurol Suppl* 1976;37:126–133.

63. McCarthy RE. Management of neuromuscular scoliosis. *Ortho Clin North Am* 1999;30:435–449.

64. Schoenmakers MAGC, Gulmans VAM, Gooskens RHJM, et al. Spinal fusion in children with spina bifida: influence on ambulation level and functional abilities. *Eur Spine J* 2005;14:415–422.

65. Muller EB, Nordwall A. Prevalence of scoliosis in children with myelomeningocele in western Sweden. *Spine* 1992;17:1097–1102.

66. Mazur J, Menelaus MB, Dickens DRV, et al. Efficacy of surgical management for scoliosis in myelomeningocele: correction of deformity and alteration of functional status. *J Pediatr Orthop* 1986;6:568–575.

67. McMaster MJ. Anterior and posterior instrumentation and fusion of thoracolumbar scoliosis due to myelomeningocele. *J Bone Joint Surg Br* 1987;69:20–25.

68. Banta JV. Combined anterior and posterior fusion for spinal deformity in myelomeningocele. *Spine* 1990;15:946–952.

69. Ward WT, Wenger DR, Roach JW. Surgical correction of myelomeningocele scoliosis: a critical appraisal of various spinal instrumentation systems. *J Pediatr Orthop* 1989;9:262–268.

70. Parsch D, Geiger F, Brocai DR, et al. Surgical management of paralytic scoliosis in myelomeningocele. *J Pediatr Orthop B* 2001;10:10–17.

71. Banit DM, Iwinski HJ, Talwalkar V, et al. Posterior spinal fusion in paralytic scoliosis and myelomeningocele. *J Pediatr Orthop* 2001;21: 117–125.

72. Sponseller PD, Young AT, Sarwark JF, et al. Anterior only fusion for scoliosis in patients with myelomeningocele. *Clin Orthop Relat Res* 1999; 364:117–124.

73. McCarthy RE, Dunn H, McCullough FL. Luque fixation to the sacral ala using the Dunn-McCarthy modification. *Spine* 1989;14:281.

74. Rodgers WB, Williams MS, Schwend RM, et al. Spinal deformity in myelodysplasia: correction with posterior pedicle screw instrumentation. *Spine* 1997;22:2435–2443.

75. Geiger F, Parsch D, Carstens C. Complications of scoliosis surgery in children with myelomeningocele. *Eur Spine J* 1999;8:22–26.

76. Carstens C, Koch H, Brocai DR, et al. Development of pathological lumbar kyphosis in myelomeningocele. *J Bone Joint Surg Br* 1996;78(6): 945–950.

77. Hoppenfeld S. Congenital kyphosis in myelomeningocele. *J Bone Joint Surg Br* 1967;49(2):276–280.

78. Lindseth RE, Stelzer L Jr. Vertebral excision for kyphosis in children with myelomeningocele. *J Bone Joint Surg Am* 1979;61(5):699–704.

79. Akbar M, Bremer R, Thomsen M, et al. Kyphectomy in children with myelodysplasia: results 1994–2004. *Spine* 2006;31:1007–1013.

80. Mintz LJ, Sarwark JF, Dias LS, et al. The natural history of congenital kyphosis in myelomeningocele: a review of 51 children. *Spine* 1991;16:S348–S350.

81. Smith JT, Novais E. Treatment of gibbus deformity associated with myelomeningocele in the young child with use of the vertical expandable prosthetic titanium rib (VEPTR). *J Bone Joint Surg Am* 2010;92: 2211–2215.

82. Lintner SA, Lindseth. RE. Kyphotic deformity in patients who have a myelomeningocele. Operative treatment and long-term follow-up. *J Bone Joint Surg Am* 1994;76:1301–1307.

83. Sharrard WJ. Spinal osteotomy for congenital kyphosis in myelomeningocele. *J Bone Joint Surg Br* 1968;50:466–471.

84. Freehafer AA, Vesseley JC, Mack RP. Iliopsoas muscle transfer in the treatment of myelomeningocele in patients with paralytic hip deformities. *J Bone Joint Surg* 1972;54A:1715.

85. Feiwell E. Surgery of the hip in myelomeningocele as related to adult goals. *Clin Orthop* 1980;148:87–93.

86. Swaroop VT, Dias LS. What is the optimal treatment for hip and spine in myelomeningocele? In: Wright JG, ed. *Evidence-based orthopaedics.* Amsterdam, the Netherlands: Elsevier Health Sciences, 2008:273–277.

87. Feiwell E, Sakai D, Blatt T. The effect of hip reduction on function in patients with myelomeningocele: potential gains and hazards of surgical treatment. *J Bone Joint Surg Am* 1978;60:169–173.

88. Ober FR. Fasciotomy for sciatic pain. *J Bone Joint Surg Am* 1941;23: 471–473.

89. Yount CC. The role of the tensor fasciae femoris in certain deformities of the lower extremities. *J Bone Joint Surg Am* 1926;8:171–193.

90. Sharrard WJW. Long-term follow-up of posterior transplant for paralytic dislocation of the hip. *J Bone Joint Surg Br* 1970;52:551–556.

91. Cruess RL, Turner NS. Paralysis of hip abductor muscles in spina bifida: results of treatment by the Mustard procedure. *J Bone Joint Surg Am* 1970;52:1364–1372.

92. Sherk HH, Ames MD. Functional results of iliopsoas transfer in myelomeningocele hip dislocations. *Clin Orthop Relat Res* 1978;137:181–186.

93. Sherk HH, Uppal GS, Lane G, et al. Treatment versus non-treatment of hip dislocations in ambulatory patients with myelomeningocele. *Dev Med Child Neurol* 1991;33:491–494.

94. Sherk HH, Ames MD. Talectomy in the treatment of the myelomeningocele patient. *Clin Orthop Relat Res* 1975;110:218–222.

95. Swaroop VT. Dias L. Orthopedic management of spina bifida. Part I: hip, knee, and rotational deformities. *J Child Orthop* 2009;3:441–449.

96. Castle ME, Schneider C. Proximal femoral resection-interposition arthroplasty. *J Bone Joint Surg Am* 1978;60:1051–1054.

97. McHale KA, Bagg M, Nason SS. Treatment of the chronically dislocated hip in adolescents with cerebral palsy with femoral head resection and subtrochanteric valgus osteotomy. *J Pediatr Orthop* 1990;10(4): 504–509.

98. Wright JG, Menelaus MB, Broughton NS, et al. Natural history of knee contractures in myelomeningocele. *J Pediatr Orthop* 1991;11:725–730.

99. Dias LS. Surgical management of knee contractures in myelomeningocele. *J Pediatr Orthop* 1982;2:127–131.

100. Marshall PD, Broughton NS, Menelaus MB, et al. Surgical release of knee flexion contractures in myelomeningocele. *J Bone Joint Surg Br* 1996;78:912–916.

101. Parsch K, Manner G. Prevention and treatment of knee problems in children with spina bifida. *Dev Med Child Neurol Suppl* 1976;37:114–116.

102. Drabu KJ, Walker G. Stiffness after fractures around the knee in spina bifida. *J Bone Joint Surg Br* 1985;67:266–267.

103. Curtis BH, Fisher RL. Congenital hyperextension with anterior subluxation of the knee: surgical treatment and long-term observations. *J Bone Joint Surg Am* 1969;51:255–269.

104. Birch R. Surgery of the knee in children with spina bifida. *Dev Med Child Neurol Suppl* 1976;37:111–113.

105. Sandhu PS, Broughton NS, Menelaus MB. Tenotomy of the ligamentum patellae in spina bifida: management of limited flexion range at the knee. *J Bone Joint Surg Br* 1995;77:832–833.

106. Williams JJ, Graham GP, Dunne KB, et al. Late knee problems in myelomeningocele. *J Pediatr Orthop* 1993;13:701–703.

107. Vankoski S, Moore C, Statler KD, et al. The influence of forearm crutches on pelvic and hip kinematics in children with myelomeningocele: don't throw away the crutches. *Dev Med Child Neurol* 1997;39:614–619.

108. Lim R, Dias L, Vankoski S, et al. Valgus knee stress in lumbosacral myelomeningocele: a gait-analysis evaluation. *J Pediatr Orthop* 1998;18:428–433.

109. Dias LS, Jasty MJ, Collins P. Rotational deformities of the lower limb in myelomeningocele. Evaluation and treatment. *J Bone Joint Surg Am* 1984;66:215–223.

110. Vankoski SJ, Michaud S, Dias L. External tibial torsion and the effectiveness of the solid ankle-foot orthoses. *J Pediatr Orthop* 2000;20:349–355.

111. Dodgin DA, De Swart RJ, Stefko RM, et al. Distal tibial/fibular derotation osteotomy for correction of tibial torsion: review of technique and results in 63 cases. *J Pediatr Orthop* 1998;18:95–101.

112. Fraser RK, Menelaus MB. The management of tibial torsion in patients with spina bifida. *J Bone Joint Surg Br* 1993;75:495–497.

113. Noonan KJ, Didelot WP, Lindseth RE. Care of the pediatric foot in myelodysplasia. *Foot Ankle Clin* 2000;5(2):281–304.

114. Torosian CM, Dias LS. Surgical treatment of severe hindfoot valgus by medial displacement osteotomy of the os calcis in children with myelomeningocele. *J Pediatr Orthop* 2000;20(2):226–229.

115. de Carvalho Neto J, Dias LS, Gabrieli AP. Congenital talipes equinovarus in spina bifida: treatment and results. *J Pediatr Orthop* 1996;16(6): 782–785.

116. Gerlach DJ, Gurnett CA, Limpaphayom N, et al. Early results of the Ponseti method for the treatment of clubfoot associated with myelomeningocele. *J Bone Joint Surg Am* 2009;91(6):1350–1359.

117. Janicki JA, Narayanan UG, Harvey B, et al. Treatment of neuromuscular and syndrome-associated (nonidiopathic) clubfeet using the Ponseti method. *J Pediatr Orthop* 2009;29(4):393–397.

118. Flynn JM, Herrera-Soto JA, Ramirez NF, et al. Clubfoot release in myelodysplasia. *J Pediatr Orthop B* 2004;13(4):259–262.

119. Lourenco AF, Dias LS, Zoellick DM, et al. Treatment of residual adduction deformity in clubfoot: the double osteotomy. *J Pediatr Orthop* 2001;21:713–718.

120. Dias LS, Stern LS. Talectomy in the treatment of resistant talipes equinovarus deformity in myelomeningocele and arthrogryposis. *J Pediatr Orthop* 1987;7:39–41.

121. Frawley PA, Broughton NS, Menelaus MB. Incidence and type of hindfoot deformities in patients with low-level spina bifida. *J Pediatr Orthop* 1998;18:312–313.

122. Kodros SA, Dias LS. Single-stage surgical correction of congenital vertical talus. *J Pediatr Orthop* 1999;19(1):42–48.

123. Dobbs MB, Purcell DB, Nunley R, et al. Early results of a new method of treatment for idiopathic congenital vertical talus. Surgical technique. *J Bone Joint Surg Am* 2007;89(Suppl 2 Pt 1):111–121.

124. Park KB, Park HW, Joo SY, et al. Surgical treatment of calcaneal deformity in a select group of patients with myelomeningocele. *J Bone Joint Surg Am* 2008;90(10):2149–2159.

125. Rodrigues RC, Dias LS. Calcaneus deformity in spina bifida: results of anterolateral release. *J Pediatr Orthop* 1992;12(4):461–464.

126. Stevens PM, Belle RM. Screw epiphysiodesis for ankle valgus. *J Pediatr Orthop* 1997;17(1):9–12.

127. Lubicky JP, Altiok H. Transphyseal osteotomy of the distal tibia for correction of valgus/varus deformities of the ankle. *J Pediatr Orthop* 2001;21(1): 80–88.

128. Koutsogiannis E. Treatment of mobile flatfoot by displacement oste-otomy of the calcaneus. *J Bone Joint Surg Br* 1971;53:96–100.

129. Coleman SS, Chesnut WJ. A simple test for hindfoot flexibility in the cavovarus foot. *Clin Orthop* 1977;123:60–62.

130. Schwend RM, Drennan JC. Cavus foot deformity in children. *J Am Acad Orthop Surg* 2003;11:201–211.

131. Mubarak SJ, Van Valin SE. Osteotomies of the foot for cavus deformities in children. *J Pediatr Orthop* 2009;29(3):294–299.

132. Gourineni P, Dias L, Blanco R, et al. Orthopaedic deformities asso-ciated with lumbosacral spinal lipomas. *J Pediatr Orthop* 2009;29:932–936.

133. Finn MA, Walker ML. Spinal lipomas: clinical spectrum, embryology, and treatment. *Neurosurg Focus* 2007;23:1–12.

134. Kanev PM, Lemire RJ, Loeser JD, et al. Management and longterm follow up review of children with lipomyelomeningocele, 1952–1987. *J Neurosurg* 1990;73:48–52.

Other Neuromuscular Disorders

Neuromuscular disorders other than cerebral palsy and myelodysplasia are less common; however, patients with these disorders do present in pediatric orthopaedic and neuromuscular clinics. These disorders include the muscular dystrophies and congenital myopathies, spinal muscular atrophy, Friedreich ataxia, hereditary motor sensory neuropathies (HMSN), and poliomyelitis. It is important that an accurate diagnosis be established so that an effective treatment program can be planned and initiated. Delaying the diagnosis of these disorders may lead to inappropriate treatment; furthermore, the mother of an affected child might have further pregnancies and give birth to another child with the genetic disorder (1). Accurate diagnosis requires a careful evaluation of history, physical examination, and appropriate diagnostic studies (2).

HISTORY

The history should include the details of pregnancy, delivery, and growth and development of the child involved. Questions should be asked regarding *in utero* activity, complications of delivery, birth weight, Apgar score, problems during the neonatal period, age at achievement of developmental motor milestones, age at onset of the current symptoms, and information that will clarify whether the condition is static or progressive. Systemic symptoms, such as cardiac disease, cataracts, seizures, or other abnormalities, should also be ascertained.

The family history is important in diagnosis because these disorders, with the exception of poliomyelitis, are genetic in origin. In order to arrive at an accurate diagnosis, family members of the child or adolescent involved may need to be examined for subtle expressions of the same disorder and may also be required to undergo hematologic or other studies.

PHYSICAL EXAMINATION

Most children who present for evaluation of a suspected neuromuscular disorder usually have one or more of the following: a delay in developmental milestones, abnormal gait, foot deformity, or spinal deformity. There is usually a history of progression. Physical examination consists of a thorough musculoskeletal and neurologic evaluation. Observing the child walking and performing simple tasks, such as rising from a sitting position on the floor, can be useful. Observation of the gait may reveal decreased arm swing, circumduction of the legs, scissoring, or short cadence. Standing posture may reveal increased lumbar lordosis or a wide base position for balance. Also, in the standing position, the appearance of the feet should be observed. Pes cavus or cavovarus deformities are common physical findings in many of these disorders. Having the child walk on the heels and toes gives a gross assessment of motor strength, and having the child run may reveal an increase in muscle tone or ataxia. There is an increased incidence of scoliosis in patients with neuromuscular disorders (3, 4).

Inspection of the skin should be performed for evidence of skin rashes or other abnormalities. Typical facies of the patient with spinal muscular atrophy and congenital myotonic dystrophy should become familiar to orthopaedic surgeons. The tongue should be examined to detect evidence of fasciculation suggestive of anterior horn cell diseases. Excessive drooling is common in both cerebral palsy and congenital myotonic dystrophy. In the latter, nasal speech may also be present. A thorough ophthalmologic examination is necessary in order to elicit external ophthalmoplegia or retinitis pigmentosa. In myotonic dystrophy, cataracts may develop during adolescence.

Muscle testing should be carefully performed. Generally, myopathic disorders selectively affect proximal limb muscles before affecting distal muscles. Early in the disease process, the muscles demonstrate proportionally greater weakness than would be expected from the degree of atrophy. The converse is true in neuropathies.

A careful neurologic evaluation usually completes the musculoskeletal examination. Sensory responses must be checked individually and recorded. Decreased vibratory sensation may be present in HMSNs such as Charcot-Marie-Tooth disease. In spinal muscular atrophy, the deep-tendon reflexes may be absent, but in cerebral palsy, they are increased. A positive Babinski sign confirms upper motor neuron disease. Abnormalities in the Romberg test and rapid alternating movements may indicate cerebellar involvement. Mental function evaluation may be necessary, because organic mental deterioration may be part of some neurologic syndromes. In many cases, the assistance of a pediatric neurologist can be invaluable in performing a careful neurologic and mental evaluation, because minor subtleties may offer clues to diagnosis.

DIAGNOSTIC STUDIES

Appropriate diagnostic studies are imperative for the accurate diagnosis of myopathic and neuropathic disorders (5, 6). These can be divided into hematologic studies, electromyography (EMG) with nerve conduction studies and needle electrode exam, muscle biopsy, and nerve biopsy. Molecular diagnostic studies have become available for many of these disorders, including Duchenne and Becker muscular dystrophies, myotonic dystrophy, the hereditary sensory motor neuropathies, and spinal muscular atrophy.

Hematologic Studies. The measurement of serum creatine phosphokinase (CPK) is the most sensitive test for demonstrating abnormalities of striated muscle function. The level of elevation parallels the rate and amount of muscle necrosis and decreases with time as the muscle is replaced by fat and fibrous tissue. The highest CPK levels are typically seen in the earliest stages of Duchenne or Becker muscular dystrophy, in which increases of 20 to 200 times the normal values may be found (6). The level of elevation of CPK does not correlate with the severity or rate of progression of the disorder. The highest levels are usually found in Duchenne muscular dystrophy. Umbilical cord blood CPK levels should be obtained in all male infants who are suspected of having this disorder (7). Birth trauma may elevate the CPK in umbilical cord blood, but in the healthy child, this elevation disappears promptly, whereas the enzyme level remains elevated in muscular dystrophy. Serum CPK may be mildly or moderately elevated in other dystrophic disorders, such as facioscapulohumeral muscular dystrophy and Emery-Dreifuss muscular dystrophy. It is also mildly elevated in female carriers of Duchenne muscular dystrophy, although they are asymptomatic. In congenital myopathies and peripheral neuropathies, the CPK levels are usually normal or only mildly elevated. In other neuromuscular disorders that do not directly affect striated muscle, the CPK levels are normal. Serum enzymes, such as aldolase and serum glutamic oxaloacetic transaminase (SGOT), are also important in the study of striated muscle function. Aldolase levels correlate well with the CPK levels.

Electromyography. EMG can differentiate between a myopathic and a neuropathic process but is rarely helpful in establishing a definitive diagnosis. Characteristics of neuropathic disorders include the presence of fibrillation potentials, increased insertional activity, and high-amplitude, increased-duration motor unit potentials (6). The fibrillation potential represents denervated individual muscle fibers firing spontaneously.

The EMG in myopathy is characterized by low-voltage, short-duration polyphasic motor unit potentials (6). Myopathies rarely demonstrate EMG changes characteristic of a neuropathy, although in an inflammatory muscle disease with significant muscle breakdown, there may be prominent fibrillations. The use of an experienced electromyographer is imperative in the accurate performance of the test and interpretation of EMG data.

Nerve Conduction Studies. Nerve conduction studies are important in the establishment of the diagnosis of peripheral neuropathy in children. Nerve conduction velocities are normal in children with anterior horn cell diseases, nerve root diseases, and myopathies. The normal value in the child older than 5 years is 45 to 65 m per second. In infants and younger children, the velocity is lower because myelination is incomplete.

Motor conduction velocity may be slowed in HMSN (e.g., Charcot-Marie-Tooth disease) before clinical deficits are present. The nerve conduction studies can help determine whether the neuropathy involves an isolated nerve or is a disseminated process.

Muscle Biopsy. Historically, muscle biopsy has been the most important test in determining the diagnosis of a neuromuscular disorder. More recently, molecular genetic testing has become equally, if not more, important. Muscle biopsy material is usually examined by routine histology, special histochemical stains, and electron microscopy. The criterion for selecting the muscle for biopsy is clinical evidence of muscle weakness. Muscles that are involved but are still functioning are selected in chronic diseases, such as Duchenne muscular dystrophy, because they demonstrate the greatest diagnostic changes. A more severely involved muscle may be chosen in an acute illness because the process has not had sufficient time to progress to extensive destruction. In patients who have proximal lower extremity muscle weakness, biopsy of the vastus lateralis is performed, whereas in those with distal weakness, a biopsy of the gastrocnemius is performed. Biopsy of the deltoid, biceps, or triceps is performed for shoulder girdle or proximal upper extremity weakness.

Muscle biopsies can be performed as an open procedure (8) or by percutaneous needle (9). The biopsies are obtained under general anesthesia, spinal anesthesia, regional nerve block, or a field block surrounding the area of incision. It is important that local anesthetic not be infiltrated into the biopsied muscle, because this may alter the morphology of the muscle. The vastus lateralis is the most common muscle chosen. A 4-cm incision is made and the underlying fascia is incised longitudinally. The muscle is directly visualized in order to avoid including normal fibrous septae in the specimens. Muscle clamps are used for obtaining three specimens. The clamps are oriented in the direction of the muscle fibers. A 2- to 3-mm piece of muscle is grasped in each end of the clamp. The muscle is cut at the outside edge of each clamp and a cylinder of muscle is excised. The use of a muscle clamp helps keep the muscle at its resting length and minimizes artifact. One specimen is quickly frozen in liquid nitrogen (–160°C) to prevent loss of soluble enzymes. This specimen is used for light microscopy with a variety of special preparations. The other specimens are used for routine histology and electron microscopy. The wound is subsequently closed in layers. Electrocautery may be used during the closure. If it is used before the biopsy, it may inadvertently damage the specimens and alter the morphology.

Nerve Biopsy. Occasionally, biopsy of a peripheral nerve is helpful in demyelinating disorders. Usually, the sural nerve is selected for biopsy because of its distal location and lack of autogenous zone of innervation. The patient notices no sensory change or only a mild sensory diminution after excision of the 3- to 4-cm segment of the nerve. Hurley et al. (8) reported a single incision for combined muscle and sural nerve biopsy. An incision over the posterolateral aspect of the calf allows access to the nerve and either the soleus or the peroneal muscle. This avoids the necessity for making two incisions. This technique was demonstrated to be useful in disorders in which both a muscle and a nerve biopsy may be necessary for arriving at a diagnosis.

Other Studies. Other studies that may be helpful in establishing the diagnosis of a neuromuscular disorder include electrocardiogram (ECG), pulmonary function studies, magnetic resonance imaging (MRI), ophthalmologic evaluation, amniocentesis, and pediatric neurology evaluation.

Duchenne muscular dystrophy, Friedreich ataxia, and myotonic dystrophy demonstrate ECG abnormalities. Duchenne muscular dystrophy is frequently associated with mitral valve prolapse secondary to papillary muscle involvement (10, 11). Arrhythmias under anesthesia have been reported with both Duchenne and Emery-Dreifuss muscular dystrophies (12, 13).

Pulmonary function studies demonstrate involvement of respiratory muscles, but they do not establish the diagnosis. If respiratory muscle involvement is present, the rate of deterioration can be followed up with periodic studies. This is important if surgery is contemplated in children or adolescents with muscular dystrophy, spinal muscular atrophy, or Friedreich ataxia. The forced vital capacity (FVC) is the most important study after arterial blood gas measurements (14).

MRI has been demonstrated to distinguish muscles affected by neuropathic disorders from those affected by myopathic disorders (15). Imaging estimates of the disease severity by degree of muscle involvement correlate well with clinical staging. MRI may also be important in selecting appropriate muscles for biopsy.

Ophthalmologic evaluation may demonstrate subtle or more obvious ocular changes associated with specific disorders.

GENETIC AND MOLECULAR BIOLOGY STUDIES

Genetic research through molecular biologic techniques has tremendously enhanced our understanding of the genetic aspects of many of these disorders (16, 17). The determination of the exact location of chromosomal and gene defects has led to the possibility of genetic engineering being used to correct these disorders. Unfortunately, genetic testing is quite costly, and for many disorders, such testing is not commercially available. Also, a negative test does not necessarily exclude certain disorders. For this reason, the decision to carry out genetic testing should be made only by a neuromuscular specialist or geneticist. In each of the various disorders, the current status of genetic and molecular biology research is discussed in this chapter.

MUSCULAR DYSTROPHIES

The muscular dystrophies are a group of noninflammatory inherited disorders with a progressive degeneration and weakness of skeletal muscle that has no apparent cause in the peripheral or the central nervous system (CNS). These have been categorized according to clinical distribution, severity of muscle weakness, and pattern of genetic inheritance (Table 16-1). An accurate diagnosis is important, both for prognosis and management of the individual patient and for identification of genetic factors that may be crucial in planning for subsequent children by the family involved.

SEX-LINKED MUSCULAR DYSTROPHIES

Duchenne Muscular Dystrophy. Duchenne muscular dystrophy is the most common form of muscular dystrophy (18).

TABLE 16-1	Classification of Muscular Dystrophies

Sex-linked muscular dystrophy
  Duchenne
  Becker
  Emery-Dreifuss
Autosomal recessive muscular dystrophy
  Limb-girdle
  Infantile facioscapulohumeral
Autosomal dominant muscular dystrophy
  Facioscapulohumeral
  Distal
  Ocular
  Oculopharyngeal

Transmission is by an X-linked recessive trait. A single gene defect is found in the short arm of the X chromosome. The disease is characterized by its occurrence exclusively in the male sex, except for rare cases associated with Turner syndrome. In this rare event, the XO karyotype who carries the defective gene may demonstrate the phenotype found in male patients with the disorder (6). This disorder is associated with a high mutation rate, and a positive family history is present in approximately 65% of the cases. Duchenne muscular dystrophy occurs in approximately 1 in 3500 live male births, with about one-third of the children involved having acquired the disease because of a new mutation.

Becker muscular dystrophy is a similar, but less common and less severe form of muscular dystrophy. It occurs in approximately 1 in 30,000 live male births, becomes apparent later in childhood, and has a more protracted and variable course than Duchenne muscular dystrophy. This disorder is discussed later but is mentioned here because of the similar inheritance pattern and molecular biology abnormality.

Clinical Features.   Duchenne muscular dystrophy is generally clinically evident when the child is at an age of between 3 and 6 years. Earlier onset may also occur. The family may have observed that the child's ability to achieve independent ambulation was delayed or that he has become a toe walker. Children at the age of 3 years or older may demonstrate frequent episodes of tripping and falling, in addition to difficulty in activities requiring reciprocal motion, such as running or climbing stairs. Inability to hop and jump normally is commonly present.

In Duchenne muscular dystrophy, there is progressive weakness in the proximal muscle groups that descend symmetrically in both lower extremities, particularly the gluteus maximus, gluteus medius, quadriceps, and tibialis anterior muscles. The abdominal muscles are involved. Involvement of the shoulder girdle muscles (i.e., trapezius, deltoid, and pectoralis major muscles) and lower facial muscles occurs later. Pseudohypertrophy of the calf muscles caused by the accumulation of fat is common but not invariably present. Most patients have cardiac involvement, most commonly a sinus tachycardia and right ventricular hypertrophy. Life-threatening dysrhythmia or heart failure ultimately develops in approximately 10% of patients. Many also have a static encephalopathy, with mild or moderate mental retardation (19). Death from pulmonary failure and occasionally from cardiac failure occurs during the second or third decades of life.

During gait the child's cadence is slow, and he or she develops compensatory changes in gait and stance as weakness progresses. Sutherland et al. (20, 21) documented disease progression by measuring the gait variables of cadence, swing phase, ankle dorsiflexion, and anterior pelvic tilt. The hip extensors, primarily the gluteus maximus, are the first muscle group to be involved. Initially, the patient compensates by carrying the head and shoulders behind the pelvis, maintaining the weight line posterior to the hip joint and center of gravity (Fig. 16-1). This produces an anterior pelvic tilt and increases

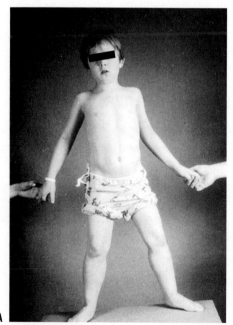
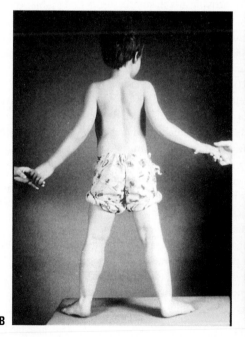
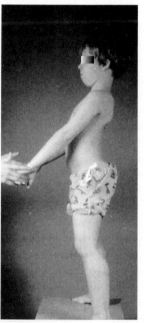

FIGURE 16-1.   **A:** A 7-year-old boy with Duchenne muscular dystrophy demonstrates precarious stance due to mild hip abduction contractures. Observe the pseudohypertrophy of the calves. **B:** Posterior view demonstrates mild ankle equinus in addition to the calf pseudohypertrophy. **C:** Side view shows an anterior tilt to the pelvis and increased lumbar lordosis, and the head and the shoulders are aligned posterior to the pelvis. This characteristic posture maintains the weight line posterior to the pelvis and center of gravity, compensates for the muscle weakness, and helps maintain balance.

lumbar lordosis. Cadence and swing-phase ankle dorsiflexion decrease, and the patient develops a waddling, wide-based gait with shoulder sway to compensate for gluteus medius weakness. Muscle weakness requires that the force line remains behind the hip joint and in front of the knee joint throughout single limb support (20–22), and hip abductors and quadriceps muscles force the patient to circumduct during the swing phase of gait while at the same time shifting the weight directly over the hip joint. The generalized pelvic weakness requires considerable forward motion to be generated by the spine for the patient to advance. Ankle plantar flexion becomes fixed, and the stance phase is reduced to the forefoot, resulting in even more difficulty with balance and cadence. Foot inversion develops as peroneal strength diminishes. The tibialis posterior muscle, which is one of the last muscles to be involved, is responsible for the inversion or varus deformity of the foot.

Weakness in the shoulder girdle, which occurs 3 to 5 years later, precludes the use of crutches to aid in ambulation. It also makes it difficult to lift the patient from under the arms. This tendency for the child to slip a truncal grasp has been termed *Meyeron sign*. As the weakness in the upper extremities increases, the child becomes unable to move his or her arms. Although the hands retain strength longer than the arms, use of the hands is limited because of weakness of the arms.

Clinical diagnosis of Duchenne muscular dystrophy is established by physical examination, including gait and specific muscle weakness, and by the absence of sensory deficits. The upper extremity and knee deep-tendon reflexes are lost early in the disease, whereas the ankle reflexes remain positive until the terminal phase. A valuable clinical sign is the *Gower sign*. The patient is placed prone or in the sitting position on the floor and asked to rise. This is usually difficult, and the patient may require the use of a chair for assistance. The patient is then asked to use his or her hands to grasp the lower legs and force the knees into extension. The patient then walks his or her hands up the lower extremities to compensate for the weakness in the quadriceps and gluteus maximus. This sign may also be found in congenital myopathies and spinal muscular atrophy. The contracture of the iliotibial band can be measured by the *Ober test*. To perform this test, the child is placed on his or her side with both hips flexed. The superior leg is then abducted and extended and allowed to fall into adduction. The degree of abduction contracture can be measured by the number of degrees the leg lacks in coming to the neutral position. Tendo-Achilles contractures also occur. Contracture of the tendo-Achilles and the iliotibial band are the most consistent deformities noted during the physical examination.

Duchenne muscular dystrophy progresses slowly but continuously. A rapid deterioration may be noted after immobilization in bed, even for short periods after respiratory infections or, perhaps, extremity fractures. Every effort should be made to maintain a daily ambulatory program. In the absence of treatment, children are usually unable to ambulate effectively by the age of 10 years (5, 23–25). The chief cause is loss of strength in the hip extensors and ankle dorsiflexors (26). These two factors can be used as a guide to predict when ambulation

will cease. With loss of standing ability, the child becomes wheelchair dependent. This results in a loss of the accentuated lumbar lordosis that protected the child from kyphoscoliosis (27). As a consequence, most patients subsequently develop a progressive spinal deformity.

Myocardial deterioration is also a constant finding. ECG changes are present in more than 90% of children with Duchenne muscular dystrophy. The average intelligence quotient of these patients has been shown to be approximately 80 (19).

Hematologic Studies.   The serum CPK is markedly elevated in the early stages of Duchenne muscular dystrophy. This may be 200 to 300 times the normal value, but decreases as the disease progresses and muscle mass is reduced. CPK levels are also elevated in female carriers of the disease (two to three times the normal value for women and girls), although not to the same extent as in affected boys. There is an 80% consistency in the results when the CPK test is repeated at three consecutive monthly intervals (28). Aldolase and SGOT levels may also be elevated, but the elevations are not unique to striated muscle disease.

Electromyography.   Although EMG will support the diagnosis of a myopathy, if the clinical findings and CPK are both suggestive of a muscular dystrophy, this test is typically not necessary. EMG shows characteristic myopathic changes with reduced amplitude, short duration, and polyphasic motor action potentials (6).

Muscle Biopsy.   The muscle biopsy specimen reveals degeneration with subsequent loss of fiber, variation in fiber size, proliferation of connective tissue and, subsequently, of adipose tissue as well (6). Increased cellularity is present, with occasional internal migration of the sarcolemmal nuclei. Histochemical testing reveals loss of clear-cut subdivisions of fiber types, especially with adenosine triphosphatase reaction, and a tendency toward type I fiber predominance. In the past, this was the diagnostic procedure of choice. However, the standard today is to first obtain blood samples for DNA polymerase chain reaction (PCR) testing for dystrophinopathies. If this is positive, there is no need for a muscle biopsy. If PCR testing is negative, then muscle biopsy is indicated for arriving at a definitive diagnosis.

Genetic and Molecular Biology Studies.   A single gene defect in the short arm of the X chromosome has been identified as being responsible for both Duchenne and Becker muscular dystrophies (16, 17, 29, 30). The status of genetic and molecular biology in Duchenne muscular dystrophy has been summarized by Shapiro and Specht (6). The gene is located at the Xp21.2 region and spans 2 million base pairs (31, 32). It includes 65 exons (i.e., coding regions) and encodes the 400-kDa protein dystrophin. The large size of the gene correlates with the high rate of spontaneous mutation. Dystrophin is a component of cell membrane cytoskeleton and represents 0.01% of skeletal muscle protein. Its distribution within skeletal, smooth, and cardiac muscle and within the brain correlates well with the clinical features in Duchenne and Becker muscular dystrophies. A structural role for the dystrophin protein is suggested by studies that demonstrate concentration of the protein in a lattice organization in the cytoplasmic membrane of skeletal muscle fibers (33, 34). Demonstrable mutations, deletions, or duplications of dystrophin are found in 70% to 80% of the affected male patients (31, 32, 35, 36). The reading frame hypothesis distinguishes the mutations that correlate with the more severe Duchenne muscular dystrophy from those that correlate with the less severe Becker muscular dystrophy. Mutations that disrupt the translational reading frame or the promoter (i.e., the specific DNA sequence that signals where RNA synthesis should begin) result in a presumably unstable protein, and this correlates with Duchenne muscular dystrophy. In contrast, mutations that do not disrupt the translational reading frame or the promoter have a lower molecular weight and semifunctional dystrophin. This correlates with the less severe Becker muscular dystrophy (31, 37).

Dystrophin testing (by dystrophin immunoblotting), DNA mutation analysis (by PCR or DNA Southern blot analysis), or both, provide methods of differentiating between Duchenne and Becker muscular dystrophies on the one hand, and other initially similar disorders [such as dermatomyositis, limb-girdle muscular dystrophy (LGMD), Emery-Dreifuss muscular dystrophy, and congenital muscular dystrophy] on the other (36, 38, 39). In the latter disorders, the dystrophin is normal. In patients with Duchenne muscular dystrophy, there is a complete absence of dystrophin, whereas in Becker muscular dystrophy, dystrophin is present, but is altered in size, decreased in amount, or both. Nicholson et al. (40) reported a positive relation between the amount of dystrophin and the age at loss of independent ambulation in 30 patients with Duchenne muscular dystrophy and in 6 patients with Becker muscular dystrophy. The researchers found that even low concentrations of dystrophin in Duchenne muscular dystrophy may have functional significance and may explain the variability of age at which ambulation ceases. The presence of partially functional dystrophin protein is sufficient to minimize the phenotypic expression, leading to the milder disorder of Becker muscular dystrophy (31, 35, 38). The same tests can be used to improve detection of female carriers (36, 39). On the basis of smaller-than-normal dystrophin protein, two atypical forms of Becker muscular dystrophy have been recognized. These are myalgia without weakness in male patients (similar to metabolic myopathy), and cardiomyopathy with little or no weakness in male patients (41).

Research studies are investigating the possibility of dystrophin replacement in diseased muscles. This involves the implantation of myoblasts, or muscle precursor cells, into the muscles of patients with Duchenne muscular dystrophy (42). This has been successful in producing dystrophin in the murine mdx model of Duchenne muscular dystrophy (43). Unfortunately, the results in human male patients have been disappointing (44–48). Perhaps the most promising evolving treatment for Duchenne's is the genetic technique of "exon skipping" or splice modulation, where there is modulation of dystrophin premessenger RNA splicing, enabling functional dystrophin protein to be produced (49).

Medication Treatments. A number of medications have been tried to improve strength and function and prolong time to disability in Duchenne dystrophy. Steroids, such as prednisone and deflazacort, have been shown to preserve or improve strength, prolong ambulation, and slow the progression of scoliosis (50–59). Thus, this has become a mainstay of therapy in many neuromuscular clinics. Unfortunately, the side effects—weight gain, osteoporosis with vertebral fractures, and myopathy—limit their usefulness (37, 52–54, 56, 60). Alternate day therapy, or pulse therapy with steroid treatment on the first 10 days of each month, may limit the side effects, slow deterioration of muscle function and not impact on patient quality of life (61, 62). Although prednisone and deflazacort appear to be equally efficacious, deflazacort appears to cause fewer side effects, especially related to weight gain (63). Creatinine supplementation has been evaluated and demonstrated an increase in handgrip strength and fat-free mass, but no improvement in functional tasks or activities of daily living (64). It did demonstrate a significant improvement in resistance to fatigue (65). Perhaps more promising is treatment with extended release albuterol, which has demonstrated increase in lean body mass, decrease in fat mass, and improved functional measures in short-term treatment of dystrophinopathy patients (66, 67). Azathioprine has also been evaluated in Duchenne muscular dystrophy but has not shown beneficial effects (68). Aminoglycoside therapy with intravenous gentamicin administration has been studied in two trials (69, 70). A decrease in serum CPK levels was demonstrated, but there was no effect on muscle strength.

Gene therapy for muscular dystrophies has proven difficult, primarily because of the size of the viral vectors and also because of the complications of immune reactions that may occur. Therefore, gene therapy is still very much in the early investigational stages. This treatment has been reviewed in detail by Chamberlain (71). Dystrophin delivery to muscle has been attempted with four primary vectors: adenovirus, retroviruses, adeno-associated viruses, and plasmids. Complications of this technology included triggering of a cellular immune response, poor integration of the vector into the host gene, and lack of a sustained response, to name only a few (72). Stem cell therapy may be a promising intervention for the dystrophinopathies. In the mdx mouse, bone marrow transplantation and injection of normal muscle-derived stem cells led to partial restoration of dystrophin expression (73).

Treatment. Orthopaedic problems in children with Duchenne muscular dystrophy include decreasing ambulatory ability, soft-tissue contractures, and spinal deformity (5, 6, 18, 74). The goals of treatment should be to improve or maintain the functional capacity of the affected child or adolescent.

The treatment modalities in Duchenne muscular dystrophy include medical therapy, physical therapy, functional testing, use of orthoses, fracture management, surgery, use of wheelchair, cardiopulmonary management, and genetic and psychological counseling.

Medical Therapy.   Recently, the use of steroids has shown promise in preserving strength, prolonging ambulation, and slowing the progression of scoliosis. However, this therapy is not in wide use because of the attendant complications as described in the earlier text.

Physical Therapy.   Physical therapy is directed toward prolongation of functional muscle strength, prevention or correction of contractures by passive stretching, gait training with orthoses and transfer techniques, ongoing assessment of muscle strength and functional capacity, and inputs regarding wheelchair and equipment measurements.

After the diagnosis of Duchenne muscular dystrophy has been established and before muscle strength has deteriorated, a program of maximum-resistance exercises should be commenced, to be performed several times a day. This may help preserve strength and delay the onset of soft-tissue contractures. Physical therapy is more effective in preventing or delaying contractures than in correcting them. Contractures develop in the ambulatory patient because the progression of muscle weakness results in the development of adaptive posturing to maintain lower extremity joint stability. A home exercise program can be effective in minimizing hip and ankle soft-tissue contractures. Exercises should be performed twice a day on a firm surface, and should include stretching of the tensor fascia lata, hamstrings, knee flexors, and ankle plantar flexors. Occasionally, serial casting may be useful in correcting existing deformities before physical therapy. Knee-flexion contractures of <30 degrees may benefit from serial or wedge casting. This enhances the use of knee–ankle–foot orthoses (KAFOs). Unless orthoses are used after casting and in conjunction with physical therapy, these contractures rapidly recur.

Functional Testing.   Functional testing predominantly involves periodic muscle testing. Muscle strength is tested by measurement of the active range of motion of a joint against gravity. This type of testing allows assessment of the rate of deterioration as well as the functional capacity of the individual.

Orthoses.   Lightweight molded plastic ankle–foot orthoses (AFOs) or KAFOs are used in independently ambulatory patients when gait becomes precarious, when early soft-tissue contractures of the knees and ankle are developing, and after surgical correction of these deformities (75–78). AFOs can also be helpful in improving tendo-Achilles contractures, especially when worn both during the day and at night (79). KAFOs are usually supplemented with a walker because of the excessive weight on the orthoses and the risk of falling. Important prescription components include partial ischial weight-bearing support, posterior thigh cuff, and a spring-loaded, drop-lock knee joint with an ankle joint set at a right angle. Ambulation may be extended for up to 3 years by the combined use of surgery and orthoses. The maintenance of a straight lower

extremity also enables the nonwalking patient to stand with support, and thereby assists in transfers.

Spinal orthoses are usually of no value in progressive spinal deformities, but wheelchair-bound patients, especially those with severe cardiopulmonary compromise and severe scoliosis, may benefit from the use of a custom wheelchair, a thoracic suspension orthosis, or a custom-made thoracic–lumbar spinal orthosis (TLSO). A mobile arm-support orthosis attached to the wheelchair may help the patient in performing personal hygiene tasks and self-feeding (80).

Fracture Management.   Fractures of the lower extremities occur frequently in children with Duchenne muscular dystrophy. This is due to decreased bone mineral density from disuse osteoporosis, steroid induced osteoporosis, or both (81–84). Fractures can result in a permanent loss of function (81, 83, 84). This occurs predominantly after ambulation has ceased and the child is wheelchair bound. These fractures are best treated by closed reduction and cast immobilization. Occasionally, open reduction and internal fixation may be needed. In children who are still ambulatory, it is important that they be placed on a program of early mobilization to allow weight bearing. This may require the use of an electrically powered circle bed. Once early healing is present, the child can be returned to the KAFO to decrease weight and enhance mobility.

Surgery.   Contractures of the lower extremities and progressive weakness impair ambulation. Surgery is indicated when independent ambulation becomes precarious and when contractures are painful or interfere with essential daily activities. The major contractures that are amenable to surgical intervention include equinus and equinovarus contractures of the ankle and foot, knee-flexion contractures, and hip-flexion and abduction contractures. In thin individuals, these contractures may be released by percutaneous techniques (74, 85). For ambulatory patients, orthotic measurements should be obtained before surgery. This allows the orthoses to be applied shortly after surgery to assist in rapid restoration of ambulation. Correction of contractures and the use of orthoses can prolong effective ambulation and assisted standing ability by a period of 1 to 3 years (5, 18, 22, 75–78, 85–90). Hsu and Furumasu (22) reported a mean prolongation of walking of 3.3 years in 24 patients with Duchenne muscular dystrophy ranging in age from 8 to 12 years at the time of surgery. It is usually not possible to restore functional ambulation once the patient has been unable to walk for more than 3 to 6 months (75). Each patient must be individually assessed to determine the functional needs and the best procedures. Common contraindications for correction of lower extremity contractures include obesity, rapidly progressive muscle weakness, or poor motivation (those who prefer to use a wheelchair rather than attempt ambulation) (6).

Foot and Ankle.   Equinus contractures occur first, followed by equinovarus contractures. This is because of a combination of tendo-Achilles contracture and muscle imbalance induced by the stronger tibialis posterior muscle. This latter muscle retains good function despite the progression of muscle weakness in other areas. These equinovarus deformities can be managed by a combination of tendo-Achilles lengthening by means of percutaneous open tenotomy (18, 74, 77, 78, 86, 87) with or without resection, or by Vulpius (5) or open Z-lengthening (89), and tibialis posterior lengthening, tenotomy, or transfer through the interosseous membrane to the dorsum of the foot (5, 6, 18, 25, 74, 76–78, 86, 87, 91–93). Scher and Mubarak have also recommended toe flexor tenotomies (94). Tibialis posterior transfer prevents recurrence of equinovarus deformities and maintains active dorsiflexion of the foot. Some orthopaedists, however, have questioned the necessity of a transfer, because it is a more extensive procedure. They prefer tenotomy, recession, or lengthening (74, 76, 86). Postoperative gait analysis has shown that the transferred tibialis posterior muscle is electrically silent (95). Greene (91) has reported that tibialis posterior myotendinous junction recession in six patients (12 ft) resulted in an increased recurrence rate when compared with transfer in nine patients (18 ft), making the former a less desirable procedure. Percutaneous tendo-Achilles lengthening under local anesthesia is usually reserved for nonambulatory patients, who typically have an equinus deformity and cannot wear shoes. The nonambulatory patient with a moderately severe equinovarus deformity may require open tenotomies of the tendo-Achilles, the tibialis posterior, and long toe flexors. Severe equinovarus contractures have been managed effectively by talectomy. Leitch et al. (96) recently studied 88 Duchenne muscular dystrophy patients and found no difference in the long-term results of those treated surgically and those who did not.

Knee. Knee-flexion contractures coexist with hip-flexion contractures and develop rapidly when the patient is wheelchair bound. These contractures limit proper positioning in bed and may lead to the development of hamstring spasm, causing considerable discomfort when the patient attempts to transfer. A Yount procedure (97) (release of the distal aspect of the tensor fascia lata and iliotibial band) is the most common procedure used in correcting knee-flexion contractures (18, 74, 76–78). Hamstring tenotomies, recession or Vulpius-type lengthening, and formal Z-lengthening may also be necessary. These procedures enhance quadriceps power and function and also relieve symptoms. Postoperatively, KAFOs are necessary in order to prevent recurrence.

Hip. Hip-flexion and -abduction contractures increase lumbar lordosis and interfere with the ability to stand and to lie comfortably supine. Patients with hip-flexion contractures may experience low back pain. Correction of flexion contractures involves release of the tight anterior muscles, including the sartorius, rectus femoris, and tensor fascia femoris (6, 18, 74). Abduction contractures are improved by release of the tensor fasciae lata proximally with use of the Ober procedure (98), modified Soutter release, the Yount procedure distally (97), or by complete resection of the entire iliotibial band.

Chan et al. (99) studied 54 patients with Duchenne muscular dystrophy and found that 15 had unilateral subluxation,

1 had bilateral subluxation, and 3 had a unilateral dislocation. They recommended serial pelvic radiographs in patients with this disorder. They also felt that any pelvic obliquity should be corrected at the time of spinal stabilization.

Upper Extremity. Upper extremity contractures are common in adolescents with Duchenne muscular dystrophy, but usually do not require treatment. These contractures include shoulder adduction, elbow flexion, forearm pronation, wrist flexion, metacarpophalangeal and proximal interphalangeal joint flexion, and others. These usually do not preclude the use of wheelchairs. Muscle weakness is the most devastating aspect of upper extremity involvement. Wagner et al. (100) demonstrated wrist ulnar deviation and flexion contractures in addition to contractures of the extrinsic and intrinsic muscles of the fingers in adolescents with Duchenne muscular dystrophy. These contractures produce boutonniere and swan neck deformities and hyperextension of the distal interphalangeal joints. The treatment of upper extremity contractures involves physical therapy with daily passive range-of-motion exercises. When passive wrist dorsiflexion is limited to neutral, a nighttime extension orthosis may be helpful. Surgery is rarely indicated for these contractures.

Spinal Deformity. Approximately 95% of patients with Duchenne muscular dystrophy develop progressive scoliosis (27, 101–108). This typically begins to occur when ambulation ceases, and it is rapidly progressive. Approximately 25% of older ambulating patients, however, have mild scoliosis (23, 109). Prolongation of ambulation by appropriate soft-tissue releases of the lower extremity contractures, thereby maintaining accentuated lumbar lordosis, can delay the onset of scoliosis (88). The curves are usually thoracolumbar, associated with kyphosis, and lead to pelvic obliquity. Scoliosis cannot be controlled by orthoses or wheelchair seating systems (102, 110–114). Although orthotic management may slow curve progression, it does not slow the systemic manifestations of Duchenne muscular dystrophy (e.g., decreasing pulmonary function and cardiomyopathy). These may complicate spinal surgery at a later time. As the scoliosis progresses, it can result in a loss of sitting balance, produce abnormal pressure, and occasionally cause the patient to become bedridden. Heller et al. (114) reported improved sitting support with an orthosis in 28 patients who either refused surgery or were considered to be inoperable.

Surgical correction of scoliosis both improves sitting balance and minimizes pelvic obliquity (102, 109, 113–116). It is usually recommended that a posterior spinal fusion be performed once the curve is >20 degrees (102, 109, 112–114, 117–119). Fusion extends from the upper thoracic spine (T2 or T4) to L5 or the pelvis. It is important to center the patient's head over the pelvis in both the coronal and sagittal planes. This usually allows complete or almost complete correction of the deformity, maintains sitting balance, improves head control, and allows more independent hand function. Although autogenous bone grafting is used in most patients, there appears to be no difference in fusion rates when allograft bone is used (120–123). Segmental spinal instrumentation techniques using Luque rod instrumentation are most commonly used (18, 74, 102, 109, 112, 116, 120, 121, 124–129) (Fig. 16-2). Other modern segmental instrumentation systems, can also be used (120, 121, 125, 130). The use of

pedicle screws and iliac bolts can improve results (131, 132) (see Fig. 16-2). All of these techniques allow sufficient fixation so that postoperative immobilization is not necessary (Fig. 16-2). Fixation to the pelvis is achieved using the Galveston or other techniques (117, 120, 124–133).

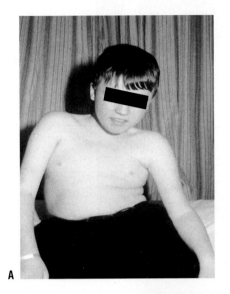
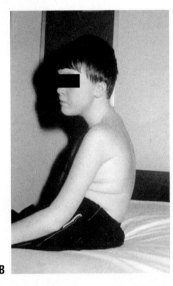
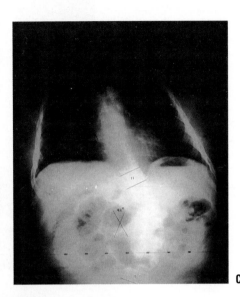
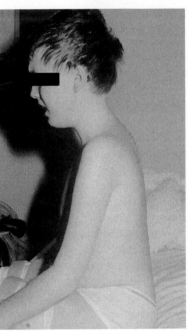

FIGURE 16-2. **A:** An 11-year-old boy with Duchenne muscular dystrophy with a rapidly progressive right thoracolumbar scoliosis and decreasing sitting balance. He uses his hands to maintain sitting balance. **B:** Side view shows an associated mild kyphotic deformity. **C:** Preoperative sitting posteroanterior radiograph demonstrates a long, sweeping, 48-degree thoracolumbar curve between T11 and L5. Six months earlier, no clinical or radiographic deformity was evident. **D:** Postoperatively, an immediate improvement in spinal alignment and sitting balance is noted. **E:** Side view demonstrates correction of the associated kyphosis. **F:** Postoperative sitting radiograph after posterior spinal fusion and Luque rod instrumentation from T4 to the sacrum. The Galveston technique, with insertion of the Luque rod into the wing of the ilium, was used for pelvic fixation. Almost complete correction of his spinal deformity was achieved. **G:** Postoperative lateral radiograph shows improved sagittal alignment.

FIGURE 16-2. *(continued)*

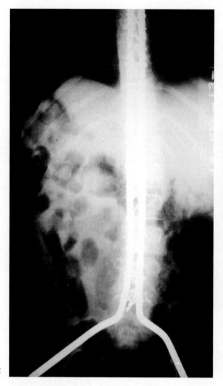
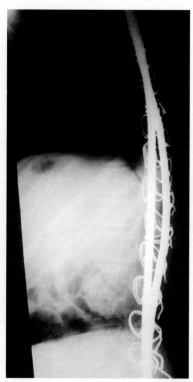

These techniques are thought to maintain better correction of pelvic obliquity. Some authors believe that fusion to L5 is sufficient, and that there will be no spinopelvic deformity throughout the remainder of the patient's life (122, 134–136). However, a postoperative spinopelvic deformity can occur and progress, and most authors recommend fusion to the pelvis (127, 129, 137). Mubarak et al. (133) recommend fusion to L5 if the curve is >20 degrees, the FVC is >40%, and the patient is using a wheelchair full time, except for occasional standing. If the patient's curve is >40 degrees or if there is pelvic obliquity >10 degrees, then fusion to the sacropelvis is recommended. In severe deformities, vertebral osteotomies may be beneficial to improve postoperative correction (138).

Careful preoperative evaluation, including pulmonary function studies and cardiology consultation, is mandatory because of the associated pulmonary and cardiac abnormalities and the risk of malignant hyperthermia (2, 3, 139–144). Children with Duchenne muscular dystrophy have a decreased FVC, commencing at approximately the age of 10 years, because of weakness of the intercostal muscles and associated contractures. There is a linear decrease over time (14, 103, 106, 119, 139). Kurz et al. (14) observed a 4% decrease in FVC for each year of age or each 10 degrees of scoliosis. It stabilizes at approximately 25% of normal until death. The presence of severe scoliosis may increase the rate of decline in the FVC. Jenkins et al. (137) reported that when the FVC is 30% or less, there is an increased risk of postoperative complication such as pneumonia and respiratory failure. Smith et al. (105) found that most patients with curves of more than 35 degrees had FVC <40% of predicted normal values. They therefore recommend that spinal arthrodesis be considered for all patients with Duchenne muscular dystrophy when they can no longer walk. Nevertheless, successful surgery can be performed in many patients with FVC as low as 20% of predicted normal valves (121). Marsh et al. (139) recently reported similar results in 17 patients with FVC >30% and 13 patients with FVC <30%. They concluded that spinal fusion could be offered to patients in the presence of a low FVC.

It is debatable whether spinal stabilization increases longevity, although it definitely increases the quality of the remaining life (102, 120, 140). In a study of 55 patients with Duchenne muscular dystrophy, of whom 32 underwent spinal fusion and 23 did not, Galasko et al. (102) found that FVC remained stable in the operated group for 36 months postoperatively and then fell slightly. In the nonoperated group, it progressively declined. The survival data showed that a significantly higher mortality rate was seen in the nonoperated group. This study indicated that spinal stabilization can increase survival for several years if it is done early, before significant progression has occurred. Velasco et al. (141) in 2007 showed that posterior spinal fusion in 56 Duchenne muscular dystrophy patients was associated with a significant decrease in the rate of respiratory decline compared with preoperative rates. Other studies, however, have shown that posterior spinal fusion has no effect on the steady decline in pulmonary function when compared with unoperated patients (118, 121, 145–147). In addition to correction and stabilization of the spine, patients experience improved quality of life, as measured by ability to function, self-image, and cosmesis (118, 124, 125, 148). Parents also reported improvement in their ability to provide care to their child.

Complications are common during and following surgery (103, 112–114, 118, 125, 134). These include excessive intraoperative blood loss, neurologic injury, cardiopulmonary compromise, postoperative infection, poor wound healing, curve progression, hardware problems, and late pseudarthrosis. Intraoperative blood loss can be minimized by early surgery and the use of hypotensive anesthesia (121). The increased intraoperative blood loss in patients with Duchenne muscular dystrophy appears to result from inadequate vasoconstriction caused by the lack of dystrophin in the smooth muscle (149). Malignant hyperthermia has been thought to be a potential complication. A recent systematic analysis by Gurnaney et al. (150) on patients with Duchenne muscular dystrophy, Becker muscular dystrophy, and other types of muscular dystrophy did not find an increased risk for malignant hyperthermia compared to the general population. Succinylcholine administration was associated with life-threatening hyperkalemia and should be avoided in those patients; tranexamic acid and epsilon aminocaproic acid (amicar) can be beneficial in decreasing intraoperative and perioperative blood loss (151, 152).

The role of intraoperative spinal cord monitoring in children with Duchenne muscular dystrophy is controversial. Noordeen et al. (149) reported that a 50% decrease in amplitude was suggestive of neurologic impairment.

Wheelchair. A wheelchair is necessary for patients who are no longer capable of independent ambulation. This is typically a motorized wheelchair that allows the patient to be independent of parents or aides, especially while attending school. The wheelchair may be fitted with a balanced mobile arm orthosis for the purpose of facilitating personal hygiene and self-feeding (80).

Cardiopulmonary Management. Respiratory failure in Duchenne muscular dystrophy is a constant threat and is the most common cause of death early in the third decade of life. Kurz et al. (14) found that the vital capacity peaks at the age when standing ceases, then declines rapidly thereafter. The development of scoliosis compounds the problems and leads to further diminution of the vital capacity (146). The complication rate in spinal surgery increases when the FVC is <30% of the normal value. Programs of vigorous respiratory therapy and the use of home negative-pressure and positive-pressure ventilators may allow patients with Duchenne muscular dystrophy to survive into the third and fourth decades of life (153–156).

Cardiac failure may occur in the second decade of life. After initially responding to digitalis and diuretics, the involved cardiac muscle becomes flabby, and the patient goes into congestive heart failure. Myocardial infarction has been reported in boys as young as 10 years. There is no correlation between the severity of pulmonary dysfunction and cardiac function, or between age and cardiac function (157). The cardiomyopathy of Duchenne muscular dystrophy exists clinically as a separate entity.

Genetic and Psychological Counseling. Proper diagnosis and early genetic counseling may help prevent the birth of additional male infants with Duchenne muscular dystrophy. It must be remembered that approximately 20% of families have already conceived and delivered a second affected male infant before the diagnosis is made in the first (78, 158). Genetic counseling with parents and family groups is important in the management of psychological problems arising when the genetic nature of the diagnosis becomes known.

Becker Muscular Dystrophy. Becker muscular dystrophy is similar to Duchenne muscular dystrophy in clinical appearance and distribution of weakness, but it is less severe (159, 160). Onset is generally after the age of 7 years and the rate of progression is slower. The patients usually remain ambulatory until adolescence or the early adult years. The Gower maneuver may occur as the weakness progresses (Fig. 16-3). Pseudohypertrophy of the calf is common, and eventually equinus and cavus foot deformities develop (Fig. 16-4). Cardiac involvement is frequent. There may be a family history of atypical muscular dystrophy. Pulmonary problems are less severe and the patient's life expectancy is greater.

Treatment. The treatment of the musculoskeletal deformities associated with Becker muscular dystrophy is essentially the same as in Duchenne muscular dystrophy. Steroid therapy (prednisone) has recently been shown to decrease serum creatine kinase levels and improve strength (161). Ankle and forefoot equinus occur commonly. Shapiro and Specht (6) have reported good outcome with the Vulpius tendo-Achilles lengthening in patients with equinus contractures. A tibialis posterior tendon transfer is performed if necessary. Forefoot equinus may require a plantar release and possibly a midfoot dorsal-wedge osteotomy for correction. The use of orthotics is also beneficial because the rate of progression is slower and the remaining muscle strength greater than in Duchenne muscular dystrophy. The incidence of scoliosis is high, especially in those adolescents who have ceased walking. These patients require careful evaluation and periodic spinal radiographs. Posterior spinal fusion and segmental instrumentation, usually Luque, are useful for patients in whom there is progression (162).

Emery-Dreifuss Muscular Dystrophy. Emery-Dreifuss muscular dystrophy is an uncommon sex-linked recessive disorder characterized by early contractures and cardiomyopathy (12). The typical phenotype is seen only in the male sex, although milder or partial phenotypes have been reported in female carriers (163–166). Affected boys show mild muscle weakness in the first 10 years of life and a tendency for toe walking. The Gower maneuver may be present in young children. The distinctive clinical criteria occur in late childhood or early adolescence. These include tendo-Achilles contractures, elbow-flexion contractures, neck-extension contracture, tightness of the lumbar paravertebral muscles, and cardiac abnormalities involving brachycardia and first-degree, and eventually complete, heart block (165, 167). The muscle weakness is slowly progressive, but there may be some stabilization in adulthood.

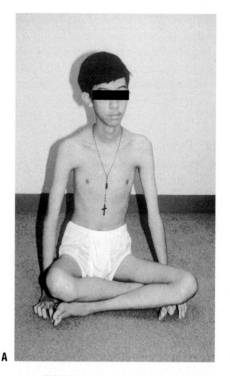
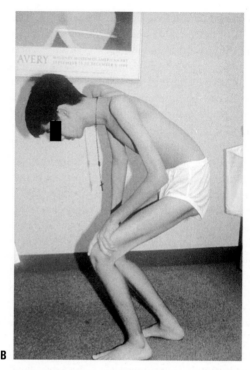
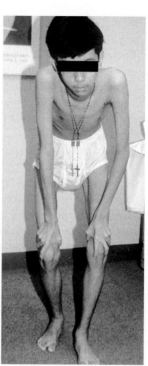

FIGURE 16-3. **A:** A 13-year-old boy with suspected Becker muscular dystrophy uses the Gower maneuver to stand from a sitting position. **B:** Manually assisted knee extension is necessary to achieve upright stance. **C:** Front view.

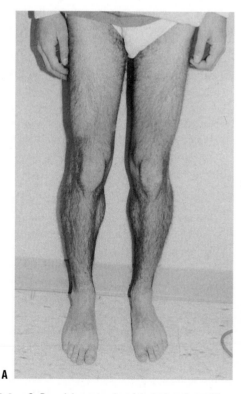
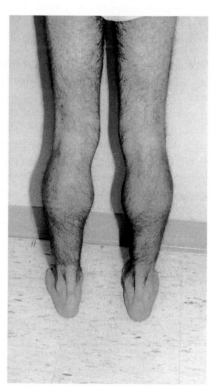

FIGURE 16-4. **A:** Pseudohypertrophy of the calves in an 18-year-old man with Becker muscular dystrophy. He is a brace-free ambulator. **B:** Posterior view.

Most patients are able to ambulate into the fifth and sixth decades of life. Obesity and untreated equinus contractures can lead to the loss of ambulatory ability at an earlier age (6).

The CPK level in patients with Emery-Dreifuss muscular dystrophy is only mildly or moderately elevated. EMG and muscle biopsy reveal myopathy. The diagnosis of this form of muscular dystrophy should be considered in patients with a myopathic phenotype, after Duchenne and Becker muscular dystrophies have been ruled out (usually by testing for dystrophin) (6). The condition should also be distinguished from scapuloperoneal muscular dystrophy and the rigid spine syndrome (167).

Genetic and Molecular Biology Studies. The gene locus for the most common variant of Emery-Dreifuss muscular dystrophy, the X-linked recessive form, has been localized, in linkage studies, to the long arm of the X chromosome at Xq28 (168–170). Rarely, an autosomal dominant form and, even less frequently, an autosomal recessive form may be seen. The autosomal dominant and autosomal recessive forms have an identified gene mutation on the lamin A/C gene on chromosome 1q21 (170). The specific type of gene testing depends on the family history and sex of the affected individual.

Treatment. The treatment for Emery-Dreifuss muscular dystrophy is similar to what is used in other forms of muscular dystrophy. The goals are to prevent or correct deformities and maximize function. Treatment modalities include physical therapy, correction of soft-tissue contractures, spinal stabilization, and cardiologic intervention.

Physical Therapy. This can be useful in the management of neck-extension contractures, elbow-flexion contractures, and tightness of the lumbar paravertebral muscles. Decreased neck flexion, which is characteristic of this disorder, can begin as early as the first decade of life, but is usually not present until the second decade. This is due to contracture of the extensor muscles and the ligamentum nuchae. According to Shapiro and Specht (6), this contracture does not progress past neutral. Lateral bending and rotation of the neck also become limited as the extensor contractures progress. Physical therapy can be helpful in maintaining limited flexion of the neck.

Soft-tissue Contractures. Tendo-Achilles lengthening and posterior ankle capsulotomy, combined with anterior transfer of the tibialis posterior tendon, can be helpful in providing long-term stabilization of the foot and ankle (6, 165). Elbow-flexion contractures usually do not require treatment. These contractures can be as severe as 90 degrees, although most do not exceed 35 degrees (6). Full flexion from this position and normal forearm pronation and supination are preserved. Physical therapy may be helpful in slowing the progress of the elbow-flexion contractures. Surgery has not been shown to be beneficial.

Spinal Stabilization. Scoliosis is common in this form of muscular dystrophy, but it shows a lower incidence of progression. This has been attributed to contractures at the lumbar and ultimately the thoracic paravertebral muscles, which seem to prevent progression (6, 165). Patients with scoliosis need to be followed closely, but most do not require treatment. Curves that progress beyond 40 degrees may require surgical stabilization.

Cardiologic Intervention. Severe brachycardia caused by complete heart block has been a major cause of sudden death in these patients. Most of them do not have cardiac symptoms preceding death. Merlini et al. (166) reported that 30 out of 73 patients with Emery-Dreifuss muscular dystrophy died suddenly, of whom only four were symptomatic. It is recommended that a cardiac pacemaker be inserted shortly after confirmation of the diagnosis (166, 171).

AUTOSOMAL RECESSIVE MUSCULAR DYSTROPHIES

Limb-Girdle Muscular Dystrophy. LGMD is common and may be more benign than the other forms of muscular dystrophy. It is a rather heterogeneous group of disorders with various classifications proposed for it over the years. The age at onset and rate of progression of muscle weakness are variable. It usually begins in the second or third decade of life. It is transmitted as an autosomal recessive trait, but an autosomal dominant pattern of inheritance has been reported in some families (172–174).

The symptoms of LGMD are similar to facioscapulohumeral muscular dystrophy, except that the facial muscles are not involved. The initial muscle weakness involves either the pelvic or shoulder girdle. The rate of progression is usually slow, with soft-tissue contractures and disability developing 20 years or more after the onset of the disease. The patients remain ambulatory for many years.

The distribution of weakness is similar to that seen in Duchenne and Becker muscular dystrophies. The iliopsoas, gluteus maximus, and quadriceps muscles are involved early in the disease process. Usually, shoulder girdle involvement occurs at about the same time. The serratus anterior, trapezius, rhomboid, latissimus dorsi, and sternal portions of pectoralis major muscles are affected most often. The disease later spreads to involve other muscles, such as the biceps brachia and the clavicular portion of the pectoralis major. Deltoid involvement may occur, but usually only later in the course of the disease. In patients with severe involvement, weakness may involve the distal muscles of the limbs, such as the wrist and finger flexors and extensors.

Two forms of LGMD are the more common pelvic-girdle type and a scapulohumeral form. The latter is rare, with symptoms involving primarily the shoulder girdle. Involvement of the pelvic girdle may not occur for many years. In the pelvic-girdle type, there is weakness of the hip extensors and abductors, resulting in accentuated lumbar lordosis, gait abnormalities, and hip instability.

The CPK level is moderately elevated in patients with LGMD. The clinical characteristics are indistinguishable from those of sporadic Becker muscular dystrophy, carriers of Duchenne or Becker muscular dystrophies, and those of childhood acid-maltase deficiency (6). Therefore, a dystrophin assay is essential in establishing the diagnosis (172).

Treatment for LGMD is similar to that for Duchenne and Becker muscular dystrophies. Significant scoliosis rarely occurs because of the late onset of the disease process. When present, it usually is mild and does not require treatment (173). Patients usually succumb to the disease process before the age of 40 years.

Genetic and Molecular Biology Studies.
Presently, a multitude of gene loci have been identified for this heterogeneous group of muscular dystrophies. The European Neuromuscular Center workshop on LGMD adopted a nomenclature to help categorize this complex and heterogeneous group of disorders. Presently, five autosomal dominant and nine autosomal recessive conditions have been identified that fit into this clinical grouping (173, 174).

Infantile Facioscapulohumeral Muscular Dystrophy.
Infantile facioscapulohumeral muscular dystrophy (IFSH MD) is being identified more frequently. It is a severe variant of the more common later-onset facioscapulohumeral muscular dystrophy (175–177). A Mobius type of facial weakness may also be present and progress asymptomatically at a relatively slow pace (178). Although many of these infants represent sporadic cases, genetic diagnosis is positive for many of them and is identical to that seen in adults (179). Facial diplegia is noted in infancy, followed by sensorineural hearing loss in childhood (mean age 5 years). Ambulation begins at a normal age, but because of progressive muscle weakness, most patients become wheelchair bound during the second decade of life. Weakness causes the child to walk with the hands and forearms folded across the upper buttocks to provide support for the weak gluteus maximus muscles (6, 175, 177). This marked lumbar lordosis is progressive and is almost pathognomonic for IFSH MD (Fig. 16-5). After the patient becomes wheelchair dependent, the lordosis leads to fixed hip flexion contractures. Equinus or equinovarus deformities and scoliosis occur less frequently.

Treatment.
The treatment of patients with IFSH MD (177) is individualized because most patients do not have significant orthopaedic deformities. These patients usually have severely compromised pulmonary functions and succumb in early adolescence. Shapiro et al. outlined the possible treatment modalities for children with IFSH MD. Flexible equinus and equinovarus deformities respond well to AFOs. Occasionally, a Vulpius-type tendo-Achilles lengthening may be necessary. Hip-flexion contractures usually do not require treatment in ambulatory patients, because treatment may decrease function. Spinal orthoses control the lordosis but do not provide correction because the spine remains flexible early in the course of the disorder. Because an orthosis interferes with ambulation, it is usually not employed. When wheelchair use is full time,

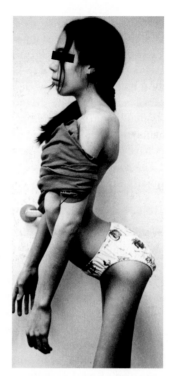

FIGURE 16-5. Marked lumbar lordosis in a 15-year-old girl with infantile facioscapulohumeral muscular dystrophy. She is still ambulatory but having increasing back pain.

a modified wheelchair with an orthosis may be useful, or perhaps a posterior spinal fusion and segmental instrumentation, depending on the severity of the deformity. Scapulothoracic stabilization is not indicated because the severity of dysfunction is so great that minimal or no improvement in shoulder function can be achieved.

AUTOSOMAL DOMINANT MUSCULAR DYSTROPHIES

Facioscapulohumeral Muscular Dystrophy.
Facioscapulohumeral muscular dystrophy is an autosomal dominant disorder having variable expression (180). The disease is characterized by muscular weakness in the face, shoulder girdle, and upper arm. It is caused by a gene defect, *FRG1*, on chromosome 4q35 (181). There is selective sparing of the deltoid, the distal part of the pectoralis major muscle, and the erector spinae muscles (182). This results in decreased scapulothoracic motion, with scapular winging and a marked decrease in shoulder flexion and abduction. Glenohumeral motion is usually preserved. The onset may occur at any age but is most common in late childhood or early adulthood. The disease occurs in both genders but is more common in women. Abortive (minimally affected) cases are common. Progression is insidious and periods of apparent arrest may occur. Cardiac and CNS involvement are absent. Life expectancy is relatively good.

Initially, the face and shoulder girdle muscles are involved, but they may be affected only mildly for many years. Facial signs, which may be present in infancy, include lack of mobility, incomplete eye closure, pouting lips with a transverse smile, and absence of eye and forehead wrinkles. It tends to produce a "pop-eye" appearance. The shoulder girdle weakness leads to scapular winging. The weight of the upper extremities, together with the weakness of the trapezius, permits the clavicles to assume a more horizontal position. It also leads to a forward-sloping appearance of the shoulders. As the disease progresses, pelvic girdle and tibialis anterior muscle involvement may also occur. Scoliosis is rare because of the late onset of the disease process.

The CPK levels in patients with facioscapulohumeral muscular dystrophy are usually normal. The diagnosis is made by physical examination and DNA confirmation. Presently, genetic testing is more than 95% sensitive and highly specific for FSHD (183).

Treatment. The winging of the scapula, with weakness of shoulder flexion and abduction, is the major orthopaedic problem in facioscapulohumeral muscular dystrophy. The deltoid, supraspinatus, and intraspinatus muscles are usually normal, however, or minimally involved. Posterior scapulocostal fusion or stabilization (scapulopexy) by a variety of techniques can be helpful in restoring mechanical advantage to the deltoid and rotator cuff muscles (184–191). This can result in increased active abduction and forward flexion of the shoulder, and improved function as well as cosmesis. Jakab and Gledhill (186) reported the results of a simplified technique for scapulocostal fusion. The technique involves wiring of the medial border of the scapula to ribs three through seven. Internal fixation is achieved with 16-gauge wire. The wires ensure firm fixation and eliminate the need for postoperative immobilization and subsequent rehabilitation. The child uses a sling for 3 to 4 days postoperatively, and then begins a physical therapy program. Jakab and Gledhill (186) found that shoulder flexion increased 28 degrees (range 20 to 40 degrees) and abduction 27 degrees (range 20 to 35 degrees) at a mean follow-up of 2.9 years. This allowed all patients to raise their arms above their heads, conferring a greater mechanical advantage. A similar technique and results were reported in 9 patients (18 shoulders) by Giannini et al. in 2006 (191). The beneficial effects do not seem to deteriorate with time (184–186, 190, 191).

Distal Muscular Dystrophy. This is a rare form of muscular dystrophy. It is also known as *Gower and M. Yoshi muscular dystrophy*. It typically begins in young adults. It is transmitted as an autosomal dominant trait. The initial involvement is in the intrinsic muscles of the hand. The disease process spreads proximally. In the lower extremities, the calves and tibialis anterior are involved first. The absence of sensory abnormalities, especially vibratory, differentiates this from Charcot-Marie-Tooth disease.

Ocular Muscular Dystrophy. Ocular muscular dystrophy, also known as *progressive external ophthalmoplegia*, is another rare form of muscular dystrophy. It typically begins in the adolescent years. The extraocular muscles are affected, resulting in diplopia and ptosis. This is followed by limitation of ocular movement (192). The upper facial muscles are often affected. The disease is slowly progressive and may involve the proximal upper extremities. The pelvis may be involved late in the disease process. Most patients with this disorder have an identifiable mitochondrial myopathy (193).

Oculopharyngeal Muscular Dystrophy. This form of muscular dystrophy is inherited in an autosomal dominant pattern with complete penetrance, and begins in the third decade of life. It is particularly common in French Canadians (194, 195).

Pharyngeal muscle involvement results in dysarthria, and in dysphasia, which leads to repetitive regurgitation and weight loss. This condition necessitates cricopharyngeal myotomy, a procedure that does not alter pharyngeal function (196). Ptosis develops in middle life.

MYOTONIA

Myotonia is a group of disorders characterized by the inability of skeletal muscle to relax after a strong contraction from either voluntary movement or mechanical stimulation. This is best demonstrated by the slowness with which a clenched fist relaxes in such patients. The most common myotonias include myotonic dystrophy, congenital myotonic dystrophy, and myotonia congenita. These are all rare disorders that are transmitted by autosomal dominant inheritance (6, 17).

Myotonic Dystrophy. Myotonic dystrophy is a systemic disorder characterized by myotonia, progressive muscle weakness, gonadal atrophy, cataracts, frontal baldness, heart disease, and dementia (197, 198). The genetic defect is located on chromosome 19q (199, 200). The distal musculature is affected first, and the myotonia begins to disappear as muscle weakness progresses. The onset occurs usually in late adolescence or early adulthood. In women, the diagnosis is frequently made only after they have given birth to a child who is more severely involved. The disease spreads slowly proximally and involves the quadriceps, hamstrings, and eventually the hip extensors. The lower extremities are more involved than the upper extremities. The most common presenting symptoms are weakness of the hands and difficulty in walking. Patients may be unable to relax their fingers after shaking hands and may need to palmar flex the hand to open the fingers. Muscles of the face, mandible, eyes, neck, and distal limbs may also be affected. The levels of serum enzymes are normal. Muscle biopsies show type I atrophy of the muscle fibers and the presence of some internal nuclei. These are nonspecific findings. The "dive-bomber" pattern on EMG is diagnostic (6). DNA testing that demonstrates a cytosine–thymine–guanine expansion affecting a protein kinase is confirmatory (199).

Examination reveals an expressionless face, ptosis, and a fish mouth that is difficult to close. There is marked wasting of the temporal, masseter, and sternocleidomastoid muscles. Deep-tendon reflexes are diminished or lost. Slit-lamp examination of the eyes reveals that most patients have lenticular opacities, cataracts, and retinopathy. Cardiac involvement is also common and includes mitral valve prolapse and arrhythmias (200, 201). Organic brain deterioration may also occur. Frontal baldness in men and glaucoma in both sexes occur in midadult life. The course of the disease is one of steady deterioration. Most patients lose the ability to ambulate within 15 to 20 years of onset of symptoms (201). There are no characteristic orthopaedic deformities, although a slight tendency toward increased hindfoot varus has been observed (6). Lifespan is shortened, and death is usually caused by pneumonia or cardiac failure.

Treatment of myotonic dystrophy is primarily orthotic because the onset is usually after skeletal maturity. An AFO may be helpful in patients with a drop foot caused by weakness of the tibialis anterior and peroneal muscles.

Congenital Myotonic Dystrophy.   This is a relatively common muscle disorder of variable expression that occurs most frequently in children whose mothers have either a forme fruste or mild clinical involvement (200–204). Although it has autosomal dominant transmission, it is predominantly transmitted from mother to child (202). This is an exception in autosomal dominant disorders and indicates additional maternal factors. Approximately 40% of patients have severe involvement or die in infancy, whereas 60% will be affected later (204). The child may have an expressionless, long, narrow face; hypotonia; delayed developmental milestones; facial diplegia; difficulty in feeding because of pharyngolaryngeal palsy; respiratory failure; and mild mental retardation. The ability to swallow improves with growth, but the hypotonia persists. Examination shows diffuse weakness and absent deep-tendon reflexes. The appearance is similar to spinal muscular atrophy. Ambulation is usually delayed. If the mother is the carrier, the child may have other organic disorders later in life. Cataracts usually occur after the age of 14 years.

The defective gene has been localized to chromosome 19, and a test for prenatal diagnosis is available (198, 205). As in the adult form, there appears to be an expansion of a highly repeated sequence of three nucleotides: cytosine, thymine, and guanine. The trinucleotide repeat is at the 3' end of a protein kinase gene on chromosome 19, which lengthens as it passes from one generation to another. The length of the sequence correlates with the severity of the disorder. DNA testing is readily available for this disorder and is the diagnostic test of choice.

Orthopaedic problems in congenital myotonic dystrophy include congenital hip dislocation and talipes equinovarus (i.e., clubfeet). There is a tendency to develop soft-tissue contractures of other major joints of the lower extremities. Clubfeet may behave like those in arthrogryposis multiplex congenita (206). Serial casting may be tried, but most require surgery, such as an extensive, complete release. If this fails, a talectomy

or Verebelyi-Ogston procedure may be useful (207). Scoliosis is also common and may require orthotic or surgical intervention (162). Spine surgery is fraught with a high incidence of complications, such as cardiac arrhythmias and postoperative infection (208). Nevertheless, because life expectancy is at least up to the early adult years, aggressive orthopaedic management improves the quality of life.

Myotonia Congenita.   Myotonia congenita is usually present at birth, but does not become clinically apparent until after the age of 10 years. In some cases, it may present as low back pain or impaired athletic ability (209–211). The severity of the myotonia varies considerably. The distribution is widespread, although it is more marked in the lower extremities than in the upper extremities (212). Myotonia is most evident during the initial movement. Repetitive movement decreases the myotonia and facilitates subsequent movements. The stiffness usually disappears within 3 to 4 minutes, and normal activities, including running, are possible. Some patients appear herculean (massively muscled) because of generalized muscle hypertrophy, particularly in the buttocks, thighs, and calves. Children with myotonia congenita have no associated weakness and no other endocrine or systemic abnormalities. The disease is compatible with a normal lifespan. A patient's disability is not great when the limits of the disease have been accepted. Procainamide and diphenylhydantoin (Dilantin) have been used with some success to decrease the myotonia, but they should be used only in severe cases (213). There are no characteristic orthopaedic deformities (6). The disorder, a chloride channelopathy, is caused by various mutations in the skeletal muscle voltage-gated chloride channel gene *ClCN1* (214, 215). To date, four mutations of the *ClCN1* gene on chromosome 7q35 have been identified with myotonia congenita (216).

CONGENITAL MYOPATHIES AND CONGENITAL MUSCULAR DYSTROPHY

Congenital myopathies and congenital muscular dystrophy cause the baby at birth or in early infancy to be "floppy" or hypotonic. When these conditions occur in an older child, they can present as muscle weakness. These disorders are not well understood clinically or at the molecular level. The diagnostic categorization is not uniform or predictive. They are defined histologically from muscle biopsies (6, 217, 218). When the biopsy findings are abnormal but not dystrophic, the patient is diagnosed as having a nonspecific myopathy (6). When considerable fibrosis is present along with necrotic fibers, congenital muscular dystrophy may be diagnosed.

CONGENITAL MYOPATHIES

The congenital myopathies include central core disease, nemaline myopathy (rod-body myopathy), myotubular myopathy (centronuclear), congenital fiber-type disproportion, and metabolic myopathies. Differentiation between these types can be accomplished through histochemical analysis and electron microscopy of muscle biopsy specimens (6, 217–219).

Central Core Disease.

Central core disease is a nonprogressive autosomal dominant congenital myopathy that frequently presents as hypotonia in infants and as delayed motor developmental milestones in young children (217, 218, 220, 221). Independent ambulation may not be achieved until the age of 4 years. The distribution of muscle involvement is similar to that found in Duchenne muscular dystrophy, with the trunk and lower extremities showing more involvement than the upper extremities, and the proximal muscles more than the distal muscle groups. The pelvic girdle shows more involvement than the shoulder. Use of the Gower maneuver is common. No deterioration in strength occurs with time; sensation is normal; and the deep-tendon reflexes are either decreased or absent. Muscle wasting is a common finding, but progression of muscle weakness is rare. Muscle biopsies show mostly type I fibers, containing central circular or oval regions that are devoid of oxidative enzymes, adenosine triphosphate activity, and mitochondria. Serum CPK and nerve conduction studies are normal, whereas EMGs show myopathic abnormalities. Scoliosis, soft-tissue contractures, neuromuscular hip subluxation and dislocation, talipes equinovarus, pes planus, and hypermobility of joints (especially the patella) are the most common musculoskeletal problems, and they may require treatment (220–223). Scoliotic deformities have patterns similar to those of idiopathic scoliosis, progress rapidly, and tend to be rigid (222). Posterior spinal fusion and segmental instrumentation yield satisfactory results. Soft-tissue contractures around the hip and knee may need to be released. Clubfeet require extensive soft-tissue releases in order to achieve correction. Congenital dislocation of the hip can be treated by open or closed reduction techniques, but the recurrence rate is high and may require osseous procedures such as pelvic or proximal femoral osteotomies (223). Central core disease is one of the disorders in which patients are susceptible to malignant hyperthermia. This association with malignant hyperthermia has led researchers to link both disorders with the long arm of chromosome 19 as the probable site of mutation (224, 225).

Nemaline Myopathy.

Nemaline, or rod-body, myopathy is a variable congenital myopathy that usually begins in infancy or early childhood, with hypotonia affecting all skeletal muscles (6, 217, 218, 226, 227). There is no involvement of cardiac muscle. Elongated facies, with a high-arched palette and a nasal, high-pitched voice, are frequently noted. Skeletal changes may resemble those seen in arachnodactyly. Martinez and Lake (226), in a review of the literature relating to 99 patients, recognized these distinct forms: neonatal (severe), congenital (moderate), and adult onset. The neonatal form is characterized by severe hypotonia, with 90% mortality in the first 3 years of life because of respiratory insufficiency. The mean survival after birth was 16 months. The moderate congenital form, which is the most common and prototypic, is diagnosed during or after the neonatal period and is characterized by mild or moderate hypotonia, weakness, and delayed developmental milestones. Most patients begin to walk at the age of 2 to 4 years, and the weakness is usually nonprogressive or only slowly progressive. The mortality rate is approximately 5% in the congenital form. Death is usually caused by severe involvement of the pharyngeal and respiratory muscles (228–230). The adult-onset form is characterized by proximal weakness that occasionally progresses acutely. There is no correlation between the number of rods and the phenotype in nemaline myopathy (227). The inheritance pattern in this disorder is variable, with autosomal recessive, autosomal dominant, and sporadic cases identified. However, all mutations identified to date follow an autosomal recessive inheritance pattern (231).

Soft-tissue contractures are uncommon in nemaline myopathy. The major musculoskeletal problems are scoliosis and lumbar lordosis. Posterior spinal fusion and segmental instrumentation may be indicated in progressive scoliotic deformities (6). Lower extremity orthoses can be helpful in providing stability to the joints and in aiding ambulation. Because of their diminished pulmonary function and the heightened risk for malignant hyperthermia, patients undergoing surgery require careful monitoring during the administration of anesthesia (232).

Centronuclear Myopathy.

Centronuclear (i.e., myotubular) myopathy is a disorder of considerable variability (217, 218, 233). Muscle biopsies demonstrate persistent myotubes that would be normal in fetal life. There are X-linked recessive, autosomal recessive, and autosomal dominant forms (234, 235). The defect in the X-linked recessive form is at the locus Xq28. The defective gene has been identified and named as *MTM1* (236). Mutation detection analysis is now available, and sensitivity of testing is up to 72% (236). These children have varying degrees of weakness, generally noted in infancy. Patients with X-linked recessive forms are usually severely involved and die in infancy. The infant with the autosomal recessive form of the disease is hypotonic at birth, but the hypotonia is not progressive and may improve with time. Most of these children are able to walk. They may have a myopathic facies, high-arched palate, and proximal muscle weakness. There is an increased incidence of cavovarus foot deformities, scoliosis, lumbar lordosis, and scapular winging. By late adolescence or early adult life, some patients lose their ability to ambulate.

Congenital Fiber-type Disproportion.

Congenital fiber-type disproportion is characterized by generalized hypotonia at or shortly after birth. The histologic findings (from muscle biopsies) that may suggest this diagnosis include a predominance of type I fibers of reduced size and relatively large type II fibers. It is recognized as a nonspecific pathologic change that occurs in many patients and has a myopathic, neuropathic, or CNS origin (237). The degree of weakness is variable, and sequential examinations determine the prognosis. Most patients become ambulatory. The most serious problem is the vulnerability to life-threatening respiratory infections during the first years of life. Proximal muscle weakness is frequently associated with acetabular dysplasia (237). To prevent postural contractures from developing, an appropriate lower extremity splint should be used until the patient achieves ambulation. Severe, rigid scoliosis can occur. Orthoses are usually ineffective, and early spinal arthrodesis may be necessary (6).

Metabolic Myopathies.

These myopathies represent a broad spectrum of metabolic abnormalities that are generally clinically evident in the first two decades of life (238). These include disorders of glycolysis, lipid metabolism, mitochondrial dysfunction, and purine nucleotide cycle defects. Myopathies caused by metabolic errors in the first step of glycolysis, for example, myophosphorylase and phosphofructokinase deficiencies, are clinically associated with cramping, weakness, and exercise intolerance with anaerobic activity (i.e., short-duration but vigorous activity). The other glycolytic disorders, such as acid maltase or debrancher enzyme deficiencies, are associated with progressive muscle weakness and wasting (239). Carnitine palmityl transferase deficiency, which is a disorder of lipid metabolism, presents with muscle cramping, weakness, and myoglobinuria following prolonged exercise. Myopathies caused by deficiencies in mitochondrial enzymes are less well defined and may be associated with severe benign exercise intolerance and progressive myopathic syndromes (239–241).

CONGENITAL MUSCULAR DYSTROPHY

Congenital muscular dystrophy is a rare disorder in which babies are "floppy," with generalized muscle weakness and with the involvement of respiratory and facial muscles (242, 243). It is a muscle disorder in which the muscle biopsy demonstrates dystrophic features characterized by considerable perimysial and endomysial fibrosis. It is different from Duchenne muscular dystrophy and Becker muscular dystrophy because it affects children of both sexes, is not associated with massively elevated levels of CPK, does not involve abnormalities of the dystrophin gene or protein, and is associated with a more variable prognosis (6). There are several forms of congenital muscular dystrophy. In one, the infant is weak at birth. Many have severe stiffness of joints, whereas others do not. A few infants have rapid progression and do not survive after the first year of life. Most, however, stabilize and survive into adulthood (243). Another type is seen in Japanese infants and has been termed *Fukuyama congenital muscular dystrophy.* It is characterized by a marked developmental defect in the CNS (244, 245). There is progressive muscle degeneration and mental retardation. Severe joint contractures develop, and many children with this condition die in the first decade of life. Three disorders are associated with congenital muscular dystrophy and CNS malformations: Fukuyama congenital muscular dystrophy,

Walker-Warburg syndrome, and muscle–eye–brain disease. Merosin-deficient congenital muscular dystrophy is associated with changes in the white matter of the brain as seen on MRI and has been linked to chromosome 6q2 (246, 247).

Common orthopaedic problems include congenital hip dislocation and subluxation, tendo-Achilles contractures, and talipes equinovarus (Fig. 16-6). Because most patients survive, aggressive orthopaedic management is warranted. This may include physical therapy, orthoses, soft-tissue releases, and perhaps osteotomy (6, 248). Early physical therapy may be helpful in preventing soft-tissue contractures. Soft-tissue releases in the treatment of congenital dislocation of the hip are characterized by a high incidence of recurrent dislocation (Fig. 16-7) (248). Progressive scoliosis may be initially treated by an orthosis, although most patients require surgical stabilization similar to the procedure used in other forms of muscular dystrophy (127).

SPINAL MUSCULAR ATROPHY

Spinal muscular atrophy is a group of disorders characterized by degeneration of the anterior horn cells of the spinal cord, and occasionally the neurons of the lower bulbar motor nuclei, resulting in muscle weakness and atrophy (249–253). They are autosomal recessive disorders that occur in approximately 1 in 6000 to 10,000 individuals. The prevalence of carriers is estimated at 1 in 40 to 1 in 50 (254). The loss of anterior horn cells is considered to be an acute event without progression. The neurologic deterioration may stabilize and remain unchanged for long periods (255, 256). The progression of muscle weakness is a reflection of normal growth that exceeds muscle reserve. Respiratory function is compromised, and atelectasis and pneumonia are the usual causes of death.

Clinical Classification.

The clinical features of spinal muscular atrophy vary widely and are based on the age at onset and the functional capacity of the child at the time of diagnosis. This has led to the disorder being classified into three types. These include Type I (severe), or acute Werdnig-Hoffman disease; Type II (intermediate), or chronic Werdnig-Hoffman disease; and Type III (mild), or Kugelberg-Welander disease (257). All three fall within the spectrum of the same disorder, but each has its specific diagnostic criteria and prognosis. There is a considerable overlap between these three disorders, however, and most authors consider them to be a single disorder, namely, spinal muscular atrophy (258). Generally, the earlier the onset, the worse the prognosis.

Type I, Acute Werdnig-Hoffman Disease.

The Type I spinal muscular atrophy is characterized by clinical onset between birth and 6 months. These children typically have severe involvement with marked weakness and hypotonia. They usually die from respiratory failure between the ages of 1 and 24 months. Because of their young age and severe involvement, orthopaedic intervention is not indicated in

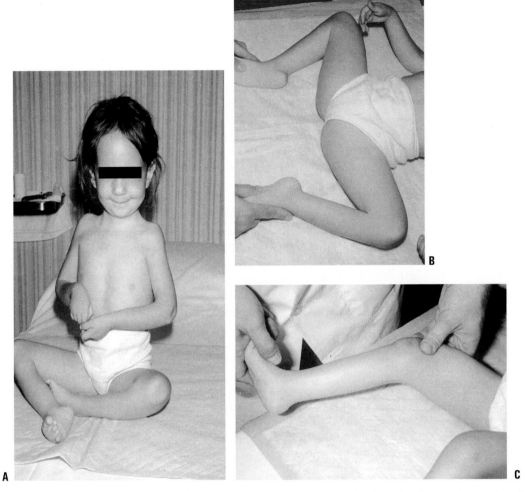

FIGURE 16-6. **A:** Clinical photograph of a 3-year-old girl with congenital muscular dystrophy. Observe the position of the upper and lower extremities. **B:** The hips are flexed, abducted, and externally rotated. **C:** Moderate knee-flexion contractures are present.

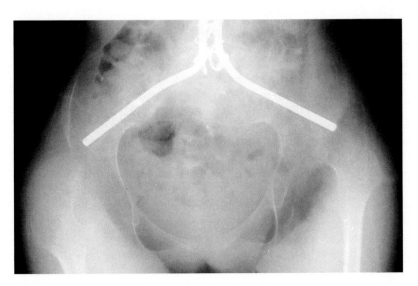

FIGURE 16-7. Pelvic radiograph of an 11-year-old girl with congenital muscular dystrophy, 3 years after posterior spinal fusion and Luque rod instrumentation, including the Galveston technique. She is wheelchair dependent and has developed bilateral asymptomatic hip dislocations despite extensive soft-tissue releases in early childhood.

these children. Pathologic fractures may occur because of *in utero* osteoporosis secondary to decreased movement at birth, thereby suggesting the presence of osteogenesis imperfecta (259). These fractures heal rapidly with immobilization.

Type II, Chronic Werdnig-Hoffman Disease.
The clinical onset of Type II spinal muscular atrophy occurs at between the ages of 6 and 24 months. These children show less severe involvement than those with Type I spinal muscular atrophy but are never able to walk. They may, however, live into the fourth and fifth decades of life.

Type III, Kugelberg-Welander Disease.
The clinical onset of Type III spinal muscular atrophy occurs after the age of 2 years and usually before the age of 10 years. Walking is usually possible until late childhood or early adolescence. These patients are usually not able to run. Their motor capacity decreases with time, and they have difficulty rising from the floor because of weakness of the pelvic-girdle muscles; this is known as the *Gower sign*. There is atrophy of the lower limbs, with pseudohypertrophy of the calves. Cranial nerve muscles are usually not affected. These patients have normal intelligence and may function effectively in society. Both the quality and quantity of life may be extended in Type II and Type III spinal muscular atrophy by the use of nighttime or full-time assisted ventilation (260).

Functional Classification.
Evans et al. (261) developed a four-group functional classification that may be useful prognostically:

Group I.
Children never sit independently, have poor head control, and develop early progressive scoliosis.

Group II.
Children have head control and the ability to sit if placed in a sitting position but are unable to stand or walk, even with orthotics.

Group III.
Children have the ability to pull to stand and to walk with external support, such as orthoses.

Group IV.
Children have the ability to walk and run independently.

Other studies have supported the use of this classification (251, 257).

Genetic and Molecular Biology Studies.
Linkage studies have established that the genetic homogeneity for the three types of spinal muscular atrophy occur at the same locus on chromosome 5q (16, 17, 249, 262). Two genes have been found to be associated with disease, the survival motor neuron (*SMN*) gene and the neuronal apoptosis inhibitory protein (*NAIP*) gene (250, 263, 264). The presence of large-scale deletions involving both genes corresponds to a more severe phenotype. Prenatal diagnosis is available with the use of PCR amplification assays. No specific gene therapy is available.

Clinical Features.
The clinical features of spinal muscular atrophy vary according to the clinical classification. The clinical characteristics common to all groups are relatively symmetric limb and trunk weakness, and muscle atrophy that affects the lower extremities more than the upper extremities and the proximal muscles more than the distal muscles. Hypotonia and areflexia are present. Sensation and intelligence are normal. In infants, gross fasciculations of the tongue and fine tremors of the fingers are commonly present (256, 265). The only muscles not involved are the diaphragm, sternothyroid, sternohyoid, and the involuntary muscles of the intestine, bladder, heart, and sphincters (249, 257).

Diagnostic Studies.
The studies used in the initial diagnosis of spinal muscular atrophy include laboratory studies, EMG, nerve conduction studies, DNA testing, and muscle biopsies. Hematologic studies in spinal muscular atrophy are not particularly useful (253). The CPK and aldolase levels are normal to only slightly elevated. In patients with spinal muscular atrophy, electrophysiologic studies such as EMG show typical neuropathic changes such as increased amplitude and duration of response (253). Denervational changes, manifest as prominent fibrillation potentials, are a hallmark of this disorder. Nerve conduction velocities are typically normal, although the compound muscle action potential amplitude is typically markedly diminished (266). Muscle biopsies are usually diagnostic, demonstrating muscle fiber degeneration and atrophy of fiber groups (253). However, with the recent advent of genetic testing for this disorder, muscle biopsy is usually not necessary. DNA testing is highly sensitive for this disorder and is readily available. DNA PCR for spinal muscular atrophy is now the diagnostic procedure of choice.

Radiographic Evaluation.
There are no specific radiographic characteristics that are useful in making the diagnosis of spinal muscular atrophy. The most common radiographic abnormalities are nonspecific and include hip subluxation or dislocation and progressive spinal deformity (253). Spinal radiographs, posteroanterior and lateral, should be obtained in the sitting position to avoid the compensations seen in the standing and supine positions.

Treatment.
The major orthopaedic abnormalities associated with spinal muscular atrophy include the presence of soft-tissue contractures of the lower extremities, hip subluxation and dislocation, and spinal deformity (252, 253).

Lower Extremity Soft-Tissue Contractures.
Soft-tissue contractures of the lower extremities are the result of progressive muscle degeneration and replacement with fibrous tissue. Ambulation may be promoted and soft-tissue contractures delayed by the use of orthoses such as KAFOs (267). Contractures tend to occur most frequently after the child becomes wheelchair bound. The prolonged sitting posture enhances hip- and knee-flexion contractures. Contractures of the soft tissues of the hip may also result in abnormal growth

of the proximal femur, predisposing the patient to coxa valga and progressive hip subluxation. Soft-tissue contractures without an associated osseous deformity usually do not require treatment. Even when they are released, the sitting posture of the child promotes their recurrence.

Hip Subluxation and Dislocation.

Progressive hip subluxation leading to dislocation occurs predominantly in spinal muscular atrophy Types II and III (268, 269). It is important that hip dislocation be prevented in order to provide comfort and sitting balance and to maintain pelvic alignment. A comfortable sitting posture is important if the adolescent or young adult is to function in society. Periodic anteroposterior radiographs of the pelvis, beginning in mid- to late childhood, are important in order to ensure early recognition of coxa valga and subluxation. Once diagnosed, it is usually progressive because of the continued muscle weakness and soft-tissue contractures. Procedures that have been used with some success include soft-tissue releases such as adductor tenotomy, iliopsoas recession, and medial hamstring lengthening. This restores some balance to the proximal musculature. A varus derotation osteotomy is frequently indicated if the hip is severely subluxated (253). If the hip is dislocated, an open reduction with capsulorrhaphy and pelvic osteotomy of the Chiari type may be of benefit to the patient. The usual pelvic rotation osteotomies (e.g., Salter, Sutherland, Steel) sacrifice posterior coverage to gain lateral (superior) and anterior coverage. In the child who will be predominantly in a sitting position, this lack of posterior coverage may predispose the patient to a posterior subluxation and pain. Therefore, the pelvic osteotomy method chosen must allow improved posterior coverage. This is usually accomplished with the Chiari osteotomy or perhaps a shelf procedure. Even after satisfactory alignment of the hip, resubluxation and dislocation can occur because of the progressive degeneration of the proximal muscles (270). These children require annual clinical and radiographic evaluation to assess the hips postoperatively. Thompson and Larsen (269) reported four cases of recurrent hip dislocation after corrective surgery. Two patients had second operations followed by recurrent dislocation. Therefore, these orthopaedists question the advisability of treatment of hip dislocations in patients with spinal muscular atrophy. Sporer and Smith (268) recently documented that patients with a hip dislocation had minimal pain or problems with sitting, and no difficulty with perineal care. They suggested observation rather than surgery for hip dislocation. Similar recommendations were recently made by Zenios et al. (271). Thus, treatment of hip subluxation and dislocation in spinal muscular atrophy is controversial. Each patient must be evaluated individually. The presence of pain, rather than the radiographic appearance of the hips, should be the main indication for treatment.

Spinal Deformity.

Most children with this condition who survive into adolescence develop a progressive spinal deformity. This occurs in 100% of the children and adolescents with Type II disease, and most of those with Type III, especially when they lose their ability to walk (261, 272–276). As in other neuromuscular disorders, the progression of the curve has an adverse effect on pulmonary function (274).

The deformity typically begins in the first decade of life because of severe truncal weakness. Once the deformity begins, it is steadily progressive and can reach a high magnitude of severity unless appropriately managed. The thoracolumbar paralytic C-shaped and single thoracic patterns, usually curved to the right, are most common. Approximately 30% of the children also have an associated kyphosis, which is also progressive (273, 276). In Type II spinal muscular atrophy, the mean expected increase in scoliosis is 8.3 degrees per year, whereas in Type III it is 2.9 degrees per year.

Orthotic Management. Bracing is ineffective in preventing or halting the progression of scoliosis or kyphosis in children with spinal muscular atrophy (252, 261, 272, 276–280). However, it can be effective in improving sitting balance and slowing the rate of progression in young ambulatory children (280). This has the advantage of allowing them to reach an older, more suitable age for undergoing surgical intervention. Orthotic treatment may help maintain overall posture, aid sitting posture, and slow the curve progression in younger nonambulatory children with deformities between 20 and 40 degrees. The TLSO is the most common orthosis used in children with spinal muscular atrophy. This orthosis must be carefully molded in order to distribute the forces over a large surface area. This is necessary for preventing skin irritation and breakdown, which is a major problem for children with neuromuscular diseases. Furumasu et al. (281) found that orthoses had the effect of decreasing the ability to function because of decreased spinal flexibility. It is also important to ensure that the TLSO does not further compromise the child's limited pulmonary functions. Occasionally, wheelchair modifications can also be effective in controlling truncal alignment and improving sitting posture (253). This may also be helpful in slowing the rate of curve progression. Unfortunately, almost all children with spinal muscular atrophy eventually require surgery for spinal deformity.

Surgery. The criteria for surgical spinal stabilization in spinal muscular atrophy include curve magnitude >40 degrees, satisfactory flexibility on supine lateral bending as seen on radiographs, and an FVC >40% of normal (251). When these criteria are met, a posterior spinal fusion with segmental spinal instrumentation techniques such as Luque rod instrumentation and sublaminar wires is used (Fig. 16-8) (116, 177, 123, 125, 126, 252, 272–275, 277–279, 281, 282). Other segmental spinal instrumentation systems can also be utilized. However, these do not usually distribute the forces of instrumentation throughout the spine as efficiently as the Luque rods with sublaminar wiring do. The spine is usually osteopenic, and there is a risk of bone failure unless the forces produced by instrumentation are minimized by extensive distribution. Fixation to the pelvis using the Galveston technique (130) or other techniques (133, 282) is common. In most children who are nonambulatory and have pelvic obliquity, fusion to the pelvis provides

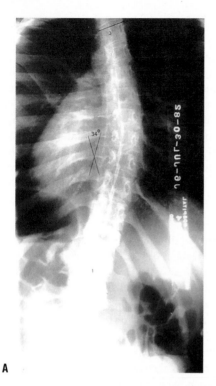

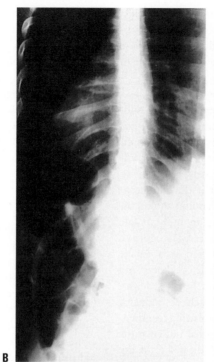

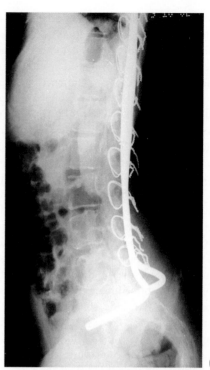

A   B   C

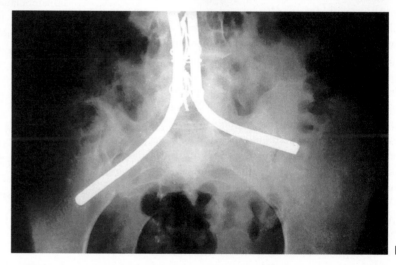

D

FIGURE 16-8. **A:** Sitting posteroanterior spinal radiograph of an 18-year-old woman with spinal muscular atrophy. A slowly progressive scoliosis has affected her wheelchair sitting balance. **B:** Postoperative radiograph after posterior spinal fusion and Luque rod instrumentation using the Galveston technique provided almost complete correction of the spinal deformity. Thirteen years postoperatively she functions independently despite the subsequent need for a tracheostomy and ventilator support. **C:** Lateral view demonstrates preservation of lumbar lordosis, which is important for proper sitting balance. **D:** Anteroposterior view of the pelvis shows proper positioning of the Luque rods in the ilium. They should penetrate as far into the ilium as possible for maximum strength.

improved spinopelvic stability and alignment. Anterior spinal fusion and instrumentation are rarely indicated in view of the compromised pulmonary status of these children, which could predispose them to pulmonary complications postoperatively (279). Anterior fusions alone are too short to adequately stabilize the entire spine. When the procedure is performed, it is combined with a simultaneous or staged posterior spinal fusion, usually with Luque rod instrumentation (116). Whatever posterior instrumentation system is used, it is important to ensure that no postoperative immobilization is necessary; this enhances sitting balance and pulmonary status and makes transfers easier.

Patients experience a decrease in function after spine fusion (272, 281). Although spinal alignment and sitting balance are improved, the loss of spinal mobility decreases the function of the upper extremities and activities of daily living such as performing transfers and maintaining personal hygiene. Askin et al. (283) recommended early surgery to preserve function. They found as well that the patient's functional ability may not improve following surgery, but the cosmetic results are gratifying, and the caregivers also find it easier to carry out their tasks. Bridwell et al. (123) reported improved function, self-image, cosmesis, and caregiver ability in 21 patients with spinal muscular atrophy followed for a mean of 7.8 years postoperatively (range 2 to 12.6 years). Growing rods or rods that can be elongated periodically may be helpful in young children with spinal muscular atrophy who have severe deformities (284). This allows definitive surgery to be delayed until an older age. Pelvic fixation can be used as a distal foundation (285).

Operative complications are similar to those in other neuromuscular disorders. These include excessive blood loss, pulmonary complications, neurologic injury, wound infection, loss of fixation (caused by osteopenia), pseudarthrosis, and even death (115, 272, 276, 277, 279, 282). The use of segmental spinal instrumentation techniques and aggressive preoperative and postoperative respiratory therapy may lead to fewer complications. Hypotensive anesthesia and intraoperative spinal cord monitoring may be helpful in decreasing intraoperative blood loss and neurologic injury. Noordeen et al. (149) reported that a 50% decrease in amplitude of motor action potential may be indicative of an impending neurologic injury.

FRIEDREICH ATAXIA

Spinocerebellar degenerative diseases are a group of relatively uncommon disorders that are hereditary and progressive. Friedreich ataxia is the most common form and has orthopaedic implications because it is associated with a high incidence of scoliosis. In whites, this disorder accounts for up to half of all cases of hereditary ataxia (286). Friedreich ataxia is characterized by slow, progressive spinocerebellar degeneration. It occurs in approximately 1 in 50,000 live births. It is autosomal recessive and occurs most commonly in North America in people of French–Canadian heritage. Both sexes are affected equally.

Clinical Features. Friedreich ataxia is characterized by a clinical triad consisting of (i) ataxia (which is usually the presenting symptom); (ii) areflexia of the knees and ankles; and (iii) a positive plantar response, or the Babinski sign (253, 286). Geoffroy et al. (287) established strict criteria for the clinical diagnosis of typical Friedreich ataxia. This has been modified by Harding (288, 289). The primary symptoms and signs that occur in all affected patients include onset before the age of 25 years; progressive ataxia of limbs and gait; absent knee and ankle deep-tendon reflexes; positive plantar response; decreased nerve conduction velocities in the upper extremities, with small or absent sensory action potentials; and dysarthria. The secondary symptoms and signs that are present in more than 90% of the cases include scoliosis, pyramidal weakness in the lower extremities, absent reflexes in the upper extremities, loss of position and vibratory sense in the lower extremities, and an abnormal ECG. Supplementary symptoms and signs are present in fewer than 50% of the cases. These include optic atrophy, nystagmus, distal weakness and wasting, partial deafness, pes cavus, and diabetes mellitus.

The mean age at onset is between 7 and 15 years, although the range is wide, from the age of 4 years to as late as 25 years (253, 286–290). Most of the patients lose their ability to walk and are wheelchair bound by the second or third decade of life. Labelle et al. (291) demonstrated that the muscle weakness is always symmetric, initially proximal rather than distal, more severe in the lower extremities, and rapidly progressive when the patients become nonambulatory. The first muscle to be involved is the hip extensor (gluteus maximus). They also demonstrated that muscle weakness is not the primary cause of loss of ambulatory function. Ataxia and other factors also play a role. Death usually occurs in the fourth or fifth decade because of progressive hypertrophic cardiomyopathy, pneumonia, or aspiration (286, 288).

Nerve conduction studies show decreased or absent sensory action potentials in the digital and sural nerves. Conduction velocity in the motor and sensory fibers of the median and tibial nerves is moderately slowed. An EMG shows a loss of motor units and an increase in polyphasic potentials. The ECG in adults typically shows a progressive hypertrophic cardiomyopathy. Hematologic tests such as CPK are normal, but there is increased incidence of clinical and chemical diabetes mellitus.

Genetic and Molecular Biology Studies.
Chamberlain et al. (292) have demonstrated that individuals with Friedreich ataxia have a defect on chromosome 9q13. Additional studies have identified two loci on chromosome 9 (*D9S5* and *D9S15*) that are linked to Friedreich ataxia (293). It is now known that this condition is caused by a trinucleotide repeat of GAA, which causes loss of expression of the frataxin protein. There is an inverse relation between the number of trinucleotide repeats and the age at onset of the disease (294). Various medications such as physostigmine, tryptophan, buspirone, and amantadine have been tried for symptomatic treatment, with generally disappointing results (295–300). DNA testing is available and is the diagnostic test of choice.

Treatment. The major orthopaedic problems in Friedreich ataxia are pes cavovarus, spinal deformity, and painful muscle spasms (253, 286).

Pes Cavovarus. Pes cavovarus is common in patients with Friedreich ataxia. It is slowly progressive and tends to become rigid. When combined with ataxia, it can result in decreased ability to stand and walk. Orthotic management is usually ineffective in preventing the deformity, but an AFO can be used after surgery to stabilize the foot and ankle and to prevent recurrent deformity. Surgical procedures can be used in ambulatory patients to improve balance and walking ability. Procedures that have been shown to be effective include tendo-Achilles lengthening and tibialis posterior tenotomy, lengthening, or anterior transfer to the dorsum of the foot (253, 286). The tibialis anterior muscle may also be involved and may require tenotomy, lengthening, or centralization to the dorsum of the foot to prevent recurrence. In fixed, rigid deformities, a triple arthrodesis may be necessary for achieving a plantigrade foot.

Spinal Deformity. Scoliosis occurs in almost all patients with Friedreich ataxia (286, 288, 301–304). The age at onset is variable and usually begins while the patient is still ambulatory. The incidence of curve progression has been shown to correlate to the age at clinical onset of the disease process. Labelle et al. (303) demonstrated that when the disease onset is before the age of 10 years and scoliosis occurs before the age of 15 years, most scoliotic curves progress to >60 degrees and require surgical intervention. When the disease onset is after the age of 10 years and the scoliosis occurs after the age of 15 years, the curve progression is not as severe; most do not reach 40 degrees by skeletal maturity, and do not progress thereafter. There was found to be no correlation between curve progression, degree of muscle weakness, level of ambulatory function, and duration of the disease process. The patterns of scoliosis in patients with Friedreich ataxia are similar to those in adolescent idiopathic scoliosis rather than to those in neuromuscular scoliosis. The pathogenesis of scoliosis in Friedreich ataxia appears to be not muscle weakness but ataxia that causes a disturbance of equilibrium and postural reflexes. Double major (i.e., thoracic and lumbar) and single thoracic or thoracolumbar curves are the most common curve patterns (301–304). Only a few patients have lumbar or long C-shaped thoracolumbar curves. About two-thirds of these patients develop an associated kyphosis >40 degrees (303). The treatment of scoliosis in Friedreich ataxia can be by either orthotic or surgical methods.

Orthoses. A TLSO may be tried in ambulatory patients having 25- to 40-degree curves. It is usually not well tolerated, but it may slow the rate of progression although it rarely stabilizes the curve (263, 276, 304). In ambulatory patients, an orthosis may interfere with walking because it prevents the compensatory truncal movement that is necessary for balance and movement.

Surgery. In progressive curves >60 degrees, especially in older adolescents confined to wheelchairs, a single-stage posterior spinal fusion stabilizes the curve and yields moderate correction. Curves between 40 and 60 degrees can be either observed or treated surgically, depending on the patient's age at clinical onset, the age when scoliosis was first recognized, and evidence of curve progression. Posterior segmental spinal instrumentation using Harrington rods and sublaminar wires or Luque rod instrumentation has been demonstrated to be effective in achieving correction and a solid arthrodesis (115, 301–303). Other segmental spinal instrumentation systems will also be effective (304). Fusions are typically from the upper thoracic (T2 or T3) to lower lumbar regions. Fusion to the sacrum is usually unnecessary, except in C-shaped thoracolumbar curves with associated pelvic obliquity (302). Autogenous bone supplemented with banked bone, when necessary, usually produces a solid fusion. Anterior surgery, with or without instrumentation, usually followed by a posterior spinal fusion and instrumentation, is limited to rigid curves that are >60 degrees and associated with poor sitting balance. Intraoperative spinal cord monitoring using somatosensory evoked potentials are usually ineffective (304). Surgery is performed only after a thorough cardiopulmonary evaluation and under careful intraoperative and postoperative monitoring. Postoperative immobilization should be avoided. Vertebral osteopenia and spinal stenosis are not problems in Friedreich ataxia.

Painful Muscle Spasms. Painful muscle spasms occur in some patients with Friedreich ataxia (253). They usually begin in the late adolescent or early adult years and worsen with time. The spasms are characterized by a sudden onset and short duration. The hip adductors and the knee extensors are commonly involved. Initial treatment is usually massage, warming, and perhaps muscle relaxants, such as diazepam and Baclofen. In adults, if the adductor or quadriceps spasms are interfering with perineal care or sitting balance, the patient may benefit from tenotomies. However, this is rarely necessary.

HEREDITARY MOTOR SENSORY NEUROPATHIES

HMSNs are a large group of variously inherited neuropathic disorders (253, 286, 305). Charcot-Marie-Tooth disease is the prototype, but there are other disorders with similar but different manifestations.

Classification. The classification system for HMSN is presented in Table 16-2 HMSN Types I, II, and III are encountered predominantly in pediatric orthopaedic and neuromuscular clinics, whereas HMSN Types IV, V, VI, and VII tend to be late-onset and occur in adults (253).

HMSN Type I is an autosomal dominant disorder, and includes disorders referred to as peroneal atrophy, Charcot-Marie-Tooth disease (hypertrophic form), or Roussy-Levy syndrome. It is a demyelinating disorder that is characterized by peroneal muscle weakness, absent deep-tendon reflexes, and slow nerve conduction velocities. HMSN Type II is the neuronal form of Charcot-Marie-Tooth disease with progressive axon loss. It is characterized by persistently normal reflexes, sensory and motor nerve conduction times that are only mildly abnormal, decreased compound motor action potentials, and variable inheritance patterns (253). These two types are clinically

TABLE 16-2	Classification of Hereditary Motor Sensory Neuropathies	
Type	**Name(s)**	**Inheritance**
I	Peroneal atrophy, Charcot-Marie-Tooth syndrome (hypertrophic form), or Roussy-Levy syndrome (areflexic dystaxia)	Autosomal dominant
II	Charcot-Marie-Tooth syndrome (neuronal form)	Variable
III	Dejerine-Sottas disease	Autosomal recessive
IV	Refsum disease	
V	Neuropathy with spastic paraplegia	
VI	Optic atrophy with peroneal muscle atrophy	
VII	Retinitis pigmentosa with distal muscle weakness and atrophy	

similar, although HMSN Type II often causes less severe weakness and has a later onset than HMSN Type I. HMSN Type III is the autosomal recessive disorder, Dejerine-Sottas disease. This disorder begins in infancy and is characterized by more severe alterations in nerve conduction and by sensory disturbances that are more extensive than in HMSN Types I and II. The HMSN Types I and III are caused by demyelinization of peripheral nerves, whereas Type II is caused by axon loss. These are characterized by muscle weakness in the feet and hands, absent deep-tendon reflexes, and diminution of distal sensory capabilities, particularly light touch position and vibratory sensation (253).

The four additional types are of late onset, and are rarely seen by pediatric orthopaedists or in pediatric neuromuscular clinics: HMSN Type IV, Refsum disease, is characterized by excessive phytanic acid; HMSN Type V is an inherited spastic paraplegia, with distal weakness in the limbs presenting in the second decade of life, and characterized by an awkward gait and equinus foot deformities; HMSN Type VI is characterized by optic atrophy in association with peroneal muscle atrophy; and HMSN Type VII is associated with retinitis pigmentosa, distal weakness in the limbs, and muscle atrophy.

Diagnostic Studies. Diagnosis of HMSN is made by physical examination, in combination with EMG, nerve conduction studies, and genetic testing. The EMG findings in HMSN show typical neuropathic changes, with increased amplitude and duration of response. Nerve conduction studies in patients with the demyelinating HMSN Types I and III show marked slowing of the rate of impulse conduction in the muscles involved. A biopsy specimen of a muscle such as the gastrocnemius demonstrates typical neuropathic findings, including atrophy of the fiber group, with all of the fibers in an abnormal group having uniformly small diameter. A biopsy specimen of a peripheral nerve, usually the sural nerve, shows typical demyelinization, confirming the diagnosis of peripheral neuropathy.

Genetic and Molecular Biology Studies. Many individuals with HMSN Type I have a DNA duplication of a portion of the short arm of chromosome 17 in the region of p11.2 to p12 (17, 306–308). Additional studies have shown a human peripheral myelin protein-22 gene to be contained within the duplication (309–311). It is thought that the abnormality in the peripheral myelin protein-22 gene, which encodes the myelin protein, has a causative role in Charcot-Marie-Tooth disease. Either a point mutation in peripheral myelin protein-22 or duplication of the region that contains the peripheral myelin protein-22 gene can result in the disorder (312).

HMSN Type II is heterogeneous in its inheritance mode, occurring either as an autosomal dominant or as an autosomal recessive trait (313). Chromosome linkage has been identified at 1p35–36 (314), at 8p21 involving the neurofilament-light gene (315), and on 7q11-q21 (316). HMSN Type III, previously referred to as Dejerine-Sottas disease, also shows genetic

heterogeneity, with multiple loci identified to date. Inheritance typically follows an autosomal recessive pattern.

Confirmatory diagnosis can be made by DNA testing.

Treatment. Children with HMSN typically present with gait disturbance or foot deformities. The severity of involvement is variable. In severe involvement, there may be proximal muscle weakness. The major orthopaedic problems include pes cavovarus, hip dysplasia, spinal deformity, and hand and upper extremity dysfunction.

Historically, the mainstay in the treatment of the HMSNs has been the orthopaedic approach. Recently, however, there have been promising results with the use of progesterone receptor antagonists. In transgenic rat studies, administration of selective progesterone receptor antagonists led to decreased overexpression of PMP22 and improved CMT phenotype (317). Presently, human studies are underway and appear promising (318).

Pes Cavovarus. The pathogenesis of cavovarus deformities in children with HMSN and other neuromuscular disorders is becoming better understood (319–325). The components of the pes cavovarus deformity include claw toes; plantar-flexed first metatarsal with adduction and inversion of the remaining metatarsals; midfoot malposition of the navicular, cuboid, and cuneiforms, leading to a high arch (cavus); and hindfoot varus malposition between the talus and calcaneus (Fig. 16-9). Initially, HMSNs affect the more distal muscles. The mildest cases show involvement of the toes and forefoot, whereas the midfoot and hindfoot are progressively affected with progression of the disease process. In a computed tomography study of 26 patients with HMSN I, II, or III, Price et al. (326) found that the interossei and lumbrical muscles of the feet demonstrated earlier and more severe involvement than the extrinsic muscles. These intrinsic muscles have the most distal innervation. Even with minimal weakness, the invertor muscles, such as the tibialis anterior and tibialis posterior muscles, are stronger than the evertors, such as the peroneus longus; this relation favors the development of adduction and varus deformities.

Pes cavovarus deformities are progressive, but the rate is variable, even among patients belonging to the same family. Initially, the deformity is flexible but later becomes rigid. Shapiro and Specht (253) identify the plantar-flexed first metatarsal as the key finding. As the first metatarsal becomes increasingly plantar flexed, increasing hindfoot varus and supination and cavus of the forefoot and midfoot follow. The block test is useful for determining the mobility of the remainder of the foot in children with a rigid plantar-flexed first metatarsal (322).

The goals in the treatment of foot deformities in children with HMSN include maintenance of a straight, plantigrade, and relatively flexible foot during growth (324, 325, 327). This maximizes function and minimizes the development of osseous deformities that may require more extensive surgery (such as a triple arthrodesis) in adolescence and early adult years.

The treatment options for the management of foot deformities include plantar release, plantar–medial release,

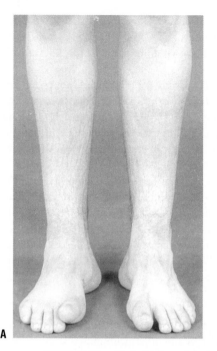
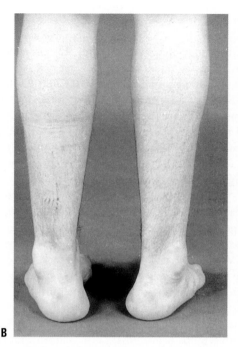
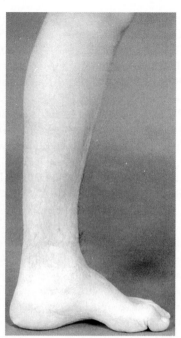

FIGURE 16-9. **A:** Front view of the lower legs and feet of a 16-year-old boy with hereditary motor sensory neuropathy Type I (i.e., Charcot-Marie-Tooth disease). His calves are thin, and he has mildly symptomatic cavus feet. Clawing of the toes is minimal. **B:** Posterior view demonstrates moderate heel varus. **C:** The cavus foot deformity is most apparent when viewed from the medial side. A mild flexion deformity of the great toe interphalangeal joint is present.

tendon transfers, calcaneal osteotomy, midtarsal osteotomy, triple arthrodesis, and correction of toe deformities (321, 322, 324, 325).

Plantar Release. In children younger than 10 years with a mild cavovarus deformity, a plantar release may be helpful in correcting the plantar-flexed first metatarsal and providing correction of the associated flexible deformities of the hindfoot and midfoot (328). In the radical plantar release described by Paulos et al. (322), selective Z-lengthening of the long toe flexor tendons and the tibialis posterior tendon are performed if there is a "bowstring" effect after plantar release.

Plantar–Medial Release. In a child younger than 10 years, if the hindfoot deformity is rigid and leading to fixed varus deformity, the plantar release may be combined with a medial release (322). The medial structures to be released include the ligamentous and capsular structures between the talus and calcaneus (except the posterior talocalcaneal ligament), and the capsule of the talonavicular joints. The navicular is then reduced onto the head of the talus and secured with a smooth Steinmann pin. The posterior ankle and subtalar joint ligaments and the tendo-Achilles are not disturbed because they are necessary for counterresistance during postoperative serial casting. Once the incision has healed, a series of corrective weight-bearing casts are applied. Excellent correction of the entire foot has been reported after this technique.

Tendon Transfers. In children and adolescents with flexible cavovarus deformities in which active inversion is associated with relative weakness of the evertor muscles, a transfer of the tibialis anterior tendon to the dorsum of the midtarsal region in line with the third metatarsal may be helpful (329). The transfer is designed to balance strength, but the foot must be aligned initially by a plantar release and perhaps the plantar–medial release.

Other tendinous procedures that may be used depend on the individual needs of the patient. These may include tendo-Achilles lengthening, anterior transfer at the tibialis posterior tendon, long toe extensors to the metatarsals or midfoot, and flexor-to-extensor tendon transfers for claw toes (322, 329). Tendo-Achilles lengthening is rarely necessary, as the equinus is due to the plantar-flexed first metatarsal and forefoot. The hindfoot is typically in a calcaneus position.

Calcaneal Osteotomy. In children who are younger than 10 years and who have mild but fixed deformity, a calcaneal osteotomy may be helpful in correcting the varus deformity of the hindfoot (253). This osteotomy does not interfere with growth because it is not made through a cartilaginous growth area. To allow lateral translation, the osteotomy is cut slightly obliquely, passing from a superior position on the lateral surface to a more inferior position on the medial surface. It is possible to translate the distal fragment by as much as one-third of its transverse diameter, thereby allowing conversion of weight bearing from varus to mild valgus. In patients who are older than 10 years or who are more severely affected, a lateral closing-wedge calcaneal osteotomy, with lateral translation of the distal and posterior fragments, is performed (Fig. 16-10) (253). In both procedures, the osteotomy is stabilized with staples or Steinmann pins.

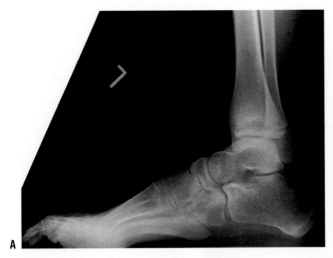
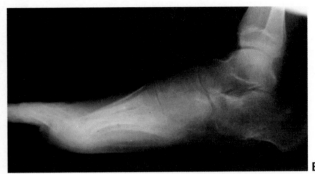

FIGURE 16-10. **A:** Moderate cavovarus deformity of the left foot in a 14-year-old boy with Charcot-Marie-Tooth disease. His condition was managed with a closing-wedge valgus osteotomy at the calcaneus, an opening-wedge, plantar-based osteotomy of the medial cuneiform, and soft-tissue balancing. **B:** Postoperatively, the cavovarus deformity has been improved. He is a brace-free ambulator because of restoration of muscle balance.

Metatarsal Osteotomy. The metatarsal osteotomy provides correction by removal of a dorsal and slightly laterally based wedge, with the proximal osteotomy cut through the acicular and cuboids, and the distal cut through the cuboids and three cuneiforms. Moderate deformities can be corrected satisfactorily with this procedure, especially if it is augmented with a plantar release, calcaneal osteotomy, and perhaps an anterior transfer of the tibialis anterior tendon. Equinus deformities of the midfoot and varus deformities of the forefoot can be corrected with appropriate wedge resections. Growth retardation and limitation of mobility are minimal when compared with the situation after a triple arthrodesis. Recently, the use of the Ilizarov external fixator and a V-osteotomy has been shown to be effective in achieving a painless plantigrade foot (330). This approach can obviate the need for a triple arthrodesis in selected patients. Recently, Ward et al. (331) reported very long-term results of 25 patients (41 ft) treated with a base at the first metatarsal osteotomy, transfer of the extensor hallucis longus to the metatarsal neck, a plantar release, transfer of the peroneus longus to the peroneus brevis, and, in a few selected cases, centralization of the tibialis anterior tendon. At a mean follow-up of 26.1 years, the feet were functioning well. They had a slight increase in hindfoot varus and low evidence of ankle degenerative osteoarthritis.

Triple Arthrodesis. In adolescents who have reached skeletal maturity and who have a severe deformity, walk with difficulty, and cannot run, a triple arthrodesis may be performed. Every attempt should be made to avoid this procedure because of the associated complications of undercorrection, overcorrection, pseudoarthrosis of the talonavicular joint, and degenerative changes in the ankle and midfoot joints (332–335).

Wetmore and Drennan (334) reported unsatisfactory results in 23 of 30 ft (16 patients) at a mean follow-up at 21 years. The progressive muscle imbalance resulted in recurrent pes cavovarus deformities. There was also an increased incidence of degenerative osteoarthritis of the ankle as a consequence of the deformity and the loss of subtalar joint motion. These surgeons were of the opinion that triple arthrodesis should be limited to patients with severe, rigid deformities. Saltzman et al. (336) reported similar results in 67 ft in 57 patients, including 6 ft in patients with Charcot-Marie-Tooth disease, at 25 and 44 years of mean follow-up. However, 95% of the patients were satisfied with the clinical results.

The Ryerson triple arthrodesis is preferred because the surfaces of the talocalcaneal, talonavicular, and calcaneal cuboids joints are removed, along with appropriate-sized wedges to correct the various components of the hindfoot and midfoot deformities (Fig. 16-11). In patients who have marked equinus of the midfoot and forefoot in relation to a relatively well-positioned hindfoot, the Lambrinudi triple arthrodesis may be performed (337). Once an arthrodesis has been performed to straighten the foot, tendon transfers to balance muscle power are of great importance.

Toe deformities in adolescent patients or in those who have undergone a triple arthrodesis may be corrected by proximal and distal interphalangeal fusion or flexor-to-extensor tendon transfer. The great toe may require an interphalangeal joint fusion and transfer of the extensor hallucis longus from the proximal phalanx to the neck of the first metatarsal (Jones procedure). The latter then serves as a foot dorsiflexor.

Hip Dysplasia. Hip dysplasia in HMSN occurs in approximately 6% to 8% of the children who are affected (338, 339). Occasionally, hips may be dislocatable at birth, although the neuropathy does not become apparent for several years. It is more likely to occur in HMSN Type I than in HMSN Type II

FIGURE 16-11.   **A:** Anteroposterior radiograph of severe cavovarus deformity of the right foot in a 14-year-old boy with Charcot-Marie-Tooth disease, in standing posture. **B:** Lateral radiograph demonstrates a varus hindfoot and midfoot, and a plantar flexed first metatarsal. **C:** Postoperative anteroposterior radiograph, taken in standing posture, following a Ryerson triple arthrodesis, soft-tissue balancing, and correction of his claw toe deformities. **D:** Lateral radiograph showing markedly improved alignment.

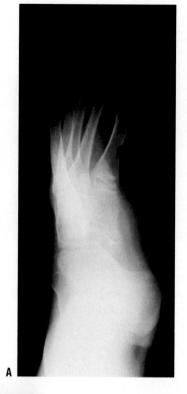
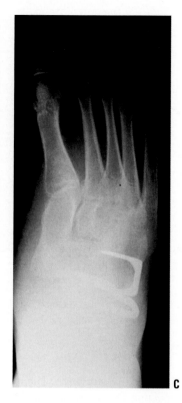
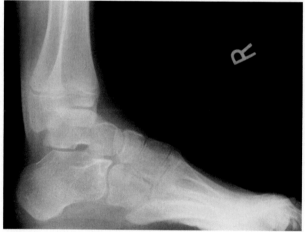
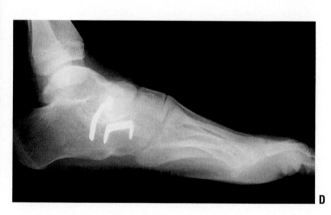

because of the more severe neurologic involvement in the former. Walker et al. (339) proposed that the slight muscle weakness about the hip in growing children with HMSN may be sufficient to distort growth and development, leading to dysplasia. Usually, hip dysplasia is diagnosed between the ages of 5 and 15 years following mild discomfort (338–341). However, dysplasia may be present in asymptomatic patients (Fig. 16-12). Annual anteroposterior radiographs of the pelvis have been recommended to allow early diagnosis and treatment. Typical radiographic findings include acetabular dysplasia, coxa valga, and subluxation. The treatment of HMSN hip dysplasia includes soft-tissue releases to correct contractures and restore muscle balance, and pelvic or proximal femoral varus derotation osteotomies, or both, to stabilize and

adequately realign the hip (338, 340–343). The type of pelvic osteotomy is determined by the patient's age and the severity of the dysplasia. Rotational osteotomies (Salter, Steel) are useful in many children with mild dysplasia, whereas periacetabular osteotomies are useful in adolescents and young adults (342), and the Chiari osteotomy (343) is used when there is severe dysplasia.

Spinal Deformity.   Scoliosis occurs in approximately 15% of children with HMSN (344, 345). These children are usually ambulatory, with age of onset of spinal deformity of approximately 12 years. A study by Walker et al. (346) found a 37% incidence of scoliosis or kyphoscoliosis in children with HMSN. A more recent large study by Karol and Elerson (345)

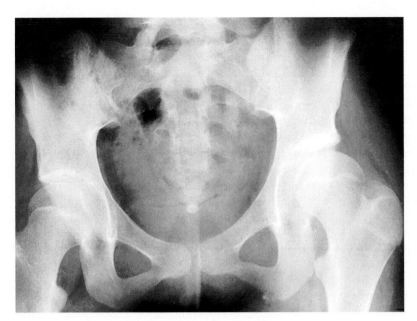

FIGURE 16-12. Anteroposterior pelvic radiograph of a 15-year-old girl with Charcot-Marie-Tooth disease. Asymptomatic acetabular dysplasia of the left hip is visible. The medial joint is slightly widened. The Shenton line is disrupted, and the center-edge angle is 16 degrees. This condition was first observed 6 years earlier and did not progress.

demonstrated a 15% incidence. The incidence increases to 50% in those who were skeletally mature. Spinal deformity is more common in girls and in HMSN Type I. Curve progression requiring orthoses or surgery is common. The curve patterns and management are similar to those in idiopathic adolescent scoliosis, except for an increased incidence of left-sided thoracic curves and associated kyphosis (345). As a consequence, orthotic management can be effective in arresting progression of the deformity. If progression reaches 45 to 50 degrees, a posterior spinal fusion and segmental spinal instrumentation similar to idiopathic scoliosis can effectively stabilize and partially correct the deformity (344, 345). Intraoperative spinal cord monitoring with somatosensory cortical-evoked potentials may show no signal transmission (345, 347). This is because of the demyelinization of the peripheral nerves and perhaps the degeneration of the dorsal root ganglion and dorsal column of the spinal cord. A wake-up test may need to be performed.

Hand and Upper Extremity Dysfunction. The upper extremities are involved in about two-thirds of individuals with HMSN (348, 349). The involvement tends to be milder, however, and does not appear until a later age. Intrinsic muscle weakness with decreased stability is a relatively common finding. In a study of 68 patients with Charcot-Marie-Tooth disease, the mean age at onset of symptoms in the hands and upper extremities was 19 years. Intrinsic muscle function was initially impaired, and patients became aware of motor weakness and a lack of dexterity. Sensory changes such as numbness are usually present concomitantly. Physical and occupational therapy may be helpful. In some patients, operative intervention, such as transfer of the flexor digitorum sublimis to restore opposition, nerve compression releases, soft-tissue contracture releases, and joint arthrodeses, may be effective in improving function. Preoperative EMG has been shown to aid in

selecting optimal forearm muscles for tendon transfers to the hand (350).

POLIOMYELITIS

Acute poliomyelitis results from an acute viral infection, with localization in the anterior horn cells of the spinal cord and certain brain stem motor nuclei. It is caused by one of three poliomyelitis viruses known as *Brunhilde* (Type 1), *Lansing* (Type 2), and *Leon* (Type 3). Humans are the natural host for poliomyelitis virus, transmitting the disease by the oropharyngeal route. The poliomyelitis viruses have varying virulence. Most poliomyelitis virus infections have an abortive course, with only mild gastrointestinal symptoms. Fewer than 1% of infections develop into the paralytic form of the disease. The development of prophylactic vaccines has greatly reduced the incidence of polio, although the disease remains a major health problem in developing countries. Fewer than 10 cases occur in the United States annually, and these most commonly result from administering the active oral polio vaccine (351, 352).

Pathology. The poliomyelitis virus invades the body through the oropharyngeal route and multiplies in the gastrointestinal tract lymph nodes before spreading to the CNS by the hematogenous route. The incubation period ranges from 6 to 20 days. Motor neurons in the anterior horn cells of the spinal cord and brain stem are acutely attacked. In the spinal cord, the lumbar and cervical regions are particularly involved. The medulla, cerebellum, and midbrain may also be involved. Except for the motor areas, the white matter of the spinal cord and the cerebral cortex are uninvolved.

Damage to the anterior horn cells may be caused directly by viral multiplication and toxic by-products of the virus, or indirectly from ischemia, edema, and hemorrhage in the glial tissues surrounding the anterior horn cells. In addition to acute inflammatory cellular reaction, edema with perivascular mononuclear cuffing occurs.

The inflammatory response gradually subsides, and the necrotic ganglion cells are surrounded and partially dissolved by macrophages and neutrophils. After 4 months, the spinal cord is left with residual areas of gliosis and lymphocytic cell collections occupying the area of the destroyed motor cells. Evidence of continuous disease activity has been found in spinal cord segments examined two decades after the onset of the disease. Histopathologic sections demonstrate a loss or atrophy of motor neurons, severe reaction gliosis, and mild-to-moderate perivascular interparenchymal inflammation, with sparing of corticospinal tracts. The skeletal muscle demonstrates gross atrophy and histologic tests show that this lost muscle has been replaced with fat and connective tissue. The percentage of motor units destroyed in an individual muscle varies markedly, and the resultant clinical weakness is proportionate to the number of lost motor units. Sharrard (353) reported that clinically detectable weakness is present only when more than 60% of the motor nerve cells supplying the muscle have been destroyed. The muscles involved may range from those of just one extremity to those of all four extremities, the trunk, and the bulbar musculature.

Muscles innervated by the cervical and lumbar segments are the ones most frequently involved. However, involvement occurs twice as frequently in the lower extremity as in the upper extremity muscles. Sharrard (354) combined clinical and histologic studies that demonstrated that muscles with short motor nerve cell columns are often severely paralyzed, whereas those with long motor cell columns are more frequently left paretic or weak. The quadriceps, tibialis anterior, medial hamstrings, and hip flexors are the lumbar innervated muscles most frequently involved. The deltoid, triceps, and pectoralis major are most frequently affected in the upper extremities. The sacral nerve roots are usually spared, resulting in the characteristic preservation of the intrinsic muscles of the foot (355).

Recovery of muscle function depends on return to function of the anterior horn cells that have been damaged but not destroyed. Clinical recovery begins during the first month after the acute illness and is nearly complete by the 6th month, although there is limited potential for additional recovery through the 2nd year. Sharrard (353) has stated that the mean final grade of a muscle is two grades above its assessment at 1 month and one grade above it at 6 months.

Disease Stages. Management of poliomyelitis varies according to the stage of the disease process. The stages are designated as acute, convalescent, or chronic. Because the acute and convalescent stages are rarely encountered in this country, orthopaedic management is usually confined to the chronic stage. Every year, most pediatric orthopaedic programs see several children with poliomyelitis in the chronic stage. These children have usually been adopted from nonindustrialized nations or from parents who have immigrated from such countries.

Acute Stage. Acute poliomyelitis may cause symptoms ranging from mild malaise to generalized encephalomyelitis with widespread paralysis. Diagnosis is based on clinical findings, because there are no diagnostic laboratory tests. This phase generally lasts 7 to 10 days. The return to normal temperature for 48 hours and the absence of progressive muscle involvement indicates the end of the acute phase. This phase is usually managed by pediatricians because there may be medical problems, especially respiratory, that may be life threatening.

The orthopedist should be familiar with the clinical signs of acute poliomyelitis. Meningismus is reflected in the characteristic flexor posturing of the upper and lower extremities. The muscles involved are tender, even to gentle palpation. Clinical examination can be difficult because of pain during the acute stage.

Orthopaedic treatment during this phase emphasizes prevention of deformity and ensuring comfort. This approach consists of physical therapy with gentle, passive range-of-motion exercises and splinting. Muscle spasms, which can lead to shortening and contractures, may respond to the application of warm, moist heat. This can relieve muscle sensitivity and discomfort. Sharrard (353) emphasized that rapid loss of elasticity, coupled with shortening of tendons, fascia, and ligaments, leads to contractures.

Convalescent Stage. The convalescent phase of poliomyelitis begins 2 days after the temperature returns to normal and progression of the paralytic disease ceases. The phase continues for 2 years, during which spontaneous improvement of muscle power occurs. The assessment of the rate of recovery in poliomyelitis is made by serial examination of the muscle strength. Muscle assessment should be performed once every month for 6 months and then at 3-month intervals during the remainder of the convalescent stage.

Any muscle that demonstrates <30% of normal strength at 3 months after the acute phase should be considered to be permanently paralyzed. Muscles showing evidence of more than 80% return of strength require no specific therapy. Muscles that fall between these two parameters retain the potential for useful function, and therapy should be directed toward recreating hypertrophy of the remaining muscle fibers.

The treatment goals during this phase include efforts to prevent contractures and deformity, restoration and maintenance of normal range of motion of the joints, and help for individual muscles to achieve maximum possible recovery. Physical therapy and orthotics are the main treatment modalities. Physical therapy is directed toward having individual muscles assume maximum capability within their pattern of normal motor activity and not permitting adaptive or substitute patterns of associated muscles to persist. Hydrotherapy can also be helpful in achieving these goals. Orthoses, both ambulatory and nighttime, are necessary for supporting the extremity during this phase.

Chronic Stage. The chronic stage of poliomyelitis begins after 2 years, and it is during this stage that the orthopedist assumes responsibility for the long-term management resulting from muscle imbalance (356).

The management goal during the chronic stage is to achieve maximal functional capacity. This is accomplished by restoring muscle balance, preventing or correcting soft-tissue contractures, correcting osseous deformities, and directing allied personnel, such as physical therapists, occupational therapists, and orthotists. Using this approach, Arora and Tandon (357) have shown that ambulation can be restored in patients who could only crawl earlier (328). Therefore, each patient requires a careful evaluation to determine what procedures may be effective in restoring ambulation, if possible, and maximizing function.

Treatment

Soft-Tissue Contractures.
Flaccid paralysis, muscle imbalance, and growth all contribute to soft-tissue contractures and fixed deformities in poliomyelitis. Contractures result from the increased mechanical advantage of the stronger muscles that continue the attenuation of their weaker antagonists. The greater the disparity in muscle balance, the sooner a contracture may develop.

Instability of a joint does not result in a fixed deformity, except in cases where it is allowed to persist over a period of years in a growing child. Static instability can be controlled readily and indefinitely by orthoses. Dynamic instability of a joint readily produces a fixed deformity, and orthotic control is difficult. Deformities are initially confined to soft tissues, but later, bone growth and joint alignment may also be affected.

The age at onset of poliomyelitis is significant. The osseous growth potential of young children makes them more vulnerable to secondary osseous deformities. The worst deformities occur in young children and those with severe muscle imbalance. Release of soft-tissue contractures and appropriate tendon transfers performed in a young child are crucial for preventing structural changes.

Tendon Transfers.
Achievement of muscle balance in patients with dynamic instability effectively halts progression of paralytic deformity. Tendon transfers are performed when dynamic muscle imbalance is sufficient to produce deformity, and when orthotic protection is required. Transfers should be delayed until the paralyzed muscle has been given adequate postural treatment to ensure that it has regained maximum strength and that the proposed tendon transfer is really required. The objectives of tendon transfer are to provide active motor power to replace function of a paralyzed muscle or muscles, to eliminate the deformity caused by a muscle when its antagonist is paralyzed, and to produce stability through better muscle balance.

The muscle to be transferred should be rated good or fair before transfer, and must have adequate strength to actively perform the desired function. On an average, one grade of motor power is lost after muscle transfer. The length and range of motion of the transferred muscle and that of the muscle being replaced must be similar. Loss of original function resulting from tendon transfers must be balanced against potential gains. Free passive range of motion is essential in the absence of deformity at the joint to be moved by the tendon transfer. A transfer as an adjunct to bony stabilization cannot be expected to overcome a fixed deformity. The smooth gliding channel for the tendon transfer is essential. A traumatic handling of the muscle tissue can prevent injury to its neurovascular supply and prevent adhesions. The tendon should be rooted in a straight line between its origin and new insertion. Attachment of the tendon transfer should be under sufficient tension to correspond to normal physiologic conditions and should allow the transferred muscle to achieve a maximum range of contraction.

Osteotomies.
Osseous deformities may produce deformities in the joints, and thereby impair the alignment of the extremities, mostly the lower extremities, and limit their ability to function. Osteotomies can be helpful in restoring alignment and improving function. Because of possible recurrence during subsequent growth, these procedures are usually postponed, if possible, until late childhood or early adolescence.

Arthrodeses.
Arthrodeses are usually performed for salvage, except in the foot where a subtalar, triple, or pantalar arthrodesis may be useful in stabilization and realignment.

Treatment Guidelines.
The basic treatment guidelines for chronic or postpoliomyelitis in children have been outlined by Watts (358). These guidelines include restoring ambulation, correcting the factors that cause deformities with growth, correcting factors that reduce dependency on orthoses, correcting upper extremity problems, and treating spinal deformities. Understandably, these guidelines allow the child or adolescent to achieve the maximum possible functional level. The specific methods of achieving each guideline are multiple, sometimes complex, and based on careful evaluation of the patient. Because children with previous poliomyelitis are infrequently encountered, specific details on the various procedures are not presented. Such information can be obtained from the references in the various sections.

The orthopedist must establish a comprehensive plan for each child on the basis of a thorough musculoskeletal examination—in particular, range of motion of the joints, existing deformities, and manual testing of the individual muscles of the extremities and trunk. The latter should be individually recorded on a worksheet that can be available for future reference. It is important to remember that a muscle normally loses one grade of power when transferred. To be functionally useful, a muscle grade of at least 4 is necessary, although a grade 3 muscle, when transferred, may be an effective tenodesis in preventing deformity by balancing an opposing muscle.

Upper Extremity.
In polio, involvement of the upper extremities tends to be less severe than that of the lower extremities. A stable upper extremity, especially the shoulder, is necessary for supporting body weight when using a walker or crutches. It is also necessary for transfers or for shifting the

trunk if the patient is wheelchair bound. A functional elbow, wrist, and hand are necessary for optimum independent functioning.

Shoulder. Shoulder stability is essential for all upper extremity activities. Satisfactory levels of functioning of the hand, forearm, and elbow are a prerequisite for any reconstructive surgery on the shoulder. The major problems affecting the shoulder are paralysis of the deltoid, pectoralis major, subscapularis, supraspinatus, and infraspinatus muscles. Rarely are all these muscles involved because they are innervated at different levels. Tendon transfers can occasionally be effective in restoring shoulder stability. When there is extensive weakness, shoulder arthrodesis may be helpful. Arthrodesis may also be indicated where there is a painful subluxation or dislocation. A strong trapezius serratus anterior muscle is necessary for allowing improved functioning after fusion. El-Gammal et al. (359) recently demonstrated that, after a shoulder fusion and a free-functioning gracilis muscle transplantation, there was improvement in upper extremity function in children and adolescents with a flail shoulder and elbow caused by poliomyelitis. The muscle was reinnervated by the spinal accessory or phrenic nerve. All transplanted muscles gained at least grade 3 power. The best results occurred with the reinnervation by the spinal accessory nerve.

Elbow. The major problem affecting the elbow is loss of flexion. When the biceps and brachialis are paralyzed, a tendon transfer may be helpful in restoring useful elbow flexion. Possible procedures include a Steindler flexorplasty, which transfers the origin of the wrist flexors to the anterior aspect of the distal humerus (360). The best functional results occur in patients whose elbow flexors are only partially paralyzed and whose fingers and wrist flexors are normal. Transfer of the sternal head of the pectoralis major may also be considered. Other possible procedures include transfer of the sternocleidomastoid and latissimus dorsi, and anterior transfer of the triceps brachii. Paralysis of the triceps brachii muscle may occur in poliomyelitis, but it seldom interferes with elbow function because gravity passively extends the elbow. The triceps brachii muscles need to function, however, for activities in which the body weight is shifted to the hands (such as in transferring from bed to wheelchair) or in crutch walking.

Forearm. Fixed deformities of the forearm seldom create major functional disabilities in children and adolescents with poliomyelitis. Pronation contractures are the most common disability. Functioning can be improved with release of the pronator teres and transfer of the flexor carpi ulnaris muscle.

Hand. Tendon transfers and fusions for improving the functioning of the hand can be considered in selected cases. The number of possible transfers is large, and each patient requires a careful evaluation in order to ensure maximum functional improvement. Carpal tunnel syndrome has also been reported as one of the long-term sequelae of poliomyelitis and is associated with prolonged use of crutches or a cane (361).

Lower Extremity. Lower extremity problems are most common in poliomyelitis. They can have a significant impact on functional ability, especially ambulation.

Lower Extremity Length Discrepancy. This is a common problem when there is asymmetrical neurologic involvement. If the discrepancy is >2 cm, it can produce a great many disturbances. An appropriately timed contralateral epiphyseodesis is the usual procedure of choice. Greater discrepancy may be treated orthotically. Lengthening is rarely considered as an option. However, D'Souze and Shah (362) recently demonstrated that circumferential periosteal sleeve resection of the distal femur and/or distal tibia can produce a transient growth stimulation that can be helpful in mild discrepancies, usually 2 to 3 cm.

Hip. Hip problems in poliomyelitis include muscle paralysis, soft-tissue contractures, internal or medial femoral torsion, coxa valga, and hip subluxation and dislocation. Periodic anteroposterior radiographs of the pelvis are necessary for assessing growth and the relation between the femoral head and the acetabulum. Functioning can be improved and subluxation–dislocation prevented, with appropriate soft-tissue releases, tendon transfers, proximal femoral varus derotation osteotomy, and pelvic osteotomy (Fig. 16-13) (363). It is important that the procedures be coordinated in order to provide as balanced a musculature as possible so that hip stability can be maintained. Lau et al. (363) reported good or satisfactory results in 70% of patients with paralytic hip instability caused by poliomyelitis. The key parameters for successful management are muscle balance, the femoral neck shaft and anteversion angles, and the acetabular geometry.

Knee. Flexion contractures, extension contractures, genu valgum, and external rotation of the tibia are the common knee deformities in poliomyelitis that can produce an adverse effect on functional ambulation. Hamstring release, distal femoral extension osteotomy, proximal femoral extension osteotomy, and rotational tibial osteotomies are common procedures (364–368). One of the most common soft-tissue procedures is that described by Yount (97), in which the distal iliotibial band, including the intermuscular septum, is released. This may be combined with an Ober (98) release proximally if hip-flexion contractures are also present. Shahcheraghi et al. (369) recently reported that anterior hamstring tendon transfer significantly improved active knee extension and function in patients with paralysis of the quadriceps femoris muscle following poliomyelitis.

Foot and Ankle. Deformities of the foot (usually cavus and cavovarus) and ankle are among the most common in adolescents with poliomyelitis (324, 370). Drennan (370) has discussed possible procedures for correcting the deformities and improving muscle balance. This is achieved by a combination of procedures: correction of soft-tissue contractures, tendon transfers, and bone-stabilizing procedures such as calcaneal osteotomy, subtalar arthrodesis, triple arthrodesis, and pantalar arthrodesis (371–377). Recently, the use of the Ilizarov external

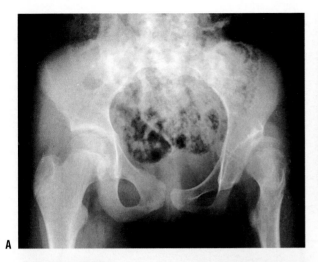

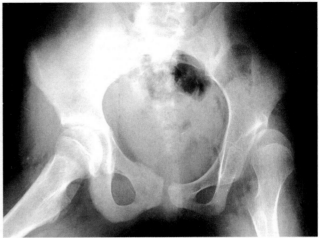

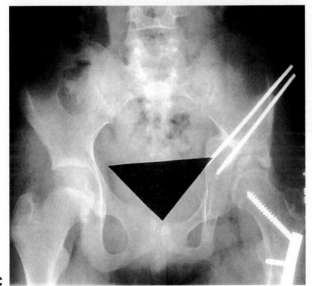

FIGURE 16-13. **A:** Anteroposterior radiograph of the pelvis of a 13-year-old Korean girl who had poliomyelitis. She has a painful subluxation of her left hip. The acetabulum is dysplastic, the center-edge angle is 6 degrees, and a coxa valga deformity of the proximal femur is present. **B:** Frog-leg or Lauenstein lateral. **C:** Two years after a proximal femoral varus derotation osteotomy and Chiari pelvic osteotomy, there is markedly improved alignment of the left hip, and she is asymptomatic.

fixator has been shown to be helpful in correction of complex foot deformities following poliomyelitis (378). A careful evaluation of the patient is required for determining the appropriate procedures. Arthrodeses produce good long-term results with a low incidence of ankle degenerative arthritis, because patients with poliomyelitis place lower functional demands and stresses on the ankle (371, 374, 375).

Spine. Scoliosis occurs in about one-third of patients with poliomyelitis. The type and severity of the curvature depends on the extent of paralysis and residual muscle power of the trunk muscles and pelvic obliquity. The most common curve patterns are the double major thoracic and lumbar curves, followed by the long paralytic C-shaped thoracolumbar curve (379). Pelvic obliquity occurs in approximately 50% of the patients with spinal deformity. Because of severe rotation, kyphosis in the lumbar spine and lordosis in the thoracic spine are also common.

The goals of treatment are to obtain a balanced, vertical torso over a level pelvis. This permits stable sitting and leaves

the hands free for activities. It also helps prevent decubiti and paralytic hip dislocation. In young children with curves of between 20 and 40 degrees, orthotic management with a TLSO can be tried. It rarely provides complete stability, but can be effective in slowing the rate of progression and allowing the child to reach a more suitable age for surgery. In severe cases in young children, segmental spinal instrumentation without fusion may be considered. Eberle (380), however, reported failure of segmental spinal instrumentation in 15 of 16 children with poliomyelitis between the ages of 5 and 12 years. Therefore, children who undergo instrumentation without fusion should be treated with TLSO and subsequently undergo a fusion procedure as soon as possible in order to prevent late complications. For adolescents with a supple spine and a curve of <60 degrees, a posterior spinal fusion with segmental instrumentation, usually Luque rod instrumentation, provides stability and a low pseudoarthrosis rate (116, 379). Other segmental spinal instrumentation systems are also effective. In severe curves of 60 to 100 degrees, a combined anterior and posterior spinal fusion is usually necessary (381). Anterior

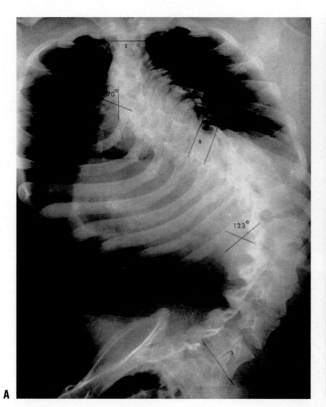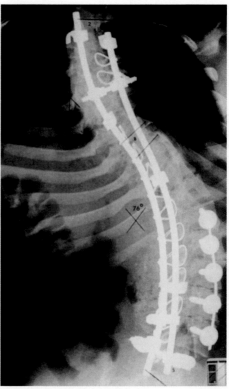

FIGURE 16-14. **A:** Anteroposterior spinal radiograph, taken in the seated position, of a 17-year-old girl from the Middle East who has a severe paralytic scoliosis. There is a 123-degree left thoracolumbar scoliosis and a 70-degree right thoracic scoliosis. She contracted poliomyelitis at the age of 2 years, which left her with flail lower extremities and essentially normal upper extremities. She is wheelchair dependent and has pain from rib-pelvis impingement. **B:** Postoperative radiograph after staged anterior spinal fusion and Zielke instrumentation and posterior spinal fusion using Isola instrumentation from T3 to the sacrum. Pain relief was complete and sitting balance improved. The left thoracolumbar curve has been reduced to 70 degrees and the right thoracic curve to 47 degrees.

spinal instrumentation with a Dwyer or Zielke system may be used in thoracolumbar and lumbar curves. Anterior discectomy and fusion is preferred for thoracic curves. The posterior spinal fusion and instrumentation may be performed the same day, or performed 1 or 2 weeks later. Leong et al. (382) and others (381, 383) have demonstrated that combined anterior and posterior spinal fusions provide excellent correction for postpoliomyelitis spinal deformity, including the associated pelvic obliquity (Fig. 16-14). Rarely is preoperative traction, or traction between staged anterior and posterior procedures, necessary for additional correction. Fusion to the pelvis or sacrum is usually necessary in patients with severe pelvic obliquity (384, 385).

POSTPOLIOMYELITIS SYNDROME

Postpoliomyelitis syndrome is a true entity occurring in adults, and is a sequela to poliomyelitis. Reactivation of the poliomyelitis virus has been mistaken for amyotrophic lateral sclerosis. Postpoliomyelitis syndrome is thought to be

an overuse syndrome (386). Diagnosis is based on five criteria and is essentially a diagnosis of exclusion. The criteria include

1. A confirmed history of previous poliomyelitis
2. Partial to fairly complete neurologic and functional recovery
3. A period of neurologic and functional stability of at least 15 years' duration
4. Onset of two or more of the following health problems since achieving a period of stability: unaccustomed fatigue, muscle and joint pain or both, new weakness in muscles previously affected or unaffected, functional loss, intolerance to cold, and new atrophy
5. No other medical diagnosis to explain the aforementioned health problems

Postpoliomyelitis syndrome is more likely to develop in those with onset later than the age of 10 years, because older children are more likely to have severe poliomyelitis. Management of these patients is conservative and consists of muscle strengthening, decreasing the duration of effort, and orthotics (386). Reconstructive surgery is rarely indicated or necessary.

REFERENCES

1. Read L, Galasko CS. Delay in diagnosing Duchenne muscular dystrophy in orthopaedic clinics. *J Bone Joint Surg Br* 1986;68:481.
2. Anderson PB, Rando TA. Neuromuscular disorders of childhood. *Curr Opin Pediatr* 1999;11:497.
3. Berven S, Bradford DS. Neuromuscular scoliosis: causes of deformity and principles for evaluation and management. *Semin Neurol* 2002;22:167.
4. Pruijs JE, van Tol MJ, van Kesteren RG, et al. Neuromuscular scoliosis: clinical evaluation pre- and postoperative. *J Pediatr Orthop B* 2000;9:217.
5. Shapiro F, Bresnan MJ. Current concepts review. Orthopaedic management of childhood neuromuscular disease. Part III: diseases of muscle. *J Bone Joint Surg Am* 1982;64:1102.
6. Shapiro F, Specht L. Current concepts review. The diagnosis and orthopaedic treatment of inherited muscular diseases of childhood. *J Bone Joint Surg Am* 1993;75:439.
7. Zellweger H, Antonik A. Newborn screening for Duchenne muscular dystrophy. *Pediatrics* 1975;55:30.
8. Hurley ME, Davids JR, Mubarak SJ. Single-incision combination biopsy (muscle and nerve) in the diagnosis of neuromuscular disease in children. *J Pediatr Orthop* 1994;14:740.
9. Mubarak SJ, Chambers HG, Wenger DR. Percutaneous muscle biopsy in the diagnosis of neuromuscular disease. *J Pediatr Orthop* 1992;12:191.
10. Sanjal SK, Leung RK, Tierney RC, et al. Mitral valve prolapse syndrome in children with Duchenne's progressive muscular dystrophy. *Pediatrics* 1979;63:116.
11. Yazawa Y. Mitral valve prolapse related to geometrical changes of the heart in cases of progressive muscular dystrophy. *Clin Cardiol* 1984;7:198.
12. Emery AEH. X-linked muscular dystrophy with early contractures and cardiomyopathy (Emery-Dreifuss type). *Clin Genet* 1987;32:360.
13. Seay AR, Ziter FA, Thompson JA. Cardiac arrest during induction of anesthesia in Duchenne muscular dystrophy. *J Pediatr* 1978;93:88.
14. Kurz LT, Mubarak SJ, Schultz P, et al. Correlation of scoliosis and pulmonary function in Duchenne muscular dystrophy. *J Pediatr Orthop* 1983;3:347.
15. Schreiber A, Smith WL, Ionasescu V, et al. Magnetic resonance imaging of children with Duchenne muscular dystrophy. *Pediatr Radiol* 1987;17:495.
16. Specht LA. Molecular basis and clinical applications of neuromuscular disease in children. *Curr Opin Pediatr* 1991;3:966.
17. Dietz FR, Mathews KD. Current concepts review. Update on genetic bases of disorders with orthopaedic manifestations. *J Bone Joint Surg Am* 1996;78:1583.
18. Sussman M. Duchenne muscular dystrophy. *J Am Acad Orthop Surg* 2002;10:138.
19. Marsh GG, Munsat TL. Evidence for early impairment of verbal intelligence in Duchenne muscular dystrophy. *Arch Dis Child* 1974;49:118.
20. Sutherland DH, Olshen R, Cooper L, et al. The pathomechanics of gait in Duchenne muscular dystrophy. *Dev Med Child Neurol* 1981;23:3.
21. Sutherland DH. Gait analysis in neuromuscular diseases. *AAOS Instr Course Lect* 1990;39:333.
22. Hsu JD, Furumasu J. Gait and posture changes in the Duchenne muscular dystrophy child. *Clin Orthop* 1993;288:122.
23. Brooke MH, Fenichel GM, Griggs RC, et al. Duchenne muscular dystrophy. Patterns of clinical progression and effects of supportive therapy. *Neurology* 1989;39:475.
24. Emery AEH. *Duchenne muscular dystrophy*, 2nd ed. New York, NY: Oxford University Press, 1988.
25. Rideau Y, Glorion B, Duport G. Prolongation of ambulation in the muscular dystrophies. *Acta Neurol* 1983;38:390.
26. Bakker JP, De Groot IJ, Beelen A, et al. Predictive factors of cessation of ambulation in patients with Duchenne muscular dystrophy. *Am J Phys Med Rehabil* 2002;81:906.
27. Wilkins KE, Gibson DA. The patterns of spinal deformity in Duchenne muscular dystrophy. *J Bone Joint Surg Am* 1976;58:24.
28. Roses AD, Roses MJ, Miller SE, et al. Carrier detection in Duchenne muscular dystrophy. *N Engl J Med* 1976;294:193.
29. Kunkel LM, Monaco AP, Hoffman E, et al. Molecular studies of progressive muscular dystrophy (Duchenne). *Enzyme* 1987;38:72.
30. Slater GR. The missing link in Duchenne muscular dystrophy. *Nature* 1987;330:693.
31. Hoffman EP, Brown RH Jr, Kunkel LM. Dystrophin. The protein product of the Duchenne muscular dystrophy locus. *Cell* 1987;51:919.
32. Hoffman EP, Kunkel LM. Dystrophin abnormalities in Duchenne/Becker muscular dystrophy. *Neuron* 1989;2:1019.
33. Darras BT. Molecular genetics of Duchenne and Becker muscular dystrophy. *J Pediatr* 1990;117:1.
34. Uchino M, Araki S, Miike T, et al. Localization and characterization of dystrophin in muscle biopsy specimens for Duchenne muscular dystrophy and various neuromuscular disorders. *Muscle Nerve* 1989;12:1009.
35. Beggs AH, Hoffman EP, Snyder JR, et al. Exploring the molecular basis for variability among patients with Becker muscular dystrophy. Dystrophin gene and protein studies. *Am J Hum Genet* 1991;49:54.
36. Specht LA, Kunkel LM. Duchenne and Becker muscular dystrophies. In: Rosenberg RN, Prusiner SB, DiMauro S, et al., eds. *The molecular and genetic basis of neurological disease*. Boston, MA: Butterworth-Heinemann, 1993:613.
37. Hoffman EP, Kunkel LM, Angelini C, et al. Improved diagnosis of Becker muscular dystrophy by dystrophin testing. *Neurology* 1989;39:1011.
38. Hoffman EP, Fischbeck KH, Brown RH, et al. Characterization of dystrophin in muscle-biopsy specimens from patients with Duchenne's or Becker's muscular dystrophy. *N Engl J Med* 1988;318:1363.
39. Specht LA, Beggs AH, Korf B, et al. Prediction of dystrophin phenotype by DNA analysis in Duchenne/Becker muscular dystrophy. *Pediatr Neurol* 1992;8:432.
40. Nicholson LVB, Johnson M, Bushby KMD, et al. Functional significance of dystrophin positive fibres in Duchenne muscular dystrophy. *Arch Dis Child* 1993;68:632.
41. Gospe SM Jr, Lazaro RP, Lava NS, et al. Familial X-linked myalgia and cramps. A nonprogressive myopathy associated with a deletion in the dystrophin gene. *Neurology* 1989;39:1277.
42. Partridge TA. Invited review. Myoblast transfer. A possible therapy for inherited myopathies? *Muscle Nerve* 1991;14:197.
43. Partridge TA, Morgan JE, Coulton GR, et al. Conversion of mdx myofibres from dystrophin-negative to -positive by injection of normal myoblasts. *Nature* 1989;337:176.
44. Gussoni E, Pavlath GK, Lanctot AM, et al. Normal dystrophin transcripts detected in Duchenne muscular dystrophy patients after myoblast transplantation. *Nature* 1992;356:435.
45. Huard J, Bouchard JP, Roy R, et al. Human myoblast transplantation; preliminary results of 4 cases. *Muscle Nerve* 1992;15:550.
46. Karpati G, Ajdukovic D, Arnold D, et al. Myoblast transfer in Duchenne muscular dystrophy. *Ann Neurol* 1993;34:8.
47. Law PK, Goodwin TG, Fang Q, et al. Feasibility, safety and efficacy of myoblast transfer therapy on Duchenne muscular dystrophy boys. *Cell Transplant* 1992;1:235.
48. Mendell JR, Kissel JT, Amato AA, et al. Myoblast transfer in the treatment of Duchenne's muscular dystrophy. *N Engl J Med* 1995;333:832.
49. Wood MJ, Gait MJ, Yin H. RNA-targeted splice-correction therapy for neuromuscular disease. *Brain* 2010;133:957–972.
50. DeSilva S, Drachman D. Prednisone treatment in Duchenne muscular dystrophy. *Arch Neurol* 1987;44:818.
51. Heckmatt J, Rodillo E, Dubowitz V. Management of children. Pharmacological and physical. *Br Med Bull* 1989;45:788.
52. Dubowitz V. Prednisone in Duchenne dystrophy [Editorial]. *Neuromuscul Disord* 1991;1:161.
53. Fenichel GM, Florence JM, Pestronk A, et al. Long-term benefit from prednisone therapy in Duchenne muscular dystrophy. *Neurology* 1991;41:1874.

54. Mendell JR, Moxley RT, Griggs RC, et al. Randomized double-blind six-month trial of prednisone in Duchenne's muscular dystrophy. *N Engl J Med* 1989;320:1592.

55. Biggar WD, Gingras M, Fehlings DL, et al. Deflazacort treatment of Duchenne muscular dystrophy. *J Pediatr* 2001;138:45.

56. Connolly AM, Schierbecker J, Renna R, et al. High dose weekly oral prednisone improves strength in boys with Duchenne muscular dystrophy. *Neuromuscul Disord* 2002;12:917.

57. Alman BA, Raza SN, Biggar WD. Steroid treatment and the development of scoliosis in makes with Duchenne muscular dystrophy. *J Bone Joint Surg Am* 2004;86-A:519.

58. Houde S, Filiatrault M, Fournier A, et al. Deflazacort use in Duchenne muscular dystrophy: an 8-year follow-up. *Pediatr Neurol* 2008;38:200–206.

59. King WM, Ruttencutter R, Nagaraja HN, et al. Orthopedic outcomes of long-term daily corticosteroid treatment in Duchenne muscular dystrophy. *Neurology* 2007;68:1607–1613.

60. Bothwell JE, Gordon KE, Dooley JM, et al. Vertebral fractures in boys with Duchenne muscular dystrophy. *Clin Pediatr* 2003;42:353.

61. Bennakker EA, Fock JM, Van Tol MJ, et al. Intermittent prednisone therapy in Duchenne muscular dystrophy: a randomized controlled trial. *Arch Neurol* 2005;62:128–132.

62. Campbell C, Jacob P. Deflazacort for the treatment of Duchenne Dystrophy: a systematic review. *BMC Neurol* 2003;8:3–7.

63. Bonfati MD, Ruzza G, Bonometto P, et al. Creatinine monohydrate enhances strength and body composition in Duchenne muscular dystrophy. *Muscle Nerve* 2000;23(9):1344.

64. Tarnopolsky MA, Mahoney DJ, Vajsar J, et al. Creatinine monohydrate enhances strength and body composition in Duchenne muscular dystrophy. *Neurology* 2004;62:1771.

65. Louis M, Lebacq J, Poortmans JR, et al. Beneficial effects of creatine supplementation in dystrophic patients. *Muscle Nerve* 2003;27:604–610.

66. Fowler EG, Graves MC, Wetzel GT, et al. Pilot trial of albuterol in Duchenne and Becker muscle dystrophy. *Neurology* 2004;62:1006.

67. Skura CL, Fowler EG, Wetzel GT, et al. Albuterol increases lean body mass in ambulatory boys with Duchenne or Becker muscular dystrophy. *Neurology* 2008;70:137.

68. Griggs RC, Moxley RT, Mendell JR, et al. Duchenne dystrophy: randomized, controlled trial of prednisone (18 months) and azathioprine (12 months). *Neurology* 1993;43:520.

69. Wagner KR, Hamed S, Hadley DW, et al. Gentamicin treatment of Duchenne and Becker muscular dystrophy due to nonsense mutations. *Ann Neurol* 2001;49:706.

70. Serrano C, Wall C, Moore SA, et al. Gentamicin treatment for muscular dystrophy patients with stop codon mutations. *Neurology* 2001;56(Suppl 3):A79.

71. Chamberlain JS. Gene therapy of muscular dystrophy. *Hum Mol Genet* 2002;11:2355.

72. Hartigan-O'Connor D, Chamberlain J. Developments in gene therapy for muscular dystrophy. *Microsc Res Tech* 2000;48:223.

73. Gussoni E. Dystrophin expression in the mdx mouse restored by stem cell transplantation. *Nature* 1999;401:390.

74. Green NE. The orthopaedic care of children with muscular dystrophy. *AAOS Instr Course Lect* 1987;36:267.

75. Heckmatt JZ, Dubowitz V, Hyde SA, et al. Prolongation of walking in Duchenne muscular dystrophy with lightweight orthoses: review of 57 cases. *Dev Med Child Neurol* 1985;27:149.

76. Spencer GE Jr, Vignos PJ Jr. Bracing for ambulation in childhood progressive muscular dystrophy. *J Bone Joint Surg Am* 1962;44:234.

77. Spencer GE Jr. Orthopaedic care of progressive muscular dystrophy. *J Bone Joint Surg Am* 1967;49:1201.

78. Vignos PJ, Wagner MB, Karlinchak B, et al. Evaluation of a program for long-term treatment of Duchenne muscular dystrophy. Experience at the University Hospitals of Cleveland. *J Bone Joint Surg Am* 1966;78:1844.

79. Hyde SA, Filytrup I, Glent S, et al. A randomized comparative study of two methods for controlling tendoAchilles contracture in Duchenne muscular dystrophy. *Neuromuscul Disord* 2000;10:257.

80. Yasuda YL, Bowman K, Hsu JD. Mobile arm supports: criteria for successful use in muscle disease patients. *Arch Phys Med Rehabil* 1986;67:253.

81. Larson CM, Henderson RC. Bone mineral density and fractures in boys in Duchenne muscular dystrophy. *J Pediatr Orthop* 2000;20:71.

82. Aparicio LF, Jurkovic M, DeLullo J. Decreased bone density in ambulatory patients with Duchenne muscular dystrophy. *J Pediatr Orthop* 2002;22:179.

83. McDonald DG, Kinali M, Gallagher AC, et al. Fracture prevalence in Duchenne muscular dystrophy. *Dev Med Child Neurol* 2002;44:695.

84. Vestergaard P, Glerup H, Steffensen BF, et al. Fracture risk in patients with muscular dystrophy and spinal muscular atrophy. *J Rehabil Med* 2001;33:150.

85. Smith SE, Green NE, Cole RJ, et al. Prolongation of ambulation in children with Duchenne muscular dystrophy by subcutaneous lower limb tenotomy. *J Pediatr Orthop* 1993;13:331.

86. Bowker JH, Halpin PJ. Factors determining success in reambulation of the child with progressive muscular dystrophy. *Ortho Clin North Am* 1978;9:431.

87. Hsu JD. The management of foot deformity in pseudohypertrophic muscular dystrophy (DMD). *Ortho Clin North Am* 1976;7:979.

88. Rodillo EB, Fernandez-Bermejo E, Heckmatt JZ, et al. Prevention of rapidly progressive scoliosis in Duchenne muscular dystrophy by prolongation of walking with orthoses. *J Child Neurol* 1988;3:269.

89. Williams EA, Read L, Ellis A, et al. The management of equinus deformity in Duchenne muscular dystrophy. *J Bone Joint Surg Br* 1984;66:546.

90. Forst J, Forst R. Lower limb surgery in Duchenne muscular dystrophy. *Neuromuscul Disord* 1999;9:176.

91. Greene WB. Transfer versus lengthening of the posterior tibial tendon in Duchenne's muscular dystrophy. *Foot Ankle* 1992;13:526.

92. Hsu JD, Hoffer MM. Posterior tibial tendon transfer through the interosseous membrane. A modification of the technique. *Clin Orthop* 1978;131:202.

93. Miller GM, Hsu JD, Hoffer MM, et al. Posterior tibial tendon transfer. A review of the literature and analysis of 74 procedures. *J Pediatr Orthop* 1982;2:33.

94. Scher DM, Mubarak SJ. Surgical prevention of foot deformity in patients with Duchenne muscular dystrophy. *J Pediatr Orthop* 2002;22:384.

95. Melkonian GJ, Cristafaro RL, Perry J, et al. Dynamic gait electromyography study in Duchenne muscular dystrophy (DMD) patients. *Foot Ankle* 1983;1:78.

96. Leitch KK, Raza N, Biggar D, et al. Should foot surgery be performed in children with Duchenne muscular dystrophy? *J Pediatr Orthop* 2005;25:95.

97. Yount CC. The role of the tensor fasciae femoris in certain deformities of the lower extremities. *J Bone Joint Surg Am* 1926;8:171.

98. Ober FR. The role of the iliotibial band and fascia lata as a factor in the causation of low back disabilities and sciatica. *J Bone Joint Surg* 1936;18:105.

99. Chan, KG, Galasko CS, Delaney C. Hip subluxation and dislocation in Duchenne muscular dystrophy. *J Pediatr Orthop B* 2001;10:219.

100. Wagner MB, Vignos PJ Jr, Carlozzi C. Duchenne muscular dystrophy: a study of wrist and hand function. *Muscle Nerve* 1989;12:236.

101. Cambridge W, Drennan JC. Scoliosis associated with Duchenne muscular dystrophy. *J Pediatr Orthop* 1987;7:436.

102. Galasko CCB, Delaney C, Morris P. Spinal stabilization in Duchenne muscular dystrophy. *J Bone Joint Surg Br* 1992;74:210.

103. Gibson, DA, Wilkins KE. The management of spinal deformities in Duchenne muscular dystrophy. A new concept in spinal bracing. *Clin Orthop* 1975;108:41.

104. Hsu JD. The natural history of spine curvature progression in the nonambulatory Duchenne muscular dystrophy patient. *Spine* 1983;8:771.

105. Smith AD, Koreska J, Moseley CF. Progression of scoliosis in Duchenne muscular dystrophy. *J Bone Joint Surg Am* 1989;71:1066.

106. Lord J, Behrman B, Varzos N, et al. Scoliosis associated with Duchenne muscular dystrophy. *Arch Phys Med Rehabil* 1990;71:13.

107. Karol L. Scoliosis in patients with Duchenne muscular dystrophy. *J Bone Joint Surg Am* 2007;89:155.

108. Kinali M, Main M, Eliahoo J, et al. Predictive factors for the development of scoliosis in Duchenne muscular dystrophy. *Eur J Paediatr Neurol* 2007;11:160.

109. Colbert AP, Craig C. Scoliosis management in Duchenne muscular dystrophy. Prospective study of modified Jewett hyperextension brace. *Arch Phys Med Rehabil* 1987;68:302.

110. Seeger BR, Sutherland AD, Clark MS. Orthotic management of scoliosis in Duchenne muscular dystrophy. *Arch Phys Med Rehabil* 1984;65:83.

111. Sussman MD. Advantage of early spinal stabilization and fusion in patients with Duchenne muscular dystrophy. *J Pediatr Orthop* 1984;4:532.

112. Swank SM, Brown JC, Perry RE. Spinal fusion in Duchenne's muscular dystrophy. *Spine* 1982;7:484.

113. Weimann, RL, Gibson DA, Moseley CF, et al. Surgical stabilization of the spine in Duchenne muscular dystrophy. *Spine* 1983;8:776.

114. Heller KD, Forst R, Forst J, et al. Scoliosis in Duchenne muscular dystrophy: aspects of orthotic treatment. *Prosthet Orthot Int* 1997;21:202.

115. Boachie-Adjei O, Lonstein JE, Winter RB, et al. Management of neuromuscular spinal deformities with Luque segmental instrumentation. *J Bone Joint Surg Am* 1989;71:548.

116. Marchesi D, Arlet V, Stricker U, et al. Modification of the original Luque technique in the treatment of Duchenne's neuromuscular scoliosis. *J Pediatr Orthop* 1997;17:743.

117. Miller F, Moseley CF, Koreska J. Spinal fusion in Duchenne muscular dystrophy. *Dev Med Child Neurol* 1992;34:775.

118. Oda T, Shimizu N, Yonenobu K, et al. Longitudinal study of spinal deformity in Duchenne muscular deformity. *J Pediatr Orthop* 1993;13:478.

119. Bridwell KH, O'Brien MF, Lenke LG, et al. Posterior spinal fusion supplemented with only allograft bone in paralytic scoliosis. Does it work? *Spine* 1994;19:2658.

120. Brook PD, Kennedy JD, Stern LM, et al. Spinal fusion in Duchenne's muscular dystrophy. *J Pediatr Orthop* 1996;16:324.

121. Fox HJ, Thomas CH, Thompson AG. Spinal instrumentation for Duchenne's muscular dystrophy: experience of hypotensive anesthesia to minimize blood loss. *J Pediatr Orthop* 1997;17:750.

122. Yazici M, Asher MA. Freeze-dried allograft for posterior spinal fusion in patients with neuromuscular spinal deformities. *Spine* 1997;22:1467.

123. Bridwell KH, Baldus C, Iffrig TM, et al. Process measures and patient/parent evaluation of surgical management of spinal deformities in patients with progressive flaccid neuromuscular scoliosis (Duchenne's muscular dystrophy and spinal muscular atrophy). *Spine* 1999;24:1300.

124. Ramirez N, Richards SB, Warren PD, et al. Complications after posterior spinal fusion in Duchenne's muscular dystrophy. *J Pediatr Orthop* 1997;17:109.

125. Broom MJ, Banta JV, Renshaw TS. Spinal fusion augmented by Luque rod segmental instrumentation for neuromuscular scoliosis. *J Bone Joint Surg Am* 1989;71:32.

126. Bentley G, Haddad F, Bull TM, et al. The treatment of scoliosis in muscular dystrophy using modified Luque and Harrington-Luque instrumentation. *J Bone Joint Surg Br* 2001;83:22.

127. Yazici M, Asher MA, Hardacker JW. The safety and efficacy of Isola-Galveston instrumentation and arthrodesis in the treatment of neuromuscular spinal deformities. *J Bone Joint Surg* 2000;82:524.

128. Heller KD, Wirtz DC, Siebert CH, et al. Spinal stabilization in Duchenne muscular dystrophy: principle of treatment and record of 31 operative treated cases. *J Pediatr Orthop B* 2001;10:18.

129. Lonstein JE. The Galveston technique using Luque or Cotrel-Dubousset rods. *Ortho Clin North Am* 1994;25:311–320.

130. McCarthy RE, Bruffett WL, McCullough FL. S rod fixation to the sacrum in patients with neuromuscular spinal deformities. *Clin Orthop* 1999;364:26.

131. Hahn F, Hauser D, Espinosa N, et al. Scoliosis correction with pedicle screws in Duchenne muscular dystrophy. *Eur Spine J* 2008;17:255.

132. Mehta SS, Modi HN, Srinivasalu S, et al. Pedicle screw-only constructs with lumbar or pelvic fixation for spinal stabilization in patients with Duchenne muscular dystrophy. *J Spinal Disord Tech* 2009;22:428.

133. Mubarak SJ, Morin WD, Leach J. Spinal fusion in Duchenne muscular dystrophy—fixation and fusion to the sacropelvis? *J Pediatr Orthop* 1993;13:752.

134. Rice JJ, Jeffers BL, Devitt AT, et al. Management of the collapsing spine for patients with Duchenne muscular dystrophy. *Ir J Med Sci* 1998;167:242.

135. Sengupta DK, Mehdian SH, McConnell JR, et al. Pelvic or lumbar fixation for the surgical management of scoliosis in Duchenne muscular dystrophy. *Spine* 2002;27:2072.

136. Alman BA, Kim HK. Pelvic obliquity after fusion of the spine in Duchenne muscular dystrophy. *J Bone Joint Surg Br* 1999;81:821.

137. Jenkins JG, Bohn D, Edmonds JF, et al. Evaluation of pulmonary function in muscular dystrophy patients requiring spinal surgery. *Crit Care Med* 1982;10:645.

138. Suh SW, Modi HN, Yang J, et al. Posterior multilevel vertebral osteotomy for correction of severe and rigid neuromuscular scoliosis: a preliminary study. *Spine* 2009;34:1315.

139. Marsh A, Edge G, Lehovsky J. Spinal fusion in patients with Duchenne's muscular dystrophy and a low forced vital capacity. *Eur Spine J* 2003;12:507.

140. Rideau Y, Jankowski LW, Grellet J. Respiratory function in the muscular dystrophies. *Muscle Nerve* 1981;4:155.

141. Velasco MV, Colin AA, Zurakowski D, et al. Posterior spinal fusion for scoliosis in Duchenne muscular dystrophy diminishes the rate of respiratory decline. *Spine* 2007;32:459.

142. Rideau Y, Delaubier A. Neuromuscular respiratory deficit. Setting back mortality. *Semin Orthop* 1987;2:203.

143. Smith PEM, Calverley PMA, Edwards RHT, et al. Practical problems in the respiratory care of patients with muscular dystrophy. *N Engl J Med* 1987;316:1197.

144. Kennedy JD, Staples AJ, Brook PD, et al. Effect of spinal surgery on lung function in Duchenne muscular dystrophy. *Thorax* 1995;50:1173.

145. Miller F, Moseley CF, Koreska J, et al. Pulmonary function and scoliosis in Duchenne dystrophy. *J Pediatr Orthop* 1988;8:133.

146. Miller RG, Chalmers AC, Dao H, et al. The effects of spine fusion on respiratory function in Duchenne muscular dystrophy. *Neurology* 1991;41:38.

147. Granata C, Merlini L, Cervellati S, Long-term results of spine surgery in Duchenne muscular dystrophy. *Neuromuscul Disord* 1996;6:61.

148. Noordeen MH, Hoddad FS, Muntoni F, et al. Blood loss in Duchenne muscular dystrophy: vascular smooth muscle dysfunction. *J Pediatr Orthop B* 1999;8:212.

149. Noordeen MHH, Lee J, Gibbons CER, et al. Spinal cord monitoring in operations for neuromuscular scoliosis. *J Bone Joint Surg Br* 1997;79:53.

150. Gurnaney H, Brown A, Litman RS. Malignant hyperthermia and muscular dystrophies. *Anes Analg* 2009;109:1043.

151. Shapiro F, Zurakowski D, Sethna NF. Tranexamic acid diminishes intraoperative blood loss and transfusion in spinal fusions for Duchenne muscular dystrophy scoliosis. *Spine* 2007;32:2278.

152. Thompson GH, Florentino-Pineda I, Poe-Kochert C, et al. The role of Amicar in surgery for neuromuscular scoliosis. *Spine* 2008;33:2623.

153. Alexander MA, Johnson EW, Petty J, et al. Mechanical ventilation of patients with late stage Duchenne muscular dystrophy. Management in the home. *Arch Phys Med Rehabil* 1979;60:289.

154. Bach JR, O'Brien J, Krolenberg R, et al. Muscular dystrophy. Management of end stage respiratory failure in Duchenne muscular dystrophy. *Muscle Nerve* 1987;10:177.

155. Curran FJ. Night ventilation by body respirators for patients in chronic respiratory failure due to late stage Duchenne muscular dystrophy. *Arch Phys Med Rehabil* 1981;62:270.

156. Hilton T, Orr RD, Perkin RM, et al. End of life care in Duchenne muscular dystrophy. *Pediatr Neurol* 1993;9:165.

157. Stewart CA, Gilgoff I, Baydur A, et al. Gated radionuclide ventriculography in the evolution of cardiac function in Duchenne's muscular dystrophy. *Chest* 1988;94:1245.

158. Emery AEH, Watt MS, Clack ER. The effects of genetic counseling in Duchenne muscular dystrophy. *Clin Genet* 1972;3:147.

159. Becker PE. Two new families of benign sex-linked recessive muscular dystrophy. *Rev Can Biol* 1962;21:551.

160. Bradley WG, Jones MZ, Mussini JM, et al. Becker-type muscular dystrophy. *Muscle Nerve* 1978;1:111.

161. Johnsen SD. Prednisone therapy in Becker's muscular dystrophy. *J Child Neurol* 2001;16:870.

162. Daher YH, Lonstein JE, Winter RB, et al. Spinal deformities in patients with muscular dystrophy other than Duchenne. A review of 11 patients having surgical treatment. *Spine* 1985;10:614.

163. Dickey RP, Ziter FA, Smith RA. Emery-Dreifuss muscular dystrophy. *J Pediatr* 1984;104:555.

164. Miller RG, Layzer RB, Mellenthin MA, et al. Emery-Dreifuss muscular dystrophy with autosomal dominant transmission. *Neurology* 1985; 35:1230.

165. Shapiro F, Specht L. Orthopedic deformities in Emery-Dreifuss muscular dystrophy. *J Pediatr Orthop* 1991;11:336.

166. Merlini L, Granata C, Dominici P, et al. Emery-Dreifuss muscular dystrophy. Report of five cases in a family and review of the literature. *Muscle Nerve* 1986;9:481.

167. Goto I, Ishimoto S, Yamada T, et al. The rigid spine syndrome and Emery-Dreifuss muscular dystrophy. *Clin Neurol Neurosurg* 1986;88:293.

168. Consalez GG, Thomas NST, Stayton CL, et al. Assignment of Emery-Dreifuss muscular dystrophy to the distal region of Xq28. The results of a collaborative study. *Am J Hum Genet* 1991;48:468.

169. Thomas N, Williams H, Elsas LJ, et al. Localization of the gene for Emery-Dreifuss muscular dystrophy to the distal long arm of the X-chromosome. *J Med Genet* 1986;23:596.

170. Bonne G, Di Barletta MR, Varnous S. Mutations in the gene encoding lamin A/C cause autosomal dominant Emery Dreifuss muscular dystrophy. *Nat Genet* 1999;21:285.

171. Hopkins LC, Jackson JA, Elsas LJ. Emery-Dreifuss humeroperoneal muscular dystrophy. An X-linked myopathy with unusual contractures and bradycardia. *Ann Neurol* 1981;10:230.

172. Arikawa E, Hoffman EP, Kaido M, et al. The frequency of patients with dystrophin abnormalities in a limb-girdle patient population. *Neurology* 1991;41:1491.

173. Bushby K. Report on the 12th ENMC sponsored international workshop—the 'limb-girdle' muscular dystrophies. *Neuromuscul Disord* 1992;2:3.

174. Bushby KM, Beckmann JS. The limb girdle muscular dystrophies—proposal for a new nomenclature. *Neuromuscul Disord* 1995;4:337.

175. Riley RO, Marzulo DC, Hans MB. Muscular dystrophy. Infantile fascioscapulohumeral muscular dystrophy. New observations. *Acta Neural Scand* 1986;74:51.

176. Korf BR, Bresnan MJ, Shapiro F, et al. Fascioscapulohumeral dystrophy presenting in infancy with facial diplegia and sensorineural deafness. *Ann Neurol* 1985;17:513.

177. Shapiro F, Specht L, Korf BR. Locomotor problems in infantile fascioscapulohumeral muscular dystrophy. Retrospective study of 9 patients. *Acta Orthop Scand* 1991;62:367.

178. Hanson PA, Rowland LP. Mobius syndrome and fascioscapulohumeral muscular dystrophy. *Arch Neurol* 1971;24:31.

179. Brouwer OF, Padberg GW, Baker E, et al. Fascioscapulohumeral muscular dystrophy in early childhood. *Arch Neurol* 1994;51:387.

180. Fisher J, Upadhyaya M. Molecular genetics of fascioscapulohumeral muscular dystrophy (FSHD). *Neuromuscul Disord* 1997;7:55.

181. Wijmenga C, Frants RR, Brouwer OF, et al. Location of fascioscapulohumeral muscular dystrophy gene on chromosome 4. *Lancet* 1990; 336:651.

182. Bodensteiner JB, Schochet SS. Fascioscapulohumeral muscular dystrophy. The choice of a biopsy site. *Muscle Nerve* 1986;9:544.

183. Orrell RW, Tawil R, Forrester J, et al. Definitive molecular diagnosis of fascioscapulohumeral muscular dystrophy. *Neurology* 1999;52:1822.

184. Bunch WH, Siegal IM. Scapulothoracic arthrodesis in fascioscapulohumeral muscular dystrophy. Review of seventeen procedures with three to twenty-one year follow-up. *J Bone Joint Surg Am* 1993;75:372.

185. Copeland SA, Levy O, Warner GC, et al. The shoulder in patients with muscular dystrophy. *Clin Orthop* 1999;368:80.

186. Jakab E, Gledhill RB. Simplified technique for scapulocostal fusion in fascioscapulohumeral dystrophy. *J Pediatr Orthop* 1993;13:749.

187. Ketenjian AY. Scapulocostal stabilization for scapular winging in fascioscapulohumeral muscular dystrophy. *J Bone Joint Surg Am* 1978;60:476.

188. Kocialkowski A, Frostick SP, Wallace WA. One-stage bilateral thoracoscapular fusion using allografts. A case report. *Clin Orthop* 1991; 273:264.

189. Letournel E, Fardeau M, Lytle JO, et al. Scapulothoracic arthrodesis for patients who have fascioscapulohumeral muscular dystrophy. *J Bone Joint Surg Am* 1990;72:78.

190. Berne D, Laude F, Laporte C, et al. Scapulothoracic arthrodesis in facioscapulohumeral muscular dystrophy. *Clin Orthop* 2003;409:106.

191. Giannini S, Ceccarelli F, Faldini C, et al. Scapulopexy of winged scapula secondary to facioscapulohumeral muscular dystrophy. *Clin Orthop* 2006;449:288.

192. Wosick WF, Alker G. CT manifestation of ocular muscular dystrophy. *Comput Radiol* 1984;8:391.

193. Olson W, Engel WK, Walsh GO, et al. Oculocraniosomatic neuromuscular disease with "ragged-red" fibers. *Arch Neurol* 1993;26:193.

194. Pratt MF, Meyers PK. Oculopharyngeal muscular dystrophy. Recent ultrastructural evidence for mitochondrial abnormalities. *Laryngoscope* 1986;96:368.

195. Dobrowski JM, Zajtchuck JT, LaPiana FG, et al. Oculopharyngeal muscular dystrophy. Clinical and histopathologic correlations. *Otolaryngol Head Neck Surg* 1986;95:131.

196. Duranceau A, Forand MD, Fautaux JP. Surgery in oculopharyngeal muscular dystrophy. *Am J Surg* 1980;139:33.

197. O'Brien TA, Harper PS. Course, prognosis and complications of childhood-onset myotonic dystrophy. *Dev Med Child Neurol* 1984;26:62.

198. Schonk D, Coerwinkel-Driessen M, van Dalen I, et al. Definition of subchromosomal intervals around the myotonic dystrophy gene region at 19q. *Genomics* 1989;4:384.

199. International Myotonic Dystrophy Consortium, New nomenclature and DNA testing guidelines for myotonic dystrophy type-1 (DM-1). *Neurology* 2000;54:1218.

200. Bell DB, Smith DW. Myotonic dystrophy in the neonate. *J Pediatr* 1972;81:83.

201. Carroll JE, Brooke MH, Kaiser K. Diagnosis of infantile myotonic dystrophy. *Lancet* 1975;2:608.

202. Hanson PA. Myotonic dystrophy in infancy and childhood. *Pediatr Ann* 1984;13:123.

203. Vanier TM. Dystrophia myotonica in childhood. *Br Med J* 1960; 2(5208):1284.

204. Zellweger H, Lonasescu V. Early onset of myotonic dystrophy in infants. *Am J Dis Child* 1973;125:601.

205. Speer MC, Pericak-Vance MA, Yamaoka L, et al. Presymptomatic and prenatal diagnosis in myotonic dystrophy by genetic linkage studies. *Neurology* 1990;40:671.

206. Bowen RS Jr, Marks HG. Foot deformities in myotonic dystrophy. *Foot Ankle* 1984;5:125.

207. Gross RH. The role of the Verebelyi-Ogston procedure: the management of the arthrogrypotic foot. *Clin Orthop* 1985;194:99.

208. Colovic V, Walker RW. Myotonia dystrophia and spinal surgery. *Paediatr Anaesth* 2002;12:351.

209. Burnham R. Unusual causes of stiffness in two hockey players. *Clin J Sport Med* 1997;7:137.

210. Haig AJ. The complex interactions of myotonic dystrophy in low back pain. *Spine* 1991;16:580.

211. Weinberg J, Curl LA, Kuncl RW, et al. Occult presentation of myotonia congenita in a 15-year-old athlete. *Am J Sports Med* 1999;27:529.

212. Winters JL, McLaughlin LA. Myotonia congenita. *J Bone Joint Surg Am* 1970;52:1345.

213. Geschwind N, Simpson JA. Procaine amide in the treatment of myotonia. *Brain* 1955;78:81.

214. Kubisch C, Schmidt-Rose T, Fontaine B, et al. ClC-1 chloride channel mutations in myotonia congenita: variable penetrance of mutations shifting the voltage dependence. *Hum Mol Genet* 1998;7:1753.

215. Plassart-Schiss E, Gervais A, Eymard B, et al. Novel muscle chloride channel (ClCN1) mutations in myotonia congenita with various modes of inheritance including incomplete dominance and penetrance. *Neurology* 1998;50:1176.

216. Lehmann-Horn F, Jurkatt-Rott K. Voltage-gated ion channels and hereditary disease. *Physiol Rev* 1999;79:1317.

217. Goebel HH. Congenital myopathies. In: Adachi M, Ser JH, eds. *Neuromuscular disorders.* New York, NY: Igaku-Shoin Medical Publishers, 1990:197.

218. Goebel HH. Congenital myopathies. Semin *Pediatr Neurol* 1996;3:152.

219. Riggs JE, Bodensteiner JB, Schochet SS Jr. Congenital myopathies/dystrophies. *Neurol Clin* 2003;21:779.

220. Gamble JG, Rinsky LA, Lee JH. Orthopaedic aspects of central core disease. *J Bone Joint Surg Am* 1988;70:1061.

221. Shuaib A, Paasuke RT, Brownell KW. Central core disease. Clinical features in 13 patients. *Medicine* 1987;66:389.

222. Kumano K. Congenital non-progressive myopathy, associated with scoliosis: clinical, histological, histochemical and electron microscopic studies of seven cases. *Nippon Seikeigeka Gakkai Zasshi* 1980;54:381.

223. Ramsey PL, Hensinger RN. Congenital dislocation of the hip associated with central core disease. *J Bone Joint Surg Am* 1975;57:648.

224. Frank JP, Harati Y, Butler IJ, et al. Central core disease and malignant hyperthermia syndrome. *Ann Neurol* 1980;7:11.

225. Haan EA, Freemantle CJ, McCure JA, et al. Assignment of the gene for central core disease to chromosome 19. *Hum Genet* 1990;86:187.

226. Martinez BA, Lake BD. Childhood nemaline myopathy: a review of clinical presentation in relation to prognosis. *Dev Med Child Neurol* 1987;29:815.

227. Shimomura C, Nonaka I. Nemaline myopathy: comparative muscle histochemistry in the severe neonatal, moderate congenital and adult-onset forms. *Pediatr Neurol* 1989;5:25.

228. Eeg-Olofsson O, Henriksson KG, Thornell LE, et al. Early infant death in nemaline (rod) myopathy. *Brain Dev* 1983;5:53.

229. Maayan C, Springer C, Armon T, et al. Nemaline myopathy as a cause of sleep hypoventilation. *Pediatrics* 1986;77:390.

230. McComb RD, Markesbery WR, O'Connor WN. Fatal neonatal nemaline myopathy with multiple congenital anomalies. *J Pediatr* 1979;95:47.

231. Pelin K, Hilpela P, Donner K, et al. Mutations in the nebulin gene associated with autosomal recessive nemaline myopathy. *Proc Natl Acad Sci U S A* 1999;96:2305.

232. Cunliffe M, Burrows FA. Anesthetic implications of nemaline rod myopathy. *Can Anaesth Soc J* 1985;32:543.

233. Wallgren-Pettersson C, Clarke A, Samson F, et al. The myotubular myopathies: differential diagnosis of the X-linked recessive, autosomal dominant and autosomal recessive forms and present state of DNA studies. *J Med Genet* 1995;32:673.

234. Darnsfors C, Larsson HEB, Oldfors A, et al. X-linked myotubular myopathy: a linkage study. *Clin Genet* 1990;37:335.

235. Laporte J, Hu LJ, Kretz C, et al. A gene mutated in X-linked myotubular myopathy defines a new putative tyrosine phosphatase family conserved in yeast. *Nat Genet* 1996;13:175.

236. Laporte J, Biancalana V, Tanner SM, et al. MTM1 mutations in X-linked myotubular myopathy. *Hum Mutat* 2000;15:393.

237. Cavanagh NPC, Lake BD, McMeniman P. Congenital fibre type disproportion myopathy. A histological diagnosis with an uncertain clinical outlook. *Arch Dis Child* 1979;54:735.

238. Gullotta F. Metabolic myopathies. *Pathol Res Pract* 1985;80:10.

239. Cornelio F, DiDonato S. Myopathies due to enzyme deficiencies. *J Neurol* 1985;232:321.

240. Kearns TP, Sayre GP. Retinitis pigmentosa, external ophthalmoplegia and complete heart block. *Arch Ophthalmol* 1958;60:280.

241. Mechler F, Mastaglia FL, Serena M, et al. Mitochondrial myopathies. A clinico-pathological study of cases with and without extra-ocular muscle involvement. *Aust NZ J Med* 1986;16:185.

242. Leyten QH, Gabreels FJ, Renier WO, et al. Congenital muscular dystrophy: a review of the literature. *Clin Neurol Neurosurg* 1996;98:267.

243. McManamin JB, Becker LE, Murphy EG. Congenital muscular dystrophy: a clinicopathologic report of 24 cases. *J Pediatr* 1982;100:692.

244. Fukuyama Y, Osawa M, Suzuki H. Congenital progressive muscular dystrophy of the Fukuyama type—clinical, genetic and pathological considerations. *Brain Dev* 1981;3:1.

245. Fukuyama Y, Osawa M. A genetic study of the Fukuyama type congenital muscular dystrophy. *Brain Dev* 1983;6:373.

246. Hillaire D, Leclerc A, Faure S, et al. Localization of merosin negative congenital muscular dystrophy to chromosome 6q2 by homozygosity mapping. *Hum Mol Genet* 1994;3:1657.

247. Philpot J, Sewry C, Pennock J, et al. Clinical phenotype in congenital muscular dystrophy: correlation with expression of merosin in skeletal muscle. *Neuromuscul Disord* 1995;5:301.

248. Jones R, Kahn R, Hughes S, et al. Congenital muscular dystrophy. The importance of early diagnosis and orthopaedic management in the long-term prognosis. *J Bone Joint Surg Br* 1979;61:13.

249. Gordon N. The spinal muscular atrophies. *Dev Med Child Neurol* 1991;33:930.

250. Iannaccone ST. Spinal muscular atrophy. *Sem Neurol* 1998;18:19.

251. Russman BS, Melchreit R, Drennan JC. Spinal muscular atrophy. The natural course of the disease. *Muscle Nerve* 1983;6:179.

252. Shapiro F, Bresnan MJ. Current concepts review. Orthopaedic management of childhood neuromuscular disease. Part I Spinal muscular atrophy. *J Bone Joint Surg Am* 1982;64:785.

253. Shapiro F, Specht L. Current concepts review. The diagnosis and orthopaedic treatment of childhood spinal muscular atrophy, peripheral neuropathy, Friedreich ataxia and arthrogryposis. *J Bone Joint Surg Am* 1993;75:1699.

254. Emery AED. Population frequencies of inherited neuromuscular diseases—a world summary. *Neuromuscul Disord* 1991;1:19.

255. McAndrew PE, Parsons DW, Simard LR, et al. Identification of proximal spinal muscular atrophy carriers and patients by analysis of SMNt and SMNc gene copy number. *Am J Hum Genet* 1997;60:1411.

256. Iannaccone ST, Browne RH, Samaha FJ, et al. Prospective study of spinal muscular atrophy before age 6 years. *Pediatr Neurol* 1993;9:187.

257. Pearn J. Classifications of spinal muscular atrophies. *Lancet* 1980;1:919.

258. Russman BS, Iannaccone ST, Buncher CR, et al. Spinal muscular atrophy. New thoughts on the pathogenesis and classification schema. *J Child Neurol* 1992;7:347.

259. Burke SW, Jameson VP, Roberts JM, et al. Birth fractures in spinal muscular atrophy. *J Pediatr Orthop* 1986;6:34.

260. Gilgoff IS, Kahlstrom E, McLaughlin E, et al. Long-term ventilatory support in spinal muscular atrophy. *J Pediatr* 1989;115:904.

261. Evans GA, Drennan JC, Russman BS. Functional classification and orthopaedic management of spinal muscular atrophy. *J Bone Joint Surg Br* 1981;63:516.

262. Brzustowicz LM, Lehner T, Castilla LH, et al. Genetic mapping of chronic childhood-onset spinal muscular atrophy to chromosome 5q 11.2. *Nature* 1990;334:540.

263. Butler P, Burglen L, Clermont O, et al. Large scale deletions of the 5ql3 region are specific to Werdnig-Hoffman disease. *J Med Genet* 1996;33:281.

264. Stewart H, Wallace A, McGaughran J, et al. Molecular diagnosis of spinal muscular atrophy. *Arch Dis Child* 1998;78:531.

265. Miles JM. Diagnosis and discussion. Type I spinal muscular atrophy (Werdnig-Hoffman disease). *Am J Dis Child* 1993;147:908.

266. Ryniewicz B. Motor and sensory conduction velocity in spinal muscular atrophy: follow-up study. *Electromyogr Clin Neurophysiol* 1977;17:385.

267. Granata C, Cornelio F, Bonfiglioli S, et al. Promotion of ambulation of patients with spinal muscular atrophy by early fitting of knee-ankle-foot orthoses. *Dev Med Child Neurol* 1987;29:221.

268. Sporer SM, Smith BG. Hip dislocation in patients with spinal muscular dystrophy. *J Pediatr Orthop* 2003;23:10.

269. Thompson CE, Larsen Q. Recurrent hip dislocation in intermediate spinal atrophy. *J Pediatr Orthop* 1990;10:638.

270. Brown CJ, Zeller JL, Swank SM, et al. Surgical and functional results of spine fusion in spinal muscular atrophy. *Spine* 1989;14:763.

271. Zenios M, Sampath J, Cole C, et al. Operative treatment for hip subluxation in spinal muscular atrophy. *J Bone Joint Surg Br* 2005;87:1541.

272. Granata C, Merlini L, Magni E, et al. Spinal muscular atrophy. Natural history and orthopaedic treatment of scoliosis. *Spine* 1989;14:760.

273. Phillips DP, Roye DP Jr, Farcy J-P, et al. Surgical treatment of scoliosis in a spinal muscular atrophy population. *Spine* 1990;15:942.

274. Rodillo E, Marini ML, Heckmaht JZ, et al. Scoliosis in spinal muscular atrophy. Review of 63 cases. *J Child Neurol* 1989;4:118.

275. Merlini L, Granata C, Bonfiglioli S, et al. Scoliosis in spinal muscular atrophy. Natural history and management. *Dev Med Child Neurol* 1989;31:301.

276. Riddick MF, Winter RB, Lutter LD. Spinal deformities in patients with spinal muscle atrophy. A review of 36 patients. *Spine* 1982;7:476.

277. Aprin H, Bowen JR, MacEwen GD, et al. Spine arthrodesis in patients with spinal muscular atrophy. *J Bone Joint Surg Am* 1982;64:1179.

278. Hensinger RN, MacEwen GD. Spinal deformity associated with heritable neurological conditions. Spinal muscular atrophy. Friedreich's ataxia, familial dysautonomia, Charcot-Marie-Tooth disease. *J Bone Joint Surg Am* 1976;58:13.

279. Piasecki JO, Mahinpour S, Lovine DB. Long-term follow-up of spinal fusion in spinal muscular atrophy. *Clin Orthop* 1986;207:44.

280. Letts M, Rathbone D, Yamashita T, et al. Soft Boston orthosis in management of neuromuscular scoliosis. *J Pediatr Orthop* 1992;12:470.

281. Furumasu J, Swank SM, Brown JC, et al. Functional activities in spinal muscular atrophy patients after spinal fusion. *Spine* 1989;14:771.

282. Daher YH, Lonstein JE, Winter RB, et al. Spinal surgery in spinal muscular atrophy. *J Pediatr Orthop* 1985;5:391.

283. Askin GN, Hallett R, Hare N, et al. The outcome of scoliosis surgery in the severely physically handicapped child. An objective and subjective assessment. *Spine* 1997;22:44.

284. Blakemore LC, Scoles PV, Thompson GH, et al. Submuscular Isola rods with or without limited apical fusion in the management of severe spinal deformities in young children: preliminary report. *Spine* 2001;26:2044.

285. Sponseller PD, Yang JS, Thompson GH, et al. Pelvic fixation of growing rods: comparison of constructs. *Spine* 2009;34:1706.

286. Shapiro F, Bresnan MJ. Current concepts review. Orthopaedic management of childhood neuromuscular disease. Part II: peripheral neuropathies, Friedreich's ataxia and arthrogryposis multiplex congenita. *J Bone Joint Surg Am* 1982;64:949.

287. Geoffroy G, Barbeau A, Breton G, et al. Clinical description and roentgenologic evaluation of patients with Friedreich's ataxia. *Can J Neurol Sci* 1976;3:279.

288. Harding AE. Friedreich's ataxia. A clinical and genetic study of 90 families with an analysis of early diagnostic criteria and intrafamilial clustering of clinical features. *Brain* 1981;104:589.

289. Harding AE. Classification of the hereditary ataxias and paraplegias. *Lancet* 1983;1:1151.

290. Filla A, DeMichele G, Caruso G, et al. Genetic data and natural history of Friedreich's disease. A study of 80 Italian patients. *J Neurol* 1990;237:345.

291. Labelle H, Beauchomp M, LaPierre Duhaime M, et al. Pattern of muscle weakness and its relation to loss of ambulatory function in Friedreich's ataxia. *J Pediatr Orthop* 1987;7:496.

292. Chamberlain S, Shaw J, Rowland A, et al. Mapping of mutation causing Friedreich's ataxia to human chromosome 9. *Nature* 1988;334:248.

293. Fujita R, Hanauer A, Vincent A, et al. Physical mapping of two loci (D9S5 and D9S15) tightly linked to Friedreich ataxia locus (FRDA) and identification of nearby CpG Islands by pulsefield gel electrophoresis. *Genomics* 1991;10:915.

294. Campuzano V, Montermini L, Motto MD, et al. Friedreich's ataxia: autosomal recessive disease caused by an intronic GAA triplet repeat expansion. *Science* 1996;271:1423.

295. Karl RA, Budelli MM, Wachsner R. Double-blind, triple-crossover trial of low doses of oral physostigmine in inherited ataxias. *Neurology* 1981;31:288.

296. Wessel K, Hermsdorfer J, Deger K, et al. Double-blind crossover study with levorotatory form of hydroxytryptophan in patients with degenerative cerebellar diseases. *Arch Neurol* 1995;52:451.

297. Trouillas P, Serratrice G, Laplane D, et al. Levorotatory form of 5-hydroxytryptophan in Friedreich ataxia. Results of a double-blind drug-placebo cooperative study. *Arch Neurol* 1995;52:456.

298. Peterson PL, Saad J, Nigro MA. The treatment of Friedreich ataxia with amantadine hydrochloride. *Neurology* 1988;38:1478.

299. Brandsema JF, Stephens D, Hartley J. Intermediate-dose idebenone and quality of life in Friedrich ataxia. *Pediatr Neurol* 2010;42:338.

300. Kearney M, Orrell RW, Fahey M, et al. Antioxidants and other pharmacological treatments for Friedrich ataxia. *Cochrane Database Syst Rev* 2009;7(4).

301. Cady RB, Bobechko WP. Incidence, natural history and treatment of scoliosis in Friedreich's ataxia. *J Pediatr Orthop* 1984;4:673.

302. Daher YH, Lonstein JE, Winter RB, et al. Spinal deformities in patients with Freidreich ataxia. A review of 19 patients. *J Pediatr Orthop* 1985;5:553.

303. Labelle H, Tohme S, Duhaime M, et al. Natural history of scoliosis in Friedreich's ataxia. *J Bone Joint Surg Am* 1986;68:564.

304. Milbrandt TA, Kunes JR, Karol LA. Friedreich's ataxia and scoliosis: the experience at two institutions. *J Pediatr Orthop* 2008;28:234.

305. Warner LE, Garcia CA, Lupski JR. Hereditary peripheral neuropathies: clinical forms, genetics, molecular mechanisms. *Annu Rev Med* 1999;50:263.

306. Lupski JR, de Oca-Luna RM, Slaugenhaupt S, et al. DNA duplication associated with Charcot-Marie-Tooth disease type IA. *Cell* 1991;66:219.

307. Vance JM, Nicholson GA, Yamaoka LH, et al. Linkage of Charcot-Marie-Tooth neuropathy type 1A to chromosome 17. *Exp Neurol* 1989; 104:186.

308. Vance JM. Hereditary motor and sensory neuropathies. *J Med Genet* 1991;28:1.

309. Patel PI, Roa BB, Welcher AA, et al. The gene for the peripheral myelin protein pmp-22 is a candidate for Charcot-Marie-Tooth disease type IA *Nat Genet* 1992;1:159.

310. Timmerman V, Nelis E, Van Hut W, et al. The peripheral myelin protein gene pmp-22 is contained within the Charcot-Marie-Tooth disease type IA duplication. *Nat Genet* 1992;1:171.

311. Valentijn LJ, Bolhuis PA, Zorn I, et al. The peripheral myelin gene PMP-22/GAS-3 is duplicated in Charcot-Marie-Tooth disease type IA. *Nat Genet* 1992;1:166.

312. Roa BB, Garcia CA, Suter U, et al. Charcot-Marie-Tooth disease type IA Association with a spontaneous point mutation in the PMP22 gene. *N Engl J Med* 1993;329:96.

313. De Jonghe P, Timmerman V, Van Broeckhoven C II. Workshop of the European CMT consortium: 53rd ENMC International Workshop on Classification and Diagnostic Guidelines for Charcot-Marie-Tooth Type 2 and Distal Hereditary Motor Neuropathy, 26–28 September 1997, Naarden, The Netherlands. *Neuromuscul Disord* 1998;8:426.

314. Ben Othmane K, Middleton LT, Loprest LJ, et al. Localization of a gene (CMT2a) for autosomal dominant Charcot-Marie-Tooth disease type 2 to chromosome 1p and evidence of genetic heterogeneity. *Genomics* 1993;17:370.

315. Mersiyanova IV, Perepelov AV, Polyakov AV, et al. A new variant of Charcot-Marie-Tooth disease type 2 is probably the result of a mutation in the neurofilament-light gene. *Am J Hum Genet* 2000;67:37.

316. Ismailov SM, Fedotov VP, Dadali EL, et al. A new locus for autosomal dominant Charcot-Marie-Tooth disease type 2 (CMT2F) maps to chromosome 7q11-q21. *Eur J Hum Genet* 2001;9:650.

317. Sereda MW, Meyer zu Horste G, Sater U, et al. Therapeutic administration of progesterone antagonist in a model of Charcot-Marie-Tooth disease. *Nat Med* 2003;9:1457.

318. Bradbury J. Antiprogesterone hope for inherited neuropathy. *Lancet Neurol* 2004;3:6.

319. Alexander TJ, Johnson KA. Assessment and management of pes cavus in Charcot-Marie-Tooth disease. *Clin Orthop* 1989;246:273.

320. Mann RA, J Missirian. Pathophysiology of Charcot-Marie-Tooth disease. *Clin Orthop* 1988;234:221.

321. McCluskey WP, Lovell WW, Cummings RJ. The cavovarus foot deformity. Etiology and management. *Clin Orthop* 1989;247:27.

322. Paulos L, Coleman SS, Samuelson KM. Pes cavovarus. Review of a surgical approach using selective soft-tissue procedures. *J Bone Joint Surg Am* 1980;62:942.

323. Sabir M, Lyttle D. Pathogenesis of Charcot-Marie-Tooth disease. Gait analysis and electrophysiologic, genetic, histopathologic, and enzyme studies in a kinship. *Clin Orthop* 1984;184:223.

324. Schwend RM, Drennan JC. Cavus foot deformity in children. *J Am Acad Orthop Surg* 2003;11:201.

325. Olney B. Treatment of the cavus foot. Deformity in the pediatric patient with Charcot-Marie-Tooth. *Foot Ankle Clin* 2000;5:305.

326. Price AE, Maisel R, Drennan JC. Computed tomographic analysis of the pes cavus. *J Pediatr Orthop* 1993;13:646.

327. Wines AP, Chen D, Lynch B, et al. Foot deformities in children with hereditary motor and sensory neuropathy. *J Pediatr Orthop* 2005;25:241.

328. Bost FC, Schottstaedt ER, Larsen LJ. Plantar dissection. An operation to release the soft tissues in recurrent or recalcitrant talipes equinovarus. *J Bone Joint Surg Am* 1960;42:151.

329. Roper BA, Tibrewal SB. Soft tissue surgery in Charcot-Marie-Tooth disease. *J Bone Joint Surg Br* 1989;71:17.

330. Kucukkaya M, Kabukcuogulu Y, Kuzgun U. Management of the neuromuscular foot deformities with the Ilizarov method. *Foot Ankle Int* 2002;23:135.

331. Ward CM, Dolan LA, Bennett DL, et al. Long-term results of reconstruction for treatment of a flexible cavovarus foot in Charcot-Marie-Tooth disease. *J Bone Joint Surg Am* 2008;90:2631.

332. Angus PD, Cowell HR. Triple arthrodesis. A critical long-term review. *J Bone Joint Surg Br* 1986;68:260.

333. Mann DC, Hsu JD. Triple arthrodesis in the treatment of fixed cavovarus deformity in adolescent patients with Charcot-Marie-Tooth disease. *Foot Ankle* 1992;13:1.

334. Wetmore RS, Drennan JC. Long-term results of triple arthrodesis in Charcot-Marie-Tooth Disease. *J Bone Joint Surg Am* 1989;71:417.

335. Wukich DK, Bowen JR. A long-term study of triple arthrodesis for correction of pes cavovarus in Charcot-Marie-Tooth disease. *J Pediatr Orthop* 1989;9:433.

336. Saltzman CL, Fehrle MJ, Cooper RR, et al. Triple arthrodesis: twenty-five and forty-four-year average follow-up of the same patients. *J Bone Joint Surg Am* 1999;81:1391.

337. Hall JE, Calvert PT. Lambrinudi triple arthrodesis. A review with particular reference to the technique of operation. *J Pediatr Orthop* 1987;7:19.

338. Pailthorpe CA, Benson MK. Hip dysplasia in hereditary motor and sensory neuropathies. *J Bone Joint Surg Br* 1992;74:538.

339. Walker JL, Nelson KR, Heavilon JA, et al. Hip abnormalities in children with Charcot-Marie-Tooth disease. *J Pediatr Orthop* 1994;14:54.

340. Kumar SJ, Marks HG, Bowen JR, et al. Hip dysplasia associated with Charcot-Marie-Tooth disease in the older child and adolescent. *J Pediatr Orthop* 1985;5:511.

341. Fuller JE, DeLuca PA. Acetabular dysplasia and Charcot-Marie-Tooth disease in a family. A report of four cases. *J Bone Joint Surg Am* 1995;77:1087.

342. Trumble, SJ, Mayo KA, Mast JW. The periacetabular osteotomy. Minimum 2-year follow-up in more than 100 hips. *Clin Orthop* 1999;363:54.

343. Osebold WR, Lester EL, Watson P. Dynamics of hip joint remodeling after Chiari osteotomy: 10 patients with neuromuscular disease followed for 8 years. *Acta Orthop Scand* 1997;68:128.

344. Daher YH, Lonstein JE, Winter RB, et al. Spinal deformities in patients with Charcot-Marie-Tooth disease. A review of 12 patients. *Clin Orthop* 1986;202:219.

345. Karol LA, Elerson E. Scoliosis in patients with Charcot-Marie-Tooth Disease. *J Bone Joint Surg Am* 2007;89:1504.

346. Walker JL, Nelson KR, Stevens DB, et al. Spinal deformity in Charcot-Marie-Tooth disease. *Spine* 1994;19:1044.

347. Krishna M, Taylor JF, Brown MC, et al. Failure of somatosensory-evoked-potential monitoring in sensorimotor neuropathy. *Spine* 1991;16:479.

348. Brown RE, Zamboni WA, Zook EG, et al. Evaluation and management of upper extremity neuropathies in Charcot-Marie-Tooth disease. *J Hand Surg* 1992;17-A:523.

349. Miller MJ, Williams LL, Slack SL, et al. The hand in Charcot-Marie-Tooth disease. *J Hand Surg Br* 1991;16:191.

350. Mackin GA, Gordon MJ, Neville HE, et al. Restoring hand function in patients with severe polyneuropathy: the role of electromyography before tendon transfer surgery. *J Hand Surg Am* 1999;24:732.

351. Gaebler JW, Kleiman MB, French ML, et al. Neurologic complications in oral polio vaccine recipients. *J Pediatr* 1986;108:878.

352. Strebel PM, Sutter RW, Cochi SL, et al. Epidemiology of poliomyelitis in the United States one decade after the last reported case of indigenous wild virus-associated disease. *Clin Infect Dis* 1992;14:568.

353. Sharrard WJW. Muscle recovery in poliomyelitis. *J Bone Joint Surg Br* 1955;37:63.

354. Sharrard WJW. The segmental innervation of the lower limb musculature in man. *Ann R Coll Surg Engl* 1964;35:106.

355. Kojima H, Furuta Y, Fujita M, et al. Onuf's motor neuron is resistant to poliovirus. *J Neurol Sci* 1989;93:85.

356. Johnson EW Jr. Results of modern methods of treatment of poliomyelitis. *J Bone Joint Surg* 1945;27:223.

357. Arora SS, Tandon H. Prediction of walking possibility in crawling children in poliomyelitis. *J Pediatr Orthop* 1999;19:715.

358. Watts HG. Management of common third world orthopaedic problems. Paralytic poliomyelitis, tuberculosis of bones and joints, Hansen's disease (leprosy), and chronic osteomyelitis. *Instr Course Lect* 1992;41:471.

359. El-Gammal TA, El-Sayed A, Kotb MM. Shoulder fusion and free-functioning gracilis transplantation in patients with elbow and shoulder paralysis caused by poliomyelitis. *Microsurgery* 2002;22:199.

360. Liu T-K, Yang R-S, Sun J-S. Long-term results of the Steindler flexorplasty. *Clin Orthop* 1993;276:104.

361. Waring WP, Werner RA. Clinical management of carpal tunnel syndrome in patients with long-term sequelae of poliomyelitis. *J Hand Surg Am* 1989;14:865.

362. D'Souze H, Shah NM. Circumferential periosteal sleeve resection: results in limb-length discrepancy secondary to poliomyelitis. *J Pediatr Orthop* 1999;19:215.

363. Lau JHK, Parker JC, Hsu LCS, et al. Paralytic hip instability in poliomyelitis. *J Bone Joint Surg Br* 1986;68:528.

364. Asirvatham R, Watts HG, Rooney RJ. Rotation osteotomy of the tibia after poliomyelitis. *J Bone Joint Surg Br* 1990;72:409.

365. Asirvatham R, Rooney RJ, Watts HG. Proximal tibial extension medial rotation osteotomy to correct knee flexion contracture. *J Pediatr Orthop* 1991;11:646.

366. Mehta SN, Mukherjee AK. Flexion osteotomy of the femur for genu recurvatum after poliomyelitis. *J Bone Joint Surg Br* 1991;73:200.

367. Men H-X, Bian C-H, Yang C-D, et al. Surgical treatment of the flail knee after poliomyelitis. *J Bone Joint Surg Br* 1991;73:195.

368. El-Said NS. Osteotomy of the tibia for correction of complex deformity. *J Bone Joint Surg Br* 1999;81:780.

369. Shahcheraghi GH, Jarid M, Zeighami B. Hamstring tendon transfer for quadriceps femoris transfer. *J Pediatr Orthop* 1996;16:765.

370. Drennan JC. Poliomyelitis. In: Drennan JC, ed. *The child's foot and ankle*. New York, NY: Rowen Press, 1992:305.

371. Adelaar RS, Dannelly EA, Meunier PA, et al. A long-term study of triple arthrodesis in children. *Orthop Clin North Am* 1996;4:895.

372. Asirvatham R, Watts HG, Rooney RJ. Tendoachilles tenodesis to the fibula. A retrospective study. *J Pediatr Orthop* 1991;11:652.

373. Westin GW, Dingeman RD, Gausewitz SH. The results of tenodesis of the tendo Achilles to the fibular for paralytic pes calcaneus. *J Bone Joint Surg Am* 1988;70:320.

374. DeHeus JAC, Marti RK, Besselaar PP, et al. The influence of subtalar and triple arthrodesis on the tibiotalar joint. A long-term follow-up study. *J Bone Joint Surg Br* 1997;79:644.

375. El-Batonty MM, Aly EI-S, El-Lakkany MR, et al. Triple arthrodesis for paralytic valgus; a modified technique: brief report. *J Bone Joint Surg Br* 1988;70:493.

376. Pandy AK, Pandy S, Prasnd V. Calcaneal osteotomy and tendon sling for the management of calcaneus deformity. *J Bone Joint Surg Am* 1989;71:1192.

377. Dhillon MS, Sandhu HS. Surgical options in the management of residual foot problems of poliomyelitis. *Foot Ankle Clin* 2000;5:327.

378. Kocaoglu M, Eralp L, Atalar AC, et al. Correction of complex foot deformities using the Ilizarov external fixator. *J Foot Ankle Surg* 2002;41:30.

379. Mayer PJ, Edwards JW, Dove J, et al. Post-poliomyelitis paralytic scoliosis. A review of curve patterns and results of surgical treatment in 118 consecutive patients. *Spine* 1981;6:573.

380. Eberle CF. Failure of fixation after segmental spinal instrumentation without arthrodesis in the management of paralytic scoliosis. *J Bone Joint Surg Am* 1988;70:696.

381. DeWald RL, Faut M. Anterior and posterior spinal surgery for paralytic scoliosis. *Spine* 1979;4:401.

382. Leong JCY, Wilding K, Mok CD, et al. Surgical treatment of scoliosis following poliomyelitis: a review of 110 cases. *J Bone Joint Surg Am* 1981;63:726.

383. O'Brien JP, Yau ACMC, Gertzbien S, et al. Combined staged anterior and posterior correction of the spine in scoliosis following postmyelitis. *Clin Orthop* 1975;110:81.

384. Eberle CF. Pelvic obliquity and the unstable hip after poliomyelitis. *J Bone Joint Surg Br* 1982;64:300.

385. Gau YL, Lonstein JE, Winter RB, et al. Luque-Galveston procedure for correction and stabilization of neuromuscular scoliosis and pelvic obliquity. A review of 68 patients. *J Spinal Disord* 1991;4:399.

386. Perry J, Barnes G, Gronley JK. The postpolio syndrome. An overuse phenomenon. *Clin Orthop* 1988;233:145.

Idiopathic Scoliosis

INTRODUCTION

Idiopathic scoliosis defines a potentially severe musculoskeletal disorder of unknown etiology that occurs most commonly in adolescents. In its milder forms, the scoliosis may produce only a change in the shape of the trunk, but when severe can be markedly disfiguring and ultimately lead to cardiopulmonary compromise (Fig. 17-1). The goal of this chapter is to present the key elements in diagnosis, natural history, and treatment of both early-onset and adolescent idiopathic scoliosis (AIS).

The etiology of typical scoliosis is not yet known, and therefore the term idiopathic remains appropriate. Scoliosis can also be classified based on associated conditions because it occurs in many neuromuscular disorders (cerebral palsy, muscular dystrophy, and others) as well as in association with generalized diseases and syndromes (neurofibromatosis, Marfan syndrome, bone dysplasia). Congenital scoliosis, caused by a failure in vertebral formation or segmentation, causes a more mechanically understandable type of scoliosis.

The etiology of a scoliotic deformity (idiopathic, neuromuscular, syndrome-related, congenital) largely dictates its natural history, including the risk for and rate of curve progression. Additionally, the age at onset has a significant effect on the natural history, since spinal growth will typically result in progression of the scoliosis. Although scoliosis includes both sagittal plane and transverse plane rotation malalignment of the spinal column, the deformity is most readily recognized on the coronal plane. A better understanding of the three-dimensional nature of scoliosis has led to many recent advances in its treatment.

THREE-DIMENSIONAL DEFORMITY OF SCOLIOSIS

The normal spine is straight in the frontal plane, but has sagittal plane contours including thoracic kyphosis averaging 30 to 35 degrees (range: 10 to 50 degrees, T5–T12) and lumbar lordosis averaging 50 to 60 degrees (range: 35 to 80 degrees, T12–S1) (1–3). The scoliotic spine deviates from midline in the frontal plane and rotates maximally at the apex of the curve (4, 5). It is this vertebral rotation at the apex of the curve, through the attached ribs that produces the typical posterior chest wall prominence (Adams sign) that allows early diagnosis (6, 7) (Fig. 17-2). The axial plane rotation can also produce anterior chest wall deformity that can be manifested as breast asymmetry, with the right breast less prominent in most patients with the typical right thoracic curve (8).

In the past, it was thought that the lateral curvature of scoliosis was also kyphotic (increased roundback). It is now understood that most thoracic idiopathic scoliosis is associated with a *decrease* in normal thoracic kyphosis (9, 10). Dickson et al. (11, 12) have added to Somerville's postulate (13) that an early evolution to lordosis in the normally kyphotic thoracic spine leads to a rotational buckling of the spinal column (Fig. 17-3). The apical thoracic lordosis is more easily seen on three-dimensional reconstructions by viewing the spine with a true lateral projection of the apical vertebra. Standard lateral radiographs overestimated the apical region kyphosis by an average of 10 degrees (14). In some case, there may be an increase in kyphosis that should raise suspicion for a nonidiopathic cause of the curvature (syringomyelia, Chiari malformation). For unknown reasons, most progressive idiopathic thoracic scoliosis in adolescents is convex to the right side (15).

The global deformity of the spine includes local deformity in both discs and vertebrae. Wedging develops in both structures, and changes in vertebral body shape are thought to follow the Hueter-Volkmann principles of bone growth (16),

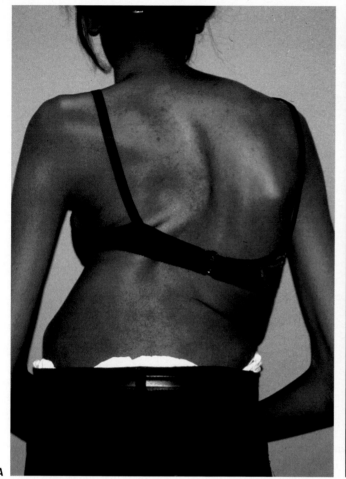
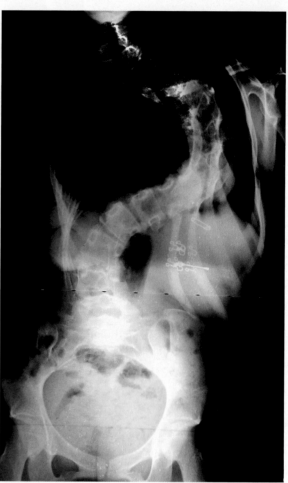

FIGURE 17-1. **A**: This 16-year-old girl with severe scoliosis refused early treatment and had severe progression. Her clinical examination demonstrated marked trunk and rib deformity, and she had reduced pulmonary function. **B**: The PA radiograph demonstrates a right thoracic curvature of 125 degrees. With proper diagnosis and early treatment, deformity such as this should be completely avoidable in AIS.

that is, reduced growth in regions of excessive compression as might occur in the concavity of a scoliotic spine. This causes asymmetric growth and/or remodeling (according to Wolff's law) of the vertebral bodies, pedicles, laminae, and facet joints, as well as of the transverse and spinous processes (Fig. 17-4). The vertebral body is noted to deform in a clockwise direction, while the spinous process deforms in a compensatory counterclockwise direction as seen on computerized tomography (CT) scan (17). Reduced concave growth accentuates the deformity, increases the compressive forces, and perpetuates the process (18).

ETIOLOGY

Despite the substantial research that has been performed, the etiology for AIS remains unknown. Many theories have been proposed including genetic factors; disorders of bone, muscle, and disc; growth abnormalities; and factors related to the central nervous system.

Genetic Factors. Several studies have demonstrated an increased incidence of scoliosis in the family members of affected individuals, thereby suggesting the existence of a genetic component to the etiology of scoliosis (19–22). Risenborough and Wynne-Davies (23) found scoliosis in 11.1% of first-degree relatives of 207 patients with idiopathic scoliosis. Examination of scoliosis in twins has further supported this with monozygotic (identical) twins demonstrating a higher concordance rate when compared to dizygotic twin (24–26). Genetic studies of families in which multiple family members are affected have suggested several sites within the genome that appear to be linked to scoliosis (27, 28); however, the exact genes remain unknown. An evaluation of the family pedigrees of 131 patients with AIS found 127 with connections to other scoliosis patients. The authors concluded that there is at least one or two major genes responsible for AIS (29). Some specific candidate genes have been ruled out (type I and II collagen, fibrillin, and elastin), while other hormone-related genes appear promising (30–32). Currently, genetic

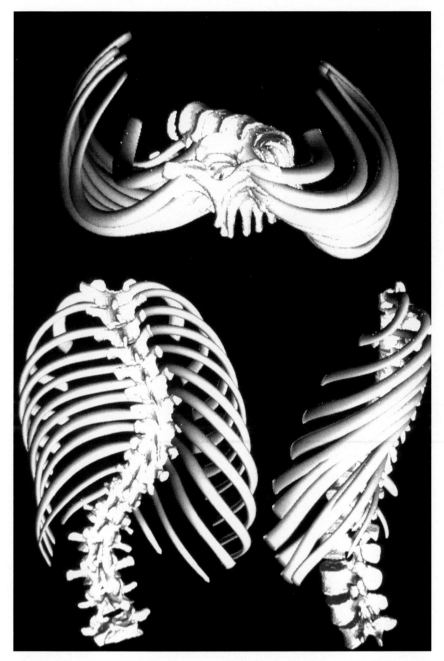

FIGURE 17-2. A three-dimensional reconstruction of the scoliotic spine and trunk demonstrates the three-plane deformity of the spine and attached ribs. The torsional deformity is maximal at the apex of the curvature. (Courtesy of St. Justine Hospital, Montreal, Quebec, Canada.)

tests are being evaluated to assess for risk of a patient with a mild curve progressing to a severe curve.

Tissue Deficiencies. Considering that scoliosis affects patients with known musculoskeletal diseases, some believe that the primary pathology involves specific structural tissues of the spine (bone, muscle, ligament, and/or disc). For example, fibrous dysplasia (bone–collagen abnormality) resulting in dysplastic, misshapen vertebrae (33), muscle disorders such as Duchenne muscular dystrophy leading to a collapsing scoliosis, and soft tissue–collagen disorders such as Marfan syndrome are all associated with the development of scoliosis. It seems plausible that subtle deficiencies in any of the tissues

of the spine could result in a predilection for collapse of the spine and idiopathic scoliosis progression (34). Some studies (35–37) have found that girls with scoliosis had a lower bone mineral density when compared to matched controls suggesting that AIS may be related to osteopenia (35, 38). Recent studies, however, have suggested that this relative decrease bone mineral density was more strongly related to the patient's body mass index (BMI) than the scoliosis (39). Therefore, the rationale for how osteopenia relates to the pathogenesis of scoliosis remains undefined.

Vertebral Growth Abnormality Theories. Considering that the development of scoliosis and its progression are

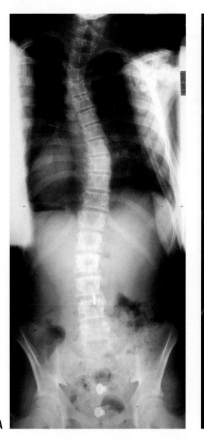
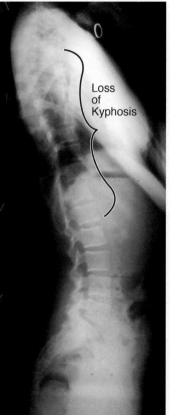
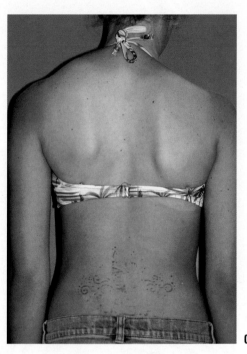

FIGURE 17-3. **A**: This PA radiograph demonstrates the appearance of a double thoracic scoliosis curve pattern. **B**: The lateral radiograph demonstrates the relatively straight sagittal profile of the thoracic spine with loss of normal thoracic kyphosis. This is a common feature of AIS. **C**: The clinical appearance of this patient demonstrates a prominent scapula. However, this is not caused by kyphosis but by the rotational deformity of the ribs, which secondarily makes the right scapula more prominent. Additionally, a left upper thoracic trapezial fullness can be appreciated in this patient, caused by the left upper thoracic curvature.

temporally related to the time of rapid adolescent growth has led many to believe that the etiology is related to abnormalities in spinal growth (40, 41). Initially, differential growth rates between the right and the left sides of the spine were thought to generate an asymmetry that would be accentuated with asymmetric biomechanical loading and the Hueter-Volkmann effect (42–45). Others have postulated that the etiology of scoliosis relates to a relative overgrowth of the anterior spinal column compared to the posterior column resulting in a relative thoracic lordosis (11, 12, 43, 46–49). If the condition is severe enough, the spine rotates laterally to maintain global sagittal balance, effectively shortening by rotation or buckling (50) the "extra" anterior column length. This theory accounts for all three planes of deformity. In addition, computer-generated finite element modeling of anterior spinal overgrowth has been able to replicate the typical three-dimensional deformity of scoliosis (51). Studies of the growth mechanism of the anterior and posterior aspects of the vertebral elements suggest a different mechanism of growth in each (endochondral growth anteriorly and intramembranous growth posteriorly) (52).

Several studies suggest that adolescents with scoliosis are taller than their peers (53–57). Increased levels of growth hormones (58, 59) and characteristic body morphometry (thin, increased arm span, physically less developed appearance) (60–62) also appear to be related to the development of scoliosis. Hormones are known to be involved in pubertal changes, and their roles in scoliosis development have been widely studied (58, 63, 64). Although the relation between scoliosis progression and skeletal growth is well recognized, the proposed alterations in the regulation of growth that could be responsible for scoliosis are not yet defined.

Central Nervous System Theories.   Disorders of the brain, spinal cord, and nerves may result in scoliosis. The role of the central nervous system in idiopathic scoliosis has been studied in detail (65–71). Goldberg et al. noted greater asymmetry of the cerebral cortices in patients with scoliosis (67). Also, abnormalities in equilibrium and vestibular function have been noted in patients with scoliosis (70, 72–76); however, it is difficult to be sure whether these findings are primary or secondary (77). A recent study, however, has suggested that idiopathic

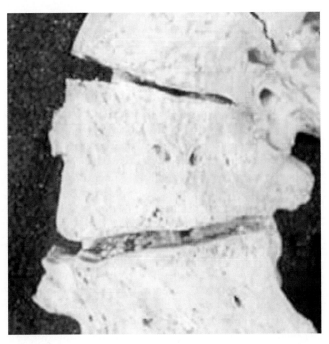

FIGURE 17-4. This anterior view of a human scoliotic specimen demonstrates the substantial wedging of the apical vertebra. These changes in shape of the vertebra are thought to be a result of altered growth, according to the Hueter-Volkmann law. This appears to be a component of the progression seen in idiopathic scoliosis during rapid phases of growth. (Courtesy of Stefan Parent, MD.)

structure whose "normal" state has multiple curves in the sagittal plane. There are likely several causes of idiopathic scoliosis, and active research continues in an attempt to find a unifying theory as to its development. The most promising clues seem to be coming from the advanced genome-wide studies that are underway.

DEFINITIONS

Scoliosis is defined as a coronal plane curvature of >10 degrees with curves less than this considered normal and called *spinal asymmetry*.

Curve Location. Scoliotic deformities assume a variety of curve patterns and several useful classification systems have been developed. The Terminology Committee of the Scoliosis Research Society (SRS) gives a detailed technical description of curve location.

The regions of the spine affected by scoliosis are defined by the location of the apical vertebrae as noted in the following list:

- Cervical: apex between C2 and C6
- Cervicothoracic: apex between C7 and T1
- Thoracic: apex between T2 and T11
- Thoracolumbar: apex between T12 and L1
- Lumbar: apex between L2 and L4
- Lumbosacral: apex at L5 or below

The *apex* of a curve defines its center and is the most laterally deviated disc or vertebra of the curve. Usually, a single vertebra can be defined. When a pair of vertebrae is at the apex, the "apical disc" is used to define the level of the apex. The apical vertebra(e) are also the most horizontal. Therefore, a patient with an apical vertebra at T8 is said to have a thoracic curve, whereas an apex at T12 is considered a thoracolumbar scoliosis. The *end vertebrae* of a curve define the proximal and distal extent of a curve and are determined by locating the vertebrae most tilted from the horizontal (these vertebrae are used for making the Cobb measurement). The *central sacral vertical line* (CSVL) is a vertical line that bisects the sacrum and is used for assessing the coronal plane balance of the spine in relation to its base (the pelvis). The *stable* vertebra is the most cephalad vertebra distal to the major curve that is bisected (or most closely bisected) by the CSVL. The *neutral* vertebra is the most cephalad vertebra that has no axial rotation associated with it. This is most easily recognized as a symmetric appearance of the pedicles with a midline appearance of the spinous process (Fig. 17-5).

scoliosis is not related to brain function (78). Syringomyelia is associated with an increased incidence of scoliosis (79–81), possibly due to direct pressure on the sensory or motor tracts of the spinal cord. Alternatively, there may be no relation to the dilation of the central canal, but instead brain-stem irritation from an associated Chiari malformation or enlargement of the fourth ventricle of the brain could be the cause.

It has also been postulated that melatonin and the pineal gland may be related to scoliosis. This theory is based on research involving pinealectomy in chickens. The procedure was found to result in a high incidence of severe scoliosis in the birds (82–84). Results of subsequent studies of primate and human melatonin levels have been conflicting and inconclusive. Machida et al. (85) found a lower-than-normal melatonin concentration in the serum of patients with progressive scoliosis compared to the serum of those with stable curves. In contrast, others have found no difference in either urine or serum melatonin levels between patients with scoliosis and age-matched controls or pinealectomized nonhuman primates (86–89). Confounding these studies is a recent report of melatonin signaling dysfunction in osteoblasts from patients with scoliosis (90). Currently, there is no confirmation that melatonin deficiency in humans is associated with scoliosis, as is seen in chickens.

In summary, the etiology of scoliosis remains unknown. As Stagnara (91) has noted, one should not be surprised that a minor disturbance in the structure, support system, or growth of the spine could lead to scoliosis, particularly in a complex

Age at Onset. Age at diagnosis is also used to define idiopathic scoliosis groups as follows:

- Infantile (0 to 3 years)
- Juvenile (4 to 10 years)
- Adolescent (11 to 17 years)
- Adult (≥ 18 years)

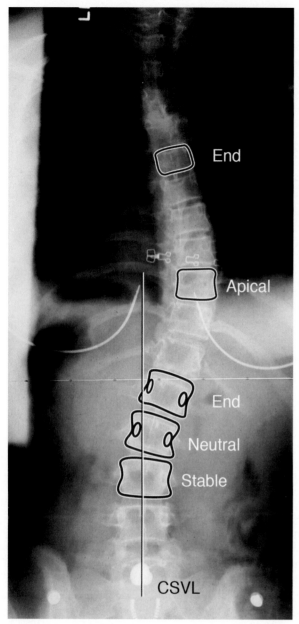

FIGURE 17-5. PA radiograph demonstrating the important vertebra and landmarks that define this curvature. The two end vertebrae of the thoracic curve are at T6 and L1, with the apex or apical vertebra at T10. The end vertebrae define the ones most tilted from the horizontal and are used for measuring the Cobb angle of the curvature. The neutral vertebra is the most cephalad vertebra that has neutrally rotated pedicles, whereas the stable vertebra is the most proximal one that remains bisected by the CSVL. The CSVL is drawn vertically from the midsacrum. These landmarks become important in ultimately defining a curvature, as well as in determining the levels for surgical treatment.

The age at which idiopathic scoliosis develops is one of the most important factors in determining the natural history of the disorder. Since younger patients have greater growth potential, the early-onset cases are more likely to be progressive. The onset of scoliosis before the adolescent growth spurt

is more likely to have an underlying spinal cord abnormality as the cause of the deformity. The incidence of such an abnormality is approximately 10% to 20% in the juvenile and infantile groups (92–94).

Major, Minor, Structural, and Nonstructural Curves. Curves may also be described as major or minor. The major curve is usually the first to develop and is the curve of greatest magnitude. However, at times, two or even three curves of equal severity exist, which make the determination of a major versus a minor curve difficult. Minor or compensatory curves develop after formation of the primary curve potentially as a means of balancing the head and the trunk over the pelvis. Similar compensation occurs in the sagittal plane where the typical lordotic thoracic curve may end both cranially and caudally with a junctional kyphosis. It is important to recognize focal and global alterations in the sagittal plane when planning surgical correction.

The terms *structural* and *nonstructural* have also been used for describing the flexibility of the minor scoliotic curves, *structural* curves being the more rigid ones (not correcting well when bent to the side). The degree of curve rigidity, which differentiates a structural from a nonstructural curve, has been debated, although Lenke et al. (95) have proposed a limit of 25 degrees on side-bending radiographs as the value above which a curve is considered to be structural.

Etiologic Classification. Scoliosis can be broadly classified according to etiology as idiopathic (or idiopathic-like), neuromuscular, syndrome related, or congenital. It is important to consider a patient presenting with scoliosis as a patient presenting with a sign (i.e., scoliosis) rather than a diagnosis— scoliosis. Although most scoliosis (approximately 80%) is idiopathic, the remaining cases are associated with a wide variety of disorders in which scoliosis is often the presenting complaint.

The SRS has classified scoliosis as being associated with each of the diagnoses seen in Table 17-1. The scoliosis associated with these conditions will be discussed in other chapters of this text. Neuromuscular disorders of either neuropathic or myopathic etiology make up a large proportion of the nonidiopathic causes of scoliosis in childhood. Intra- or extraspinal tumors or abnormalities must also be considered as possible causes of scoliosis. Congenital scoliosis and kyphosis as well may lead to progressive spine deformity. An awareness of each potentially associated condition helps when analyzing the various proposed etiologic factors in idiopathic scoliosis. More importantly, the diagnosis of idiopathic scoliosis requires the exclusion of these other conditions.

EVALUATION OF THE PATIENT WITH SCOLIOSIS

In North America, a screening examination either in a school or at a routine primary care visit often leads to referral to a specialist. Many of these patients, therefore, have no symptoms

TABLE 17-1	SRSs Diagnoses by Which Scoliosis Can Be Classified

Idiopathic	Fiber-type disproportion	Osteochondrodystrophies
Infantile	Congenital hypotonia	Achondroplasia
Resolving	Myotonia dystrophica	Spondyloepiphyseal dysplasia
Progressive	Other	Diastrophic dwarfism
Juvenile	Congenital	Mucopolysaccharidoses
Adolescent	Failure of formation	Other
Muscular	Wedge vertebra	Tumor
Neuropathic	Hemivertebra	Benign
Upper motor neuron	Failure of segmentation	Malignant
Cerebral palsy	Unilateral bar	Rheumatoid disease
Spinocerebellar degeneration	Bilateral (fusion)	Metabolic
Friedreich disease	Mixed	Rickets
Charcot-Marie-Tooth disease	Associated with neural tissue defect	Juvenile osteoporosis
Roussy-Levy disease	Myelomeningocele	Osteogenesis imperfecta
Syringomyelia	Meningocele	Related to lumbosacral area
Spinal cord tumor	Spinal dysraphism	Spondylolysis
Spinal cord trauma	Diastematomyelia	Spondylolisthesis
Other	Other	Other
Lower motor neuron	Neurofibromatosis	Thoracogenic
Poliomyelitis	Mesenchymal	Post-thoracoplasty
Other viral myelitides	Marfan syndrome	Post-thoracotomy
Traumatic	Homocystinuria	Other
Spinal muscular atrophy	Ehlers-Danlos syndrome	Hysterical
Werdig-Hoffmann disease	Other	Functional
Kugelberg-Welander disease	Traumatic	Postural
Myelomeningocoele (paralytic)	Fracture or dislocation (nonparalytic)	Secondary to short leg
Dysautonomia (Riley-Day syndrome)	Postirradiation	Due to muscle spasm
Other	Other	Other
Myopathic	Soft-tissue contractures	
Arthrogryposis	Postempyema	
Muscular dystrophy	Burns	
Duchenne (pseudohypertrophic)	Other	
Limb-girdle		
Facioscapulohumeral		

and are completely unaware of their potential spinal deformity. Evaluating a patient with scoliosis requires the physician to assess the patient for all conditions (Table 17-1) that are associated with scoliosis. While most adolescents presenting with scoliosis will be diagnosed as idiopathic, a careful history and physical examination are required in order to be certain no other causes exist that may affect their management.

History. While recording the patient's history, the physician should include questions about family history of scoliosis, the patient's recent growth, and the physical changes of puberty (breast budding, axillary/pubic hair, onset of menses in girls, and voice change in boys). When compared to the rates of occurrence in the general population, scoliosis occurs three times more frequently in a child whose parent is similarly affected and seven times more frequently if a sibling is affected (21). Additionally, if the patient's parents or sibling has been treated for scoliosis, this may suggest a greater likelihood of

progression in the patient. A record of increases in height over the prior few years is important in predicting remaining spinal growth and the risk for curve progression (96, 97). This information may be available from the primary care physician, or sometimes from measurements on the wall/door in the family's home. Breast development and the onset of menses are important maturational time points in females (98, 99). The past surgical history is important in identifying scoliosis associated with congenital heart disease and/or a prior thoracotomy. The family history as well as a review of body systems should identify disorders known to be associated with scoliosis (Table 17-1).

The presence or absence of severe back pain is important because most patients with idiopathic scoliosis have little or no discomfort. After scoliosis has been diagnosed (in a screening setting), patients often develop "pain" that continues until the diagnosis and prognosis have been clarified by an orthopaedic consultant who can provide reassurance. Despite the common belief among physicians that mild idiopathic scoliosis is never painful, Ramirez et al. (100) noted back pain (generally mild) in 23% of 2442 patients with "idiopathic" scoliosis. Only 9% of those with pain were subsequently found to have an underlying pathologic condition to explain it (diagnoses such as spondylolysis/spondylolisthesis, Scheuermann kyphosis, syringomyelia, herniated disc, tethered cord, and intraspinal tumor). Therefore when evaluating a child with scoliosis, a significant complaint of back pain should make one question, "Is this truly an idiopathic curve?" A child or an adolescent who presents with *severe* back pain and is subsequently found to have scoliosis requires a very carefully taken history, a physical examination, and a radiographic study [a bone scan and/or magnetic resonance imaging (MRI) study may be required] because an underlying etiologic cause is more likely (100–102). However, the clinician must distinguish between the "severe pain" (requiring further workup) and the mild fatigue pain (as described earlier), reported by Ramirez et al. (100) and Fairbank et al. (103). During adolescence, activity-related musculoskeletal low back pain occurs at a frequency greater than in childhood but less than in adulthood (104, 105).

Age at onset, rate of curve progression, and the presence of neurologic symptoms and signs are the most useful findings in identifying nonidiopathic scoliosis. In younger patients (<10 years) with an unrecognized neurologic cause, actual neurologic findings are often absent on physical examination, and the spinal curvature itself must be considered as the initial sign of a neural axis abnormality (92, 93, 106–108). The most common intraspinal abnormality found in this age group is syringomyelia (dilation of the central spinal canal) often with an associated Chiari malformation (brain stem below the level of the foramen magnum) (Fig. 17-6).

The rapid development of a severe curve suggests a nonidiopathic type of scoliosis. Neurologic symptoms such as weakness, sensory changes (upper and lower extremities), and balance/gait disturbance suggest intraspinal pathology (syringomyelia, tethered cord, tumor, etc.) as the cause of spinal curvature (101, 106, 107). The neurologic history should therefore focus on information about the patient's difficulties with grasping, walking, running, and stair climbing. A history of radiating pain, numbness, tingling in the limbs, and difficulties with bowel or bladder control should also be sought.

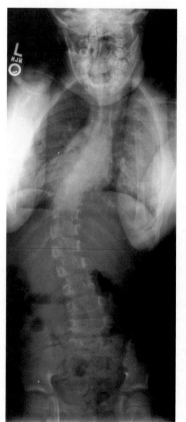
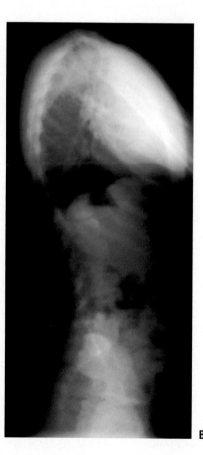
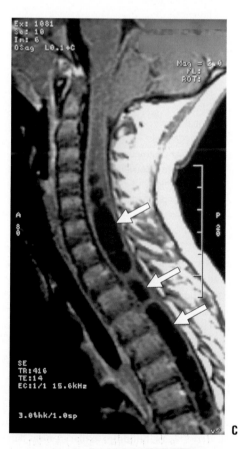

FIGURE 17-6. **A**: PA radiograph of a juvenile patient with a left thoracic curve. **B**: The lateral radiograph demonstrates relatively normal or even slightly increased thoracic kyphosis. Because the patient is in the juvenile age group and the curve is left side with an increased rather than decreased thoracic kyphosis, a spinal magnetic resonance imaging (MRI) was ordered. **C**: MRI of the midsagittal section of the cervicothoracic spine demonstrates a large syringomyelia (*arrows*) with significant dilatation of the central spinal canal. The syringomyelia was treated with suboccipital decompression.

Physical Examination.

Physical examination of a patient with scoliosis includes evaluation of trunk shape, trunk balance, the neurologic system, limb length, skin markings, and skeletal abnormalities. Assessment of pubertal development includes assessment of the stages of breast development and the presence of axillary/pubic hair (Tanner stages). This can be done discreetly without fully undressing the patient. Girls can be asked to wear a two-piece swimsuit for the physical examination (the instruction regarding this can be given at the time of fixing the appointment). This reduces the patient's anxiety and apprehension, yet allows assessment of breast and overall development.

With the patient standing, the back and the trunk are inspected for asymmetry of shoulder height, scapular position, and shape of the waist viewed from both front and rear. Potential pelvic tilt (an indicator of limb-length difference) is determined by palpating the iliac crests and the posterior inferior iliac spines bilaterally in the standing patient with both hips and knees fully extended. Lateral translation of the head can be measured in centimeters of deviation from the gluteal cleft by dropping a plumb line from C7. Deviation of the chest cage (trunk shift) should also be assessed because patients can have full head compensation (return of the head and neck back to midline) yet have marked lateralization of the trunk (Fig. 17-7).

Forward Bend Test.

The forward bend test, first described by Adams in Britain (109), has the patient bend forward at the waist with the knees straight and the palms together. This examination should be performed from behind (to assess lumbar and midthoracic rotation) and from the front (to assess upper thoracic rotation), as well as from the side (to assess kyphosis). Any asymmetry of the upper thoracic, midthoracic, thoracolumbar, and lumbar regions should be quantitated with a scoliometer (110) [to determine the angle of trunk rotation (ATR)] or by measuring the height of the prominence in centimeters (Fig. 17-8). This prominence reflects the rotational deformity of the spine associated with scoliosis (111, 112). Although there is not always an exact correlation, in general an ATR of 5 to 7 degrees is associated with a radiographic Cobb angle measurement of 15 to 20 degrees. [This is only an approximate guideline—occasionally patients may have little trunk rotation and yet have significant radiographic scoliosis, and *vice versa* (113).]

An inability to bend directly forward at the waist or a decreased range during forward/side bending may be caused by pain, lumbar muscle spasm, and/or hamstring tightness; any of these should suggest underlying pathology. These findings plus abnormalities in straight-leg-raise testing suggest irritation of the lumbar roots caused by spondylolysis, disc herniation, infection, neoplasm, or other factors.

Neurologic Examination.

The neurologic examination should evaluate balance, motor strength in the major muscle groups of all four extremities, and sensation. Watching the patient's gait, toe-and-heel walk, tandem walk, deep squat, and

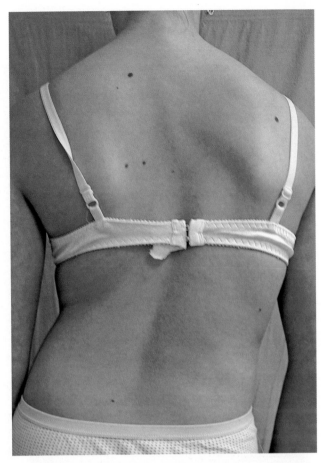

FIGURE 17-7. Careful examination of the back is required in order to identify the physical features of scoliosis. These include asymmetry of the scapulae, shift of the trunk, and asymmetry of the waistline, as well as asymmetry in the level of the shoulders.

single-leg hop allows rapid assessment of balance and motor strength. The presence of a cavus deformity of the feet, especially if it is unilateral, suggests an abnormality of the neurologic system/spinal cord. Testing for reflexes should include deep tendon reflexes of the upper and lower extremities as well as the Babinksi test for long tract signs. Abdominal reflexes are obtained by lightly stroking the abdominal wall with a blunt instrument (end of reflex hammer) adjacent to the umbilicus with the patient supine and relaxed. The expected brisk and symmetrical unilateral contraction of the abdominal musculature pulling the umbilicus toward the side being stroked indicates normalcy. When the reflex is persistently abnormal (reflex absent on one side and present on the other), intraspinal disorders, particularly syringomyelia, should be considered. The lower cranial nerves and the upper extremity examination should not be ignored because cervical-level pathology (particularly syringomyelia) presents here (81, 114).

Further Assessment, Limb Length.

Additional components of a comprehensive scoliosis examination include inspection of the skin (both on the back and elsewhere) for

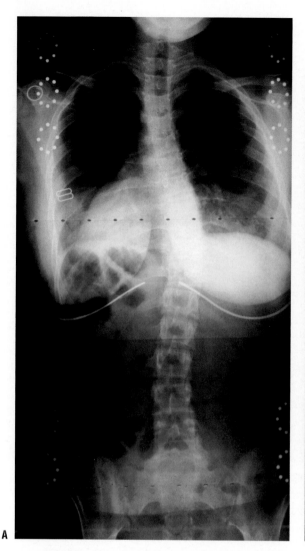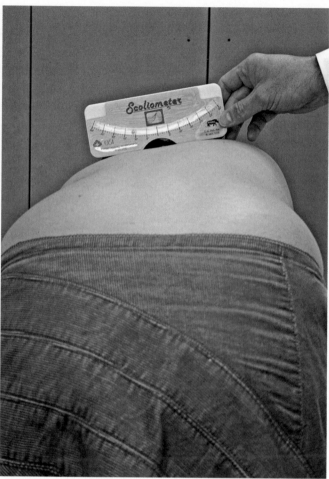

FIGURE 17-8. **A**: A 28-degree right thoracic scoliosis as seen on the PA radiograph. **B**: The Adams forward bend test demonstrated an 11-degree scoliometer measurement, indicating a corresponding measure for the ATR associated with this scoliosis. The forward bend test remains one of the most reliable means of detecting early scoliosis, other than a radiograph. Scoliometer measurements >7 degrees generally warrant a screening PA radiograph.

cutaneous evidence of an associated disease. Café-au-lait spots and/or axillary freckles suggest possible neurofibromatosis, whereas dimpling or a hairy patch in the lumbosacral area may suggest an underlying spinal dysraphism. Excessive laxity of skin or joints may be related to a connective tissue disorder such as Marfan syndrome or Ehlers-Danlos syndrome.

Limb length should also be measured in the supine position if pelvic tilt is noted during the standing examination. A spinal curvature that results from a limb-length difference is usually compensatory and serves to rebalance the trunk over the pelvis. A short right leg results in a compensatory right lumbar curve. There is no rotational deformity of the spine with these curves, and in the lumbar region the prominence noted on the forward bend test is on the concave side of the curve (the long leg makes the iliac crest and the lumbar spine

more prominent on that side). This is the opposite of what is seen in true lumbar scoliosis, where the rotational prominence noted on the bending test is found on the side of the curve convexity. The presence of the bending test rotational prominence on the "wrong" side in a lumbar curve is almost always diagnostic of spinal asymmetry caused by limb-length discrepancy rather than true scoliosis. The prominence disappears if the pelvis is leveled with an appropriately sized block underneath the short leg.

Radiographic Assessment. The ideal screening radiographs for scoliosis are upright (standing) posteroanterior (PA) and lateral projections of the entire spine exposed on a single cassette. The radiograph must be taken with the patient standing because diagnostic and treatment standards developed over the years are based on films in the upright posture. In very young patients, or in those with severe neuromuscular involvement, radiographs taken in the sitting or even supine position may be the only ones possible. The magnitude of the curve is greater when the patient is upright (compared to supine), and this is of particular importance in infantile and congenital curves when radiographs are taken before and after walking age. "Curve progression" may mistakenly be noted with the first upright-position radiograph as compared to prior supine views, when in fact one has simply documented that gravity causes a curve to be more severe. The sagittal balance varies with the method of arm positioning (the arms must be flexed for the spine to be clearly visualized). With the arms held straight forward, the trunk shifts posteriorly, and therefore the best position for viewing relaxed standing is with the arms flexed as little as possible to clear the spine (115). A lateral view of the lumbosacral junction is often performed in lumbar scoliosis to assess for spondylolysis/spondylolisthesis as a possible cause (Fig. 17-9).

Radiographic techniques that are used for minimizing radiation exposure of sensitive tissue (e.g., breast, thyroid, ovaries, and bone marrow) include taking only the required number of x-rays, utilizing rare earth radiographic enhancing screens with fast film, and a posterior-to-anterior exposure (116–118). The lifetime risk for developing breast or thyroid cancer has been suggested to increase by 1% to 2% in patients who are exposed to multiple x-rays during the course of treatment of scoliosis; however, these data relate to the 1960s and 1970s, before new radiation-reducing techniques became available. The greatest reduction in breast and thyroid exposure is associated with the PA exposure [compared to the anteroposterior (AP)]; this reduces breast/thyroid exposure three- to sevenfold (118). AP projection can shield the breasts; this is, however, not recommended because this projection increases thyroid exposure (shielding the thyroid obstructs the view of the upper spine). A new x-ray detection system that requires roughly one-eighth the radiation has been developed by Charpak, which has the potential to substantially reduce radiation for this population (116, 117). Doctors counsel their patients by assuring them that during the radiographic procedure, the exposure to the x-rays required to treat the disorder correctly will be minimal and that the benefit of undergoing the procedure outweighs the risk of not knowing the type and severity of the scoliosis.

When surgical treatment is being considered, lateral-bend radiographs (to assess curve flexibility) are required. Radiographs of side bending allow one to determine the degree of curve flexibility, and to decide what levels to include in the instrumented and fused segments. Controversy remains regarding the best method of obtaining AP films of side bending. Supine-position side-bending views (patient maximally bent to the right and left) are standard at many institutions, whereas others believe that a standing-position bend film is a better indicator, particularly in the lumbar spine. Lateral bending over a bolster provides somewhat greater correction and has been proposed as a more accurate predictor of the cor-

rection obtainable with the more powerful modern surgical instrumentation methods (87, 119) (Fig. 17-10). In curves >60 to 70 degrees, longitudinal traction films may also be helpful in evaluating curve flexibility (120, 121). There is no universal standard for how to obtain radiographs of bending. Additionally, there is little agreement on how to make use of the information gained. Flexible minor curves may be spared arthrodesis in many cases, and this flexibility information has been utilized (yet not necessarily standardized) in surgical decision making. More severe cases of scoliosis, that is, curves that do not straighten to <50 to 60 degrees, have been suggested as benefiting from an anterior release procedure prior to posterior instrumentation.

The Stagnara oblique view, taken perpendicular to the rib prominence rather than in the PA direction, provides a more accurate picture of large curves that have a large rotational component. From this angle, the true magnitude of the scoliosis can be measured more accurately (14, 122). Similarly, an oblique lateral may show the true sagittal alignment at the apex.

Reading Scoliosis Films. Assessment of the standing PA film begins by looking for soft-tissue abnormalities, congenital bony abnormalities (wedge vertebrae, etc.), and then by assessing curvature (coronal plane deviation). Bone assessment includes looking for wedged or hemivertebrae (Fig. 17-11) and bar formation bridging a disc space as well as midline irregularities such as spina bifida or a bony spike suggesting diastematomyelia. The pedicles should be inspected in order to verify that they are present bilaterally and that the interpedicular distance is not abnormally increased, which would suggest an intraspinal mass (123, 124). Absent pedicles or vertebral body lucency are associated with lytic processes, such as tumor or infection. If a curve is noted, the symmetry and the levelness of the pelvis are analyzed. A limb-length discrepancy can be estimated by determining height differences between iliac wing and hip joint, assuming the patient had hips and knees fully extended when the film was exposed.

Curve measurement using the Cobb method (125) allows quantification of the curve. A protractor or digital software tool allows for accurate measurements. The caudal and cranial end vertebrae to be measured are the vertebrae that are the most tilted, with the degree of tilt between these two vertebrae defining the Cobb angle (in a normal spine this angle is 0 degrees). One should outline the superior end plate of the cranial end vertebra and the inferior end plate of the caudal end vertebra. If measuring by hand, construct a perpendicular to each of these lines and then measure the angle at which the lines cross. When more than one curve exists, a Cobb angle measurement should be made for each curve (Fig. 17-12). The wide variation of inter- and intraobserver error (approximately 5 degrees for any curve measurement) should be understood by the surgeon and the anxious parents (and patient) (126). Therefore, a 6-degree difference is accepted by most surgeons as the criterion for determining curve progression in idiopathic scoliosis.

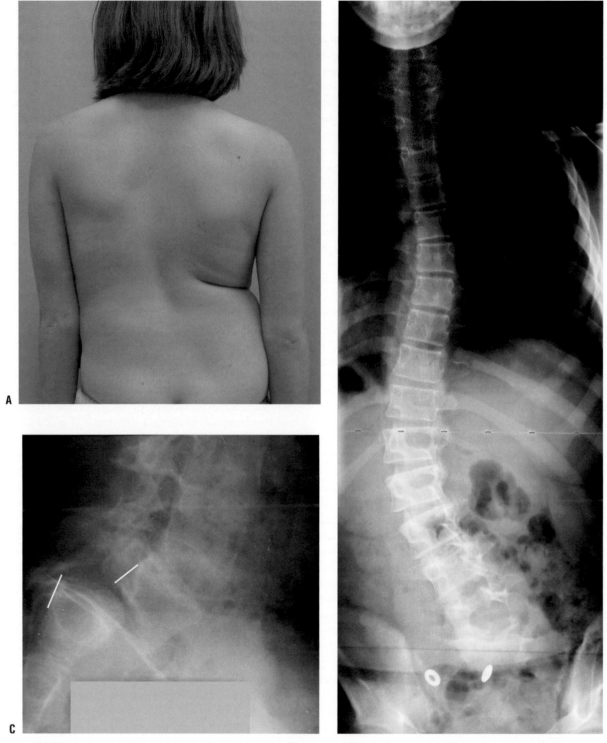

FIGURE 17-9. **A**: This 10-year-old girl presented with symptoms of increasing trunk decompensation, as well as low back pain and posterior thigh discomfort. She has an obvious trunk shift to the left, suggesting scoliosis. The PA rather than the AP view is preferred because there is reduced radiation exposure. **B**: The standing-position PA radiograph confirms a 43-degree left lumbar scoliosis. **C**: Standing-position lateral view focused at the L5–S1 level demonstrates severe spondylolisthesis. Most of this patient's lumbar deformity is related to an asymmetric forward slipping of L5 on S1, with rotational deformity translated to the lumbar spine above. Following correction of her spondylolisthesis with fusion from L4 to the sacrum, her scoliosis reduced to <15 degrees.

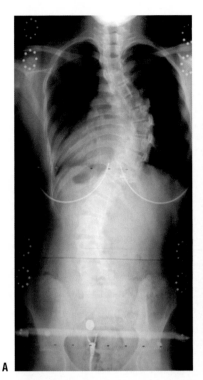

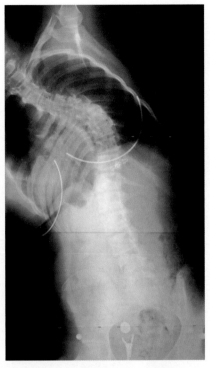

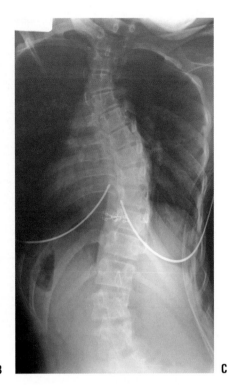

A   B   C

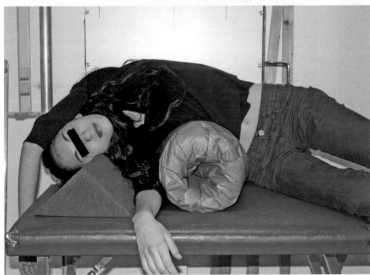

D

FIGURE 17-10. **A**: This standing-position preoperative PA radiograph demonstrates right thoracic scoliosis with moderate left lumbar scoliosis. **B**: The flexibility of the left upper thoracic and left lumbar curves was assessed via the left-side-bending radiograph. **C**: The flexibility of the right thoracic curve was evaluated using the bolster side-bending technique. **D**: The bolster side-bending film is taken with the trunk laterally flexed on a bolster positioned under the ribs that correspond to the apex of the deformity.

Vertebral rotation, maximal at the apex of a curve, is demonstrated on radiographic film by asymmetry of the pedicles and a shift of the spinous processes toward the concavity. Two methods are available for quantifying this rotation, one suggested by Nash and Moe (127) and the other by Perdriolle (128). Vertebral rotation is not routinely measured clinically, however, and both methods have substantial inaccuracies, which limit their usefulness (129).

Skeletal maturity should be assessed radiographically in order to estimate remaining spinal growth, an important predictor of risk for curve progression. The most widely used method in patients with scoliosis, although probably the least reliable, is that of Risser (130), who noted that the iliac crest apophysis ossifies in a predictable fashion from lateral to medial, and that

its fusion to the body of the ilium mirrors the fusion of the vertebral ring apophysis, signifying completion of spinal growth. The lateral-to-medial ossification of the iliac crest apophysis occurs over a period of 18 to 24 months, finally capping the entire iliac wing. Risser classified the extent of apophyseal ossification in stages, ranging from Risser 0, indicating absence of ossification in the apophysis, to Risser V, indicating fusion of the fully ossified apophysis to the ilium (spinal growth complete) (131). Risser I through IV are assigned to the intermediate levels of maturity as seen in Figure 17-13.

Risser originally described this finding on AP radiographs, which place the iliac apophysis close on the x-ray film. This is in contrast to the common current practice of PA projections and may explain some of the difficulties in reading this sign

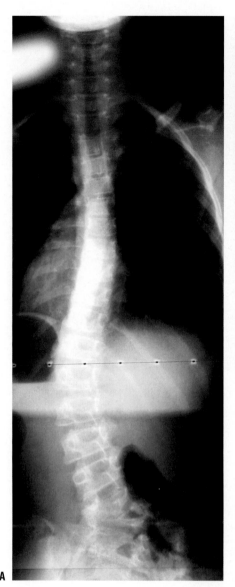

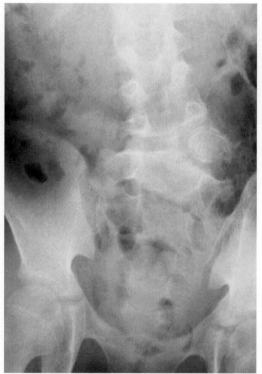

FIGURE 17-11. **A**: This adolescent patient presented with spinal deformity. The standing-position PA radiograph demonstrates an obvious left thoracolumbar deformity. On careful examination, an abnormality at the lumbosacral junction is suggested. **B**: A cone-down radiograph of the lumbosacral junction demonstrates a clear hemivertebra. This congenital malformation is the primary deformity, and the thoracolumbar deformity above is a compensatory curve. It is certainly important to recognize this because treatment of the thoracolumbar curve would lead to marked decompensation to the left.

(132). Despite the common reporting of the Risser sign as a measure of maturity, the appearance of the iliac apophysis generally occurs after the most important period of rapid growth (97, 99). Little and Sussman (133) have suggested that the Risser sign is no more accurate at predicting scoliosis progression than chronologic age.

The status of the triradiate cartilage of the acetabulum also provides a landmark for assessing growth potential. The triradiate growth cartilage usually closes before the iliac apophysis appears (Risser 0), at about the time of maximal spinal growth (134, 135) (Fig. 17-14). Skeletal age can also be measured using the Greulich and Pyle atlas (136) to compare hand radiographs against illustrated standards, although these readings become less accurate (large standard deviations) in the juvenile age group. Some authors have recommended using the maturation of the olecranon to determine skeletal age (137). Sanders has recently reported on the "digital skeletal age," which provides information about growth potential par-

ticularly useful during the Risser 0 phase (138). This system uses the progressive development of the epiphysis of the metacarpal and phalanges to determine skeletal age.

Specialized Imaging Studies. Most idiopathic scoliosis cases do not require imaging beyond plain radiography. Specialized imaging methods that can be used to evaluate cases with unusual features include MRI, CT, and bone scintigraphy, each with specific indications and advantages.

MRI has almost completely replaced myelography in the study of the neural elements in spine disorders. An exception is the patient who has had prior placement of stainless steel implants (making MRI visualization nearly impossible) and who continues to have symptoms or develops new ones that have to be studied.

MRI study of the spine is indicated for all patients with idiopathic scoliosis in the infant and juvenile age groups (92, 93, 139, 140) and also for those with congenital bony anoma-

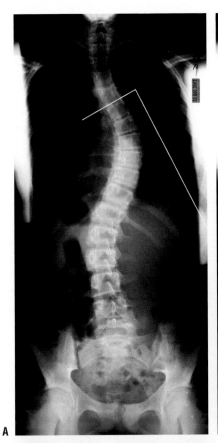

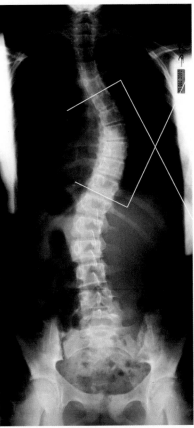

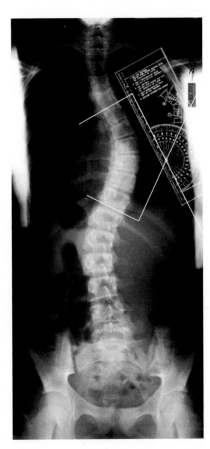

A

B

C

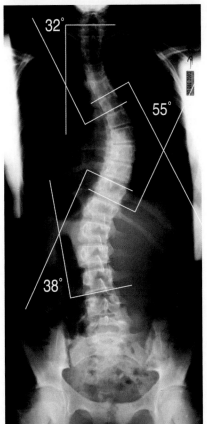

D

FIGURE 17-12.   **A**: Measurement of the Cobb angle. The end vertebrae of each curve must be selected before any measurement can be made. The end vertebrae of the curve are those which are most tilted from the horizontal. **B**: The endplates of the superior and inferior end vertebrae of the thoracic curve are marked on this figure. Perpendicular lines are constructed. **C**: The angle between the two lines is measured with a protractor and defined as the Cobb angle measure of the scoliosis. **D**: This method is used for quantifying the magnitude of scoliosis at each of the three regions: upper thoracic, main thoracic, and lumbar.

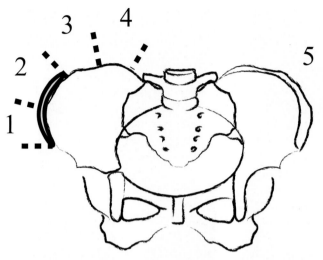

FIGURE 17-13. Risser sign. The iliac apophysis ossifies in a predictable manner beginning laterally and progressing medially. The capping of the iliac wing is correlated with slowing and completion of spinal growth, generally occurring over a period of 18 to 24 months.

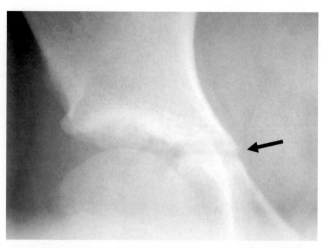

FIGURE 17-14. The triradiate cartilage of the acetabulum is seen here (*arrow*). The closure of this growth cartilage signifies completion of the most rapid phase of adolescent growth. However, at least 2 years of growth may be remaining following closure of the triradiate cartilage.

lies if surgical correction is planned (141, 142). Left thoracic curves have been shown to have an increased association with spinal cord anomalies and may be an indication for MRI study (140, 143). It has also been suggested that all male patients should have a screening MRI, although no studies exist to substantiate this. Indications are not clear for routine MRI prior to corrective surgery in patients with typical idiopathic scoliosis (for whom clinical neurologic examination has shown normal results) (144). Several prospective studies have been completed (145–147) of routine MRI screening for preoperative assessment (spine and brain) of all patients with idiopathic scoliosis. There is no evidence that an MRI is helpful in an otherwise normal adolescent with scoliosis. Clearly, however, patients with an abnormality in the neurologic examination (140) or with cutaneous findings (suggestive of dysraphism or neurofibromatosis) should have an MRI study of the spine and/or brain. Additionally, Ouellet et al. (148) have suggested that a hyperkyphotic sagittal alignment of the thoracic spine should raise suspicion of a syringomyelia and trigger an MRI study. Severe angular and rotational deformities may be difficult to analyze with an MRI because the spinal canal deviates into and out of the planar cuts of the sagittal and coronal images. CT myelography that produces a dye column may be better for revealing stenosis or an intraspinal filling defect in extremely severe cases of scoliosis.

The workup of patients with substantial back pain with no obvious cause may require a bone scan and/or MRI to evaluate for possible tumor, infection, or spondylolysis. The bone scan is an excellent screening test for studying the patient with scoliosis who is experiencing pain. The test allows one to screen for conditions ranging from osteoid osteoma to hydronephrosis. A single-photon emission computed tomography type of bone scan (computerized tomographic enhancement)

is very useful in identifying spondylolysis and its varying presentations (unilateral, bilateral, cold scan, hot scan, etc.). If an area of increased activity is noted on the bone scan, additional imaging (either MR or CT) may be required. An MRI may also be used as a screening tool for patients who are in pain, although cortical lesions (spondylolysis) may be harder to identify, and benign osteoid osteomas have been overinterpreted as malignancies. A screening MRI should include the entire length from the brain stem/posterior fossa to the sacrum. Individual MRI sequences for the brain, cervical, thoracic, and lumbar regions are not required. A limited number of images, primarily in the sagittal and coronal planes, are sufficient to identify a tumor, Chiari malformation, syringomyelia, or tethered cord. All aspects of the evaluation of a patient with scoliosis (history, physical examination, imaging studies) should be focused first on identifying possible nonidiopathic causes of the deformity, and only secondarily on characterizing the specific features of the curve. If one assumes an idiopathic etiology, an underlying spinal cord abnormality or associated syndrome will be very difficult to identify. One cannot recognize what one does not look for.

NATURAL HISTORY OF IDIOPATHIC SCOLIOSIS

Idiopathic scoliosis makes up the largest subset of patients with spinal deformity and, because its etiology is unknown, this diagnosis is one of exclusion made only after a careful evaluation has ruled out other causes of scoliosis. The natural history of nonidiopathic scoliosis along with the appropriate choice of treatment (and associated risks of treatment) may deviate substantially from that of idiopathic scoliosis. The history,

TABLE 17-2	Prevalence of Scoliosis				
		(% of patients with curves of this magnitude)			
Authors	No. of patients	>5 degrees	>10 degrees	>20 degrees	>30 degrees
Stirling et al. (155)	15,799	2.7	0.5	—	—
Bruszewski and Kamza (149)	15,000	3.8	3.0	0.5	0.15
Rogala et al. (153)	26,947	5.3	2.2	—	—
Shands and Eisberg (154)	50,000	1.9	1.4	0.5	0.29
Kane and Moe (151)	75,290	—	—	—	0.13
Huang (112)	33,596	—	1.5	0.2	0.04
Morais et al. (156)	29,195	—	1.8	0.3	—
Soucacos et al. (99)	82,901	—	1.7	0.2	0.04

examination, and imaging studies should be focused both on evaluating the severity of the deformity and on identifying its cause. Clinical features and treatment of idiopathic scoliosis also vary according to the age group to which the patient belongs (infantile, juvenile, adolescent). These are summarized in the subsequent text.

Prevalence of Idiopathic Scoliosis.
The prevalence of idiopathic scoliosis (with a curve of >10 degrees) in the childhood and adolescent population has been reported as ranging from 0.5 to 3 per 100 (149–155). The reported prevalence of larger curves (>30 degrees) ranges from 1.5 to 3 per 1000 (156, 157). Therefore, small-to-moderate curves are the more common ones, and severe (life-threatening) curves are rare (Table 17-2).

The percentage of cases seen in each age group demonstrates a strong predominance of adolescent scoliosis, with a series from Boston showing 0.5% infantile, 10.5% juvenile, and 89% adolescent incidence (23). The natural history for each group varies substantially.

Although classically idiopathic scoliosis has been divided into three groups according to the age of onset (infantile, juvenile, adolescent), there is a movement to simplify this to "early-onset scoliosis" (before age 10 years) and "late-onset scoliosis" (typical adolescent scoliosis) (155). Dickson and Weinstein (158) and Weinstein et al. (159) believe that only early-onset scoliosis has the potential for evolution into severe thoracic deformity with cardiac and pulmonary compromise.

Infantile Idiopathic Scoliosis.
Infantile idiopathic scoliosis (IIS) cases have been more commonly reported from Britain than North America (23, 160, 161). More recent reports, however, suggest a decrease in the frequency of infantile cases, more closely paralleling the North American experience (162).

IIS presents as a left thoracic curve in approximately 90% of cases, with a male:female ratio of 3:2 (160, 161, 163, 164). The curvature is often accompanied by plagiocephaly, hip dysplasia, congenital heart disease, and mental retardation (21, 165).

The series from Britain suggests that the vast majority (up to 90%) of these curves are self-limiting and resolve spontaneously (164); however, the few that are progressive can be difficult to manage, often resulting in lasting deformity and pulmonary impairment (166).

Prediction of Progression in Infantile Curves.
Risk factors that predict a high likelihood for curve progression have been identified by Mehta (167) who, in a study of 135 patients with IIS, determined certain radiographic prognostic parameters: (a) rib vertebral angle difference (RVAD) and (b) phase of the rib head. The difference in the obliquity between the two ribs attaching to the apical vertebra (right versus left) is known as the *RVAD*. The RVAD is the most commonly utilized measure and is determined at the apical vertebra on an AP radiograph. The ribs in the concavity of progressive infantile scoliosis are relatively horizontal, whereas those on the convex side are more vertically aligned (Fig. 17-15). Eighty-three percent of Mehta's reported cases resolved when the RVAD was

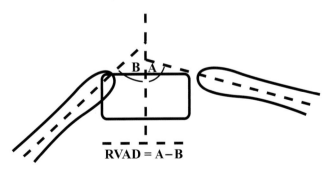

FIGURE 17-15. In IIS, the RVAD helps in predicting curve progression. The RVAD is constructed by first determining the angle of the right and left ribs at the apical vertebral level of the deformity. The slope of the ribs relative to the transverse plane is measured for each rib. The difference in the angle between the right and left sides is the RVAD. A difference of more than 20 degrees suggests a high likelihood of a progressive form of IIS, according to Mehta.

<20 degrees, compared to 84% progressing when the RVAD was >20 degrees (167, 168).

Juvenile Idiopathic Scoliosis.

Juvenile idiopathic scoliosis (JIS), defined as scoliosis with an onset at the ages of 4 to 10 years, accounts for approximately 8% to 16% of childhood idiopathic scoliosis (25, 169, 170), and in many respects represents a transitional group between the infantile and adolescent groups. Curves with onset in this age group are often progressive, with potential for severe trunk deformity and eventual cardiac and pulmonary compromise. Many patients who present in adolescence (previously undiagnosed and untreated) with severe thoracic curves requiring immediate surgery had the onset of their curves in the juvenile age period, making the differentiation between juvenile and adolescent grouping problematic.

In JIS, boys seem to be affected earlier than girls (171, 172). In a series of 109 patients evaluated by Robinson and McMaster, the boys presented at a mean age of 5 years 8 months compared to a mean age of 7 years 2 months for the girls. The ratio of girls to boys was 1:1.6 for those younger than 6 years and 2.7:1 for those older than 6 years at presentation. Additionally, there were equal numbers of right- and left-side curves in the younger group (<6 years) with a preponderance of right-side curves (3.9:1) in the patients older than 6 years (171). When curves reach 30 degrees, they are nearly always progressive if left untreated (172). The rate of progression is 1 to 3 degrees per year before the age of 10 years, and this increases sharply to 4.5 to 11 degrees per year after that age (171). This is particularly true of thoracic curves that, despite treatment with braces, require arthrodesis in more than 90% of the patients (169, 171). The surgical treatment of JIS is similar to that for AIS; however, anterior growth ablation (fusion) in addition to posterior instrumentation and fusion is more commonly indicated to prevent "crankshaft" rotational growth following posterior fusion (see subsequent text). In very young patients, instrumentation involving a system that can be periodically

lengthened is sometimes used (instrumentation without fusion or fusion only at proximal and distal hook sites).

Adolescent Idiopathic Scoliosis.

Patients with this most common category of scoliosis theoretically develop a curve after the age of 10 years, corresponding to the rapid growth phase of adolescence. Again, the separation of adolescent and juvenile curves is somewhat arbitrary because an 11-year-old girl who presents with a 70-degree scoliosis almost certainly had the onset of scoliosis in the juvenile age period. As noted previously, the data indicate that the prevalence of curves of 10 degrees or greater ranges between 0.5% and 3%. These data have been collected from a variety of sources including screening chest x-rays and school-screening programs. Roughly 2% of adolescents have a scoliosis of 10 degrees or greater, but only 5% of these cases experience progression of the curve to >30 degrees. The ratio of boys to girls is equal among patients with minor curves, but girls predominate as the curve magnitude increases, with the ratio reaching 1:8 among those requiring treatment (170).

Risk Factors for Progression.

Knowledge of which curves will likely worsen and which will not is critical in deciding which patients need treatment. The parameters that are significant in assessing the risk for scoliosis progression include gender, remaining skeletal growth, curve location, and curve magnitude. Scoliosis progression is most rapid during peak skeletal growth (early infancy and adolescence). The peak growth velocity of adolescence averages 8 to 10 cm of overall height gain per year (40, 135), with half of this growth coming from the trunk (spine) (25) (Fig. 17-16). Several determinants are useful in predicting the remaining growth. The age of the patient is one such obvious determinant. However, substantial variations in skeletal growth are seen among patients of the same chronologic age; therefore, bone age is a more consistent indicator (173). Menarchal status helps determine the growth spurt in girls (the onset of menses generally follows approximately

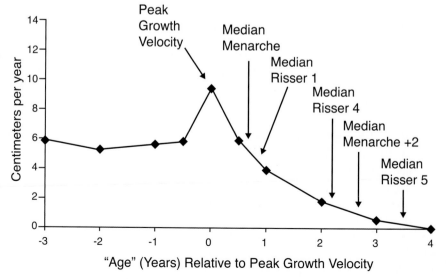

FIGURE 17-16. During the adolescent growth spurt, the rate of increase in height rises from approximately 6 cm per year to as much as 10 cm per year. The age at peak height velocity or the time of most rapid growth occurs before the onset of menses or appearance of the Risser sign. It is during this phase of growth that scoliosis progression is most likely. (From Little DG, Song KM, Katz D, et al. Relationship of peak height velocity to other maturity indicators in idiopathic scoliosis in girls. *J Bone Joint Surg Am* 2000;82:685–693, with permission.)

12 months after the most rapid stage of skeletal growth). (For additional information on growth, see Chapter 2.)

The Risser sign, which is associated with the inaccuracies noted in the preceding text, has been used for assessing the risk for curve progression. When the Risser sign is 1 or less the risk for progression is up to 60% to 70%, whereas if the patient is Risser 3 the risk is reduced to <10% (4, 174).

Unfortunately, many of the readily identifiable markers of maturity (menarcheal status, Risser sign) are quite variable and appear just after the adolescent growth spurt. If there is no accurate record of prior growth performance, it is impossible to tell whether a premenarcheal, Risser 0 patient is approaching, in the midst of, or past the time of most rapid growth and consequent risk for scoliosis progression. Closure of the triradiate cartilage of the acetabulum as well as capping of the digital epiphysis has been identified as radiographic signs that more closely approximate the time of peak growth velocity (137, 143).

The curve pattern has also been identified as an important variable for predicting the probability of progression. Curves with an apex above T12 are more likely to progress than isolated lumbar curves (174). Curve magnitude at initial diagnosis also appears to be a factor associated with progression (41, 175) (Fig. 17-17). In a series of skeletally immature patients (Risser 0 or 1), curve progression occurred in 22% of cases with a curve at initial diagnosis of 5 to 19 degrees, compared with 68% incidence of curve progression when the initial curve was 20 to 29 degrees (40). The rate of curve progression increased to 90% when the initial curve was 30 to 59 degrees (159, 176).

Natural History in Adulthood. The long-term effects of idiopathic scoliosis in adults should be understood when considering treatment in childhood and adolescence. The risk of

curve progression is greatest during the rapid phases of growth as discussed in the preceding text; however, not all curves stabilize after growth stops. In the long-term studies performed at the University of Iowa, more than two-thirds of the patients experienced curve progression even after skeletal maturity. Thoracic curves of <30 degrees tended not to progress, with the most marked progression occurring in curves between 50 to 75 degrees at the completion of growth (continuing to progress at a rate of approximately 1 degree per year). Lumbar curves generally progressed if they were >30 degrees at skeletal maturity (177, 178). Several studies provide insights into what the future holds for affected individuals. Early studies of patients with untreated scoliosis whose cases were followed for up to 50 years reported a mortality rate twice that expected in the general population, with cardiopulmonary problems being cited as the most common cause of death (179, 180). Disability and back pain were common among the patients (180, 181). Unfortunately, the etiology of the scoliosis in these studies was mixed (idiopathic, congenital, neuromuscular), and the severity of the scoliosis was not known in the cases of many of the patients, making correlations to those with idiopathic scoliosis impossible.

In more recent studies, in which only patients with AIS were included, the increased mortality rate reported previously has not been confirmed (159, 182). Mortality from cor pulmonale and right heart failure was seen only in severe thoracic curves (>90 to 100 degrees) (183, 184).

Pulmonary function becomes limited as thoracic scoliosis becomes more severe (>70 degrees) (159, 182, 185–187). The incidence of mild-to-moderate impairment in forced vital capacity and forced expiratory volume in 1 second (FEV1) increases with curve magnitude (183, 188) (Fig. 17-18). The associated deformity of the chest cavity causes restrictive lung disease.

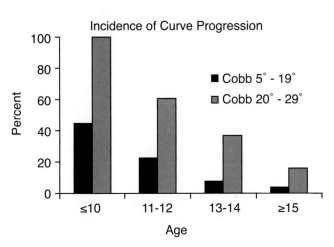

FIGURE 17-17. The incidence of scoliosis curve progression is greatest for younger ages and for larger curves. (From Lonstein JE, Carlson JM. The prediction of curve progression in untreated idiopathic scoliosis during growth. *J Bone Joint Surg Am* 1984;66:1061–1071, with permission.)

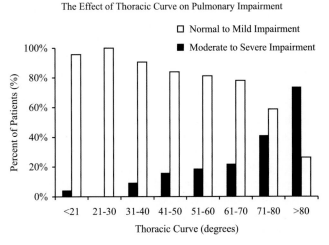

FIGURE 17-18. Pulmonary function as it relates to thoracic curve severity. As can be seen, a greater thoracic Cobb magnitude is associated with a greater risk of moderate-to-severe pulmonary impairment. (From Newton PO, et al. Results of preoperative pulmonary function testing of adolescents with idiopathic scoliosis. *J Bone Joint Surg Am* 2005;87:1937–1946, with permission.)

Thoracic lordosis also decreases lung volume and increases the deleterious effects of scoliosis on pulmonary function (183).

Estimates regarding the frequency of back pain and associated disability in adults with scoliosis vary, but most studies have demonstrated slightly higher rates of back pain compared to control groups (182, 184, 189, 190). The 1476 patients with AIS surveyed in Montreal had more frequent and more severe back pain than did 1755 control subjects (184). Disability rates have been higher in some series (180, 184) and similar in others (182). After 50-year follow-up, 65% of patients with late-onset idiopathic scoliosis reported chronic back pain compared with 35% of the controls (159).

The social impact of scoliosis varies with the individual and with the cultural setting. Nowadays, many patients are seriously concerned about the appearance of their backs and seek medical treatment to correct their deformities (188). Some studies report that the rate of marriage is lower among women with scoliosis; this implies a psychosocial impact of the deformity (179, 180). Many modern parents are unwilling to accept significant deformity of any type in their child, whether it is dental, dermatologic, or orthopaedic, particularly if there is a reasonable and safe way to correct the condition. However, as safe as scoliosis surgery has become, it carries with it finite risks and lasting consequences, most notably loss of spinal motion within the treated segments. Balancing these risks against current and/or future deformity challenges the decision-making skills of the treating surgeon.

SCHOOL SCREENING FOR SCOLIOSIS

School-screening programs have been instituted in many countries to detect scoliosis at an early stage. The goal is to detect childhood scoliosis early enough to allow brace treatment rather than in its late stages when surgical correction and fusion would be needed (191–193). Screening programs for any disease are indicated if effective early treatment methods exist, and if the disorder is frequent enough to justify the cost. Although screening programs for scoliosis are widespread in North America, the variable sensitivity and specificity of the screening exam and the questioned efficacy of brace treatment have caused some to suggest that school screening is not justified (158, 192, 194–196).

Despite these concerns, scoliosis screening is commonly performed on school children between the fifth and the sixth grades (age 10 to 12 years) (110). The Adams forward bend test is employed in combination with scoliometer (110) measurement of the maximum ATR (Fig. 17-8). A referral and a radiograph are recommended when the ATR is >7 degrees (25, 170). The 7-degree ATR standard detects nearly all curves >30 degrees, but leads to a large number of patient referrals (2 to 3 per 100 children screened) (110, 111) for radiographs in adolescents who have only spinal asymmetry (Cobb angle <10 degrees) or mild scoliosis (Cobb angle <25 degrees) not needing treatment. Overall, in school-screening programs, the incidence of curves of Cobb angle >10 degrees is approximately 3%, and of curves >25 degrees, about 0.3%.

Despite the criticism leveled at school screening (cost, over-referral), many experts believe that the emphasis placed on screening for early diagnosis has greatly increased awareness of scoliosis, not only in the lay public but also among primary care physicians. It appears that the combination of increased awareness plus the efficacy of screening programs has reduced the number of patients who do not see a physician until they have a marked deformity (191, 193, 197, 198). This theory remains controversial, and others have presented longitudinal data (following the institution of a screening program) that contradict this opinion (157, 194, 199).

TREATMENT OF IDIOPATHIC SCOLIOSIS

In considering the treatment options of idiopathic scoliosis, one must understand the natural history of the untreated condition. Improved understanding of three-dimensional deformity and advances in surgical techniques and instrumentation have dramatically changed the management of idiopathic scoliosis in the past half century. Therefore, the short-term outcomes of the most modern treatment are reasonably well known; however, the long-term results are less well defined. Because of this lack of knowledge, there may be continuing controversy regarding treatment choices in any individual patient.

Nonoperative Treatment of Idiopathic Scoliosis.
Most patients with spinal curves <15 degrees are referred back to their pediatrician to continue routine yearly screening. If there is a concern for progression based on growth remaining or family history, a repeat exam can be done in 12 months. Idiopathic curves of 15 to 25 degrees should be monitored with clinical and radiographic examination every 6 to 12 months (depending on the age and growth rate of the patient) with clinical and radiographic examination. Those in the rapid phases of growth are seen at more frequent intervals (every 4 to 6 months). Curves >30 degrees should be monitored for progression after skeletal maturity, with radiographs obtained approximately every 5 years. Curve progression in the mature patient (when it occurs) is slow enough (approximately 1 degree per year) that more frequent follow-up is not indicated.

Indications for Orthotic (Brace) Treatment.
In growing children, a spinal orthosis (brace) may be considered when a curve progresses to 25 degrees (200–206). Some surgeons insist that curve progression of more than 5 degrees be documented before using bracing in curves of <30 degrees. Others will consider bracing early at 20 degrees when there is a strong family history for progressive scoliosis (for instance, if the mother or a sibling has required surgical treatment for scoliosis) (205). Scoliosis braces of many different styles and corrective mechanical principles have been developed, the common goal being to modify spinal growth by applying an external force (203). Because brace treatment depends

on spinal growth modulation, treatment is prescribed only for patients with substantial spinal growth remaining (Risser 2 or less). The upper limit of curve magnitude that is amenable to brace treatment is approximately 40 to 45 degrees. Most studies have confirmed that, even in the most cooperative patients, the final result of brace treatment is merely maintenance of the curve at the degree of severity present at the onset of bracing. Many families will be excited by the improvement seen within the brace and anticipate this to be the outcome of using a brace, but when the brace is discontinued the curve will generally settle to its pretreatment level of severity (204, 207, 208). Patients with scoliosis and their parents should be advised of this limitation.

In the patient with early-onset scoliosis (infantile and JIS), braces are also commonly used as a primary form of treatment or utilized between periods of casting. While the hope is to prevent the need for surgery, the primary goal is to slow progression, delay surgical intervention, and allow continued spinal growth before intervening surgically. Similar to adolescent patients, the threshold to begin bracing in these patients is 20 to 25 degrees. The indications for surgery in early-onset patients are less clear, and, therefore, brace wear is typically used beyond the 40-degree limit utilized in adolescent patients.

Brace Types.   The Milwaukee brace, developed by Walter Blount at Milwaukee Children's Hospital in the 1940s, became the standard against which other designs were compared (209). This brace remained popular into the 1980s (210), but due to its poor tolerance by many patients, it is not routinely prescribed. The original design provided longitudinal traction between the skull and the pelvis with lateral translational forces directed through pads on the chest wall.

An underarm brace or a thoracolumbarsacral orthosis (TLSOs) [e.g., Boston (211, 212) and Wilmington (213, 214)] (Fig. 17-19) has replaced the Milwaukee brace in most centers because of more ready acceptance by the patients. Because no cervical extension is used, the brace is less conspicuous. The wearing of a visible scoliosis brace is seen as a stigma by many teenage patients, and consequently produces a negative self-image (215, 216). Despite improvements in the appearance of the brace (worn under the clothes, no visible neckpiece), many teenagers will not cooperate with brace wear. Reasons for failure include pain (217), poor fit, discomfort from the heat, family environment, and concerns about self-esteem. The use of such underarm braces is limited to curves with an apex below T7.

The Charleston and Providence nighttime bending braces (218, 219) attempt to create a more complete correction of the curve by producing a maximal trunk bend, so severe that

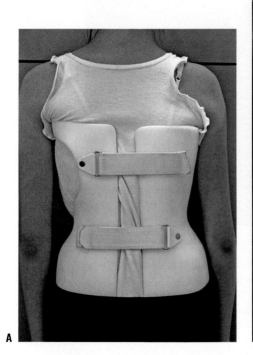
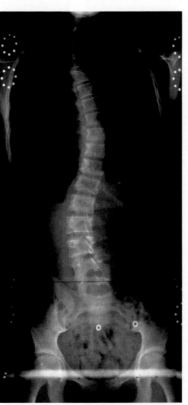
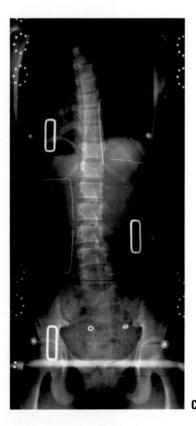

A   B   C

FIGURE 17-19.   **A**: Boston brace. **B**: This PA radiograph demonstrates a right thoracic left lumbar curve pattern in an adolescent patient with remaining growth. **C**: The in-brace radiograph demonstrates a reduction of both the thoracic and the lumbar curves.

it precludes walking (Fig 17-20). These braces are therefore prescribed only for nighttime wear.

There have also been attempts to design nonrigid braces with straps specifically placed to provide to corrective forces on each curve. By being flexible, the belief is that they provide dynamic curve correction (220, 221). These braces have not been as extensively tested as their more rigid counterparts and are less commonly prescribed (206, 222).

Wearing Schedule. The correction achieved by a brace is thought to be caused by the constant corrective molding of the trunk and spine during growth. As such, full-time (23 hours

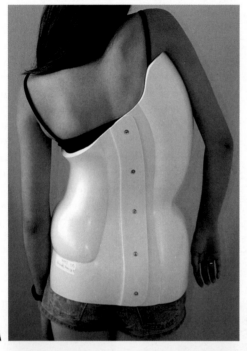

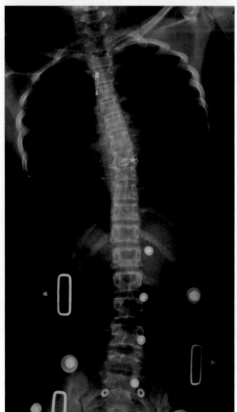

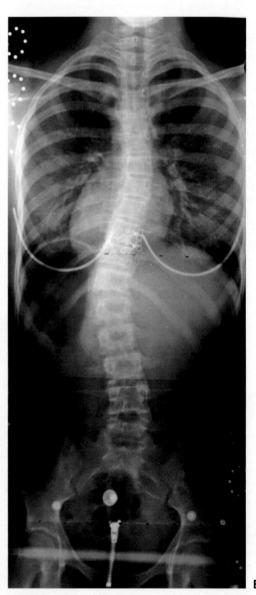

FIGURE 17-20. **A**: Charleston nighttime bending brace. **B**: This thoracolumbar curve is one that appears amenable to treatment with a nighttime bending brace. **C**: The in-brace radiograph demonstrates nearly complete correction of the thoracolumbar curvature.

per day) brace wear was first advised by Blount and continues to be recommended by many who prescribe scoliosis braces. Certain centers began to treat patients for only 16 hours per day, allowing the child to go to school without the brace, hoping that the abbreviated schedule would lead to greater compliance by the patient (213, 223). This schedule is popular with many surgeons (and patients).

A meta-analysis performed by the SRS Prevalence and Natural History Committee found a dose-dependent relation between the number of in-brace hours per day and success in preventing curve progression (224), thereby suggesting that ensuring more hours of brace wear per day provides more effective correction. This contradicted a study with the Wilmington brace that did not demonstrate a difference in efficacy between part-time and full-time bracing (213). A recent publication from Katz et al. suggests a dose-dependent effect of bracing (225). They prospectively evaluated patients treated with a Boston brace and measured brace wear using a heat sensor. Curves did not progress in 82% of patients that wore their brace >12 hours compared with only 31% that wore their brace <7 hours.

Brace Efficacy. The effectiveness of bracing for idiopathic scoliosis has been presumed for many years, yet well-controlled treatment trials with and without bracing have not been completed (200, 226). Earlier studies reporting high success rates for brace treatment were subsequently noted to have included many patients who were at low risk for progression. Lonstein and Winter evaluated 1020 patients treated with a Milwaukee brace, over half of whom were at substantial risk for progression, and for whom the natural history was known. In the group with an initial curve between 20 and 29 degrees and at high risk for progression, the brace was found to be effective compared to natural history data pertaining to the untreated state (210). This is in contrast to the findings of Noonan et al. (227) who have recently called into question the efficacy of the Milwaukee brace.

In 1995, the results of a prospective, controlled (but not randomized) study of bracing by the SRS were published. Results were compared in 286 patients, with an initial curve of 25 to 35 degrees: 129 were observed but received no treatment, 111 were treated with an underarm brace, and 46 were treated with nighttime electrical stimulation (46 patients). Curve progression at the end of bracing (skeletal maturity) was limited to <5 degrees in 74% of those treated with a brace, compared with 34% in those who received no treatment. The group treated with electrical stimulation had a success rate of only 33% (200). Critics cite flaws in this study related to it being nonrandomized, nonblinded, with baseline differences between groups and a lack of reporting on surgical rates (158, 205). A recent Cochrane review reported that there is very low-quality evidence in support of bracing (222). Many concerns regarding these studies have been related to the compliance of brace wear (228). Objective compliance devices using temperature sensors have been developed to determine compliance (229, 230). Currently, a randomized

multicenter study supported by the National Institutes of Health is being undertaken to assess the effectiveness of brace wear for AIS (230).

Data regarding the efficacy of various brace designs are mixed, with differing inclusion criteria making direct comparisons difficult (223, 224). However, in two studies, a full-time underarm brace was more successful than a nighttime Charleston bending brace both in preventing curve progression and in preventing surgery (201, 231). Both of these studies were retrospective with potential biases, and no prospective comparison of various braces has been performed to confirm these conclusions. One study did suggest that the nighttime Charleston brace equaled the efficacy of a Boston brace for single-lumbar and thoracolumbar curves (201).

In summary, although brace treatment for progressive curves is considered the standard of care in many centers, the scientific basis for brace efficacy is not powerful. When to intervene remains a difficult decision to make that requires an active discussion between the treating physician, the patient and the parents. This is because although very mild curves appear to be more effectively controlled with a brace, a blanket application of this policy would lead to many children being braced unnecessarily. Waiting until the curve reaches 30 degrees allows one to brace the smallest number of patients, yet the margin between a curve of 30 degrees (brace instituted) and 40 to 50 degrees (surgery indicated) is distressingly small. Finally, many adolescents strongly resist brace wear and such resistance is understandable (232, 233). Compliance is thought to be a major factor in why there is less success with bracing in teenage boys who might have to wear a brace for as long as 5 years (skeletal maturity is often reached only at age 18 or greater). Karol (234) reported a bracing failure rate of 74% in boys. Each of these factors makes orthotic (brace) treatment of scoliosis a continuing challenge.

Once a patient has been prescribed a brace, the patient should then have an in-brace PA radiograph to determine effectiveness. The goal is to achieve at least 50% curve correction in fulltime braces and >75% correction in bending braces. Patients are subsequently monitored similar to nonbraced patients every 6 months with radiographs out of the brace to document possible progression. Any decision to either discontinue the brace or recommend surgery is based on curve magnitude and progression out of the brace as well as skeletal maturity.

Corrective Casting. In some cases, bracing may not provide sufficient corrective force, and a molded body cast may be indicated. In the years before the advent of posterior instrumentation, this was the primary means of obtaining curve correction prior to fusion. Today it is used to aid in immobilizing patients who are too small for rigid instrumentation prior to fusion, or in those with severe deformities who are too young to undergo fusion. Progressive IIS is currently the most common indication for a well-molded corrective body cast (235). In these young patients, rib deformity associated with the cast pressure is almost certain to occur. However, this approach may delay the repeated surgeries that will follow application of a growing rod instrumentation system in such a patient. The complications associated with growth rod constructs make them a method of last resort. Risser-type casting is a good choice in patients with progressive IIS, either before moving to a brace or after a bracing failure has occurred. Similar to other forms of treatment, there are many techniques for applying the cast to obtain three-dimensional spinal deformity correction (Fig. 17-21). Mehta (236) has reported on the outcomes of her casting method which focuses on elongation and derotation of the trunk.

Surgical Correction of Idiopathic Scoliosis

Indications. The goals for surgical treatment of idiopathic scoliosis include the prevention of further curve progression, obtaining three-dimensional realignment, while maximizing coronal and sagittal balance. Corrective instrumentation plus arthrodesis (fusion) provides the best method for achieving lasting correction. This can be done either anteriorly, posteriorly, or in severe cases via both anterior and posterior methods. Current techniques rely on the development of a stable fusion to maintain the correction over time, with the rods serving as internal struts while fusion proceeds. Application of a rod system without a bony fusion predictably leads to eventual rod fracture and loss of correction; instrumentation without fusion (as in growing rod constructs) can be useful as a temporizing method.

The indications for surgical correction of scoliosis are based on curve magnitude, clinical deformity, risk for progression, skeletal maturity, and curve pattern. In general, thoracic curves of Cobb angle >40 to 50 degrees in skeletally immature patients should be surgically corrected, whereas surgical correction is reserved for curves of 50 degrees or more in mature patients (in whom there is a lower risk of progression). These

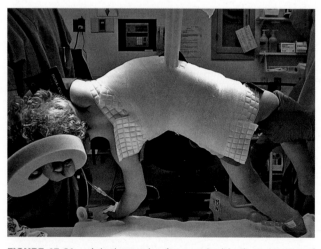

FIGURE 17-21. A body cast is often required in the treatment of progressive IIS. This demonstrates a method of applying a bending force by suspending the trunk with muslin before rolling a Goretex-lined fiberglass cast.

Cobb angle ranges are meant as guidelines rather than absolute indications and are based on the natural history of untreated scoliosis. Factors other than Cobb angle should be strongly considered when deciding between operative and nonoperative treatment. Trunk deformity (rotation) and trunk balance are important factors in deciding when to advise surgical correction. A patient with a lumbar curve of 35 degrees may have such a severe lateral trunk shift that surgical correction is indicated (Fig. 17-22). The curve pattern has a great impact on the deformity of the trunk associated with the scoliosis; long, single curves can produce a more noticeably unbalanced trunk requiring surgical intervention at a lower absolute Cobb angle (Fig. 17-23). In contrast, two well-balanced 50-degree curves (double major pattern) in a skeletally mature patient may be reasonably monitored for progression. It is not absolutely clear whether a long instrumented fusion has improved long-term outcomes compared with two initially stable balance curves.

When recommending surgical treatment of scoliosis, it is implied that both immediate and long-term outcomes will be improved as compared to nonoperative treatment. The short-term results of surgical treatment are well known, with a variety of surgical techniques having been studied for most curve types. Midterm (5 to 10 years) outcomes of modern corrective surgery are becoming available (237–241) but, like all advancing technologies, the surgical methods tend to change faster than the results can be collected. The 20-year follow-up study by Dickson et al. (242) of Harrington's surgically treated patients showed good long-term results.

Posterior Spinal Instrumentation. Harrington (243) of Houston introduced posterior spinal instrumentation in the early 1960s to make spine fusions more predictable. Prior to this, *in situ* fusions with body cast correction were performed (244) to correct the deformity and to immobilize the spine while the fusion progressed. The addition of Harrington's instrumentation improved scoliosis correction and greatly reduced the incidence of pseudarthrosis following scoliosis surgery.

Harrington Instrumentation. The Harrington instrumentation system consists of a ratcheted concave distraction rod with a hook at either end and a threaded compression rod attached to the transverse processes on the convex side of the curve. Coronal plane improvement provided by the Harrington distraction rod was often gained at the expense of decreased thoracic kyphosis and flattening of the lumbar spine (the so-called *flat-back deformity*), as noted in the sagittal plane (Fig. 17-24). The lower the instrumentation extended into the lumbar spine, the greater the loss in lordosis as well as the higher the likelihood of experiencing low back pain (245, 246). Subsequent modifications of the Harrington concept included the use of sublaminar wires or a square-ended rod to allow rod contouring (in an attempt to maintain thoracic kyphosis and lumbar lordosis) while preventing rod rotation with distraction (247).

The trend toward protecting normal lumbar contour was greatly advanced by Moe's clarification that most scoliosis

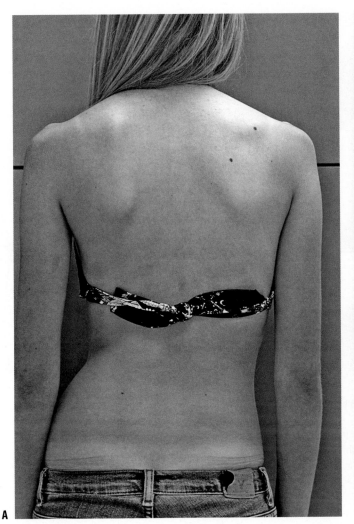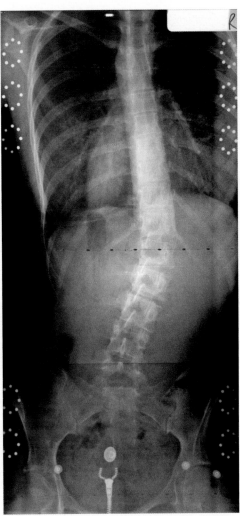

FIGURE 17-22. **A**: This photography demonstrates relatively substantial trunk decompensation to the right associated with thoracolumbar scoliosis. **B**: A relatively great length of the spine is involved in the deformity, and this may in some way be responsible for the fairly sizable trunk decompensation despite a Cobb angle measurement of 35 degrees. Other thoracolumbar deformities of similar Cobb angle magnitude are often associated with much less clinical deformity. This highlights the shortcomings of using only the Cobb angle measure in determining appropriate treatment.

(with apparent double curves) requiring surgical correction may *not* require fusion of the lumbar curve. He noted that the lumbar curve is very often secondary and does not require fusion (the so-called *King-Moe type 2 curve*). Application of the King-Moe curve classification will be emphasized later in this chapter (248).

Cotrel-Dubousset and Other Double-Rod, Multiple-Hook Systems. Nearly 20 years after Harrington's method was introduced, Cotrel and Dubousset (265) in France introduced a multihook system, which allowed distraction and compression on the same rod. Sagittal plane contouring of the rods and segmental hook fixation improved curve correction and postoperative stability. Many other segmental fixation posterior instrumentation systems utilizing similar concepts are now available for surgical correction of scoliosis. Current options for attach-

ment to the posterior spine include hooks (for attachment to the transverse processes, laminae, and pedicles), sublaminar wires (Luque), spinous process wires, and pedicle screws (250, 251).

Pedicle Screw Systems. The use of pedicle screws has become increasingly popular for the management of idiopathic scoliosis through a posterior approach. Initially, surgeons were concerned about the size of thoracic pedicles and the safety in placement of pedicle screws, especially on the concave side (249, 252). Pioneered by Suk, it has been shown that pedicle screws can be safely placed in the thoracic spine (253–255).

The benefits provided by three-column pedicle screw fixation included greater coronal Cobb correction, improved vertebral derotation (axial plane correction) resulting in greater rib prominence reduction, decreased need for anterior releases

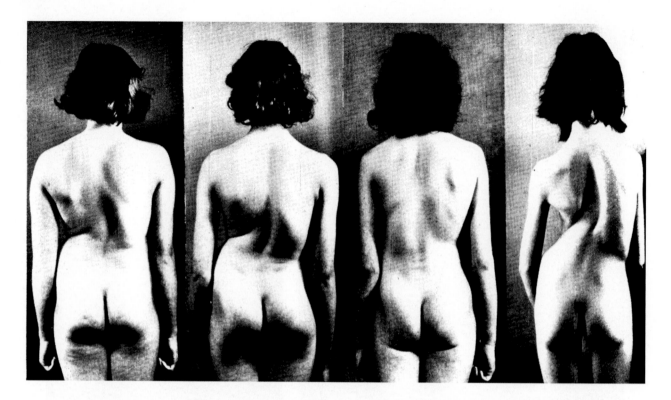

Lumbar   Thoraco-lumbar   Double Major   Thoracic

FIGURE 17-23. This classic series of photographs from James demonstrates the clinical appearance of four patients, each with a 70-degree magnitude scoliotic curve, although with different curve patterns. The clinical deformity is greater in single curves, particularly in the thoracic spine. (From Montgomery F, Willner S. The natural history of idiopathic scoliosis. Incidence of treatment in 15 cohorts of children born between 1963 and 1977. *Spine* 1997;22:772–774, with permission.)

in large, stiff curves and potentially saving of fusion levels (250, 256–258). It has also been suggested that the three-column fixation may help prevent the crankshaft phenomenon seen in skeletally immature patients. The concerns regarding pedicle screws include increased cost, inability to accurately place in dysplastic pedicles, safety concerns, and a common secondary reduction in thoracic kyphosis (253, 259, 260). Since their introduction, pedicle screws have also evolved from a fixed device (monoaxial screw) to a multiaxial screw that can simplify rod reduction but has decreased correctional control, to a uniplanar screw (screw head motion limited to the sagittal plane) that has been suggested to have the benefits of both screws types (261, 262).

It must be emphasized that it is still important to understand how to utilize hooks and wires in the management of scoliosis. Even among surgeons skilled at pedicle screw instrumentation, hooks and wires continue to be used. In situations where a pedicle screw cannot be placed and a fixation point is needed, a hook or a wire (cable) can be a safe and effective alternative (263). Proximally, it also has been postulated that transverse process hooks may minimize the risk of junctional kyphosis by limiting the soft-tissue dissection needed to place pedicle screws (264).

Mechanisms of Correction.   The advances in instrumentation have allowed for the development of multiple techniques to achieve scoliosis correction through a posterior approach. The use of compression and distraction has long been used to manage scoliosis since the time of Harrington instrumentation. Distraction on the concave rod decreases scoliosis. In the thoracic spine, posterior distraction also increases kyphosis, which is desired in the typical hypokyphotic idiopathic curve. Compression on the convex rod can aid in reducing the coronal curve. This maneuver also increases lordosis, which is useful when correcting a lumbar scoliosis. These are the principles that created the common patterns for hook placement with multihook systems (Fig. 17-25), and that continue to be utilized even with modern pedicle screw systems to segmentally enhance spinal deformity correction. It is important to remember, however, the effect of compression and distraction on kyphosis and lordosis so as not to inadvertently negatively affect the sagittal balance.

Frontal plane realignment of the spine can be accomplished by translating the vertebra. This translational movement may be performed by connecting the concave rod, precontoured to the desired sagittal profile (anticipating some rod flattening), to each fixation site along the spine and then

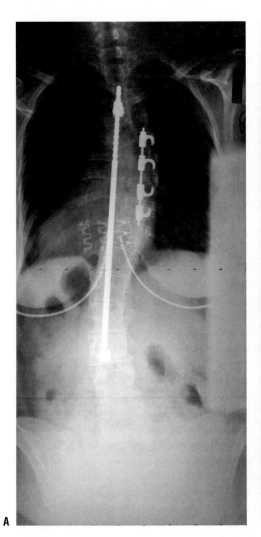

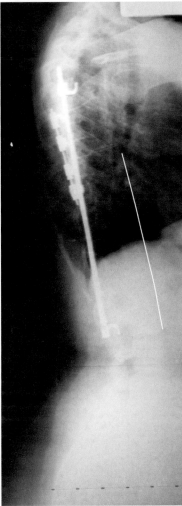

FIGURE 17-24. A: Harrington distraction rod is seen on the left, combined with a smaller threaded compression rod on the right. **B:** Distraction into the lumbar spine associated with this system unfortunately often leads to a reduction in lumbar lordosis, creating a flat-back deformity.

rotating the rod into the sagittal plane. This rod "derotation" maneuver, popularized by Dubousset, remains an effective method for translating the apex of the curve into a more normal position, thereby improving both the coronal and the sagittal deformity (265). Another method for translating the apex in space involves locking the concave rod into the position of anticipated correction and then sequentially drawing the spine to the rod (Fig. 17-26). Both translation techniques require a rod stiff and strong enough to maintain its contour as well as bony fixation sufficient to withstand the corrective forces. Otherwise, a stiff curve will cause a weak rod to "bend out" or an implant (screw, wire, or hook) to pull out of the bone.

The transverse plane correction of vertebral rotation (particularly at the apex of the curve) has traditionally not been addressed by translation, rod derotation, compression, and distraction techniques (266, 267). Differential rod contouring in the sagittal plane between the convex and concave side rods can apply some derotational forces to the apical vertebrae. By overcontouring kyphosis into the concave rod and undercontouring the convex rod, this can produce a rotational moment across a vertebra (Fig. 17-27). The concave rod is placed initially causing the deeper (more anteriorly displaced)

concave apical vertebrae to be drawn (rotated) more posteriorly. The convex rod is then placed on the proximal vertebra. By cantilevering this convex rod and progressively engaging each caudal vertebra, it produces the desired rotational moment and correction. Since the convex side of the apex vertebra is the most elevated, this differential contouring produces the greatest rotational correction where the axial rotation is greatest. The heads of pedicle screws can also be directly manipulated with specialized derotation instruments. En bloc vertebral derotation involves application of force on three to four apical segments from the convex side and rotating each vertebra around the axis of the concave rod. It is similar to the technique of differential rod contouring except that the force is applied on all vertebrae simultaneously with temporary instruments. In the technique of segmental direct vertebral-body rotation, the derotation maneuver is applied to individual segments (268). Utilizing the neutral vertebra as the reference point, each vertebra is derotated to this neutral axial rotational alignment (Fig. 17-28). Since monoaxial screws and uniplanar screws are fixed in the direction of the axial plane, they have been shown to be the best at maximizing correction of axial plane vertebral rotation (261).

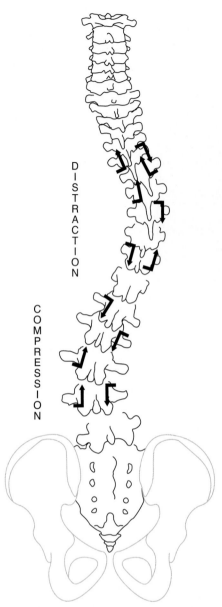

FIGURE 17-25. This hook pattern represents the commonly used method for achieving correction of a right thoracic left lumbar scoliosis curve pattern. The left-side rod would be placed first, with distraction in the thoracic spine being an appropriate force to correct both scoliosis and restore thoracic kyphosis, whereas compression in the lumbar spine is used for correcting the scoliosis as well as for maintaining lumbar lordosis. The right-side rod is placed secondarily for additional stabilization. This sequence applies in most cases in which the thoracic spine has lost normal thoracic kyphosis. In patients with increased kyphosis, a right-side thoracic compression rod should ideally be placed first.

Posterior Releases/Osteotomies. The amount of correction during scoliosis surgery is not only dependent on the instrumentation and techniques utilized but also dependent on the flexibility of the spine. For many flexible AIS cases, the releases provided by the surgical exposure and the face-

tectomies needed for the fusion provide enough for a well-balanced and acceptable correction. Recently, more aggressive posterior-based osteotomies (Ponte, Smith-Petersen, pedicle subtraction) are more commonly being used to increase the flexibility of the spine in order to maximize coronal, sagittal, and rotation correction (269, 270) (Fig. 17-29). These releases in combination with modern segmental pedicle screw instrumentation have allowed larger and more rigid curves to be addressed from a posterior-only approach (257). In extreme cases, experienced surgeons will perform a vertebral column resection to obtain a desired correction (271). When utilizing any of these correction techniques, proper intraoperative neurologic spinal cord monitoring becomes even more critical to minimize risk of spinal cord injury.

Anterior Release and Fusion. There is no consensus about the modern indications for a combined anterior and posterior approach in idiopathic scoliosis. Historic recommendations have been for patients with large (>75 degrees) rigid curves (bend correction <50 degrees) and those at risk for post-fusion crankshaft deformity. As mentioned above, the use of aggressive posterior releases combined with segmental pedicle screw instrumentation has led several to question the threshold of what is considered a "large" curve (257). Curve flexibility is increased by anterior disc excision, allowing greater correction with posterior instrumentation. The bone graft used anteriorly leads to a very stable fusion (anterior and posterior). The procedure involves anterior disc excision with release of the anterior longitudinal ligament, removal of the annulus fibrosis and nucleus pulposus, excision of the vertebral endplate cartilage, and occasionally (in severe cases) excision of the rib head at the costovertebral joint and posterior longitudinal ligament.

Crankshaft deformity (134, 256, 272–274) is caused when anterior spinal growth continues despite successful posterior fusion, resulting in worsening rotational deformity (Fig. 17-30). The problem occurs only in skeletally immature patients (Risser 0, triradiate cartilage open). Measuring crankshaft growth is difficult, although it has been defined as an increase in the Cobb angle of more than 10 degrees, or an increase in apical rotation despite successful posterior fusion. This largely axial rotational deformity is difficult to measure with routine radiography. It does appear that an anterior fusion arrests the anterior growth center and limits the development of this late deformity in young patients who are at risk (275).

An additional advantage of anterior release and fusion is the increased area for arthrodesis (vertebral endplates), presumably reducing the risk of pseudarthrosis. The thoracoscopic approach provides a means of accomplishing anterior disc excision and fusion with minimally invasive methods (276–278), thereby reducing the approach-related morbidity of a thoracotomy (277, 279, 280).

Anterior Spinal Instrumentation. While posterior spinal instrumentation has remained the standard for treating most AIS curves, anterior spinal instrumentation continues to be

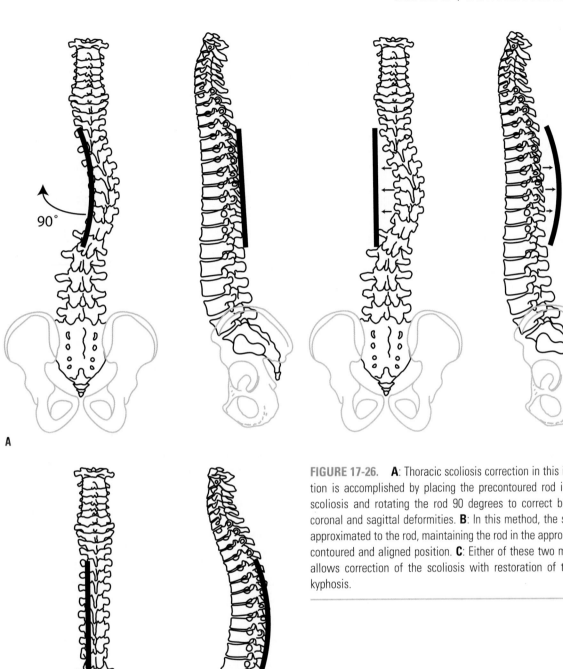

FIGURE 17-26. **A**: Thoracic scoliosis correction in this illustration is accomplished by placing the precontoured rod into the scoliosis and rotating the rod 90 degrees to correct both the coronal and sagittal deformities. **B**: In this method, the spine is approximated to the rod, maintaining the rod in the appropriately contoured and aligned position. **C**: Either of these two methods allows correction of the scoliosis with restoration of thoracic kyphosis.

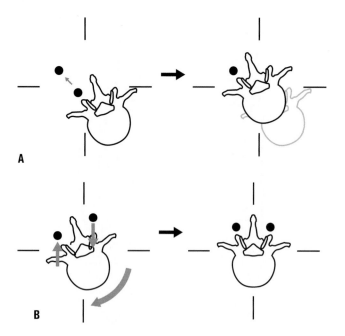

FIGURE 17-27. **A**: Translation of the thoracic apex to the corrected position, either by rod derotation or translation of the vertebra to a stationary rod, does not necessarily correct vertebral rotation. **B**: To address the rotational deformity of the apical vertebra, it is often desirable to use differential rod contouring between the left-side and the right-side rods. The left-side rod, contoured into a greater degree of kyphosis, provides a posteriorly directed translational force on the left while a slightly undercontoured sagittal alignment on the right-side rod provides an opposite direction of anterior translation reducing apical vertebral rotation.

used in select cases. The first anterior instrumentation systems introduced by Dwyer (281) and then by Zielke and Berthet (282) were both flexible compression systems that generated kyphosis within the instrumented segments. This production

of kyphosis may be desirable in the scoliotic hypokyphotic thoracic spine, but is generally undesirable in the lumbar region. Subsequently, more rigid solid-rod anterior systems were developed in an attempt to improve the sagittal alignment, particularly when treating thoracolumbar and lumbar curves.

Scoliotic curve patterns that are amenable to corrective anterior instrumentation and fusion generally include those with a single structural deformity. The most experience with correcting anterior scoliosis has been gained in the treatment of thoracolumbar and lumbar scoliosis (283–289). Direct access to the vertebral bodies and intervertebral discs is possible through an open anterior thoracoabdominal approach. Anterior disc excision creates mobility (290), which enhances correction in the frontal and axial planes, but decreases sagittal plane lordosis. Special attention to the sagittal plane is required when anterior compression instrumentation is used distal to the thoracolumbar junction so as to avoid production of an iatrogenic flat-back deformity. Structural interbody support in the form of a structural bone graft or an interbody "cage" has been advocated as a means of maintaining sagittal alignment (288, 291). Double-rod, double-screw anterior systems provide additional control of the sagittal plane (284, 292, 293) and overall construct stability (294) (Fig. 17-31). Traditionally, anterior instrumentation was thought to achieve similar or greater correction than posterior instrumentation for the same curve, often with fewer levels requiring instrumentation (295, 296). Recent data, however, suggest that with the use of pedicle screws and posterior osteotomies, one can provide similar or greater correction over similar fusion levels as compared to anterior instrumentation methods (297).

Instrumentation Without Fusion. Instrumentation without fusion, a technique utilized in young children with curves that progress relentlessly despite aggressive cast and/ or brace treatment, includes a subcutaneously or subfascially positioned growing construct that spans the deformity (298,

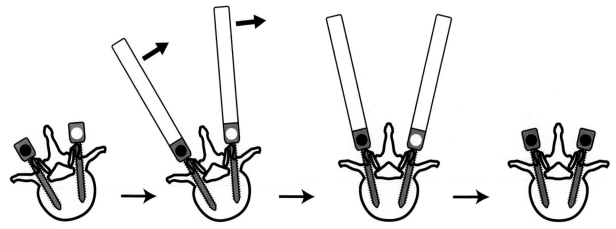

FIGURE 17-28. Use of pedicle screws offers a more powerful means of correcting axial plane vertebral rotation. Fixed-head pedicle screws placed segmentally can be manipulated around the concave rod to provide a means of apical derotation.

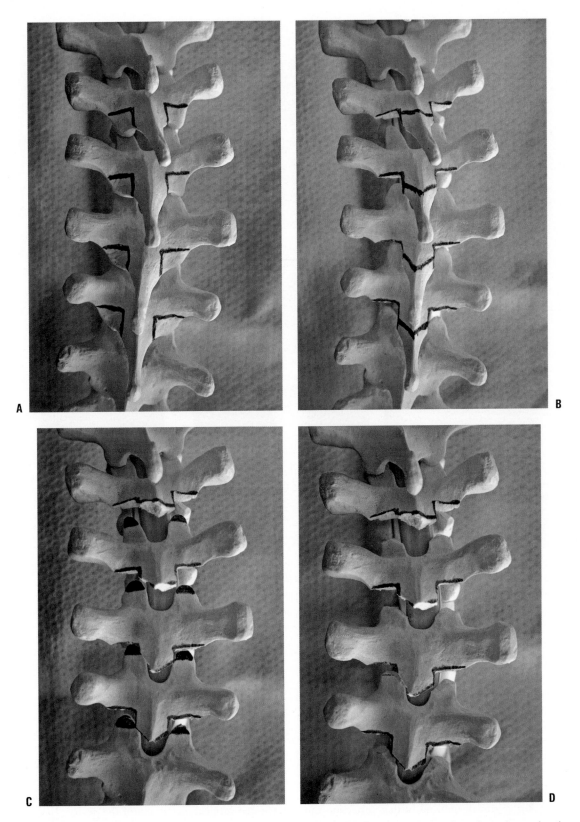

FIGURE 17-29.   Ponte release to increase flexibility in thoracic scoliosis **A**: First a facetectomy is performed removing the caudal facet from the superior vertebra exposing the articular surface. **B**: The spinous process including the intervening supra-spinous and interspinous ligament are removed. This exposes the ligamentum flavum, which is removed as well. **C**: The superior portion of the superior facet as well as facet capsule is removed. **D**: The posterior elements are no longer connected across the released segments, thereby increasing the flexibility across the deformity apex.

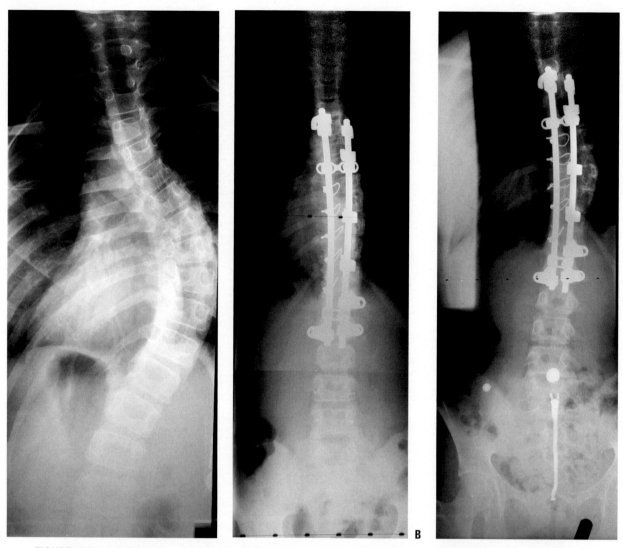

FIGURE 17-30. A: This 8-year, 9-month-old girl presented with a 60-degree right thoracic scoliosis. **B**: She underwent an isolated posterior instrumentation and fusion, which reduced the deformity to 22 degrees. **C**: Because of continued anterior spinal growth, a crankshaft deformity developed with curve progression. The trunk decompensated, and increased thoracic prominence developed despite a successful posterior fusion. Two years postoperatively, the curve had progressed to 43 degrees.

299). The purpose is to allow truncal growth and lung maturation while attempting to control the spinal deformity. In "growing rods," a limited fusion is performed at the proximal and distal foundation sites to secure either pedicle screws or hooks to the spine. In the intervening segments, one or two rods are placed without stripping the spine because exposure alone may lead to spontaneous fusion in a young child (this is the rationale for the concept of a "subcutaneous" or "subfascial" rod). Sequential distraction is performed every 6 to 12 months during growth until no further correction can be obtained (Fig. 17-32). The height gained with these procedures is usually modest, and complications are common (infection, rod breakage, spontaneous fusion, and screw/hook pullout) (298, 300, 301). A short convex hemiepiphyseodesis (anterior and posterior fusion) over the apical levels was advocated by some, but this has not been shown to be any more

effective than the growing rod by itself (256, 302). Another option for correction without fusion is the vertical expandable prosthetic titanium rib (VEPTR). This device attaches to the ribs proximally, while distally it can attach to the ribs, spine, or pelvis. While initially described for "thoracic insufficiency syndrome," which is commonly associated with scoliosis, its role in idiopathic early-onset scoliosis has been expanded at some centers (303, 304).

Growing rods and the VETPR allow for growth by repeated surgical distraction of the device. To avoid the need for repeated surgery, some are now using the concept of guiding growth. Initially described by McCarthy (305), the "Shilla" technique utilizes a short instrumented apical fusion to correct the deformity that then has rods extended to pedicle screws placed proximally and distally. These end screws while fixed to bone are allowed to slide along extra long rods.

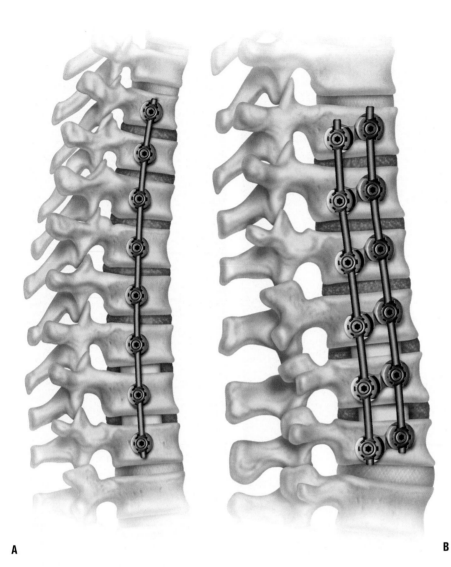

FIGURE 17-31. **A**: This schematic demonstrates the single-rod anterior construct used in thoracic scoliosis correction. Note the structural grafting of the lower two levels. **B**: This dual-rod construct is generally preferred for management of thoracolumbar scoliosis. Structural grafting may also be required in this construct to aid in maintaining lumbar lordosis. This construct offers greater construct rigidity compared to the single-rod constructs.

A   **B**

Ideally, as the patient grows, the screws and rods result in "guided growth." In most cases of growing rods, VEPTR, and the Shilla technique, it is anticipated that a final definitive fusion will be performed at or near the end of skeletal growth.

Another evolving technique for manipulating spinal growth involves anterior convex side implants designed to limit growth, but without resulting in a fusion. Methods under investigation include the use of various staples/plates and flexible tethering elements (306–308). It is hoped that one day such may be applied to a moderate-sized curve and result in resolution of the deformity with growth similar to the way limb alignment is presently manipulated with hemiepiphyseal devices.

POSTERIOR EXPOSURE OF THE THORACIC AND THE LUMBAR SPINE

Many techniques have been developed for exposure of the spine posteriorly. The technique illustrated here is that taught by John E. Hall (Figs. 17-33 to 17-41). There are two goals to this

exposure: The structures that are a part of the procedure must be seen clearly, without bits of shredded soft tissue remaining, and the blood loss should be minimal. This exposure, like all others, is based on the anatomy of the area. The exposure follows the same principles for exposure of the radius or the tibia: Muscles and ligaments are released from their attachments and the bone is exposed subperiosteally. When performed in this manner, the blood loss for the exposure of the thoracic and the lumbar spine for fusion of a double curve should not exceed 100 mL in the routine patient. To minimize blood loss, the surgeon should expose each segment completely at the outset and not leave soft tissue behind on the bone with a view to remove it later.

Surgical Correction According to Curve Pattern.

Idiopathic scoliosis takes on several typical and distinct curve patterns, the most common being a right thoracic curve. Classification systems were developed based on these patterns to assist the surgeon in selecting the appropriate curve or vertebral levels to include in the fusion. The first significant attempt

Text continued on page 668

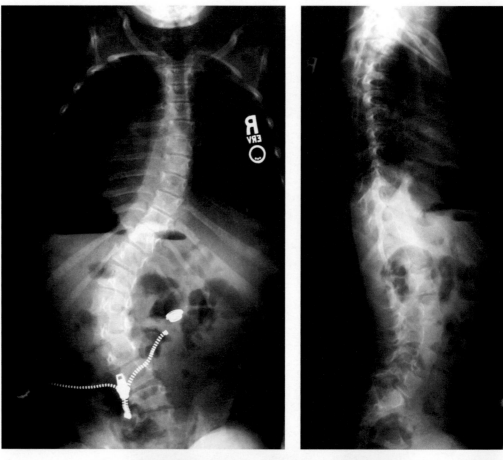

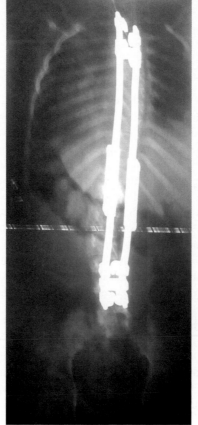

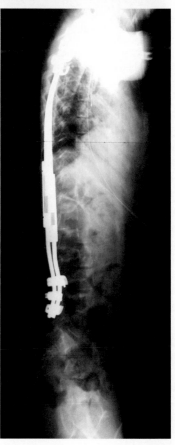

FIGURE 17-32. **A**: This juvenile patient presented with progressive lumbar scoliosis. The curve progressed despite attempts at bracing. **B**: The lateral radiograph demonstrates reasonable sagittal alignment. **C**: This patient underwent growing dual-rod instrumentation with fusion performed only at the proximal and distal hook sites. **D**: The sagittal profile is maintained and the growth connectors allow periodic lengthening with growth.

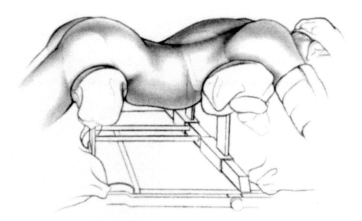

FIGURE 17-33. **Posterior Exposure of the Thoracic and the Lumbar Spine.** The patient is positioned on a frame such as the Relton-Hall frame or the Jackson table so that the abdomen is free. This reduces the pressure on the abdomen and reduces the intraoperative blood loss (1, 2). Care should be taken to ensure that the cephalad bolsters are not impinging on the axilla and that they are pressing against the lateral chest wall. The breasts should be "tucked" between the bolsters to minimize pressure. Likewise, it is important to be certain that the iliac crests are padded and that a good deal of the pressure from the bolsters is on the proximal portion of the thigh below the bolsters. The arms should not be hyperabducted, and the ulnar nerves should be free. It is important to check the preoperative radiograph for a cervical rib. Improper arm positioning in these patients may result in a C8 or T1 palsy. The entire back, as well as the posterior pelvis, is in the operative field so that bone from the posterior iliac crest can be obtained for arthrodesis.

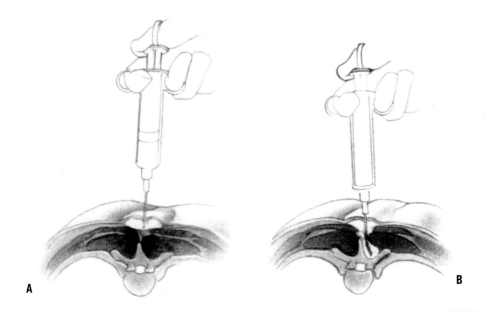

A

B

FIGURE 17-34. It is usually necessary to make this incision from the spinous process above the most proximal vertebra to be instrumented to the spinous process of the most caudal vertebra to be instrumented. The incision should be a straight line between these two points so that the scar lies in the midline and will be nearly straight after correction of the curve. If, however, the curve is severe and the correction is not anticipated to approach 30 degrees, the incision can be made in a curved manner following the shape of the deformity. If the fusion is to end in the region of L1 or L2, a separate incision can be used to obtain the iliac graft (see Figs. 17-42 to 17-48). If the L3 or lower vertebrae are to be fused, however, it is easier to extend the incision to the sacrum remaining in the midline (see Fig. 17-43). After a slight cut partly through the dermis, the tissues can be infiltrated with a solution of adrenaline and saline (1:500,000). This is injected into the dermis to produce a *peau d'orange* effect. Sufficient volume should be injected **(A)** to swell the tissues. If desired, the same solution can be injected deeply. The needle follows the spinous process down to the lamina **(B)**, and 5 mL of the same solution is injected at each level and on each side.

FIGURE 17-35. The incision is deepened down to the tips of the spinous processes. It is important to identify and stay in the midline so that muscle is not cut, with consequent bleeding. The midline is identified by a thin line, which is actually the interspinous ligaments connecting the spinous processes. In severe cases of scoliosis with marked rotation, the muscles on the concave side are rolled up and over the midline, requiring that the knife (or cautery tip) be angled under it to reach the midline. After the apophysis of each spinous process is identified, it is split down to the bone with a knife or a cautery.

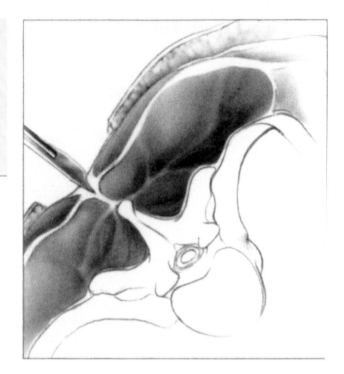

FIGURE 17-36. The exposure begins at the cranial end. The spinous process of the lamina above the one to be instrumented is exposed by pulling the cartilaginous tip of the spinous process off **(A)**, turning the elevator with flat surface against the spinous process and sliding it down in the direction of the spinous process onto the lamina and the base of the transverse process. This is done in order to gain better exposure of the vertebra below. Care should be taken to follow the direction of the spinous process to avoid entering muscle and also to prevent unnecessary bleeding. This procedure is then performed on the vertebra below so that the spinous process, the lamina, and the base of the transverse process of that vertebra are stripped of periosteum. These structures, however, are obscured by the muscle tissue on top of the elevator. The attachment of this muscle **(B)** to the caudal edge of the more superior lamina (the first one exposed) is not obvious. Using a knife (or a cautery tip), these attachments are divided from the bone. The cut starts laterally or medially, but it should go from the tip of the spinous process to the lateral edge of the facet joint (*dotted line*). Division of these attachments is aided by placing the tissue under tension with the elevator.

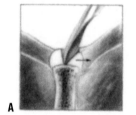

A

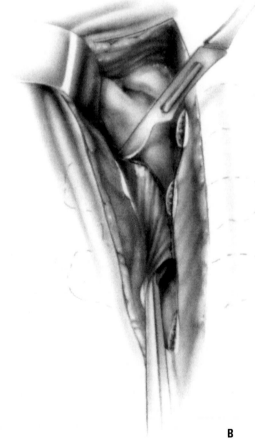

B

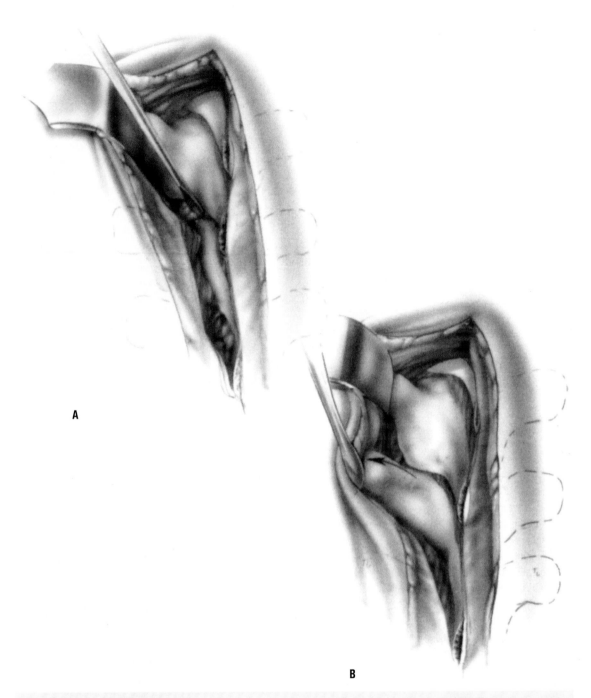

FIGURE 17-37. After the cut has been completed and the loose fatty tissue cleared from between the spinous processes, the elevator is placed in the cut that was made over the facet joint **(A)**. From here, the elevator is drawn up the cephalad aspect of the transverse process **(B)**. This should clear all of the tissue from the facet. The remainder of the transverse process is cleared to its tip. The very tip of the transverse process is obscured by the ligamentous attachment to the rib and, in most circumstances, can be left undisturbed provided that sufficient bone is exposed.

FIGURE 17-38. Before repeating these steps on the next vertebra, it is important to expose carefully the caudal edge of the vertebra just cleaned. This is accomplished by starting on the transverse process. With a small twisting motion of the elevator, the periosteum is cleared until the rounded edge of the bone can be seen. This is of particular importance in the region of the facet. If this is not accomplished, it will not be possible to view the facet clearly to cut the capsule, and the result will be shreds of soft tissue remaining on the bone. If a curette is used to remove the soft tissue from the facet joints, it should be used in a lateral-to-medial direction to avoid inadvertent penetration of the ligamentum flavum and possible spinal cord injury.

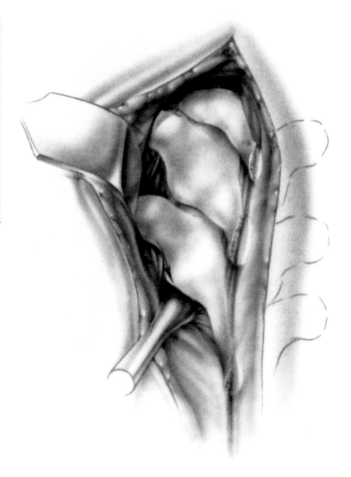

FIGURE 17-39. In the lumbar spine the anatomy is different, and therefore, the technique is different. In the lumbar spine the spinous processes are farther apart. The space between these processes is filled with a thick ligament that cannot be divided as easily as in the thoracic spine. Using the elevator to place the tissues under tension, this ligament is divided by cutting between the two spinous processes (*A*). This cut should extend down to the lamina. With a little care, it is not difficult to avoid entering the spinal canal. Although the anatomy appears different in this region, the principles are the same. Because the ligamentous attachments are on the caudal edge of the more cephalad lamina (*B*), they are divided sharply as the elevator applies tension and continues the subperiosteal dissection of the lamina. This brings the dissection to the capsule of the facet joint.

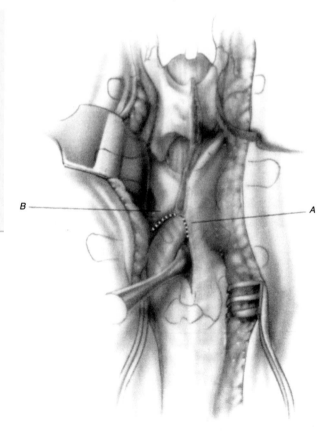

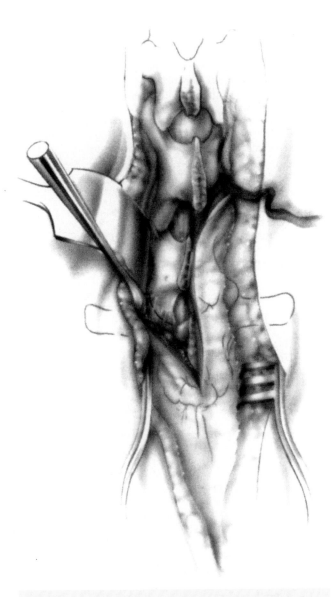

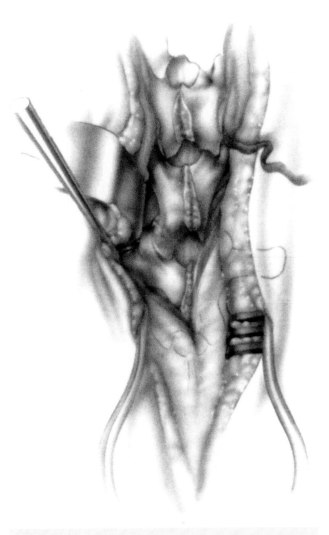

FIGURE 17-40. The easiest way to expose the facet joint is to follow the lamina out to the point where there is no more bone. Proceeding in a cranial direction from here is the inferior articular process, which in turn leads to the inferior facet. With the inferior articular process and the capsule of the facet exposed, a knife or an electrocautery is used to divide the capsule, starting on the inferior articular process and going in a cranial direction across the facet capsule (*dotted line*). At this point, the elevator can easily clean the capsule from both sides of the facet.

FIGURE 17-41. The transverse process is usually found just caudal to the level of the facet. By coming off the side of the inferior facet with the elevator, staying in contact with bone, the dissection follows onto the transverse process. Care should be taken with the elevator to pull laterally and upward to expose the transverse process. After the transverse processes are exposed, a laparotomy sponge is packed into this area lateral to the facet joints and over the spinous processes. This not only tamponades venous bleeding but also stretches the tissues, making exposure and decortication easier when the surgeon returns to the area.

FIGURE 17-42. The features of the King-Moe classification. (From King HA, Moe JH, Bradford DS, et al. The selection of fusion levels in thoracic idiopathic scoliosis. *J Bone Joint Surg Am* 1983;65:1302–1313, with permission.)

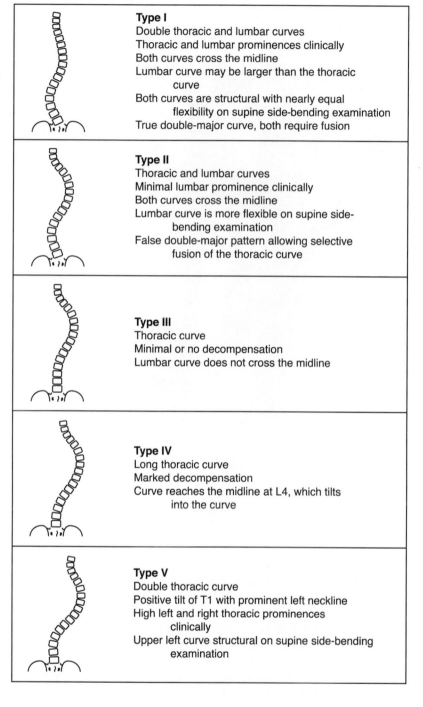

Type I
Double thoracic and lumbar curves
Thoracic and lumbar prominences clinically
Both curves cross the midline
Lumbar curve may be larger than the thoracic
    curve
Both curves are structural with nearly equal
    flexibility on supine side-bending examination
True double-major curve, both require fusion

Type II
Thoracic and lumbar curves
Minimal lumbar prominence clinically
Both curves cross the midline
Lumbar curve is more flexible on supine side-
    bending examination
False double-major pattern allowing selective
    fusion of the thoracic curve

Type III
Thoracic curve
Minimal or no decompensation
Lumbar curve does not cross the midline

Type IV
Long thoracic curve
Marked decompensation
Curve reaches the midline at L4, which tilts
    into the curve

Type V
Double thoracic curve
Positive tilt of T1 with prominent left neckline
High left and right thoracic prominences
    clinically
Upper left curve structural on supine side-bending
    examination

to classify AIS was developed by Moe and reported by King et al. (King-Moe classification) (Fig. 17-42) (248). Based on coronal radiographs, it was designed primarily to decide when to instrument the thoracic curve alone (in patients with apparent double curves) and when to instrument both the thoracic and the lumbar curves. Despite its routine use, the system was not designed as a comprehensive classification of idiopathic scoliosis curve patterns.

Primary lumbar and thoracolumbar curves, and also triple curves, were not included in the King-Moe classification. Others have designed classification systems that are more com-

prehensive (95, 309). The system proposed by Lenke et al. considers both frontal and sagittal plane deformity and is designed to guide surgical treatment decision making for all curve patterns. This classification system is a triad system including a description of the curve type (1–6), lumbar curve size (A,B,C), and sagittal plane alignment (hyperkyphotic, normal, hypokyphotic) (Fig. 17-43). The perceived utility of the Lenke et al. system was its comprehensive, biplanar nature and, most importantly, its ability to suggest regions of the spine that theoretically require fusion. Specific criteria for establishing "structural" minor curves were set forth. Although not perfect in predicting

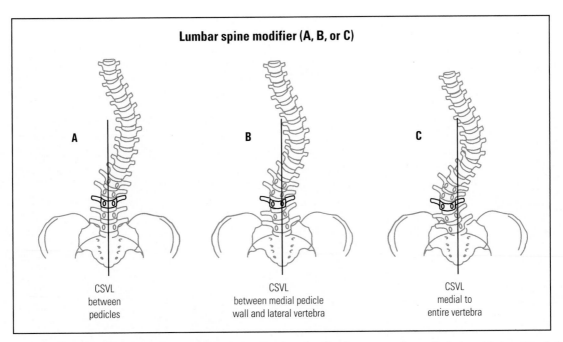

Lumbar spine modifier (A, B, or C)

A

B

C

CSVL
between
pedicles

CSVL
between medial pedicle
wall and lateral vertebra

CSVL
medial to
entire vertebra

FIGURE 17-43. The Lenke classification. This comprehensive classification system for scoliosis is a triad system that involves curve-type, lumbar spine modifier, and thoracic sagittal modifier.

which curves experienced surgeons will choose to instrument, the classification system correlated approximately 85% of the time with what was actually done by surgeons (310, 311).

Right Thoracic Curve Pattern (Lenke 1; King II, III). The right thoracic curve is the most common idiopathic scoliosis curve pattern, occurring in roughly one-half of operative cases. While the fusion can be performed through either an anterior or a posterior approach, a posterior-based instrumentation and fusion is more common. The extent of fusion is generally limited to the thoracic curve, although the lowest-instrumented vertebra is chosen largely on the basis of the features of the lumbar deformity. The Lenke 1A curves has the least apically translated lumbar curves and is routinely instrumented distally to 1 (or 2) level(s) proximal to the stable vertebra (vertebra bisected by the CSVL) when treated posteriorly, and to the lower end Cobb vertebra when instrumented anteriorly (Fig. 17-44). Recently, two distinct Lenke 1A curve patterns were identified based on the direction of L4 tilt (Fig. 17-45) (312). Lenke 1A-L curves (i.e., L4 tilts to the left) appear to be behave like smaller versions of 1B curves with similar fusion-level selection, while 1A-R curves where L4 tilts to the right appear more like King IV curves. The 1A-R curves require a more distal fusion than 1A-L/1B curves to maintain balance and avoid "adding on" of the curve distally. The 1B curve pattern is amenable to either approach (anterior or posterior), with the lower instrumented vertebra being usually the stable vertebra between the thoracic and lumbar curves (Fig. 17-46). Lenke 1C curves present with a substantial lumbar curve, with the lumbar apical vertebra completely deviated lateral to the CSVL. The surgi-

cal treatment approach in this type of curve in the King-Moe classification (type II) has been associated with substantial controversy regarding the appropriateness of sparing lumbar motion with an isolated (selective) thoracic fusion. In most cases of Lenke 1C curves, a selective thoracic fusion can be performed while maintaining frontal plane balance. The larger the thoracic deformity (Cobb angle, apical translation, rotation) compared to the lumbar curve, the more likely the success of selective thoracic instrumentation (313–316) (Fig. 17-47). However, the clinical appearance of the patient should also be a determinant. A dominant lumbar rotational prominence, even if highly flexible, likely requires inclusion in the fusion (Fig. 17-48). In large lumbar curves, vigorous selective correction of the thoracic curve with a posterior instrumentation system may result in postoperative truncal decompensation to the left (317, 318). If selective fusion is decided upon in such patients, it has been recommended to balance the correction of the thoracic curve with the anticipated spontaneous lumbar curve correction to minimize the chance of residual trunk imbalance (313). If selective fusion is chosen, the procedure can be performed through either an anterior or a posterior approach (319). When deciding to perform a selective thoracic fusion, it is important to evaluate the lateral x-ray as well. If a "junctional kyphosis" is noted between the two curves, then consideration should be given to extending the fusion distal to this kyphosis, thereby incorporating the lumbar curve into the surgical treatment (Fig. 17-49).

Double Thoracic Curve Pattern (Lenke 2; King V). The double thoracic curve pattern consists of two structural

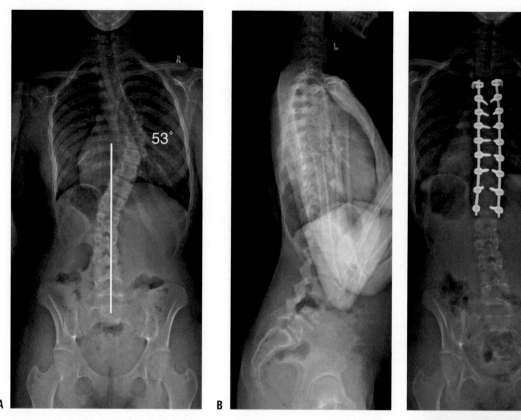

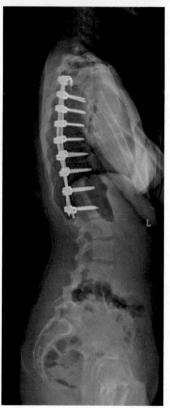

FIGURE 17-44. **A**: The PA radiograph demonstrates a Lenke 1A curve. **B**: Lateral radiograph demonstrates hypokyphosis. **C, D**: Posterior instrumentation was performed, stopping distally at L1, which is the vertebra substantially touched by the CSVL.

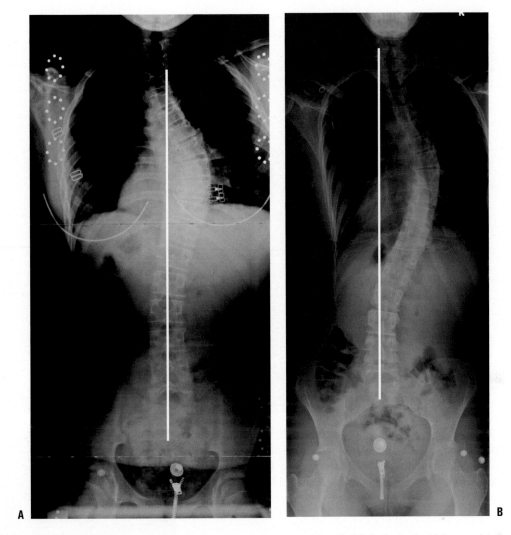

FIGURE 17-45. Two distinct patterns for the Lenke 1A curve have been identified **A**: In the Lenke 1A-L curve, L4 tilts to the left. This curve behaves like a smaller Lenke 1B. **B**: In the Lenke 1A-R, L4 tilts to the right. This curve behaves more like a King IV curve.

thoracic curves (right main thoracic and left upper thoracic) and is usually recognized clinically by the presence of an elevated left shoulder. An isolated right thoracic curve is typically associated with an elevated right shoulder. A left upper thoracic curve that results in left shoulder elevation and/or is relatively rigid (remains >20 to 25 degrees on side-bending film) generally requires instrumentation that includes the curve typically beginning proximally at T2 (320) (Fig. 17-50). If the double pattern is not recognized and the right thoracic curve alone is straightened, the left shoulder elevation is often worse following the surgery (321–324). Other radiographic measures such as the tilt of T1 and the clavicular angle have also been used to determine whether the proximal thoracic curve should be instrumented (321). Ultimately, the ability to control the postoperative balance of the shoulders is not absolute and is dependent not only on the level selected but also on the amounts of main thoracic and upper thoracic curve correction obtained. With greater degrees of main thoracic curve

correction, inclusion of part or all of the upper thoracic curve (irrespective of side bending to <25 degrees) is often performed to achieve/maintain shoulder balance. The sagittal alignment of the upper thoracic region also requires careful assessment. This is an area that (as in the thoracolumbar spine) may also be found to be hyperkyphotic. If this region just proximal to the thoracic curve is locally kyphotic (>20 degrees, T2–T5), the instrumentation should extend proximally to cover this area in an attempt to avoid aggravating a proximal junctional kyphosis (PKJ) (Fig. 17-51).

Right Thoracic, Left Lumbar Curve Pattern (Lenke 3, 6; King I, II).

The lumbar curve (usually convex to the left) that often presents in association with a right thoracic curve may vary substantially in both magnitude (Cobb angle) and severity of rotation. Either the thoracic or lumbar curve may dominate such a double-major curve pattern, although the thoracic curve is more often the primary one. In deciding on

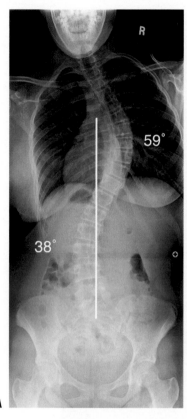
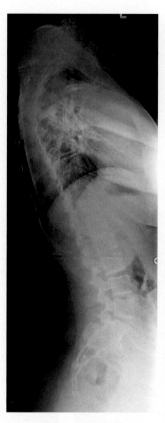
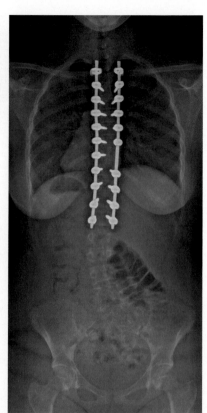
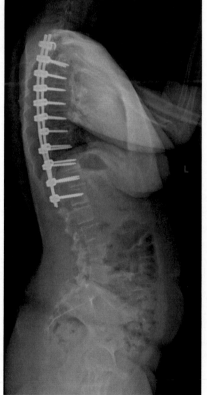

FIGURE 17-46. **A**: This PA radiograph demonstrates a Lenke 1B curve. The lumbar curve corrected to 22 degrees on side bending. **B**. The lateral demonstrates no junctional kyphosis between the thoracic and the lumbar curve. **C,D**: Postoperative radiographs demonstrate a posterior instrumented fusion from T3 to L1.

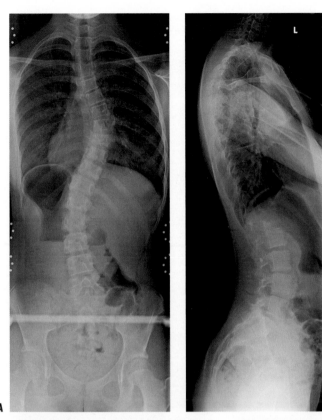

FIGURE 17-47. **A**: This Lenke 1C curve demonstrates a lumbar curve that corrects to just <12 degrees on side bend. The lumbar curve flexibility and differences in apical translation makes a selective thoracic fusion the optimal treatment choice. **B**: The lateral demonstrates no junctional kyphosis. **C,D**: Postoperative radiographs demonstrate a posterior instrumented fusion from T4 to T12.

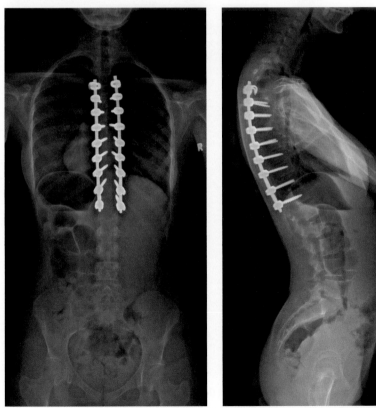

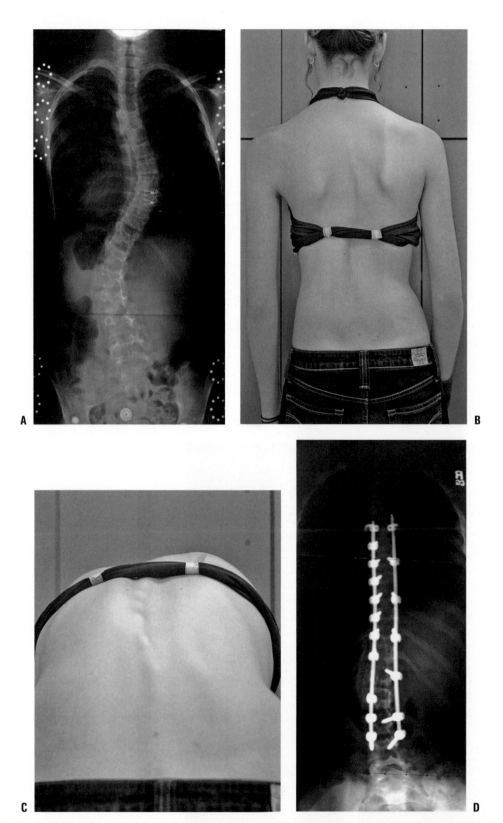

FIGURE 17-48.   A: This PA radiograph demonstrates relatively well-balanced right thoracic and left lumbar curves. The thoracic curve measures slightly larger, and the lumbar curve on side bending corrects to 20 degrees. This classifies as a Lenke 1C curve. **B**: The clinical appearance of this patient demonstrates nearly equal deformity of the thoracic and lumbar regions. **C**: On forward bending, however, the lumbar prominence (ATR: 19 degrees) was larger than the thoracic prominence (ATR: 9 degrees), confirming the greater rotational deformity present in the lumbar spine. **D**: Based largely on the greater lumbar rotation, this patient was not felt to be a candidate for selective thoracic fusion and underwent instrumentation of both thoracic and lumbar curves.

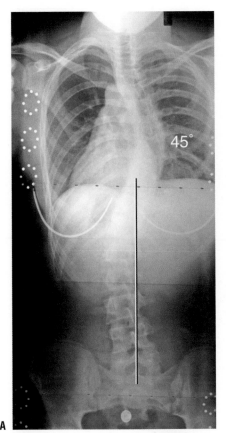

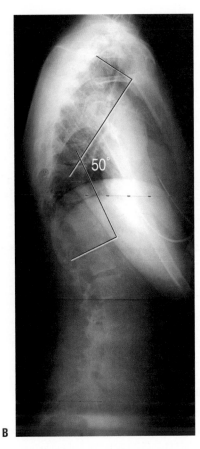

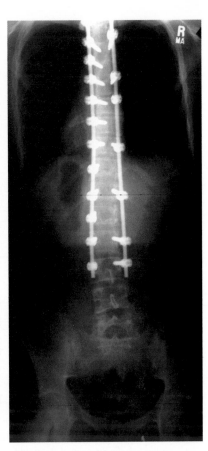

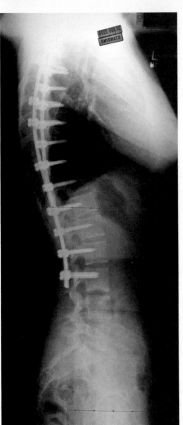

FIGURE 17-49. A: This PA radiograph demonstrates a Lenke 1C deformity. **B**: The lateral radiograph, however, demonstrates hyperkyphosis, making this a 1B+ curve pattern. In addition, the patient had 26 degrees of junctional kyphosis between the thoracic and lumbar curve. **C,D**: Because of the substantial kyphosis associated with this deformity, the posterior instrumentation was extended proximally and distally to control the sagittal deformity in addition to the coronal deformity.

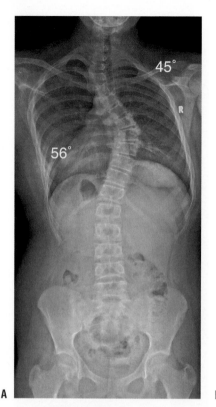
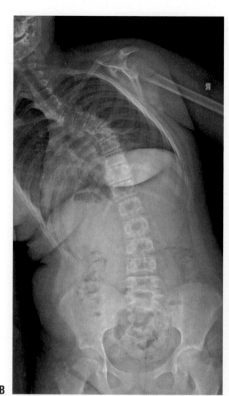
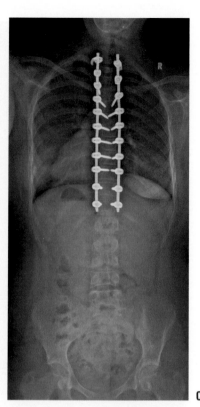

A   B   C

FIGURE 17-50. **A**: PA view of double thoracic scoliosis (Lenke 2B). **B**: On side bending, the upper demonstrates no significant change. In many cases, this apparent lack of flexibility is because of the patients desire to keep the head upright as seen in this radiograph. **C**: Because of the rigidity of the upper thoracic curve, both the upper thoracic and main thoracic curves underwent instrumented fusion. Even with instrumentation of the upper thoracic curve, the patient still had residual elevation of the left shoulder postoperatively.

surgical treatment, one must determine which of the curves requires instrumentation and fusion (thoracic, lumbar, or both). In a Lenke 3 curve (both curves "structural"), the thoracic curve is larger and/or more rigid than the lumbar curve. Generally, both curves are instrumented; however, similar to a Lenke 1C curve, selective fusion of only the thoracic curve can be considered for occasional Lenke 3C curves where the thoracic curve is substantially larger and the lumbar deformity relatively mild (248, 314). In most cases of Lenke 3C curves, however, the lumbar curve is large enough to require fusion in order to achieve a well-balanced spine after correction. In Lenke 6 curves, the lumbar curve is by definition dominant and always should be included in the fusion.

When instrumentation of both the thoracic and lumbar curves is required, the approach is posterior, and the distal extent is usually to the L3 or L4 level. Ideally, the distal extent of the fusion should be as proximal as possible in order to preserve lumbar motion segments, yet long enough to avoid creating trunk imbalance. Choosing between L3 and L4 can be difficult. The most predictable spinal balance occurs when the fusion/instrumentation extends distally to the stable vertebra (the vertebra best bisected by the CSVL). In a patient with a large lumbar curve, this may be L4 or even L5. Fusion to a level proximal to the stable vertebra, such as L3, may be

considered if there is minimal axial rotation of L3 as noted on the side-bend film to the left for a left lumbar curve, and if L3 becomes parallel to the pelvis with side bending to the right. Others may consider choosing the lower end of the instrumentation as the end Cobb vertebra (the caudal vertebra that results in the largest Cobb angle). This is less obvious when both L3 and L4 are parallel to each other on the standing coronal radiograph. Again, the surgical goal is to achieve improved spinal alignment with global truncal balance with both C7 and the trunk well centered over the pelvis in both the sagittal and the coronal planes (Fig. 17-52).

Lumbar or Thoracolumbar Curve Pattern (Lenke 5C).

A primary lumbar or thoracolumbar curve pattern does not have a significant thoracic component and may be convex to the left or right (the left being the more common). In such cases, isolated fusion of a lumbar or thoracolumbar curve is appropriate and can be accomplished by either anterior or posterior methods. Correction with posterior hook constructs has not been as successful as anterior instrumentation in achieving derotation of the lumbar curve. Limited anterior instrumentation of the apical three or four vertebrae has been proposed by Bernstein and Hall (295) with satisfactory early outcomes in most patients. Longer anterior constructs (325) that include all the measured Cobb angle levels, some with

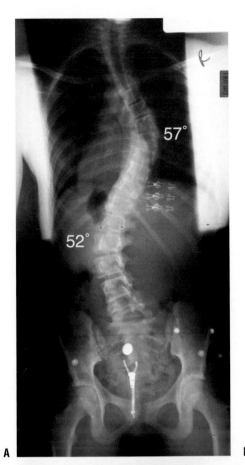

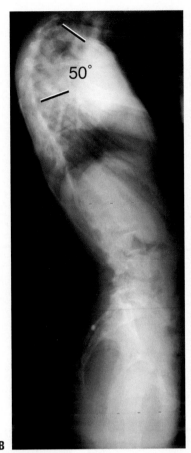

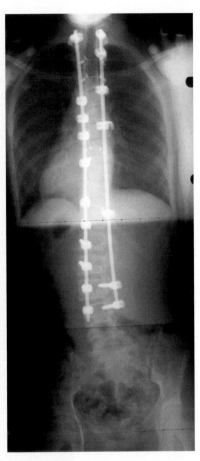

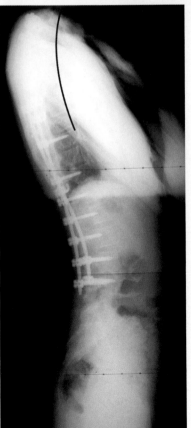

FIGURE 17-51. **A,B**: These radiographs demonstrate right thoracic, left lumbar scoliosis with substantial upper thoracic kyphosis. **C,D**: In this case, the instrumentation was extended proximally to correct the kyphotic aspect of the deformity.

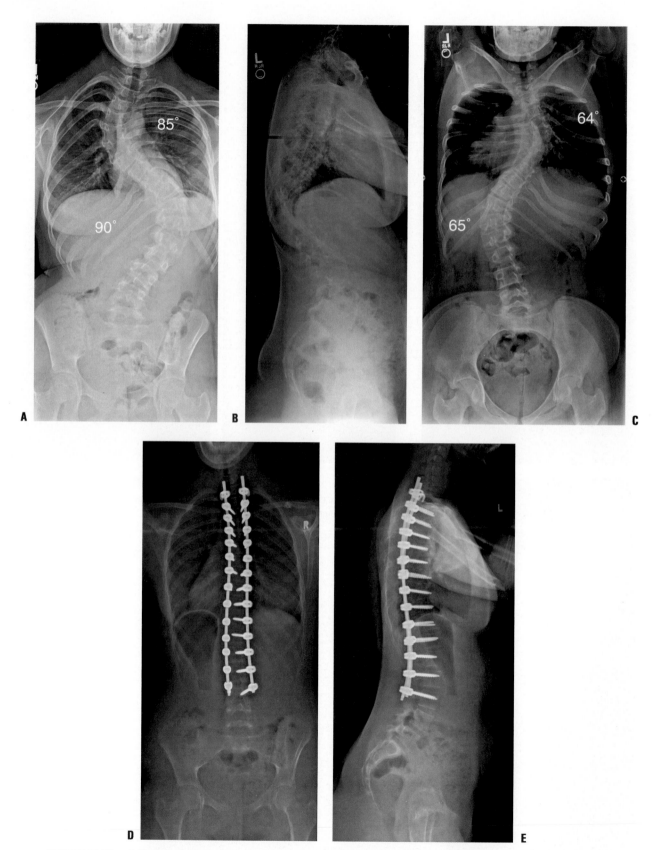

FIGURE 17-52. **A,B**: This double-major scoliosis has Lenke 6C curve pattern. Note the junctional kyphosis between the thoracic and the lumbar curve **C**: Due to the magnitude of the curve, a supine traction film was obtained that demonstrated similar flexibility between the thoracic curve and the lumbar curve, 64 and 65 degrees, respectively. **D,E**: On the basis of the structural features of the right thoracic and left lumbar curves, instrumented correction was performed from T2 to L3.

the use of bone graft or a structural cage in the disc space (288, 326), have traditionally been done in the treatment of these curves (Fig. 17-53). Pedicle screw fixation has allowed better control and correction of these curves when corrected with posterior instrumentation (270). Segmental pedicle screw fixation in combination with wide posterior facet excision has become popular with reportedly greater correction and shorter hospital stays than those associated with anterior methods (297) (Fig. 17-54).

Triple Curve Pattern (Lenke 4). The Lenke 4 or triple curve pattern includes curves in all three locations: left upper thoracic, right thoracic, and left lumbar/thoracolumbar and is the least common curve type. Determination of the proximal extent of the fusion is similar to Lenke 2 or double thoracic curve. The desired effect on the postoperative shoulder balance should guide the decision to fuse the proximal curve. The caudal fusion level requires the same analysis needed for Lenke 3 and 6 curve patterns. First it is important to evaluate if the lumbar curve needs to be fused—generally it does. If so, then the appropriate lower end vertebra (L3 or L4) for fusion needs to be determined.

OUTCOMES OF SURGICAL TREATMENT

Given that the methods used for surgical correction of AIS [Harrington instrumentation in the 1960s, Cotrel-Dubousset (CD) instrumentation in the 1980s] are fairly recent, very long-term outcome data are not yet available. Spinal instrumentation techniques continue to undergo modification and improvement almost faster than outcome studies can be performed. The SRS has developed an outcome assessment system that attempts to more precisely evaluate the functional outcomes in patients with scoliosis (327–329). Recently, a questionnaire was also developed to measure patients' perceptions of their clinical deformity associated with their scoliosis.

Outcome After Posterior Surgery. The longest follow-up data are available for patients treated with Harrington instrumentation and fusion. An average coronal plane improvement of the Cobb angle by 14% to 48% has been reported (266, 330). The analysis of long-term functioning after long posterior fusions has focused on the incidence of late-onset low back pain. Conflicting results have been reported regarding the prevalence of pain and the correlation of pain with the caudal level of instrumentation. Cochran et al. (331) noted an increased frequency of pain in patients fused at L4 or L5 compared to those fused at L3 or above, but several other studies have not been able to correlate the levels of fusion with subsequent back pain (189, 332–335).

Despite conflicting results regarding the increased potential for low back pain with more caudal levels of instrumentation and fusion, it seems intuitive that one should minimize the caudal extent of a fusion. Winter et al. (336) demonstrated

a significant loss of global spinal motion when arthrodeses included L4 compared to arthrodeses fused only inferiorly to upper- or midlumbar levels. Fusion to more caudal levels has also been associated with higher rates of radiographically visible degenerative changes in the unfused distal levels (332, 337, 338). A recent prospective study demonstrated increasing motion at L4/L5 the more caudal a fusion extended into the lumbar spine (339). It is possible this increased motion may ultimately lead to increase wear and risk degeneration at this level.

Another concern with the use of Harrington rods that extended into the lumbar spine was the loss of lumbar lordosis associated with distraction instrumentation. Known as flat-back syndrome, the resulting positive sagittal balance has been shown to be quite disabling as patients lose their ability to compensate by hyperextension through the remaining discs and hips with age (245, 333, 340, 341). The relation of alignment and degenerative changes to the development of low back pain requires additional follow-up and analysis (342).

The early (318, 343) and the midterm (239) (5- to 15-year follow-up) results of CD instrumentation (multihook system) suggest improved coronal and sagittal plane correction, compared to Harrington instrumentation (344). An average coronal correction of 41% to 61% can be expected (256, 330, 345). Despite the early expectation that systems such as the CD type would substantially derotate the spine, little improvement in vertebral rotation deformity has been seen (266, 267, 346–348). Requirements for postoperative immobilization in a brace or cast significantly decreased as compared to Harrington instrumentation. Additionally, pseudarthrosis rates and loss of correction have been reduced with multisegmental systems (239, 256, 266, 344). However, early in the experience with CD instrumentation, truncal decompensation to the left was commonly noted in King type II curves when selective thoracic fusion was performed (237, 315, 318, 349). Several techniques have been suggested to avoid this difficulty including avoidance of thoracic curve overcorrection, proper fusion-level selection, and selective placement of hooks (314, 316, 317).

Asher et al. (237) reported the results after an average follow-up of 5 years of a consecutive series of 185 patients with idiopathic scoliosis treated with Isola instrumentation. Correction of the largest curve averaged 65% while rib hump rotation decreased 39%. These results are generally better than those reported with original CD constructs. Features of the Isola construct that likely contributed to these improved radiographic outcomes are the segmental fixation, particularly in the apical segments. Other hybrid systems with largely segmental fixation have resulted in comparable degrees of deformity correction (350).

The use of pedicle screw fixation rather than hooks has led to improved degrees of correction. This was first demonstrated with the application of screw fixation in lumbar scoliosis that was a component of a double-major curve (255, 350). Dislodgement of distal hooks with consequent loss of correction, although not common, does occur with some

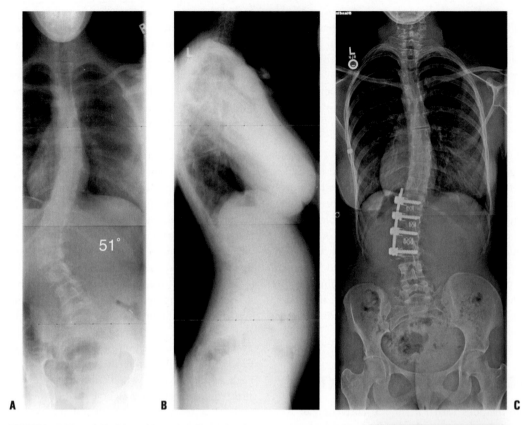

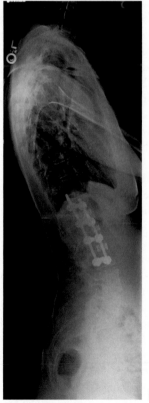

FIGURE 17-53. **A,B**: PA and lateral radiographs demonstrate a Lenke 5C thoracolumbar scoliosis. **C,D**: This deformity was addressed by double anterior rod correction through a thoracoabdominal approach. Interbody structural support consisted of cages to prevent loss of lumbar lordosis.

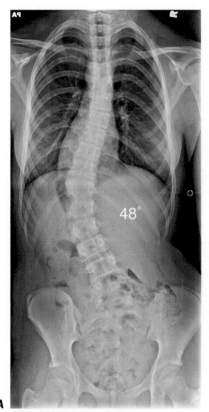

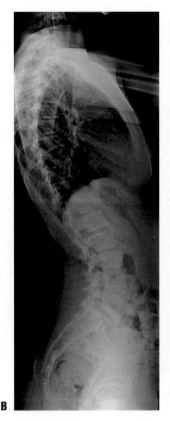

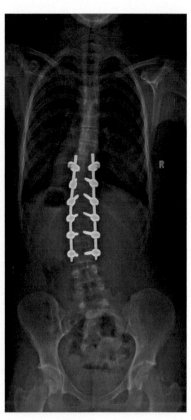

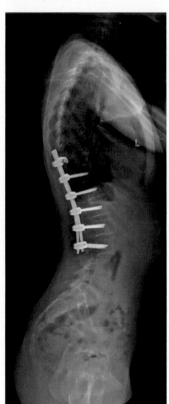

FIGURE 17-54. **A,B**: PA and lateral radiographs demonstrate a Lenke 5C thoracolumbar scoliosis. **C,D**: Postoperative radiographs demonstrate improved coronal balance following segmental pedicle screw fixation in combination with wide posterior facet excision or releases.

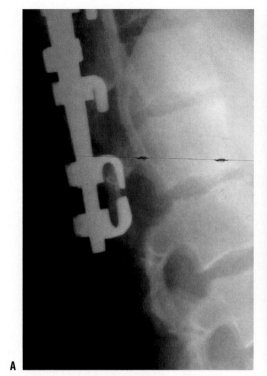
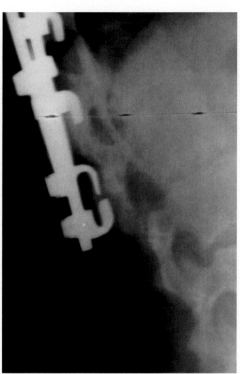

A

B

FIGURE 17-55. **A:** Laminar hook fixation is common in the lower constructs for thoracic and lumbar curves. **B:** They can, however, on rare occasion, dislodge with fracture of the lamina. Pedicle screw fixation offers a method of salvaging such a situation and of reducing the incidence of such failure to begin with.

frequency (255) (Fig. 17-55). Similar loss of distal fixation is much less common when pedicle screws are utilized.

The placement of pedicle screws throughout the thoracic and the lumbar spine has become routine throughout North America. In 1995 Suk et al. (350) reported greater correction of thoracic deformity with segmental pedicle screws than with hooks, and other surgeons have also adopted this approach with similar outcomes (250, 255, 260, 351, 352). In these reports, the percentage coronal correction with thoracic hook constructs ranged from 50% to 55% compared to the results with screw fixation that approached or exceeded 70% correction.

In addition to improved coronal correction, greater transverse plane (rib hump) correction has been demonstrated especially when used in conjunction with vertebral body derotation techniques (268). For many, this has reduced the need for thoracoplasty and its associated morbidity on pulmonary function. Others continue to perform thoracoplasty to maximize rib hump correction and suggest minimal effects on clinical pulmonary function (353).

Maximizing the correction of the scoliotic curve is one of the goals of surgical treatment, but this must not compromise the additional goals of surgery: preventing progression, attaining coronal and sagittal balance, and maximizing residual spinal flexibility (354). Coronal decompensation after surgical correction has been described by numerous authors in and has been attributed to a variety of causes including overcorrection of the thoracic curve (355, 356). In fact, the impressive

outcomes of segmental thoracic pedicle screw correction have led Suk et al. (357) to suggest expanding the fusion into the proximal thoracic spine (up to T2) in many patients so as to avoid shoulder imbalance (elevation of the left shoulder) postoperatively.

In the sagittal plane, recent studies have suggested that high correction with pedicle screw instrumentation results in decreased thoracic kyphosis and thereby risk decreasing lordosis in the uninstrumented lumbar spine (250, 351, 358). The cause for this lost kyphosis is believed to be the improved coronal and axial correction as discussed above. As discussed in the etiology section, the typical main thoracic curve is hypokyphotic from the relative overgrowth of the anterior column that is responsible for the curve development. Greater correction would return this increased length anteriorly. Without increasing length posteriorly, this would lordose the spinal column. Currently, techniques to allow lengthening of the posterior column during deformity correction are being investigated to allow maximal correction in all three planes.

Outcome After Anterior Surgery. Until recently, anterior correction of scoliosis had been the primary method used for the treatment of lumbar and thoracolumbar scoliosis. The percentage of frontal plane correction with Dwyer, Zielke, Texas Scottish Rite Hospital (TSRH), or Kaneda instrumentation has been reported as being between 67% and

98% (283, 285, 287–289, 295, 359). Similar to other techniques, there was a learning process in how to best utilize the instrumentation. Fusion and correction required performing a disc excision followed by anterior compression. This has the potential to reduce sagittal plane lumbar lordosis, which in most cases is undesirable (360, 361). Sweet et al. (288) have reported that sagittal alignment in the lumbar spine can be maintained if interbody structural support is added blocking open the disc space anteriorly. Another concern with anterior instrumentation was the higher rate of pseudarthrosis with eventual rod breakage and loss of correction compared to posterior methods. This was thought to be secondary to the use of a single fixation rod. Many surgeons recommended their patients wear a brace postoperatively. The subsequent development and the introduction of two-rod anterior systems provided more rigid fixation and resulted in decreased pseudarthrosis rates while maintaining high degrees of correction in both the sagittal and coronal planes (292, 325, 362, 363) (Fig. 17-56). A recent study demonstrated good long-term results at an average of 16 years following anterior fusion for either a thoracolumbar or lumbar idiopathic curve (364). Interestingly, most patients did have radiographic evidence of early degenerative changes.

The use of an anterior approach to the thoracic spine has also seen a significant decline in popularity. When compared with multisegmental posterior hook systems, open anterior instrumentation and fusion demonstrated similar coronal correction with improved sagittal profile across less fusion segments (average of 2.5 vertebrae less). The single-rod anterior systems were associated with a greater incidence of rod breakage. It was also suggested that anterior instrumentation should not be used in hyperkyphotic spines because of their tendency to increase kyphosis (296). A subsequent paper also reported a greater spontaneous improvement of the uninstrumented portion of the lumbar spine (293). Recently, the 5-year follow-up on patients that had open instrumented anterior fusion was published. The study demonstrated approximately 50% correction in both the instrumented thoracic spine and the uninstrumented lumbar spine as well as 9-degree improvement (increase) in thoracic kyphosis. The main downside was the lasting reduction in pulmonary function tests (specifically, FEV1) even after 5 years. The decrease in pulmonary function following open thoracic spine surgery compared with posterior surgery is one of the reasons for the decline in this approach (365, 366).

The thoracoscopic-instrumented anterior approach has many of the advantages of the open approach without the significant impact to the chest wall and pulmonary function. While compared to a posterior approach, the thoracoscopic procedure demonstrated a minor decline in pulmonary function, it was not as significant and lasting as an open anterior approach (366–368). The main advantages of this procedure are the minimal muscle dissection and the appearance of the scar compared with either an open anterior or a posterior approach (369). A 5-year follow-up study on patients treated with thoracoscopic-instrumented anterior fusion demonstrated results similar to open anterior with a 50% curve correction

(240). The concern reported by the authors was the risk of rod breakage and pseudoarthrosis. Another drawback to the procedure was the learning curve needed to master the technique (370). Given these limitations and the powerful corrections obtained with modern posterior segmental instrumentation, a decline in the use of the anterior approach, both open and thoracoscopic, for moderately sized thoracic and thoracolumbar/lumbar curves has occurred over the past decade.

COMPLICATIONS

The complications of scoliosis surgery can be serious, although over the last 20 to 30 years these procedures have become much safer. The remarkable corrective power of the new instrumentation methods, coupled with better surgical skills, spinal cord monitoring, methods to minimize blood loss, and advances in anesthesia, has altered the way one advises patients regarding possible complications following scoliosis surgery.

Neurologic Deficits. A postoperative neurologic deficit is one of the most feared complications that can occur during idiopathic scoliosis surgery. The majority of literature on neurologic injury present pooled data of patients with many underlying diagnoses and report an incidence between 0.3% and 1.4% (371–374). The most recent data from the SRS were published in 2006, which reported 31 neurologic injuries in just over 6000 patients with idiopathic scoliosis (372). None of the cases had a complete injury and full recovery was documented in 61% of patients.

The etiology of spinal cord dysfunction can be classified as a result of direct trauma (contusion) to the cord by misplaced implants, excessive traction to the neural elements caused by scoliosis correction, and vascular insufficiency to the cord. The blood supply to the spinal cord is segmental and enters through the neural foramina. There has been some controversy as to the risk of vascular insufficiency to the cord associated with ligation of the anterior segmental blood vessels in anterior spine surgery. Winter et al. (375) reported 1197 cases in which segmental vessels were divided with no neurologic sequelae noted. There have, however, been other reports suggesting a possible vascular cause of spinal cord dysfunction postoperatively after segmental vessel ligation. Those at greatest risk appear to be patients with congenital malformations and hyperkyphosis (376, 377). If an anterior procedure requires division of the segmental vessels, they should be ligated in the midvertebral body area rather than near the neural foramen. In high-risk cases (congenital, kyphosis, revision surgery) temporary clamping of the vessels with concomitant spinal cord monitoring has been suggested by some as a means of detecting a potentially critical source of spinal cord blood supply (376).

Induced hypotension is a well-accepted approach to minimize operative blood loss in surgery for scoliosis; however, the mean arterial pressure must be maintained at a safe level in order to ensure adequate blood flow to the spinal cord. In extremely complex corrections (kyphosis, osteotomies, revision

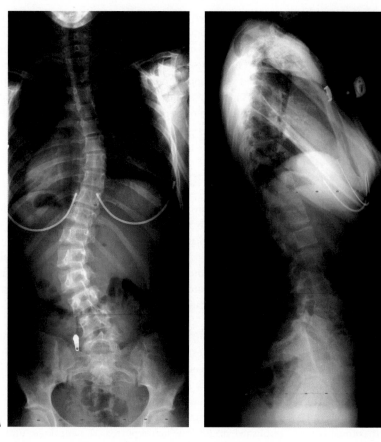

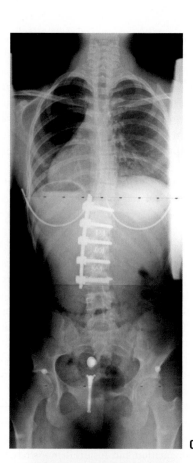

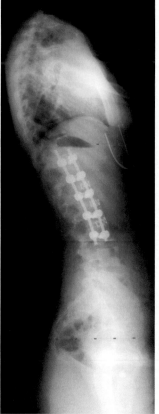

FIGURE 17-56. **A,B**: This demonstrates a typical left thoracolumbar scoliosis. **C,D**: In cases with a dual-rod interior construct, we utilize two screws in each vertebra with a two-hole vertebral staple that provides excellent postoperative stability. Interbody support is utilized to maintain lumbar lordosis while compression between the screws is performed to correct the scoliosis. No bracing is required following such instrumentation.

surgery) where the risk for cord ischemia is greater, the surgeon may elect to keep the blood pressure higher, even though blood loss will be greater, to ensure cord perfusion (378).

Spinal Cord Monitoring.

The wake-up test described by Stagnara (91) was the first widely used method for monitoring spinal cord function after deformity correction. This technique includes decreasing the level of anesthesia intraoperatively to a level that allows the patient to follow commands. The patient is instructed to move his or her feet/toes, confirming the competency of the spinal cord motor tracts (379).

Continuous electrical spinal cord monitoring has become almost standard in surgical correction of spine deformity. Currently, options for spinal cord monitoring include somatosensory-evoked potentials (SSEPs), transcranial motor–evoked potentials (TcMEPs), and H-reflexes. SSEPs are obtained by stimulating distally (legs) and measuring the response proximally (brain), and have been considered reliable in detecting changes in spinal cord function (380). The concern with SSEPs has been the lag time that can occur between the insult to the spinal cord and the resulting signal changes. Changes in motor pathway monitoring or TcMEPs have been shown to be more sensitive to spinal cord dysfunction especially vascular insults. These changes are also detected earlier than SSEPs allowing for a more rapid intervention (381). Because TcMEPs requires higher stimulating voltage to the brain, there had been some concern about their use in patients at risk of having a seizure. Triggered electromyographic (EMG) monitoring is also used to assess placement of

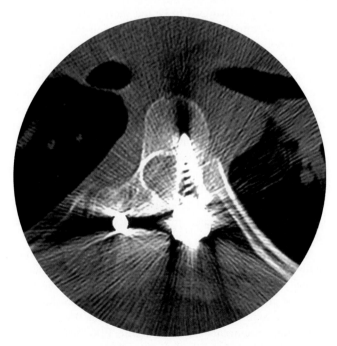

FIGURE 17-57. This pedicle screw was misdirected, reaching the medial aspect of the spinal canal. While there were no neurologic deficits associated with this, triggered EMG monitoring, if done, would have most likely demonstrated a threshold below 6 mA.

pedicle screws (382). While absolute thresholds have not been established, thresholds below 6 mA have been associated with a higher incidence of medial breach (Fig. 17-57). In general, the greater the number, the less likely the screw is in contact with neural elements. This method is less reliable in detecting lateral screw misplacement.

Additional factors have been found to affect the quality and presence of spinal cord monitoring responses, resulting in false-positive indications of spinal cord deficit. These include hypotension, hypothermia, dislodgment of the monitoring leads, and other technical malfunctions in the system. When critical neuromonitoring changes are noted, these potential causes should be sought and corrected. If the monitoring abnormalities persist, any corrective maneuvers performed should be undone and a wake-up test conducted to actively assess the neurologic status (378). If the spine remains stable, complete removal of the implants should be considered as soon as a deficit is confirmed. Concomitantly, the patient's mean arterial blood pressure should be maintained at 80 mm Hg, and adequate blood volume should be given to maximize oxygen delivery to the spinal cord. Institution of the methylprednisolone steroid spinal cord injury protocol (383) may also be considered, although the efficacy in this specific group of patients with spinal cord injury has not been carefully studied.

Blood Loss, Transfusion.

Scoliosis surgery may be associated with blood loss requiring transfusion. This requires appropriate anticipation by the surgeon based on the type of deformity and the extent of the planned surgery. Preoperative autologous donation may be the most reliable way to avoid exposure to allogenic blood products, although this is not possible in all patients (reasons include small size of patient, psychological stress of donating, long distance to the blood bank, preoperative anemia, congenital heart disease, expense). Intraoperative red blood cell salvage systems or cell savers are commonly used in scoliosis surgery and, depending on the specific case, have been shown to decrease the need for allogenic blood transfusions (384). Antifibrinolytic agents given at the time of surgery that enhance clotting are also becoming more popular. Aminocaproic acid, tranexamic acid, and aprotinin have all demonstrated reduced blood loss and the amount of blood transfused for scoliosis surgery (385). Recently, the use of aprotinin was suspended in the US over safety concerns generated in adult cardiac patients. Other alternatives to minimize allogenic blood exposure include preoperative erythropoietin administration (386), intraoperative hemodilution (387), and controlled hypotensive anesthesia (388). Currently, these methods are less commonly used because of their effects on neuromonitoring except in cases where a patient's belief may prevent the ability to give blood transfusions (389).

Early Postoperative Complications.

Complications in the early postoperative period include respiratory compromise, wound infection, and delayed-onset neurologic deficit. The incidence of respiratory complications in idiopathic scoliosis is approximately 1%, whereas wound complications (infections and seromas/hematomas) occur in approximately 2% of cases (390). These rates are affected by the type of procedure performed with anterior procedures having greater respiratory problems and posterior procedures more commonly having wound concerns. Independent of the approach used, blood loss, anesthesia time, and a history of renal disease also significantly increase the rate of complications (390).

Delayed-onset neurologic deficit has been seen following surgery for idiopathic scoliosis. Therefore, careful neurologic monitoring of the upper and lower extremity function for the 48 hours following corrective surgery must be emphasized. Cases have been reported that confirmed that the patient had intact neurologic function after the surgery but suffered loss of motor and sensory function in the days following surgery (371, 391, 392). The etiology of delayed-onset paraplegia is unclear. It may be vascular, resulting from postoperative hypotension, or mechanical, resulting from a compressive hematoma. Patients with delayed-onset neurologic deficit should undergo advanced imaging (MRI and/or CT) to determine if a compressive lesion exist and as quickly as possible have the corrective instrumentation removed or the corrective forces removed (if the instrumentation is required for spinal stability as may be required after a three-column osteotomy). Similar to intraoperative deficits, the patient's mean arterial pressure and blood volume should be increased, and consideration given to administering steroids (378).

Implant-Related Complications.
Complications related to the implants may present early or late in the postoperative period. Loss of implant fixation may occur if excessive corrective forces are applied to the bone anchors. The strength by which a rod exerts force on the spine is influenced by the rod contour as well as by its material properties (stainless steel, titanium, or cobalt chrome) (393). Fracture as a result of poor bone quality can cause an implant to loosen (394). Biomechanical comparison has also demonstrated different pullout strength between pedicle screws, laminar hooks, and wiring (395), which vary based on the direction of loading. Implant malpositioning is a relatively common complication that while can result in catastrophic complication, typically causes little clinical sequelae. A study evaluating the placement of pedicle screws with postoperative CT demonstrated significant medial or lateral pedicle breaches in 10.5% of the screws (396) (Fig. 17-58). None of the patients demonstrated any clinical consequences from these misplaced screws. This should not, however, lessen one's vigilance in placing pedicle screws in the pediatric spinal deformity population. The use of triggered EMG and intraoperative fluoroscopy can aid in ensuring proper pedicle screw placement (397). Anterior instrumentation malpositioning can also place patients at risk. In addition to spinal canal penetration, one must consider the proximity of the aorta to the vertebral column when placing both anterior and posterior screws (398).

Late implant problems include broken implants and painful or prominent fixation (399). A late broken implant typically implies the presence of a nonunion or a pseudoarthrosis. Motion at the pseudoarthrosis site ultimately causes the stabilizing implant (rod or screw) to fatigue and break. The time period before implant failure occurs depends on the size, material, and number of the rods used. In the presence of a pseudoarthrosis, small single-rod systems may become fatigued and fracture within a year, while a double-rod system may not fail for several years. Interestingly, a rod fracture or pseudoarthrosis may not result in clinical symptoms; therefore, revision surgery is generally indicated for pain or deformity progression.

Patients that present with delayed pain around their instrumentation or surgical site may represent the development of a delayed infection (400–402). Evaluation of tissue surrounding instrumentation removed for late pain has demonstrated particulate wear debris (403). In cases where either pain or infection necessitate instrumentation removal, there should be concern for loss of deformity correction even when a pseudoarthrosis has not been identified (404). It may be wise to re-instrument the spine to prevent loss of correction. In cases of infection, titanium implants may be associated with a lower incidence of surgical-site infection in some published reports (405), although definitive data to support this concept are lacking.

Other Complications.
Additional complications that can present in a delayed fashion relate to progression of deformity and spinal imbalance. These problems usually occur in patients that had surgery at a young age and/or had fusions that were later determined to be too short. Crankshaft is an example of postoperative scoliosis progression through residual anterior growth following a posterior fusion in a skeletally immature patient (272). Lumbar curve or thoracic curve progression can occur following a selective thoracic or selective lumbar fusion, respectively. "Adding on," defined as progression or extension of the primary curve, typically is seen as progressive wedging in the disc below the lowest-instrumented vertebra or as an increase in the number of vertebra in the measured Cobb (406). Minor degrees of radiographic deformity progression rarely significantly alter the clinical appearance of the patient and should merely be monitored. However, in cases where significant progression results in further clinical deformity or imbalance, an extension of the fusion may be indicated.

Similar to coronal plane problems, progressive deformity in the sagittal plane can also occur. PJK, defined as a 10-degree change between the end-instrumented vertebra and the adjacent one or two uninstrumented vertebra, has been shown to be relative common with an incidence between 9% and 27% (407, 408). Factors that correlated with PJK included large preoperative thoracic kyphosis, a loss of thoracic kyphosis in the instrumented segments, the use of pedicle screws, and a higher BMI (408). In most patients, this is no more than a radiographic concern as few patients complain of their junctional deformity.

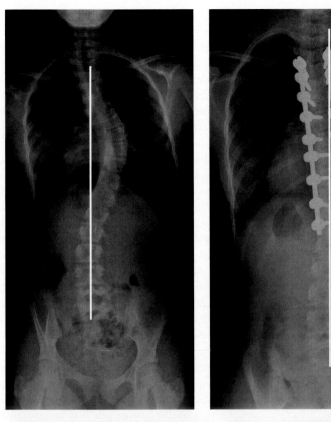

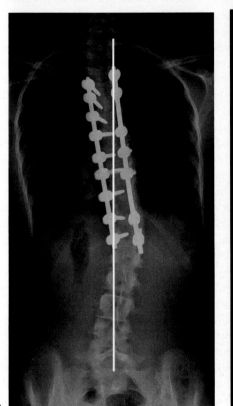

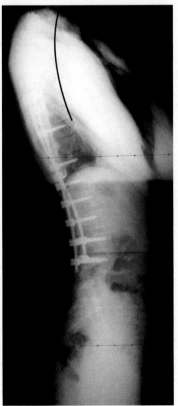

FIGURE 17-58. A: PA radiograph demonstrates a Lenke 1A curve. **B**: Distally, the patient was fused to T12, which was the vertebra last touched by the CSVL as seen on the first erect radiograph. **C**: At 2-year follow-up, the patient has developing "adding on" as demonstrated by both the progressive wedging in the disc below the lowest-instrumented vertebra and an increase in the number of vertebra in the measured Cobb. **D**: Lateral view at 2 years post-operatively.

FUTURE TREATMENT

Concerns regarding the long-term effects of decreased spinal mobility following spinal fusion have led to investigations into novel methods to manage the progressive curve. Methods actively being explored include vertebral body stapling and anterior tethering. The goal is to use these devices as a fusionless method to alter a patient's remaining spinal growth to achieve correction of the curve. By exploiting the effects of the Hueter-Volkmann law, the hope is that compressing the convex anterior growth plates will inhibit their growth, while allowing the continued posterior and concave growth to ultimately reverse the deformity. One day we hope patients will have opportunities for spinal deformity correction without the effects of lost spinal mobility that is associated with our current corrective techniques of fusion (306–308).

AUTHORS' PREFERRED TREATMENT

Our preferences for treating scoliosis are based on our individual biases; some are founded on facts, some on intuition, and some on past experiences/mistakes. Our choices for a given patient's treatment have evolved and are continually being assessed. The recommendations that follow reflect our current approaches to bracing and surgical treatment of AIS.

Brace Treatment. We generally believe that brace treatment has the potential to modify the natural history of a select few patients with scoliosis. We understand the challenges of such therapy for many teenaged patients as well as the desires of many for some chance to avoid surgical treatment. We offer a thoracic-lumbar spinal orthosis (TLSO) to female patients whom we believe to be at risk for progression and are willing to commit to a wearing schedule of at least 16 hours per day. Rarely do we prescribe a TLSO for a male teenager with scoliosis other than to occasionally delay an inevitable fusion in a boy with many years of remaining growth. In general, a custom-made underarm TLSO is the type of brace we use; however, a nighttime bending brace is considered when the patient has only a thoracolumbar curve.

Surgical Treatment. The complexity of surgical decision making in scoliosis makes generalizations regarding preferred methods difficult. In general, most cases are treated with posterior instrumentation, and we make every effort to spare as many motion segments of the lumbar spine as possible. Our primary goal is to prevent curve progression and obtain coronal, sagittal, and axial balance. In nearly all cases, we utilize pedicle screws (thoracic and lumbar) to maximize three-dimensional correction.

While not every curve is treated according to the Lenke classification system, we are in general agreement with its recommendations. The clinical appearance of the patient also influences the decisions to instrument a particular curve. All patients with more than one structural curve are instrumented

posteriorly. The majority of single thoracic curves (Lenke 1A-C) are also currently treated posteriorly. Historically, some patients were treated with thoracoscopic anterior instrumentation; however, the challenges with thoracoscopic instrumentation without a lasting demonstrable benefit to the outcome have led to decreased use of this technique. A thoracoscopic release may be performed in large, rigid curves or in those with substantial risk for crankshaft (open triradiate cartilage).

We nearly treat all thoracolumbar curves with posterior spinal instrumentation as well. In the past, anterior instrumentation was our preferred technique. A relatively short anterior fusion, ending distally at L3 in most cases, had yielded consistent results. However, the use of aggressive posterior releases along with segmental pedicle screws has provided similar results and typically can be accomplished across the same levels as an anterior procedure. We still consider an anterior approach for those patients with very small pedicles in which segmental screw fixation may not be possible.

Thus, in general, posterior pedicle screw instrumentation has become our preferred method of fixation with hooks (transverse process, pedicle, and lamina) and sublaminar wires added as required. Segmental fixation throughout the concave thoracic curve is sought in order to maximize fixation so that correction forces required to achieve ideal three-dimensional balance can be attained with less concern for screw pullout. Pedicle screw fixation on the convex side may be less critical for maximal correction, yet these pedicle screws are often easier and safer to place than those on the concavity. We utilize EMG pedicle screw stimulation to assess cortical integrity of the pedicle and remove or replace screws with values <4 to 6 mAmps. Radiographic confirmation of screw position is also assessed with the image intensifier intraoperatively (Fig. 17-59). We often place two thoracic transverse process hooks (when transverse process is large enough) at the cephalad end of our construct. These require less dissection to place than a screw and may minimize the risk of proximal junctional kyphosis. To increase the flexibility of the spine and improve thoracic kyphosis, we will frequently perform Ponte-type releases at the lordotic apex of the curve. We believe these releases allow the posterior column to lengthen during the correction and accommodate the relatively excessive anterior column length seen in AIS (discussed in the etiology section).

When screws have been successfully placed in a segmental fashion, they offer a powerful means to achieve deformity correction. To maximize three-dimensional correction, we utilize steel rods with a high yield point (200 ksi) aggressive differential rod contouring, compression/distraction, and segmental vertebral derotation. With appropriate level selection, we hope to achieve a balanced correction that minimizes deformity (reduces the coronal deformity, increases the thoracic kyphosis, and decreases the axial plane rotation) and maximizes spinal flexibility. Currently, we do not routinely perform thoracoplasty in association with our thoracic curve corrections and reserve this procedure for the most deformed chest cages.

Our choice for bone graft had traditionally been iliac crest autograft. However, with the use of pedicle screw fixation, the

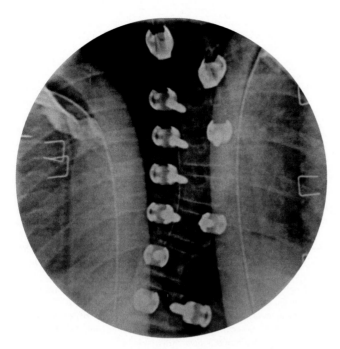

FIGURE 17-59. This intraoperative intensifier view demonstrates the appearance of pedicle screws placed in the thoracic apex. There is a gradual transition in the rotation of the left-sided apical screws, maximal at the apex. The lateral view should also confirm appropriate screw length.

lamina and facet joints are free of obstructing instrumentation, and the augmentation of local bone with allograft when combined with aggressive midline decortication seems adequate in most cases.

The surgical management of AIS has undergone a significant evolution from the time of treatment with bone grafting and corrective casting. Our surgical approaches, which 10 years ago relied heavily on anterior procedures, have now been replaced primarily with posterior spinal instrumentation and fusion procedures. Interestingly, the prospect of fusionless surgery as discussed above may once again increase anterior spinal surgery, especially thoracoscopic methods, in the future.

REFERENCES

1. Bernhardt M, Bridwell KH. Segmental analysis of the sagittal plane alignment of the normal thoracic and lumbar spines and thoracolumbar junction. *Spine* 1989;14:717–721.
2. Propst-Proctor SL, Bleck EE. Radiographic determination of lordosis and kyphosis in normal and scoliotic children. *J Pediatr Orthop* 1983;3:344–346.
3. Vedantam R, Lenke LG, Keeney JA. Comparison of standing sagittal spinal alignment in asymptomatic adolescents and adults. *Spine* 1998;23:211–215.
4. Stokes IA, Bigalow LC, Moreland MS. Measurement of axial rotation of vertebrae in scoliosis. *Spine* 1986;11:213–218.
5. Perdriolle R, Borgne PL, Dansereau J. Idiopathic scoliosis in three dimensions: a succession of two-dimensional deformities? *Spine* 2001;26:2719–2726.
6. Stokes IA, Armstrong JG, Moreland MS. Spinal deformity and back surface asymmetry in idiopathic scoliosis. *J Orthop Res* 1988;6:129–137.
7. Asher MA, Cook LT. The transverse plane evolution of the most common adolescent idiopathic scoliosis deformities. A cross-sectional study of 181 patients. *Spine* 1995;20:1386–1391.
8. Denoel C, et al. Idiopathic scoliosis and breast asymmetry. *J Plast Reconstr Aesthet Surg* 2009;62(10):1303–1308.
9. Lawton JO, Dickson RA. The experimental basis of idiopathic scoliosis. *Clin Orthop* 1986;210:9–17.
10. Ohlen G, Aaro S, Bylund P. The sagittal configuration and mobility of the spine in idiopathic scoliosis. *Spine* 1988;13:413–416.
11. Dickson RA. The aetiology of spinal deformities. *Lancet* 1988;1:1151–1155.
12. Dickson RA, Lawton JO, Archer IA. The pathogenesis of idiopathic scoliosis. Biplanar spinal asymmetry. *J Bone Joint Surg Br* 1984;66:8–15.
13. Somerville EW. Rotational lordosis: the development of the single curve. *J Bone Joint Surg Br* 1952;34:421–427.
14. Hayashi K, et al. Three-dimensional analysis of thoracic apical sagittal alignment in adolescent idiopathic scoliosis. *Spine (Phila Pa 1976)* 2009; 34(8):792–797.
15. Goldberg CJ, Dowling FE, Fogarty EE. Left thoracic scoliosis configurations. Why so different? *Spine* 1994;19:1385–1389.
16. Stokes IA. Idiopathic scoliosis: terminology. In: Burwell G, Dangerfield PH, Margulies JY, eds. *Spine: state of the art reviews.* Philadelphia, PA: Hanley & Belfus, 2000:349.
17. Kotwicki T, Napiontek M. Intravertebral deformation in idiopathic scoliosis: a transverse plane computer tomographic study. *J Pediatr Orthop* 2008;28(2):225–229.
18. Stokes IA, Burwell RG, Dangerfield PH. Biomechanical spinal growth modulation and progressive adolescent scoliosis—a test of the 'vicious cycle' pathogenetic hypothesis: summary of an electronic focus group debate of the IBSE. *Scoliosis* 2006;1:16.
19. Robin GC, Cohen T. Familial scoliosis. A clinical report. *J Bone Joint Surg Br* 1975;57:146–148.
20. Miller NH. Cause and natural history of adolescent idiopathic scoliosis. *Orthop Clin North Am* 1999;30:343–352.
21. Wynne-Davies R. Familial (idiopathic) scoliosis. A family survey. *J Bone Joint Surg Br* 1968;50:24–30.
22. Wynne-Davies R. Genetic aspects of idiopathic scoliosis. *Dev Med Child Neurol* 1973;15:809–811.
23. Risenborough EJ, Wynne-Davies R. A genetic survey of idiopathic scoliosis in Boston, Massachusetts. *J Bone Joint Surg Am* 1973;55:974–982.
24. Kesling KL, Reinker KA. Scoliosis in twins. A meta-analysis of the literature and report of six cases. *Spine* 1997;22:2009–2014.
25. Anderson M, Hwang SC, Green WT. Growth of the normal trunk in boys and girls during the second decade of life. Related to age, maturity, and ossification of the iliac epiphyses. *J Bone Joint Surg Am* 1965;47:1554–1564.
26. Inoue M, Minami S, Kitahara H. Idiopathic scoliosis in twins studied by DNA fingerprinting: the incidence and type of scoliosis. *J Bone Joint Surg Br* 1998;80:212–217.
27. Gurnett CA, et al. Genetic linkage localizes an adolescent idiopathic scoliosis and pectus excavatum gene to chromosome 18 q. *Spine (Phila Pa 1976)* 2009;34(2):E94–E100.
28. Ward K, et al. Polygenic inheritance of adolescent idiopathic scoliosis: a study of extended families in Utah. *Am J Med Genet A* 2010; 152A(5):1178–1188.
29. Ogilvie JW, et al. The search for idiopathic scoliosis genes. *Spine (Phila Pa 1976)* 2006;31(6):679–681.
30. Carr AJ, Ogilvie DJ, Wordsworth BP. Segregation of structural collagen genes in adolescent idiopathic scoliosis. *Clin Orthop* 1992;274:305–310.
31. Miller NH, Mims B, Child A. Genetic analysis of structural elastic fiber and collagen genes in familial adolescent idiopathic scoliosis. *J Orthop Res* 1996;14:994–999.
32. Zhang HQ, et al. Association of estrogen receptor beta gene polymorphisms with susceptibility to adolescent idiopathic scoliosis. *Spine (Phila Pa 1976)* 2009;34(8):760–764.
33. Guille JT, Bowen JR. Scoliosis and fibrous dysplasia of the spine. *Spine* 1995;20:248–251.

34. Ponseti IV, Pedrini V, Wynne-Davies R. Pathogenesis of scoliosis. *Clin Orthop* 1976;120:268–280.

35. Cheng JC, Guo X. Osteopenia in adolescent idiopathic scoliosis. A primary problem or secondary to the spinal deformity? *Spine* 1997;22:1716–1721.

36. Burner WL, Badger VM, Sherman FC. Osteoporosis and acquired back deformities. *J Pediatr Orthop* 1982;2:383–385.

37. Cook SD, Harding AF, Morgan EL. Trabecular bone mineral density in idiopathic scoliosis. *J Pediatr Orthop* 1987;7:168–174.

38. Cheng JC, Qin L, Cheung CS. Generalized low areal and volumetric bone mineral density in adolescent idiopathic scoliosis. *J Bone Miner Res* 2000;15:1587–1595.

39. Szalay EA, et al. Adolescents with idiopathic scoliosis are not osteoporotic. *Spine (Phila Pa 1976)* 2008;33(7):802–806.

40. Loncar-Dusek M, Pecina M, Prebeg Z. A longitudinal study of growth velocity and development of secondary gender characteristics versus onset of idiopathic scoliosis. *Clin Orthop* 1991;270:278–282.

41. Lonstein JE, Carlson JM. The prediction of curve progression in untreated idiopathic scoliosis during growth. *J Bone Joint Surg Am* 1984;66:1061–1071.

42. Roaf R. Rotation movements of the spine with special reference to scoliosis. *J Bone Joint Surg Br* 1958;40:312–332.

43. Roaf R. The basic anatomy of scoliosis. *J Bone Joint Surg Br* 1966;48:786–792.

44. Stokes IA, Laible JP. Three-dimensional osseo-ligamentous model of the thorax representing initiation of scoliosis by asymmetric growth. *J Biomech* 1990;23:589–595.

45. Stokes IA, Spence H, Aronsson DD. Mechanical modulation of vertebral body growth. Implications for scoliosis progression. *Spine* 1996;21:1162–1167.

46. Cruickshank JL, Koike M, Dickson RA. Curve patterns in idiopathic scoliosis. A clinical and radiographic study. *J Bone Joint Surg Br* 1989;71:259–263.

47. Millner PA, Dickson RA. Idiopathic scoliosis: biomechanics and biology. *Eur Spine J* 1996;5:362–373.

48. Murray DW, Bulstrode CJ. The development of adolescent idiopathic scoliosis. *Eur Spine J* 1996;5:251–257.

49. Smith RM, Dickson RA. Experimental structural scoliosis. *J Bone Joint Surg Br* 1987;69:576–581.

50. Azegami H, Murachi S, Kitoh J. Etiology of idiopathic scoliosis. Computational study. *Clin Orthop* 1998;357:229–236.

51. Villemure I, Aubin CE, Grimard G. Evolution of 3D deformities in adolescents with progressive idiopathic scoliosis. *Stud Health Technol Inform* 2002;91:54–58.

52. Guo X, Chau WW, Chan YL. Relative anterior spinal overgrowth in adolescent idiopathic scoliosis. Results of disproportionate endochondral-membranous bone growth. *J Bone Joint Surg Br* 2003;85:1026–1031.

53. Archer IA, Dickson RA. Stature and idiopathic scoliosis. A prospective study. *J Bone Joint Surg Br* 1985;67:185–188.

54. Buric M, Momcilovic B. Growth pattern and skeletal age in school girls with idiopathic scoliosis. *Clin Orthop* 1982:238–242.

55. Nordwall A, Willner S. A study of skeletal age and height in girls with idiopathic scoliosis. *Clin Orthop* 1975;110:6–10.

56. Willner S. A study of growth in girls with adolescent idiopathic structural scoliosis. *Clin Orthop* 1974;101:129–135.

57. Drummond DS, Rogala EJ. Growth and maturation of adolescents with idiopathic scoliosis. *Spine* 1980;5:507–511.

58. Skogland LB, Miller JA. Growth related hormones in idiopathic scoliosis. An endocrine basis for accelerated growth. *Acta Orthop Scand* 1980;51:779–780.

59. Willner S, Nilsson KO, Kastrup K. Growth hormone and somatomedin A in girls with adolescent idiopathic scoliosis. *Acta Paediatr Scand* 1976;65:547–552.

60. LeBlanc R, Labelle H, Forest F. Morphologic discrimination among healthy subjects and patients with progressive and nonprogressive adolescent idiopathic scoliosis. *Spine* 1998;23:1109–1115.

61. LeBlanc R, Labelle H, Rivard CH. et al. Relation between adolescent idiopathic scoliosis and morphologic somatotypes. *Spine* 1997;22:2532–2536.

62. Normelli H, Sevastik J, Ljung G. et al. Anthropometric data relating to normal and scoliotic Scandinavian girls. *Spine* 1985;10:123–126.

63. Ahl T, Albertsson-Wikland K, Kalen R. Twenty-four-hour growth hormone profiles in pubertal girls with idiopathic scoliosis. *Spine* 1988;13:139–142.

64. Inoue M, Minami S, Nakata Y. Association between estrogen receptor gene polymorphisms and curve severity of idiopathic scoliosis. *Spine* 2002;27:2357–2362.

65. Burwell RG, Cole AA, Cook TA. Pathogenesis of idiopathic scoliosis. The Nottingham concept. *Acta Orthop Belg* 1992;5 8:33–58.

66. Dretakis EK. Scoliosis associated with congenital brain-stem abnormalities. A report of eight cases. *Int Orthop* 1984;8:37–46.

67. Goldberg CJ, Dowling FE, Fogarty EE. et al. An examination of a nonspinal perceptual system. *Spine* 1995;20:1685–1691.

68. Gregoric M, Pecak F, Trontelj JV. Postural control in scoliosis. A statokinesimetric study in patients with scoliosis due to neuromuscular disorders and in patients with idiopathic scoliosis. *Acta Orthop Scand* 1981;52:59–63.

69. Thomsen M, Steffen H, Sabo D, et al. *J Pediatr Orthop* 1996;5B:185–189.

70. Wiener-Vacher SR, Mazda K. Asymmetric otolith vestibulo-ocular responses in children with idiopathic scoliosis. *J Pediatr* 1998;132:1028–1032.

71. Wyatt MP, Barrack RL, Mubarak SJ. Vibratory response in idiopathic scoliosis. *J Bone Joint Surg Br* 1986;68:714–718.

72. Herman R, Mixon J, Fisher A. Scoliosis Research Society. Idiopathic scoliosis and the central nervous system: a motor control problem. The Harrington lecture, 1983. *Spine* 1985;10:1–14.

73. Keessen W, Crowe A, Hearn M. Proprioceptive accuracy in idiopathic scoliosis. *Spine* 1992;17:149–155.

74. Lidstrom J, Friberg S, Lindstrom L. Postural control in siblings to scoliosis patients and scoliosis patients. *Spine* 1988;13:1070–1074.

75. Sahlstrand T, Ortengren R, Nachemson A. Postural equilibrium in adolescent idiopathic scoliosis. *Acta Orthop Scand* 1978;49:354–365.

76. Woods LA, Haller RJ, Hansen PD. Decreased incidence of scoliosis in hearing-impaired children. Implications for a neurologic basis for idiopathic scoliosis. *Spine* 1995;20:776–780.

77. O'Beirne J, et al. Equilibrial dysfunction in scoliosis—cause or effect? *J Spinal Disord* 1989;2(3):184–189.

78. Lee JS, et al. Adolescent idiopathic scoliosis may not be associated with brain abnormalities. *Acta Radiol* 2009;50(8):941–946.

79. Inoue M, Nakata Y, Minami S. Idiopathic scoliosis as a presenting sign of familial neurologic abnormalities. *Spine* 2003;28:40–45.

80. Samuelsson L, Lindell D. Scoliosis as the first sign of a cystic spinal cord lesion. *Eur Spine J* 1995;4:284–290.

81. Zadeh HG, Sakka SA, Powell MP. Absent superficial abdominal reflexes in children with scoliosis. An early indicator of syringomyelia. *J Bone Joint Surg Br* 1995;77:762–767.

82. Machida M, Dubousset J, Imamura Y. An experimental study of chickens for the pathogenesis of idiopathic scoliosis. *Spine* 1993;18:1609–1615.

83. Machida M, Dubousset J, Imamura Y. Role of melatonin deficiency in the development of scoliosis in pinealectomised chickens. *J Bone Joint Surg Br* 1995;77:134–138.

84. Wang X, Jiang H, Raso J. Characterization of the scoliosis that develops after pinealectomy in the chicken and comparison with adolescent idiopathic scoliosis in humans. *Spine* 1997;22:2626–2635.

85. Machida M, Dubousset J, Imamura Y. Melatonin. A possible role in pathogenesis of adolescent idiopathic scoliosis. *Spine* 1996;21:1147–1152.

86. Bagnall KM, Raso VJ, Hill DL. Melatonin levels in idiopathic scoliosis. Diurnal and nocturnal serum melatonin levels in girls with adolescent idiopathic scoliosis. *Spine* 1996;21:1974–1978.

87. Cheung KM, Luk KD. Prediction of correction of scoliosis with use of the fulcrum bending radiograph. *J Bone Joint Surg Am* 1997;79:1144–1150.

88. Fagan AB, Kennaway DJ, Sutherland AD. Total 24-hour melatonin secretion in adolescent idiopathic scoliosis. A case-control study. *Spine* 1998;23:41–46.

89. Hilibrand AS, Blakemore LC, Loder RT. The role of melatonin in the pathogenesis of adolescent idiopathic scoliosis. *Spine* 1996;21:1140–1146.

90. Moreau A, da SW, Forget S. Melatonin signaling dysfunction in adolescent idiopathic scoliosis. *Spine* 2004;29:1772–1781.

91. Stagnara P. *Spinal deformity*. London, UK: Butterworth & Co. Ltd, 1988.

92. Dobbs MB, Lenke LG, Szymanski DA. Prevalence of neural axis abnormalities in patients with infantile idiopathic scoliosis. *J Bone Joint Surg Am* 2002;84-A:2230–2234.

93. Gupta P, Lenke LG, Bridwell KH. Incidence of neural axis abnormalities in infantile and juvenile patients with spinal deformity. Is a magnetic resonance image screening necessary? *Spine* 1998;23:206–210.

94. Pahys JM, Samdani AF, Betz RR. Intraspinal anomalies in infantile idiopathic scoliosis: prevalence and role of magnetic resonance imaging. *Spine (Phila Pa 1976)* 2009;34(12):E434–E438.

95. Lenke LG, Betz RR, Harms J. Adolescent idiopathic scoliosis: a new classification to determine extent of spinal arthrodesis. *J Bone Joint Surg Am* 2001;83-A:1169–1181.

96. Duval-Beaupere G, Lamireau T. Scoliosis at less than 30 degrees. Properties of the evolutivity (risk of progression). *Spine* 1985;10:421–424.

97. Little DG, Song KM, Katz D. Relationship of peak height velocity to other maturity indicators in idiopathic scoliosis in girls. *J Bone Joint Surg Am* 2000;82:685–693.

98. Dimeglio A. Growth in pediatric orthopaedics. *J Pediatr Orthop* 2001;21:549–555.

99. Soucacos PN, Zacharis K, Gelalis J. Assessment of curve progression in idiopathic scoliosis. *Eur Spine J* 1998;7:270–277.

100. Ramirez N, Johnston CE, Browne RH. The prevalence of back pain in children who have idiopathic scoliosis. *J Bone Joint Surg Am* 1997;79:364–368.

101. Barnes PD, Brody JD, Jaramillo D. Atypical idiopathic scoliosis: MR imaging evaluation. *Radiology* 1993;186:247–253.

102. Mehta MH. Pain provoked scoliosis. Observations on the evolution of the deformity. *Clin Orthop* 1978:58–65.

103. Fairbank JC, Pynsent PB, Poortvliet JAV. Influence of anthropometric factors and joint laxity in the incidence of adolescent back pain. *Spine* 1984;9:461–464.

104. Mierau D, Cassidy JD, Yong-Hing K. Low-back pain and straight leg raising in children and adolescents. *Spine* 1989;14:526–528.

105. Turner PG, Green JH, Galasko CS. Back pain in childhood. *Spine* 1989;14:812–814.

106. Baker AS, Dove J. Progressive scoliosis as the first presenting sign of syringomyelia. Report of a case. *J Bone Joint Surg Br* 1983;65:472–473.

107. Citron N, Edgar MA, Sheehy J. Intramedullary spinal cord tumours presenting as scoliosis. *J Bone Joint Surg Br* 1984;66:513–517.

108. Lewonowski K, King JD, Nelson MD. Routine use of magnetic resonance imaging in idiopathic scoliosis patients less than eleven years of age. *Spine* 1992;17:S109–S116.

109. Adams W. *Lectures on pathology and treatment of lateral and other forms of curvature of the spine*. London, UK: Churchill Livingstone, 1865.

110. Bunnell WP. Outcome of spinal screening. *Spine* 1993;18:1572–1580.

111. Grossman TW, Mazur JM, Cummings RJ. An evaluation of the Adams forward bend test and the scoliometer in a scoliosis school screening setting. *J Pediatr Orthop* 1995;15:535–538.

112. Huang SC. Cut-off point of the scoliometer in school scoliosis screening. *Spine* 1997;22:1985–1989.

113. Korovessis PG, Stamatakis MV. Prediction of scoliotic Cobb angle with the use of the scoliometer. *Spine* 1996;21:1661–1666.

114. Yngve D. Abdominal reflexes. *J Pediatr Orthop* 1997;17:105–108.

115. Marks MC, Stanford CF, Mahar AT. Standing lateral radiographic positioning does not represent customary standing balance. *Spine* 2003;28:1176–1182.

116. Deschenes S, et al. Diagnostic imaging of spinal deformities: reducing patients radiation dose with a new slot-scanning X-ray imager. *Spine (Phila Pa 1976)* 2010;35(9):989–994.

117. Kalifa G, et al. Evaluation of a new low-dose digital x-ray device: first dosimetric and clinical results in children. *Pediatr Radiol* 1998;28(7):557–561.

118. Levy AR, Goldberg MS, Mayo NE. Reducing the lifetime risk of cancer from spinal radiographs among people with adolescent idiopathic scoliosis. *Spine* 1996;21:1540–1547.

119. Luk KD, Cheung KM, Lu DS. Assessment of scoliosis correction in relation to flexibility using the fulcrum bending correction index. *Spine* 1998;23:2303–2307.

120. Takahashi S, Passuti N, Delecrin J. Interpretation and utility of traction radiography in scoliosis surgery. Analysis of patients treated with Cotrel-Dubousset instrumentation. *Spine* 1997;22:2542–2546.

121. Vaughan JJ, Winter RB, Lonstein JE. Comparison of the use of supine bending and traction radiographs in the selection of the fusion area in adolescent idiopathic scoliosis. *Spine* 1996;21:2469–2473.

122. Stagnara P. Medical observation and tests for scoliosis. *Rev Lyon Med* 1968;17:391–401.

123. Larsen JL. The lumbar spinal canal in children. Part II: the interpedicular distance and its relation to the sagittal diameter and transverse pedicular width. *Eur J Radiol* 1981;1:312–321.

124. Papp T, Porter RW, Aspden RM. The growth of the lumbar vertebral canal. *Spine* 1994;15:2770–2773.

125. Cobb J. Outline for the study of scoliosis. *Instr Course Lect* 1948;5:261.

126. Carman DL, Browne RH, Birch JG. Measurement of scoliosis and kyphosis radiographs. Intraobserver and interobserver variation. *J Bone Joint Surg Am* 1990;72:328–333.

127. Nash CL, Moe JH. A study of vertebral rotation. *J Bone Joint Surg Am* 1969;51:223–229.

128. Perdriolle R. *La scoliose: son etude tridimensionnelle*. In: Maloine SA, ed. Paris, France: 1979.

129. Richards BS. Measurement error in assessment of vertebral rotation using the Perdriolle torsionmeter. *Spine* 1992;17:513–517.

130. Risser JC. The iliac apophysis: an invaluable sign in the management of scoliosis. *Clin Orthop* 1958;11:111–119.

131. Noordeen MH, Haddad FS, Edgar MA. Spinal growth and a histologic evaluation of the Risser grade in idiopathic scoliosis. *Spine* 1999;24:535–538.

132. Izumi Y. The accuracy of Risser staging. *Spine* 1995;20:1868–1871.

133. Little DG, Sussman MD. The Risser sign: a critical analysis. *J Pediatr Orthop* 1994;14:569–575.

134. Sanders JO, Herring JA, Browne RH. Posterior arthrodesis and instrumentation in the immature (Risser-grade-0) spine in idiopathic scoliosis. *J Bone Joint Surg Am* 1995;77:39–45.

135. Sanders JO, Little DG, Richards BS. Prediction of the crankshaft phenomenon by peak height velocity. *Spine* 1997;22:1352–1356.

136. Greulich W, Pyle S. *Radiographic atlas of skeletal development of the hand and wrist*. 2nd ed. Stanford, CA: Stanford University Press, 1959.

137. Charles YP, et al. Skeletal age assessment from the olecranon for idiopathic scoliosis at Risser grade 0. *J Bone Joint Surg Am* 2007;89(12):2737–2744.

138. Sanders JO, et al. Predicting scoliosis progression from skeletal maturity: a simplified classification during adolescence. *J Bone Joint Surg Am* 2008;90(3):540–553.

139. Evans SC, Edgar MA, Hall-Craggs MA. MRI of 'idiopathic' juvenile scoliosis. A prospective study. *J Bone Joint Surg Br* 1996;78:314–317.

140. Schwend RM, Hennrikus W, Hall JE. Childhood scoliosis: clinical indications for magnetic resonance imaging. *J Bone Joint Surg Am* 1995;77:46–53.

141. Bradford DS, Heithoff KB, Cohen M. Intraspinal abnormalities and congenital spine deformities: a radiographic and MRI study. *J Pediatr Orthop* 1991;11:36–41.

142. McMaster MJ. Occult intraspinal anomalies and congenital scoliosis. *J Bone Joint Surg Am* 1984;66:588–601.

143. Mejia EA, Hennrikus WL, Schwend RM. A prospective evaluation of idiopathic left thoracic scoliosis with magnetic resonance imaging. *J Pediatr Orthop* 1996;16:354–358.

144. Cheng JC, Guo X, Sher AH. Correlation between curve severity, somatosensory evoked potentials, magnetic resonance imaging in adolescent idiopathic scoliosis. *Spine* 1999;24:1679–1684.

145. Brien MFO, Lenke LG, Bridwell KH. Preoperative spinal canal investigation in adolescent idiopathic scoliosis curves. *Spine* 1994;19:1606–1610.

146. Do T, Fras C, Burke S. Clinical value of routine preoperative magnetic resonance imaging in adolescent idiopathic scoliosis. A prospective

study of three hundred and twenty-seven patients. *J Bone Joint Surg Am* 2001;83-A:577–579.

147. Maenza RA. Juvenile and adolescent idiopathic scoliosis: magnetic resonance imaging evaluation and clinical indications. *J Pediatr Orthop B* 2003;12:295–302.

148. Ouellet JA, LaPlaza J, Erickson MA. Sagittal plane deformity in the thoracic spine: a clue to the presence of syringomyelia as a cause of scoliosis. *Spine* 2003;28:2147–2151.

149. Bruszewski J, Kamza A. Czestosc wystepowania skolioz na podstawie anacizy zdec maxoobrakowych. *Chir Narzadow Ruchu Ortop Pol* 1957; 22:115.

150. Dickson RA. Scoliosis in the community. *Br Med J* 1983;286: 615–618.

151. Kane WJ, Moe JH. A scoliosis-prevalence survey in Minnesota. *Clin Orthop* 1970;69:216–218.

152. Morais T, Bernier M, Turcotte F. Age- and sex-specific prevalence of scoliosis and the value of school screening programs. *Am J Public Health* 1985;75:1377–1380.

153. Rogala EJ, Drummond DS, Gurr J. Scoliosis: incidence and natural history. A prospective epidemiological study. *J Bone Joint Surg Am* 1978;60:173–176.

154. Shands AR, Eisberg HB. The incidence of scoliosis in the state of Delaware. A study of 50,000 minifilms of the chest made during a survey for tuberculosis. *J Bone Joint Surg Am* 1955;37:1243–1249.

155. Stirling AJ, Howel D, Millner PA. Late-onset idiopathic scoliosis in children six to fourteen years old. A cross-sectional prevalence study. *J Bone Joint Surg Am* 1996;78:1330–1336.

156. Kane WJ. Scoliosis prevalence: a call for a statement of terms. *Clin Orthop* 1977;126:43–46.

157. Montgomery F, Willner S. The natural history of idiopathic scoliosis. Incidence of treatment in 15 cohorts of children born between 1963 and 1977. *Spine* 1997;22:772–774.

158. Dickson RA, Weinstein SL. Bracing (and screening)—yes or no? *J Bone Joint Surg Br* 1999;81:193–198.

159. Weinstein SL, Dolan LA, Spratt KF. Health and function of patients with untreated idiopathic scoliosis: a 50-year natural history study. *JAMA* 2003;289:559–567.

160. James JIP, Lloyd-Roberts GC, Pilcher MF. Infantile structural scoliosis. *J Bone Joint Surg Br* 1959;41:719–735.

161. Scott JC, Morgan TH. The natural history and prognosis of infantile idiopathic scoliosis. *J Bone Joint Surg Br* 1955;37:400–413.

162. McMaster MJ. Infantile idiopathic scoliosis: can it be prevented? *J Bone Joint Surg Br* 1983;65:612–617.

163. James JIP. Idiopathic scoliosis: the prognosis, diagnosis, and operative indications related to curve patterns and the age of onset. *J Bone Joint Surg Br* 1954;36:36–49.

164. Lloyd-Roberts GC, Pilcher MF. Structural idiopathic scoliosis in infancy. *J Bone Joint Surg Br* 1965;47:520–523.

165. Hooper G. Congenital dislocation of the hip in infantile idiopathic scoliosis. *J Bone Joint Surg Br* 1980;62-B:447–449.

166. Goldberg CJ, Gillic I, Connaughton O. Respiratory function and cosmesis at maturity in infantile-onset scoliosis. *Spine* 2003;28:2397–2406.

167. Mehta MH. The rib vertebral angle in the early diagnosis between resolving and progressive infantile scoliosis. *J Bone Joint Surg Br* 1972;54:230–243.

168. Ceballos T, Ferrer-Torrelles M, Castillo F. Prognosis in infantile idiopathic scoliosis. *J Bone Joint Surg Am* 1980;62:863–875.

169. Tolo VT, Gillespie R. The characteristics of juvenile idiopathic scoliosis and results of its treatment. *J Bone Joint Surg Br* 1978;60-B:181–188.

170. Bunnell WP. The natural history of idiopathic scoliosis. *Clin Orthop* 1988;229:20–25.

171. Robinson CM, McMaster MJ. Juvenile idiopathic scoliosis. Curve patterns and prognosis in one hundred and nine patients. *J Bone Joint Surg Am* 1996;78:1140–1148.

172. Mannherz RE, Betz RR, Clancy M. Juvenile idiopathic scoliosis followed to skeletal maturity. *Spine* 1988;13:1087–1090.

173. Biondi J, Weiner DS, Bethem D. Correlation of Risser sign and bone age determination in adolescent idiopathic scoliosis. *J Pediatr Orthop* 1985;5:697–701.

174. Peterson LE, Nachemson AL. Prediction of progression of the curve in girls who have adolescent idiopathic scoliosis of moderate severity. Logistic regression analysis based on data from the Brace Study of the Scoliosis Research Society. *J Bone Joint Surg Am* 1995;77:823–827.

175. Karol LA, Johnston CE, Browne RH. Progression of the curve in boys who have idiopathic scoliosis. *J Bone Joint Surg Am* 1993;75:1804–1810.

176. Nachemson A, Lonstein R, Weinstein S. Report of the prevalence and Natural History Committee of the Scoliosis Research Society. Presented at the Annual Meeting of the Scoliosis Research Society; 1982: Denver, CO.

177. Weinstein SL, Ponseti IV. Curve progression in idiopathic scoliosis. *J Bone Joint Surg Am* 1983;65:447–455.

178. Weinstein SL. Idiopathic scoliosis. Natural history. *Spine* 1986;11: 780–783.

179. Nachemson A. A long term follow-up study of non-treated scoliosis. *Acta Orthop Scand* 1968;39:466–476.

180. Nilsonne U, Lundgren KD. Long-term prognosis in idiopathic scoliosis. *Acta Orthop Scand* 1968;39:456–465.

181. Fowles JV, Sliman N, Nolan B. The treatment of idiopathic scoliosis in Tunisia. A review of the first five years. *Acta Orthop Belg* 1978;44: 416–423.

182. Weinstein SL, Zavala DC, Ponseti IV. Idiopathic scoliosis: long-term follow-up and prognosis in untreated patients. *J Bone Joint Surg Am* 1981;63:702–712.

183. Winter RB, Lovell WW, Moe JH. Excessive thoracic lordosis and loss of pulmonary function in patients with idiopathic scoliosis. *J Bone Joint Surg Am* 1975;57:972–977.

184. Mayo NE, Goldberg MS, Poitras B. The Ste-Justine Adolescent Idiopathic Scoliosis Cohort Study. Part III: back pain. *Spine* 1994;19:1573–1581.

185. Pehrsson K, Danielsson A, Nachemson A. Pulmonary function in adolescent idiopathic scoliosis: a 25 year follow up after surgery or start of brace treatment. *Thorax* 2001;56(5):388–393.

186. Upadhyay SS, Mullaji AB, Luk KD. Relation of spinal and thoracic cage deformities and their flexibilities with altered pulmonary functions in adolescent idiopathic scoliosis. *Spine* 1995;20:2415–2420.

187. Newton PO, et al. Results of preoperative pulmonary function testing of adolescents with idiopathic scoliosis. A study of six hundred and thirty-one patients. *J Bone Joint Surg Am* 2005;87(9):1937–1946.

188. Payne WK, Ogilvie JW, Resnick MD. Does scoliosis have a psychological impact and does gender make a difference? *Spine* 1997;22:1380–1384.

189. Dickson JH, Erwin WD, Rossi D, et al. A twenty-one-year follow-up. *J Bone Joint Surg Am* 1990;72:678–683.

190. Collis DK, Ponseti IV. Long-term follow-up of patients with idiopathic scoliosis not treated surgically. *J Bone Joint Surg Am* 1969;51:425–445.

191. Soucacos PN, Soucacos PK, Zacharis KC. School-screening for scoliosis. A prospective epidemiological study in northwestern and central Greece. *J Bone Joint Surg Am* 1997;79:1498–1503.

192. Pruijs JE, van der Meer R, Hageman MA. The benefits of school screening for scoliosis in the central part of The Netherlands. *Eur Spine J* 1996;5:374–379.

193. Lonstein JE, Bjorklund S, Wanninger MH. Voluntary school screening for scoliosis in Minnesota. *J Bone Joint Surg Am* 1982;64:481–488.

194. Goldberg CJ, Dowling FE, Fogarty EE. School scoliosis screening and the United States Preventive Services Task Force. An examination of long-term results. *Spine* 1995;20:1368–1374.

195. Morrissy RT. School screening for scoliosis. A statement of the problem. *Spine* 1988;13:1195–1197.

196. US Preventive Services Task Force. Screening for adolescent idiopathic scoliosis. Review article. *JAMA* 1993;269(20):2667–2672.

197. Winter RB. The pendulum has swung too far. Bracing for adolescent idiopathic scoliosis in the 1990s. *Orthop Clin North Am* 1994;25: 195–204.

198. Winter RB. Adolescent idiopathic scoliosis [Editorial]. *N Engl J Med* 1986;314:1379–1380.

199. Velezis MJ, Sturm PF, Cobey J. Scoliosis screening revisited: findings from the District of Columbia. *J Pediatr Orthop* 2002;22:788–791.

200. Nachemson AL, Peterson LE. Effectiveness of treatment with a brace in girls who have adolescent idiopathic scoliosis. A prospective, controlled study based on data from the Brace Study of the Scoliosis Research Society. *J Bone Joint Surg Am* 1995;77:815–822.

201. Katz DE, Richards BS, Browne RH. A comparison between the Boston brace and the Charleston bending brace in adolescent idiopathic scoliosis. *Spine* 1997;22:1302–1312.

202. Nash CL. Current concepts review: scoliosis bracing. *J Bone Joint Surg Am* 1980;62:848–852.

203. Castro FP. Adolescent idiopathic scoliosis, bracing, and the Hueter-Volkmann principle. *Spine J* 2003;3:180–185.

204. Willers U, Normelli H, Aaro S. Long-term results of Boston brace treatment on vertebral rotation in idiopathic scoliosis. *Spine* 1993;18: 432–435.

205. Dolan LA, Weinstein SL. Surgical rates after observation and bracing for adolescent idiopathic scoliosis: an evidence-based review. *Spine (Phila Pa 1976)* 2007;32(19 Suppl):S91–S100.

206. Weinstein SL, et al. Adolescent idiopathic scoliosis. *Lancet* 2008; 371(9623):1527–1537.

207. Carr WA, Moe JH, Winter RB. Treatment of idiopathic scoliosis in the Milwaukee brace. *J Bone Joint Surg Am* 1980;62:599–612.

208. Mellencamp DD, Blount WP, Anderson AJ. Milwaukee brace treatment of idiopathic scoliosis: late results. *Clin Orthop* 1977;126:47–57.

209. Blount W, Schmidt A. The Milwaukee brace in the treatment of scoliosis. *J Bone Joint Surg Am* 1957;37:693.

210. Lonstein JE, Winter RB. The Milwaukee brace for the treatment of adolescent idiopathic scoliosis. A review of one thousand and twenty patients. *J Bone Joint Surg Am* 1994;76:1207–1221.

211. Emans JB, Kaelin A, Bancel P. The Boston bracing system for idiopathic scoliosis. Follow-up results in 295 patients. *Spine* 1986;11:792–801.

212. Watts HG, Hall JE, Stanish W. The Boston brace system for the treatment of low thoracic and lumbar scoliosis by the use of a girdle without superstructure. *Clin Orthop* 1977;29:87–92.

213. Allington NJ, Bowen JR. Adolescent idiopathic scoliosis: treatment with the Wilmington brace. A comparison of full-time and part-time use. *J Bone Joint Surg Am* 1996;78:1056–1062.

214. Piazza MR, Bassett GS. Curve progression after treatment with the Wilmington brace for idiopathic scoliosis. *J Pediatr Orthop* 1990;10: 39–43.

215. Apter A, Morein G, Munitz H. The psychosocial sequelae of the Milwaukee brace in adolescent girls. *Clin Orthop* 1978;131:156–159.

216. MacLean WE, Green NE, Pierre CB. Stress and coping with scoliosis: psychological effects on adolescents and their families. *J Pediatr Orthop* 1989;9:257–261.

217. Ramirez N, Johnston CE, Browne RH. Back pain during orthotic treatment of idiopathic scoliosis. *J Pediatr Orthop* 1999;19:198–201.

218. D'Amato CR, Griggs S, McCoy B. Nighttime bracing with the Providence brace in adolescent girls with idiopathic scoliosis. *Spine (Phila Pa 1976)* 2001;26(18):2006–2012.

219. Price CT, Scott DS, Reed FR. Nighttime bracing for adolescent idiopathic scoliosis with the Charleston bending brace: long-term follow-up. *J Pediatr Orthop* 1997;17:703–707.

220. Coillard C, et al. SpineCor—a non-rigid brace for the treatment of idiopathic scoliosis: post-treatment results. *Eur Spine J* 2003;12(2): 141–148.

221. Coillard C, et al. Effectiveness of the SpineCor brace based on the new standardized criteria proposed by the scoliosis research society for adolescent idiopathic scoliosis. *J Pediatr Orthop* 2007;27(4):375–379.

222. Negrini S, et al. Braces for idiopathic scoliosis in adolescents. *Cochrane Database Syst Rev* 2010(1):CD006850.

223. Green NE. Part-time bracing of adolescent idiopathic scoliosis. *J Bone Joint Surg Am* 1986;68:738–742.

224. Rowe DE, Bernstein SM, Riddick MF. A meta-analysis of the efficacy of non-operative treatments for idiopathic scoliosis [see Comments]. *J Bone Joint Surg Am* 1997;79:664–674.

225. Katz DE, et al. Brace wear control of curve progression in adolescent idiopathic scoliosis. *J Bone Joint Surg Am* 2010;92(6):1343–1352.

226. Fernandez-Feliberti R, Flynn J, Ramirez N. Effectiveness of TLSO bracing in the conservative treatment of idiopathic scoliosis. *J Pediatr Orthop* 1995;15:176–181.

227. Noonan KJ, Weinstein SL, Jacobson WC. Use of the Milwaukee brace for progressive idiopathic scoliosis. *J Bone Joint Surg Am* 1996;78: 557–567.

228. Takemitsu M, et al. Compliance monitoring of brace treatment for patients with idiopathic scoliosis. *Spine (Phila Pa 1976)* 2004;29(18): 2070–2074; discussion 2074.

229. Nicholson GP, et al. The objective measurement of spinal orthosis use for the treatment of adolescent idiopathic scoliosis. *Spine (Phila Pa 1976)* 2003;28(19):2243–2250; discussion 2250–2251.

230. Schiller JR, Thakur NA, Eberson CP. Brace management in adolescent idiopathic scoliosis. *Clin Orthop Relat Res* 2010;468(3):670–678.

231. Howard A, Wright JG, Hedden D. A comparative study of TLSO, Charleston, and Milwaukee braces for idiopathic scoliosis. *Spine* 1998;23:2404–2411.

232. Climent JM, Sanchez J. Impact of the type of brace on the quality of life of adolescents with spine deformities. *Spine* 1999;24:1903–1908.

233. Wickers FC, Bunch WH, Barnett PM. Psychological factors in failure to wear the Milwaukee brace for treatment of idiopathic scoliosis. *Clin Orthop* 1977;126:62–66.

234. Karol LA. Effectiveness of bracing in male patients with idiopathic scoliosis. *Spine* 2001;26:2001–2005.

235. Sanders JO, et al. Derotational casting for progressive infantile scoliosis. *J Pediatr Orthop* 2009;29(6):581–587.

236. Mehta MH. Growth as a corrective force in the early treatment of progressive infantile scoliosis. *J Bone Joint Surg Br* 2005;87(9): 1237–1247.

237. Asher M, Lai SM, Burton D. Safety and efficacy of Isola instrumentation and arthrodesis for adolescent idiopathic scoliosis: two- to 12-year follow-up. *Spine* 2004;29:2013–2023.

238. Edgar MA, Mehta MH. Long-term follow-up of fused and unfused idiopathic scoliosis. *J Bone Joint Surg Br* 1988;70:712–716.

239. Lenke LG, Bridwell KH, Blanke K. Radiographic results of arthrodesis with Cotrel-Dubousset instrumentation for the treatment of adolescent idiopathic scoliosis. A five to ten-year follow-up study. *J Bone Joint Surg Am* 1998;80:807–814.

240. Newton PO, et al. Surgical treatment of main thoracic scoliosis with thoracoscopic anterior instrumentation. a five-year follow-up study. *J Bone Joint Surg Am* 2008;90(10):2077–2089.

241. Tis JE, et al. Adolescent idiopathic scoliosis treated with open instrumented anterior spinal fusion: five-year follow-up. *Spine (Phila Pa 1976)* 2010;35(1):64–70.

242. Dickson JH, Mirkovic S, Noble PC. Results of operative treatment of idiopathic scoliosis in adults. *J Bone Joint Surg Am* 1995;77: 513–523.

243. Harrington PR. Treatment of scoliosis: correction and internal fixation by spine instrumentation. *J Bone Joint Surg Am* 1962;44:591–610.

244. Hibbs RA. A report of fifty-nine cases of scoliosis treated by the fusion operation. By Russell A. Hibbs, 1924. *Clin Orthop* 1988;229:4–19.

245. Swank SM, Mauri TM, Brown JC. The lumbar lordosis below Harrington instrumentation for scoliosis. *Spine* 1990;15:181–186.

246. Bartie BJ, Lonstein JE, Winter RB. Long-term follow-up of adolescent idiopathic scoliosis patients who had Harrington instrumentation and fusion to the lower lumbar vertebrae: is low back pain a problem? *Spine (Phila Pa 1976)* 2009;34(24):E873–E878.

247. Winter RB. Harrington instrumentation into the lumbar spine: technique for preservation of normal lumbar lordosis. *Spine* 1986;11: 633–635.

248. King HA, Moe JH, Bradford DS. The selection of fusion levels in thoracic idiopathic scoliosis. *J Bone Joint Surg Am* 1983;65: 1302–1313.

249. Parent S, Labelle H, Skalli W. Morphometric analysis of anatomic scoliotic specimens. *Spine* 2002;27:2305–2311.

250. Clements DH, et al. Correlation of scoliosis curve correction with the number and type of fixation anchors. *Spine (Phila Pa 1976)* 2009;34(20):2147–2150.

251. Herrera-Soto JA, et al. The use of multiple anchors for the treatment of idiopathic scoliosis. *Spine (Phila Pa 1976)* 2007;32(18):E517–E522.

252. Liljenqvist UR, Link TM, Halm HF. Morphometric analysis of thoracic and lumbar vertebrae in idiopathic scoliosis. *Spine* 2000;25:1247–1253.

253. Kim YJ, et al. Free hand pedicle screw placement in the thoracic spine: is it safe? *Spine (Phila Pa 1976)* 2004;29(3):333–342; discussion 342.

254. Suk SI, et al. Thoracic pedicle screw fixation in spinal deformities: are they really safe? *Spine (Phila Pa 1976)* 2001;26(18):2049–2057.

255. Hamill CL, Lenke LG, Bridwell KH. The use of pedicle screw fixation to improve correction in the lumbar spine of patients with idiopathic scoliosis. Is it warranted? *Spine* 1996;21:1241–1249.

256. Andrew T, Piggott H. Growth arrest for progressive scoliosis. Combined anterior and posterior fusion of the convexity. *J Bone Joint Surg Br* 1985;67:193–197.

257. Dobbs MB, et al. Anterior/posterior spinal instrumentation versus posterior instrumentation alone for the treatment of adolescent idiopathic scoliotic curves more than 90 degrees. *Spine (Phila Pa 1976)* 2006;31(20):2386–2391.

258. Suk SI, et al. Selective thoracic fusion with segmental pedicle screw fixation in the treatment of thoracic idiopathic scoliosis: more than 5-year follow-up. *Spine (Phila Pa 1976)* 2005;30(14):1602–1609.

259. Belmont PJ Jr, et al. In vivo accuracy of thoracic pedicle screws. *Spine (Phila Pa 1976)* 2001;26(21):2340–2346.

260. Kim YJ, et al. Comparative analysis of pedicle screw versus hybrid instrumentation in posterior spinal fusion of adolescent idiopathic scoliosis. *Spine (Phila Pa 1976)* 2006;31(3):291–298.

261. Kuklo TR, et al. Monoaxial versus multiaxial thoracic pedicle screws in the correction of adolescent idiopathic scoliosis. *Spine (Phila Pa 1976)* 2005;30(18):2113–2120.

262. Lonner BS, et al. Treatment of thoracic scoliosis: are monoaxial thoracic pedicle screws the best form of fixation for correction? *Spine (Phila Pa 1976)* 2009;34(8):845–851.

263. Senaran H, et al. Difficult thoracic pedicle screw placement in adolescent idiopathic scoliosis. *J Spinal Disord Tech* 2008;21(3):187–191.

264. Helgeson MD, et al. Evaluation of proximal junctional kyphosis in adolescent idiopathic scoliosis following pedicle screw, hook, or hybrid instrumentation. *Spine (Phila Pa 1976)* 2010;35(2):177–181.

265. Dubousset J, Cotrel Y. Application technique of Cotrel-Dubousset instrumentation for scoliosis deformities. *Clin Orthop Relat Res* 1991(264):103–110.

266. Helenius I, Remes V, Yrjonen T. Harrington and Cotrel-Dubousset instrumentation in adolescent idiopathic scoliosis. Long-term functional and radiographic outcomes. *J Bone Joint Surg Am* 2003;85-A:2303–2309.

267. Labelle H, Dansereau J, Bellefleur C. Perioperative three-dimensional correction of idiopathic scoliosis with the Cotrel-Dubousset procedure. *Spine* 1995;20:1406–1409.

268. Lee SM, Suk SI, Chung ER. Direct vertebral rotation: a new technique of three-dimensional deformity correction with segmental pedicle screw fixation in adolescent idiopathic scoliosis. *Spine (Phila Pa 1976)* 2004;29(3):343–349.

269. Pizones J, et al. Does wide posterior multiple level release improve the correction of adolescent idiopathic scoliosis curves? *J Spinal Disord Tech* 2010;23(7):e24–e30.

270. Shufflebarger H, Geck M, Clark C. The posterior approach for lumbar and thoracolumbar adolescent idiopathic scoliosis: posterior shortening and pedicle screws. *Spine* 2004;29:269–276.

271. Lenke LG, et al. Posterior vertebral column resection for severe pediatric deformity: minimum two-year follow-up of thirty-five consecutive patients. *Spine (Phila Pa 1976)* 2009;34(20):2213–2221.

272. Dubousset J, Herring JA, Shufflebarger H. The crankshaft phenomenon. *J Pediatr Orthop* 1989;9:541–550.

273. Roaf R. Vertebral growth and its mechanical control. *J Bone Joint Surg Br* 1960;42:40–59.

274. Roberto RF, Lonstein JE, Winter RB. Curve progression in Risser stage 0 or 1 patients after posterior spinal fusion for idiopathic scoliosis. *J Pediatr Orthop* 1997;17:718–725.

275. Lapinksy AS, Richards BS. Preventing the crankshaft phenomenon by combining anterior fusion with posterior instrumentation. Does it work? *Spine* 1995;20:1392–1398.

276. Crawford AH, Wall EJ, Wolf R. Video-assisted thoracoscopy. *Orthop Clin North Am* 1999;30:367–385.

277. Newton PO, Wenger DR, Mubarak SJ. Anterior release and fusion in pediatric spinal deformity. A comparison of early outcome and cost of thoracoscopic and open thoracotomy approaches. *Spine* 1997;22:1398–1406.

278. Regan JJ, Mack MJ, Picetti GD. A technical report on video-assisted thoracoscopy in thoracic spinal surgery. Preliminary description. *Spine* 1995;20:831–837.

279. Newton PO, Marks M, Faro F. Use of video-assisted thoracoscopic surgery to reduce perioperative morbidity in scoliosis surgery. *Spine* 2003;28:S249–S254.

280. Newton PO, Shea KG, Granlund KF. Defining the pediatric spinal thoracoscopy learning curve: sixty-five consecutive cases. *Spine* 2000;25:1028–1035.

281. Dwyer AF. Experience of anterior correction of scoliosis. *Clin Orthop* 1973;93:191–214.

282. Zielke K, Berthet A. VDS—ventral derotation spondylodesis—preliminary report on 58 cases. *Beitr Orthop Traumatol* 1978;25:85–103.

283. Kaneda K, Fujiya N, Satoh S. Results with Zielke instrumentation for idiopathic thoracolumbar and lumbar scoliosis. *Clin Orthop* 1986:195–203.

284. Kaneda K, Shono Y, Satoh S. Anterior correction of thoracic scoliosis with Kaneda anterior spinal system. A preliminary report. *Spine* 1997;22:1358–1368.

285. Luk KD, Leong JC, Reyes L. The comparative results of treatment in idiopathic thoracolumbar and lumbar scoliosis using the Harrington, Dwyer, and Zielke instrumentations. *Spine* 1989;14:275–280.

286. Sanders AE, Baumann R, Brown H. Selective anterior fusion of thoracolumbar/lumbar curves in adolescents: when can the associated thoracic curve be left unfused? *Spine* 2003;28:706–713.

287. Suk SI, Lee CK, Chung SS. Comparison of Zielke ventral derotation system and Cotrel-Dubousset instrumentation in the treatment of idiopathic lumbar and thoracolumbar scoliosis. *Spine* 1994;19:419–429.

288. Sweet FA, Lenke LG, Bridwell KH. Maintaining lumbar lordosis with anterior single solid-rod instrumentation in thoracolumbar and lumbar adolescent idiopathic scoliosis. *Spine* 1999;24:1655–1662.

289. Turi M, Johnston CE, Richards BS. Anterior correction of idiopathic scoliosis using TSRH instrumentation. *Spine* 1993;18:417–422.

290. Haher TR, Bergman M, Brien MO. The effect of the three columns of the spine on the instantaneous axis of rotation in flexion and extension. *Spine* 1991;16:S312–S318.

291. Lenke LG, Bridwell KH. Mesh cages in idiopathic scoliosis in adolescents. *Clin Orthop* 2002;394:98–108.

292. Hopf CG, Eysel P, Dubousset J. Operative treatment of scoliosis with Cotrel-Dubousset-Hopf instrumentation. New anterior spinal device. *Spine* 1997;22:618–627; discussion.

293. Lenke LG, Betz RR, Bridwell KH. Spontaneous lumbar curve coronal correction after selective anterior or posterior thoracic fusion in adolescent idiopathic scoliosis. *Spine* 1999;24:1663–1671.

294. Fricka KB, Kim C, Newton PO. Spinal lordosis with marked opisthotonus secondary to dystonia musculorum deformans: case report with surgical management. *Spine* 2001;26:2283–2288.

295. Bernstein RM, Hall JE. Solid rod short segment anterior fusion in thoracolumbar scoliosis. *J Pediatr Orthop B* 1998;7:124–131.

296. Betz RR, Harms J, Clements DH. Comparison of anterior and posterior instrumentation for correction of adolescent thoracic idiopathic scoliosis. *Spine* 1999;24:225–239.

297. Geck MJ, et al. Comparison of surgical treatment in Lenke 5C adolescent idiopathic scoliosis: anterior dual rod versus posterior pedicle fixation surgery: a comparison of two practices. *Spine (Phila Pa 1976)* 2009;34(18):1942–1951.

298. Moe JH, Kharrat K, Winter RB. Harrington instrumentation without fusion plus external orthotic support for the treatment of difficult curvature problems in young children. *Clin Orthop* 1984;185:35–45.

299. Thompson GH, et al. Comparison of single and dual growing rod techniques followed through definitive surgery: a preliminary study. *Spine (Phila Pa 1976)* 2005;30(18):2039–2044.

300. Fisk JR, Peterson HA, Laughlin R. Spontaneous fusion in scoliosis after instrumentation without arthrodesis. *J Pediatr Orthop* 1995;15:182–186.

301. Bess S, et al. Complications of growing-rod treatment for early-onset scoliosis: analysis of one hundred and forty patients. *J Bone Joint Surg Am* 2010;92(15):2533–2543.

302. Marks DS, Iqbal MJ, Thompson AG. Convex spinal epiphysiodesis in the management of progressive infantile idiopathic scoliosis. *Spine* 1996;21:1884–1888.

303. Campbell R, Smith M, Hell-Vocke A. Expansion thoracoplasty; the surgical technique of opening-wedge thoracotomy. *J Bone Joint Surgery Am* 2004;86:51–64.

304. Smith JT. Bilateral rib-to-pelvis technique for managing early-onset scoliosis. *Clin Orthop Relat Res* 2011;469(5):1349–1355.

305. McCarthy RE, et al. Shilla growing rods in a caprine animal model: a pilot study. *Clin Orthop Relat Res* 2010;468(3):705–710.

306. Betz RR, et al. Vertebral body stapling: a fusionless treatment option for a growing child with moderate idiopathic scoliosis. *Spine (Phila Pa 1976)* 2010;35(2):169–176.

307. Crawford CH III, Lenke LG. Growth modulation by means of anterior tethering resulting in progressive correction of juvenile idiopathic scoliosis: a case report. *J Bone Joint Surg Am* 2010;92(1):202–209.

308. Newton PO, et al. Spinal growth modulation with use of a tether in an immature porcine model. *J Bone Joint Surg Am* 2008;90(12):2695–2706.

309. Coonrad RW, Murrell GA, Motley G. A logical coronal pattern classification of 2,000 consecutive idiopathic scoliosis cases based on the Scoliosis Research Society–defined apical vertebra. *Spine* 1998;23:1380–1391.

310. Lenke LG, Betz RR, Clements D. Curve prevalence of a new classification of operative adolescent idiopathic scoliosis: does classification correlate with treatment? *Spine* 2002;27:604–611.

311. Newton PO, Faro FD, Lenke LG. Factors involved in the decision to perform a selective versus nonselective fusion of Lenke 1B and 1C (King-Moe II) curves in adolescent idiopathic scoliosis. *Spine* 2003;28:S217–S223.

312. Miyanji F, et al. Is the lumbar modifier useful in surgical decision making?: defining two distinct Lenke 1A curve patterns. *Spine (Phila Pa 1976)* 2008;33(23):2545–2551.

313. Bridwell KH, McAllister JW, Betz RR. Coronal decompensation produced by Cotrel-Dubousset "derotation" maneuver for idiopathic right thoracic scoliosis. *Spine* 1991;16:769–777.

314. Lenke LG, Bridwell KH, Baldus C. Preventing decompensation in King type II curves treated with Cotrel-Dubousset instrumentation. Strict guidelines for selective thoracic fusion. *Spine* 1992;17:S274–S281.

315. Thompson JP, Transfeldt EE, Bradford DS. Decompensation after Cotrel-Dubousset instrumentation of idiopathic scoliosis. *Spine* 1990;15:927–931.

316. Richards BS. Lenke 1C, King type II curves: surgical recommendations. *Orthop Clin North Am* 2007;38(4):511–520, vi.

317. Richards BS. Lumbar curve response in type II idiopathic scoliosis after posterior instrumentation of the thoracic curve. *Spine* 1992;17:S282–S286.

318. Richards BS, Birch JG, Herring JA. Frontal plane and sagittal plane balance following Cotrel-Dubousset instrumentation for idiopathic scoliosis. *Spine* 1989;14:733–737.

319. Patel PN, et al. Spontaneous lumbar curve correction in selective thoracic fusions of idiopathic scoliosis: a comparison of anterior and posterior approaches. *Spine (Phila Pa 1976)* 2008;33(10):1068–1073.

320. Cil A, et al. The validity of Lenke criteria for defining structural proximal thoracic curves in patients with adolescent idiopathic scoliosis. *Spine (Phila Pa 1976)* 2005;30(22):2550–2555.

321. Kuklo TR, Lenke LG, Graham EJ. Correlation of radiographic, clinical, and patient assessment of shoulder balance following fusion versus nonfusion of the proximal thoracic curve in adolescent idiopathic scoliosis. *Spine* 2002;27:2013–2020.

322. Kuklo TR, Lenke LG, Won DS. Spontaneous proximal thoracic curve correction after isolated fusion of the main thoracic curve in adolescent idiopathic scoliosis. *Spine* 2001;26:1966–1975.

323. Lenke LG, Bridwell KH, Brien MFO. Recognition and treatment of the proximal thoracic curve in adolescent idiopathic scoliosis treated with Cotrel-Dubousset instrumentation. *Spine* 1994;19:1589–1597.

324. Winter RB. The idiopathic double thoracic curve pattern. Its recognition and surgical management. *Spine* 1989;14:1287–1292.

325. Kaneda K, Shono Y, Satoh S. New anterior instrumentation for the management of thoracolumbar and lumbar scoliosis. Application of the Kaneda two-rod system. *Spine* 1996;21:1250–1261.

326. Sweet FA, Lenke LG, Bridwell KH. Prospective radiographic and clinical outcomes and complications of single solid rod instrumented anterior spinal fusion in adolescent idiopathic scoliosis. *Spine* 2001;26:1956–1965.

327. Haher TR, Gorup JM, Shin TM. Results of the Scoliosis Research Society instrument for evaluation of surgical outcome in adolescent idiopathic scoliosis. A multicenter study of 244 patients. *Spine* 1999;24:1435–1440.

328. Haher TR, Merola A, Zipnick RI. Meta-analysis of surgical outcome in adolescent idiopathic scoliosis. A 35-year English literature review of 11,000 patients. *Spine* 1995;20:1575–1584.

329. Merola AA, Haher TR, Brkaric M. A multicenter study of the outcomes of the surgical treatment of adolescent idiopathic scoliosis using the Scoliosis Research Society (SRS) outcome instrument. *Spine* 2002;27:2046–2051.

330. Stasikelis PJ, Pugh LI, Ferguson RL. Distraction instrumentation outcomes in scoliosis. *J Pediatr Orthop B* 1998;7:106–110.

331. Cochran T, Irstam L, Nachemson A. Long-term anatomic and functional changes in patients with adolescent idiopathic scoliosis treated by Harrington rod fusion. *Spine* 1983;8:576–584.

332. Connolly PJ, Schroeder HPV, Johnson GE. Adolescent idiopathic scoliosis. Long-term effect of instrumentation extending to the lumbar spine. *J Bone Joint Surg Am* 1995;77:1210–1216.

333. Danielsson AJ, Nachemson AL. Radiologic findings and curve progression 22 years after treatment for adolescent idiopathic scoliosis: comparison of brace and surgical treatment with matching control group of straight individuals. *Spine* 2001;26:516–525.

334. Danielsson AJ, Nachemson AL. Back pain and function 23 years after fusion for adolescent idiopathic scoliosis: a case-control study—part II. *Spine* 2003;28:E373–E383.

335. Poitras B, Mayo NE, Goldberg MS. The Ste-Justine Adolescent Idiopathic Scoliosis Cohort Study. Part IV: surgical correction and back pain. *Spine* 1994;19:1582–1588.

336. Winter RB, Carr P, Mattson H. A study of functional spinal motion in women after instrumentation and fusion for deformity or trauma. *Spine* 1997;22:1760–1764.

337. Helenius I, Remes V, Yrjonen T. Comparison of long-term functional and radiologic outcomes after Harrington instrumentation and spondylodesis in adolescent idiopathic scoliosis: a review of 78 patients. *Spine* 2002;27:176–180.

338. Willner S, Johnsson B. Thoracic kyphosis and lumbar lordosis during the growth period in boys and girls. *Acta Paediatr Scand* 1983;72:873–878.

339. Marks M, et al. Postoperative segmental motion of the unfused spine distal to the fusion in 100 adolescent idiopathic scoliosis patients. *Spine (Phila Pa 1976)* 2012;37(10):826–832.

340. Potter BK, Lenke LG, Kuklo TR. Prevention and management of iatrogenic flatback deformity. *J Bone Joint Surg Am* 2004;86-A:1793–1808.

341. Sarwahi V, Boachie-Adjei O, Backus SI. Characterization of gait function in patients with postsurgical sagittal (flatback) deformity: a prospective study of 21 patients. *Spine* 2002;27:2328–2337.

342. Perez-Grueso FS, Fernandez-Baillo N, Arauz de Robles S. The low lumbar spine below Cotrel-Dubousset instrumentation: long-term findings. *Spine* 2000;25:2333–2341.

343. Lenke LG, Bridwell KH, Baldus C. Cotrel-Dubousset instrumentation for adolescent idiopathic scoliosis. *J Bone Joint Surg Am* 1992;74:1056–1067.

344. Humke T, Grob D, Scheier H. Cotrel-Dubousset and Harrington instrumentation in idiopathic scoliosis: a comparison of long-term results. *Eur Spine J* 1995;4:280–283.

345. Remes V, Helenius I, Schlenzka D. Cotrel-Dubousset (CD) or Universal Spine System (USS) instrumentation in adolescent idiopathic scoliosis (AIS): comparison of midterm clinical, functional, radiologic outcomes. *Spine* 2004;29:2024–2030.

346. Aronsson DD, Stokes IA, Ronchetti PJ. Surgical correction of vertebral axial rotation in adolescent idiopathic scoliosis: prediction by lateral bending films. *J Spinal Disord* 1996;9:214–219.

347. Sawatzky BJ, Tredwell SJ, Jang SB. Effects of three-dimensional assessment on surgical correction and on hook strategies in multi-hook instrumentation for adolescent idiopathic scoliosis. *Spine* 1998;23:201–205.

348. Willers U, Transfeldt EE, Hedlund R. The segmental effect of Cotrel-Dubousset instrumentation on vertebral rotation, rib hump and the thoracic cage in idiopathic scoliosis. *Eur Spine J* 1996;5:387–393.

349. Benli IT, Tuzuner M, Akalin S. Spinal imbalance and decompensation problems in patients treated with Cotrel-Dubousset instrumentation. *Eur Spine J* 1996;5:380–386.

350. Suk SI, Lee CK, Kim WJ. Segmental pedicle screw fixation in the treatment of thoracic idiopathic scoliosis. *Spine* 1995;20:1399–1405.

351. Lowenstein JE, et al. Coronal and sagittal plane correction in adolescent idiopathic scoliosis: a comparison between all pedicle screw versus hybrid thoracic hook lumbar screw constructs. *Spine (Phila Pa 1976)* 2007;32(4):448–452.

352. Barr SJ, Schuette AM, Emans JB. Lumbar pedicle screws versus hooks. Results in double major curves in adolescent idiopathic scoliosis. *Spine* 1997;22:1369–1379.

353. Suk SI, et al. Thoracoplasty in thoracic adolescent idiopathic scoliosis. *Spine (Phila Pa 1976)* 2008;33(10):1061–1067.

354. Majdouline Y, et al. Scoliosis correction objectives in adolescent idiopathic scoliosis. *J Pediatr Orthop* 2007;27(7):775–781.

355. Arlet V, et al. Decompensation following scoliosis surgery: treatment by decreasing the correction of the main thoracic curve or "letting the spine go." *Eur Spine J* 2000;9(2):156–160.

356. Dobbs MB, et al. Can we predict the ultimate lumbar curve in adolescent idiopathic scoliosis patients undergoing a selective fusion with undercorrection of the thoracic curve? *Spine (Phila Pa 1976)* 2004;29(3):277–285.

357. Suk SI, et al. Indications of proximal thoracic curve fusion in thoracic adolescent idiopathic scoliosis: recognition and treatment of double thoracic curve pattern in adolescent idiopathic scoliosis treated with segmental instrumentation. *Spine (Phila Pa 1976)* 2000;25(18):2342–2349.

358. Newton PO, et al. Preservation of thoracic kyphosis is critical to maintain lumbar lordosis in the surgical treatment of adolescent idiopathic scoliosis. *Spine (Phila Pa 1976)* 2010;35(14):1365–1370.

359. Kohler R, Galland O, Mechin H. The Dwyer procedure in the treatment of idiopathic scoliosis. A 10-year follow-up review of 21 patients. *Spine* 1990;15:75–80.

360. Kostuik JP, Carl A, Ferron S. Anterior Zielke instrumentation for spinal deformity in adults. *J Bone Joint Surg Am* 1989;71:898–912.

361. Lowe TG, Peters JD. Anterior spinal fusion with Zielke instrumentation for idiopathic scoliosis. A frontal and sagittal curve analysis in 36 patients. *Spine* 1993;18:423–426.

362. Hurford RK Jr, et al. Prospective radiographic and clinical outcomes of dual-rod instrumented anterior spinal fusion in adolescent idiopathic scoliosis: comparison with single-rod constructs. *Spine (Phila Pa 1976)* 2006;31(20):2322–2328.

363. Lowe TG, et al. Single-rod versus dual-rod anterior instrumentation for idiopathic scoliosis: a biomechanical study. *Spine (Phila Pa 1976)* 2005;30(3):311–317.

364. Kelly DM, et al. Long-term outcomes of anterior spinal fusion with instrumentation for thoracolumbar and lumbar curves in adolescent idiopathic scoliosis. *Spine (Phila Pa 1976)* 2010;35(2):194–198.

365. Newton PO, et al. Predictors of change in postoperative pulmonary function in adolescent idiopathic scoliosis: a prospective study of 254 patients. *Spine (Phila Pa 1976)* 2007;32(17):1875–1882.

366. Yaszay B, Jazayeri R, Lonner B. The effect of surgical approaches on pulmonary function in adolescent idiopathic scoliosis. *J Spinal Disord Tech* 2009;22(4):278–283.

367. Kim YJ, et al. Pulmonary function in adolescent idiopathic scoliosis relative to the surgical procedure. *J Bone Joint Surg Am* 2005;87(7):1534–1541.

368. Kishan S, et al. Thoracoscopic scoliosis surgery affects pulmonary function less than thoracotomy at 2 years postsurgery. *Spine (Phila Pa 1976)* 2007;32(4):453–458.

369. Newton PO, et al. Surgical treatment of main thoracic scoliosis with thoracoscopic anterior instrumentation. Surgical technique. *J Bone Joint Surg Am* 2009;91(Suppl 2):233–248.

370. Lonner BS, et al. The learning curve associated with thoracoscopic spinal instrumentation. *Spine (Phila Pa 1976)* 2005;30(24):2835–2840.

371. Bridwell KH, Lenke LG, Baldus C. Major intraoperative neurologic deficits in pediatric and adult spinal deformity patients. Incidence and etiology at one institution. *Spine* 1998;23:324–331.

372. Coe JD, et al. Complications in spinal fusion for adolescent idiopathic scoliosis in the new millennium. A report of the Scoliosis Research Society Morbidity and Mortality Committee. *Spine (Phila Pa 1976)* 2006;31(3):345–349.

373. Diab M, Smith AR, Kuklo TR. Neural complications in the surgical treatment of adolescent idiopathic scoliosis. *Spine (Phila Pa 1976)* 2007;32(24):2759–2763.

374. Winter RB. Neurologic safety in spinal deformity surgery. *Spine (Phila Pa 1976)* 1997;22(13):1527–1533.

375. Winter RB, Lonstein JE, Denis F. Paraplegia resulting from vessel ligation. *Spine* 1996;21:1232–1233.

376. Apel DM, Marrero G, King J. Avoiding paraplegia during anterior spinal surgery. The role of somatosensory evoked potential monitoring with temporary occlusion of segmental spinal arteries. *Spine* 1991;16:S365–S370.

377. Glassman SD, Johnson JR, Shields CB. Correlation of motor-evoked potentials, somatosensory-evoked potentials, and the wake-up test in a case of kyphoscoliosis. *J Spinal Disord* 1993;6:194–198.

378. Pahys JM, et al. Neurologic injury in the surgical treatment of idiopathic scoliosis: guidelines for assessment and management. *J Am Acad Orthop Surg* 2009;17(7):426–434.

379. Hall JE, Levine CR, Sudhir KG. Intraoperative awakening to monitor spinal cord function during Harrington instrumentation and spine fusion. Description of procedure and report of three cases. *J Bone Joint Surg Am* 1978;60:533–536.

380. Szalay EA, Carollo JJ, Roach JW. Sensitivity of spinal cord monitoring to intraoperative events. *J Pediatr Orthop* 1986;6:437–441.

381. Schwartz DM, et al. Neurophysiological detection of impending spinal cord injury during scoliosis surgery. *J Bone Joint Surg Am* 2007;89(11):2440–2449.

382. Raynor BL, et al. Can triggered electromyograph thresholds predict safe thoracic pedicle screw placement? *Spine (Phila Pa 1976)* 2002;27(18):2030–2035.

383. Bracken MB. Methylprednisolone in the management of acute spinal cord injuries. *Med J Aust* 1990;153:368.

384. Bowen RE, et al. Efficacy of intraoperative cell salvage systems in pediatric idiopathic scoliosis patients undergoing posterior spinal fusion with segmental spinal instrumentation. *Spine (Phila Pa 1976)* 2010;35(2):246–251.

385. Tzortzopoulou A, et al. Antifibrinolytic agents for reducing blood loss in scoliosis surgery in children. *Cochrane Database Syst Rev* 2008(3):CD006883.

386. Vitale MG, Stazzone EJ, Gelijns AC. The effectiveness of preoperative erythropoietin in averting allogenic blood transfusion among children undergoing scoliosis surgery. *J Pediatr Orthop B* 1998;7:203–209.

387. Olsfanger D, Jedeikin R, Metser U. Acute normovolemic haemodilution and idiopathic scoliosis surgery: effects on homologous blood requirements. *Anaesth Intensive Care* 1993;21:429–431.

388. McNeill TW, DeWald RL, Kuo KN. Controlled hypotensive anesthesia in scoliosis surgery. *J Bone Joint Surg Am* 1974;56:1167–1172.

389. Joseph SA Jr, et al. Blood conservation techniques in spinal deformity surgery: a retrospective review of patients refusing blood transfusion. *Spine (Phila Pa 1976)* 2008;33(21):2310–2315.

390. Carreon LY, et al. Non-neurologic complications following surgery for adolescent idiopathic scoliosis. *J Bone Joint Surg Am* 2007;89(11): 2427–2432.

391. Johnston CE, Happel LT, Norris R. Delayed paraplegia complicating sublaminar segmental spinal instrumentation. *J Bone Joint Surg Am* 1986;68:556–563.

392. Mineiro J, Weinstein SL. Delayed postoperative paraparesis in scoliosis surgery. A case report. *Spine* 1997;22:1668–1672.

393. Pienkowski D, et al. Multicycle mechanical performance of titanium and stainless steel transpedicular spine implants. *Spine (Phila Pa 1976)* 1998;23(7):782–788.

394. Okuyama K, et al. Influence of bone mineral density on pedicle screw fixation: a study of pedicle screw fixation augmenting posterior lumbar interbody fusion in elderly patients. *Spine J* 2001;1(6):402–407.

395. Coe JD, et al. Influence of bone mineral density on the fixation of thoracolumbar implants. A comparative study of transpedicular screws, laminar hooks, and spinous process wires. *Spine (Phila Pa 1976)* 1990;15(9):902–907.

396. Lehman RA Jr, et al. Computed tomography evaluation of pedicle screws placed in the pediatric deformed spine over an 8-year period. *Spine (Phila Pa 1976)* 2007;32(24):2679–2684.

397. Kuntz CT, et al. Prospective evaluation of thoracic pedicle screw placement using fluoroscopic imaging. *J Spinal Disord Tech* 2004;17(3):206–214.

398. Sucato DJ, Kassab F, Dempsey M. Analysis of screw placement relative to the aorta and spinal canal following anterior instrumentation for thoracic idiopathic scoliosis. *Spine (Phila Pa 1976)* 2004;29(5):554–59; discussion 559.

399. Flynn JM, et al. Radiographic classification of complications of instrumentation in adolescent idiopathic scoliosis. *Clin Orthop Relat Res* 2010;468(3):665–669.

400. Clark CE, Shufflebarger HL. Late-developing infection in instrumented idiopathic scoliosis. *Spine* 1999;24:1909–1912.

401. Richards BS. Delayed infections following posterior spinal instrumentation for the treatment of idiopathic scoliosis. *J Bone Joint Surg Am* 1995;77:524–529.

402. Wimmer C, Gluch H. Aseptic loosening after CD instrumentation in the treatment of scoliosis: a report about eight cases. *J Spinal Disord* 1998;11:440–443.

403. Senaran H, et al. Ultrastructural analysis of metallic debris and tissue reaction around spinal implants in patients with late operative site pain. *Spine (Phila Pa 1976)* 2004;29(15):1618–1623; discussion 1623.

404. Potter BK, et al. Loss of coronal correction following instrumentation removal in adolescent idiopathic scoliosis. *Spine (Phila Pa 1976)* 2006;31(1):67–72.

405. Arens S, et al. Influence of materials for fixation implants on local infection. An experimental study of steel versus titanium DCP in rabbits. *J Bone Joint Surg Br* 1996;78(4):647–651.

406. Suk SI, et al. Determination of distal fusion level with segmental pedicle screw fixation in single thoracic idiopathic scoliosis. *Spine (Phila Pa 1976)* 2003;28(5):484–491.

407. Hollenbeck SM, et al. The prevalence of increased proximal junctional flexion following posterior instrumentation and arthrodesis for adolescent idiopathic scoliosis. *Spine (Phila Pa 1976)* 2008;33(15): 1675–1681.

408. Kim YJ, et al. Proximal junctional kyphosis in adolescent idiopathic scoliosis after 3 different types of posterior segmental spinal instrumentation and fusions: incidence and risk factor analysis of 410 cases. *Spine (Phila Pa 1976)* 2007;32(24):2731–2738.

Suken A. Shah
Kit Song

Congenital Scoliosis

INTRODUCTION

Congenital scoliosis is defined as a lateral deviation of the spine associated with one of a broad range of congenital vertebral malformations (CVMs) that can form during *in utero* development. It is distinct from other spinal deviations in which malformations do not occur and can present as an isolated spine anomaly or be associated with a large number of visceral organ and syndromic abnormalities. In Smith's "Recognizable Patterns of Human Malformation," over 40 syndromes have CVMs listed as one of the presenting features (1).

The malformations are always present at birth, but the development of the scoliosis may occur over time. They can occur in any part of the spinal column and are believed to be a result of the disruption of the process of somatogenesis that occurs between the 5th and 8th weeks of gestation (2–8). These malformations are not unique to humans as several other species develop such abnormalities in response to teratogenic exposures or from genetic predispositions (9–14).

Of great importance is the high incidence of associated abnormalities in other organ systems that can lead to significant adverse impacts upon the health and well-being of affected individuals. In addition to this is the realization that management of the developing deformity is often extremely challenging and, due to the variation of presentation, highly individualized. This chapter focuses upon children with congenital vertebral anomalies. We do not discuss infantile scoliosis or other conditions where there may be deformity without malformations.

INCIDENCE/PREVALENCE

The true incidence and prevalence of congenial vertebral malformations is unknown. Many individuals without visible deformity are undoubtedly not found, and many series intermix patients with syndromic or other neuromuscular conditions. Large population studies utilizing screening chest x-rays for tuberculosis suggested a thoracic spine incidence of 0.5 to 1:1,000 live births (15), with more recent ultrasound screening studies finding an incidence of 0.1 to 0.3:1,000 live births with many of these children having other complex birth defects (16, 17). In general, the incidence should be considered to be rare, with kyphotic CVMs even rarer.

MECHANISM OF SPINE FORMATION

It is useful to review the evolving knowledge and understanding of spine formation and development as it may relate to the formation of CVMs. Much of this knowledge has been gained from the observation of human embryonic development (18) and study of murine models of spine formation. During gastrulation, four identified *Hox* gene clusters containing 39 genes (*Hox A, B, C,* and *D*) are believed to determine positional information along the rostrocaudal axis of developing vertebrates (11, 18, 19). They are expressed in cells of the developing mesoderm and ectoderm that later form the somites, which in turn form the vertebrae, ribs, and muscles. Vertebrae are derived from the paraxial mesoderm that forms from the superficial epiblast cells growing into the primitive streak during gastrulation forming the paraxial mesoderm. These develop into the segmental units of the somite, which then subdivide into ventral sclerotome (vertebral precursor) and dorsal dermatomyotome (muscle, skin, rib precursors) units (3, 18, 20). Induction of the sclerotome is signaled by the notochord and the floor plate of the neural tube. This involves the Sonic Hedgehog protein (21). Subsequent fusion of the ventral and dorsal sclerotomes then forms vertebrae (3, 18, 20). It is believed that a molecular segmentation clock that is mediated through the Notch signaling pathways controls vertebrate segmentation (3, 10, 12, 22) with formation of somites in a rostral to caudal sequence. This involves periodic expression of 50 to 100 cyclic genes. Genes that are believed to impact this pathway are lunatic fringe (*LFNG*), *DLL3*, and *MESP2* (23, 24) (Fig. 18-1).

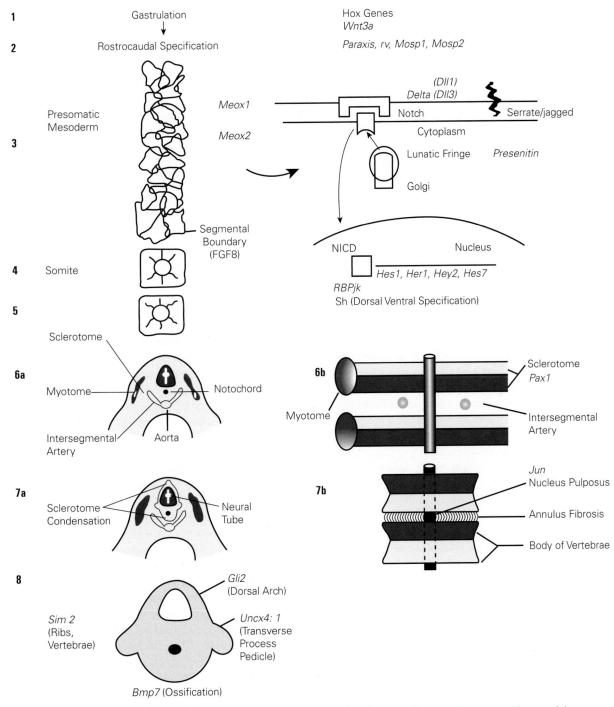

FIGURE 18-1. Schematic diagram showing pathway of murine embryologic development of somites with potential gene interactions highlighted. Segmentation is operated through a molecular clock operating through the Notch signaling pathway. Segment boundary formation is mediated by fibroblast growth factor 8. Sclerotome formation and subdivision into dorsal and ventral halves is mediated by *Pax 1* and *Meox1*.

ETIOLOGY

The true etiology of the development of CVMs is unknown. The spectrum of the disorder is very large, ranging from syndromic cases such as Jarcho-Levin syndrome to isolated hemivertebrae, and a number of environmental and genetic associations have been identified, suggesting that both genetic factors and teratogenic effects from the environment play a role in the disturbances of normal spine formation.

Anoxia created by carbon monoxide exposure to mouse and chick models at a critical time and specific dose has been demonstrated to cause CVMs very similar to those found in humans (9, 25–27). Similar outcomes in humans due to exposure to carbon monoxide have been postulated, but not clearly established (28). Other environmental factors have been clinically associated with the development of CVM. Alcohol exposure with fetal alcohol syndrome (29), anticonvulsant medications Valproic acid and Dilantin (30–33), retinoic acid (31), hyperthermia (34), maternal insulin-dependent diabetes (35, 36), and folate deficiency (37) have all been implicated in abnormalities of the spine in humans.

Model organisms such as the chick and mouse strongly suggest that there is a genetic contribution to the development of CVM (3, 11, 12, 38). In humans, the heterogeneous clinical manifestations, variety of morphologic features, and phenotypic presentations described as failures of formation or failures of segmentation had led to the belief that the majority of cases were sporadic events (39). Recent evidence suggests that there is a strong role for genetic factors in the development of human CVMs. The genetic transmission of some cases of CVM has been shown to have a familial recurrence rate of 3% (20, 40), and an increasing number of vertebral malformation syndromes have identifiable genetic etiologies. Spondylocostal dysostosis patients have a loss of normal vertebral morphology throughout the entire spine and have been shown to have mutations in *delta-like 1 (DLLS), mesoderm posterior 2 (MESP2),* and *LFNG.* Mutations in these affect the Notch signaling pathway and highlight the importance of Notch in vertebral column formation in humans (3, 41, 42). Spondylothoracic dysostosis (commonly referred to as Jarcho-Levin syndrome) is a confusing array of CVMs, all of which have rib anomalies with fusion of all ribs. A homozygous recessive nonsense mutation in *MESP2* has been identified. Alagille syndrome is an autosomal dominant condition with bile duct paucity, cardiac, eye, kidney, pancreas, and vertebral anomalies in 22% to 87% of affected individuals. Mutations in *JAG1* and *NOTCH2* have been found in these patients (2, 3). Klippel-Feil syndrome was first reported in 1894 (43) and described in 1912 (44). Most cases have been found to be sporadic in families, but autosomal dominant, recessive, and X-linked forms have been reported. There has been recent evidence that *PAX1* mutation and notch pathway mutations can be found in patients with Klippel-Feil syndrome (8, 45–47). As isolated CVM are often sporadic occurrences with a given family, candidate gene analysis has been used. Using mouse–human synteny analysis, 27 eligible loci have been identified, of which 21 cause

vertebral malformations in the mouse. Six of these—*PAX1, WNT3A, DLL3, SLC35A3, T(Brachyury),* and *TBX6*—have been studied in some detail and show promise as potential loci for the formation of CVMs in humans (3, 13, 14, 46–48).

ASSOCIATED CONDITIONS

CVMs do not occur in isolation. As they develop during a critical stage of organogenesis, as many as 61% have other associated malformations (49), and the development of progressive deformity may lead to secondary organ involvement. The malformations seen are in general neurologic and visceral, with most tied to the level of the CVM.

Neurologic abnormalities have been described in 18% to 38% of patients with CVM (50–54). A prospective evaluation of consecutive patients with CVM found that 38% had an intraspinal anomaly, with higher concentrations among patients with cervical and thoracic CVM, mixed patterns of segmentation and formation, and congenital kyphosis (50). Half of these patients had physical findings to suggest that they had an intraspinal lesion. Diastematomyelia was the most common finding followed by intraspinal lipoma, tethered cord, Chiari malformation with or without associated syringomyelia, dermoid cyst, and epidermoid cyst (Figs. 18-2 to 18-4). For patients with an isolated hemivertebrae, there may also be a high incidence of intraspinal anomalies. Belmont found that of their 76 patients with C3VM, 29 had an isolated hemivertebrae, and of these, 8 (28%) had an MRI abnormality (55). Thirteen had abnormal clinical findings. A review of these patients and published series of similar patients suggests that an abnormal finding on the history of physical examination had an accuracy of 65%, sensitivity of 59%, specificity of 87%, a negative predictive value of 72%, and a positive predictive value of 74% (45, 50, 51, 56, 57).

For patients with known congenital cardiac abnormalities, the incidence of scoliosis has been found to be as high as 10% (58), but most of these are normally segmented (26, 58). Farley found that only 11/48 children (23%) with congenital heart disease (CHD) who had scoliosis had congenital scoliosis. The converse relationship of a higher incidence of CHD (baseline incidence 0.5% in the general population) in patients primarily found to have a congenital scoliosis has not been demonstrated, but it is believed that there is a higher incidence. Basu et al. (50) found cardiac abnormalities in 26% of patients with CVM. Two-thirds of these had knowledge of the cardiac abnormality before they presented for evaluation of their spine. Of those who did not have prior knowledge, of the cardiac defect, 2/10 (20%) did proceed to active management.

The incidence of renal anomalies in CVM has been reported as 26% to 37% (49, 50, 54, 59–61). The most common anomalies have been unilateral renal agenesis, urinary duplication, ectopic kidney, reflux, and a horseshoe kidney. The incidence of renal anomalies may be higher if there is an associated rib anomaly in addition to the CVM (52). In most of the series, the renal anomalies were unsuspected, leading to general recommendations to screen children for these problems.

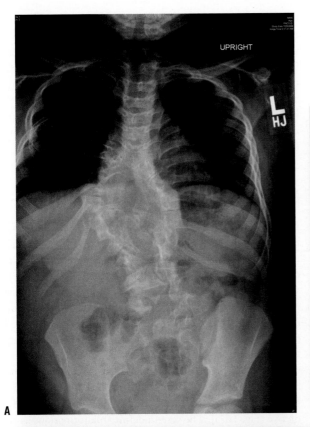

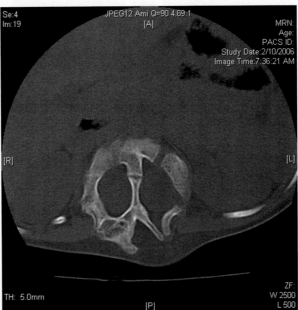

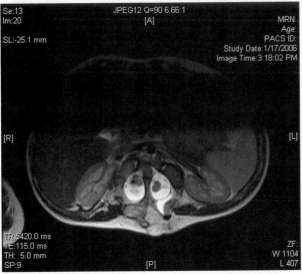

FIGURE 18-2. **A:** Example of diastematomyelia—plain radiographs may reveal a central canal bony process as the child matures. **B:** Plain radiographs. **C:** MRI findings.

Morbidity associated with large progressive increases in deformity has largely been related to the development of restrictive lung disease and is believed to be a function of both altered alveolar multiplication and altered dynamics of breathing due to constriction of the thorax (62–72). As compared to idiopathic scoliosis, the loss in vital capacity for a given Cobb angle is believed to be 15% greater for individuals with CVM (73). Several series have shown a progressive loss in vital capacity for progressive curves but have shown that if there is no progression and no associated severe rib anomalies, the vital capacity average for individuals with CVM is 87% of predicted (67, 69,

73–75). Similarly, diffusion capacity for nonprogressive CVM has been found to be normal, suggesting that congenital scoliosis without fused ribs may not be associated with pulmonary hypoplasia or thoracic insufficiency syndrome (TIS) (72). Overall, however, the greater the deformity and the more proximal the deformity, the greater the apparent long-term impact upon spirometry (62, 63, 66, 69). For severe progressive curves, body mass index (BMI) less than the 5th percentile can be common, and this may create a higher risk situation for the operative management of these children. One of the primary clinical correlates to measurable declines in functional vital capacity

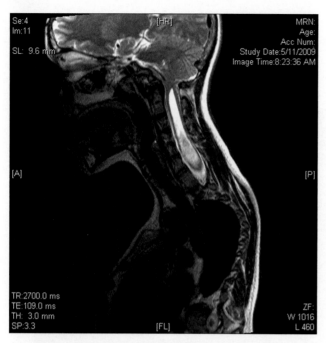

FIGURE 18-3. Example of syrinx with Chiari I malformation.

(FVC) in CVM is an altered BMI (74). Another is increased asymmetry of ventilation/perfusion (V/Q), which occurs in about 50% of children with TIS and congenital scoliosis (75).

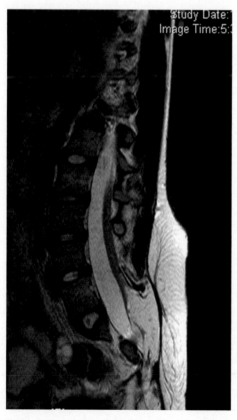

FIGURE 18-4. Example of a tethered spinal cord with an intraspinal lipoma.

Coupled with this is the observation that diffusion capacity does decline with worsening deformity presumably due to a reduction in the total alveolar surface area (72). Cobb angle has not been correlated to either FVC changes or to altered function as measured by V/Q scans (68, 71). Surgical interventions aimed at stabilizing the chest/spine in patients with TIS have been shown to preserve growth-related changes in vital capacity over time but do not appear to be able to catch up for lost function (68, 70).

CLASSIFICATION/NATURAL HISTORY

Early reports of CVM suggested a benign natural history (76), but subsequent reports by Winter and Moe (77) and MacEwen et al. (78) identified severe deformities from high-risk patterns of deformity. Subsequent classifications for CVM have been several (77, 79–83). Most have focused upon trying to assign a risk of progression by study of the natural history of deformities presenting to surgeons. Despite new knowledge gained by three-dimensional (3D) imaging using computed tomographic (CT) scans (79) and information about genetic mechanisms by which CVMs may form, the classification schemes proposed by Winter and Moe (77) and Nasca et al. (82) and modified by McMaster and Ohtsuka (80) remains the most useful and predictive (Fig. 18-5). The system defines malformations as either failures of formation, failures of segmentation, or combinations of these. The malformations can occur in frontal, sagittal, or both planes. The likelihood of progression is predicted by the anticipated potential for either unbalanced growth created by uneven growth potential due to failures of formation (hemivertebrae, wedge vertebrae) or growth retardation due to tethering created by failures of segmentation (bar). Approximately 10% of patients have patterns of CVM that are not definable by this classification scheme. The highest risk of progression was shown by McMaster to be in situations where there is unbalanced growth opposite an asymmetric tether as in a unilateral unsegmented bar with a contralateral hemivertebrae. The average annual rate of progression was found to be from 5 degrees to >10 degrees per year. The next highest risk of progression was in those with a unilateral unsegmented bar followed by double hemivertebrae (80) (Fig. 18-6). Reports of untreated patients followed in surgical clinics document a risk of progression to curves >40 degrees at maturity from 37% to 84% (76, 77, 80). For any given deformity type, there is variability in progression that may be due to the fact that it is difficult to account for variation in anterior and posterior CVMs at any given level. The most rapid times of progression were in the first 5 years of life and from ages 10 to 14 years. If there were clinically evident deformities in the first year of life, a worse overall prognosis was found (84, 85). The risk of progression has been predicated upon the belief that there is no growth potential of involved segments with CVM, leading to deformity and a shortened trunk (85). Campbell and Hell-Vocke (86) have questioned this with evidence of growth in CVM segments used forced growth techniques.

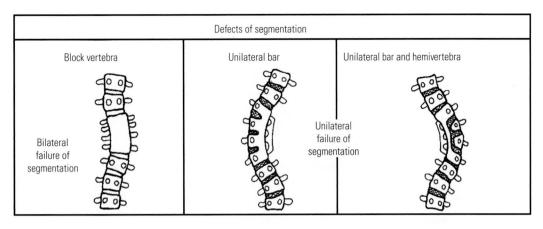

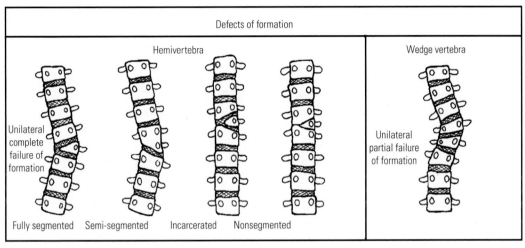

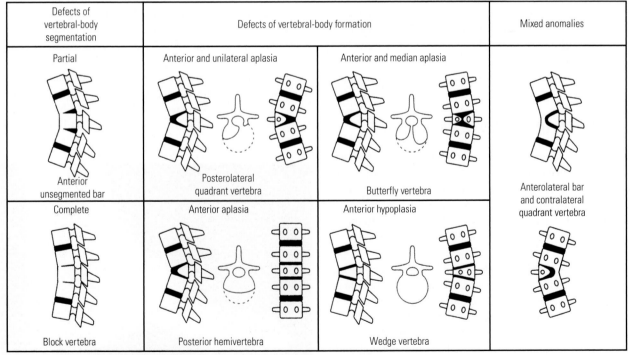

FIGURE 18-5. **A:** Classification of congenital scoliosis showing failures of formation and segmentation. Incarcerated hemivertebrae have compensatory deformities proximal and distal to it. The highest risk for progression lies with a hemivertebrae opposite a unilateral bar. **B:** Classification of congenital kyphosis. A high percentage of true congenital kyphosis deformities will progress and can lead to paraplegia especially if in the thoracic spine.

Site of curvature	Type of congenital anomaly					
	Block vertebra	Wedge vertebra	Hemivertebra		Unilateral unsegmented bar	Unilateral unsegmented bar and contralateral hemivertebrae
			Single	Double		
Upper thoracic	<1°–1°	★–2°	1°–2°	2°–2.5°	2°–4°	5°–6°
Lower thoracic	<1°–1°	2°–3°	2°–2.5°	2°–3°	5°–6.5°	6°–7°
Thoracolumbar	<1°–1°	1.5°–2°	2°–3.5°	5°–★	6°–9°	>10°–★
Lumbar	<1°–★	<1°–★	<1°–1°	★	>5°–★	★
Lumbosacral	★	★	<1°–1.5°	★	★	★

▣ No treatment required ▦ May require spinal surgery ☐ Require spinal fusion ★ Too few or no curves

Ranges represent the degree of derotation before and after 10 years of age

FIGURE 18-6. Risk of progression of types of CVM as compiled by McMaster. Highest rates of progression were in unilateral unsegmented bar and contralateral hemivertebrae.

The clinical impact of progressive deformities associated with CVM has focused historically on respiratory consequences and more recently upon quality-of-life measures. There is no clear association that has been established between classifications of CVM and mortality or morbidity. Patients with severe progressive deformities have been demonstrated to have severe restrictive lung disease and significant morbidity with early death (62–64, 85, 86). They have also been found to have a significantly diminished quality of life as measured by the Child Health Questionnaire in the domains of physical limitations and caregiver burdens, but not in psychosocial domains (87). Surgical intervention for these deformities has not yet been shown to alter these natural histories. It appears that pulmonary function decline can be stabilized with surgical treatment in some cases, but improvement in depressed vital capacity has not been observed (68, 70). Similarly, diminished quality of life does not appear to be improved after intervention (88).

EVALUATION OF PATIENTS WITH CVM

The wide range of presentations and the high incidence of visceral anomalies that can be present in patients with CVMs mandate that all evaluations include a careful history and physical examination. Presentations will range from severely involved children with obvious visceral and structural anomalies to those with nonprogressive and asymptomatic malformations.

Neurologic. Many relatively uninvolved children will be referred due to incidental findings on imaging studies obtained for other reasons. Growth charts should be reviewed as children with CVMs may have altered growth velocities and can present with disproportionate growth retardation. Delays in developmental milestones such as walking and running and potty training can be important signs of an underlying spinal dysraphism as can symptoms of back pain in very young children. Physical findings of posterior midline trunk hairy patches, large nevi, or hemangiomas, atrophy of extremities,

a cavus foot (Figs. 18-7 and 18-8), or any neurologic abnormalities (weakness, balance difficulties, sensory, hyperreflexia, asymmetric abdominal reflexes) can indicate an underlying spinal dysraphism in 50% to 80% of cases (19, 50, 51). It is widely recommended that an MRI of the neural axis be obtained prior to surgical intervention for CVM (45, 50–53, 56, 78, 89–91). Less clear is whether there is benefit to the routine ordering of spine MRI scans for asymptomatic children with CVM who are not to undergo surgery. The positive and negative predictive value of physical examination and clinical history is 74% and 72% respectively for determination of MRI abnormalities (45, 50). As many younger children will require an anesthetic for a spine MRI, in asymptomatic nonprogressive deformities in children, observation to an older age is recommended. Intrauterine MRI has been tested for defining neural axis lesions in CVM. It has been found to be better than intrauterine ultrasound, but its overall accuracy and role in managing CVM are as yet unknown (92–95). For neonates with a suspected abnormality of the neural axis, ultrasound has been shown to be an effective screening tool and can be used

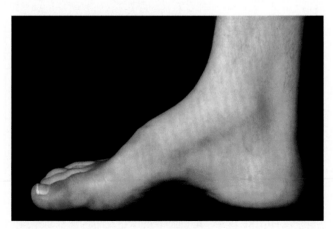

FIGURE 18-7. Cavus foot. High incidence of neurologic abnormalities associated with this finding.

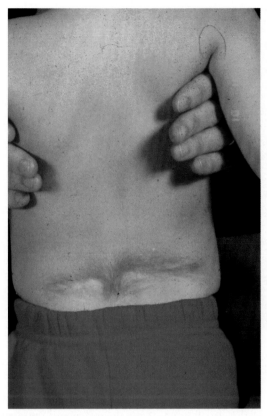

FIGURE 18-8. Midline hairy patch consistent with an underlying spinal dysraphism.

in a cost-effective manner depending upon the expertise of the individual performing it (8, 47, 54).

Renal.   As up to one-third of patients may have an underlying renal anomaly and many will be asymptomatic, evaluation of the urinary system is generally advised (29, 49, 50, 52, 59, 69). Renal ultrasound has replaced contrast intravenous pyelogram as the imaging study of choice (60, 89). For patients who are undergoing MRI for evaluation of the neural axis, renal anomalies can be well-visualized when a modified spine MRI is ordered (96).

Cardiac.   As many as two-thirds of patients with cardiac abnormalities and CVM will have had diagnosis made by their primary care provider or a cardiologist prior to presentation for evaluation of their CVM (50, 58). For those who have not had prior evaluation and who are asymptomatic, the majority of the cardiac anomalies that may be present will not require active treatment. Cardiac screening is recommended for patients who are to undergo surgical treatment (89).

Pulmonary.   Children with progressive and severe deformities are at risk for developing significant restrictive lung disease (62, 69, 73, 75, 82). The linkage between the spine, thorax, and lung growth and function has been brought to light by Campbell et al. (64) through their definition of TIS as the

inability of the thorax to support normal lung growth and function. It is recommended that children who are to undergo surgical intervention for progressive disease have a pulmonary evaluation prior to surgery. There are currently no established guidelines related to respiratory function that guide decisions for surgical intervention.

The assessment of lung function in children is made difficult by their inability to cooperate with pulmonary function testing (97). For very young children, CT lung volumes have been offered as a surrogate (98–100), but correlation between measured changes in volume and change in respiratory function as measured by physiologic testing has not been established for these populations of normal children. Right lung CT volumes have been found to highly correlate with preoperative right lung function as measured by ventilation perfusion scans, but to have poor correlation after surgery for patients with TIS (101). This implies that alterations in volume alone do not predict impact upon respiratory function. Current concerns related to the risk of radiation exposure to children from CT scans should bring to light risk–benefit questions when ordering these tests (102–104). Recently, dynamic chest and diaphragm motion has been evaluated using ultrafast dynamic MRI in an effort to define how chest wall perturbations may affect respiratory efforts through their impact upon chest wall compliance and diaphragm motion. Correlation with spirometry data has been done in healthy, normal subjects, with the technique showing great promise for the assessment of individuals with pathologic conditions (105, 106).

Children with TIS will manifest with hypercarbia and hypoxemia in advanced stages of their disorder (62–65, 67, 74). Serologic evaluation with capillary blood gases looking for elevation of serum bicarbonate indicating CO_2 retention and of serum hemoglobin levels that would indicate hypoxemia is recommended at the time of initial evaluation (64, 65).

Radiographic.   Biplanar radiographs have been the main mechanism for evaluation and guidance of decisions related to the surgical intervention for patients with CVM. For complex CVM, inter- and intraobserver reliability of the Cobb angle appears to be 10 degrees (107–109). Campbell et al. has developed the techniques of space available for the lung (SAL) and the interpedicular line ratio as alternatives for measuring deformity (64, 110). The reliability of these measures has not yet been established and correlation to respiratory changes has not been made. As pointed out earlier, the risk of curve progression is not always predicted by classification schemes utilizing biplanar radiographs. This coupled with the increasing use of pedicle screw fixation has prompted 3D evaluation of CVM prior to surgery using CT (111–113) and interest in developing classification systems based upon CT data (79) (Fig. 18-9). No consistent threshold value has been established at which intervention should be performed, but it has generally been recommended that documentable progression at a prepubertal age should be strongly considered for surgery

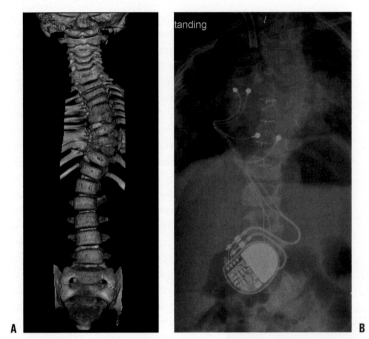

FIGURE 18-9. Three-dimensional CT scan **(A)** of a complex CVM **(B)**. Note the mix of posterior and anterior defects.

(38, 77, 90, 114). As patients with CVM often have deformity at multiple levels, it is recommended that all patients have radiographic evaluation of their entire spine upon presentation, with special attention given to cervical spine abnormalities prior to surgery (89).

SUMMARY

Patients who present with CVM have identifiable defects in segmentation during early fetal development. They will present with a wide range of phenotypic expressions and have varying degrees of risk for progression and morbidity. Careful evaluation of these patients for associated visceral and neural axis abnormalities is advised upon initial presentation and before surgical intervention. Consistent criteria for surgical intervention have not been identified, but in general rapid progression of deformity at a prepubertal age carries a poor prognosis and surgical intervention is recommended. Three-dimensional imaging is rapidly becoming a standard in preoperative evaluation and planning. The remainder of this chapter focuses on the evolving techniques for intervention.

TREATMENT

Nonoperative Treatment

Observation. The child with a congenital vertebral anomaly requires close observation during growth until maturity. The anomaly, although present at birth, may not manifest itself as a clinically visible deformity until many years later,

after sufficient asymmetric growth has resulted in scoliosis. Hence, the classification of the deformity and the predicted natural history is crucial to determining the prescribed treatment. The patient can be monitored with radiographs at 6- to 12-month intervals depending on the type of malformation, location of the anomaly(ies), prior curve behavior, and the age of the child relative to spinal growth. Changes in the congenital deformity can be rapid in infancy and again in the preadolescent growth spurt, but relatively quiescent in middle childhood (5 to 10 years of age) (115). The location of the CVM is also important. Progressive cervical CVMs produce significant shoulder asymmetry and neck deformities (Fig. 18-10), and progressive limbosacral CVMs can produce a truncal shift or pelvic obliquity and coronal imbalance (Fig. 18-11). Some thought should be given to avoidance of radiographs at frequent, routine intervals just as a reflex reaction due to the cumulative nature of radiation to a young person over her lifetime (116). It can be very helpful to obtain the initial radiographs of a child, for example, a chest x-ray in the newborn nursery, in order to identify hemivertebrae, congenital bars, or fused ribs and then compare to films that are more contemporary in order to gain an understanding of the sometimes-complex pathology (Fig. 18-12). In a child <2 years, supine films are adequate, but after standing age, erect, full-length radiographs should be obtained in the posterior–anterior projection and lateral, when necessary. Clinicians should be aware that positional changes when x-rays are obtained during this development phase (sitting to standing) may drastically change the measured Cobb angle.

This archive of films should be carefully evaluated for changes not only in the congenital area and its associated curve but also in the compensatory (noncongenital) areas,

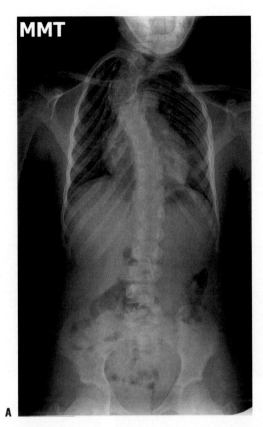
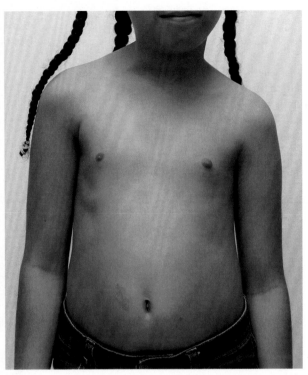

FIGURE 18-10. Progressive congenital kyphoscoliosis in an 8-year-old female. **A:** Erect radiograph with multiple vertebral anomalies centered at the cervicothoracic area including hemivertebra, wedge vertebrae, and a vertebral bony bar. **B:** Clinical photo illustrating the child's head tilt, neck and shoulder asymmetry.

truncal shift, or shoulder asymmetry as proxies for progression in the primary congenital curve. Small, subtle changes can be missed if one only examines the most recent studies; errors compounded and the window for optimal intervention can be missed. Due to the malformations, identification of the landmarks used to measure the Cobb angle(s) can be troublesome and inaccurate among and between observers (117). Consistency of the end points used must be maintained when measuring the radiographs over time; carefully remeasure the prior studies when necessary to determine if progression has occurred (107). The vertebral endplates are most commonly used as endpoints to calculate the Cobb angle, but pedicles may be used if endplate anatomy is unclear.

If there is progression of the compensatory, noncongenital scoliosis, without a change in the congenital primary curve, the possibility of spinal cord dysraphism needs to be investigated with an MRI scan of the entire spine. Spinal cord tethering, thickened filum terminale, syrinx, or lipoma may be present. However, as mentioned previously, given the fairly high rate of intraspinal anomalies noted on MRI in patients with congenital scoliosis, even isolated hemivertebra, routine use for all cases of congenital scoliosis may be justified (118).

Nonsurgical Treatment. There is little evidence that bracing is effective for congenital scoliosis; the congenital portion

of the curve is usually short and inflexible. However, Winter et al. (119) reported that an orthosis may be useful in certain congenital circumstances: compensatory curves above or below the congenital segment, long sweeping congenital curves with a flexible component, and for maintaining truncal and spinal balance following localized fusion during growth. A brace can be used in a young child as a supplement to surgery to curtail activities and protect instrumentation in soft bone. Bracing is not appropriate for congenital kyphosis, lordosis, or scoliosis with a known poor prognosis, such as a unilateral bar with a contralateral hemivertebra.

Halo Traction. Previously viewed as only of historical interest, halo-gravity traction is a viable adjunct in the modern treatment of severe scoliosis and is safe for congenital patients, in general. The exception is a patient with a short, sharp angular deformity associated with kyphosis—proceed with caution or avoid traction altogether. Used preoperatively before posterior correction and fusion or between staged anterior release procedures, halo-gravity traction is effective at maximizing correction of stiff deformities and well tolerated by patients, since they are allowed out of bed to a wheelchair or walker in traction. This treatment also has medical benefits; in the week(s) preceding surgery, patients can perk up nutritionally, gain weight, and improve pulmonary function and bone density.

FIGURE 18-11. Progressive lumbosacral congenital scoliosis in a 2-year-old male. **A:** Erect posterior–anterior (PA) radiograph of the child at 18 months showing ipsilateral hemivertebrae at L2 and L5/S1. **B:** Erect PA radiograph at 2 years of age showing progression of the lumbosacral scoliosis, truncal shift, coronal imbalance and pelvic obliquity. **C:** Lateral radiograph with mildly decreased lumbar lordosis. **D:** Coronal reconstructed computed tomography (CT) scan illustrating lumbar hemivertebra and lumbosacral hemivertebra with oblique sacrum.

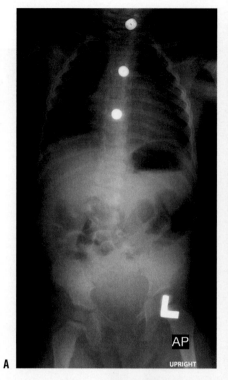

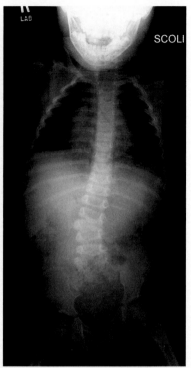

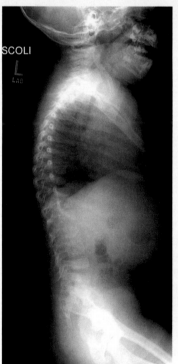

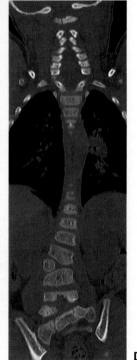

Initially, traction should start with light weight and increase slowly while the patient is monitored for complaints or neurologic changes, and the maintenance of traction is variable from 2 weeks to many months. Clinical studies are hard to analyze since a small group of congenital patients are reported within a group of other etiologies of severe scoliosis, but most authors agree that there is improvement of the Cobb angle (28% to

35%), truncal height and balance, SAL, frontal and sagittal alignment, and avoidance of neurologic injury (120–123).

Surgical Treatment

Management Themes. After a thorough analysis of the deformity, the natural history or documentation of progression may be an indication for surgery. A multimodality evaluation

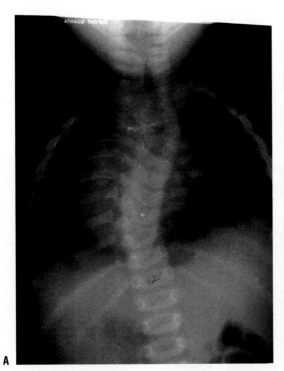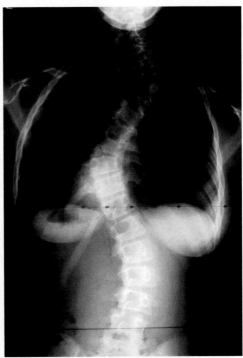

A   **B**

FIGURE 18-12. Progressive congenital scoliosis with development of compensatory thoracolumbar curve. **A:** Chest radiograph in the newborn nursery of an infant female showing contralateral thoracic hemivertebrae (hemimetameric shift). **B:** PA erect radiograph 14 years later showing the natural history: progression of both congenital curves and development of a compensatory lumbar curve.

of the patient is necessary to assess and manage any associated anomalies, pulmonary function, and nutritional status. The surgical treatment of congenital scoliosis can generally be divided into procedures that will prevent or control further deformity, gradually correct deformity, or ones that acutely correct the deformity. Fusion *in situ* is the classic example of a procedure for prevention or control; convex anterior hemiepiphysiodesis and posterior hemiarthrodesis may gradually correct congenital scoliosis when done at the appropriate time, with the remaining growth and hemivertebrae resection or spinal osteotomy having the potential to acutely correct even severe deformities.

Historically, experts have asserted that it is easier to prevent a deformity than to correct one, and this reiterates the principles of vigilance in observation and knowledge of the natural history of the type of anomaly (124, 125). However, the ability to predict the natural history of many mixed, complex anomalies seen in congenital scoliosis is variable and sometimes an irrelevant issue if the patient presents when the deformity is severe (Figs. 18-13 and 18-14) or previous procedures have proved to be unsuccessful. The armamentarium of surgical options, therefore, must include a spectrum of techniques from the simple to the complex procedure for salvage when there is no other option. The goals of management of patients with congenital scoliosis are that at skeletal maturity, the patient should have a balanced spine, maximized pulmonary function, optimized spinal height, and no deterioration of neurologic function.

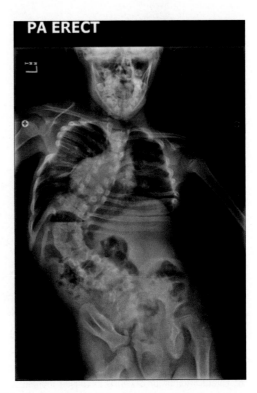

FIGURE 18-13. Progressive congenital scoliosis and associated anomalies in a 9-year-old female. The mixed anomalies include hemivertebrae, block vertebrae, wedge vertebrae, a vertebral bony bar, and fused ribs. She also has congenital short femur and a tethered cord.

***In Situ* Fusion.** If a curve is predicted to worsen or progression has been documented, an *in situ* fusion can halt progression and is ideal for stabilizing a small curve, provided it is done at the proper time in a young child. The classic anomaly appropriate for this treatment is a unilateral bar or a unilateral bar with a contralateral hemivertebra that is diagnosed early with no associated deformity, since there is thought to be little potential growth on the concavity of the deformity. *In situ* fusions are safe from a complication standpoint and technically simple to perform even in small children, but may be unreliable to control progression due to crankshaft and add-on phenomenon. The growth potential of the anterior column of the spine must be assessed as minimal by MRI or CT before a posterior tether (fusion) is applied in a young child, or progression of the curvature may result even in the case of a solid arthrodesis (126–128).

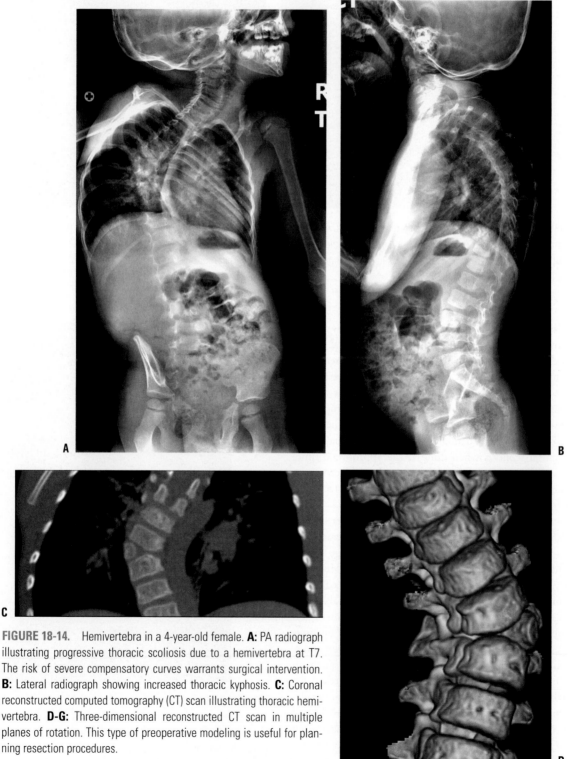

FIGURE 18-14. Hemivertebra in a 4-year-old female. **A:** PA radiograph illustrating progressive thoracic scoliosis due to a hemivertebra at T7. The risk of severe compensatory curves warrants surgical intervention. **B:** Lateral radiograph showing increased thoracic kyphosis. **C:** Coronal reconstructed computed tomography (CT) scan illustrating thoracic hemivertebra. **D-G:** Three-dimensional reconstructed CT scan in multiple planes of rotation. This type of preoperative modeling is useful for planning resection procedures.

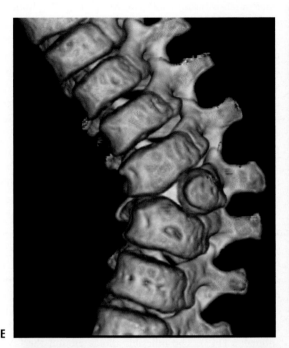

E

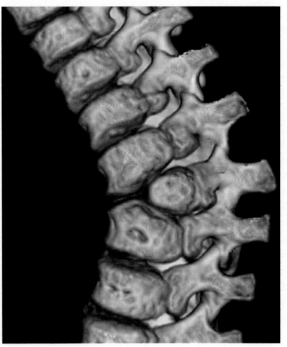

F

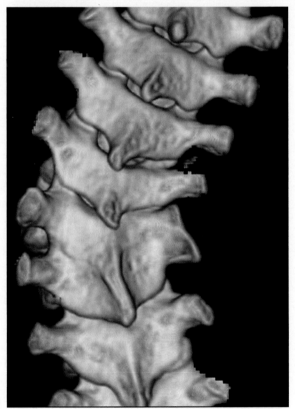

G

FIGURE 18-14.   (*Continued*)

When the potential for anterior growth exists, the patient should have an anterior growth cessation procedure (epiphysiodesis or fusion) performed, open or thoracoscopically, in the thoracic spine. Occasionally, an *in situ* fusion may offer correction over time—if there is growth potential on the concavity of a scoliosis or anteriorly for kyphosis—but more often, it is meant to prevent progression of a relatively short congenital deformity in an otherwise balanced spine.

Most commonly performed posteriorly for a kyphosing scoliosis, the procedure can be performed anteriorly as well, as a lordosing deformity would dictate. The fusion levels selected must include all of the vertebrae in the measured Cobb angle and typically extend at least to a level above and below the anomalous segment(s) (129) or the entire length on the contralateral side of a bar (130). Classically described for small children, postoperative immobilization is provided by a cast, but newer, downsized instrumentation may be implanted safely to provide more stable fixation (131), reduce the chance of pseudarthroses, and limit the immobilization time (132). The concern over an extensive fusion of the spine in a young child is that it stops growth. Inhibition of spinal growth can lead to a disproportionate posture, lead to a shortened trunk, hinder lung development, and lead to TIS (133–135).

Convex Hemiepiphysiodesis/Hemiarthrodesis. This procedure offers partial growth arrest on the convex side of the deformity with remaining growth, and thus, little or no concave growth should be expected. Most commonly applied to isolated hemivertebra in young children, unilateral failures of formation with modest curves are the deformities that are most appropriate for this technique. Some correction can be achieved over time, depending on the age and growth potential of the child at the time of the procedure; some correction is also initially obtained in the postoperative cast. Long-term results show that <15 degrees of total correction can be achieved, with some patients obtaining no correction of the curve or truncal imbalance (136–138). The procedure is generally conducted with an anterior approach (open or thoracoscopic), extirpation of the disks and cartilaginous growth plates, anterior spinal fusion and a posterior spinal hemiarthrodesis on the convexity over the same segments (the concave side is not exposed since it could lead to spontaneous fusion), and postoperative immobilization in a cast or a brace in a somewhat corrected position.

Results are variable, but the best outcomes seem to be in patients younger than 5 years with an isolated lumbar hemivertebra with a progressive curve <40 to 50 degrees (139, 138). One of the complications is failure to achieve correction. Roaf (124) reported that 60% of his patients had correction of at least 10 degrees, whereas Keller et al. (140), with a transpedicular approach showed that 37% of curves improved, 42% remained the same, 16% progressed 10 to 15 degrees, and 5% progressed more than 15 degrees. Thompson et al. (138), in their series of 30 patients showed that 76% had an improvement of the Cobb angle; the best corrections were obtained in the lumbar spine rather than in the high thoracic or thoracic spine. This procedure was not recommended in cases with associated kyphosis,

since anterior fusion could contribute to the kyphotic component (141), but more recent refinement of the technique by Cil et al. (142), with extension of the anterior hemiarthrodesis all the way to the posterior longitudinal ligament may avoid sagittal deterioration. Convex hemiepiphysiodesis and *in situ* fusion are low-risk procedures, but due to the limited correction and unpredictability of future correction with growth, other methods are more reproducible for treatment of congenital scoliosis.

HEMIVERTEBRA EXCISION

Excision of the hemivertebrae offers immediate correction of the congenital deformity and restoration of truncal balance over a short segment. The ideal indication is a young patient (<5 years of age), with an isolated hemivertebrae in the thoracolumbar, lumbar, or lumbosacral area with progression and/or associated coronal imbalance. Cervicothoracic hemivertebrae can cause marked shoulder and neck imbalance and are amenable to excision but obviously carry with them an increased risk of neurologic deficit due to the manipulation of the column around the spinal cord needed to perform the procedure and associated vertebral artery anomalies (143). The inflexible thorax around the CVM may pose limits to the correction. The spectrum of the technique of hemivertebrae excision ranges from staged anterior and posterior resection procedures, simultaneous anterior and posterior resection, and posterior-only excision. Small stature instrumentation, multimodality neurophysiologic monitoring, advances in surgical techniques, and proper experience have lowered the complication rate and improved outcomes (Figs. 18-15 to 18-21).

The excision of hemivertebrae, first described by Bradford and Boachie-Adjei (144) and then subsequently by Klemme et al. (145), was outlined as a sequential anterior, then posterior excision, which offered a safe, circumferential exposure of the spine and allowed removal of the disks above and below the hemivertebra, in addition to the bone itself. Then, the corresponding lamina and pedicle can be removed, the convexity compressed posteriorly, and a small area fused with instrumentation, and the bone that is removed can be used for graft. In an effort to save the operative time needed to reposition the patient and drape again between the anterior and posterior procedures, both can be performed simultaneously. This allows proper control of the sagittal plane and the ability to titrate the excision for the proper correction, better visualization, reduced risk of crankshaft, and pseudarthrosis since the disks are completely removed (146, 147). In a series reported by Hedequist et al. (147a), 18 patients underwent simultaneous exposures with excision and instrumentation at an average age of 3 years, and the authors achieved 70% correction without any neurologic complications or pseudarthroses.

Hemivertebra excision performed as a posterior-only procedure is growing in popularity since the report of Ruf and Harms (148) in 2002. They described excellent results in patients younger than 6 years who underwent posterior-only hemivertebrae excision and segmental transpedicular screw instrumentation for curves with an average Cobb angle of 45 degrees. Curve correction to 14 degrees (75%) was

Text continued on page 718

Hemivertebra Excision (Figs. 18-15 to 18-21)

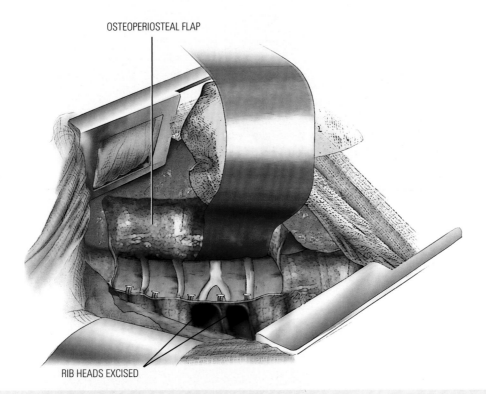

OSTEOPERIOSTEAL FLAP

RIB HEADS EXCISED

FIGURE 18-15. **Hemivertebra Excision.** The patient is taken to the operating room and placed on a standard operating table in the lateral decubitus position with the hemivertebra side facing up. Standard lateral decubitus positioning is used with an axillary roll and padding under the peroneal nerve, between the legs, under the down arm, and between the arms. In general, we prefer to flex the operating table to allow maximal visualization and opening up of the disk spaces. The patient's hemithorax and hemiabdomen are prepped from just beyond the midline anteriorly to just beyond the midline posteriorly.

Spinal cord monitoring should be done throughout the procedure and can be supplemented by a wake-up test.
If a thoracic hemivertebra is to be excised, a standard thoracotomy incision is made, removing the rib one or two levels above the hemivertebra. If the hemivertebra is at the thoracolumbar junction, a standard thoracoabdominal approach through the 11th or 10th rib may be used. This allows exposure and excision of a hemivertebra down to the L2 or L3 level. For lumbosacral junction hemivertebrae, a standard retroperitoneal approach is used. It is good practice to identify the hemivertebra to be excised with radiographic markers, such as a Keith needle, before exposure, to ensure that the correct level is approached.

In exposing the hemivertebra, after segmental vessel ligation, either an extraperiosteal or subperiosteal exposure can be used. We prefer to use a subperiosteal exposure to allow a flap with osteogenic potential to overlay the resection site. The spine must be subperiosteally exposed from the inferior aspect of the vertebral body above to the superior aspect of the vertebral body below. The osteoperiosteal flap must be elevated all the way around to the opposite side as shown. The flap allows protection of the great vessels on the concavity of the curvature.

In the thoracic spine, the rib head at the level of the hemivertebra should be removed to allow exposure of the transverse process and the disk space. The rib head at the next inferior vertebra in the thoracic spine may also need to be removed to allow for adequate exposure of the disk space. Bleeding can be controlled with bone wax.

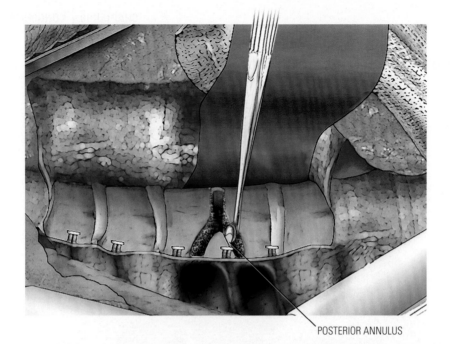

POSTERIOR ANNULUS

FIGURE 18-16. All disk materials above and below the hemivertebra are excised back to the posterior annulus using knife, curette, and rongeurs. We tend to use the rongeurs at the more superficial levels and then curettes as one approaches the posterior annulus.

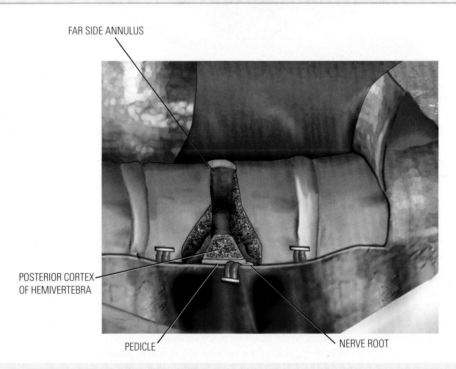

FAR SIDE ANNULUS

POSTERIOR CORTEX
OF HEMIVERTEBRA

PEDICLE

NERVE ROOT

FIGURE 18-17. The inferior end plate of the vertebra above and the superior end plate of the vertebra below must also be excised. This can be done with curettes or Cobb elevators.

It is important to leave a portion of the most lateral annulus intact to act as a stabilizing tether during the posterior hemivertebra removal and closure of the gap. It is important to excise all of the soft tissues opposite to the hemivertebra. This may appear as disk material or fibrocartilage. Failure to excise all of this tissue except for the most lateral annulus will result in ineffective closure of the gap.

After the disk material has been removed, the hemivertebra excision is begun. This can be accomplished with a burr, rongeur, or curette. We prefer to use rongeurs and curettes. The bone removed is saved to be used as bone graft in filling some of the gap anteriorly and also posteriorly. We use rongeurs to remove the bulk of the hemivertebrae and then curettes, curetting from the concave to the convex side toward the surgeon. All the cancellous bone is removed back to the posterior cortex. In the thoracic spine, the transverse process is subperiosteally dissected anteriorly and rongeured off at its base.

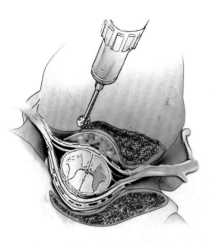

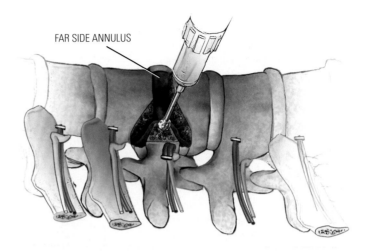

FAR SIDE ANNULUS

FIGURE 18-18. Final removal of the posterior vertebral cortex can be done in one of several ways. We prefer to use a diamond-tipped dental burr to enter the spinal canal in the midline. After a small hole is made, a small Harper-Kerrison rongeur may be used to remove the entire posterior cortex of the hemivertebra.

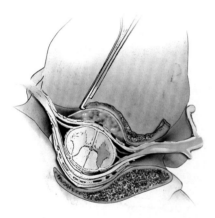

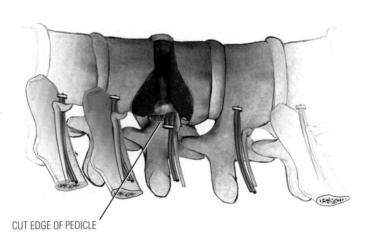

CUT EDGE OF PEDICLE

FIGURE 18-19. After the cortical bone is removed from the apex of the hemivertebra all the way back to the pedicle, the annular tissues superiorly and inferiorly can also be removed. The neural foramina both above and below the hemivertebra must be opened completely and the nerve roots visualized. Any bleeding that is encountered should be addressed with bipolar cautery or packing with thrombin-soaked Gelfoam.

The final structure removed anteriorly is the pedicle of the hemivertebra. The pedicle can be removed in several ways. It can be gradually nibbled away with narrow-nosed rongeurs or, as we prefer, the central portion drilled until decancellated followed by the outer walls being removed with either rongeurs or curettage toward the pedicle center.

The pedicle bone should be nibbled away as far posteriorly as possible.

The dura is covered with a Gelfoam or Oxycel pad or fat graft, and then bone chips from the excised hemivertebra are loosely placed into the space. The osteoperiosteal flap is then sutured back down loosely, and in the chest the pleura is repaired. The wound is then closed in the standard fashion.

The second portion of the procedure can be done in the lateral decubitus position.

However, we prefer to roll the patient prone and transfer the patient to a spine frame (e.g., Jackson table, Relton-Hall frame). In some children, we prefer to use two laminectomy rolls (made of rolled bath blankets or foam), one under the chest and one under the iliac crests, leaving the abdomen free.

FIGURE 18-20. In the posterior approach, the spine is exposed from a standard midline exposure overlying the area of the hemivertebra. A radiograph is taken to determine the appropriate level for excision. The spine is then exposed subperiosteally. The ligamentum flavum above and below the hemilamina is carefully incised and removed with the Kerrison rongeur. Any bleeding is controlled by bipolar cautery or packing with thrombin-soaked Gelfoam. After the ligamentum flavum has been removed, the hemilamina is gradually removed from the midline to its lateral aspect. We generally do this with standard narrow-nosed rongeurs or Harper-Kerrison rongeurs. It is much easier to remove the posterior arch from the posterior approach when more of the pedicle has been removed by the anterior procedure.

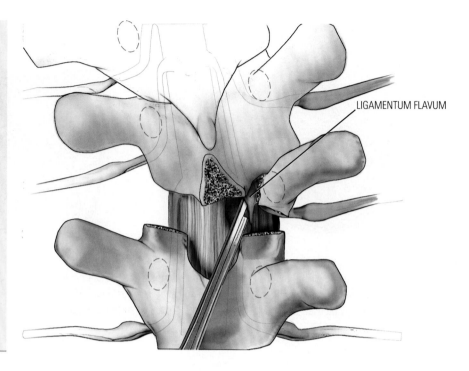

LIGAMENTUM FLAVUM

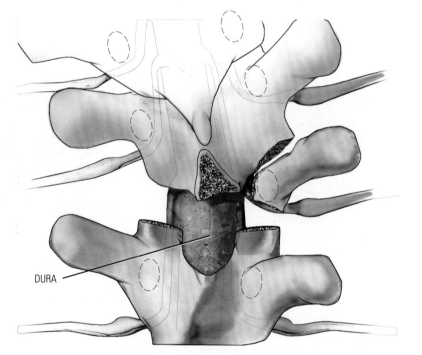

DURA

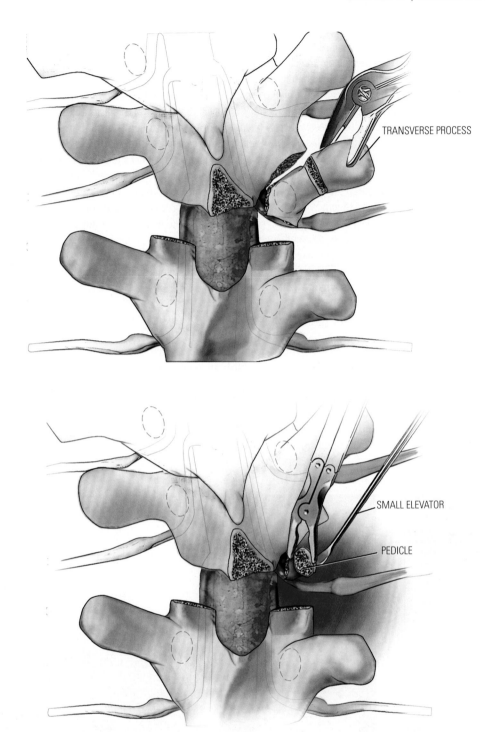

TRANSVERSE PROCESS

SMALL ELEVATOR

PEDICLE

FIGURE 18-21. In the lumbar spine, the transverse process is transected at its base with a narrow-nose or Kerrison rongeur. In the thoracic spine, if the transverse process was left intact in the anterior approach, it must be removed at this point. After the lamina, facets, and transverse processes have been completely removed, the pedicle can be grasped with a rongeur or hemostat; with one prong inside the center of the pedicle and one on the cortical margin, the pedicle is slowly removed. If resistance is encountered, it is most important to use a small elevator to free the margin of the pedicle and remove it either *in toto* or piecemeal with narrow-nose rongeurs or curettes.

After all the bone is removed, the surgeon can easily visualize the dural sac with the nerve roots above and below the hemivertebra. The surgeon must take great care when watching the closure of the apical wedge osteotomy to make certain that the downgoing pedicle does not impinge on the two nerve roots going through the single neural foramen. If there is any concern about pedicle impingement, the superior pedicle must be thinned or even excised to prevent nerve root impingement. The laminae above and below can then be decorticated and the portions of the rib removed from the anterior portion of the procedure; the morselized hemivertebrae can be used for bone graft.

FIGURE 18-21. (*Continued*) When the hemivertebra to be excised is at the lumbosacral junction, a separate incision may be necessary to expose the iliac crest and obtain cortical and cancellous bone.

In very young patients, internal fixation is generally not possible, and the defect is closed and maintained in that position by casting. In toddlers and older children, small compression devices may be applied using the rod and hook configuration. Another alternative in older patients is the use of pedicle screws in the pedicle above and below the hemivertebra, with a small rod connecting the two screw heads. If no internal fixation is used, after wound closure, the patient must be turned carefully onto a pediatric spica table and a body spica cast that includes both legs down to the ankles applied. The cast should extend proximally up to the clavicle line. The patient's torso should be bent into the convexity of the curvature to maintain correction. Radiographs should be obtained in the operating room to ensure that the wedge is closed and that adequate correction has been obtained. It is also important to make certain that pressure is applied to the apex of the deformity posteriorly while the plaster is drying, to prevent the spine from drifting into kyphosis. If adequate correction has not been obtained, the cast can be wedged while the patient is still under anesthesia. If internal fixation is used, the surgeon will decide whether casting is necessary. If the surgeon believes that the internal fixation was very stable at surgery, the patient may be placed either in a cast or a thoracolumbar spinal orthosis after surgery, with a single-leg extension, depending on the surgeon's preference. In our opinion, external immobilization is important regardless of the stability of the internal fixation.

maintained at an average 3.5 years follow-up with no neurologic complications (Fig. 18-22). The purported advantages were the avoidance of an anterior surgery with similar correction of local deformities. The use of transpedicular instrumentation at this age may raise eyebrows due to concern over the risk of closure of the neurocentral synchondrosis (NCS) and iatrogenic spinal stenosis. The NCS closes at 3 to 6 years of age,

but the spinal canal diameter at birth is already roughly two-thirds of adult size (149–151). In subsequent reports of the technique by Ruf and Harms (152, 153), no canal stenosis was found in young children upon follow-up imaging years later. However, somewhat contradictory to these findings, transpedicular instrumentation in compression mode across the NCS

Text continued on page 723

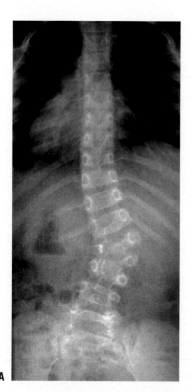
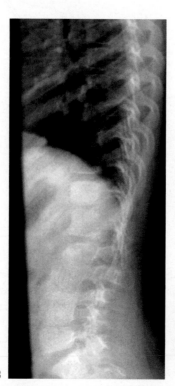
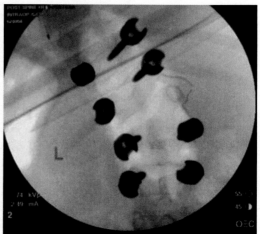

FIGURE 18-22. Posterior-only hemivertebra resection in a 5-year-old female. **A:** PA erect radiograph illustrating L1 hemivertebra. **B:** Lateral erect radiograph showing mild thoracolumbar kyphosis. **C:** Intraoperative fluoroscopy after posterior exposure to localize CVM and place pedicle screws.

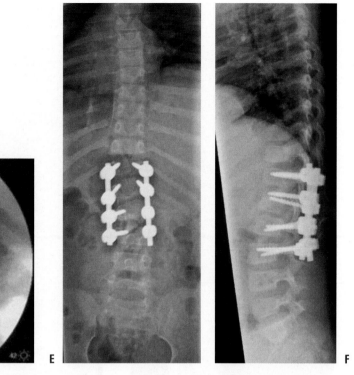

D   E   F

FIGURE 18-22.   (*Continued*) **D:** Intraoperative fluoroscopy after resection of hemivertebra and compression of pedicle screw and rod instrumentation across the convex defect and correction of scoliosis. **E:** Postoperative PA radiograph showing maintenance of correction and excellent coronal balance. **F:** Lateral erect view showing restoration of thoracolumbar lordosis.

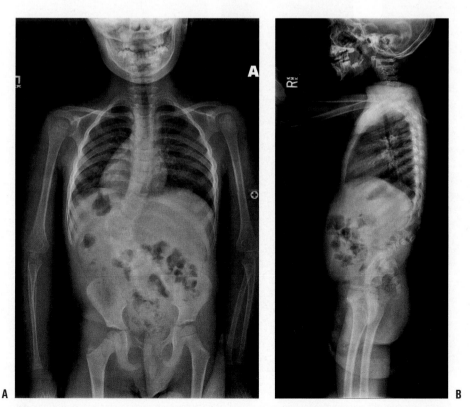

A   B

FIGURE 18-23.   Posterior-only hemivertebra excision, asymmetric pedicle subtraction osteotomy and multilevel fusion in a 4.5-year-old boy with progressive congenital kyphoscoliosis. **A:** PA erect radiograph illustrating thoracolumbar congenital scoliosis. **B:** Lateral radiograph showing thoracolumbar kyphosis near the apex of the scoliosis. **C:** Sagittal MRI scan.

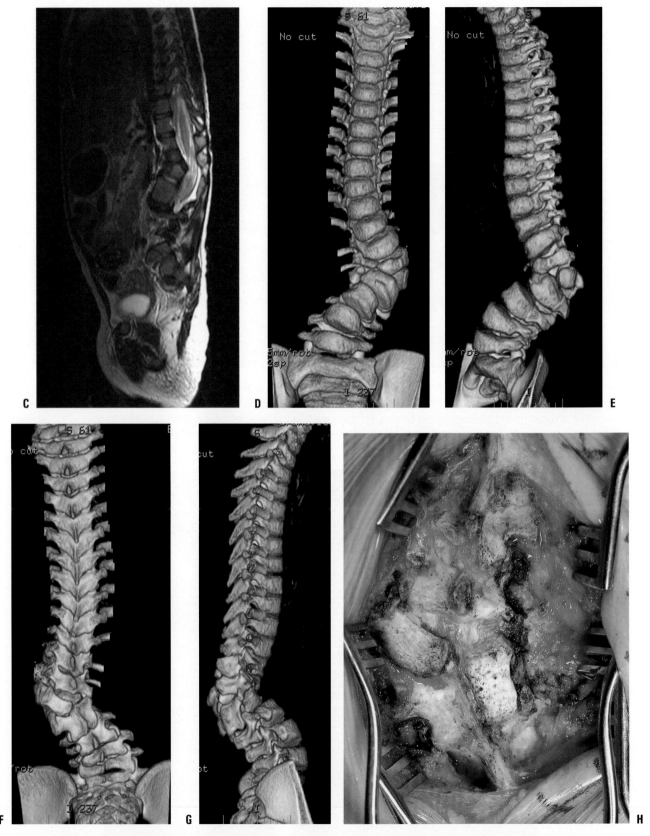

FIGURE 18-23. (*Continued*) **D-G:** Three-dimensional reconstructed CT scan in multiple planes of rotation. This type of preoperative modeling is useful for planning resection procedures in complex deformities since it identifies anatomy, confirms relationships between and anterior and posterior elements and visualizes the sagittal plane with great clarity. **H:** Intraoperative photograph after subperiosteal exposure of the levels to be treated. The posterior elements and landmarks can be correlated with the CT-scan images to confirm the level of resection.

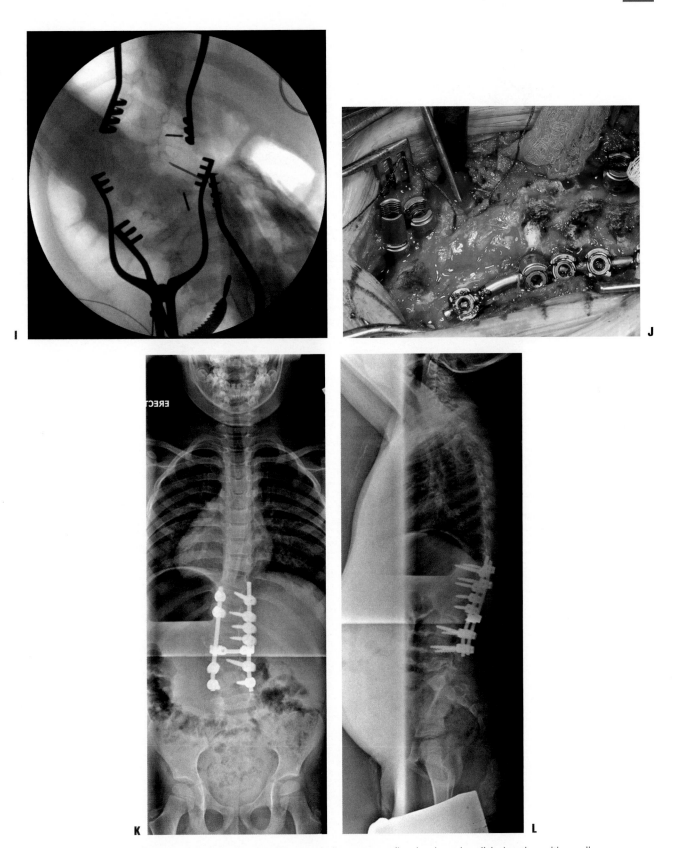

FIGURE 18-23. (*Continued*) **I:** Intraoperative fluoroscopic image to confirm levels and pedicle location with needles or Kwires. **J:** Intraoperative photograph after pedicle screw insertion, during hemivertebra resection and stabilization with temporary rod. **K,L:** PA and lateral radiographs 2 years postoperatively showing maintenance of correction and balance in both planes.

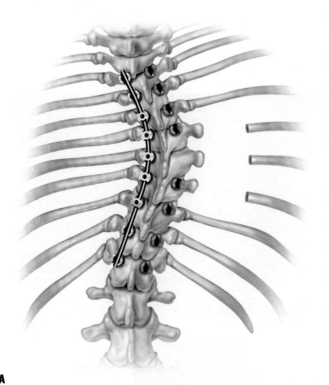

A

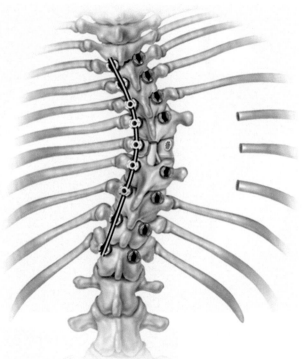

B

FIGURE 18-24. Thoracic hemivertebra resection or asymmetric vertebral column resection. **A:** Pedicle screws are inserted and temporary stabilizing rod is secured. Vertebra to be resected is identified and confirmed and corresponding rib is resected with one above and below. **B:** Laminectomy is performed with pedicle resected to base, preserving the medial wall of the pedicle (thoracic nerve root may be tied off). **C:** Osteotome is used to remove the body.

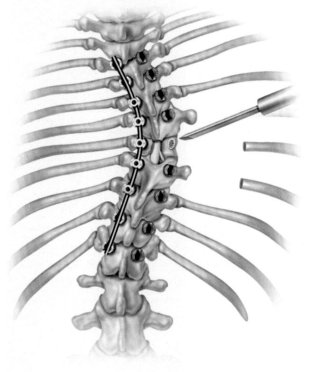

C

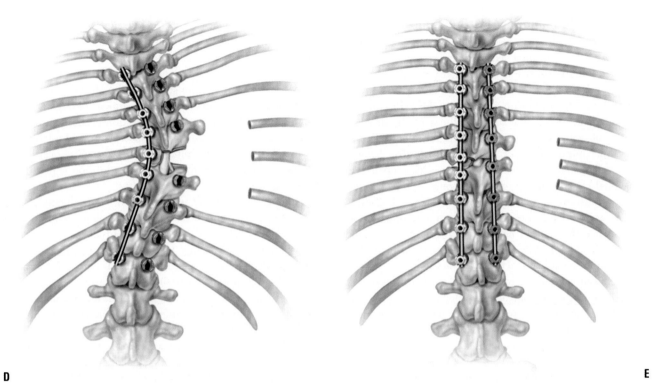

D   E

FIGURE 18-24.   (*Continued*) **D:** Pituitary rongeurs and curettes are used to remove the disks above and below. The resection must reach the concave side in order to allow the convexity to close. **E:** Temporary working rods are exchanged for the final construct, the convexity is compressed and the resection is closed (a structural cage may be necessary for anterior column support). Care is taken to avoid subluxation of the spinal column, excessive buckling of the dura or laminar impingement. (Images courtesy of James Millerick.)

(and subsequent closure) did produce canal narrowing on the ipsilateral side in a porcine study (154).

Suk et al. (155) prefers the posterior-only procedure as well, due to its decreased operative time, ability to address the deformity at the apex, and correction by controlled shortening across the resection gap. Shono et al. (156) reported obtaining 64% correction with posterior-only techniques in 12 adolescent patients and no complications. In a multicenter comparison of three techniques (hemiepiphysiodesis or *in situ* fusion, instrumented correction and fusion or instrumented hemivertebra resection) in 76 patients, Yaszay et al. (157) and the Harms Study Group showed that the resection group had better correction, shorter fusions, less blood loss, and shorter operative times, but a slightly higher complication rate.

Posterior-only resection is technically easier in a kyphotic deformity than a lordotic situation, since the apex of the deformity in kyphoscoliosis presents itself posteriorly (Fig. 18-23). Hemivertebra resection should include a costotransversectomy when performed in the thoracic spine for added exposure and visualization of the disks above and below the hemivertebra; furthermore, rib head excision creates flexibility in a stiff thoracic deformity that may become important in the correction (Fig. 18-24). Sacrifice of a thoracic nerve root is sometimes necessary for adequate exposure for resection or insertion of a structural cage.

Adequate resection of the hemivertebra is of paramount importance since excising the anomalous vertebra just to the midline, where the bony portion may end, without extension to the concave side with adequate release and division of a bar, for instance, will not result in sufficient correction of the curve. A "wedge" resection to the concave edge is usually necessary to achieve full correction of a single congenital deformity, which will theoretically prevent progression of secondary, longer curves in the noncongenital portion of the spine (158).

The ideal time for resection is dependent on many factors, but early resection is favorable before secondary structural curves develop and a longer fusion is necessary. Resection before age 2 poses challenges for stabilization with instrumentation, but casting is an option for external immobilization in the youngest patients. Early resection seems to make neurologic deficit less likely, as numerous reports advocate (148, 159). Neurologic complications are typically due to direct manipulation or contusion of the spinal cord or nerve root, or stretching (distraction) on the concave side with correction.

Contraindications to hemivertebra excision include spinal dysraphism at the same segment, inability to stabilize the resection with instrumentation or rigid external support, the presence of rigid deformities above or below the planned resection, which may not correct and cause spinal imbalance, and vascular anomalies associated with the CVM.

Fusion with Correction and Instrumentation. This procedure is commonly performed when correction of multiple segments in the congenital deformity and or secondary curves is desired and the principle of balancing the spine is most important. It should be noted that correction of the congenital part of the curve carries with it significant difficulty compared to idiopathic scoliosis due to the stiffness of the deformity and risk of neurologic deficit, but with meticulous technique and proper monitoring, safe correction is possible. Standing x-rays will define the stable zones, truncal decompensation, congenital curves, and compensatory ones. With the use of bending and/or traction x-rays, we can define the flexibility of these respective deformities and then begin to formulate a plan to rebalance the spine. Choosing levels for instrumentation can be difficult, especially in scenarios when there are multiple noncontiguous anomalies (160). The entire curve must be included, but areas above or below the congenital curve may not behave in the same manner as idiopathic scoliosis. Rigid unbalanced curves may cause shoulder imbalance or truncal decompensation and an unhappy patient. Traction x-rays may be helpful in determining how much correction will still keep reasonable balance.

The use of instrumentation allows correction and stabilization until the arthrodesis heals, and the use of titanium instrumentation allows further imaging of the spinal cord, if needed. Proper preoperative planning of the levels to be included, anatomical challenges, and instrumentation needs are paramount. The surgeon should choose a versatile system with a robust inventory of proper size implants to fit the patient and take into account the biomechanics of different rod diameters and materials when planning the correction, especially in small children.

In segmented congenital deformities, facetectomy, ligamentum flavum resection, posterior osteotomies (or resections), and anterior discectomies are useful strategies to make a long, severe, rigid curve more flexible. Patients with significant growth remaining may be candidates for anterior discectomies and fusion to obtain better rotational correction and decrease the risk of crankshaft.

The correction of severe deformities is a challenging endeavor fraught with increased neurologic risk. Osteotomies of congenital fusions or bars will aid in correction, but inherent in this arena are complications of bleeding, cord or nerve root manipulation, and frequently inadequate pedicles to obtain segmental anchorage. Whenever possible, the osteotomy should shorten the spine and rely on compression correction rather than lengthening with distraction. In the most rigid, deformed, fused, or unsegmented areas, when there is no other option, vertebral column resection (VCR) is a technique to obtain profound correction over a short segment (see below).

Osteotomy of Prior Fusion or Revision Surgery. Occasionally, patients may present with a history of previous treatment such as an *in situ* fusion, and with subsequent growth and/or progression of the deformity, they have severe, rigid curves with pain, truncal decompensation, pelvic obliquity,

or neurologic deficit. Reconstructive surgery is indicated for these patients and may be achieved by anterior or posterior osteotomies of the previous fusion including VCR to rebalance the spine and instrumentation to restore spinal imbalance and provide the best chance for stable arthrodesis (Fig. 18-25). The basic principles are similar to the treatment of large deformities mentioned above, in which resection is effective for focal correction, anterior release and/or posterior-based osteotomies are used to correct the spine or induce flexibility over longer segments, and rebalancing the spine and fusion is performed with segmental instrumentation.

Leatherman (160a) is credited with introducing a two-stage corrective procedure for severe congenital deformities in 1969. He recognized that a posterior fusion alone in a rapidly progressing deformity may not prevent further progression, particularly in cases with unilateral bars. Furthermore, he taught the principle that in order to avoid the danger of traction paraplegia (which had resulted from Harrington distraction instrumentation around that time), the spine must be shortened as well as straightened. As such, a two-stage resection of the vertebral column was described by Leatherman and Dickson (129) in 60 patients with congenital spinal deformities for whom a two-stage corrective procedure provided excellent results. The first stage was anterior resection of the vertebral body, and the second stage was posterior resection, fusion of the curve, and instrumentation. In patients with congenital scoliosis and a mean age of 11 years (2+3 years to 16+8 years), an average correction of 47% was achieved, with no significant complications including paresis. These results are especially impressive considering that nonsegmental compression and distraction instrumentation was used and surgeries were performed without contemporary monitoring.

For the rigid, focal deformities, in either a primary or revision situation, where there is no other option, VCR can obtain dramatic correction over a short segment, but even the experienced surgeon should be prepared for excessive bleeding and assume the substantial risk of neurologic deficit. Multimodality intraoperative neurologic monitoring is mandatory since more than a quarter will have intraoperative neurologic events, and transcranial motor-evoked potentials are the most sensitive for prediction of postoperative neurologic deficit and allow prompt action intraoperatively to reduce the risk of permanent injury (161). Adequate laminectomy for visualization, stabilization with temporary working rods, undercutting the ends of the resection, and anterior structural grafting with a cage (to avoid shortening) may avert spinal subluxation and cord impingement. In a prospective, multicenter study of 147 patients who underwent VCRs for pediatric spinal deformity, the overall postoperative neurologic deficit rate was 13% (0.7% permanent), most of them at the spinal cord level, and common risk factors included kyphosis, congenital abnormalities, and revision surgery (162). The overall radiographic correction rate was excellent for kyphoscoliosis (51%) and for congenital deformity (46%), and Scoliosis Research Society (SRS) scores were significantly improved in the self-image, satisfaction domains, and total scores (163) (Fig. 18-26).

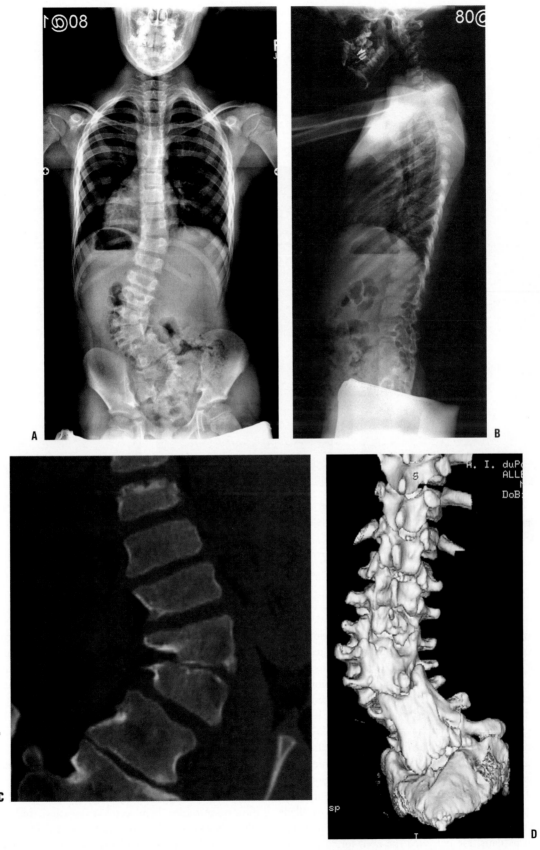

FIGURE 18-25. Osteotomy of prior fusion and revision surgery in a 10-year-old male with lumbosacral congenital scoliosis. **A,B:** PA and lateral radiographs of the boy who presented with a history of prior *in situ* fusion at age 4 with progression of the deformity, coronal and sagittal imbalance. **C,D:** CT scans showing the congenital elements and presumed pseudarthrosis.

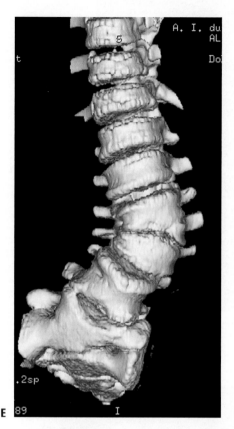

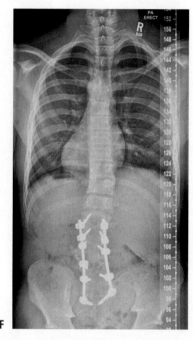

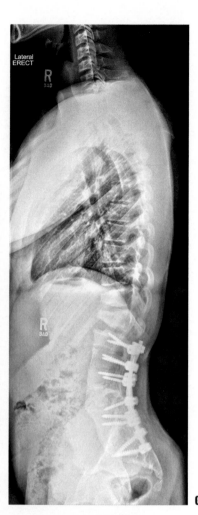

FIGURE 18-25. (*Continued*) **E:** CT scans showing the congenital elements and presumed pseudarthrosis. **F,G:** Postoperative radiographs 5 years after surgery showing excellent maintenance of correction and reconstruction of lumbar lordosis and sagittal balance.

Current segmental instrumentation has allowed earlier mobilization of the patient and improved correction, but has not decreased the technical complexity of the resection operation or the possible complications. In an effort to reduce the operative time and morbidity of staged or simultaneous anterior/posterior procedures, single posterior resections were devised. Suk et al.'s (164) series of posterior VCRs in an adult group of 38 congenital scoliosis patients described 63% correction of the scoliosis, but described major complications including paralysis, root injuries, fixation failures, infections, and hemopneumothoraces. Lenke's report of posterior VCR procedures for severe spinal deformities in 43 patients (heterogeneous group of adults and children) described excellent results with no permanent neurologic deficits in this challenging group of patients. He reiterated the need for spinal cord monitoring to prevent neurologic deficits since 18% patients lost intraoperative motor-evoked responses and promptly returned to baseline with surgical intervention (165).

The ability to treat severe deformities through an all-posterior vertebral resection has obviated the need for a circumferential approach in both primary and revision surgery except in special situations of lordotic deformities. Lenke et al. (166) reported on 35 consecutive pediatric patients who underwent posterior VCR of one to three levels; the average OR time was 460 minutes and average estimated blood loss (EBL) was 691 mL. Twelve patients had congenital scoliosis and had an average correction of 24 degrees (60%).

Considerable experience and skill are necessary to achieve results as described above and a stepwise progression with Ponte or Smith Peterson osteotomies, pedicle subtraction osteotomies, hemivertebra resection, and subsequently VCR is a reasonable approach. Careful preoperative planning, localization, and identification of complex anatomy are paramount to proper decision making for osteotomy and execution of the planned procedure. The authors have found 3D CT scans and even scaled models of the spine

Text continued on page 740

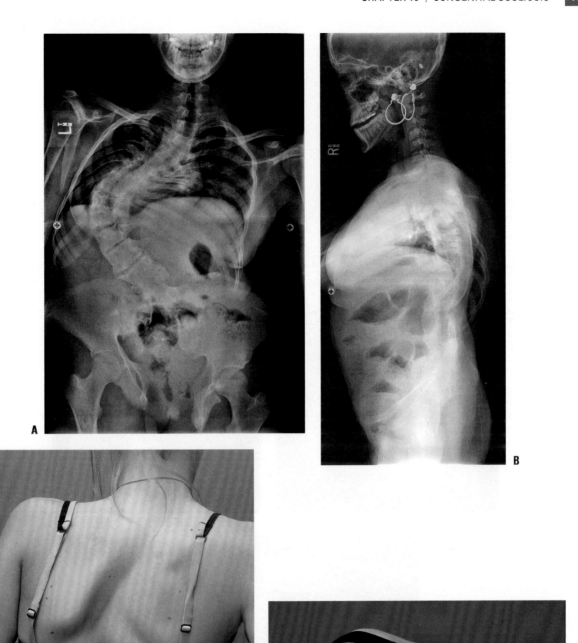

FIGURE 18-26.   Multiple vertebral column resections in a 16-year-old female with congenital scoliosis and cloacal exstrophy. **A,B:** Preoperative PA and lateral radiographs showing a scoliosis of 105 degrees 11 years after a previous *in situ* fusion of the lumbo sacral area. **C,D:** Clinical photos of the patient showing severe truncal decompensation and chest wall deformity with forward bend.

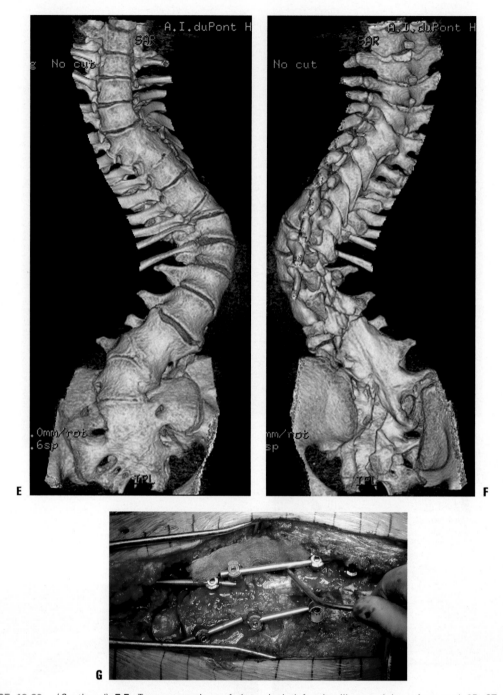

FIGURE 18-26. (*Continued*) **E,F:** Two perspectives of the spinal deformity illustrated by reformatted 3D CT scans. **G:** Intraoperative photo of the procedure showing two level VCR (L5 and T11) with temporary stabilizing rods prior to final correction.

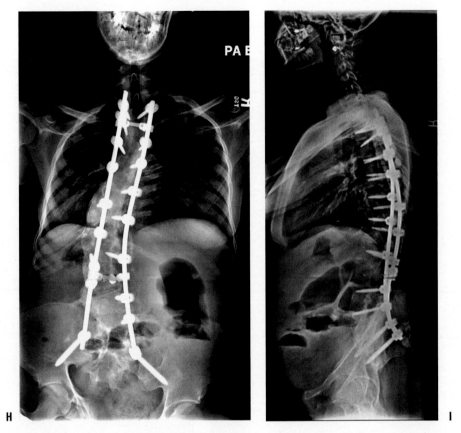

FIGURE 18-26. (*Continued*) **H,I:** PA and lateral radiographs 2 years after surgery.

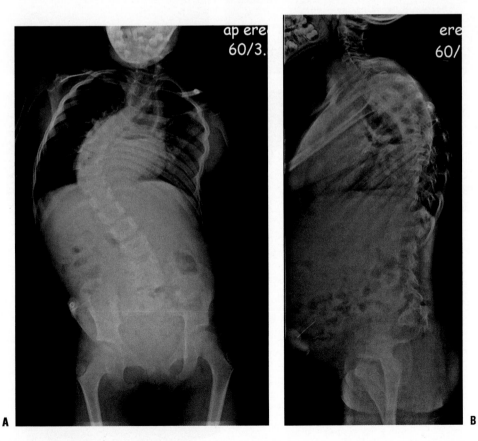

FIGURE 18-27. Growth rods in the management of congenital scoliosis in a 6-year-old female with vertebral-anus-cardio-vascular-trachea-esophagus-renal-limb-bud (VACTERL) syndrome. **A:** Erect PA radiograph showing a progressive scoliosis of 82 degrees and significant chest wall deformity. **B:** Lateral erect radiograph; note proximal thoracic kyphosis.

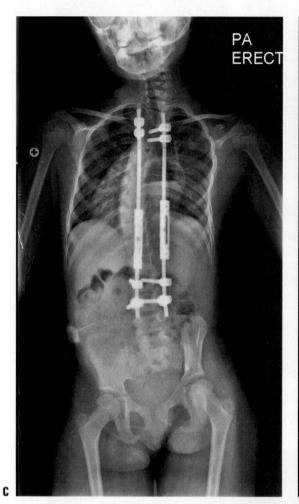

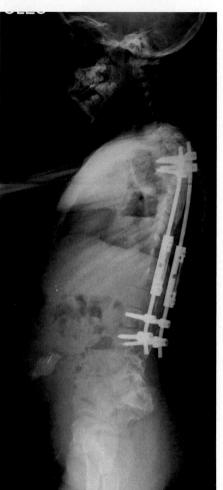

FIGURE 18-27. (*Continued*) **C,D:** Erect PA and lateral radiographs 18 months after dual growing rod implantation with fusion only at the proximal and distal anchor levels. The intervening tandem connectors at the thoracolumbar junction are lengthened every 6 months to maintain longitudinal spinal growth. **E:** Postoperative clinical photo of the patient.

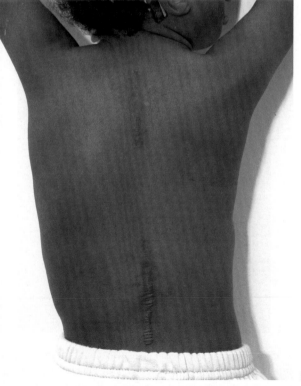

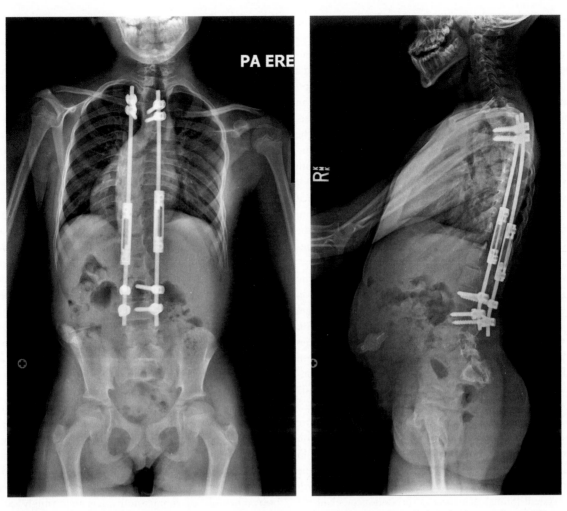

FIGURE 18-27. (*Continued*) **F,G:** Erect radiographs 4 years after initial implantation: six lengthenings and over 8.5 cm increase in T1-S1 height.

constructed from these scans to be very useful in resection and osteotomy procedures. Not infrequently, important information can be gleaned from this step in planning. The risk of substantial bleeding in any osteotomy is to be expected, and the risk of neurologic deficit (at the spinal cord level or nerve root compromise) is considerable. The surgeon's most trusted team should be present, and communication should be open and clear to prevent an intraoperative complication.

Growth Modulation and Future Directions.   An alternative to fusion techniques is the use of growing rod techniques that correct the deformity but allow for spinal growth (Fig. 18-27). Preserving growth with control of the spinal deformity in a young child is an attractive concept that may be an option in some patients, especially when the deformity is recognized and referred early in its evolution. In very young children, long

sections of the spine involved with CVMs or compensatory curves should not be fused whenever possible, especially in the thoracic spine, to avoid a significant reduction in pulmonary function (135, 167). Congenital scoliosis is associated with short stature and decreased truncal height; combining this with a multilevel spinal arthrodesis can have a further detrimental effect on spinal growth, truncal height, and pulmonary function, leading to TIS (134). The growth of the spine is the greatest in the first 5 years of life, and sitting height is about 60% of that of an adult by age 5 years (115), so growth should be encouraged in this period without sacrificing control of the curve. The use of interval lengthening of posterior spinal instrumentation without fusion, the "growing-rod" technique, has a role in the management of early-onset scoliosis, including congenital scoliosis (145) without rib fusions. The growing rod technique is effective and reliable for treating congenital deformities in growing children if the CVM segments are somewhat flexible, the anomalous segment is too large for resection, or other definitive treatment or is accompanied by a long, structural compensatory curve. The most commonly used dual rod systems have been described by Akbarnia and Thompson with moderate success; modest gains in spinal length of 3 to 7 cm (1.2 cm per year); improvement in SAL; and an acceptable complication rate of superficial infections, dislodged implants, and broken rods (168, 138). The technique involves anchorage at the proximal and distal stable zones with hooks or screws after subperiosteal dissection; fusion is desirable in these small areas away from the apex for anchor stability. Rods are then tunneled submuscularly joined by tandem connectors placed at the thoracolumbar junction, where the interval distraction is performed for lengthening the spine. An apical fusion, excision, or osteotomy for the congenital portion of the curve can be performed and then growing rods implanted to lengthen the spine and accommodate growth in the compensatory curve(s) (169). Apical fusions in patients with single-rod growing systems do create challenges such as increased force to lengthen and smaller gains (170, 171) as well as crankshaft, but with dual rods these difficulties may be obviated. The vertical expandable prosthetic titanium rib (VEPTR) device is indicated for use in patients with congenital scoliosis and fused ribs to address thoracic hypoplasia and prevent TIS when a large amount of growth remains (172) (see below). Unfortunately, both of these approaches require a scheduled operative lengthening recommended at 6-month intervals and ultimately are treated with a spinal fusion in most cases when no further lengthening can be achieved or the accelerative phase of growth is over. An alternative is a growth guidance system (Shilla) that corrects the scoliotic apex of the curve with a limited fusion and allows for continued guided growth at the proximal and distal portions of the spine, avoiding the need for routine operative lengthenings. Clinical data are limited, but McCarthy et al. (173) caprine animal model showed an average of 48 mm of growth at the ends of the rods near the sliding screws over 6 months. There were no implant failures, but minor wear debris was observed.

VEPTR (VERTICAL EXPANDABLE PROSTHETIC TITANIUM RIB)

The VEPTR was developed by Campbell (174) for the management of TIS. This heterogeneous group of conditions is defined as those in which the function of the thorax is insufficient to support normal growth and development. These conditions may be naturally occurring or can be iatrogenic. All forms of early onset scoliosis, many skeletal dysplasias, and congenital or acquired chest wall deformities including early spinal fusions are included. VEPTR devices currently are used under a humanitarian device exemption status by the FDA after undergoing an IDE trial in the early 2000s. This status requires institutions using the device to have an active institutional review board approval and restricts its use to neuro-

muscular scoliosis conditions, congenital scoliosis, constricted hemithorax conditions such as fused ribs or costal dysplasias, and acquired severe chest wall deficiencies.

Historically, it was believed that growth of vertebral segments within a region of congenital malformations did not occur. As such, treatments focused on short-segment fusions and convex hemiepiphysiodesis that would include segments outside of the malformed segment in an effort to gain compensatory correction. The notion that guided or forced growth management of congenital scoliosis deformities could not be done in congenital abnormalities was challenged by Campbell et al. (175) with their use of rib-based systems using the VEPTR (Fig. 18-28). In an uncontrolled and nonselective group of patients with congenial scoliosis with and without rib fusions, application of rib–to-rib– or rib-to-spine–based distraction devices with an expansion thoracoplasty (174) led to elongation of the concave side of the deformity by an average of 8 mm/year and of the convex side by 8.3 mm/year over mean follow-up of 4 years. Stabilization of the spinal deformity and secondary overall increase in lung volumes has been reported (175), leading many to believe that the combination of congenital spinal malformations and rib fusions is the ideal situation under which to use VEPTR devices (176–182).

The technique of VEPTR for congenital scoliosis and fused ribs has been described in detail by Campbell et al. (174, 175). The key components are an opening wedge thoracostomy through the fused rib segments, a lateral rib-to-rib–based strut, and a medial rib-to-rib– or rib-to-spine–based hybrid construct (Fig. 18-28A–D). In the absence of fused ribs, the role of thoracostomy has increasingly come into question due to concerns about altered chest wall compliance with the scarring created by the procedure. Rib anchors are recommended to be just lateral to the rib heads and avoidance of anchors above the 2nd rib is recommended due to the risk of brachial plexus injuries by proximal migration of the anchors (176, 183). Subperiosteal dissection of the ribs is done for placement of the rib cradles, and with the introduction of VEPTR II, multiple anchor points and ribs can now be used. Distal spine anchors are designed to be via laminar hooks. The off-label use of pedicle screw anchors has been introduced with recommendations to have at least two distal anchors to decrease the incidence of screw migration through the pedicles. We have found that use of a ventriculoperitoneal shunt passer and chest tube facilitates submuscular passage of the hybrid rod for cases that will have a distal spine anchor. No standard exists for the frequency of expansions. Borrowing from the experience of "growing rod" systems, recommendations have been for intervals of 6 months to optimize spinal growth (178, 184).

The incidence of complications related to the use of VEPTR implants has paralleled that of other growth preservation systems. Anchor migration, implant failure, wound infections, and loss of control of the deformity have all been reported (185–187).

VEPTR (Vertical Expandable Prosthetic Titanium Rib) (Fig. 18-28)

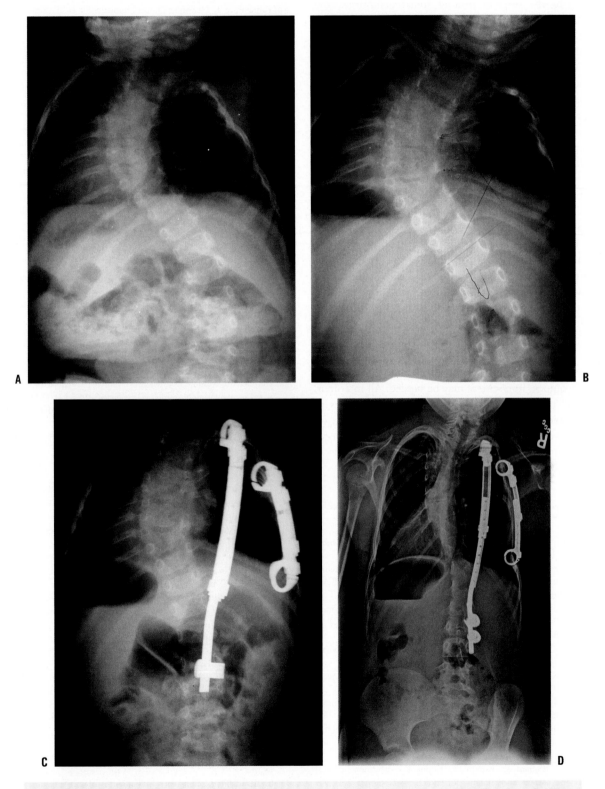

FIGURE 18-28. Congenital scoliosis with multiple fused ribs **A:** 6-month-old female. **B:** Age 20 months. **C:** VEPTR implantation age; 23 months **D:** Age 11 years.

CONCLUSIONS

The treatment of congenital scoliosis is among the most interesting to the surgeon treating spinal deformities and focuses on early diagnosis and surgical treatment before large curves develop. The authors cannot emphasize enough the importance of the observational period of the treatment of patients with congenital scoliosis, namely giving thought to the evolution of the deformity with growth and acting at the appropriate time if surgery is necessary. Vertebral anomalies with a progressive natural history need to be managed aggressively. Outcomes are generally better with simple procedures with a favorable complication profile. *In situ* fusion or hemiepiphysiodesis are viable options if there is little to no deformity present, but the potential for progression is high. For moderate deformities, correction with instrumentation and arthrodesis will provide satisfactory results. Young children with an isolated hemivertebra are excellent candidates for resection if progression is noted; this keeps the area of arthrodesis small and avoids the development of compensatory curves. Extensive spinal arthrodesis should be avoided, especially before age 5, and growing rods can be used in children with long segmented areas of the spine to modulate growth and control the curve. TIS and congenital scoliosis with fused ribs seems to be best managed by the VEPTR device and expansion thoracostomy. For severe, rigid deformities in older children, osteotomies or resections to rebalance the spine with attention to the more structural compensatory curves may be needed. All too often, in a referral practice, we have seen missed opportunities in which a simpler procedure could have been performed, saving the patient and family from a much larger, complicated procedure and protracted recovery.

REFERENCES

1. Jones K, Smith DW. *Smith's recognizable patterns of human malformation,* Edited 857. Philadelphia, PA: Saunders, 1997.
2. Erol B, Tracy MR, Dormans JP, et al. Congenital scoliosis and vertebral malformations: characterization of segmental defects for genetic analysis. *J Pediatr Orthop* 2004;24(6):674–682.
3. Giampietro PF, et al. Progress in the understanding of the genetic etiology of vertebral segmentation disorders in humans. *Ann N Y Acad Sci* 2009;1151:38–67.
4. Hedequist D, Emans J. Congenital scoliosis: a review and update. *J Pediatr Orthop* 2007;27(1):106–116.
5. Hensinger RN. Congenital scoliosis: etiology and associations. *Spine (Phila PA 1976)* 2009;34:1745–1750.
6. Tanaka T, Uhthoff HK. Significance of resegmentation in the pathogenesis of vertebral body malformation. *Acta Orthop Scand* 1981;52:331–338.
7. Tanaka T, Uhthoff HK. The pathogenesis of congenital vertebral malformations: a study based on observations made in 11 human embryos and fetuses. *Acta Orthop Scand* 1981;52:413–425.
8. Tracy MR, Dormans JP, Kusumi K. Klippel-Feil syndrome: clinical features and current understanding of etiology. *Clin Orthop Relat Res* 2004;424:183–190.
9. Alexander PG, Tuan RS. Carbon monoxide-induced axial skeletal dysmorphogenesis in the chick embryo. *Birth Defects Res A Clin Mol Teratol* 2003;67(4):219–230.
10. Dequeant M, Pourquie O. Segmental patterning of the vertebrate embryonic axis. *Nat Rev Genet* 2008;9:370–382.
11. Kessel M, Gruss P. Murine developmental control genes. *Science* 1990;249:374–379.
12. Palmeirium I, Henrique D, Ish-Horowicz D, et al. Avian hairy gene expression identifies a molecular clock linked to vertebrate segmentation and somitogenesis. *Cell* 1997;91:639–648.
13. Shinkai Y, Tjuji T, Kawamoto Y, et al. New mutant mouse with skeletal deformities caused by mutation in delta like 3 (DLL3) gene. *Exp Anim* 2004;53:129–136.
14. Thomsen B, et al. A missense mutation in the bovine SLC35A3 gene, encoding a UDP-N-acetylglucosamine transporter, causes complex vertebral malformation. *Genome Res* 2006;16:97–105.
15. Shands AR, Eisberg HB. The incidence of scoliosis in the state of Delaware; a study of 50,000 minifilms of the chest made during a survey for tuberculosis. *J Bone Joint Surg Am* 1955;37:1243–1249.
16. Forrester MB, Merz RD. Descriptive epidemiology of hemivertebrae, Hawaii, 1986–2002. *Congenit Anom (Kyoto)* 2006;46(4):172–176.
17. Goldstein I, Makhoul IR, Weissman A, et al. Hemivertebra: prenatal diagnosis, incidence and characteristics. *Fetal Diagn Ther* 2005;20(2):121–126.
18. Ganey TM, Ogden JA. Development and maturation of the axial skeleton. In: Weinstein SL, ed. *The pediatric spine.* Philadelphia, PA: Lippincott Williams & Wilkins, 2001:3–54.
19. Mark M, Rijli FM, Chambon P. Homeobox genes in embryogenesis and pathogenesis. *Pediatr Res* 1997;42:421–429.
20. Giampietro PF, et al. Congenital and idiopathic scoliosis: clinical and genetic aspects. *Clin Med Res* 2003;1(2):125–136.
21. Fan C, Porter JA, Chiang C, et al. Long-range sclerotome induction by sonic hedgehog: direct role of the amino-terminal cleavage product and modulation by the cyclic AMP signaling pathway. *Cell* 1995;81:457–465.
22. Conlon RQ, Reaume AG, Rossant J. Notch 1 is required for the coordinated segmentation of somites. *Development* 1995;121:1533–1545.
23. Pourquie O. Building the spine: the vertebrate segmentation clock. *Cold Spring Harb Symp Quant Biol* 2007;72:445–449.
24. Pourquie O, Kusumi K. When body segmentation goes wrong. *Clin Genet* 2001;60:409–416.
25. Farley FA, Loder RT, Nolan BT, et al. Mouse model for thoracic congenital scoliosis. *J Pediatr Orthop* 2001;21(4):537–540.
26. Farley FA, Phillips WA, Herzenberg JE, et al. Natural history of scoliosis in congenital heart disease. *J Pediatr Orthop* 1991;11(1):42–47.
27. Loder RT, Hernandez MJ, Lerner AL, et al. The induction of congenital spinal deformities in mice by maternal carbon monoxide exposure. *J Pediatr Orthop* 2000;20(5):662–666.
28. Norman CA, Halton DM. Is carbon monoxide a workplace teratogen? A review and evaluation of the literature. *Am Occup Hyg* 1990;34:335–347.
29. Tredwell SJ, Smith DF, Macleod PJ, et al. Cervical spine anomalies in fetal alcohol syndrome. *Spine (Phila Pa 1976)* 1982;7:331–334.
30. Bantz EW. Valproic acid and congenital malformations. A case report. *Clin Pediatr (Phila)* 1984;23:352–353.
31. Giavini E, Menegola E. Gene-teratogen interactions in chemically induced congenital malformations. *Biol Neonate* 2004;85:73–81.
32. Hanold KC. Teratogenic potential of valproic acid. *J Obstet Gynecol Neonatal Nurs* 1986;15:111–116.
33. Wide K, Winbladh B, Kallen B. Major malformations in infants exposed to antiepileptic drugs in utero, with emphasis on carbamazepine and valproic acid: a nation-wide, population-based register study. *Acta Paediatr* 2004;93(2):174–176.
34. Edwards MF. Hyperthermia as a teratogen: a review of experimental studies and their clinical significance. *Teratog Carcinog Mutagen* 1986;6:563–582.
35. Ewart-Toland A, Yankowitz J, Winder A, et al. Oculoauriculovertebral abnormalities in children of diabetic mothers. *Am J Med Genet* 2000;90:303–309.
36. Lowy C, Beard RW, Goldschmidt J. Congenital malformations in babies of diabetic mothers. *Diabet Med* 1986;3(5):458–462.

37. De Wals P, et al. Reduction in neural-tube defects after folic acid fortification in Canada. *N Engl J Med* 2007;357:135–142.

38. Huppert SS, Le A, Schroeter EH, et al. Embryonic lethality in mice homozygous for a processing-deficient allele of Notch-1. *Nature* 2000;405:966–970.

39. McMaster MJ. Congenital scoliosis caused by a unilateral failure of vertebral segmentation with contralateral hemivertebrae. *Spine (Phila Pa 1976)* 1998;23(9):998–1005.

40. Wynne-Davies R. Congenital vertebral anomalies: aetiology and relationship to spina bifida cystica. *J Med Genet* 1975;12:280–288.

41. Bulman MP, et al. Mutations in the human delta homologue, DLL3, cause axial skeletal defects in spondylocostal dysostosis. *Nat Genet* 2000;24:438–441.

42. Giampietro PF, et al. DLL3 as a candidate gene for vertebral malformations. *Am J Med Genet A* 2006;140(22):2447–2453.

43. Hutchinson J. Deformity of shoulder girdle. *Br Med J* 1894;1:634.

44. Klippel M, Feil A. Un cas d'absence des vertebres cervicales. *Nouv Icon Salpet* 1912;25:223.

45. Clarke RA, Singh S, McKenzie H, et al. Familial Klippel-Feil syndrome and paracentric inversion inv(8)(q22.2q23.3). *Am J Hum Genet* 1995;57:1364–1370.

46. McGaughran JA, Oates D, Donnai D, et al. Mutations in PAX1 may be associated with Klippel-Feil syndrome. *Eur J Hum Genet* 2003;11:468–474.

47. Thomsen MB, Schneider U, Weber M, et al. Scoliosis and congenital anomalies associated with Klippel-Feil syndrome types I-III. *Spine (Phila Pa 1976)* 1997;22(4):396–401.

48. Auleha A, Wehrle C, Brand-Sberi B, et al. Wnt3a plays a major role in the segmentation clock controlling somitogenesis. *Dev Cell* 2003;4(3):407–418.

49. Beals RK, Robbins JR, Rolfe B. Anomalies associated with vertebral malformations. *Spine (Phila Pa 1976)* 1993;18(10):1329–1332.

50. Basu PS, Elsebaie H, Noordeen MH. Congenital spinal deformity: a comprehensive assessment at presentation. *Spine (Phila Pa 1976)* 2002;27(20):2255–2259.

51. Bradford DS, Heithoff KB, Cohen M. Intraspinal abnormalities and congenital spine deformities: a radiographic and MRI study. *J Pediatr Orthop* 1991;11:36–41.

52. McMaster MJ. Occult intraspinal anomalies and congenital scoliosis. *J Bone Joint Surg Am* 1984;66(4):588–601.

53. Prahinski JR, Polly DW, McHale KA, et al. Occult intraspinal anomalies in congenital scoliosis. *J Pediatr Orthop* 2000;20(1):59–63.

54. Tori JA, Dickson JH. Association of congenital anomalies of the spine and kidneys. *Clin Orthop Relat Res* 1980;148:259–262.

55. Belmont PJ, Kuko TR, Taylor KF, et al. Intraspinal anomalies associated with isolated congenital hemivertebra: the role of routine magnetic resonance imaging. *J Bone Joint Surg Am* 2004;86-A:1704–1710.

56. Cardoso M, Keating RF. Neurosurgical management of spinal dysraphism and neurogenic scoliosis. *Spine (Phila Pa 1976)* 2009;34:1775–1782.

57. Fribourg D, Delgado E. Occult spinal cord abnormalities in children referred for orthopedic complaints. *Am J Orthop* 2004;33(1):18–25.

58. Reckles LN, Peterson HA, Weidman WH, et al. The association of scoliosis and congenital heart defects. *J Bone Joint Surg Am* 57(4):449–55:1975.

59. MacEwen GD, Winter RB, Hardy JH, et al. Evaluation of kidney anomalies in congenital scoliosis. *Clin Orthop Relat Res* 1972;434:4–7.

60. Rai AS, Taylor TK, Smith GH, et al. Congenital abnormalities of the urogenital tract in association with congenital vertebral malformations. *J Bone Joint Surg Br* 2002;84(6):891–895.

61. Vitko RJ, Cass AS, Winter RB. Anomalies of the genitourinary tract associated with congenital scoliosis and congenital kyphosis. *J Urol* 108:655–659.

62. Berend N, Marlin GE. Arrest of alveolar multiplication in kyphoscoliosis. *Pathology* 1979;11:485–491.

63. Bergofsky EH. Respiratory failure in disorders of the thoracic cage. *Am Rev Respir Dis* 1979;119:643–669.

64. Campbell RM Jr, et al. The characteristics of thoracic insufficiency syndrome associated with fused ribs and congenital scoliosis. *J Bone Joint Surg Am* 2003;85-A(3):399–408.

65. Caubet JF, et al. Increased hemoglobin levels in patients with early onset scoliosis. *Spine (Phila Pa 1976)* 2009;34:2534–2536.

66. Davies G, Reid L. Effect of scoliosis on growth of alveoli and pulmonary arteries and on right ventricle. *Arch Dis Child* 1971;46:623–632.

67. Day GA, Upadhyay SS, Ho EK, et al. Pulmonary functions in congenital scoliosis. *Spine(Phila Pa 1976)* 1994;19(9):1027–1031.

68. Mayer OH, Redding G. Early changes in pulmonary function after vertical expandable prosthetic titanium rib insertion in children with thoracic insufficiency syndrome. *J Pediatr Orthop* 2009;29:35–38.

69. McMaster MJ, Glasby MA, Singh H, et al. Lung function in congenital kyphosis and kyphoscoliosis. *J Spinal Disord Tech* 2007;20(3):203–208.

70. Motoyama EK, Deeney VF, Fine GF, et al. Effects on lung function of multiple expansion thoracoplasty in children with thoracic insufficiency syndrome: a longitudinal study. *Spine(Phila Pa 1976)* 2006;31(3):284–290.

71. Redding G, Song K, Inscore S, et al. Lung function asymmetry in children with congenital and infantile scoliosis. *Spine J* 2008;8(4):639–644.

72. Siegler D, Zorab PA. The influence of lung volume on gas transfer in scoliosis. *Br J Dis Chest* 1982;76:44–50.

73. Owange-Iraka JW, Harrison A, Warner JO. Lung function in congenital and idiopathic scoliosis. *Eur J Pediatr* 1984;142:198–200.

74. Bowen RE, Scaduto AA, Banuelos S. Decreased body mass index and restrictive lung disease in congenital thoracic scoliosis. *J Pediatr Orthop* 2008;28(6):665–668.

75. Muirhead A, Conner AN. The assessment of lung function in children with scoliosis. *J Bone Joint Surg Br* 1985;67(5):699–702.

76. Kuhns JG, Hormell RS. Management of congenital scoliosis; review of one hundred seventy cases. *AMA Arch Surg* 1952;65:250–263.

77. Winter RB, Moe JH. Congenital scoliosis a study of 234 patients treated and untreated. Part I: natural history. *J Bone Joint Surg Am* 1968;50-A:1–47.

78. MacEwen GD, Conway JJ, Miller WT. Congenital scoliosis with a unilateral bar. *Radiology* 1968;90:711–715.

79. Kawakami N, Tsuji T, Imagama S, et al. Classification of congenital scoliosis and kyphosis: a new approach to the three-dimensional classification for progressive vertebral anomalies requiring operative treatment. *Spine (Phila Pa 1976)* 2009;34:1756–1765.

80. McMaster MJ, Ohtsuka K. The natural history of congenital scoliosis. *J Bone Joint Surg Am* 1982;64:1128–1147.

81. McMaster MJ, Singh H. Natural history of congenital kyphosis and kyphoscoliosis. A study of one hundred and twelve patients. *J Bone Joint Surg Am* 1999;81(10):1367–83.

82. Nasca RJ, Stilling FH III, Stell HH. Progression of congenital scoliosis due to hemivertebrae and hemivertebrae with bars. *J Bone Joint Surg Am* 1975;57(4):456–466.

83. Winter RB, Moe JH, Wang JF. Congenital kyphosis: its natural history and treatment as observed in a study of one hundred thirty patients. *J Bone Joint Surg Am* 1973;55:223–256.

84. Batra S, Ahuja S. Congenital scoliosis: management and future directions. *Acta Orthop Belg* 2008;74(2):147–160.

85. Goldberg CJ, Moore DP, Fogarty EE, et al. The natural history of early onset scoliosis. *Stud Health Technol Inform* 2002;91:68–70.

86. Campbell RM Jr, Hell-Vocke AK. Growth of the thoracic spine in congenital scoliosis after expansion thoracoplasty. *J Bone Joint Surg Am* 2003;85-A(3):409–420.

87. Pehrsson K, Larsson S, Oden A, et al. Long-term follow-up of patients with untreated scoliosis. A study of mortality, causes of death and symptoms. *Spine (Phila Pa 1976)* 1992;17:1091–1096.

88. Vitale MG, et al. Health-related quality of life in children with thoracic insufficiency syndrome. *J Pediatr Orthop* 2008;28:239–243.

89. Chan G, Dormans JP. Update on congenital spinal deformities: preoperative evaluation. *Spine (Phila Pa 1976)* 2009;34:1766–1774.

90. McMaster MJ, Singh H. The surgical management of congenital kyphosis and kyphoscoliosis. *Spine (Phila Pa 1976)* 2001;26(19):2146–2154; discussion 2155.

91. Suh SW, Sarwark JF, Vora A, et al. Evaluating congenital spine deformities for intraspinal anomalies with magnetic resonance imaging. *J Pediatr Orthop* 2001;21(4):525–531.

92. von Koch CS, Orit AG, Goldstein RB, et al. Fetal magnetic resonance imaging enhances detection of spinal cord anomalies in patients with sonographically detected bony anomalies of the spine. *J Ultrasound Med* 2005;24:781–789.

93. Lowe LH, Johanek AJ, Moore CW. Sonography of the neonatal spine: part 2, spinal disorders. *AJR Am J Roentgenol* 2007;188:739–744.

94. Lowe LH, Johanek AJ, Moore CW. Sonography of the neonatal spine: part I, normal anatomy, imaging pitfalls, and variations that may simulate disorders. *AJR Am J Roentgenol* 2007;188:733–738.

95. Medina LS. Spinal dysraphism: categorizing risk to optimize imaging. *Pediatr Radiol* 2009;39(Suppl 2):S242–S246.

96. Riccio AI, Guille JT, Grissom L, et al. Magnetic resonance imaging of renal abnormalities in patients with congenital osseous anomalies of the spine. *J Bone Joint Surg Am* 2007;89:2456–2459.

97. Beydon N. et al. An official American thoracic society/European respiratory society statement: pulmonary function testing in preschool children. *Am J Respir Crit Care Med* 2007;175:1304–1345.

98. De Jong PA, Long FR, Wong JC, et al. Computed tomographic estimation of lung dimensions throughout the growth period. *Eur Respir J* 2006;27:261–267.

99. Emans JB, Caubet JF, Ordonez CL, et al. The treatment of spine and chest wall deformities with fused ribs by expansion thoracostomy and insertion of vertical expandable prosthetic titanium rib: growth of thoracic spine and improvement of lung volumes. *Spine (Phila Pa 1976)* 2005;30(Suppl 17):S58–S68.

100. Gollogly S, Smith JT, White SK, et al. The volume of lung parenchyma as a function of age: a review of 1050 normal CT scans of the chest with three-dimensional volumetric reconstruction of the pulmonary system. *Spine (Phila Pa 1976)* 2004;29:2061–2066.

101. Redding G, Song KM, Swanson J, et al. V/Q asymmetry changes following treatment of TIS. In: Proceedings of the 44th Annual Meeting of the Scoliosis Research Society. San Antonio, TX, 2009.

102. O'Daniel JC, Stevens DM, Cody DD. Reducing radiation exposure from survey CT scans. *AJR Am J Roentgenol* 2005;185:509–515.

103. Paterson A, Frush DP. Dose reduction in paediatric MDCT: general principles. *Clin Radiol* 2007;62:507–517.

104. Paterson A, Frush DP, Donnelly LF. Helical CT of the body: are settings adjusted for pediatric patients? *AJR Am J Roentgenol* 2001;176:297–301.

105. Swift AJ, Woodhouse N, Fichele S, et al. Rapid lung volumetry using ultrafast dynamic magnetic resonance imaging during forced vital capacity maneuver: correlation with spirometry. *Invest Radiol* 2007;42:37–41.

106. Voorhees A, An J, Berger KI, et al. Magnetic resonance imaging-based spirometry for regional assessment of pulmonary function. *Magn Reson Med* 2005;54:1146–1154.

107. Facanha-Filho FAM, Winter RB, Lonstein JE, et al. Measurement accuracy in congenital scoliosis. *J Bone Joint Surg Am* 2001;83(1):42–45.

108. Heckman JD, et al. Statistical differences: consider the methodology. *J Bone Joint Surg Am* 2002;84:1078.

109. Loder RT, Urguhart A, Steen H, et al. Variability in cobb angle measurements in children with congenital scoliosis. *J Bone Joint Surg Br* 1995;77:768–770.

110. Campbell RM Jr, et al. The effect of opening wedge thoracostomy on thoracic insufficiency syndrome associated with fused ribs and congenital scoliosis. *J Bone Joint Surg Am* 2004;86-A(8):1659–1674.

111. Hedequist DJ, Emans JB. The correlation of preoperative three-dimensional computed tomography reconstructions with operative findings in congenital scoliosis. *Spine (Phila Pa 1976)* 2003;28(22):2531–2534; discussion 1.

112. Newton PO, Hahn GW, Fricka KB, et al. Utility of three-dimensional and multiplanar reformatted computed tomography for evaluation of pediatric congenital spine abnormalities. *Spine (Phila Pa 1976)* 2002;27(8):844–850.

113. Hedequist DJ. Surgical treatment of congenital scoliosis. *Orthop Clin North Am* 2007;38(4): 497–509, vi.

114. Marks DS, Qaimkhani SA. The natural history of congenital scoliosis and kyphosis. *Spine (Phila Pa 1976)* 2009;34(17):1751–1755.

115. Dimeglio A. Growth of the spine before age 5 years. *J Pediatr Orthop B* 1993;1(2):102–107.

116. Doody MM, Lonstein JE, Stovall M, et al. Breast cancer mortality after diagnostic radiography: findings from the U.S. Scoliosis Cohort Study. *Spine (Phila Pa 1976)* 2000;25(16):2052–2063.

117. Loder RT, Urquhart A, Steen H, et al. Variability in Cobb angle measurements in children with congenital scoliosis. *J Bone Joint Surg Br* 1995;77(5):768–770.

118. Prahinski JR, Polly DW Jr, McHale KA, et al. Occult intraspinal anomalies in congenital scoliosis. *J Pediatr Orthop* 2000;20(1):59–63.

119. Winter RB, Moe JH, MacEwen GD, et al. The Milwaukee brace in the nonoperative treatment of congenital scoliosis. *Spine* 1976;1:85–96.

120. Sink EL, Karol LA, Sanders J, et al. Efficacy of perioperative halo-gravity traction in the treatment of severe scoliosis in children. *J Pediatr Orthop* 2001;21(4):519–524.

121. Rinella A, Lenke L, Whitaker C, et al. Perioperative halo-gravity traction in the treatment of severe scoliosis and kyphosis. *Spine (Phila Pa 1976)* 2005;30(4):475–482.

122. Sponseller PD, Takenaga RK, Newton P, et al. The use of traction in the treatment of severe spinal deformity. *Spine (Phila Pa 1976)* 2008;33(21):2305–2309.

123. Watanabe K, Lenke LG, Bridwell KH, et al. Efficacy of perioperative halo-gravity traction for treatment of severe scoliosis. *J Orthop Sci* 2010;15(6):720–730.

124. Roaf R. The treatment of progressive scoliosis by unilateral growth-arrest. *J Bone Joint Surg Br* 1963;45:637–651.

125. Hall JE, Herndon WA, Levine CR. Surgical treatment of congenital scoliosis with or without Harrington instrumentation. *J Bone Joint Surg Am* 1981;63:608–619.

126. Dubousset J, Herring JA, Shufflebarger H. The crankshaft phenomenon. *J Pediatr Orthop* 1989;9(5):541–550.

127. Terek RM, Wehner J, Lubicky JP. Crankshaft phenomenon in congenital scoliosis: a preliminary report. *J Pediatr Orthop* 1991;11(4):527–532.

128. Kesling KL, Lonstein JE, Denis F, et al. The crankshaft phenomenon after posterior spinal arthrodesis for congenital scoliosis: a review of 54 patients. *Spine (Phila Pa 1976)* 2003;28(3):267–271.

129. Leatherman KD, Dickson RA. Two-stage corrective surgery for congenital deformities of the spine. *J Bone Joint Surg Br* 1979;61:324–328.

130. McMaster M. Congenital scoliosis caused by unilateral failure of vertebral segmentation with contralateral hemivertebrae. *Spine (Phila Pa 1976)* 1998;23:998–1005.

131. Hedequist DJ, Hall JE, Emans JB. The safety and efficacy of spinal instrumentation in children with congenital spine deformities. *Spine (Phila Pa 1976)* 2004;29(18):2081–2086.

132. Kim YJ, Otsuka NY, Flynn JM, et al. Surgical treatment of congenital kyphosis. *Spine (Phila Pa 1976)* 2001;26(20):2251–2257.

133. Thompson GH, Akbarnia BA, Kostial P, et al. Comparison of single and dual growing rod techniques followed through definitive surgery: a preliminary study. *Spine (Phila Pa 1976)* 2005;30(18):2039–2044.

134. Campbell RM Jr, Smith MD, Mayes TC, et al. The characteristics of thoracic insufficiency syndrome associated with fused ribs and congenital scoliosis. *J Bone Joint Surg Am* 2003;85-A:399–408.

135. Karol LA, Johnston C, Mladenov K, et al. Pulmonary function following early thoracic fusion in non-neuromuscular scoliosis. *J Bone Joint Surg Am* 2008;90(6):1272–1281.

136. Winter R. Convex anterior and posterior hemiarthrodesis and hemiepiphyseodesis in young children with progressive congenital scoliosis. *J Pediatr Orthop* 1981;1(4):361–366.

138. Thompson AG, Marks DS, Sayampanathan SR, et al. Long-term results of combined anterior and posterior convex epiphysiodesis for congenital scoliosis due to hemivertebrae. *Spine (Phila Pa 1976)* 1995;20(12):1380–1385.

139. Marks DS, Sayampanathan SR, Thompson AG, et al. Long-term results of convex epiphysiodesis for congenital scoliosis. *Eur Spine J* 1995;4(5):296–301.

140. Keller PM, Lindseth RE, DeRosa GP. Progressive congenital scoliosis treatment using a transpedicular anterior and posterior convex hemiepiphysiodesis and hemiarthrodesis: a preliminary report. *Spine (Phila Pa 1976)* 1994;19(17):1933–1939.

141. Andrew T, Piggott H. Growth arrest for progressive scoliosis: combined anterior and posterior fusion of the convexity. *J Bone Joint Surg Br* 1985;67:193–197.

142. Cil A, Yazici M, Alanay A, et al. The course of sagittal plane abnormality in the patients with congenital scoliosis managed with convex growth arrest. *Spine (Phila Pa 1976)* 2004;29:547–552.

143. Ruf M, Jensen R, Harms J. Hemivertebra resection in the cervical spine. *Spine (Phila Pa 1976)* 2005;30(4):380–385.

144. Bradford DS, Boachie-Adjei O. One-stage anterior and posterior hemivertebral resection and arthrodesis or congenital scoliosis. *J Bone Joint Surg Am* 1990;72:536–540.

145. Klemme WR, Denis F, Winter RB, et al. Spinal instrumentation without fusion for progressive scoliosis in young children. *J Pediatr Orthop* 1997;17(6):734–742.

146. Bollini G, Docquier PL, Viehweger E. Lumbar hemivertebra resection. *J Bone Joint Surg Am* 2006;88:1043–1052.

147. Lazar RD, Hall JE. Simultaneous anterior and posterior hemivertebra excision. *Clin Orthop Relat Res* 1999;364:76–84.

147a. Hedequist DJ, Hall JE, Emans JB. Hemivertebra excision in children via simultaneous anterior and posterior exposures. *J Pediatr Orthop* 2005;25:60–63.

148. Ruf M, Harms J. Hemivertebra resection by a posterior approach: innovative operative technique and first results. *Spine (Phila Pa 1976)* 2002;27, 1116–1123.

149. Maat GJ, Matricali B, van Persijn van Meerten EL. Postnatal development and structure of the neurocentral junction. Its relevance for spinal surgery. *Spine (Phila Pa 1976)* 1996;21(6):661–666.

150. Wang JC, Nuccion SL, Feighan JE. Growth and development of the pediatric cervical spine documented radiographically. *J Bone Joint Surg Am* 2001;83-A:1212–1218.

151. Jeffrey JE, Campbell DM, Golden MH, et al. Antenatal factors in the development of the lumbar vertebral canal: a magnetic resonance imaging study. *Spine (Phila Pa 1976)* 2003;28(13):1418–1423.

152. Ruf M, Harms J. Pedicle screws in 1- and 2-year-old children: technique, complications and effect on further growth. *Spine (Phila Pa 1976)* 2002;27:E460–E466.

153. Ruf M, Harms J. Posterior hemivertebra resection with transpedicular instrumentation: early correction in children aged 1 to 6 years. *Spine (Phila Pa 1976)* 2003;28(18):2132–2138.

154. Cil A, Yazici M, Daglioglu K, et al. The effect of pedicle screw placement with or without application of compression across the neurocentral cartilage on the morphology of the spinal canal and pedicle in immature pigs. *Spine (Phila Pa 1976)* 2005;30(11):1287–1293.

155. Suk S-I, Chung ER, Kim JH, et al. Posterior vertebral column resection for severe rigid scoliosis. *Spine* 2005;30:1682–1687.

156. Shono Y, Abumi K, Kaneda K. One-stage posterior hemivertebra resection and correction using segmental posterior instrumentation. *Spine* 2001;26(7):752–7.

157. Yaszay B, O'Brien M, Shufflebarger HL, et al. The efficacy of hemivertebra resection for congenital scoliosis: a multicenter retrospective comparison of three surgical techniques. *Spine* 2011;36(24):2052-2060.

158. Ruf M, Jensen R, Letko L, et al. Hemivertebra resection and osteotomies in congenital spinal deformity. *Spine* 2009;34(17):1791–1799.

159. Klemme WR, Polly DW Jr, Orchowski JR. Hemivertebral excision for congenital scoliosis in very young children. *J Pediatr Orthop* 2001;21(6):761–764.

160. Hedden D. Management themes in congenital scoliosis. *J Bone Joint Surg Am* 2007;89-A(Suppl 1):72–78.

160a. Leatherman K. Resection of vertebral bodies. *J Bone Joint Surg Am* 1969;51-A:206.

161. Sucato DJ, Shah SA, Lenke LG, et al. Prompt response to critical spinal cord monitoring changes during vertebral column resection results in a low incidence of permanent neurologic deficit. *Proceedings of the 45th Annual Meeting of the Scoliosis Research Society.* Kyoto, Japan, 2010:109.

162. Shah SA, Sucato DJ, Newton, PO, et al. Perioperative neurologic events from a multicenter consecutive series of pediatric vertebral column resection: nature, frequency and outcomes. *Proceedings of the 17th International Meeting on Advanced Spine Techniques.* Toronto, Ontario, Canada, 2010:97.

163. Lenke LG, Newton PO, Sucato DJ, et al. Complications following 147 consecutive vertebral column resections for severe pediatric spinal deformity: a multicenter analysis. *Spine* 2012 Jul 20. [Epub ahead of print]

164. Suk S-I, Chung ER, Lee SM, et al. Posterior vertebral column resection in fixed lumbosacral deformity. *Spine* 2005;30(23):E703–E710.

165. Lenke LG, Sides BA, Koester LA, et al. Vertebral column resection for the treatment of severe spinal deformity. *Clin Orthop Relat Res* 2010;468(3):687–699.

166. Lenke LG, O'Leary PT, Bridwell KH, et al. Posterior vertebral column resection for severe pediatric deformity: minimum two-year follow up of thirty-five consecutive patients. *Spine* 2009;34(20):2213–2221.

167. Canavese F, Dimeglio A, Volpatti D, et al. Dorsal arthrodesis of thoracic spine and effects on thorax growth in prepubertal New Zealand white rabbits. *Spine* 2007;32:E443–E450.

168. Akbarnia BA, Marks DS, Boachie-Adjei O, et al. Dual growing rod technique for the treatment of progressive early-onset scoliosis: a multicenter study. *Spine* 2005;30:S46–S57.

169. Blakemore LC, Scoles PV, Poe-Kochert C, et al. Submuscular Isola rod with or without limited apical fusion in the management of severe spinal deformities in young children: preliminary report. *Spine* 2001;26:2044–2048.

170. Noordeen HM, Shah SA, Elsebaie HB, et al. In vivo distraction force and length measurements of growing rods: which factors influence on the ability to lengthen? *Spine* 2011;36(26):2299-303.

171. Farooq N, Garrido E, Altaf F, et al. Minimizing complications with single submuscular growing rods: a review of technique and results on 88 patients with minimum two-year follow-up. *Spine* 2010;35(25):252–258.

172. Yazici M, Emans J. Fusionless instrumentation systems for congenital scoliosis: expandable spinal rods and vertical expandable prosthetic titanium rib in the management of congenital spine deformities in the growing child. *Spine* 2009;34(17):1800–1807.

173. McCarthy RM, Sucato D, Turner JL, et al. Shilla growing rods in a caprine animal model: a pilot study. *Clin Orthop Relat Res* 2010;468(3):705–710.

174. Campbell RM Jr, Smith MD, Hell-Vocke AK. Expansion thoracoplasty: the surgical technique of opening-wedge thoracostomy. Surgical technique. *J Bone Joint Surg Am* 2004;86-A(Suppl 1):51–64.

175. Campbell RM Jr, Hell-Vocke AK. Growth of the thoracic spine in congenital scoliosis after expansion thoracoplasty. *J Bone Joint Surg Am* 2003;85-A(3):409–420.

176. Nassr A, Larson AN, Crane B, et al. Iatrogenic thoracic outlet syndrome secondary to vertical expandable prosthetic titanium rib expansion thoracoplasty: pathogenesis and strategies for prevention/treatment. *J Pediatr Orthop* 2009;29(1):31–34.

177. Ramirez N, Flynn JM, Serrano JA, et al. The Vertical Expandable Prosthetic Titanium Rib in the treatment of spinal deformity due to progressive early onset scoliosis. *J Pediatr Orthop B* 2009;18(4):197–203.

178. Thompson GH, Akbarnia BA, Campbell RM Jr. Growing rod techniques in early-onset scoliosis. *J Pediatr Orthop* 2007;27(3):354–361.

179. Samy MA, Al Zayed ZS, Shaheen MF. The effect of a vertical expandable prosthetic titanium rib on shoulder balance in patients with congenital scoliosis. *J Child Orthop* 2009.

180. Smith JT. The use of growth-sparing instrumentation in pediatric spinal deformity. *Orthop Clin North Am* 2007;38(4):547–552, vii.

181. Smith JT, Jerman J, Stringham J, et al. Does expansion thoracoplasty improve the volume of the convex lung in a windswept thorax? *J Pediatr Orthop* 2009;29(8):944–947.

182. Yazici M, Emans J. Fusionless instrumentation systems for congenital scoliosis: expandable spinal rods and vertical expandable prosthetic titanium rib in the management of congenital spine deformities in the growing child. *Spine (Phila Pa 1976)* 2009;34(17):1800–1807.

183. Skaggs DL, Choi PD, Rice C, et al. Efficacy of intraoperative neuro-logic monitoring in surgery involving a vertical expandable prosthetic titanium rib for early-onset spinal deformity. *J Bone Joint Surg Am* 2009;91(7):1657–1663.
184. Akbarnia BA, Marks DS, Boachie-Adjei O, et al. Dual growing rod technique for the treatment of progressive early-onset scoliosis: a multicenter study. *Spine* 2005;30(17 Suppl):S46–S57.
185. Campbell RM Jr, et al. The effect of opening wedge thoracostomy on thoracic insufficiency syndrome associated with fused ribs and congenital scoliosis. *J Bone Joint Surg Am* 2004;86-A(8):1659–1674.

186. Emans JB, Caubet JF, Ordonez CL, et al. The treatment of spine and chest wall deformities with fused ribs by expansion thoracostomy and insertion of vertical expandable prosthetic titanium rib: growth of thoracic spine and improvement of lung volumes. *Spine (Phila Pa 1976)* 2005;30(17 Suppl):S58–S68.
187. Shah SC, Birknes JK, Sagoo S, et al. Vertical Expandable Prosthetic Titanium Rib (VEPTR): indications, technique, and management review. *Surg Technol Int* 2009;18:223–229.

Kyphosis

Kyphosis is a curvature of the spine in the sagittal plane in which the convexity of the curve is directed posteriorly. Lordosis is a curvature of the spine in the sagittal plane in which the convexity of the curve is directed anteriorly. The thoracic spine and the sacrum normally are kyphotic, and the cervical spine and the lumbar spine normally are lordotic (1). Although several authors have tried to define normal kyphosis of the thoracic spine and normal lordosis of the lumbar spine, these studies have shown much variability in what is considered normal (2–8). The ranges of normal kyphosis and lordosis change with increasing age and vary according to the gender and the area of the spine involved (2–5). The degree of kyphosis or lordosis that is considered normal or abnormal depends on the location of the curvature and the age of the patient. For example, 30 degrees of kyphosis is normal in the thoracic spine but abnormal at the thoracolumbar junction.

The normal range of thoracic kyphosis is considered to be 19 to 45 degrees and that of lumbar lordosis, 30 to 60 degrees (9). Measurements of kyphosis and lordosis are made from standard scoliosis radiographs with the patient standing with his or her knees locked, feet shoulder width apart, elbows bent, and knuckles in the supraclavicular fossa bilaterally. This will place the patient's arms at approximately a 45-degree angle from the vertical axis of the body (10). Thoracic kyphosis is measured on a lateral radiograph as the angle between the superior end plate of T2 and the inferior end plate of T12. Proximal thoracic kyphosis is measured from the superior end plate of T2 to the inferior end plate of T5. Middle and lower thoracic kyphosis is measured from the superior end plate of T5 to the inferior end plate of T12.

The apex of normal thoracic kyphosis is the T6–T7 disc space (11, 12). The thoracolumbar junction should have no kyphosis or lordosis (11). Lumbar lordosis begins at L1–L2 and increases gradually until the L3–L4 disc space. There is a reciprocal relationship between the orientation of the sacrum, sacral slope, and the pelvic incidence and the characteristics of lumbar lordosis and location of the apex of lumbar lordosis (Fig. 19-1) (13–16). A sacral slope of <35 degrees and a low pelvic incidence are associated with a relatively flat, short lumbar lordosis. A sacral slope of more than 45 degrees and a high pelvic incidence are associated with a long, curved lumbar lordosis (14).

Initially, during fetal and intrauterine development, the entire spine is kyphotic. During the neonatal period, the thoracic, lumbar, and sacral portions of the spine remain in a kyphotic posture. Cervical lordosis begins to develop when a child starts holding his or her head up. When an upright posture is assumed, the primary and secondary curves begin to develop. The primary curves are thoracic and sacral kyphosis, and the secondary or compensatory curves in the sagittal plane are cervical and lumbar lordosis. These curves balance each other so that the head is centered over the pelvis (2, 17, 18).

The ranges of normal thoracic kyphosis and lumbar lordosis are dynamic, progressing gradually with growth (19). During the juvenile and adolescent growth periods, thoracic kyphosis and lumbar lordosis become more pronounced and take on a more adult appearance. Mac-Thiong et al. (13) showed that pelvic incidence and tilt increased with growth but sacral slope remained stable.

Differences also exist between male and female spines (6), and thoracic kyphosis and spine mobility are different in boys and girls: during the juvenile and adolescent periods (ages 8 to 16 years), girls have less thoracic kyphosis and thoracic spinal mobility than do boys of the same age (3, 12). Thoracic kyphosis also tends to progress with age: from 30 to 70 years of age, women have a progressive increase in kyphosis, from a mean of 25 degrees to a mean of 40 degrees (19). Men also show a definite progression with age, but at a lower rate.

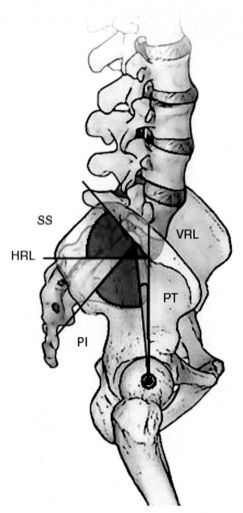

FIGURE 19-1. Radiographic measurements of pelvic incidence (a), sacral slope (b), and pelvic tilt (c). SS, sacral slope; HRL, horizontal reference line; PI, pelvic incidence; PT, pelvic tilt; VRL, vertical reference line. (From MF, Kuklo TR, Blanke KM, et al. *Radiographic measurement manual: Spinal Deformity Study Group (SDSG)*. Memphis, TN: Medtronic Sofamor Danek, Fall 2004.)

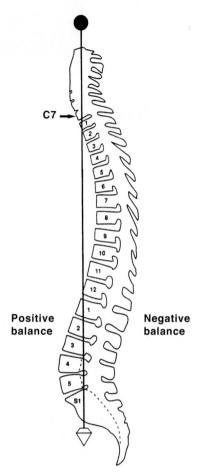

FIGURE 19-2. A plumb line is dropped from the middle of the C7 vertebral body to the posterosuperior corner of the S1 vertebral body. (From Bernhardt M. Normal spinal anatomy: normal sagittal plane alignment. In: Bridwell KH, DeWald RL, eds. *The textbook of spinal surgery*, 2nd ed. Philadelphia, PA: Lippincott-Raven, 1997:185.)

Normal sagittal balance is defined as a plumb line dropping from C7 and intersecting the posterosuperior corner of the S1 vertebral body (Fig. 19-2). Positive sagittal balance occurs when the plumb line falls in front of the sacrum, and negative sagittal balance occurs when the plumb line falls behind the sacrum (20).

Different forces are exerted on the spine, depending on the presence of kyphosis or lordosis. In the upright position, the spine is subjected to the forces of gravity, and several structures maintain its stability: the disc complex (nucleus pulposus and annulus), the ligaments (anterior longitudinal ligament, posterior longitudinal ligament, ligamentum flavum, apophyseal joint ligaments, and interspinous ligament), and the muscles (the long spinal muscles, the short intrinsic spinal muscles,

and the abdominal muscles). Alteration in function resulting from paralysis, surgery, tumor, infection, or alteration in growth potentials can cause a progressive kyphotic deformity in a child (21). Both compressive and tensile forces are produced by the action of gravity on an upright spine (Fig. 19-3). In normal thoracic kyphosis, the compressive forces borne by the anterior elements are balanced by the tensile forces borne by the posterior elements. In a lordotic spine, the compressive forces are posterior and the tensile forces are anterior. These forces of compression and tension on the spinal physes can cause changes in normal growth, and a growth deformity can be added to a biomechanical deformity to cause a pathologic kyphosis (21, 22).

Voutsinas and MacEwen (23) suggested that relative differences in forces applied to the spine are reflected more accurately by the length and width of a kyphotic curve than by just the degree of the curve. For example, curves that are longer and wider (farther from the center of gravity) are more likely to cause deformity in an immature spine (Fig. 19-4). Winter

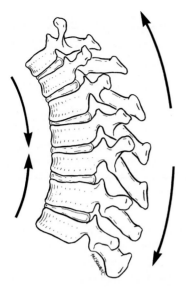

FIGURE 19-3. Forces that contribute to kyphotic deformity of the thoracic spine. The anterior vertebral bodies are in compression, and the posterior vertebral elements are in tension. (From White AA III, Panjabi MM. Practical biomechanics of scoliosis and kyphosis. In: White AA, Panjabi MM, eds. *Clinical biomechanics of the spine.* Philadelphia, PA: JB Lippincott, 1990:127.)

and Hall (24) classified disorders that result in kyphosis of the spine. Only the more common causes are presented in this chapter; the other causes are discussed elsewhere in this book (Table 19-1).

POSTURAL KYPHOSIS

Postural kyphosis is a flexible deformity of the spine and is common in juvenile and adolescent patients. Usually, the parents are more concerned about the postural roundback deformity than the adolescent is, and these parental concerns typically are what bring the patient to the physician's office. The physician's role in this situation is to rule out more serious causes of kyphosis. Postural kyphosis should be differentiated from pathologic types of kyphosis, such as Scheuermann disease, and from congenital kyphosis. When observed from the side, patients with postural roundback have a gentle rounding of the back while bending forward (Fig. 19-5). Patients with Scheuermann disease and congenital kyphosis have a sharp angular kyphosis or gibbus on forward bending when observed from the side. Radiographs usually are necessary to rule out pathologic types of kyphosis. Patients with postural kyphosis do not have radiographic vertebral-body changes, and the deformity is completely correctable by changes in position or posture. This deformity is common in patients who are taller than their peers and in young adolescent girls undergoing early breast development who tend to stoop because they are self-conscious about their bodies (25).

No active medical treatment is necessary. Bracing is not indicated. Exercises have been suggested and may help maintain better posture, but adherence to such a therapy program is difficult for juveniles and young adolescents. This problem is best treated by educating the patient and, more important, the parents and by observation (26).

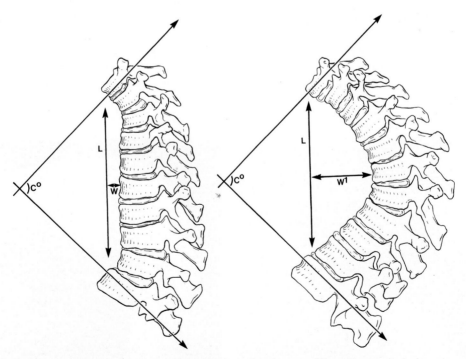

FIGURE 19-4. The two spinal curvatures represented by these drawings are different in magnitude; however, using cobb's method to measure the deformities, the degrees of curvature are identical. The differences in the curves are more accurately reflected when the length of the curves (*L*) and their respective widths (*W* and *W*¹) are taken into consideration. (From Voutsinas SA, MacEwen GD. Sagittal profiles of the spine. *Clin Orthop* 1986;210:235.)

TABLE 19-1	Disorders Affecting the Spine and Resulting in Kyphosis

I. Postural disorders
II. Scheuermann kyphosis
III. Congenital disorders
  a. Defect of formation
  b. Defect of segmentation
IV. Paralytic disorders
  a. Poliomyelitis
  b. Anterior horn cell disease
V. Myelomeningocele
VI. Posttraumatic
  a. Acute
  b. Chronic
  c. With/without cord damage
VII. Inflammatory
  a. Tuberculosis
  b. Other infection
VIII. Postsurgical
  a. Postlaminectomy
  b. Postbody (tumor) excision

IX. Inadequate fusion
  a. Too short
  b. Pseudoarthrosis
X. Postirradiation
  a. Neuroblastoma
  b. Wilms tumor
XI. Metabolic
  a. Osteoporosis
    1. Senile
    2. Juvenile
  b. Osteogenesis imperfecta
XII. Developmental
  a. Achondroplasia
  b. Mucopolysaccharidosis
  c. Other
XIII. Collagen disease (e.g., Marie-Strumpell)
XIV. Tumor
  a. Benign
  b. Malignant
XV. Neurofibromatosis

From Winter RB, Hall JE. Kyphosis in childhood and adolescence. *Spine* 1978;3:285.

CONGENITAL KYPHOSIS

Congenital kyphosis is an uncommon deformity, but, despite its rare occurrence, neurologic deficits resulting from this deformity are frequent.

Congenital kyphosis occurs because of abnormal development of the vertebrae, including a failure of developing segments of the spine to form or to separate properly (27). The spine may be either stable or unstable, or it may become

TABLE 19-2	Winter's Classification of Congenital Deformity

Type	Description
I	Failure of formation of all or part of the vertebral body
II	Failure of segmentation of one or multiple vertebral levels
III	Mixed form, with elements of both failure of formation and failure of segmentation

unstable with growth (28). Spinal deformity in congenital kyphosis usually progresses with growth, and the amount of progression is directly proportional to the number of vertebrae involved, the type of involvement, and the amount of remaining normal growth in the affected vertebrae (28, 29).

Van Schrick in 1932 (30) and Lombard and LeGenissel in 1938 (31) initially described two basic types of congenital kyphosis: a failure of formation of part or all of the vertebral body and a failure of segmentation of part or all of the vertebral body. Winter et al. (27, 32) developed the most useful classification of congenital kyphosis, which divides the deformity into three types (Table 19-2). Type I is failure of formation of all or part of the vertebral body (Fig. 19-6A); type II is failure of segmentation of one or multiple vertebral levels (Fig. 19-6B); and type III is a mixed form, with elements of both failure of formation and failure of segmentation.

McMaster and Singh (33) further subdivided this classification into types of vertebral-body deformity. Defects of vertebral-body segmentation consist of a partial (anterior unsegmented bar) or a complete (block vertebrae) failure of segmentation. Defects of vertebral-body formation are divided into four types: (a) posterolateral quadrant vertebrae, (b) butterfly

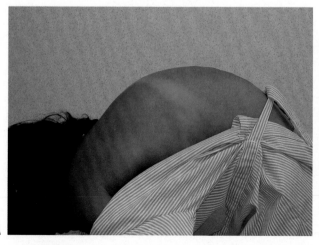
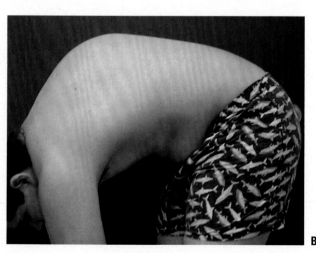

FIGURE 19-5. **A**: Lateral view of normal spinal contour on forward bending. **B**: Lateral view of a patient with Scheuermann disease on forward bending. Note the break in the normal contour and sharp angular nature of the spine.

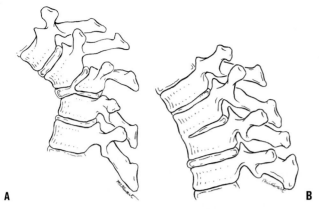

FIGURE 19-6. **A**: Congenital kyphosis caused by failure of formation of the vertebral body (type I). **B**: Congenital kyphosis caused by failure of segmentation (type II). (Courtesy of Robert Winter, MD, Minneapolis.)

vertebrae, (c) posterior hemivertebrae, and (d) wedged vertebrae (Fig. 19-7). Dubousset (34) and Zeller et al. (35) added a rotary dislocation of the spine, and Shapiro and Herring (36) further divided type III displacement into types A (sagittal plane only) and B (rotary, transverse, and sagittal planes). Any classification can be subdivided further into deformities with or without neurologic compromise; this is useful for making treatment decisions because each type of congenital kyphosis has a distinct natural history and risk of progression.

Most of the vertebral malformations that cause spinal deformity occur between the 19th and the 30th days of fetal development (28, 32, 37). The somatic mesoderm, which is devoted to the formation of the vertebral column and the rib cage, undergoes segmentation into 38 to 44 pairs of discrete, bilateral somites. The formation of a vertebra depends on contributions of cells from two separate and successive pairs of sclerotomes. This condensation of the paired sclerotomes occurs at approximately 5 weeks of gestation. If one side of the pair of sclerotomes fails to develop, a hemivertebra is formed, resulting in congenital scoliosis (38, 39).

Tsou (40) concluded that congenital kyphosis and congenital scoliosis occur during different periods of spinal development. He divided the development of the spine into an embryonic period (the first 56 days) and a fetal period (from day 57 to birth). During the embryonic period, failure of segmentation and aplasia of part of the vertebrae, resulting in hemivertebra formation, cause scoliosis, while congenital kyphosis occurs in the fetal period, during the cartilaginous phase of development (40). Failure of formation occurs in this phase when the cartilaginous centrum of the vertebral body forms a functionally inadequate growth cartilage.

Failure of formation varies from complete aplasia (which involves the pars and the facet joints and makes the spine unstable) to involvement of only the anterior one-third to one-half of the vertebral body. This abnormal development is

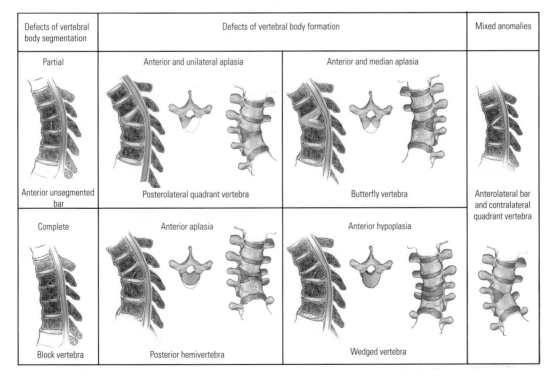

FIGURE 19-7. Drawings showing the different types of vertebral anomalies that produce congenital kyphosis or kyphoscoliosis. (From McMaster MJ, Singh H. Natural history of congenital kyphosis and kyphoscoliosis. *J Bone Joint Surg* 1999;81A:1367–1383.)

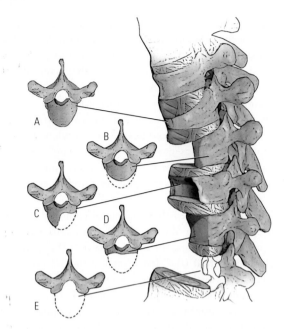

FIGURE 19-8. The five most common patterns of congenital vertebral hypoplasia and aplasia are illustrated in lateral and transverse views. Types *B* and *E* tend to produce pure congenital kyphosis. (From Tsou PM. Embryology of congenital kyphosis. *Clin Orthop* 1977;128:18.)

thought to be the result of inadequate vascularization of the vertebral body during the fetal period, leading to hypoplasia or aplasia of the anterior vertebral body. If one side of the vertebra is involved more than the other side, scoliosis also may occur (Fig. 19-8). Unlike hemivertebral anomalies that occur in the embryonic period because of maldevelopment of corresponding pairs of somites causing congenital scoliosis, posterior arch anomalies usually are absent in pure congenital kyphosis.

Failure of segmentation has been described as an osseous metaplasia of the annulus fibrosus (40, 41) that acts as a tether against normal growth and causing spinal deformity. The height of the vertebral bodies is relatively normal, but the depth of the ossification of the annulus fibrosus varies. Ossification may be delayed, with a period of normal growth followed by spontaneous ossification. Kyphosis caused by a "segmentation defect" is believed to represent a developmental defect of the perivertebral structures (the annulus fibrosis, the ring apophysis, and the anterior longitudinal ligament) rather than a true intervertebral bar (42).

The natural history of congenital kyphosis is well known and based on the type of kyphosis: failure of formation (type I), failure of segmentation (type II), or mixed anomalies (type III). Congenital kyphosis tends to be progressive, with the greatest rate of progression occurring during the time of most rapid growth of the spine (birth to 3 years of age) and during the adolescent growth spurt. Winter et al. (32) found that failure of formation (type I deformity)

produces a much more severe kyphosis, with a rate of progression that averages 7 degrees per year, whereas type II deformities progress an average of 5 degrees per year. McMaster and Singh found the most rapid progression in type III kyphosis, followed by type I, because of involvement of posterolateral quadrant vertebrae. In their study, a type III kyphosis progressed at a rate of 5 degrees per year before 10 years of age and 8 degrees per year thereafter until the end of growth. Type I (failure of formation) kyphosis progressed 2.5 degrees per year before 10 years of age and 5 degrees per year thereafter (33). Type I and III deformities are associated with a much higher incidence of neurologic involvement and paraplegia than are type II deformities. Neurologic problems occur more frequently in patients with type I and III deformities because they tend to have an acute angular kyphosis over a short segment, which places the spinal cord at higher risk for compression at the level of acute angulation. Type II deformities (failure of segmentation) rarely result in neurologic problems because involvement of several segments produces a more gradual kyphosis, and vertebral-body height usually is maintained with little or no vertebral-body wedging. The most frequent location of congenital kyphosis is T10–L1 (32).

Patients with congenital kyphosis may have other anomalies. Intraspinal abnormalities have been reported to occur in 5% to 37% of patients with congenital kyphosis and congenital scoliosis (43–46). A study by Bradford et al. (47) indicated that this incidence may be even greater. They found that six of eight patients with congenital kyphosis had spinal cord abnormalities visible on magnetic resonance imaging (MRI). Although the proposed time of development of the deformity may be different from that of congenital scoliosis, other nonskeletal anomalies such as cardiac, pulmonary, renal, and auditory disorders or Klippel-Feil syndrome (48, 49) can be associated with congenital kyphosis. McMaster et al. (50) found an adverse effect on lung development and function caused by an increasing constriction of the rib cage and impairment of diaphragmatic movement. The more cranial the level of the congenital kyphosis, especially above T10, the more significant the effect on respiratory impairment.

Patient Presentation. The diagnosis of a congenital spine problem usually is made by a pediatrician before the patient is seen by an orthopaedist. The deformity may be detected before birth on prenatal ultrasonography (51) or noted as a clinical deformity in a newborn. If the deformity is mild, congenital kyphosis can be overlooked until a rapid growth spurt makes the condition more obvious. Some mild deformities are found by chance on radiographs that are obtained for other reasons. Clinical deformities seen in a newborn tend to have a worse prognosis than those discovered as incidental findings on plain radiographs. Physical examination usually reveals a kyphotic deformity at the thoracolumbar junction or in the lower thoracic spine. An attempt should be made to determine the rigidity of the deformity by flexion and extension of the spine. A detailed neurologic examination should be done, looking for any subtle signs of neurologic compromise. Associated musculoskeletal and nonmusculoskeletal anomalies should be sought on physical examination.

High-quality, detailed anteroposterior and lateral radiographs provide most information in the evaluation of congenital kyphosis (Fig. 19-9). Failure of segmentation and the true extent of failure of formation may be difficult to detect on early films because of incomplete ossification. Flexion and extension lateral radiographs are helpful in determining the rigidity of the kyphosis and possible instability of the spine. Computerized tomography (CT) with three-dimensional reconstructions can identify the amount of vertebral-body involvement and can determine whether more kyphosis or scoliosis might be expected (Fig. 19-10). CT scans can identify only the nature of the bony deformity and the size of the cartilage anlage. They do not show the amount of growth potential in the cartilage anlage, and therefore only an estimate of possible progression can be made. MRI should be obtained in most cases because of the significant incidence of intraspinal abnormalities. In addition, the location of the spinal cord and any areas of spinal

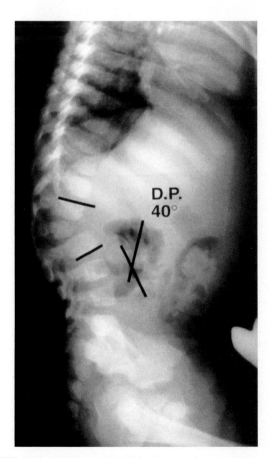

FIGURE 19-9. A 2-year-old child with type I congenital kyphosis measuring 40 degrees. Radiograph demonstrates failure of formation of the anterior portion of the first lumbar vertebra.

cord compression caused by the kyphosis can be seen on MRI. The cartilage anlage will be well defined by MRI in patients with failure of formation (Fig. 19-11); however, as with CT scans and plain radiographs, MRI cannot reveal how much growth potential is present in the cartilage anlage and can only help estimate the probability of a progressive deformity.

Congenital kyphosis, as well as associated renal problems, can be seen on routine prenatal ultrasonography as early as 19 weeks of gestation (51). Myelograms have been used for documenting spinal cord compression but have been mostly replaced by MRI. If myelography is used, images should be taken with the patient prone and supine. Myelograms obtained in only the prone position may miss information about spinal cord compression because of pooling of dye around the apex of the deformity. Myelography can be used in conjunction with CT scanning to add to the diagnostic information obtained.

Treatment. Because the natural history of this condition usually is one of continued progression with an increased risk of neurologic compromise, surgery usually is the preferred method of treatment (27). If the deformity is mild or if the diagnosis is uncertain, close observation may be a treatment option. However, observation of a congenital kyphotic deformity must be used with caution, and the physician must not be lulled into a false sense of security if the deformity progresses only 3 to 5 degrees over a 6-month period. If the deformity is observed over 2 to 3 years, it will have progressed 18 to 30 degrees and cannot thereafter be easily corrected. Bracing has no role in the treatment of congenital kyphosis, unless compensatory curves are being treated above or below the congenital kyphosis (27, 48, 52). Bracing a rigid structural deformity, such as congenital kyphosis, neither corrects the deformity nor stops the progression of kyphosis. To document that there has been a significant change in kyphosis, radiographs should be taken by a standardized method, and the same end vertebral bodies should be measured. This will ensure that any change that has occurred since the previous radiograph is accurately measured.

Surgery is the recommended treatment for congenital kyphosis. The type of surgery depends on the type and size of the deformity, the age of the patient, and the presence of neurologic deficits. Procedures can include posterior fusion, anterior fusion, both anterior and posterior fusions, and anterior osteotomy with posterior fusion. Fusion can be done with or without instrumentation.

Treatment of Type I Deformities. The treatment of type I deformities depends on the stage of the disease: early with mild deformity, late with moderate or severe deformity, and late with severe deformity and spinal cord compression.

Early Treatment of Mild Deformities. For type I deformities, the best treatment is early posterior fusion. If the deformity is

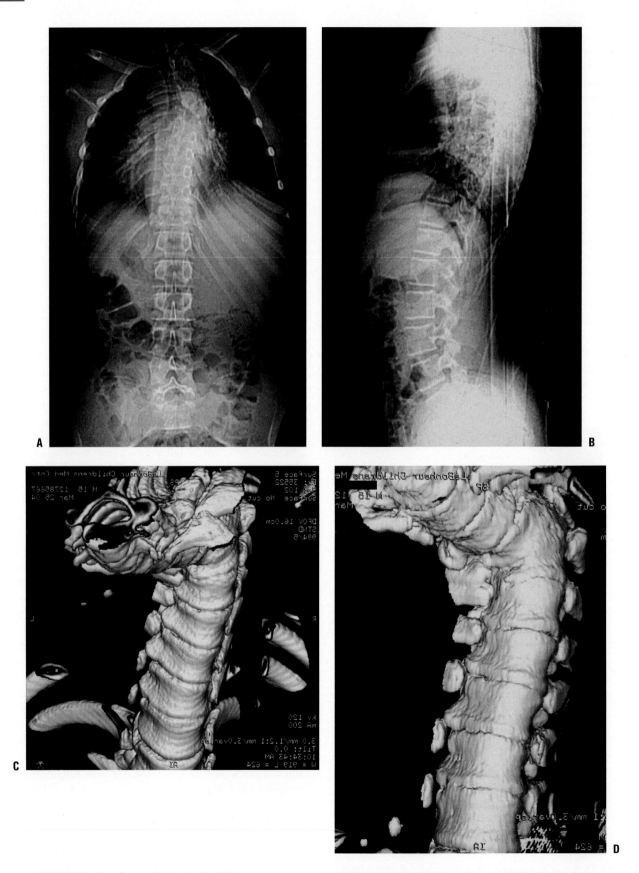

FIGURE 19-10.   Congenital kyphosis. **A,B**: Anteroposterior and lateral radiographs. Note inadequate detail of kyphosis on lateral radiograph of spine. **C–E**: CT three-dimensional reconstruction views that clearly demonstrate the bony anatomy of congenital kyphosis.

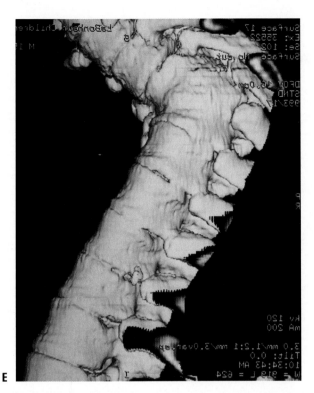

FIGURE 19-10. *(Continued)*

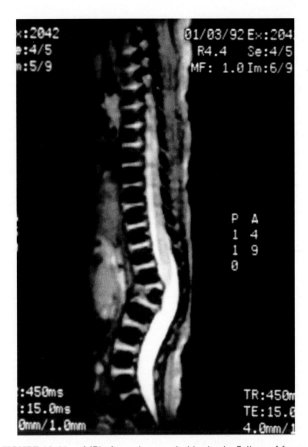

FIGURE 19-11. MRI of type I congenital kyphosis. Failure of formation of the anterior vertebral body is demonstrated, but the growth potential of the involved vertebra cannot be determined. Note the pressure on the dural sac.

<50 or 55 degrees and the patient is younger than 5 years of age, posterior fusion alone, extending from one level above the kyphotic deformity to one level below, is recommended (27, 32, 48, 53). This may allow for some improvement in the kyphotic deformity because of continued growth anteriorly from the anterior end plates of the vertebrae one level above and one level below the congenital kyphotic vertebrae that are included in the posterior fusion. McMaster and Singh (54) reported 15 degrees of correction in nine of 11 patients treated with this technique. Kim et al. (55) reported that after posterior fusion alone correction of kyphosis occurred with growth only in patients younger than 3 years of age and with type II and III deformities. Anterior and posterior spinal fusions at least one level above and one level below the congenital kyphosis are indicated in curves of more than 60 degrees (55). Anterior and posterior fusions predictably halt the progression of the kyphotic deformity but, because of ablation of the anterior physes (35, 53, 55), do not allow for the possibility of some correction of the deformity with growth.

Late Treatment of Moderate to Severe Deformities. In older patients with type I kyphotic deformities, posterior arthrodesis alone may be successful if the kyphosis is <50 to 55 degrees (32, 56). If the deformity is more than 55 degrees (which usually is the case in deformities detected late), anterior and posterior fusion produces more reliable results (32, 56). Anterior arthrodesis alone will not correct the deformity. Any correction of the deformity requires anterior strut grafting with temporary distraction and posterior fusion, with or without posterior

compression instrumentation. The posterior instrumentation may allow for some correction of the kyphosis but should be regarded more as an internal stabilizer than as a correction device (27). Instrumentation has been reported to decrease the pseudoarthrosis rate (55). Correction by instrumentation should be used with caution in rigid, angular curves because of the high incidence of neurologic complications. If anterior strut grafting is done, the strut graft should be placed anteriorly under compression. If no correction is attempted and the goal of surgery is just to stop progression of the kyphosis, a simple anterior interbody fusion combined with a posterior fusion can be used. Smith et al. (57) described simultaneous anterior and posterior approaches through a costotransversectomy that allowed resection of the posterior hemivertebra and correction of the kyphosis with posterior compression instrumentation. Correction of the kyphosis could be obtained safely once the posterior hemivertebra was removed and the thecal sac could be observed during corrections. The use of skeletal traction (halo-pelvic, halo-femoral, or halo-gravity) to correct the deformity is tempting, but is not recommended because of the risk of paraplegia (58). In a patient with a rigid gibbus deformity, traction pulls the spinal cord against the apex of the rigid kyphosis and can lead to neurologic compromise (Fig. 19-12).

FIGURE 19-12. The effect of traction on a rigid congenital kyphosis. **A**: The apical area does not change with traction, but the adjacent spine is lengthened. **B**: As the spine lengthens, so does the spinal cord, producing increased tension in the cord and aggravating existing neurologic deficits. (From Lonstein JE, Winter RB, Moe JH, et al. Neurologic deficit secondary to spinal deformity. *Spine* 1980;5:331.)

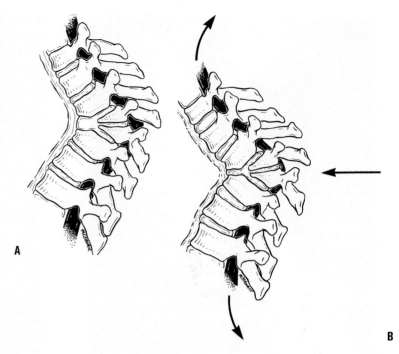

A

B

ANTERIOR STRUT GRAFT FOR KYPHOSIS.

Strut grafts are most often used for patients with severe kyphotic deformities with or without associated scoliosis. Strut grafts can also be used in cases of tumor resections and/or vertebral-body collapse secondary to infections and/or trauma. Anterior strut grafting with a free graft is generally used for a kyphosis without neurologic deficits in order to prevent further progression of the deformity (Figs. 19-13 to 19-17). It can be used either by an *in situ* fusion technique or fusion with minimal intraoperative correction. If intraoperative correction is anticipated, the kyphosis must be mobile at its apex. There must be no fusions posteriorly or, if there are, these must be released prior to any attempt at correction. Distraction of a rigid kyphosis carries a high risk of neurologic injury for the patient and therefore should never be attempted. The struts can be from the fibula or rib, or both. Vascularized or free vascularized grafts may also be used for these procedures. Nonvascularized fibular grafts are the most commonly used structural grafts for kyphotic deformities, as they provide the greatest structural support. The fibula is ideal because one can obtain a large length (up to 26 cm) in mature patients. The disadvantage, however, of using free fibula is that the graft may take a long time to incorporate (up to 2 years). These free fibular grafts are at their weakest point 6 months postoperatively (creeping substitution) and hence subject to fracture, particularly when the graft is placed more than 4 cm anterior to the apex of the kyphosis.

Although rib can be used, it is structurally a very weak graft. Rib is most often used to supplement a fibular autograft (58).

The strut graft generally extends from one end vertebra of the kyphosis to the other. It should lie as far anteriorly and as close to the midline as possible to allow for maximum structural support. Strut grafting has the advantage of being able to stabilize the kyphotic deformity by placing a compression arthrodesis in the line of axial stress of the spine. A vascularized rib graft is a useful alternative when rapid incorporation (6 to 8 weeks) is desired and ligation of segmental vessels is contraindicated. This may be used in kyphosis with preexisting neurologic lesions and especially in cases where fusion *in situ* is indicated to prevent further curve progression. Vascularized grafts are not subjected to creeping substitution. When a vascularized rib graft is planned, it is obtained by swinging a portion of the rib down with a vascular pedicle to provide an anterior strut for a kyphotic deformity. The rib selected is chosen to best fit with the level to be bridged. For kyphosis with an apex between T2 and T5, a rib two or three segments below the apex of the kyphosis is the ideal rib to use. If the apex of the kyphosis is at T6 or below, a rib two or three segments proximal to the kyphosis apex is the one to be selected. The rib is rotated on a muscle pedicle flap. This technique requires meticulous dissection with preservation of the vasculature. Firm incorporation is achieved within 6 to 8 weeks; hence, this technique is ideally suited for fusion *in situ* as the grafts have a low mechanical load capacity.

Strut grafting is contraindicated when a second procedure is planned that may produce enough correction to dislodge the anterior strut graft. If this is anticipated, the strut grafting should be done after the corrective posterior procedure is completed. Other contraindications include conditions where the bone is so soft that the strut graft may penetrate the posterior cortex and cause spinal cord injury.

Text continued on page 752

Anterior Strut Graft for Kyphosis (Figs. 19-13 to 19-17)

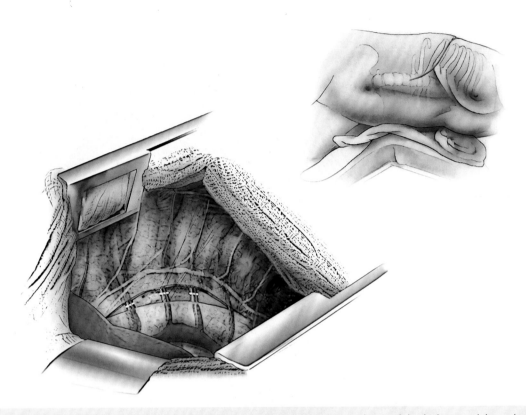

FIGURE 19-13.   Anterior Strut Graft for Kyphosis. A standard thoracotomy or thoracoabdominal approach is used over the rib to be excised. The rib to be excised is at the upper end vertebra of the kyphotic deformity. Another way to select the appropriate rib is to identify the apex of the kyphosis and draw a line to the midaxillary line. This line will intersect the appropriate rib to be removed. The resected rib is excised subperiosteally and cut off at the costal transverse joint. Appropriate retractors are placed. The parietal pleura is incised and opened from the most proximal disc space to be exposed and then opened distally to the distal end vertebra. The segmental vessels are isolated in the midline and tied with interrupted 2-0 silk sutures. The vessels and the parietal pleura are bluntly dissected off the entire spine, exposing the entire spine throughout the length of the intended fusion. As the next step, we prefer to expose the spine subperioste-ally by the development of a periosteal flap beginning at the rib head of the most proximal vertebra to be incorporated in the fusion and ending at the rib head (or transverse process in the lumbar spine) of the most distal included vertebra. This subperiosteal flap is developed as far to the opposite side of the spine as possible; this is especially important if a scoliotic deformity is present. In scoliosis, deformity exposure must include the concavity of the curve. This periosteal flap is protec-tive of the soft tissues on the opposite side; it also provides an excellent bed for bony fusion. Some surgeons may prefer extraperiosteal dissection.

FIGURE 19-14. All exposed intervertebral discs are then removed back to the
posterior longitudinal ligament with rongeurs and curettes of varying sizes and
shapes. In congenital deformities, large
amounts of cartilaginous material may be
present in the apex of the kyphosis or the
apex of the kyphoscoliosis. All this cartilaginous material and the vertebral end
plates should be removed completely, as
far back as the posterior longitudinal ligament, leaving this ligament intact.

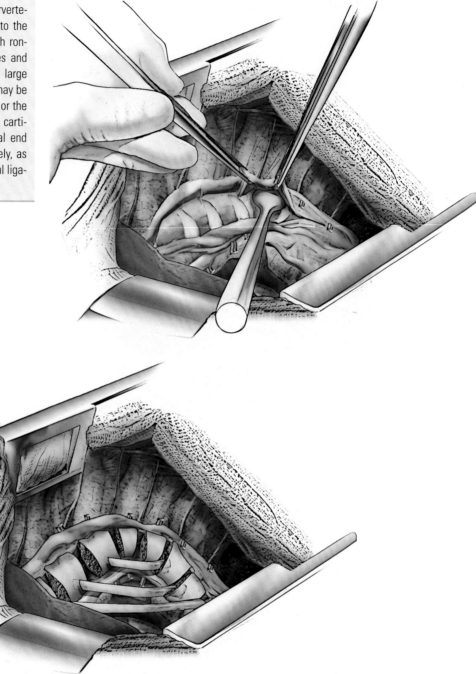

FIGURE 19-15. The fibular graft is harvested in the standard fashion. The fibular strut should lie as far anteriorly and as
close to the midline as possible. A suture or a ruler can be used to measure the length of the most anterior strut. It is important not to overly shorten this strut prior to actual insertion. The anchoring holes for the fibular strut may be made in one of
several ways. A burr can be used to develop anchoring holes in the anterior cortices of the vertebral body, or a trough can
be prepared with curettes and gouges in the inferior aspect of the end vertebral body above and the superior aspect of the
end vertebral body below. In this technique, a small notch is made in the cortex with a rongeur to allow the graft to be keyed
into place during manual curve correction. For *in situ* fusion, mild correction will be obtained by use of manual compression
over the apex of the kyphotic deformity. Manual pressure is applied over the apex of the kyphosis and the appropriate length
graft keyed into position in one end vertebra and then the other. The end of the fibula may require some tapering, which is
best done with a burr prior to insertion into the vertebral body. When the external pressure is relieved, the graft should be
secure. If more than one structural graft is to be used, those closest to the apex must be inserted prior to insertion of the
primary (most anterior) graft. Rib may be used for these secondary grafts and then morselized rib or iliac crest, or both, are
packed into the intervening spaces.

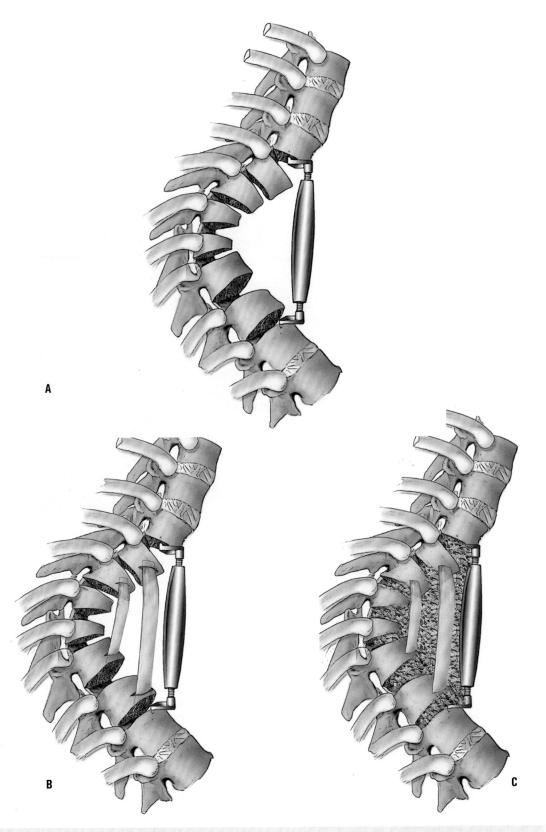

FIGURE 19-16.   **A–C**: Although the procedure is not often done today, if correction is to be attempted anteriorly, one of several types of distractors must be placed in the furthest anterior position and gradually elongated. The distractor should be gradually spread over time with careful monitoring of spinal cord function by electrophysiologic (motor and sensory) monitoring. Once maximal distraction is obtained, grafts are inserted in a manner similar to the aforementioned technique.

FIGURE 19-17. With the vascularized rib technique, the skin incision is made approximately at the level of the rib selected for the fusion. The intercostal musculature cranial to the rib is divided with the rib exposed subperiosteally at the costochondral margin and resected. The intercostal musculature is cut about 0.5 cm caudal to the selected rib leaving the neurovascular bundle intact. The appropriate length of rib is determined. The rib is subperiosteally exposed at the level of sectioning and the neurovascular bundle carefully ligated and sectioned. The intercostal musculature is then divided and the interspace opened further to allow exposure of the surgical area. The neurovascular bundle is then followed from the point of rib resection to the intervertebral foramen. The periosteum is freed on both ends of the ribs by approximately 1 cm to allow for insertion into the ends of the kyphotic segment. The fusion area can either be exposed as discussed above through subperiosteal dissection, or the graft can be keyed into position at the end vertebra as illustrated, without extensive subperiosteal dissection. I prefer to expose the bed for vascularized rib in the same fashion as for a free fibular graft.

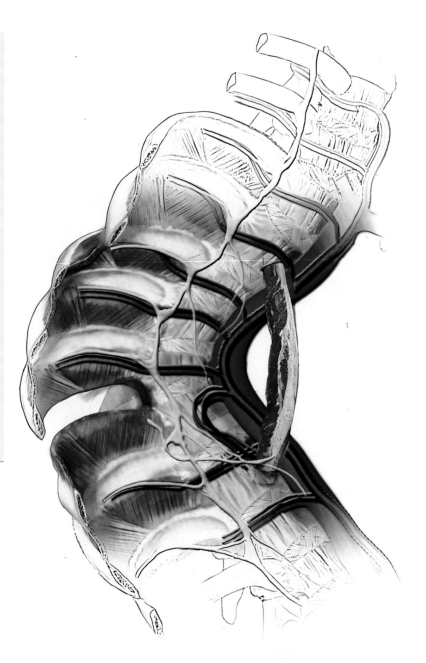

Technique. The patient is placed in a standard lateral decubitus position. If the kyphotic deformity is associated with scoliosis, the kyphosis is approached from the convex side of the curvature. If, however, it is a pure kyphotic deformity, then in the thoracic region, a right-sided thoracotomy is preferred, whereas if the kyphosis apex is at the thoracolumbar junction, then a left-sided thoracotomy is preferred.

Late Treatment of Severe Deformities with Cord Compression. It is difficult to attempt late treatment of a severe congenital kyphotic deformity that is accompanied by spinal cord compression. If congenital kyphosis causes spinal cord compression, anterior decompression is indicated. The compression is created by bone or disc material pressing into the front of the spinal cord, and this can be decompressed only by an anterior procedure; laminectomy has no role in the treatment of this condition (24). If associated with scoliosis, the anterior approach for decompression may be on the concavity of the scoliosis to allow the spinal cord to move both forward and into the midline after decompression. After adequate decompression has been achieved, the vertebrae involved are fused with an anterior strut graft. This is followed by a posterior fusion, with or without posterior stabilizing instrumentation. Postoperative support with a cast, brace, or halo cast may be required.

Treatment of Type II Deformities. Treatment of type II deformities can be divided into early treatment of mild deformities and late treatment of severe deformities as outlined by

Mayfield et al. (59). If a type II kyphosis is mild and detected early, posterior fusion with compression instrumentation can be done. The kyphosis should be <50 degrees for a posterior fusion alone to have a good chance of success. The posterior fusion should include all the involved vertebrae, plus one vertebra above and one vertebra below the congenital kyphosis.

Compression instrumentation can be used more safely in type II deformities, because the kyphosis is more rounded and affects several segments, instead of being sharply angular as in type I deformities. If the deformity is severe and detected late, correction can be obtained only with anterior osteotomies and fusion, followed by posterior fusion and compression instrumentation (59).

Complications of Treatment. Some of the more frequent complications of treatment of congenital kyphosis are pseudarthrosis, progression of kyphosis, and paralysis. Pseudarthrosis and progression of the kyphotic deformity can be minimized by using anterior and posterior fusions for deformities of more than 50 degrees. The posterior fusion should extend from one level above to one level below the involved vertebrae. This may allow for some correction with growth.

Paralysis is perhaps the most feared complication of spinal surgery. The risk of this complication can be lessened by not attempting to maximally correct the deformity with instrumentation. Instrumentation should be used only for stabilization of rigid deformities unless simultaneous anterior vertebral-body resection and posterior fusion and instrumentation are done through a costotransversectomy approach as described by Smith et al. (57). The use of halo traction in rigid congenital kyphotic deformities has been associated with an increased risk of neurologic compromise (58). Another long-term problem, occurring in approximately 38% of patients with kyphosis, is low back pain caused by increased lumbar lordosis, which is needed to compensate for the kyphotic deformity (60).

PROGRESSIVE ANTERIOR VERTEBRAL FUSION

Progressive anterior vertebral fusion (PAVF) is rare and is an uncommon cause of kyphosis in pediatric patients; however, if discovered late it may be confused with type II congenital kyphosis. Knutsson (61), in 1949, was the first to describe PAVF in the English-language literature, and fewer than 100 cases have since been reported (62–68). Because the largest reported series (26 patients) was from the University Hospital of Copenhagen (68), some have named this the Copenhagen syndrome. This condition is distinguishable from type II congenital kyphosis because the disc spaces and vertebral bodies are normal at birth and later become affected with an anterior fusion. Although the etiology is unknown, PAVF is probably a distinct clinical condition; however, it may represent a delayed type II congenital kyphosis.

Dubousset (34) suggested that certain forms of type II congenital kyphosis (failure of segmentation) may be inher-

ited. The patients have a failure of segmentation, with delayed fusion of the anterior vertebral elements, which is not visible on radiographs until 8 or 10 years of age. He described one family in which three individuals had delayed ossification and congenital kyphosis, and another family in which the grandmother, mother, and two sisters had the deformity. Kharrat and Dubousset (62) also found this condition to be familial in 6 of 15 patients, and Van Buskirk et al. (63) reported associated anomalies in 7 of 15 patients, including heart defects, tibial agenesis, foot deformities, Klippel-Feil syndrome, Ito syndrome, pulmonary artery stenosis, and hemisacralization of L5.

Neurologic deficits are usually not seen in patients with PAVF, but Smith (63) reported one case of spinal cord compression resulting from an acutely angled kyphosis. Van Buskirk et al. (63) and Dubousset (28, 34) described five stages of PAVF: stage 1 is disc space narrowing, which occurs to a greater extent anteriorly than posteriorly; stage 2 is increased sclerosis of the vertebral end plates of the anterior and middle columns; stage 3 is fragmentation of the anterior vertebral end plates; stage 4 is fusion of the anterior and sometimes the middle columns; and stage 5 is development of a kyphotic deformity. Hughes and Saifuddin (67) described the MRI appearance of PAVF in three patients: early anterior disc narrowing (Fig. 19-18A), significant end-plate edema and fatty marrow changes (Fig. 19-18B), and finally multilevel anterior fusion and disc obliteration (Fig. 19-18C–E)

Kyphosis is the last stage in PAVF and is caused by the anterior disc space fusing while part of the posterior disc space remains open, allowing for continued growth in the posterior disc space and the posterior column. Bollini et al. (65) found that patients with thoracic PAVF had a relatively good prognosis, whereas those with lumbar involvement had a poor prognosis. Involvement of the thoracic spine is better tolerated by patients than is involvement of the lumbar area because of the normal kyphotic posture of the thoracic spine. Therefore, nonoperative treatment is recommended for most thoracic PAVF deformities. For PAVF in the lumbar spine, a posterior spinal fusion is indicated in stages 1, 2, and 3. In stages 4 and 5, the kyphotic deformity has already occurred in a normally lordotic lumbar spine. Posterior fusion will only stop progression of kyphotic deformity. If normal sagittal alignment is to be obtained, an anterior osteotomy followed by posterior fusion and instrumentation is recommended (61–68).

INFANTILE LUMBAR HYPOPLASIA

Campos et al. (69) reported thoracolumbar kyphosis secondary to lumbar hypoplasia in seven normal infants; the thoracolumbar kyphosis resolved spontaneously with growth. Patients presented with a clinically apparent kyphotic deformity in the first year of life. Radiographically, the patients had a relatively sharply angled kyphosis, with the apex at the affected vertebra (Fig. 19-19A). The affected vertebra had a wedge shape with an anterosuperior indentation, giving it a

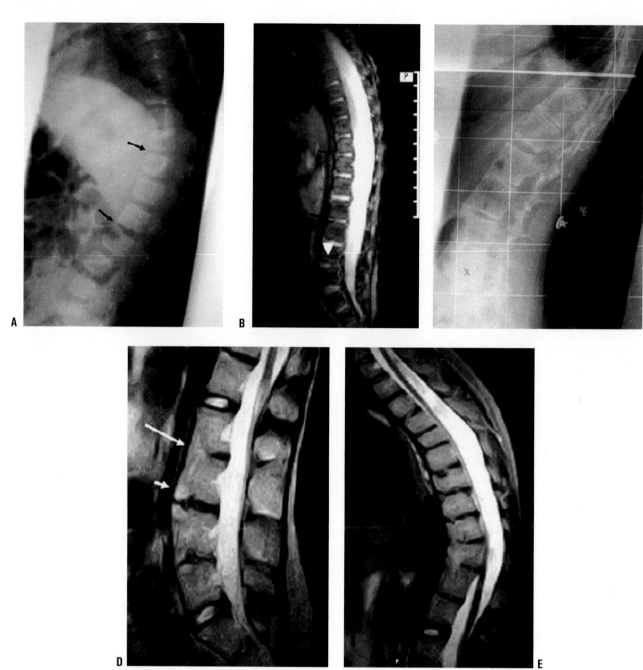

FIGURE 19-18. Progressive anterior vertebral fusion. **A**: Lateral radiograph of the thoracolumbar spine at age 12 months. Note narrowing at the T11/T12 and L2/L3 disc spaces anteriorly (*arrows*). **B**: MR imaging at age 12 months with sagittal STIR sequences through the thoracolumbar spine demonstrates early loss of anterior disc height at the T11/T12 and L2/L3 levels (*black arrows*). The horizontal high-signal intensity STIR abnormality (*white arrowhead*) at multiple end-plate levels is likely to represent normal physeal appearance at this age. **C**: Lateral radiograph (with gridlines for alignment) at age 12 years shows anterior fusion at multiple levels. **D**: MR image at age 12 years. Sagittal T2 FE sequences through the lumbar spine. Note solid fusion at the L2/L3 level (*long white arrow*), discovertebral anterior corner SI changes at the L3/L4 level (*short white arrow*), and fusion with the posterior elements. **E**: MR sagittal scanning through the thoracolumbar levels with T2 FSE sequences demonstrates T10/T11 and T11/T12 fusion and multilevel anterior disc space obliteration. (From Hughes RJ, Saifuddin A. Progressive non-infectious anterior vertebral fusion (Copenhagen syndrome) in three children: features on radiographs and MR imaging. *Skeletal Radiol* 1906;35:397–401.)

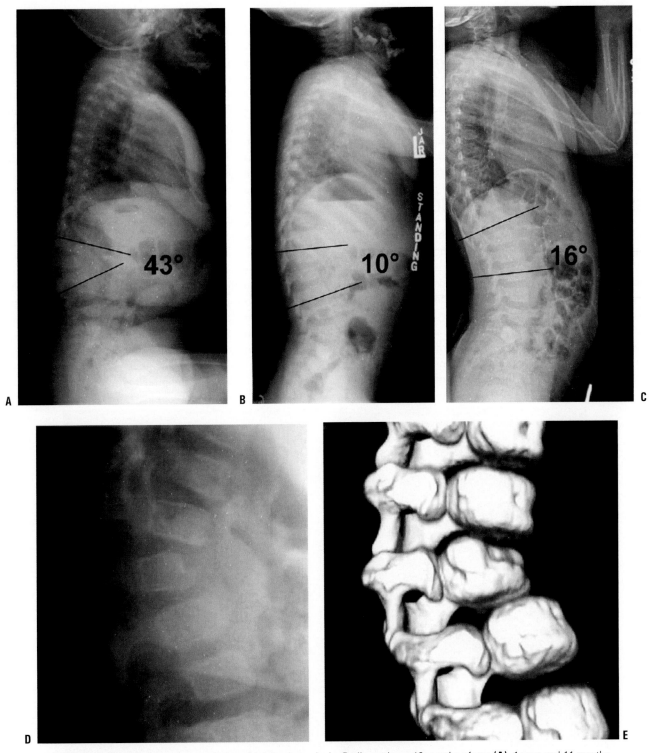

FIGURE 19-19. Spontaneous resolution of lumbar hypoplasia. Radiographs at 13 months of age **(A)**, 1 year and 11 months of age **(B)**, and 4 years and 6 months of age **(C)**. Radiograph **(D)** and computed tomographic three-dimensional reconstruction **(E)** show "beaked" L2 vertebra. (From Campos MA, Fernandes P, Dolan LA, et al. Infantile thoracolumbar kyphosis secondary to lumbar hypoplasia. *J Bone Joint Surg Am* 1908; 90:1726–1729.)

"beaked" appearance (Fig. 19-19B,C). Only one vertebra was involved in all seven infants, either at L1 or L2. The average initial kyphosis was 34 degrees. The kyphosis spontaneously improved after walking age and had corrected to normal by 6 years of age (Fig. 19-19D,E). Campos et al. recommended an initial period of observation for most patients with this type of congenital kyphosis to get a better assessment of the anomaly as ossification progresses and avoid overtreatment of lumbar hypoplasia that spontaneously improves with growth.

SEGMENTAL SPINAL DYSGENESIS

Segmental spinal dysgenesis is a congenital anomaly of the lumbar or thoracolumbar spine, consisting of focal agenesis or dysgenesis of the spine, and resulting in severe spinal stenosis and instability (70). A progressive kyphosis occurs at the site of segmental spinal dysgenesis. This condition often is confused with other spinal anomalies such as type I congenital kyphosis, sacral agenesis, lumbosacral agenesis, and lumbar agenesis. Faciszewski et al. (71) gave detailed radiographic and clinical definitions of this condition. Segmental spinal dysgenesis is characterized by severe focal stenosis of the spinal canal at the involved segment and is associated with significant narrowing of the thecal sac and absence of adjacent nerve roots. At the involved level, a ring of bone encircles the posteriorly positioned spinal canal, causing stenosis. The spinal canal is hourglass-shaped with no neurocentral junctions. There is limited potential for enlargement with growth because of the absence of neurocentral junctions, where growth occurs (Fig. 19-19). No pedicles or spinous or transverse processes are present at this level. Anterior to the bony ring is a fat-filled space. The distal bony anatomy and the spinal canal are usually normal, although spina bifida has been noted in a few cases (72). Neurologic function can range from normal to complete paraplegia. Associated anomalies are common, and there is a high incidence of neurogenic bladder (Fig. 19-20).

The etiology of segmental spinal dysgenesis is unknown. The diagnosis can be made on the basis of plain radiographs, but MRI and CT scans and three-dimensional reconstructions are usually needed to fully show the extent of this condition. Tortori-Donati et al. found that the patient's clinical status correlated with the amount of neural tissue seen on MRI at the level of the lesion (73). Progressive kyphosis occurs with this condition, and progressive neurologic deterioration was noted by Flynn et al. (74) and Faciszewski et al. (71). Early anterior and posterior fusions, with or without

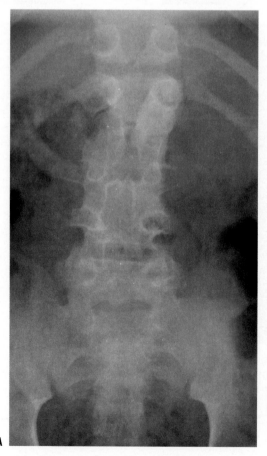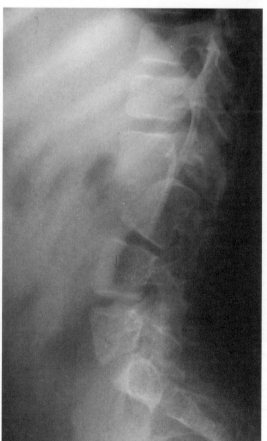

FIGURE 19-20.   Segmental spinal dysgenesis. Anteroposterior **(A)** and lateral **(B)** radiographs show narrowing of spinal canal and absence of L1 and part of L2 vertebral bodies.

decompression, are recommended. The use of spinal instrumentation is controversial because of the small size of the patient. Hughes et al. (72) recommended that treatment be directed toward the establishment and maintenance of spinal stability first and toward decompression of the cord secondarily. Bristol et al. recommended rigid spinal immobilization for 12 to 18 months to allow growth and development before spinal fusion (75).

SACRAL AGENESIS

Sacral agenesis consists of a complete or partial absence of the sacrum (76–79). Rarely is it associated with absence of the most caudal segment of the lumbar spine. The association with maternal diabetes has been well documented (76–79). Kyphosis may occur with this condition, although it usually is not progressive and does not require treatment (80, 81).

SCHEUERMANN DISEASE

Scheuermann disease is a common cause of structural kyphosis in the thoracic, thoracolumbar, and lumbar spine. Scheuermann originally described this rigid juvenile kyphosis in 1919; it is characterized by vertebral-body wedging that is believed to be caused by a growth disturbance of the vertebral end plates (82, 83) (Fig. 19-21).

Classification.   Scheuermann disease can be divided into two distinct groups: a typical form and an atypical form. These two types are determined by the location and natural history of the kyphosis, including symptoms occurring during adolescence and after growth is completed. Typical Scheuermann disease usually involves the thoracic spine, with a well-established natural history during adolescence and after skeletal maturity (84). In this classic form of Scheuermann kyphosis three or more consecutive vertebrae, each wedged 5 degrees or more (Sorensen criteria), produce a structural kyphosis. In contrast, atypical Scheuermann disease usually is located in the thoracolumbar junction or in the lumbar spine, and its natural history is well defined. The atypical type is characterized by vertebral end-plate changes, disc space narrowing, and anterior Schmorl nodes but does not necessarily fulfill Sorensen's criteria of three consecutively wedged vertebrae of 5 degrees. Thoracic Scheuermann is the more common form, with the atypical form less frequently seen.

Epidemiology.   Typical Scheuermann disease consists of a rigid thoracic kyphosis in a juvenile or adolescent spine. The apex of kyphosis is located between T7 and T9 (11). The reported incidence of Scheuermann deformities in the general population ranges from 0.4% to 10% (85–89). Reported male-to-female ratios vary in the literature. Scheuermann originally reported a male preponderance of 88% (82). Most reports in the literature note either a slight male preponderance

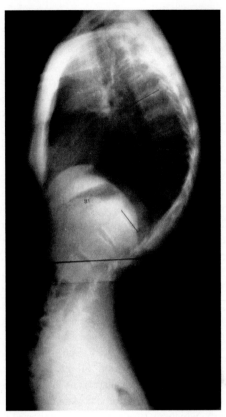

FIGURE 19-21.   Lateral radiograph of a patient with Scheuermann disease and an 81-degree kyphotic deformity. Note the narrowing of the intervertebral disc spaces and the irregularity of the vertebral end plates. There is an associated increase in lumbar lordosis below the kyphotic deformity.

or an equal male-to-female ratio (87–92). Bradford et al. (86) have been the only ones to report an increased incidence of Scheuermann disease in women.

The age at onset of Scheuermann kyphosis is during the prepubertal growth spurt, between 10 and 12 years of age. Sorensen (88) described a Scheuermann prodrome in patients who had a lax, asthenic posture from the age of approximately 4 to 8 years, and in whom, within a few years, a fixed kyphosis developed. The clinical detection of Scheuermann disease occurs at approximately 10 to 12 years of age. Wedging of apical vertebrae has not been reported before 10 years of age (93). Radiographic evidence of Scheuermann disease usually is not detectable in patients younger than 10 years of age because the ring apophysis is not yet ossified. Until the ring apophysis ossifies, vertebral-body wedging and irregularity of the end plate are difficult to measure on radiographs.

Etiology.   Many possible etiologies have been suggested for Scheuermann disease, but the true cause remains unknown. Genetic, vascular, hormonal, metabolic, and mechanical factors have been suggested as causes of Scheuermann kyphosis. Sorensen (88) noted a high familial predilection, and Halal et al. (94), in a study of five families, and McKenzie and

Sillence (95), in a study of 12 families, suggested that the disease may be inherited in an autosomal dominant fashion with a high degree of penetrance. Additional support for a genetic basis for this condition is provided by Carr et al. (96, 97) in a report of Scheuermann disease occurring in identical twins and by Damborg et al. (98), who found an almost 3% prevalence and 74% heritability in a large group of twins (over 35,000 individuals). Halal et al. (94), McKenzie and Sillence (95), and Carr et al. (97) reported possible autosomal dominant inheritance of Scheuermann kyphosis.

Scheuermann believed that the kyphosis was caused by a form of avascular necrosis of the ring apophysis, which led to a growth disturbance resulting in a progressive kyphosis with growth (82, 83). The problem with this theory is that the ring apophysis contributes little, if at all, to the longitudinal growth of the vertebrae (97, 99). Bick and Copel (99) demonstrated that the ring apophysis lies outside the true cartilaginous physis and contributes nothing to the longitudinal growth of the vertebral body. Therefore, a disturbance in the ring apophysis should not affect growth of the vertebrae or cause vertebral wedging.

Schmorl (100) described a herniation of disc material through the cartilaginous end plate, known as *Schmorl nodes*. He believed that the herniation of disc material occurred because of a weakened end plate. The disc herniation was thought to damage the anterior end plate, resulting in abnormal growth, which in turn caused the kyphosis. There is a definite increased incidence of Schmorl nodes in patients with Scheuermann kyphosis, but the problem with this theory is that Schmorl nodes are found outside the area of kyphosis and also are present in individuals who have asymptomatic, normal spines and do not have a kyphotic deformity.

Ferguson (101) suggested that persistence of an anterior vascular groove altered the anterior growth of the vertebral body, but Aufdermaur and Spycher (102, 103) and Ippolito and Ponseti (104) were unable to document growth disturbances around the anterior vascular groove and concluded that persistence of an anterior vascular groove is a sign of immaturity of the spine. Lambrinudi (105) postulated that Scheuermann disease resulted from upright posture and a tight anterior longitudinal ligament. The fact that no cases of Scheuermann disease have been found in quadruped animals lends support to this theory (106). This has led to the more popular belief that the anterior end-plate changes are caused by mechanical forces in response to Wolff's law or the Hueter-Volkmann principle. Compression forces in the anterior physis cause a decrease in growth in the area of the kyphosis. Indirect support for this argument can be found in the changes in the wedging of the involved vertebral bodies and the reversal of these changes when bracing or casting is used in the immature spine. Scoles et al. (106) also supported this theory by demonstrating disorganized endochondral ossification in the involved vertebrae, similar to that seen in Blount disease. They concluded that the changes in endochondral ossification resulted from increased pressure on the vertebral physis.

Ascani et al. (107, 108) found that patients who have Scheuermann disease tend to be taller than normal for their chronologic and skeletal ages with bone age more advanced than their chronologic age. Because they found increased growth hormone levels in these patients, they suggested that the increased height and the advanced skeletal age could be caused by the increased growth hormone. The increased height and the more rapid growth may make the vertebral end plates more susceptible to increased pressure and result in the changes seen in Scheuermann disease. The increased growth hormone levels noted by Ascani et al. may also lead to a relative osteoporosis of the spine, which, in turn, may predispose the spine to the development of Scheuermann disease.

Bradford et al. (85, 109), Burner et al. (110), and Lopez et al. (111) reported in the 1980s that Scheuermann kyphosis may be caused by a form of juvenile osteoporosis. However, using quantitative CT scans, Gilsanz et al. (112) found no evidence of osteoporosis in patients with Scheuermann kyphosis compared with normal research subjects. The authors suggested that the technique used to determine osteoporosis might account for the differences between their report and those that show osteoporosis. In a study using single-photon absorptiometric analysis of cadaver vertebrae from patients with Scheuermann kyphosis, Scoles et al. (106) also found no evidence of osteoporosis.

What is shown by the histologic studies of Ascani et al. (107), Ippolito et al. (104, 113), and Scoles et al. (106) is that an alteration in endochondral ossification occurs. Whether this altered endochondral ossification is the cause or result of kyphosis is not known. Ippolito and Ponseti (104) found a decrease in the number of collagen fibers, which were thinner than normal, and an increase in proteoglycan content. Some areas of the altered end plate showed direct bone formation from cartilage instead of the normal physeal sequences of ossification. These studies help support the belief that Scheuermann kyphosis is an underlying growth problem of the anterior vertebral end plates.

Atypical Scheuermann kyphosis, or thoracolumbar and lumbar kyphosis, is believed to be caused by trauma to the immature spine, resulting in irregularities of the end plate (114).

Natural History. Many early studies suggested an unfavorable natural history for Scheuermann disease and recommended early treatment to prevent severe deformity, pain, impaired social functioning, embarrassment about physical appearance, myelopathy, degeneration of the disc spaces, spondylolisthesis, and cardiopulmonary failure. Despite these reports, few long-term follow-up studies of Scheuermann disease were performed until that of Murray et al. (87). Findings by Travaglini and Conti (39, 115), Murray et al. (87), and Lowe (116) suggest that the natural history of the disease tends to be benign.

The kyphotic deformity progresses rapidly during the adolescent growth spurt. Bradford et al. (117) noted that, among the patients who required brace treatment, more than half had progression of their deformities during this growth spurt before brace treatment was begun. Little is known about progression of the kyphosis after growth is completed, and whether it is similar to that in scoliosis. It is not well documented whether the kyphosis will continue to progress beyond a certain degree during adulthood.

Travaglini and Conte (39) found that the kyphosis did progress during adulthood, but few patients developed severe deformities. What is known is that patients with Scheuermann kyphosis have more intense back pain, jobs that require relatively little physical activity, less range of motion of the trunk in extension, and different localization of back pain than the general population who do not have Scheuermann kyphosis (87). Even with these findings, when compared with normal individuals, patients with Scheuermann kyphosis have no significant differences in self-esteem, social limitations, or level of recreational activities. The number of days they miss from work because of back pain also is similar.

The data regarding the natural history of Scheuermann disease suggest that, although patients may have some functional limitations, their lives are not seriously restricted and they have few clinical or functional problems. Pulmonary function actually increases in these patients, probably because of the increased diameter of the chest cavity, until their kyphosis is more than 100 degrees. Patients with kyphosis of more than 100 degrees have restricted pulmonary function. Another finding in patients with Scheuermann kyphosis was that disc degeneration was five times more likely to be seen on MRI in patients with Scheuermann compared with controls (118). The clinical significance of this finding is not known (76).

Associated Conditions. Mild-to-moderate scoliosis is present in about one-third of patients with Scheuermann disease (116), but the curves tend to be small, approximately 10 to 19 degrees. Scoliosis associated with Scheuermann disease usually has a benign natural history. The scoliotic curve rarely is progressive and usually does not require treatment. Deacon et al. (118, 119, 120) divided scoliotic curves in patients with Scheuermann disease into two types, based on the location of the curve and the rotation of the vertebrae into or away from the concavity of the scoliotic curve. In the first type of curves, the apices of scoliosis and kyphosis are the same and the curve is rotated toward the convexity. The rotation of the scoliotic curve is opposite to that normally seen in idiopathic scoliosis. Deacon et al. (101, 119) suggested that the difference in direction of rotation is caused by scoliosis occurring in a kyphotic spine, instead of the hypokyphotic or the lordotic spine that is common in idiopathic scoliosis. In the second type of curves, the apex of the scoliosis is above or below the apex of the kyphosis and the scoliotic curve is rotated into the concavity of the scoliosis, more like idiopathic scoliosis. This type of scoliosis seen with Scheuermann kyphosis is the more common, and it rarely progresses or requires treatment.

Lumbar spondylolysis is a frequently associated finding in Scheuermann kyphosis (Fig. 19-22). The suggested reason

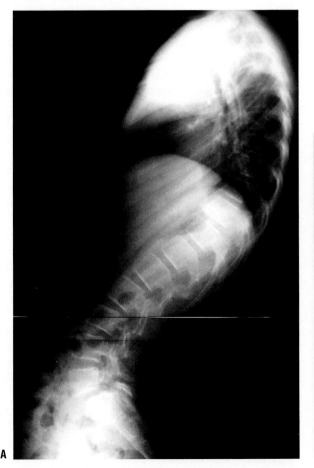
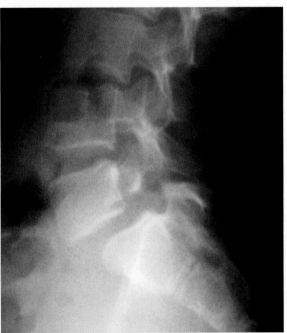

FIGURE 19-22. **A,B**: Lateral radiographs demonstrating spondylolisthesis with kyphosis.

for the increased incidence of spondylolysis is that increased stress is placed on the pars interarticularis because of the associated compensatory hyperlordosis of the lumbar spine in Scheuermann disease. This increased stress causes a fatigue fracture at the pars interarticularis, resulting in spondylolysis. Ogilvie and Sherman (121) found a 50% incidence of spondylolysis in the 18 patients they reviewed. Stoddard and Osborn reported a 54% incidence of spondylolysis in their patients with Scheuermann kyphosis (122).

Other conditions reported in patients with Scheuermann disease include endocrine abnormalities (123), hypovitaminosis (124), inflammatory disorders (122, 123), and dural cysts (106, 125).

Clinical Presentation.
Clinical signs of Scheuermann disease occur around the time of puberty. The clinical feature that distinguishes postural kyphosis from Scheuermann kyphosis is rigidity. Often, mild Scheuermann disease is believed to be postural because the kyphosis may be more flexible in the early stages than in later stages. Usually, the patient seeks treatment because of a parent's concern about poor posture. Sometimes the poor posture has been present for several months or longer, or the parents may have noticed a recent change during a growth spurt. Attributing kyphotic deformity in a child to poor posture often causes a delay in diagnosis and treatment.

Pain may be the predominant clinical complaint rather than deformity. The pain generally is located over the area of the kyphotic deformity, but also occurs in the lower lumbar spine if compensatory lumbar lordosis is severe. Back pain usually is aggravated by standing, sitting, or physical activity. The distribution and intensity of the pain vary according to the age of the patient, the stage of the disease, the site of the kyphosis, and the severity of the deformity. Pain usually subsides with the cessation of growth, although pain in the thoracic spine can sometimes continue even after the patient is skeletally mature (87, 126). More commonly, after growth is completed patients complain of low back pain caused by the compensatory or exaggerated lumbar lordosis.

Most symptoms relating to Scheuermann disease occur during the rapid growth phase. During the growth spurt, pain is reported by 22% of patients, but as the end of the adolescent growth spurt approaches, this figure reaches 60%. Some authors believe that when growth is complete the pain recedes completely, except for well-circumscribed paraspinal discomfort (127–129). In adult patients with Scheuermann disease, pain may be located in and around the posterior iliac crest. This pain is thought to result from arthritic changes at T11 and T12, because the posterior crest is supplied by this dermatome. Stagnara (130) suggested that the mobile areas above and below the rigid segment are the source of pain.

Symptoms also depend on the apex of kyphosis. Murray et al. (87) noted that if the apex of kyphosis is in the upper thoracic spine, patients have more pain with everyday activities. The degree of kyphosis has also been correlated with symptoms. It seems logical that the larger the kyphosis, the more likely it is to be symptomatic, but Murray et al. found that curves between 65 and 85 degrees produced the most symptoms, whereas curves of more than 85 degrees and <65 degrees produced fewer symptoms. However, in patients with thoracolumbar or lumbar kyphosis (atypical Scheuermann disease), activity decreased as the degree of kyphosis increased.

Lumbar Scheuermann Disease.
Patients with lumbar Scheuermann disease differ from those with thoracic deformity. These patients usually have low back pain but, unlike patients with the more common form of Scheuermann disease, their kyphotic deformity is not as noticeable. Pain is associated with spinal movement. Lumbar Scheuermann is especially common in men involved in competitive sports and in farm laborers, suggesting that the cause may be an injury to the vertebral physes from repeated trauma (131).

Physical Examination.
In a patient with Scheuermann disease, a thorough examination of the back and a complete neurologic evaluation are essential. With the patient standing, the shoulders appear to be rounded and the head protrudes forward. The anterior bowing of the shoulders is caused by tight pectoralis muscles. Angular kyphosis is seen most clearly when the patient is viewed from a lateral position and is asked to bend forward. Normally, the back exhibits a gradual rounding with forward bending, but in patients with Scheuermann disease an acute increase is evident in the kyphosis of the thoracic spine or at the thoracolumbar junction. Stagnara et al. (132) found cutaneous pigmentation to be common at the most protruding spinous process at the apex of the kyphosis, probably the result of friction exerted by the backs of chairs and clothing. Compensatory lumbar and cervical lordosis, with forward protrusion of the head, further increases the anterior flexion of the trunk. Associated hamstring and hip flexor muscle tightness often is present.

The kyphotic deformity has some rigidity and will not correct completely with hyperextension. Larger degrees of kyphosis are not necessarily more rigid, and the amount of rigidity will vary with the age of the patient (87).

The neurologic evaluation usually is normal but must not be overlooked. Spinal cord compression has been reported occasionally in patients with Scheuermann disease (133–137). Three types of neural compression have been reported: ruptured thoracic disc (138), intraspinal extradural cyst, and mechanical cord compression at the apex of kyphosis; however, spinal cord compression and neurologic compromise are rare (139). Hughes et al. (67) found that only 1% of patients with a paralyzing disc herniation had Scheuermann disease. Ryan and Taylor (136) suggested that the factors influencing the onset of cord compression in patients whose cord compression is caused by the kyphosis alone are the angle of kyphosis, the number of segments involved, and the rate of change of the angle of kyphosis. This may be why neurologic findings are rare in Scheuermann kyphosis: the kyphosis occurs gradually, over several segments, and without acute angulation.

Radiographic Examination. The most important radiographic views are anteroposterior and lateral views of the spine with the patient standing. The amount of kyphosis present is determined by the Cobb method on a lateral radiograph of the spine. This is accomplished by selecting the cranial- and caudal-most tilted vertebrae in the kyphotic deformity. A line is drawn along the superior end plate of the most cranial vertebra and the inferior end plate of the most caudal vertebra. Lines are drawn perpendicular to the lines along the end plates, and the angle they form where they meet is the degree of kyphosis (140).

The criterion for diagnosis of Scheuermann disease on a lateral radiograph is more than 5 degrees of wedging of at least three adjacent vertebrae (88). The degree of wedging is determined by drawing one line parallel to the superior end plate and another line parallel to the inferior end plate of the vertebra, and measuring the angle formed by their intersection. Bradford and Garcia (141) suggested that three wedged vertebrae are not necessary for the diagnosis, but rather an abnormal, rigid kyphosis is indicative of Scheuermann disease.

The vertebral end plates are irregular, and the disc spaces are narrowed. The anteroposterior diameter of the apical vertebra frequently is increased (106) (Fig. 19-23). Associated Schmorl nodes often are seen in the vertebrae in the kyphosis.

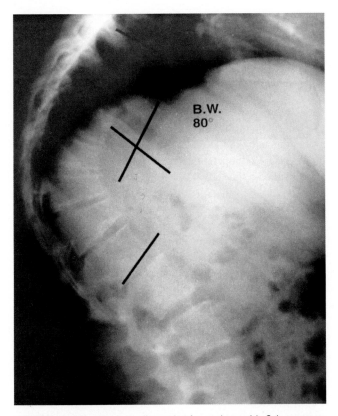

FIGURE 19-23. Lateral radiograph of a patient with Scheuermann disease demonstrates the kyphotic deformity seen in this disorder. Note the irregularity of the vertebral end plates and the anterior vertebral wedging.

Flexibility is determined by taking a lateral radiograph with the patient lying over a bolster placed at the apex of the deformity to hyperextend the spine and maximize the amount of correction seen on a hyperextension radiograph. On the lateral radiographs, most patients will be in negative sagittal balance (142). Sagittal balance is measured on the radiographs by dropping a plumb line from the center of the C7 vertebral body and measuring the distance from this line to the sacral promontory; a positive value indicates that the plumb line lies anterior to the promontory of the sacrum. Normal sagittal balance values are ±2 cm to the sacral promontory. On a lateral radiograph of lumbar Scheuermann kyphosis, irregular end plates, Schmorl nodes, and disc-space narrowing will be seen, but vertebral-body wedging is not as common. MRI and CT scans are necessary only if the patient has unusual symptoms or positive neurologic findings. An anteroposterior or a postero-anterior radiograph of the spine should be obtained to look for associated scoliosis or vertebral anomalies. The patient's skeletal maturity can be estimated from a radiograph of the left hand and wrist or from the Risser sign on the anteroposterior radiograph of the spine.

Treatment. The indications for the treatment of patients with Scheuermann kyphosis can be grouped into five general categories: pain, progression of deformity, neurologic compromise, cardiopulmonary compromise, and cosmesis.

Treatment options include observation, nonoperative methods, and surgery. Observation is an active form of treatment. If the deformity is mild and nonprogressive, the kyphosis can be observed every 4 to 6 months with lateral radiographs. The parents and the patient must understand the need for regular follow-up visits. If the deformity begins to progress, another form of treatment, such as bracing, casting, or surgery, may be indicated.

Nonoperative methods of treatment include exercise, physical therapy, bracing, and casting. Exercise and physical therapy alone will not permanently improve kyphosis that is caused by skeletal changes. The improvement seen with these methods is due to improved muscle tone and correction of bad posture. The goals of physical therapy are to increase flexibility of the spine, correct lumbar hyperlordosis, strengthen extensor muscles of the spine, and stretch tight hamstring and pectoralis muscles. The efficacy of this treatment method has not been proven, and although it may improve the postural component of Scheuermann disease, its effect on a rigid kyphosis is questionable.

Other nonoperative treatment methods can be divided into active correction systems (braces) and passive correction systems (casts). For either a brace or a cast to be effective, the kyphotic curve must be flexible enough to allow correction of at least 40% to 50% (93, 108, 143).

The Milwaukee brace is the brace recommended for the treatment of Scheuermann disease (144) (Fig. 19-24). The Milwaukee brace functions as a dynamic three-point orthosis that promotes extension of the thoracic spine. The neck ring maintains proper alignment of the upper thoracic spine,

FIGURE 19-24. A: Patient with Scheuermann kyphosis has thoracic kyphosis, compensatory lumbar lordosis, anterior protrusion of the head, and rotation of the pelvis. **B**: Patient with Scheuermann kyphosis in a Milwaukee brace. The placement of the pelvic girdle, posterior thoracic pads, occipital pads, and neck ring encourages correction of the kyphosis. **C**: Correction of kyphosis after Milwaukee brace treatment. (Courtesy of Robert Winter, MD, Minneapolis, Minnesota.)

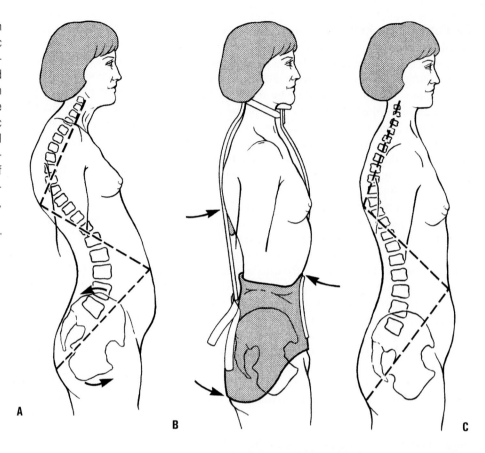

and the padded poster uprights apply pressure over the apex of the kyphosis. The pelvic girdle stabilizes the lumbar spine by flattening the lumbar lordosis. A low-profile brace, without a chin ring and with anterior shoulder pads, can be used for curves with an apex at the level of T9 or lower. The indications for brace treatment are an immature spine (at least 1 year of growth remaining in spine), some flexibility of the curve, and kyphosis of more than 50 degrees. The brace is initially worn full time for an average of 12 to 18 months. If the curve is stabilized and no progression is noted after this time, a part-time brace program can be used until skeletal maturity is reached. Gutowski and Renshaw (145) reported that part-time bracing (16 hours per day) was as effective as full-time bracing and was associated with improved patient compliance. In this study, a Boston lumbar orthosis was used to treat the kyphosis. The rationale for correction with this orthosis is that reduction of the lumbar lordosis causes the patient to dynamically straighten the thoracic kyphosis to maintain an upright posture. This presupposes a flexible thoracic kyphosis, a normal neurovestibular axis, and the absence of hip-flexion contractures.

Several orthopaedists have noted that, after initial improvement, there is a significant loss of correction after the discontinuation of brace treatment (56, 146). Montgomery and Erwin (92) stated that, if permanent correction of kyphosis is possible, a change in vertebral-body wedging should be seen before bracing is discontinued. Although some loss of correction can occur after bracing is discontinued, it still is effective in obtaining some correction of the kyphosis and possibly

in reversing vertebral-body wedging, or at least preventing progression of the kyphotic deformity (92) (Fig. 19-25). Poor results with brace treatment have been reported in patients in whom the kyphosis exceeded 75 degrees or wedging of the vertebral bodies was more than 10 degrees and in patients near or past skeletal maturity (141).

Antigravity and localizer casts have been used extensively in Europe for nonoperative treatment of Scheuermann kyphosis, with good results (130, 147–149). De Mauroy and Stagnara (147) developed a therapeutic regimen that uses serial casts for correction. This method consists of three stages. First, a physical therapy program is started in preparation for the casts. Next, three sequential antigravity casts, changed at 45-day intervals, are applied to obtain gradual correction of the deformity. The third stage involves the use of a plastic maintenance brace that is worn until skeletal maturity is reached. With this regimen the deformity was reported to improve by 40%, and there was less loss of correction after this form of nonoperative treatment was discontinued (130, 148, 149).

The indications for surgical correction remain unclear because of various opinions about pain, disability, trunk deformity, and importance of cosmesis. Therefore, the decision for surgery must be made on an individual basis. The current indications for surgery are a progressive kyphosis of more than 75 degrees and significant kyphosis associated with pain that is not alleviated by nonoperative treatment methods. The biomechanical principles of correction of kyphosis secondary to Scheuermann disease include

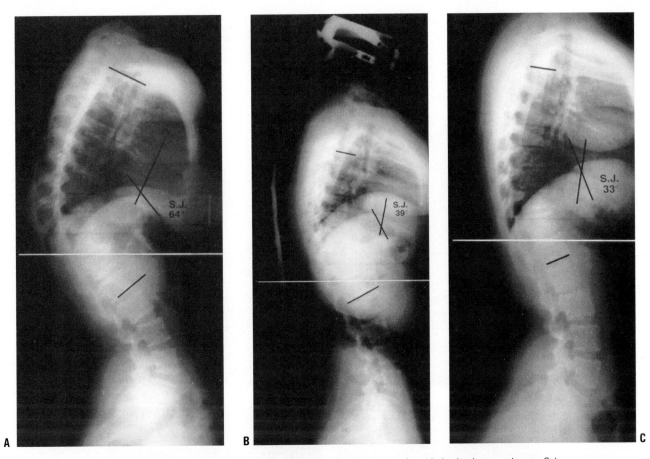

FIGURE 19-25.   A: Lateral radiograph of a 15-year-old girl with a 64-degree thoracic kyphosis secondary to Scheuermann disease. **B:** Lateral radiograph of the patient in a Milwaukee brace with the kyphotic deformity improved to 39 degrees. **C:** Lateral radiograph obtained after the patient completed brace treatment; the kyphotic deformity has improved to 33 degrees.

lengthening the anterior column (anterior release), providing anterior support (interbody fusion), and shortening and stabilizing the posterior column (compression instrumentation and arthrodesis) (150). Surgical correction of kyphosis can be achieved by a posterior approach (Fig. 19-26), an anterior approach, or a combined anterior and posterior approach. The combined anterior and posterior approach has been the most frequently recommended and reported procedure (151–154). With the development of pedicle screw fixation and posterior spinal osteotomy techniques, such as the Ponte procedure (Fig. 19-27), there has been renewed interested in posterior-only surgery. A standard posterior procedure without osteotomy can be considered if the kyphosis can be corrected to, and maintained at, <50 degrees while a posterior fusion occurs (146–148, 155, 156). Historically, the use of Harrington compression rods was common, but these rarely are used now because of the frequent complications, including rod breakage, and the need for postoperative immobilization. Anterior instrumentation for Scheuermann disease was described by Kostuik (157); it consists of anterior interbody fusion and anterior instrumentation with a Harrington distraction system augmented by postoperative bracing. Although Kostuik reported good results with

this technique, the anterior-only instrumentation approach for treatment of Scheuermann kyphosis is not widely used.

The Ponte osteotomy (Fig. 19-27) is performed using Kerrison rongeurs and begins by completely excising the ligamentum flavum, which allows for maximal mobilization of the spine. The osteotomy involves the complete resection of the inferior articular process of the cranial vertebra and the superior articular process of the caudal vertebra laterally to the neural foramen at each level. The osteotomies can be widened cranially and caudally at each level, typically in the range of 4 to 6 mm, depending on the amount of correction required. Typically, 5 to 10 degrees of correction at each level can be achieved (158).

When anterior and posterior surgeries together are used for Scheuermann disease, the anterior release and fusion are done first. The anterior release can be done through an open anterior exposure or by thoracoscopy. While thoracoscopic release may offer advantages over open thoracotomy, such as decreased postoperative pain, scarring, and impact on pulmonary function, the technique is technically challenging and has a high complication rate. Herrera-Soto et al. showed good sagittal correction, with no loss of

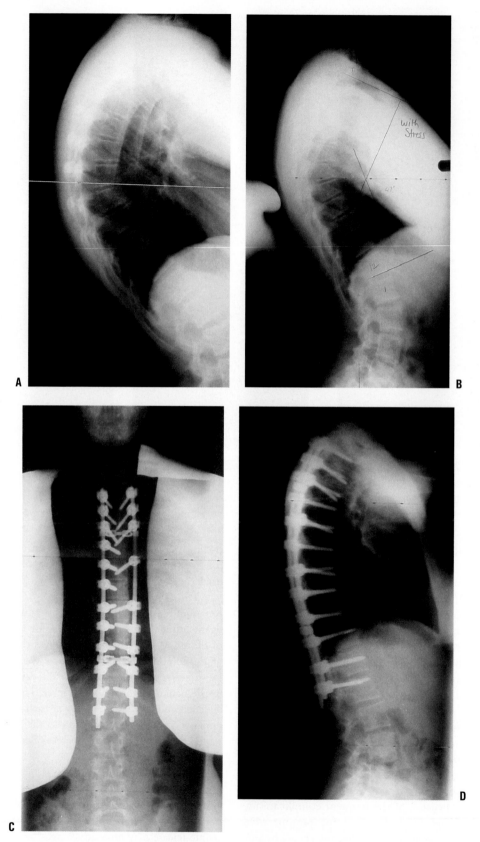

FIGURE 19-26. **A:** Thoracic Scheuermann kyphosis. **B:** After posterior fusion and instrumentation with pedicle screws. **C** and **D:** Postoperative status of posterior instrumentation and fusion with pedicle screws. (Courtesy of Dr. Anant Kumar.)

correction or junctional kyphosis using this technique; however, they had 11 complications in 9 of 19 patients, including 2 pneumothoraces and a deep venous thrombosis leading to a pulmonary embolus (159). Interbody cages have been used in an effort to improve sagittal correction (160, 161); however, Arun et al. (160) found no difference in outcomes between patients with anterior fusions using interbody cages compared to those with anterior fusions using autogenous rib graft.

The posterior fusion and instrumentation usually are done on the same day as the anterior release and fusion, but they can be done in a staged manner. For the posterior spinal fusion, a segmental instrumentation system using multiple hooks or pedicle screws or a hybrid of hooks and screws is used. Lowe (153) and Coscia et al. (162) reported high complication rates after using Luque rods and wires for posterior fixation, because this system does not allow for any compression. The use of posterior spinal osteotomies such as the Ponte

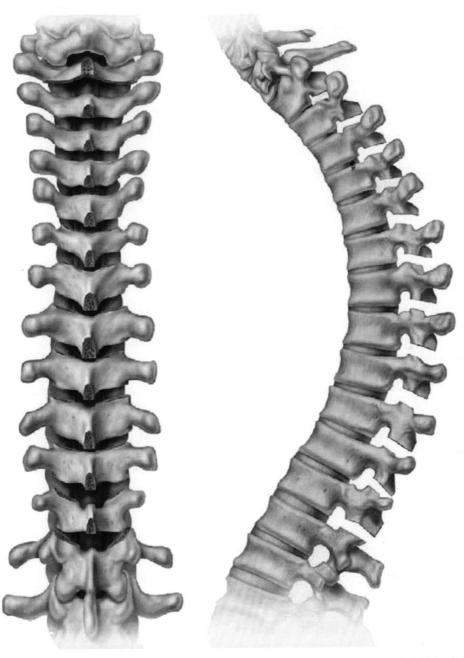

A

FIGURE 19-27. Ponte procedure: posterior-only osteotomies. **A**: Osteotomies. **B**: Anchor placement. **C**: Initial rod placement with proximal anchor compression. **D**: Final rod placement with final rod compression and deformity correction. (From Geck MJ, Macagno A, Ponte A, et al. The Ponte procedure: Posterior only treatment of Scheuermann's kyphosis using segmental posterior shortening and pedicle screw instrumentation. *J Spinal Disord Tech* 1907;19:586–593.)

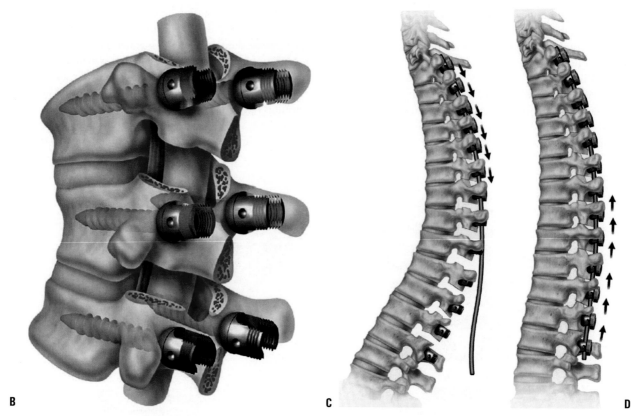

FIGURE 19-27   *(continued)*

osteotomy allows relative shortening of the posterior column, which allows greater correction of the kyphosis. Several studies have shown similar outcomes in terms of sagittal correction between patients with combined anterior–posterior release and those with posterior-only procedures with Ponte osteotomies (158, 163–165). In addition, patients with combined anterior–posterior release have more complications, longer surgical times, and more blood loss than those with posterior osteotomy and fusion alone (164, 165).

Regardless of the type of instrumentation used and whether or not other procedures such as anterior release or spinal osteotomy are done, posterior instrumentation should include at least three fixation points above the apex and at least two fixation points below the apex of the kyphosis. The fusion and instrumentation should include the proximal vertebra in the measured kyphotic deformity and the first lordotic disc distally (114, 142, 150, 166). If the fusion and instrumentation end in the kyphotic deformity, a junctional kyphosis at the end of the instrumentation is likely to develop (165).

POSTERIOR HOOK INSTRUMENTATION   This procedure has several attractive features for the treatment of kyphosis (Figs. 19-28 to 19-30). It is very rigid and requires no postoperative immobilization. In patients who have significant scoliosis in addition to kyphosis, it has the ability to correct both the kyphosis and the scoliosis. The hooks can be placed independent of the rod

(unlike the classic Harrington compression rod); it is not a problem to insert the hooks on the other side of the spine after the first hooks have been placed and tightened.

There are also disadvantages. The rods must be contoured to the desired correction, which means that most of the correction is obtained at once. This makes it difficult to get the rod into the inferior hooks in closed-hook systems after they have been placed in the superior hooks. The use of pedicle screws at the bottom of the instrumentation or a hybrid construct obviates this to a large extent.

The area of the spine that is to be fused is exposed, and the hook sites are prepared.

Two methods of hook purchase can be used in the instrumentation of kyphosis. They differ in the method used to place the hooks on the thoracic vertebrae (Figs. 19-31).

Regardless of the technique used, junctional decompensation has been reported to occur in as many as 30% of patients (142, 165). Lowe (150, 153) emphasized that overcorrection of the deformity should be avoided to prevent junctional kyphosis. He recommended that no more than 50% of the preoperative kyphosis be corrected and that the final kyphosis should never be <40 degrees. He also found that patients with Scheuermann disease tend to be in negative sagittal balance and become further negatively balanced after surgery, which may predispose them to the development of junctional kyphosis (142). Lonner et al. (165) found

Text continued on page 770

Posterior Hook Instrumentation (Figs. 19-28 to 19-30)

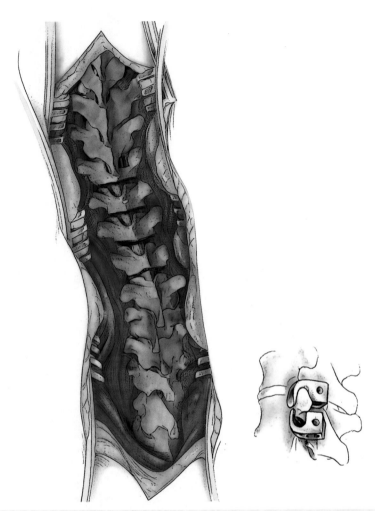

FIGURE 19-28. Posterior Hook Instrumentation. The method of hook purchase illustrated here uses the claw configuration on the thoracic vertebrae. On the cephalad side of the kyphosis, there should be at least three purchase sites on each side of the spine. These purchase sites may be of several combinations of claws, supralaminar hooks, and transverse process hooks, all depending on the bone strength, the rigidity of the curve, and the surgeon's choice. Some surgeons prefer to use supralaminar hooks as purchase sites, as opposed to the transverse processes. Others prefer to place the pedicle hook component of the claw one level distal. In this case, two claw configurations were used. The third hook was a simple transverse process hook. An alternative method on the cephalad portion of the kyphosis is the use of lamina hooks inserted into every other lamina. These can be staggered on either side of the spine. For example, a lamina hook may be inserted on the lamina of T3, T5, and T7 on one side of the spine and on the lamina of T4, T6, and T8 on the other side of the spine. These hooks are inserted on the cephalad aspect of the lamina to provide compression. Three hook sites should be prepared on each side of the spine inferior to the kyphosis. It is important when selecting levels to extend the instrumentation into the normal lordosis. These hook sites are prepared easily by removing the inferior edge of the lamina and then the ligamentum flavum to allow the lamina hook to be seated within the spinal canal. The hook sites should be prepared on both sides of the spine before any hooks or rods are placed. If this is not done, the closing of the interlaminar spaces as a result of placing the first rod makes it more difficult to prepare the sites on the opposite side. The use of pedicle screws at the lower end of the kyphosis makes insertion of the rod easier, although they may not make the correction any better. After this is completed, a radical facetectomy, with removal of a significant portion of the inferior part of the lamina, is performed in the area of the kyphosis to permit correction. This can be accomplished by entering the spinal canal in the midline and using a Kerrison rongeur to remove the bone. The bone that is removed includes the inferior portion of the lamina and the superior facet, as well as a portion of the inferior facet.

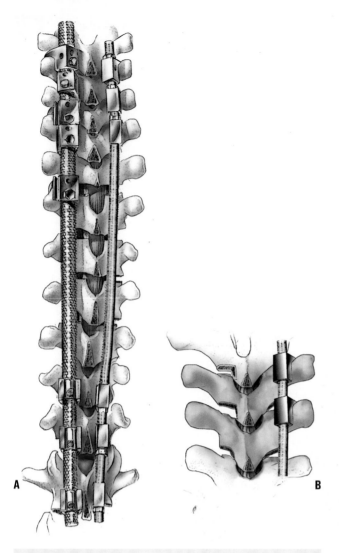

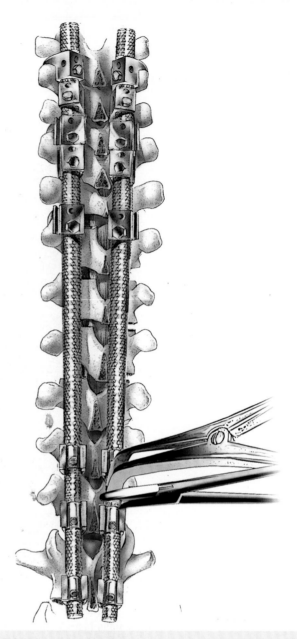

FIGURE 19-29. Now comes the most difficult part of this technique: placing the rods and the hooks. This is difficult because the rods must first be contoured to the desired final degree of correction; therefore, when they are inserted, most of the correction is gained at that time. If all the hooks and the rods are placed cephalad to the kyphosis, it is not easy to push them down into the caudal hooks. In a patient with severe kyphosis, the surgeon has the distinct impression that something will break with continued pushing. Several tricks have been suggested to deal with this problem, such as having an assistant push on the apex of the kyphosis, trying to lift the pelvis, or placing one rod in the cephalad hooks and one rod in the caudal hooks and pushing both down toward their corresponding empty hooks at the same time, as in a double-lever system. These methods may work in the case of flexible curves. Another method is to apply a small Harrington compression rod to one side, tighten it to gain correction, and then place the rigid rod system on the opposite side. The Harrington compression rod is then removed and replaced with the second rod **(A)**. In the thoracic region, the Harrington compression rod **(B)** can be placed on the transverse processes. These are usually strong enough for this temporary correction, and the hooks can be inserted rapidly. Below the kyphosis, the Harrington hooks can be placed in the holes that have been prepared for the hooks of the rigid rod system. With the newer top-opening systems, the rod can be secured in the hooks proximal to the kyphosis apex and then cantilevered into the hooks below. Compressive forces are then applied to continue the kyphosis correction.

FIGURE 19-30. After both rods are placed, most of the correction would have been obtained if the rods were contoured correctly. Some additional correction may be obtained by tightening the hooks in compression, as was done with the Harrington compression rod, spreading between the hook and a rod holder clamped onto the rod. This has the additional advantage of tightening the hook against the bone and should be performed for each hook. To complete the operation, all possible decortication is accomplished and a large amount of bone graft is added.

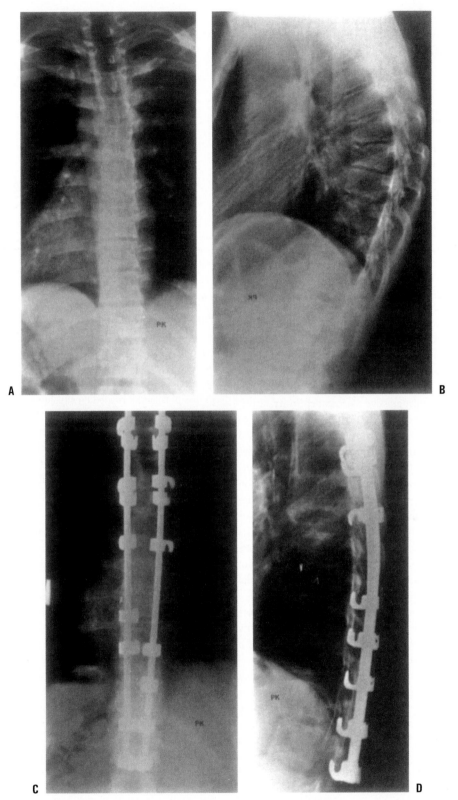

FIGURE 19-31. **A,B:** Anteroposterior and lateral radiographs of a 17-year-old boy with persisting pain secondary to Scheuermann kyphosis. **C,D:** Anteroposterior and lateral radiographs hook instrumentation in place. The upper hooks skipped a level to permit easier insertion, and the lower hooks were staggered to facilitate better decortication.

that pelvic incidence may be related to the amount of proximal junctional kyphosis and that distal junctional kyphosis was related to fusion that ended cranial to the neutral sagittal vertebra.

POSTLAMINECTOMY KYPHOSIS

A laminectomy or multiple laminectomies are needed most often in children for the diagnosis and treatment of spinal cord tumors, but also may be needed for other conditions such as neurofibromatosis, Arnold-Chiari malformation, and syringomyelia (167, 168). Although deformity after laminectomy is unusual in adults, it is common in children because of the unique and dynamic nature of the growing spine (138, 169–173). Younger age appears to be the most significant risk factor for the development of postlaminectomy cervical spine deformities (174). Postlaminectomy deformities usually result in kyphotic deformity, but a scoliotic deformity also may occur (170).

The pathophysiology of postlaminectomy kyphotic deformity can be multifactorial. Deformity of the spine after multiple laminectomies can be caused by (a) skeletal deficiencies (facet joint, laminae, and associated anterior column defects), (b) ligamentous deficiencies, (c) neuromuscular imbalance, (d) effects of gravity, and (e) progressive osseous deformity resulting from growth disturbances (167, 175). Panjabi et al. (176) showed that with loss of posterior stabilizing structures caused by removal of the interspinous ligaments, spinous processes, and laminae, the normal flexion forces placed on the spine will produce kyphosis. Gravity places a flexion moment on the spine, producing compression force on the anterior vertebrae and discs and a tensile force on the remaining posterior structures. This may explain why postlaminectomy deformities occur most often in the cervical and thoracic spine and less often in the lumbar spine. Gravity tends to cause a kyphosis in the cervical and thoracic spine, whereas it accentuates the usual lordosis of the lumbar spine.

Skeletal deficiencies also can produce deformity. An important factor influencing the development of postlaminectomy deformity is the integrity of the facet joint (170, 176–178). If the facet joint is removed or damaged during surgery, deformity is likely to develop. Raynor et al. (179) and Zdeblick et al. (180) found that, if more than 50% of the cervical facet was removed, instability and deformity of the cervical spine occurred. In addition, any secondary involvement of the anterior column, by tumor or surgical resection, adds to the risk of instability and deformity after laminectomy. Also, multiple laminectomies increase the risk of deformity when compared to single-level laminectomies (181, 182).

Insufficient soft-tissue restraints and paralysis of muscles that help stabilize the spine also can add to a postlaminectomy deformity. The spine is unable to resist the normal flexion forces placed on it by gravity and by the normal flexor muscles (183). Yasuoka et al. (184) noted increased wedging of the vertebrae and excessive motion after laminectomy in children, but not in adults. This increased wedging is caused

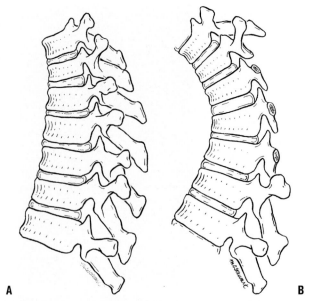

FIGURE 19-32. Drawings of the thoracic spine before and after repeated laminectomy demonstrate the effects on growth of the vertebral bodies. **A**: Before laminectomy, the anterior vertebral bodies are rectangular in configuration. **B**: The spine that has had multiple laminectomies will have increased compression anteriorly because of loss of posterior supporting structures. This compression results in less growth in the anterior portion of the vertebral body than in the posterior portion. In time, this will result in wedging of the vertebral bodies, causing a kyphotic deformity. (From Peterson HA. Iatrogenic spinal deformities. In: Weinstein SL, ed. *The pediatric spine: principles and practice.* New York, NY: Raven, 1994:651.)

by increased pressure on the cartilaginous end plates of the vertebral bodies. With time, the increased pressure causes a decrease in growth of the anterior portion of the vertebrae, according to the Hueter-Volkmann principle (Fig. 19-32). Excessive spinal motion in children after laminectomy can be attributed to the facet joint anatomy in the cervical spine and the greater ligamentous laxity of growing children. The orientation of the cervical facet joint in children is more horizontal than in adults. This horizontal orientation offers less resistance to forces that tend to cause kyphosis in the cervical spine.

Kyphosis is the most common deformity, although scoliosis also may occur, either as the primary deformity or in association with kyphosis. The incidence of postlaminectomy kyphotic deformity ranges from 33% to 100% (185), and depends on the age of the patient and the level of the laminectomy. Generally, the deformity is more likely in younger patients and after more cephalad laminectomy. For example, Yasuoka et al. (184) found that spinal deformity occurred in 46% of patients younger than 15 years of age, but in only 6% of patients 15 to 24 years of age. All the patients between 15 and 24 years of age in whom deformity developed were 18 years of age or younger. Yasuoka et al. (184) and Fraser et al. (186) found that higher levels of laminectomy were associated with a greater chance of deformity. In their studies, deformity occurred after 100% of cervical spine laminectomies, after 36% of thoracic laminectomies, and in none of the lumbar laminectomies. Yeh et al. (182) and Papagelopoulos et al. (187) found that the greater the number of laminae removed, the greater the risk is for developing kyphosis.

Kyphosis in the cervical and thoracic spine is the most common postlaminectomy deformity (188). The lumbar spine is normally in lordosis, and this may protect it from developing kyphosis after multiple lumbar laminectomies. Papagelopoulos et al. (187) reported that hyperlordosis occurred in children who had lumbar laminectomies for intraspinal tumors. If the laminectomies extended into the thoracolumbar junction, kyphosis at the thoracolumbar junction occurred in 33% of their patients. Peter et al. (189) found that most of their patients did not develop a significant deformity after multiple lumbar laminectomies for selective posterior dorsal root rhizotomy; however, 9% developed spondylolysis. This may be the result of increased lordosis in this patient population (190).

Postlaminectomy deformity can occur early in the postoperative period or gradually over time. Kyphotic deformities have been reported to occur as late as 6 years after surgery (169, 190). Progression can be either sudden or gradual, or the deformity may progress significantly only during the adolescent growth spurt.

The natural history of postlaminectomy spinal deformity is varied and depends on the age of the patient at the time of surgery, the location of the laminectomy or laminectomies, and the integrity of the facet joint. Three types of postlaminectomy kyphosis have been described in children: (a) instability after facetectomy, (b) hypermobility between vertebral bodies associated with gradual rounding of the spine, and (c) wedging of vertebral bodies caused by growth disturbances (185).

Kyphosis from instability after facetectomy tends to be sharp and angular and usually occurs in the immediate or early postoperative period, causing associated loss of neurologic function (Fig. 19-33). Gradual rounding of the kyphotic deformity is seen more often when the facet joints are preserved. Kyphosis increases gradually over time because of the stress placed on the remaining posterior structures. If the spine is immature when the laminectomy is performed, the resulting kyphosis can inhibit the growth of the anterior physes of the involved vertebrae. Unequal growth results in wedge-shaped vertebrae and a progressive kyphotic deformity that is accelerated during the adolescent growth spurt.

Other associated conditions that also may add to or cause kyphotic deformities include persistent spinal cord tumors, neurologic deficits, intraspinal pathology (hydromyelia), and radiation therapy (191, 192).

Evaluation. The evaluation of a postlaminectomy deformity should focus on (a) the flexibility of the deformity, (b) loss of spinal structures, and (c) determination of future deformity with growth. The flexibility of a deformity can be estimated by flexion and extension lateral radiographs. If these cannot be obtained, a lateral traction film can be used. CT scans and three-dimensional reconstruction views may better delineate which bony elements are missing. MRI may be used

but gives more information about the spinal cord, disc, and surrounding soft tissue than about the bony elements. To aid in preoperative planning, Lonstein (167) recommended drawing the spine preoperatively. The lines should represent the spinous processes and intact laminae and facet joints. This may aid in predicting progression of a postlaminectomy deformity.

Treatment. Treatment of postlaminectomy kyphosis is difficult, and it is best to prevent the deformity from occurring (193). The facet joints should be preserved whenever possible during laminectomy. Localized fusion at the time of facetectomy or laminectomy may help prevent progressive deformity (194). Because of the loss of bone mass posteriorly, however, localized fusion may not produce a large enough fusion mass to prevent kyphosis. Even so, this approach is advocated because it may produce enough bone mass posteriorly to stabilize what otherwise would be a severe progressive deformity.

The surgical technique of laminoplasty to expose the spinal cord may lessen the chance of progressive deformity. This approach involves suturing the laminae back in place after removal or removing just one side of the laminae and allowing them to hinge open like a book to expose the spinal cord, then suturing that side of the laminae back in place (195–197). This procedure may provide only a fibrous tether connecting the laminae to the spine, but studies have shown a decreased incidence of postlaminectomy kyphosis when it has been used (198, 199). Another technique is to hinge the laminae open in a lateral direction after dividing the laminae in the midline. This provides a lateral trough for the placement of bone graft for a lateral fusion (190, 191, 200, 201). The use of these techniques has been reported to decrease the incidence of postlaminectomy deformity, although there also have been reports of postlaminectomy deformity occurring even when laminoplasty was done (182, 192, 193, 202).

After surgery in which the laminae have been removed, bracing has been suggested to prevent deformity (194, 195, 203, 204), although no studies have documented the efficacy of this form of treatment. After the deformity has occurred and started to progress, bracing is ineffective in preventing further progression (167, 170).

For progressive or marked deformity, spinal fusion is recommended, although the patient's long-term prognosis should be considered before making definitive treatment plans. If the prognosis for survival is poor, spinal fusion may not be appropriate. However, given the availability of effective treatment protocols for tumors and the improved survival rates, fusion is usually indicated for progressive deformity. Combined anterior and posterior spinal fusion is preferred in most patients (196, 205) because the frequency of pseudarthrosis is greater if either procedure is done alone.

Lonstein (167) reported pseudarthrosis in 57% of patients after posterior fusion and in 15% of patients after anterior fusion. Anterior and posterior fusion can be done on the same day or as staged procedures. When the anterior procedure is done, care must be taken to remove all the physes back to the posterior longitudinal ligament. Leaving some of the physes in the vertebral body can cause an increase in

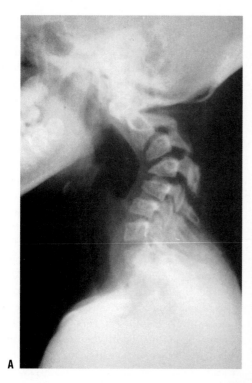

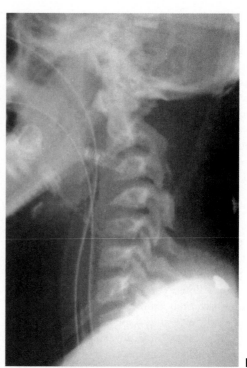

FIGURE 19-33. Radiographs of a 13-year-old girl treated for a low-grade astrocytoma. She underwent resection of the tumor, a portion of the occiput, and the laminae of C1–C4, followed by radiotherapy at a dose of 5400 cGy. **A**: A progressive cervical kyphosis developed. Note wedging of the anterior vertebral body. **B**: Radiograph in halo traction demonstrates partial reduction of the kyphosis. **C**: Postoperative radiograph after anterior and posterior fusion.

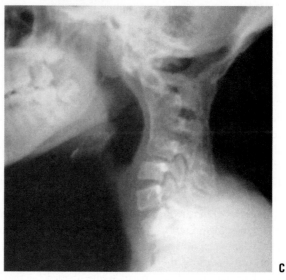

the deformity. When the posterior procedure is done, instrumentation of the involved spine is desirable, but not always possible, because of the absence of posterior elements. The development of pedicle screw fixation has been helpful in allowing the use of posterior instrumentation for postlaminectomy kyphosis. When it can be performed safely, this procedure provides secure fixation while the spinal fusion is maturing. Torpey et al. (206) recommended a posterior fusion using titanium rod instrumentation at the time of laminectomy. The instrumentation provides stability postoperatively, and the titanium rods allow for postoperative MRI to evaluate spinal cord tumors. In certain cases, anterior instrumentation with rod and bone screws or plates can be used to obtain stability and correction of the deformity (197). If the deformity

is severe or long-standing, anterior release followed by halo traction or a halo cast with an Ilizarov device can be used for obtaining gradual correction (198, 199, 207, 208).

RADIATION KYPHOSIS

The relative radiosensitivity of growing cartilage was discovered by investigators during the 1940s, and animal studies documented radiation-induced growth inhibition in growing cartilage and bone (209–214). The longitudinal growth of a vertebral body takes place through normal endochondral ossification, similar to the longitudinal growth of the metaphyses of long bones. Bick and Copel (98, 99) demonstrated this on histologic sections in fresh autopsy specimens of vertebral bodies taken from research subjects ranging in age from 14 weeks of fetal development to 23 years. This endochondral ossification at the physis is radiosensitive (98, 99, 209–211, 214, 215). Engel (209, 210) and Arkin and Simon (216) were able to produce spinal deformities in experimental animals using radiation. Arkin et al. (217) were the first to report spinal deformity in humans that was caused by radiation. After these reports, it has become clear that exposing an immature spine to radiation can produce spinal deformity, including scoliosis, kyphoscoliosis, lordoscoliosis, and kyphosis.

The three most common solid tumors of childhood for which radiation therapy is part of the treatment regimen, and in which the vertebral column is included in the radiation fields, are neuroblastoma, Wilms tumor, and medulloblastoma. Early in the history of radiation therapy, survival rates were poor and spinal deformities were not as prevalent. With improved treatment protocols and survival rates, the incidence of spinal deformities has increased. The degree of growth inhibition of the spine is related to the accumulated radiation dose and the age of the child when the spine is irradiated. Progression is directly dependent on the remaining growth potential in the irradiated vertebrae. The younger the child and the greater the accumulated radiation dose, the greater the chance of deformity (218–223). The most severe growth changes occur in patients who are 2 years of age or younger at the time of irradiation. Initial vertebral changes usually occur 6 months to 2 years after radiation exposure (224), but the deformity may not become apparent until years later, after a period of growth (218, 222).

Reports of radiation involving the spinal column show that an accumulated dose of <1000 cGy (centigray) does not produce a detectable inhibition of vertebral growth, whereas a dose of 1000 to 1900 cGy causes a temporary inhibiting effect on growth. Sometimes, this is manifested as a transverse growth arrest line in the vertebra, which gives the appearance of a bone within a bone. A dose of radiation between 1900 and 3000 cGy causes irregularity or scalloping of vertebral end plates and diminution of axial height and sometimes leads to a flattened, beaked vertebra (218, 220, 222, 224–228). A dose of 5000 cGy causes bone necrosis (192). The effect that radiation has on soft tissue also affects the progression of spinal deformity. The soft tissue anterior to the spine and the abdominal muscle can become fibrotic and act as a tether with growth, adding to the deformity of the spine as the child grows (229).

The incidence of spinal deformity after irradiation of the spine has been reported to range from 10% to 100% (218, 222, 223, 225, 230–233). These rates are decreasing because of shielding of growth centers, symmetric field selection, and decreased total accumulated radiation doses. The last of these changes has resulted from an increase in the use and effectiveness of chemotherapeutic regimens that reduce the need for large doses of radiation. Early reports showed an increased incidence of scoliotic deformities with the use of asymmetric radiation fields, and the incidence of kyphotic postirradiation deformities has increased with the use of symmetric radiation fields (234).

Any child who has received irradiation of the spine should be observed carefully for the development of spinal deformity. Because the development of deformity is related to the amount of disordered growth in the vertebral bodies that were affected by irradiation, it depends to a large extent on the amount of growth left in the spine when the irradiation was started and the amount of damage to the physes caused by irradiation (which correlates directly with the accumulated radiation dose). If the dose of radiation is large enough to cause permanent damage to the physes, the deformity will be progressive. Both postirradiation scoliosis and kyphosis progress more rapidly during times of rapid growth such as the adolescent growth period (222, 223, 226, 234). Before the adolescent growth spurt, the deformity may remain relatively stable or progress at a steady rate. Severe curves can continue to progress even after skeletal maturity, and these patients may require continued observation (Fig. 19-34).

Radiographic evaluation of a postirradiation deformity should include standard posteroanterior and lateral radiographs of the spine. Occasionally, CT scans with sagittal or coronal reconstruction are needed for better delineation of the vertebral-body deformities. The spinal cord and the surrounding soft tissue are evaluated best with MRI. Neuhauser et al. (220) described the radiographic changes seen in irradiated spines. The earliest changes were alterations in the vertebral bodies within the irradiated section of the spine caused by impairment of endochondral growth at the vertebral end plates. Growth arrest lines produced a bone-within-a-bone picture. This occurred in 28% of the 81 patients in the study by Riseborough et al. (222). Other radiographic changes were end-plate irregularity with an altered trabecular pattern and decreased vertebral-body height. This pattern was the most common radiographic change reported by Riseborough et al. (222) (83%). Contour abnormalities causing anterior narrowing and beaking of the vertebral bodies, much like those seen in patients with conditions that affect endochondral ossification (e.g., Morquio syndrome, achondroplasia), were the third type of radiographic change noted by Neuhauser et al. (220).

Treatment. Milwaukee brace treatment has been recommended for progressive curves, but generally has been ineffective for postirradiation kyphosis (222, 234), especially in patients with soft-tissue contractures contributing to the deformity. The irradiated skin also may be of poor quality, making long-term brace wear difficult. If progression occurs, spinal fusion, with or without instrumentation, should be done regardless of the age of the patient. Because bone quality is poor, fusion can be difficult to obtain after a single attempt. Anterior and posterior fusions are recommended and should extend at least one or two levels above and below the end of the kyphosis (185, 197, 222, 234, 236). The posterior fusion mass may require reexploration and repeated bone grafting after 6 months, and immobilization may need to be prolonged for 6 to 12 months. Posterior instrumentation should be used whenever feasible, because it adds increased stability while the fusion mass is maturing and may allow some limited correction of the kyphotic deformity (Fig. 19-34). Anterior instrumentation can be used in certain

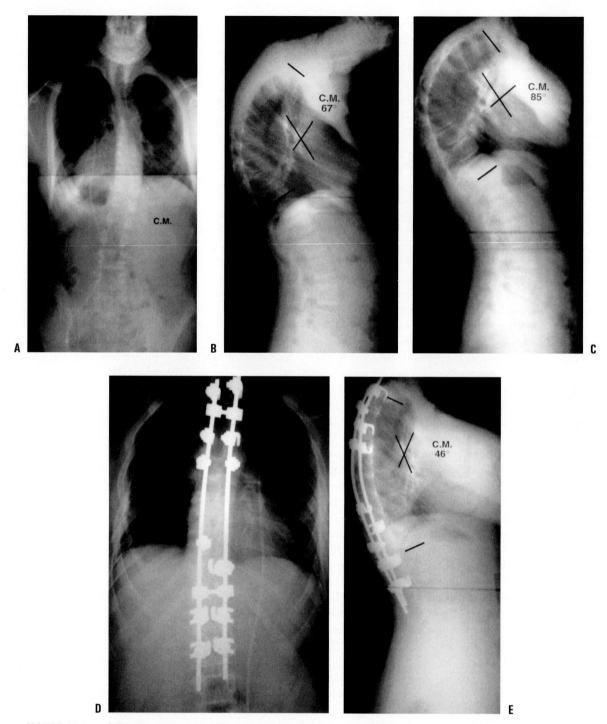

FIGURE 19-34. **A,B**: Anteroposterior and lateral radiographs of a 16-year-old child with a suprasellar germinoma treated with resection and 3400 cGy of radiation to the base of the skull and the entire spine. Radiographs demonstrate a 67-degree kyphosis with associated scoliosis. **C**: The kyphosis progressed to 85 degrees over 18 months despite bracing. **D,E**: Anteroposterior and lateral radiographs after anterior and posterior fusion with posterior instrumentation. The kyphosis has been corrected to 46 degrees.

cases; however, because of the radiation, the vertebral bodies usually remain in an infantile form, and instrumentation with bone screws may be difficult.

Correction of postirradiation kyphosis is difficult. Typically, these curves are rigid, and soft-tissue scarring and contractures often further hamper correction. Healing can be prolonged, and pseudarthrosis is common. Infection is a frequent complication

in these patients because of poor vascularity of the irradiated tissue (222). Riseborough et al. (222) reported a pseudarthrosis rate of 37% and an infection rate of 23% in their patients after surgery. King and Stowe (234) also reported a high complication rate in patients who were treated surgically. Because viscera also can be damaged by irradiation, bowel obstruction, perforation, and fistula formation may occur after spinal fusion.

This can be difficult to differentiate from postoperative cast syndrome, and the treating physician should be aware of this complication (237). Radiation myelopathy also may occur in this patient population (238). King and Stowe (234) reported postoperative paraplegia in two of seven patients who had undergone radiation treatment for neuroblastoma and surgery for correction of their kyphotic spine deformity. King and Stowe concluded that these two patients had a subclinical form of radiation myelopathy and that spinal correction compromised what little vascular supply there was to the cord. Therefore, the surgeon should be aware of this possibility and try to avoid overcorrection.

MISCELLANEOUS CAUSES OF KYPHOTIC DEFORMITIES

Spinal deformity in the sagittal plane can occur in patients with skeletal dysplasia (239, 240). The natural history of spinal deformity varies with the type of deformity and the type of dysplasia. Some sagittal plane deformities that appear severe at birth or in infancy improve spontaneously with growth, whereas others continue to progress and eventually can cause paraplegia. A knowledge of the various skeletal dysplasias and the natural history of sagittal plane deformities in each is necessary to prevent overtreatment and undertreatment.

Achondroplasia. Treatment of spinal problems often is required in patients with achondroplasia. The most common sagittal plane deformity in achondroplastic dwarfs is thoracolumbar kyphosis (241–243). The kyphosis usually is detected at birth and is accentuated when the child is sitting because of

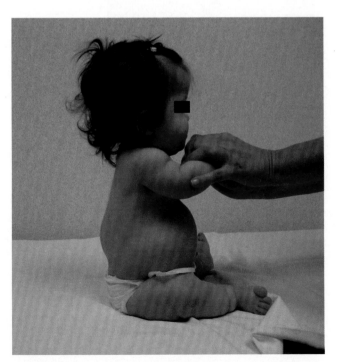

FIGURE 19-35. Achondroplastic dwarf with thoracolumbar kyphosis.

the associated hypotonia in these infants (244) (Fig. 19-35). Ambulation is delayed until approximately 18 months of age, but after ambulation begins, the thoracolumbar kyphosis tends to improve. The kyphosis usually does not resolve in children who have more hypotonia. According to Lonstein (245), thoracolumbar kyphosis resolves in 70% of achondroplastic dwarfs and persists in 30%. In one-third of these patients, or 10% of achondroplastic dwarfs, the thoracolumbar kyphosis is progressive (245) (Fig. 19-36).

A lateral radiograph of the thoracolumbar spine during infancy shows anterior wedging of the vertebrae at the apex of the kyphosis (243). In patients whose thoracolumbar kyphosis resolves, the anterior vertebral-body wedging also improves. When the kyphosis is progressive, anterior vertebral-body wedging persists.

Sponseller listed three reasons why thoracolumbar kyphosis should be corrected: (a) it may cause pressure on the conus and result in neurologic symptoms; (b) it results in an increase in the compensatory lumbar lordosis, which can increase problems from an already stenotic lumbar spine; and (c) it may increase significantly if decompressive laminectomies are needed for lumbar stenosis in the future (44).

If no improvement in the thoracolumbar kyphosis is evident once a child begins walking, a thoracolumbosacral orthosis (TLSO) is recommended to try to prevent progression of the kyphosis (246–249). Early treatment to prevent the development of a progressive kyphosis was recommended by Pauli et al. (250). They developed an algorithm for treatment of young achondroplastic patients, first counseling the parents against unsupported sitting and continuing with close follow-up. If kyphosis develops and is >30 degrees, TLSO bracing is begun and continued until the child is walking independently and there is evidence of improvement in vertebral-body wedging and kyphosis. Using this form of early intervention, Pauli et al. (250) reported no occurrences of progressive kyphosis in 66 patients. Sponseller recommended serial hyperextension casting if the kyphosis does not respond to bracing. If there is a satisfactory response to serial casting (50% or more correction in 3 to 4 months), brace treatment can be resumed (244).

Indications for surgery are documented progression of a kyphotic deformity, kyphosis of more than 40 degrees in a child older than 5 or 6 years of age, and neurologic deficits relating to the spinal deformity (242, 244, 251). Distinguishing between neurologic deficits that result from a kyphotic deformity and those associated with lumbar stenosis (which is common in achondroplastic dwarfs) can be difficult. A thorough physical examination and diagnostic studies such as CT scan and MRI may be necessary to determine appropriate treatment. The infant should be evaluated for foramen magnum stenosis, because this may be the underlying cause for the hypotonia and delayed ambulation in achondroplastic patients with kyphosis. If present, the stenosis should be treated by decompression of the foramen magnum (252). Most patients with progressive thoracolumbar kyphosis require combined anterior and posterior fusion. Instrumentation that uses hooks or wires that go into the spinal canal is not recommended in these patients

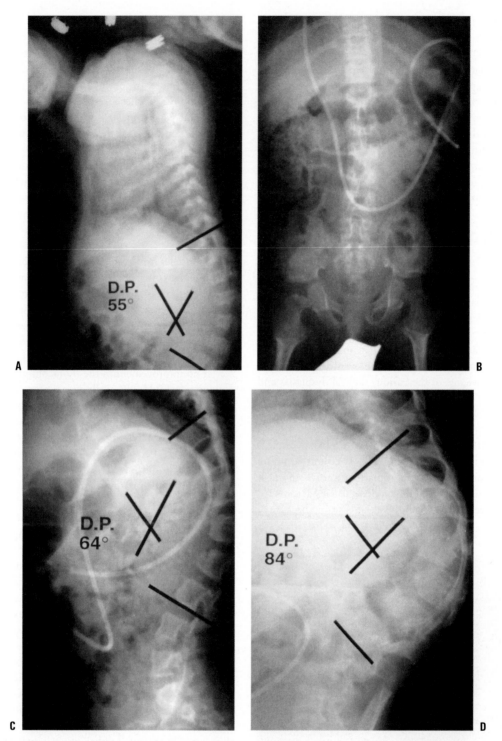

FIGURE 19-36. Achondroplastic dwarf with progressive thoracolumbar kyphosis. **A**: Lateral radiograph at 1 year of age shows a 55-degree thoracolumbar kyphosis. **B**: Anteroposterior radiograph at 5 years of age shows narrowing of the lumbar interpedicular distance characteristic of achondroplasia. **C**: Lateral radiograph at 5 years of age reveals a 64-degree kyphosis. **D**: Lateral radiograph at 9 years of age shows an 84-degree thoracolumbar kyphotic deformity.

because the small size of the spinal canal and the lack of epidural fat make instrumentation hazardous. If pedicle screws can be placed safely, this will allow for posterior instrumentation. This has the advantage of not entering an already stenotic spinal canal and giving secure fixation to aid in spinal fusion. Ain and

Shirley reported (253) good results with anterior fusion and instrumentation combined with posterior fusion.

Postlaminectomy kyphosis has been reported to occur after decompression for spinal stenosis of the skeletally immature achondroplastic spine (254, 255). Ain et al. reported that all 10 of their skeletally immature patients who had laminectomies and preservation of more than 50% of the facet joints developed progressive kyphotic deformities even though more than 50% of the facet joints were preserved. They recommended the addition of posterior instrumentation with pedicle screws and fusion when decompressive laminectomies are done in skeletally immature achondroplastic patients (255).

Pseudoachondroplasia.   Kyphotic deformities also can occur in children with pseudoachondroplasia and are caused by wedging of multiple vertebral bodies in the thoracolumbar and thoracic spine. The kyphotic deformity in patients with pseudoachondroplasia differs from that in patients with achondroplasia. In patients with pseudoachondroplasia, the kyphosis involves multiple levels and is less acutely angular than the deformity in patients with achondroplasia, which involves only one or two levels. Bracing may prevent progression of this deformity, but surgery is indicated if progression occurs despite bracing. Spinal fusion with instrumentation can be performed safely in patients with pseudoachondroplasia because there is no associated stenosis of the spinal canal as in patients with achondroplasia (256, 257).

Spondyloepiphyseal Dysplasia Congenita.   Thoracolumbar kyphotic deformities occur in approximately half of the patients with congenital spondyloepiphyseal dysplasia; these deformities usually respond to a modified TLSO (244). If surgery is needed for a progressive kyphosis, anterior and posterior fusions are recommended (257).

Diastrophic Dwarfism.   Spinal deformity is a common finding in diastrophic dysplasia (258). These spinal deformities consist of cervical kyphosis, thoracic kyphoscoliosis, and lumbar hyperlordosis. Midcervical kyphosis occurs in 15% to 33% of patients with diastrophic dwarfism (244, 259, 260); however, Remes et al. (259, 260) and Herring (261) reported spontaneous improvement Progressive cervical kyphosis (more than 60 degrees) can be stabilized with a spinal fusion (228, 238, 239). If a posterior fusion is to be done, the increased incidence of cervical spina bifida in diastrophic dwarfism must be considered during dissection (259, 260, 262).

Mucopolysaccharidosis.   Mucopolysaccharidoses are inherited lysosomal storage disorders caused by deficiency of the enzymes that are necessary for the degradation of glycosaminoglycans. There are at least 13 types of mucopolysaccharidoses. The more common names of this condition are Hurler, Hunter, Sanfilippo, Morquio, and Maroteux-Lamy syndromes. Bone marrow transplantation has increased the life expectancy of these patients. Before this treatment method became available, most children did not survive long enough to require intervention for spinal deformities. With increased survival, progressive kyphotic deformities of the spine with neurologic compromise have been reported (Fig. 19-37) (263–265). Despite bone marrow transplantation, the deposition of metabolites in bone is not reversed to the same extent as that in soft tissue (266).

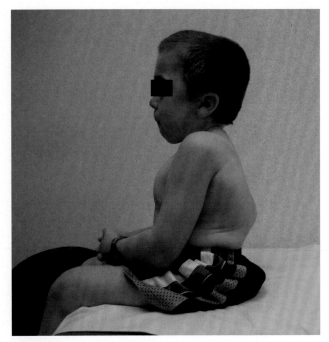

FIGURE 19-37.   Progressive kyphotic deformity in a child with mucopolysaccharidosis.

Children with mucopolysaccharidosis develop thoracolumbar kyphosis, with anterior beaking and flattening of the vertebral bodies at the level of the kyphotic deformity. Swischuk (267) suggested a mechanical cause for the anterior beaking. He postulated that hypotonia results in thoracolumbar kyphosis, resulting in herniation of the nucleus pulposus into the anterior vertebral body, which causes the anterior beaking of the vertebral body. Field et al. (266), however, examined two specimens at postmortem and found that the end-plate formation was normal, but there was a failure of ossification in the anterosuperior part of the vertebral body.

Bracing can be used to prevent progression of the kyphotic deformity, but the effectiveness of this form of treatment has not been documented. Spinal fusion is recommended for progressive kyphosis in patients with mucopolysaccharidosis. Tandon et al. (264) reported good results with posterior spinal fusion, and Dalvie et al. (263) reported good results with anterior fusion and instrumentation. Further studies are needed to determine which approach is best, but the goal of surgery is to obtain a stable fusion of the involved area to prevent any further progression of the kyphosis (244, 257, 268).

Gaucher Disease.   Gaucher disease is an uncommon hereditary glycolipid storage disorder characterized by the accumulation of glucocerebroside in the lysosomes of macrophages of the reticuloendothelial system. Splenomegaly with associated pancytopenia is the most common clinical manifestation. The skeletal manifestations are caused by infiltration of the bone marrow by Gaucher cells and include bone crisis, pathologic fracture, osteopenia, osteonecrosis, and osteomyelitis. Progressive kyphosis of the spine has been reported in these patients (269, 270). The proposed etiology of the kyphosis

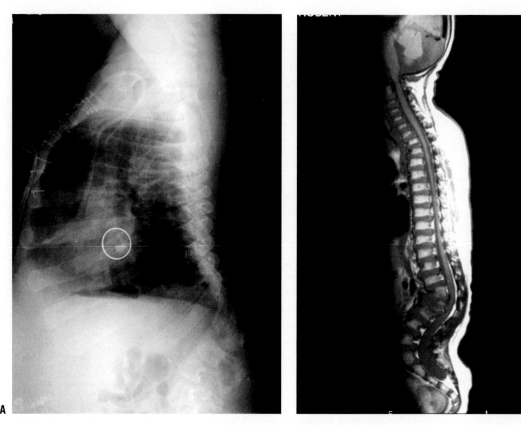

FIGURE 19-38. Lateral radiograph **(A)** and MRI **(B)** demonstrate progressive thoracolumbar kyphosis in a patient with Gaucher disease.

is infiltration of the bone marrow by Gaucher cells, resulting in bone crisis, osteopenia, and osteonecrosis that lead to vertebral-body collapse, often on multiple levels. Kyphosis can be progressive because of continued vertebral-body collapse or growth abnormalities secondary to vertebral-body collapse. If a progressive kyphosis develops, surgical intervention is recommended. If the spine is still flexible, posterior fusion and instrumentation are adequate, but if the deformity is rigid, anterior and posterior fusion and instrumentation are needed (Fig. 19-38) (269, 270).

Marfan Syndrome.   Marfan syndrome is a generalized disorder of connective tissue that affects the supporting structures of the body, especially those in the musculoskeletal system. This syndrome is caused by mutations in coding of the genes for the glycoprotein fibrillin (271, 272). Spinal deformity is the most common skeletal abnormality in Marfan syndrome, and scoliosis is the most common of these spinal deformities (245, 273–278). Thoracic lordosis has been traditionally reported as the most common sagittal plane deformity (279, 280). In some patients, the thoracic lordosis becomes severe enough to compromise respiration. With the lordotic posture of the thoracic spine, an associated kyphosis or a relative kyphosis may develop in the lumbar spine. A third common spinal deformity associated with Marfan syndrome is thoracolumbar kyphosis, which affects approximately 10% of patients (Fig. 19-39). These spinal deformities usually occur during the juvenile growth period, before the adolescent growth spurt

(280). Sponseller et al. (281) found that 41% of their patients with Marfan syndrome had a kyphotic deformity of more than 50 degrees, with a tendency toward longer kyphoses extending through the thoracolumbar junction.

Brace treatment has been recommended to try to halt the progression of spinal deformity but has been found to be ineffective (282, 283). Correction of kyphotic deformities requires anterior and posterior spinal fusion with segmental instrumentation (282). Thoracic lordosis is corrected by posterior segmental instrumentation to correct the lordotic deformity, followed by posterior fusion (284). Because dural ectasia erodes pedicles, a CT scan of the pedicles should be obtained to plan fixation. In addition, fusion should be extended to one level above and below the end vertebrae and include all curves. Complications are more frequent after surgical correction of spinal deformity in patients with Marfan syndrome than after spinal surgery in other patients and include infection (10%), dural tears (8%), instrumentation failure (21%), and pseudarthrosis (10%) (282).

Cervical spine abnormalities also are common in patients with Marfan syndrome, but clinical problems from these abnormalities are rare. Basilar impression and focal cervical kyphosis are the most frequently reported cervical spine abnormalities. Focal cervical kyphosis usually is associated with a lordotic thoracic spine (285).

Because of the increased incidence of cervical spine abnormalities, Hobbs et al. (285) recommended that patients with

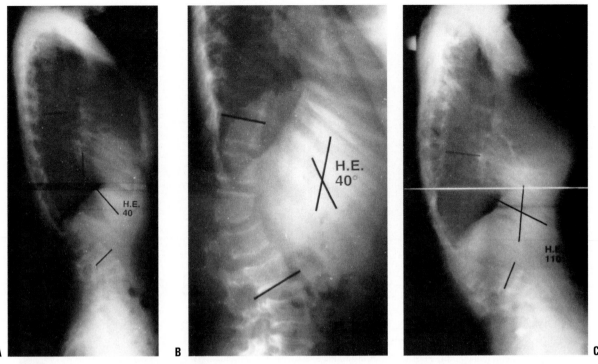

FIGURE 19-39. **A,B:** Lateral radiographs of a 17-year-old child with Marfan syndrome and a 40-degree progressive thoraco-lumbar kyphosis. **C:** Lateral radiograph of the same patient 3 years later shows that the thoracolumbar kyphosis has progressed to 110 degrees.

Marfan syndrome avoid sports that involve risks of high-impact loading of the cervical spine.

Larsen Syndrome. In 1950, Larsen et al. (286) described a congenital malformation syndrome (287) consisting of facial dysmorphism and hyperelasticity of the joints, with congenital dislocation of the knees and frequent dislocation of the hips and elbows (129, 288–291). Equinovarus or valgus foot deformities and ancillary calcaneal nuclei also are characteristic features of this syndrome. Abnormalities of the cervical spine, specifically cervical kyphosis, were not emphasized in the original description, and often this life-threatening finding is overlooked (198, 288, 292). Johnston et al. (287) reported cervical kyphosis and vertebral-body anomalies in five of nine patients with Larsen syndrome. The apex of the kyphosis usually occurs at the fourth or fifth cervical vertebra, with marked hypoplasia of one or two of the vertebral bodies (Fig. 19-40). Cervical kyphosis is present in infants with Larsen syndrome. Developmental delay may be attributed to hypotonia and dislocation of the knees or hips, but the underlying cause for developmental delay may be a chronic myelopathy from the cervical kyphosis. Cervical kyphosis and vertebral hypoplasia are easily demonstrated on lateral C-spine radiographs. Flexion and extension views usually are not needed and may be difficult to obtain safely in an infant. MRI scans will demonstrate spinal cord compression or compromise.

The recommended treatment recommendation for cervical kyphosis in Larsen syndrome is early posterior arthrodesis to stabilize the spine. An *in situ* posterior arthrodesis with autogenous iliac crest bone graft, followed by immobilization in either a halo or Minerva cast or custom orthosis, is recommended. Reduction of the kyphosis is obtained only in the postoperative halo or Minerva cast or orthosis stage of the treatment. Johnston et al. (287) found that, over a period of time following a solid posterior arthrodesis, a gradual correction of the kyphosis occurred because of continued anterior vertebral-body growth. Because the posterior arthrodesis is done at a young age, the patient must be followed for potential complications from continued anterior growth, which would result in lordosis. Johnston and Schoenecker (293) described a patient who developed neurologic symptoms from this growth-related lordosis.

Posttraumatic Deformities. Kyphosis can occur as a direct result of trauma to the spinal column or the spinal cord. Deformity can occur at a fracture site from a malunion, chronic instability leading to progressive deformity, paralysis after spinal cord injury, or from anterior growth arrest (294–298). Kyphosis at the fracture site is acute and spans a short segment of vertebrae. Paralytic kyphosis is a long, C-shaped deformity that spans many vertebral segments. Progressive kyphosis also may occur after development of a posttraumatic syrinx (299).

Kyphosis at a fracture site requires surgical intervention for correction. Anterior, posterior, and combined anterior and posterior procedures have been described for correction of posttraumatic kyphosis (300–304). Brace treatment has been ineffective for progressive paralytic kyphosis (294), and surgery is indicated for paralytic kyphosis of more than 60 degrees. If the kyphosis is flexible and can be reduced to <50 degrees, posterior fusion with segmental instrumentation can be done. If

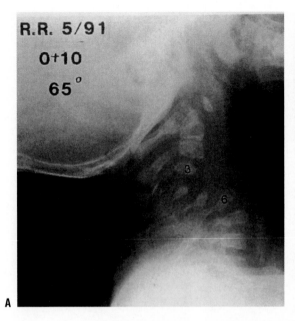

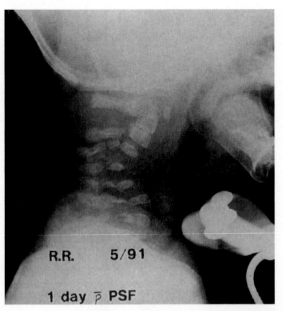

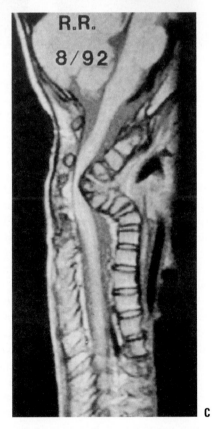

FIGURE 19-40. Larsen syndrome. **A**: Lateral radiograph of a 10-month-old patient showing kyphosis of 65 degrees, with correction to only 48 degrees in extension. **B**: Lateral radiograph immediately after posterior arthrodesis, showing the patient with orthosis and correction of kyphosis to 39 degrees. **C**: T2-weighted magnetic resonance image 15 months postoperatively shows severe impingement on spinal cord. Kyphosis had progressed to 110 degrees, and the patient was quadriplegic after a fall. (From Johnston CE, Birch JG, Daniels JL. Cervical kyphosis in patients who have Larsen syndrome. *J Bone Joint Surg Am* 1996;78:538.)

the kyphosis is rigid and cannot be reduced to <50 degrees on preoperative bending radiographs, anterior release and fusion should be (performed) followed by posterior fusion and segmental instrumentation (294, 298).

Neurofibromatosis. Kyphoscoliosis is common in patients with neurofibromatosis, although kyphosis may be the predominant deformity (305, 306). Funasaki et al. (307) found that 50% of their patients with neurofibromatosis and spinal

deformity had an abnormal sagittal curve. The vertebral bodies are frequently deformed and attenuated at the apex of the kyphosis. Dystrophic vertebral-body changes may develop over time (308, 309). Crawford (308) and Durrani et al. (310) described this as modulation of the deformity, from a nondystrophic curve to a dystrophic curve. The kyphosis typically is sharp and angular over a relatively small number of vertebral segments. Severely angular kyphosis can cause neurologic compromise (311, 312). Lonstein et al. (313) found that cord compression due to spinal curvature from neurofibromatosis was second only to congenital kyphosis as a cause of spinal cord compression. The kyphosis in patients with neurofibromatosis typically involves the thoracic spine or the upper thoracic spine. Involvement of the cervical and cervicothoracic vertebrae also has been reported (311, 314–318).

Kyphotic deformities with dystrophic changes tend to be progressive, and they more commonly lead to neurologic compromise.

Treatment of kyphoscoliosis in patients with neurofibromatosis begins with a thorough physical examination for neurologic abnormalities. MRI scans should be obtained to demonstrate any intraspinal lesions, such as pseudomeningocele, dural ectasia, or neurofibroma, which may cause impingement on the spinal cord (319). Any intraspinal lesions should be treated appropriately before spinal fusion and instrumentation are undertaken. Because posterior fusion alone has resulted in a high rate of pseudarthrosis (65%) (319), combined anterior and posterior spinal fusions combined with posterior instrumentation are recommended (320). Titanium instrumentation is preferred to allow for future MRI studies of the spine. Abundant autogenous bone grafts and prolonged immobilization may be required to obtain a solid fusion in these patients, and repeated bone grafting may be required 6 months after the initial surgery. Vascularized fibular or rib grafts also can be used for anterior fusion and structural support (109, 308, 314, 317, 321, 323).

Tuberculosis.
The spine is involved in 50% of patients with skeletal tuberculosis (324). Spinal tuberculosis is the most dangerous form of skeletal tuberculosis because of its ability to cause bone destruction, deformity, and paraplegia. In childhood spinal tuberculosis, the extent and degree of abscess formation are greater than those in adult tuberculosis, but paraplegia is less common in children than in adults with spinal tuberculosis (325). The most frequent site of spinal tuberculosis in children is the thoracolumbar junction and its adjacent segments. Tuberculosis infection usually destroys the anterior elements of the spine and results in a significant angular kyphosis at the infected site. The involved anterior vertebral bodies usually fuse once the infection is adequately treated. In young children, continued growth of the intact posterior element can cause a late increase in kyphosis in an already kyphotic spine (325).

All forms of active spinal tuberculosis are treated with a complete course of chemotherapy. First-line drugs are streptomycin, isoniazid, and rifampin, and second-line drugs are ethambutol and pyrazinamide (326). Medical therapies for spinal tuberculosis will adequately treat the tuberculum infection in most cases (324, 327–330). Bracing or casting has been used along with medical therapy to try to prevent progression of kyphosis during therapy. Rajasekaran found an average increase in deformity of 15 degrees in all patients who were treated nonsurgically (331). The greatest increase in deformity occurred during the first 6 months of treatment.

Indications for surgery in spinal tuberculosis are spinal instability, neurologic involvement, prevention or correction of spinal deformity, drainage of significant abscesses, and diagnostic biopsy (327). Neurologic involvement and present or impending paraplegia are more obvious indications for surgical intervention than the other indications. Rajasekaran described four prognostic signs to predict spinal instability and late increase in deformity. When more than two signs are present, this is a reliable predictor of progressive deformity and spinal instability. These prognostic signs are (a) dislocation of the facets, (b) posterior retropulsion of the diseased fragments, (c) lateral translation of the vertebrae in the anteroposterior view, and (d) toppling of the superior vertebra (Figs. 19-41 and 19-42) (332). Other factors that lead to a significant increase in kyphosis in children who are not treated surgically are involvement of three or more vertebral bodies, initial kyphosis of more than 30 degrees, and age younger than 15 years (333–335).

Several different surgical approaches have been used in the treatment of spinal tuberculosis (336–340). Anterior debridement and strut grafting, with or without a posterior fusion and instrumentation, have the most consistent long-term results (326, 340–352). Good results have been reported with the use of allografts for structural support anteriorly (353–355). Anterior debridement and fusion with anterior instrumentation of the spine also have had positive results in the treatment of spinal tuberculosis (356, 357). Some correction of the kyphosis may be obtained at the time of surgery. Kyphosis also can be a problem in patients with healed spinal tuberculosis (358). The infected area of the anterior spine usually fuses, and continued growth posteriorly causes progressive kyphosis that can result in paraplegia. The presence of neurologic symptoms is an indication for anterior decompression and fusion, which can be followed by posterior fusion and instrumentation.

Juvenile Osteoporosis.
Idiopathic juvenile osteoporosis is an acquired systemic condition that consists of generalized osteoporosis in otherwise normal prepubertal children (359). Although idiopathic juvenile osteoporosis is uncommon, associated kyphosis and back pain are common in patients with this condition.

Schippers (360) first described this condition in 1939 and, since that time, other authors have described its clinical findings and natural history (153, 360–367). The etiology of idiopathic juvenile osteoporosis is unknown. Laboratory values of serum calcium, phosphorus, alkaline phosphatase, parathyroid hormone, and osteocalcin are normal. The collagen type and ratios from skin biopsy samples also are normal. There have been some reports of a slight decrease in 1,25-dihydroxyvitamin D (365, 368, 369), but the significance of this finding is not known. Low serum calcitonin levels also have been reported, but treatment with calcitonin has not proven to be beneficial (342, 349). In contrast, Saggese et al. (366) noted normal serum calcitonin levels in their patients. Green (370) suggested that a mild deficiency of 1,25-dihydroxyvitamin D can explain most of the findings in idiopathic juvenile osteoporosis. During rapid growth phases, the deficiency is discovered because growth requirements cannot keep pace, causing a relative osteoporosis. When puberty occurs, the increase in sex hormone overcomes

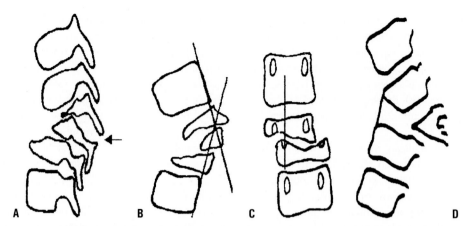

FIGURE 19-41. Radiologic signs for the spine at risk. **A**: *Separation of the facet joint.* The facet joint dislocates at the level of the apex of the curve, causing instability and loss of alignment. In severe cases, the separation can occur at two levels. **B**: *Posterior retropulsion.* This is identified by drawing two lines along the posterior surface of the first normal vertebrae above and below the curve. The diseased segments are found to be posterior to the intersection of the lines. **C**: *Lateral translation.* This is confirmed when a vertical line drawn through the middle of the pedicle of the first lower normal vertebra does not touch the pedicle of the first upper normal vertebra. **D**: *Toppling sign.* In the initial stages of collapse, a line drawn along the anterior surface of the first lower normal vertebra intersects the inferior surface of the first upper normal vertebra. "Tilt" or "toppling" occurs when the line intersects higher than the middle of the anterior surface of the first normal upper vertebra. (Reproduced with permission and copyright of the British Editorial Society of Bone and Joint Surgery. Rajasekaran S. The natural history of post-tubercular kyphosis in children. *J Bone Joint Surg* 1901;83B:954.)

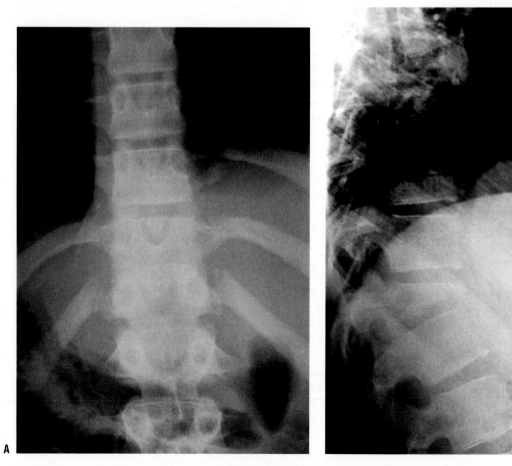

FIGURE 19-42. Anteroposterior and lateral radiographs **(A,B)** and a CT scan

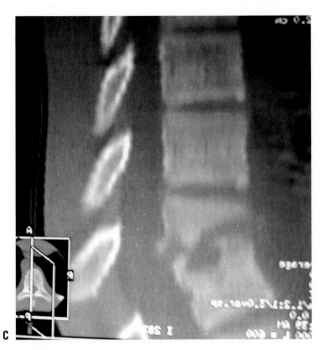

FIGURE 19-42. (*continued*) **(C)** demonstrating vertebral body collapse secondary to tuberculosis.

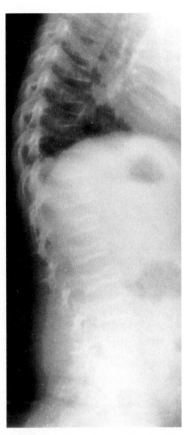

FIGURE 19-43. Lateral radiograph taken of a standing 10-year-old girl with idiopathic juvenile osteoporosis shows diffuse osteopenia, *multiple "codfish" vertebrae* in the thoracic and lumbar spine, and "coin" vertebrae in the upper thoracic spine secondary to extreme collapse. (From Green WB. *Idiopathic juvenile osteoporosis.* New York, NY: Raven, 1994.)

the deficit in 1,25-dihydroxyvitamin D, and the relative osteoporosis improves. This theory has yet to be proved.

Clinically, these patients complain of insidious onset of back pain (371), lower extremity pain or fractures, and difficulty in walking (64, 271, 372, 373). Difficulty in walking may sometimes be the only finding. This condition occurs during the prepubertal period and is slightly more common in boys than in girls. Vertebral collapse or wedging, with resulting kyphosis, is common. Brenton and Dent (374) classified idiopathic juvenile osteoporosis as mild, moderate, and severe. Patients with the mild type have only back pain and vertebral fractures; those with the moderate type have back and lower extremity pain and fractures, with some limitation of activities but eventual return to normal function; and those with the severe form have back and lower extremity pain and fractures. Both metaphyseal and diaphyseal fractures can occur in the lower extremities. Patients with severe disease improve clinically but do not return to normal activity after puberty.

Plain radiographs show wedging or collapse of the vertebral bodies. A "codfish" appearance of the vertebral bodies can occur, with the superior and inferior borders of the vertebrae becoming biconcave (Fig. 19-43). Other studies that can be useful for following the progress of this disease are single-photon absorptiometry, dual-photon absorptiometry, and quantitative CT scanning (363, 365, 366). The problem with these tests is that normal ranges for adolescents and children are variable and have not been standardized.

Idiopathic juvenile osteoporosis is a diagnosis of exclusion. Other diseases that must be considered include metabolic bone diseases, leukemia, Cushing syndrome, lysinuric protein intolerance, type I homocystinuria, and osteogenesis imper-

fecta. The natural history of this condition is spontaneous improvement or remission at the onset of puberty. Associated kyphosis tends to improve after the onset of puberty.

Treatment of idiopathic juvenile osteoporosis involves modification of activities, possible calcium and vitamin D supplementation, and supportive treatment of spinal deformities. It must be ensured that there is sufficient restriction of activities to prevent fractures, but not so much restriction as to cause an increase in osteoporosis. If a significant progressive kyphosis develops, the Milwaukee brace is the treatment of choice (364). The brace is to be worn until there is evidence of improvement of the osteoporosis. Operative therapy for this condition has been associated with a high complication rate because the poor bone quality makes instrumentation and fusion difficult (375).

REFERENCES

1. O'Rahilly R, Benson D. The development of the vertebral column. In: Bradford DS, Hensinger RN, eds. *The pediatric spine*. New York, NY: Thieme, 1985:3.
2. DiMeglio A, Bonnel F. Growth of the spine. In: Raimondi AJ, Choux M, Di Rocco C, eds. *The pediatric spine*. Vol. 1. New York, NY: Springer-Verlag, 1989:39.

3. Mellin G, Harkonen H, Poussa M. Spinal mobility and posture and their correlations with growth velocity in structurally normal boys and girls aged 13 to 14. *Spine* 1988;3:152.

4. Mellin G, Poussa M. Spinal mobility and posture in 8- to 16-year-old children. *J Orthop Res* 1992;10:211.

5. Propst-Proctor SL, Bleck EE. Radiographic determination of lordosis and kyphosis in normal and scoliotic children. *J Pediatr Orthop* 1983;3:344.

6. Schultz AB, Sorensen SE, Andersson GBJ. Measurements of spine morphology in children, ages 10–16. *Spine* 1984;9:70.

7. Stagnara P, DeMauroy JC, Dran G, et al. Reciprocal angulation of vertebral bodies in the sagittal plane: approach to references in the evaluation of kyphosis and lordosis. *Spine* 1982;7:335.

8. Willner S, Johnson B. Thoracic kyphosis and lumbar lordosis during the growth period in children. *Acta Paediatr Scand* 1983;72:873.

9. Fon GT, Pitt MJ, Thies AC Jr. Thoracic kyphosis: range in normal subjects. *AJR Am J Roentgenol* 1980;134:979.

10. O'Brien MF, Kuklo TR, Blanke KM, et al. *Radiographic measurement manual: Spinal Deformity Study Group (SDSG)*. Memphis, TN: Medtronic Sofamor Danek, Fall 1904.

11. Bernhardt M, Bridwell KH. Segmental analysis of the sagittal plane alignment of the normal thoracic and lumbar spines and the thoracolumbar junction. *Spine* 1989;14:717.

12. Hammerberg KW. Kyphosis. In: Bridwell KH, DeWald RL, eds. *The textbook of spinal surgery*. Philadelphia, PA: JB Lippincott, 1991:501.

13. Mac-Thiong JM, Labelle H, Berthonnaud E, et al. Sagittal spinopelvic balance in normal children and adolescents. *Eur Spine J* 1907;16:227.

14. Roussouly P, Gollogly S, Berthonnaud E, et al. Classification of the normal variation in the sagittal alignment of the human lumbar spine and pelvic in the standing position. *Spine (Phila Pa 1976)* 1905;30:346.

15. Vaz G, Roussouly P, Berthonnaud E, et al. Sagittal morphology and equilibrium of pelvis and spine. *Eur Spine J* 2002;11(1):80–87.

16. Vialle R, Levassor N, Rillardon L, et al. Radiographic analysis of the sagittal alignment and balance of the spine in asymptomatic subjects. *J Bone Joint Surg Am* 2005;87(2):260–267.

17. LeMire RJ. Intrauterine development of the vertebrae and spinal cord. In: Raimondi AJ, Choux M, DiRocco C, eds. *The pediatric spine*. Vol. 1. New York, NY: Springer-Verlag, 1989:19.

18. Schijman E. Comparative anatomy of the spine in the newborn infant and toddler. In: Raimondi AJ, Choux M, Di Rocco C, eds. *The pediatric spine*. Vol. 1. New York, NY: Springer-Verlag, 1989:1.

19. Cutler WB, Friedman E, Genovese-Stone E. Prevalence of kyphosis in a healthy sample of pre- and postmenopausal women. *Am J Phys Med Rehabil* 1993;72:219.

20. Bernhardt M. Normal spinal anatomy: normal sagittal plane alignment. In: Bridwell KH, DeWald RL, eds. *The textbook of spinal surgery*, 2nd ed. Philadelphia, PA: Lippincott-Raven, 1997:185.

21. White AA III, Panjabi MM. Practical biomechanics of scoliosis and kyphosis. In: White AA, Panjabi MM, eds. *Clinical biomechanics of the spine*. Philadelphia, PA: JB Lippincott, 1990:127.

22. Roaf R. Vertebral growth and its mechanical control. *J Bone Joint Surg* 1960;42B:40.

23. Voutsinas SA, MacEwen GD. Sagittal profiles of the spine. *Clin Orthop* 1986;210:235.

24. Winter RB, Hall JE. Kyphosis in childhood and adolescence. *Spine* 1978;3:285.

25. Wenger DR. Roundback. In: Wenger DR, Rang M, eds. *The art and practice of children's orthopaedics*. New York, NY: Raven, 1993:422.

26. Winter RB. Spinal problems in pediatric orthopaedics. In: Morrissy RT, ed. *Lovell & Winter's pediatric orthopaedics*, 3rd ed. Philadelphia, PA: JB Lippincott, 1990:673.

27. Winter R. Congenital kyphosis. *Clin Orthop* 1977;128:26.

28. Dubousset J. Congenital kyphosis and lordosis. In: Weinstein SL, ed. *The pediatric spine: principles and practice*. New York, NY: Lippincott Williams & Wilkins, 1900:179.

29. McMaster MJ, Ohtsuk AK. The natural history of congenital scoliosis: a study of two hundred and fifty-one patients. *J Bone Joint Surg Am* 1982;64:1128.

30. Van Schrick FG. Dir angeborene kyphose. *Zietr Orthop Chir* 1932;56:238.

31. Lombard P, LeGenissel M. Cyphoses congenitales. *Rev Orthop* 1938;22:532.

32. Winter RB, Moe JH, Wang JF. Congenital kyphosis: its natural history and treatment as observed in a study of one hundred and thirty patients. *J Bone Joint Surg Am* 1973;55:223.

33. McMaster MJ, Singh H. Natural history of congenital kyphosis and kyphoscoliosis. *J Bone Joint Surg* 1999;81A:1367–1383.

34. Dubousset J. Congenital kyphosis. In: Bradford DS, Hensinger RM, eds. *The pediatric spine*. New York, NY: Thieme, 1985:196.

35. Zeller RD, Ghanem I, Dubousset J. The congenital dislocated spine. *Spine* 1996;21:1235.

36. Shapiro J, Herring J. Congenital vertebral displacement. *J Bone Joint Surg Am* 1993;75:656.

37. Rivard CH, Narbaitz R, Uhthoff HK. Congenital vertebral malformations: time of induction in human and mouse embryo. *Orthop Rev* 1979;8:135.

38. Philips MF, Dormans J, Drummond D. Progressive congenital kyphosis: report of five cases and review of the literature. *Pediatr Neurosurg* 1997;26:130.

39. Travaglini F, Conte M. Cifosi 25 anni. Progressi in patologia vertebrate. In: Goggia A, ed. *Le cifosi*. Vol. 5. Bologna: Goggia, 1982:163.

40. Tsou PM. Embryology of congenital kyphosis. *Clin Orthop* 1977;128:18.

41. Tsou PM, Yau A, Hodgson AR. Embryogenesis and prenatal development of congenital vertebral anomalies and their classification. *Clin Orthop* 1980;152:211.

42. Morin B, Poitras B, Duhaime M, et al. Congenital kyphosis by segmentation defect: etiologic and pathogenic studies. *J Pediatr Orthop* 1985;5:309.

43. Blake NS, Lynch AS, Dowling FE. Spinal cord abnormalities in congenital scoliosis. *Ann Radiol (Paris)* 1986;29:377.

44. Basu PS, Elsebaie H, Noordeen ChM. Congenital spinal deformity. A comprehensive assessment at presentation. *Spine* 1902;27:2255–2259.

45. Prahinski JR, Polly DW Jr, Mchale KA, et al. Occult intraspinal anomalies in congenital scoliosis. *J Pediatr Orthop* 1900;19:59–63.

46. Suh S-W, Sarwark JF, Vora A, et al. Evaluating congenital spine deformities for intraspinal anomalies with magnetic resonance imaging. *J Pediatr Orthop* 1901;21:525–531.

47. Bradford DS, Heithoff KB, Cohen M. Intraspinal abnormalities and congenital spine deformities: a radiographic and MRI study. *J Pediatr Orthop* 1991;11:36.

48. Guille JT, Forlin E, Bowen JR. Congenital kyphosis. *Orthop Rev* 1993;22:235.

49. Winter RB, Moe JH, Lonstein JE. The incidence of Klippel-Feil syndrome in patients with congenital scoliosis and kyphosis. *Spine* 1984;9:363.

50. McMaster MJ, Singh H. Natural history of congenital kyphosis and kyphoscoliosis. *J Bone Joint Surg* 1999;81A:1367–1383.

51. Broekman BA, Dorr JP. Congenital kyphosis due to absence of two lumbar vertebral bodies. *J Clin Ultrasound* 1991;19:303.

52. Lubicky JP, Shook JE. Congenital spinal deformity. In: Bridwell HK, DeWald RL, eds. *The textbook of spinal surgery*. Philadelphia, PA: JB Lippincott, 1991:365.

53. Winter RB, Moe JH. The results of spinal arthrodesis for congenital spinal deformity in patients younger than five years old. *J Bone Joint Surg Am* 1982;64:419.

54. McMaster MJ, Singh H. The surgical management of congenital kyphosis and kyphoscoliosis. *Spine (Phila Pa 1976)* 1901;26:2146.

55. Kim Y-J, Otsuka NY, Flynn JM, et al. Surgical treatment of congenital kyphosis. *Spine* 1901;26:2251–2257.

56. Montgomery SP, Hall JE. Congenital kyphosis. *Spine* 1982;7:360.

57. Smith JT, Gollogly S, Dunn HK. Simultaneous anterior-posterior approach through a costotransversectomy for the treatment of congenital kyphosis and acquired kyphoscoliotic deformities. *J Bone Joint Surg Am* 1905;87:2281.

58. Winter RB, Moe JH, Lonstein JE. Congenital kyphosis: a review of 94 patients age 5 years or older with 2 years or more follow up in 77 patients. *Spine* 1985;10:224–235.

59. Mayfield JK, Winter RB, Bradford DS, et al. Congenital kyphosis due to defects of anterior segmentation. *J Bone Joint Surg Am* 1980;62:1291.

60. Winter RB. Congenital kyphosis. In: Bridwell KH, DeWald RL, eds. *The textbook of spinal surgery*, 2nd ed. Philadelphia, PA: Lippincott-Raven, 1997:1077.

61. Knutsson F. Fusion of vertebrae following noninfectious disturbance in the zone of growth. *Acta Radiol* 1949;32:404.

62. Kharrat K, Dubousset J. Bloc vertebral anterieur progress if ches 1?enfant. *Rev Chir Orthop* 1980;66:485.

63. Van Buskirk CS, Zeller RD, Dubousset JF. Progressive anterior vertebral fusion; a frequently missed diagnosis. Presented at Scoliosis Research Society, New York, 1998.

64. Smith R. Idiopathic juvenile osteoporosis: experience of twenty-one patients. *Br J Rheumatol* 1995;34:68.

65. Bollini G, Jowe JL, Zeller R. Progressive spontaneous anterior fusion of the spine. A study of seventeen patients. Presented at 15th Meeting of the European Pediatric Orthopaedic Society, Prague, 1996.

66. Andersen J, Rostgaard-Christensen E. Progressive noninfectious anterior vertebral fusion. *J Bone Joint Surg Br* 1991;73:859.

67. Hughes RJ, Saifuddin A. Progressive non-infectious anterior vertebral fusion (Copenhagen syndrome) in three children: features on radiographs and MR imaging. *Skeletal Radiol* 1906;35:397.

68. Smith JRG, Martin IR, Shaw DG, et al. Progressive noninfectious anterior vertebral fusion. *Skeletal Radiol* 1986;15:599.

69. Campos MA, Fernandes P, Dolan LA, et al. Infantile thoracolumbar kyphosis secondary to lumbar hypoplasia. *J Bone Joint Surg Am* 1908;90:1726.

70. Scott RM, Wolpert SM, Bartoshesky LE, et al. Segmental spinal dysgenesis. *Neurosurgery* 1988;22:739.

71. Faciszewski T, Winter RB, Lonstein JE. Segmental spinal dysgenesis. A disorder different from spinal agenesis. *J Bone Joint Surg Am* 1995;77:530.

72. Hughes LO, McCarthy RE, Glasier CM. Segmental spinal dysgenesis: a report of three cases. *J Pediatr Orthop* 1998;18:227.

73. Tortori-Donati P, Fondelli MP, Rossi A, et al. Segmental spinal dysgenesis: neurologic findings with clinical and embryologic correlation. *Am J Neuroradiol* 1999;19:445.

74. Flynn JM, Otsuka NY, Emans JB, et al. Segmental spinal dysgenesis: early neurologic deterioration and treatment. *J Pediatr Orthop* 1997;17:100.

75. Bristol RE, Theodore N, Rekate HL. Segmental spinal dysgenesis: report of four cases and proposed management strategy. *Childs Nerv Syst* 2007;23(3):359–364.

76. Andrish J, Kalamchi A, MacEwen GD. Sacral agenesis: a clinical evaluation of its management, heredity, and associated anomalies. *Clin Orthop* 1979;139:52.

77. Blumel J, Evans ER, Eggers GWN. Partial and complete agenesis or malformation of the sacrum with associated anomalies. Etiologic and clinical study with special reference to heredity. A preliminary report. *J Bone Joint Surg Am* 1959;41:497.

78. Rusnak SL, Driscoll SG. Congenital spinal anomalies in infants of diabetic mothers. *Pediatrics* 1965;35:989.

79. Banta JV, Nichols O. Sacral agenesis. *J Bone Joint Surg Am* 1969;51:693.

80. Pang D. Sacral agenesis and caudal spinal cord malformations. *Neurosurgery* 1993;32:755.

81. Phillips WA, Cooperman DR, Lindquist TC, et al. Orthopaedic management of lumbosacral agenesis. *J Bone Joint Surg Am* 1964;64:1282.

82. Scheuermann HW. Kyphosis dorsalis juvenilis. *Zietr Orthop Chir* 1921;41:305.

83. Scheuermann HW. Kyphosis dorsalis juvenilis. *Ugeskr Laeger* 1919;82:385.

84. Bradford DS. Juvenile kyphosis. *Clin Orthop* 1977;128:45.

85. Bradford DS, Ahmed KB, Moe JH, et al. The surgical management of patients with Scheuermann's disease: a review of twenty-four cases managed by combined anterior and posterior spine fusion. *J Bone Joint Surg Am* 1980;62:705.

86. Bradford DS, Moe JH, Winter RB. Kyphosis and postural roundback deformity in children and adolescents. *Minn Med* 1973;56:114.

87. Murray PM, Weinstein SL, Spratt KF. The natural history and long-term followup of Scheuermann kyphosis. *J Bone Joint Surg Am* 1993;75:236.

88. Sorensen KH. *Scheuermann's juvenile kyphosis. Clinical appearances, radiography, aetiology and prognosis.* Copenhagen, Denmark: Munksgaard, 1964.

89. Robin GC. The etiology of Scheuermann's disease. In: Bridwell KH, DeWald RL, eds. *The textbook of spinal surgery*, 2nd ed. Philadelphia, PA: Lippincott-Raven, 1997.

90. Fisk JW, Raigent ML, Hill PD. Incidence of Scheuermann's disease. Preliminary report. *Am J Phys Med Rehabil* 1982;61:32.

91. Fisk JW, Baigent ML, Hill PD. Scheuermann's disease. Clinical and radiological survey of 17 and 18 year olds. *Am J Phys Med Rehabil* 1984;63:18.

92. Montgomery SP, Erwin WE. Scheuermann's kyphosis: long-term results of Milwaukee brace treatment. *Spine* 1981;6:5.

93. Ascani E, La Rosa G, Ascani C. Scheuermann kyphosis. In: Weinstein SL, ed. *The pediatric spine: principles and practice*, 2nd ed. Philadelphia, PA: Lippincott Williams & Wilkins, 1901.

94. Halal F, Gledhill RB, Fraser FC. Dominant inheritance of Scheuermann's juvenile kyphosis. *Am J Dis Child* 1978;132:1105.

95. McKenzie L, Sillence D. Familial Scheuermann disease: a genetic and linkage study. *J Med Genet* 1992;29:41.

96. Carr AJ. Idiopathic thoracic kyphosis in identical twins. *J Bone Joint Surg Br* 1990;72:144.

97. Carr AJ, Jefferson RJ, Turner-Smith AR, et al. Surface stereophotogrammetry of thoracic kyphosis. *Acta Orthop Scand* 1989;60:177.

98. Damborg F, Engell V, Andersen M, et al. Prevalence, concordance, and heritability of Scheuermann kyphosis based on a study of twins. *J Bone Joint Surg Am* 2006;88(10):2133–2136.

99. Bick EM, Copel JW. The ring apophysis of the human vertebra. Contribution to human osteogeny II. *J Bone Joint Surg Am* 1951;33:783.

100. Schmorl G. Die pathogenese der juvenilen kyphose. *Fortschr Roentgen* 1930;41:359.

101. Ferguson AB Jr. The etiology of preadolescent kyphosis. *J Bone Joint Surg Am* 1956;38:149.

102. Aufdermaur M. Juvenile kyphosis (Scheuermann's disease): radiology, histology and pathogenesis. *Clin Orthop* 1981;154:166.

103. Aufdermaur M, Spycher M. Pathogenesis of osteochondrosis juvenilis Scheuermann. *J Orthop Res* 1986;4:452.

104. Ippolito E, Ponseti IV. Juvenile kyphosis: histological and histochemical studies. *J Bone Joint Surg Am* 1981;63:175.

105. Lambrinudi L. Adolescent and senile kyphosis. *BMJ* 1934;2:800.

106. Scoles PV, Latimer BM, Diglovanni BF, et al. Vertebral alterations in Scheuermann's kyphosis. *Spine* 1991;16:509.

107. Ascani E, Borelli P, Larosa G, et al. Malattia di Scheuermann. I: studio ormonale. In: Gaggia A, ed. *Progresi in patologia vertebrale*. Vol. 5. Bologna: Le Cifosi, 1982:97.

108. Ascani E, LaRossa G. *Scheuermann's kyphosis.* New York, NY: Raven, 1994.

109. Bradford DS, Daher YH. Vascularized rib grafts for stabilisation of kyphosis. *J Bone Joint Surg Br* 1986;68:357.

110. Burner WL, Badger VM, Shermann FC. Osteoporosis and acquired back deformities. *J Pediatr Orthop* 1982;2:383.

111. Lopez RA, Burke SW, Levine DB, et al. Osteoporosis in Scheuermann's disease. *Spine* 1988;13:1099.

112. Gilsanz V, Gibbens DT, Carlson M, et al. Vertebral bone density in Scheuermann disease. *J Bone Joint Surg Am* 1989;71:894.

113. Ippolito E, Bellocci M, Montanaro A, et al. Juvenile kyphosis: an ultrastructural study. *J Pediatr Othop* 1985;5:315.

114. Wenger DR, Frick S. Scheuermann kyphosis. *Spine* 1999;29:2630.

115. Travaglini F, Conte M. Untreated kyphosis: 25 years later. In: Gaggi A. ed. *Kyphosis*. Bologna: Italian Scoliosis Research Group, 1984:21.

116. Lowe TG. Current concepts review, Scheuermann disease. *J Bone Joint Surg Am* 1990;72:940.

117. Bradford DS, Moe JH, Montalvo FJ, et al. Scheuermann's kyphosis. Results of surgical treatment by posterior spine arthrodesis in twenty-two patients. *J Bone Joint Surg Am* 1975;57:439.

118. Paajanen H, Alanen A, Erkintalo BM, et al. Disc degeneration in Scheuermann disease. *Skeletal Radiol* 1989;18:523.

119. Deacon P, Flood BM, Dickson RA. Idiopathic scoliosis in three dimensions: a radiographic and morphometric analysis. *J Bone Joint Surg Br* 1984;66:509.

120. Deacon P, Berkin C, Dickson R. Combined idiopathic kyphosis and scoliosis. An analysis of the lateral spinal curvature associated with Scheuermann's disease. *J Bone Joint Surg Br* 1985;67:189.

121. Ogilvie JW, Sherman J. Spondylolysis in Scheuermann's disease. *Spine* 1987;12:251.

122. Stoddard A, Osborn JF. Scheuermann's disease or spinal osteochondrosis. Its frequency and relationship with spondylosis. *J Bone Joint Surg Br* 1979;61:56.

123. Muller R, Gschwend N. Endokrine störungen und morbus Scheuermann. *Acta Med Scand* 1969;65:357.

124. Kemp FH, Wilson DC. Some factors in the aetiology of osteochondritis of the spine. *Br J Radiol* 1947;19:410.

125. Cloward RB, Bucy PC. Spinal extradural cyst and kyphosis dorsalis juvenilis. *AJR Am J Roentgenol* 1937;38:681.

126. Roland M, Morris R. A study of the natural history of back pain. Part I: development of a reliable and sensitive measure of disability in low-back pain. *Spine* 1983;8:141.

127. Greene TL, Hensinger RN, Hunter LY. Back pain and vertebral changes simulating Scheuermann's disease. *J Pediatr Orthop* 1985;5:1.

128. Huskisson EC. Measurement of pain. *Lancet* 1974;9:1127.

129. Kaijser R. Obert kongenitale kniegelenksluxationen. *Acta Orthop Scand* 1935;6:119.

130. Stagnara P. Cyphoses thoraciques regulieres pathologiques. In: Gaggi A, ed. *Modern trends in orthopaedics.* Bologna: A Gaggi, 1982.

131. Blumenthal SL, Roach J, Herring JA. Lumbar Scheuermann's. A clinical series and classification. *Spine* 1987;12:929.

132. Stagnara P, Fauchet R, Dupeloux J, et al. Maladie des Scheuermann. *Pediatrics* 1966;21:361.

133. Bhojraj SY, Dandawate AV. Progressive cord compression secondary to thoracic disc lesions in Scheuermann's kyphosis managed by posterolateral decompression, interbody fusion, and pedicular fixation. A new approach to management of a rare clinical entity. *Eur Spine J* 1994;3:66.

134. Klein DM, Weiss RL, Allen JE. Scheuermann's dorsal kyphosis and spinal cord compression: case report. *Neurosurgery* 1986;18:628.

135. Lesoin F, Leys D, Rousseaux M, et al. Thoracic disk herniation and Scheuermann's disease. *Eur Neurol* 1987;26:145.

136. Ryan MD, Taylor TKF. Acute spinal cord compression in Scheuermann's disease. *J Bone Joint Surg Br* 1982;64:409.

137. Yablon JD, Kasdon DL, Levine H. Thoracic cord compression in Scheuermann's disease. *Spine* 1988;13:896.

138. Chiu KY, Luk KDK. Cord compression caused by multiple disc herniations and intraspinal cyst in Scheuermann's disease. *Spine* 1995;19:1075.

139. Bradford DS, Garcia A. Neurological complications in Scheuermann's disease. *J Bone Joint Surg Am* 1969;51:567.

140. Cobb J. Outline for the study of scoliosis. *Instr Course Lect* 1948;5:261.

141. Bradford DS. Vertebral osteochondrosis (Scheuermann's kyphosis). *Clin Orthop* 1981;158:83.

142. Lowe TG, Kasten MD. An analysis of sagittal curves and balance after Hook instrumentation for kyphosis secondary to Scheuermann's disease. A review of 32 patients. *Spine* 1994;19:1680.

143. Sachs B, Bradford D, Winter R, et al. Scheuermann kyphosis: followup of Milwaukee brace treatment. *J Bone Joint Surg Am* 1987;69:50.

144. Bradford DS, Moe JH, Montalvo FJ, et al. Scheuermann's kyphosis and roundback deformity: results of Milwaukee brace treatment. *J Bone Joint Surg Am* 1974;56:740.

145. Gutowski WT, Renshaw TS. Orthotic results in adolescent kyphosis. *Spine* 1988;13:485.

146. Farsetti P, Tudisco C, Caterini R, et al. Juvenile and idiopathic kyphosis. Long-term followup of 19 cases. *Arch Orthop Trauma Surg* 1991;110:165.

147. De Mauroy JC, Stagnara P. Resultats a long terme du traitement orthopedique. Aix-en-Provence, 1978:60.

148. Michel CR, Caton J. Etude des resultants a long term d'une seie de cyphoses regulieeres traitees pariorset de Livet a charniers. Presented at The Reunion of the Group d'Etude de la Scoliose, Aix-en-Provence, 1978.

149. Ponte A, Gebbia F, Eliseo F. Nonoperative treatment of adolescent hyperkyphosis: a 30 years experience in over 3000 treated patients. *Orthop Trans* 1990;14:766.

150. Lowe TG. Scheuermann's disease. *Orthop Clin North Am* 1999;30:475.

151. Bradford DS, Brown DM, Moe JH, et al. Scheuermann's kyphosis. A form of osteoporosis? *Clin Orthop* 1976;118:10.

152. Herndon WA, Emans JB, Micheli LG, et al. Combined anterior and posterior fusion for Scheuermann's kyphosis. *Spine* 1981;6:125.

153. Lowe TG. Double L-rod instrumentation in the treatment of severe kyphosis secondary to Scheuermann's disease. *Spine* 1987;12:336.

154. Nerubay J, Katznelson A. Dual approach in the surgical treatment of juvenile kyphosis. *Spine* 1986;11:101.

155. Speck GR, Chopin DC. The surgical treatment of Scheuermann's kyphosis. *J Bone Joint Surg Br* 1986;68:189.

156. Sturm PF, Dobson JC, Armstrong GWD. The surgical management of Scheuermann's disease. *Spine* 1993;18:685.

157. Kostuik JP. Anterior Kostuik-Harrington distraction systems. *Orthopedics* 1985;11:1379.

158. Geck MJ, Macagno A, Ponte A, et al. The Ponte procedure: posterior only treatment of Scheuermann's kyphosis using segmental posterior shortening and pedicle screw instrumentation. *J Spinal Disord Tech* 2007;20(8):586–593.

159. Herrera-Soto JA, Parikh SN, Al-Sayyad MJ, et al. Experience with combined video-assisted thoracoscopic surgery (VATS) anterior spinal release and posterior spinal fusion in Scheuermann's kyphosis. *Spine (Phila Pa 1976)* 2005;30(19):2176–2181.

160. Arun R, Mehdian SM, Freeman BJ, et al. Do interbody cages have a potential value in comparison to autogenous rib graft in the surgical management of Scheuermann's kyphosis. *Spine J* 2006;6(4):413–420.

161. Moquin RR, Rosner MK, Cooper PB. Combined anterior-posterior fusion with laterally placed threaded interbody c ages and pedicle screws for Scheuermann kyphosis. Case report and review of the literature. *Neurosurg Focus* 2003;14(1):e10.

162. Coscia MF, Bradford DS, Ogilvie JW. Scheuermann's kyphosis: results in 19 cases treated by spinal arthrodesis and L-rod instrumentation. *Orthop Trans* 1988;12:255.

163. Johnston CE II, Elerson E, Dagher G. Correction of adolescent hyperkyphosis with posterior-only threaded rod compression instrumentation: is anterior spinal fusion still necessary? *Spine (Phila Pa 1976)* 2005;30(13):1528–1534.

164. Koptan WM, Elmiligui YH, Elsebaie HB. All pedicle screw instrumentation for Scheuermann's kyphosis correction: is it worth it? *Spine J* 2009;9(4):296–302.

165. Lonner BS, Newton P, Betz R, et al. Operative management of Scheuermann's kyphosis in 78 patients: radiographic outcomes, complications, and technique. *Spine (Phila Pa 1976)* 2007;32(24):2644–2652.

166. Otsuka NY, Hall JE, Mah JY. Posterior fusion for Scheuermann's kyphosis. *Clin Orthop* 1990;251:134.

167. Lonstein JE. Post-laminectomy kyphosis. *Clin Orthop* 1977;128:93.

168. McLaughlin MR, Wahlig JB, Pollack IF. Incidence of postlaminectomy kyphosis after Chiari decompression. *Spine* 1997;22:613.

169. Haft H, Ransohoff J, Carter S. Spinal cord tumors in children. *Pediatrics* 1959;23:1152.

170. Lonstein JE, Winter RB, Moe JH, et al. Post-laminectomy spine deformity. *J Bone Joint Surg Am* 1976;58:727.

171. Mikawa Y, Shikata J, Yamamuro T. Spinal deformity and instability after multilevel cervical laminectomy. *Spine* 1987;12:6.

172. Tachdijian MO, Matson DD. Orthopaedic aspects of intraspinal tumors in infants and children. *J Bone Joint Surg Am* 1965;47:223.

173. Katsumi Y, Honma T, Nakamura T. Analysis of cervical instability resulting from laminectomies for removal of spinal cord tumor. *Spine* 1989;14:1171.

174. Fassett DR, Clark R, Bockemeyer DL, et al. Cervical spine deformity associated with resection of spinal cord tumors. *J Neurosurg Focus* 2006;20(2):E2.

175. Cattell HS, Clark GL Jr. Cervical kyphosis and instability following multiple laminectomies in children. *J Bone Joint Surg Am* 1967;49:713.

176. Panjabi MN, White AAI, Johnson RM. Cervical spine mechanics as a function of transection of components. *J Biomech* 1975;8:327.

177. Butler MS, Robertson WW Jr, Rate W, et al. Skeletal sequelae of radiation therapy for malignant childhood tumors. *Clin Orthop* 1990;251:235.

178. Saito T, Yamamuro T, Shikata J, et al. Analysis and prevention of spinal column deformity following cervical laminectomy I. Pathogenetic analysis of postlaminectomy deformities. *Spine* 1991;16:494.

179. Raynor RB, Pugh J, Shapiro I. Cervical facetectomy and its effect on spine strength. *J Neurosurg* 1985;63:278.

180. Zdeblick TA, Zou D, Warden KE, et al. Cervical instability after foraminotomy. A biomechanical in vitro analysis. *J Bone Joint Surg Am* 1992;74:22.

181. Bell DF, Walker JL, O'Connor G, et al. Spinal deformity after multiple-level cervical laminectomy in children. *Spine* 1994;19:406.

182. Yeh JS, Sgouros S, Walsh AR, et al. Spinal sagittal malalignment following surgery for primary intramedullary tumours in children. *Pediatr Neurosurg* 2001;35(6):318–324.

183. Albert TJ, Vacarro A. Postlaminectomy kyphosis. *Spine* 1998;23:2738.

184. Yasuoka S, Peterson HA, Laws ER Jr, et al. Pathogenesis and prophylaxis of postlaminectomy deformity of the spine after multiple level laminectomy: difference between children and adults. *Neurosurgery* 1981;9:145.

185. Perra JH. Iatrogenic spinal deformities. In: Weinstein SL, ed. *The pediatric spine: principles and practice*, 2nd ed. New York, NY: Lippincott Williams & Wilkins, 1900:491.

186. Fraser RD, Paterson DC, Simpson DA. Orthopaedic aspects of spinal tumours in children. *J Bone Joint Surg Br* 1977;59:143.

187. Papagelopoulos PJ, Peterson HA, Ebersold MJ, et al. Spinal column deformity and instability after lumbar or thoracolumbar laminectomy for intraspinal tumors in children and young adults. *Spine* 1997;22:442.

188. Amhaz HH, Fox BD, Johnson KK, et al. Postlaminoplasty kyphotic deformity in the thoracic spine: case report and review of the literature. *Pediatr Neurosurg* 2009;45(2):151–154.

189. Peter JC, Hoffman EB, Arens LJ, et al. Incidence of spinal deformity in children after multiple level laminectomy for selective posterior rhizotomy. *Childs Nerv Syst* 1990;6:30.

190. Yasuoka S, Peterson HA, MacCarty CS. Incidence of spinal column deformity after multilevel laminectomy in children and adults. *J Neurosurg* 1982;57:441.

191. Donaldson DH. Scoliosis secondary to radiation. In: Bridwell HK, DeWald RL, eds. *The textbook of spinal surgery*. Philadelphia, PA: JB Lippincott, 1991:485.

192. Whitehouse WM, Lampe I. Osseous damage in irradiation of renal tumors in infancy and childhood. *AJR Am J Roentgenol* 1953;70:721.

193. Butler JC, Whitecloud TS. Postlaminectomy kyphosis: causes and surgical management. *Orthop Clin North Am* 1992;23:505.

194. Callahan RA, Johnson RM, Margolis RN, et al. Cervical facet fusion for control of instability following laminectomy. *J Bone Joint Surg Am* 1977;59:991.

195. Ishida Y, Suzuki K, Ohmori K, et al. Critical analysis of extensive cervical laminectomy. *Neurosurgery* 1989;24:215.

196. Raimondi AJ, Gutierrez FA, Di Rocco C. Laminotomy and total reconstruction of the posterior spinal arch for spinal canal surgery in childhood. *J Neurosurg* 1976;45:555.

197. Rama B, Markakis E, Kolenda H, et al. Reconstruction instead of resection: laminotomy and laminoplasty. *Neurochirurgia (Stung)* 1990;33(Suppl 1):36.

198. Kehrli P, Bergamaschi R, Maitrot D. Open-door laminoplasty in pediatric spinal neurosurgery. *Childs Nerv Syst* 1996;12:551.

199. Mimatsu K. New laminoplasty after thoracic and lumbar laminectomy. *J Spinal Disord* 1997;10:19.

200. Shikata J, Yamamuro T, Shimizu K, et al. Combined laminoplasty and posterolateral fusion for spinal canal surgery in children and adolescents. *Clin Orthop* 1990;259:92.

201. Shimamura T, Kato S, Toba T, et al. Sagittal splitting laminoplasty for spinal canal enlargement for ossification of the spinal ligaments (OPLL and OLF). *Semin Musculoskelet Radiol* 2001;5(2):203–206.

202. Inoue A, Ikata T, Katoh S. Spinal deformity following surgery for spinal cord tumors and tumorous lesions: analysis based on an assessment of spinal functional curve. *Spinal Cord* 1996;34:536.

203. Sim FH, Svien JH, Bickel WH, et al. Swan-neck deformity following extensive cervical laminectomy: a review of twenty one cases. *J Bone Joint Surg Am* 1974;56:564.

204. Steinbok P, Boyd M, Cochrane D. Cervical spinal deformity following craniotomy and upper cervical laminectomy for posterior fossa tumors in children. *Childs Nerv Syst* 1989;5:25.

205. Otsuka NY, Hey L, Hall JE. Postlaminectomy and postirradiation kyphosis in children and adolescents. *Clin Orthop Relat Res* 1998;354:189.

206. Torpey BM, Dormans JP, Drummond DS. The use of MRI-compatible titanium segmental spinal instrumentation in pediatric patients with intraspinal tumor. *J Spinal Disord* 1995;8:76.

207. Francis WR Jr, Noble DP. Treatment of cervical kyphosis in children. *Spine* 1988;13:883.

208. Graziano GP, Herzenberg JE, Hensinger RN. The halo-Ilizarov distraction cast for correction of cervical deformity. *J Bone Joint Surg Am* 1993;75:996.

209. Engel D. An experimental study on the action of radium on developing bones. *Br J Radiol* 1938;11:779.

210. Engel D. Experiments on the production of spinal deformities by radium. *AJR Am J Roentgenol* 1939;42:217.

211. Gall EA, Luigley JR, Hilken JA. Comparative experimental studies of 190 kilovolt and 1000 kilovolt roentgen rays. I. The biological effects on the epiphyses of the albino rat. *Am J Pathol* 1940;16:605.

212. Hinkel CL. The effect of roentgen rays upon the growing long bones of albino rats. Quantitative studies of the growth limitation following irradiation. *AJR Am J Roentgenol* 1942;47:439.

213. Barr JS, Lingley JR, Gall EA. The effect of roentgen irradiation on epiphyseal growth. I. Experimental studies upon the albino rat. *AJR Am J Roentgenol* 1943;49:104.

214. Reidy JA, Lingley JR, Gall EA, et al. The effect of roentgen irradiation on epiphyseal growth. II. Experimental studies upon the dog. *J Bone Joint Surg* 1947;29:853.

215. Hinkel CL. The effect of roentgen rays upon the growing long bones of albino rats II. Histopathological changes involving endochondral growth centers. *AJR Am J Roentgenol* 1943;49:321.

216. Arkin AM, Simon N. Radiation scoliosis: an experimental study. *J Bone Joint Surg Am* 1950;32:396.

217. Arkin AM, Pack GT, Ransohoff NS, et al. Radiation-induced scoliosis: a case report. *J Bone Joint Surg Am* 1950;32:401.

218. Katz LD, Lawson JP. Radiation-induced growth abnormalities. *Skeletal Radiol* 1990;19:50.

219. Katzman H, Waugh T, Berdon W. Skeletal changes following irradiation of childhood tumors. *J Bone Joint Surg Am* 1969;51:825.

220. Neuhauser EBD, Wittenborg MH, Berman CZ, et al. Irradiation effects of roentgen therapy on the growing spine. *Radiology* 1952;59:637.

221. Rate WR, Butler MS, Robertson WWJ, et al. Late orthopaedic effects in children with Wilms' tumor treated with abdominal irradiation. *Med Pediatr Oncol* 1991;19:265.

222. Riseborough EH, Grabias SL, Burton RI, et al. Skeletal alterations following irradiation for Wilms' tumor: with particular reference to scoliosis and kyphosis. *J Bone Joint Surg Am* 1976;58:526.

223. Wallace WHB, Shalet SM, Morris-Jones PH, et al. Effect of abdominal irradiation on growth in boys treated for a Wilms tumor. *Med Pediatr Oncol* 1990;18:441.

224. Rutherford H, Dodd GD. Complications of radiation therapy: growing bone. *Semin Roentgenol* 1974;9:15.

225. Riseborough EJ. Irradiation induced kyphosis. *Clin Orthop* 1977;128:101.

226. Smith R, Daviddson JK, Flatman GE. Skeletal effects of ortho-voltage and megavoltage therapy following treatment of nephroblastoma. *Clin Radiol* 1982;33:601.

227. Vaeth JM, Levitt SH, Jones MD, et al. Effects of radiation therapy in survivors of Wilms' tumor. *Radiology* 1962;79:560.

228. Paulino AC, Wen B-C, Brown CK, et al. Late effects in children treated with radiation therapy for Wilms' tumor. *Int J Radiat Oncol Biol* 2000;46(5):1239–1246.

229. Makipernaa A, Heikkila JT, Merikanto J, et al. Spinal deformity induced by radiotherapy for solid tumors in childhood: a long-term followup study. *Eur J Pediatr* 1993;152:197.

230. Barrera M, Roy LP, Stevens M. Long-term followup after unilateral nephrectomy and radiotherapy for Wilms' tumour. *Pediatr Nephrol* 1989;3:430.

231. Butler RW. The nature and significance of vertebral osteochondritis. *Proc R Soc Med* 1955;48:895.

232. Pastore G, Antonelli R, Fine W, et al. Late effects of treatment of cancer in infancy. *Med Pediatr Oncol* 1982;10:369.

233. Rubin P, Duthie RB, Young LW. The significance of scoliosis in postir-radiated Wilms' tumor and neuroblastoma. *Radiology* 1962;79:539.

234. King J, Stowe S. Results of spinal fusion for radiation scoliosis. *Spine* 1982;7:574.

235. Donaldson WF, Wissinger HA. Axial skeletal changes following tumor dose radiation therapy. *J Bone Joint Surg Am* 1967;49:1469.

236. Mayfield JK. Post-radiation spinal deformity. *Orthop Clin North Am* 1979;10:829.

237. Shah M, Eng K, Engler GL. Radiation enteritis and radiation scoliosis. *N Y State J Med* 1980;80:1611.

238. Eyster EF, Wilsin CB. Radiation myelopathy. *J Neurosurg* 1970;32:414.

239. Hensinger RN. Kyphosis secondary to skeletal dysplasias and metabolic disease. *Clin Orthop Relat Res* 1977;128:113.

240. Tolo VT. Spinal deformity in short-stature syndromes. *Instr Course Lect* 1990;39:399.

241. Herring JA. Kyphosis in an achondroplastic dwarf. *J Pediatr Orthop* 1983;3:250.

242. Tolo VT. Surgical treatment of kyphosis in achondroplasia. In: Nicoletti B, Kopits SE, Ascani E, et al., eds. *Human achondroplasia: a multidisciplinary approach.* New York, NY: Plenum, 1988:257.

243. Eulert J. Scoliosis and kyphosis in dwarfing conditions. *Arch Orthop Trauma Surg* 1983;102:45.

244. Sponseller PD. Spinal deformity in skeletal dysplasia. In: Weinstein SL, ed. *The pediatric spine: principles and practice*, 2nd ed. New York, NY: Lippincott Williams & Wilkins, 1900:279.

245. Lonstein JE. Treatment of kyphosis and lumbar stenosis in achondroplasia. *Basic Life Sci* 1986;48:283.

246. Kopits SE. Thoracolumbar kyphosis and lumbosacral hyperlordosis in achondroplastic children. In: Nicoletti B, Kopits SE, Ascani E, et al., eds. *Human achondroplasia: a multidisciplinary approach.* New York, NY: Plenum, 1988:241.

247. Siebens AA, Hungerford DS, Kirby NA. Achondroplasia: effectiveness of an orthosis in reducing deformity of the spine. *Arch Phys Med Rehabil* 1987;68:384.

248. Siebens AA, Kirby N, Hungerford DS. Orthotic correction of sitting abnormality in achondroplastic children. In: Nicoletti B, Kopits SE, Acsani E, et al., eds. *Human achondroplasia: a multidisciplinary approach.* New York, NY: Plenum, 1988:313.

249. Winter RB, Hall JE. Kyphosis in an achondroplastic dwarf. *J Pediatr Orthop* 1983;3:250.

250. Pauli RM, Breed A, Horton VK, et al. Prevention of fixed, angular kyphosis in achondroplasia. *J Pediatr Orthop* 1997;17:726.

251. Shikata J, Yamamuro T, Iida H, et al. Surgical treatment of achondroplastic dwarfs with paraplegia. *Surg Neurol* 1988;29:125.

252. Pauli RM, Horton VK, Glinski LP, et al. Prospective assessment of risks for cervicomedullary-junction compression in infants with achondroplasia. *Am J Hum Genet* 1995;56:732.

253. Ain MC, Shirley ED. Spinal fusion for kyphosis in achondroplasia. *J Pediatr Orthop* 2004;24(5):541–545.

254. Agabegi SS, Antekeier DP, Crawford AH, et al. Postlaminectomy kyphosis in an achondroplastic adolescent treated for spinal stenosis. *Orthopedics* 2008;31(2):168.

255. Ain MC, Shirley ED, Pirouzmanesh A, et al. Postlaminectomy kyphosis in the skeletally immature achondroplast. *Spine (Phila PA 1976)* 2006;31(2)197–201.

256. Cooper RR, Ponseti IV, Maynard JA. Pseudoachondroplastic dwarfism. *J Bone Joint Surg Am* 1973;55:475.

257. Jones ET, Hensinger RN. Spinal deformity in individuals with short stature. *Orthop Clin North Am* 1979;10:877.

258. Matsuyama Y, Winter RB, Lonstein JE. The spine in diastrophic dysplasia. The surgical arthrodesis of thoracic and lumbar deformities in 21 patients. *Spine* 1999;24:2325.

259. Remes V, Tervahartiala P, Poussa M, et al. Cervical spine in diastrophic dysplasia: an MRI analysis. *J Pediatr Orthop* 2000;20(1):48–53.

260. Remes V, Marttinen E, Poussa M, et al. Cervical kyphosis in diastrophic dysplasia. *Spine* 1999;24:1990.

261. Herring JA. The spinal disorders in diastrophic dwarfism. *J Bone Joint Surg Am* 1978;60:177.

262. Poussa M, Merikanto J, Ryoppy S, et al. The spine in diastrophic dysplasia. *Spine* 1991;16:881.

263. Dalvie SS, Noordeen MHH, Vellodi A. Anterior instrumented fusion for thoracolumbar kyphosis in mucopolysaccharidosis. *Spine* 2001;26(23):E539–541.

264. Tandon V, Williamson JB, Cowie RA, et al. Spinal problems in mucopolysaccharidosis I (Hurler syndrome). *J Bone Joint Surg* 1996; 78B:938.

265. Levin TL, Berdon WE, Lachman RS, et al. Lumbar gibbus in storage diseases and bone dysplasias. *Pediatr Radiol* 1997;27:289.

266. Field RE, Buchanan JAF, Copplemans MGJ, et al. Bone marrow transplantation in Hurler's syndrome: effect on skeletal development. *J Bone Joint Surg* 1994;76B:975.

267. Swischuk LE. The beaked, notched or hooked vertebra: its significance in infants and young children. *Radiology* 1970;95:661.

268. Benson PF, Button LR, Fensom AH, et al. Lumbar kyphosis in Hunter's disease (MPS II). *Clin Genet* 1979;16:317.

269. Kocher MS, Hall JE. Surgical management of spinal involvement in children and adolescents with Gaucher's disease. *J Pediatr Orthop* 2000;20(3):383–388.

270. Wiesner L, Niggemeyer O, Kothe R, et al. Severe pathologic compression of three consecutive vertebrae in Gaucher's disease: a case report and review of the literature. *Eur Spine J* 2003;12(1):97–99.

271. Dietz HC, Cutting GR, Pyeritz RE, et al. Marfan syndrome caused by a recurrent de novo missense mutation in the fibrillin gene. *Nature* 1991;352:337.

272. Dietz HC, Pyeritz RE, Hall BD, et al. The Marfan syndrome locus: confirmation of assignment to chromosome 15 and identification of tightly-linked markers at 15 q 15-921.3. *Genomics* 1991;9:355.

273. Amis J, Herring JA. Iatrogenic kyphosis: a complication of Harrington instrumentation in Marfan syndrome. *J Bone Joint Surg Am* 1984; 66:460.

274. Beneux J, Rigault P, Poliquen JC. Les deviations rachidiennes de la maladie de Marfan chez 1?enfant. Etude de 10 cas. *Rev Chir Orthop Reparatrice Appar Mot* 1978;64:471.

275. Joseph KN, Kane HA, Milner RS, et al. Orthopaedic aspects of the Marfan phenotype. *Clin Orthop* 1992;277:251.

276. Robins PR, Moe JH, Winter RB. Scoliosis in Marfan syndrome: its characteristics and results of treatment in thirty-five patients. *J Bone Joint Surg Am* 1975;57:358.

277. Savini R, Cervellati S, Beroaldo E. Spinal deformities in Marfan syndrome. *Ital J Orthop Traumatol* 1980;6:19.

278. Taneja DK, Manning CW. Scoliosis in Marfan syndrome and arachnodactyly. In: Zorab PA, ed. *Scoliosis.* London, UK: Academic, 1977:261.

279. Goldberg MJ. Marfan and the marfanoid habitus. In: Goldberg MJ, ed. *The dysmorphic child: an orthopaedic perspective.* New York, NY: Raven, 1987:83.

280. Kumar SJ, Guille JT. Marfan syndrome. In: Weinstein SL, ed. *The pediatric spine: principles and practice*, 2nd ed. New York, NY: Lippincott Williams & Wilkins, 1900:505.

281. Sponseller PD, Hobbs W, Riley LE, et al. The thoracolumbar spine in Marfan syndrome. *J Bone Joint Surg Am* 1995;77:867.

282. Birch JG, Herring JA. Spinal deformity in Marfan syndrome. *J Pediatr Orthop* 1987;7:546.

283. Jones KB, Drkula G, Sponseller PD, et al. Spine deformity correction in Marfan syndrome. *Spine* 1902;18:1903.

284. Winter RB. Thoracic lordoscoliosis in Marfan syndrome: report of two patients with surgical correction using rods and sublaminar wires. *Spine* 1990;15:233.

285. Hobbs WR, Sponseller PD, Weiss A-PC, et al. The cervical spine in Marfan syndrome. *Spine* 1997;22:983.

286. Larsen LJ, Schottstaedt ER, Bost FC. Multiple congenital dislocations associated with characteristic facial abnormality. *J Pediatr* 1950;37:574.

287. Johnston CE, Birch JG, Daniels JL. Cervical kyphosis in patients who have Larsen syndrome. *J Bone Joint Surg Am* 1996;78:538.

288. Muzumdar AS, Lowry RB, Robinson CE. Quadriplegia in Larsen syndrome. *Birth Defects* 1977;13:192.

289. Harris R, Cullen CH. Autosomal dominant inheritance in Larsen's syndrome. *Clin Genet* 1971;2:87.

290. Dudding BA, Gorlin RJ, Langer LD. The oto-palato-digital syndrome. A new symptom-complex consisting of deafness, dwarfism, cleft palate, characteristic facies, and generalized bone dysplasia. *Am J Dis Child* 1967;113:214.

291. McKusick VA. *Mendelian inheritance in man*, 4th ed. Baltimore, MD: Johns Hopkins University Press, 1975.

292. Micheli LJ, Hall JE, Watts HG. Spinal instability in Larsen's syndrome. Report of three cases. *J Bone Joint Surg Am* 1976;58:562.

293. Johnston CE II, Schoenecker PL. Correspondence to the editor. *J Bone Joint Surg Am* 1997;79:1590.

294. Renshaw TS. Spinal cord injury and posttraumatic deformities. In: Weinstein SL, ed. *The pediatric spine: principles and practice*, 2nd ed. New York, NY: Lippincott Williams & Wilkins, 1900:585.

295. Dearolf WWI, Betz RR, Vogel LC, et al. Scoliosis in pediatric spinal cord–injured patients. *J Pediatr Orthop* 1990;10:214.

296. Malcolm BW. Spinal deformity secondary to spinal injury. *Orthop Clin North Am* 1979;10:943.

297. Mayfield JK, Erkkila JC, Winter RB. Spine deformity subsequent to acquired childhood spinal cord injury. *J Bone Joint Surg Am* 1981;63:1401.

298. Renshaw TS. Paralysis in the child: orthopaedic management. In: Bradford DS, Hensinger RM, eds. *The pediatric spine*. New York, NY: Thieme, 1985:118.

299. Griffiths EF, McCormick CC. Post-traumatic syringomyelia (cystic myelopathy). *Paraplegia* 1981;19:81.

300. Bohm H, Harms J, Donk R, et al. Correction and stabilization of angular kyphosis. *Clin Orthop Relat Res* 1990;258:56.

301. Gertzbein SD, Harris MB. Wedge osteotomy for the correction of post-traumatic kyphosis. *Spine* 1992;17:374.

302. McAfee PC, Bohlman HH, Yuan HA. Anterior decompression of traumatic thoracolumbar fractures with incomplete neurological deficit using a retroperitoneal approach. *J Bone Joint Surg Am* 1985;67:89.

303. Roberson JR, Whitesides TF Jr. Surgical reconstruction of late post-traumatic thoracolumbar kyphosis. *Spine* 1985;10:307.

304. Wu SS, Hwa SY, Lin LC, et al. Management of rigid post-traumatic kyphosis. *Spine* 1996;21:2260.

305. Craig JB, Govender S. Neurofibromatosis of the cervical spine. A report of eight cases. *J Bone Joint Surg Br* 1992;74:575.

306. Winter RB, Moe JH, Bradford DS, et al. Spine deformities in neurofibromatosis. *J Bone Joint Surg Am* 1979;61:677.

307. Funasaki H, Winter RB, Lonstein JB, et al. Pathophysiology of spinal deformities in neurofibromatosis. *J Bone Joint Surg Am* 1994;76:692.

308. Crawford AH. Pitfalls of spinal deformities associated with neurofibromatosis in children. *Clin Orthop* 1989;245:29.

309. Hsu LCS, Lee PC, Leong JCY. Dystrophic spinal deformities in neurofibromatosis, treated by anterior and posterior fusion. *J Bone Joint Surg Br* 1984;66:495.

310. Durrani AA, Crawford AH, Chouhdry SN, et al. Modulation of spinal deformities in patients with neurofibromatosis type I. *Spine* 2000;25(1):69–75.

311. Crawford AH. Neurofibromatosis. In: Weinstein SL, ed. *The pediatric spine: principles and practice*. New York, NY: Raven, 1994:619.

312. Curtis BH, Fisher RL, Butterfield WL, et al. Neurofibromatosis with paraplegia: report of 8 cases. *J Bone Joint Surg Am* 1969;51:843.

313. Lonstein JE, Winter RB, Moe JH, et al. Neurologic deficit secondary to spinal deformity. *Spine* 1980;5:331.

314. Asazuma T, Yamagishi M, Nemoto K, et al. Spinal fusion using a vascularized fibular bone graft for a patient with cervical kyphosis due to neurofibromatosis. *J Spinal Disord* 1997;10:537.

315. Gioia G, Mandelli D, Capaccioni B, et al. Postlaminectomy cervical dislocation in von Recklinghausen's disease. *Spine* 1998;23:273.

316. Kokubun S, Ozawa H, Sakurai M, et al. One-stage anterior and posterior correction of severe kyphosis of the cervical spine in neurofibromatosis. A case report. *Spine* 1993;18:2332.

317. Nijland EA, van den Berg MP, Wuisman PIJM, et al. Correction of a dystrophic cervicothoracic spine deformity in Recklinghausen's disease. *Clin Orthop Relat Res* 1998;349:149.

318. Ward BA, Harkey L, Parent AD, et al. Severe cervical kyphotic deformities in patients with plexiform neurofibromas: case report. *Neurosurgery* 1994;35:960.

319. Schorry EK, Stowens DW, Crawford AH, et al. Summary of patient data from a multidisciplinary neurofibromatosis clinic. *Neurofibromatosis* 1989;2:129.

320. Halmai V, Doman I, de Jonge T, et al. Surgical treatment of spinal deformities associated with neurofibromatosis type I. Report of 12 cases. *J Neurosurg Spine* 2002;97(3 Suppl):310–316.

321. Bradford DS. Anterior vascular pedicle bone grafting for the treatment of kyphosis. *Spine* 1980;5:318.

322. Bradford DS, Ganjavian S, Antonious D, et al. Anterior strut-grafting for the treatment of kyphosis. *J Bone Joint Surg Am* 1982;64:680.

323. Rose GK, Sanderson JM. Transposition of rib with blood supply for the stabilisation of a spinal kyphos. *J Bone Joint Surg Br* 1975;57:112.

324. Moon M-S. Tuberculosis of the spine. *Spine* 1977;22:1791.

325. Ho EKW, Leong JCY. Tuberculosis of the spine. In: Weinstein SL, ed. *The pediatric spine: principles and practice*. New York, NY: Raven, 1994:837.

326. Antituberculosis Regimens of Chemotherapy. Recommendations from the Committee on Treatment of the International Union against Tuberculosis and Lung Disease. *Bull Int Union Tuberc Lung Dis* 1988;63:60.

327. Khoo LT, Mikawa K, Fessler RG. A surgical revisitation of Pott distemper of the spine. *Spine J* 2003;3(2):130–145.

328. Moon M-S, Moon Y-W, Moon J-L, et al. Conservative treatment of tuberculosis of the lumbar and lumbosacral spine. *Clin Orthop* 1902;398:40.

329. Moon MS, Kim I, Woo YK, et al. Conservative treatment of tuberculosis of the thoracic and lumbar spine in adults and children. *Int Orthop* 1987;11:315.

330. Wimmer C, Ogon M, Sterzinger W, et al. Conservative treatment of tuberculous spondylitis: a long-term follow-up study. *J Spinal Disord* 1997;10:417.

331. Rajasekaran S. The problem of deformity in spinal tuberculosis. *Clin Orthop* 2002;(398):85–92.

332. Rajasekaran S. The natural history of post-tubercular kyphosis in children. *J Bone Joint Surg* 2001;83(7):954–962.

333. Mushkin AY, Kovalenko KN. Neurological complications of spinal tuberculosis in children. *Int Orthop (SICOT)* 1999;23:210.

334. Klöckner C, Valencia R. Sagittal alignment after anterior debridement and fusion with or without additional posterior instrumentation in the treatment of pyogenic and tuberculous spondylodiscitis. *Spine* 1903;28:1036.

335. Parthasarathy R, Sriram K, Santha T, et al. Short-course chemotherapy for tuberculosis of the spine. *J Bone Joint Surg* 1999;81B:464.

336. Schulitz KP, Kothe R, Leong JC, et al. Growth changes of solidly fused kyphotic block after surgery for tuberculosis. Comparison of four procedures. *Spine* 1997;22:1150.

337. Medical Research Council Working Party on Tuberculosis of the Spine. A controlled trial of anterior spinal fusion and debridement in the surgical management of tuberculosis of the spine in patients on standard chemotherapy: studies in Hong Kong. *Br J Surg* 1974;61:853.

338. Medical Research Council Working Party on Tuberculosis of the Spine. A controlled trial of debridement and ambulatory treatment in the management of tuberculosis of the spine in patients on standard chemotherapy. *J Trop Med Hyg* 1974;77:72.

339. Medical Research Council Working Party on Tuberculosis of the Spine. Five-year assessments of controlled trials of ambulatory treatment, debridement and anterior spinal fusion in the management of tuberculosis of the spine: studies in Bulaway (Rhodesia) and in Hong Kong. *J Bone Joint Surg Br* 1978;60:163.

340. Medical Research Council Working Party on Tuberculosis of the Spine. A ten-year assessment of a controlled trial comparing debridement and anterior spinal fusion in the management of tuberculosis of the spine in patients on standard chemotherapy in Hong Kong. *J Bone Joint Surg Br* 1982;64:393.

341. Altman GT, Altman DT, Frankovitch KF. Anterior and posterior fusion for children with tuberculosis of the spine. *Clin Orthop Relat Res* 1996;325:225.

342. Bailey HL, Gabriel M, Hodgson AR, et al. Tuberculosis of the spine in children: operative findings and results in one hundred consecutive patients treated by removal of the lesion and anterior grafting. *J Bone Joint Surg Am* 1972;54:1633.

343. Hsu LCS, Leong JCY. Tuberculosis of the lower cervical spine (C2–7): a report on forty cases. *J Bone Joint Surg Br* 1984;66:1.

344. Ito H, Tsuchiya J, Asami G. A new radical operation for Pott's disease. *J Bone Joint Surg* 1934;16:499.

345. Moon M-S. Spine update. Tuberculosis of the spine. Controversies and a new challenge. *Spine* 1997;22:1791.

346. Moon M-S, Woo Y-K, Lee K-S. Posterior instrumentation and anterior interbody fusion for tuberculous kyphosis of dorsal and lumbar spines. *Spine* 1995;19:1910.

347. Medical Research Council Working Party on Tuberculosis of the Spine. A controlled trial of ambulant outpatient treatment and inpatient rest in bed in the management of tuberculosis of the spine in young Korean patients on standard chemotherapy: a study in Masan, Korea. *J Bone Joint Surg Br* 1973;55:678.

348. Medical Research Council Working Party on Tuberculosis of the Spine. A ten-year assessment of controlled trials of inpatient and outpatient treatment and plaster-of-Paris jackets for tuberculosis of the spine in children on standard chemotherapy: studies in Masan and Pusan, Korea. *J Bone Joint Surg Br* 1985;67:103.

349. Upadhyay SS, Saji MJ, Sell P, et al. The effect of age on the change in deformity after anterior debridement surgery for tuberculosis of the spine. *Spine* 1996;21:2356.

350. Upadhyay SS, Saji MJ, Sell P, et al. Spinal deformity after childhood surgery for tuberculosis of the spine. A comparison of radical surgery and debridement. *J Bone Joint Surg Br* 1994;76:91.

351. Upadhyay SS, Saji MJ, Sell P, et al. The effect of age on the change in deformity after radical resection and anterior arthrodesis for tuberculosis of the spine. *J Bone Joint Surg Am* 1994;76:701.

352. Upadhyay SS, Sell P, Saji MJ, et al. 17-Year prospective study of surgical management of spinal tuberculosis in children. Hong Kong operation compared with debridement surgery for short- and long-term outcome of deformity. *Spine* 1993;18:1704.

353. Govender S. The outcome of allografts and anterior instrumentation in spinal tuberculosis. *Clin Orthop* 1902;398:60.

354. Govender S, Kumar KPS. Cortical allografts in spinal tuberculosis. *Int Orthop (SICOT)* 2003;27(4):244–248.

355. Govender S, Parbhoo AH. Support of the anterior column with allografts in tuberculosis of the spine. *J Bone Joint Surg* 1999;81B:106.

356. Yilmaz C, Selek HY, Gürkan I, et al. Anterior instrumentation for the treatment of spinal tuberculosis. *J Bone Joint Surg* 1999;81A:1261.

357. Benli I, Acaroglu E, Akalin S, et al. Anterior radical debridement and anterior instrumentation in tuberculosis spondylitis. *Eur Spine J* 1903;12:224.

358. Hsu LCS, Cheng CL, Leong JCY. Pott's paraplegia of late onset: the cause of compression and results after anterior decompression. *J Bone Joint Surg Br* 1988;70:534.

359. Dent CE, Friedman M. Idiopathic juvenile osteoporosis. *Q J Med* 1965;134:177.

360. Schippers JC. Over een geval van "spontane" algemeene osteoporose bij een klein meisje. *Maandschr Kindergeneeskd* 1939;8:108.

361. Evans BA, Dunstan CR, Hills E. Bone metabolism in idiopathic juvenile osteoporosis: a case report. *Calcif Tissue Int* 1983;35:5.

362. Hoekman K, Papapoulos SE, Peters ACB, et al. Characteristics and bisphosphonate treatment of a patient with juvenile osteoporosis. *J Clin Endocrinol Metab* 1985;61:952.

363. Jackson EC, Strife CF, Tsang RC, et al. Effect of calcitonin replacement therapy in idiopathic juvenile osteoporosis. *Am J Dis Child* 1988;142:1237.

364. Jones ET, Hensinger RN. Spinal deformity in idiopathic juvenile osteoporosis. *Spine* 1981;6:1.

365. Marder HK, Tsang RC, Hug G, et al. Calcitriol deficiency in idiopathic juvenile osteoporosis. *Am J Dis Child* 1982;136:914.

366. Saggese G, Bartelloni S, Baroncelli GI, et al. Mineral metabolism and calcitriol therapy in idiopathic juvenile osteoporosis. *Am J Dis Child* 1991;145:457.

367. Smith R. Idiopathic osteoporosis in the young. *Bone Joint Surg Br* 1980;62:417.

368. Rosskamp R, Sell G, Emmons D, et al. Idiopathische juvenile osteoporose—Bericht aber zwei Falle. *Klin Padiatr* 1987;199:457.

369. Samuda GM, Cheng MY, Yeung CY. Back pain and vertebral compression: an uncommon presentation of childhood acute lymphoblastic leukemia. *J Pediatr Orthop* 1987;7:175.

370. Green WB. *Idiopathic juvenile osteoporosis.* New York, NY: Raven, 1994.

371. Dimar JRII, Campbell M, Glassman SD. Idiopathic juvenile osteoporosis. An unusual cause of back pain in an adolescent. *Am J Orthop* 1995;11:865.

372. Marhaug G. Idiopathic juvenile osteoporosis. *Scand J Rheumatol* 1993;22:45.

373. Villaverde V, De Inocencio J, Merino R, et al. Difficulty walking. A presentation of idiopathic juvenile osteoporosis. *J Rheumatol* 1998;25:173.

374. Brenton DP, Dent CE. Idiopathic juvenile osteoporosis. In: Bickel H, Stern J, eds. *Inborn errors of calcium and bone metabolism.* Baltimore, MD: University Park Press, 1976:222.

375. Bartal E, Gage J. Idiopathic juvenile osteoporosis and scoliosis. *J Pediatr Orthop* 1982;2:295.

CHAPTER 20

Alexander K. Powers
Lawrence G. Lenke
Scott J. Luhmann

Spondylolysis and Spondylolisthesis

DEFINITION

Spondylolysis is a term used to refer to an isolated defect in the neural arch of the vertebra, specifically the pars interarticularis. The term originates from the Greek roots *spondylos*, which means "vertebra," and *lysis*, meaning "break" or "defect." The spondylotic defect is most common at the L5 vertebra in the pediatric and adolescent patients; however, it can be found throughout the entire spine. Spondylolysis can secondarily result in spondylolisthesis.

Early obstetricians provided the first description of spondylolisthesis after describing a difficult delivery in a woman with slippage of the 5th lumbar vertebra on the sacrum (1). The actual term *spondylolisthesis* was not coined until 1854 by Kilian (2). The word *spondylolisthesis* arises from the Greek roots *spondylos*, which means "vertebra," and *listhesis*, meaning "slippage" or "movement," referring to the forward slipping of one vertebra on the adjacent caudal vertebra.

EPIDEMIOLOGY

Of the multiple types of spondylolisthesis (Tables 20-1 and 20-2), two are found in children and adolescents. Of these two,

the congenital or dysplastic group is the less common. This type of spondylolisthesis occurs in a 2:1 ratio of girls to boys (3, 4) and accounts for between 14% and 21% of the overall cases, according to several published reports (3, 5). Children with congenital/dysplastic spondylolistheses are at higher risk for neurologic injury (e.g., cauda equina syndrome) than are those with isthmic spondylolisthesis because the intact neural arch can cause severe spinal canal stenosis beginning at approximately 50% slippage.

Isthmic spondylolisthesis is the more common type. Although most published series combine both types of spondylolisthesis (isthmic and congenital/dysplastic) with spondylolysis, most data in the literature refer to the isthmic type of spondylolisthesis. Some have suggested that the isthmic spondylolytic defect may be caused by congenital factors. With one exception (6), a defect in the pars interarticularis has never been found at birth (7–12). In fact, the pathology seems to be rare in patients younger than 5 years, with only a few cases reported in children younger than 2 years (9, 10, 12, 13). Fredrickson et al. reported on the natural history of spondylolysis and spondylolisthesis in a review of 500 children in the first grade. The prevalence of spondylolysis was 4.4% at 6 years of age, increasing to the adult rate of 6% at 14 years of age (7). In addition, they documented and associated spondylolisthesis in 68% of the 5-year-old children, which increased to 74% in adulthood; the authors also implied that the development of spondylolisthesis after the age of 6 years in children with spondylolysis is infrequent. Only seven patients in this series developed further slippage; all slippages were minimal, and none of the patients complained of pain. Virta et al. (14) identified a 2:1 ratio of occurrence in boys and girls. In their review of 1100 individuals in Finland ranging in age from 45 to 64 years, Virta et al. reported a 7% incidence of spondylolisthesis in a population of individuals who had radiographic evaluation for back pain.

TABLE 20-1 Classification of Spondylolisthesis by Wiltse et al.

Type	Description
I	Congenital (dysplastic)
II	Isthmic—defect in the pars interarticularis
IIA	Spondylolytic—stress fracture of the pars interarticularis region
IIB	Pars interarticularis—elongation of pars interarticularis
IIC	Acute pars interarticularis—traumatic fracture of pars interarticularis
III	Degenerative—due to a long-standing intersegmental instability
IV	Posttraumatic—acute fractures in the posterior elements beside the pars interarticularis region
V	Pathologic—destruction of the posterior elements from generalized or localized bone pathology

From Wiltse LL, Newman PH, Macnab I. Classification of spondylolysis and spondylolisthesis. *Clin Orthop Relat Res* 1976;117:23–29.

The prevalence of spondylolisthesis appears to be influenced by the racial or genetic background of the population studied. African Americans have the lowest rate of spondylolisthesis, 1.8%, whereas Inuit Eskimos have a prevalence of 50%. South Africans and whites fall in an intermediate range, 3.5% and 5.6%, respectively (15–17). Rowe and Roche report a difference in the incidence of spondylolisthesis depending on sex and race: for the male sex, the incidence is 6.4% in whites and 2.8% in African Americans, and in the female sex, it is 2.3% in whites and 1.1% in African Americans (18). The role that gender plays in the natural history of spondylolisthesis is illustrated by the fact that, despite the twofold higher frequency in men, the high-grade slips are four times more common in women. Osterman et al. (16) noted in their report that the lower grades of spondylolisthesis are far more common at the time of presentation: grade I, 79%; grade II, 20%; and grade III, 1%.

In lytic spondylolisthesis, the osteolysis occurs at L5 in 87% of the patients, at L4 in 10%, and at L3 in 3% (19, 20). There is also an increasing prevalence of spondylolisthesis in individuals who participate in active sports, especially in physical activities that accentuate lumbar lordosis (Table 20-3). Gymnasts have long been identified as an at-risk group for development of spondylolisthesis. Jackson et al. (21) noted an 11% incidence of bilateral pars interarticularis defects in 100 female gymnasts. An even higher rate of spondylolysis or spondylolisthesis has been identified in a similar population of Asian female gymnasts.

ETIOLOGY

The etiology of spondylolysis and spondylolisthesis remains unclear. A truly congenital etiology seems unlikely because, with one exception (6), no evidence exists for the presence of the lytic pars interarticularis defect in the newborn (7–11). Studies by Vaz et al. (22), Legaye et al. (23), and Labelle et al. (24) suggest that the intrinsic architecture of the pelvis may be an important parameter, modulating the mechanical stresses experienced by the lumbosacral junction. This is confirmed by the higher incidence of spondylolysis in certain sports, previously mentioned, and in Scheuermann disease (25). In addition, spondylolysis has not been reported in adults (average age of 27 years) who have never walked (26), suggesting that mechanical factors associated with upright posture may play a role.

TABLE 20-2 Classification of Spondylolisthesis by Marchetti and Bartolozzi

1982 Group	Pathology	1994 Type	Form	Condition
Developmental		Developmental		
	Lysis		High dysplastic	Interarticular lysis
	Elongation of the pars interarticularis			Elongation of the pars interarticularis
	Trauma			
	Acute fracture		Low dysplastic	Interarticular lysis
	Stress fracture			Elongation of the pars interarticularis
Acquired		Acquired		
	Iatrogenesis		Traumatic	Acute fracture
	Pathology			Stress fracture
	Degeneration		Postsurgical	Direct effect of surgery
				Indirect effect of surgery
			Pathologic	Local pathology
				Systemic pathology
			Degenerative	Primary Secondary

From Marchetti PC, Bartolozzi P. Classification of spondylolisthesis as a guideline for treatment. In: Bridwell KH, DeWald RL, Hammerberg KW et al., eds. *The textbook of spinal surgery*, 2nd ed., vol. 2. Philadelphia, PA: Lippincott–Raven Publishers, 1997:1211–1254.

TABLE 20-3	Sports Commonly Associated with Repetitive Lumbar Hyperextension
Gymnastics	Cheer leading
Figure skating	Football (Linemen)
Javelin throw	Butterfly stroke
Weightlifting	Volleyball

The absence of pars interarticularis defects at birth, along with the increased prevalence of spondylolysis and spondylolisthesis among athletes who participate in sports involving hyperextension, strongly suggests a mechanical etiology to the development of spondylolisthesis (27–32). Several authors have postulated that a fracture is the underlying pathomechanical event in the development of a lytic spondylolisthesis (29, 33–37). This may be either an acute traumatic event or secondary to an insidious fatigue failure during repetitive stress (38). Wiltse et al. (39) theorized that spondylolysis is a stress fracture in the pars interarticularis, specifically due to repetitive microtrauma or microstresses, with inadequate healing. Biomechanical studies have suggested that the pars interarticularis is the weakest part of the posterior neural arch (21, 34–36). During flexion and extension, the pars interarticularis is cycled through alternating compressive and tensile loads. During extension, the pars interarticularis experiences posterior compressive forces and anterior tensile forces (Fig. 20-1) (40). The ability of the pars interarticularis to resist the compressive and tensile forces during flexion and extension depends on the thickness of the cortical bone (41). The overall resilience of the pars interarticularis is undoubtedly high, as evidenced by the generally low prevalence of spondylolisthesis in the population.

The importance of the pars interarticularis and its ability to resist shear stress has been well documented; in contrast, the role of the intervertebral disk is less well understood. In the intact, morphologically normal spinal motion segment, the intervertebral disc contributes 60% of the total shear resistance (42). A skeletally immature animal model of shear load forces demonstrated that, in spines with pars interarticularis defects, the end plate (apophyseal ring) most likely was responsible for the anterior listhesis (42, 43). Kajiura et al. (44) confirmed these findings and demonstrated that the increasing strength of the growth plate during skeletal maturity is the likely reason for the infrequent occurrence of further slippage after the completion of growth.

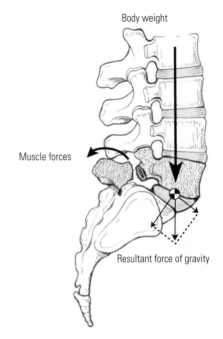

FIGURE 20-2. Forces that affect distraction of spondylolytic defect at L5.

Once the pars interarticularis defect has been created, anatomic and biomechanical forces conspire to prevent spontaneous healing of the fracture (Fig. 20-2). The shear forces created by the body's center of gravity tend to cause anterior displacement of L5 on the sacrum because of the effects of gravity, muscular activity, and body movement. The posterior muscular forces tend to extend the posterior elements, thereby tending to open the spondylolytic defect and create the spondylolisthesis. These initial events tend to precipitate a cascade of worsening biomechanics as the center of gravity moves progressively anterior, causing a vector that increases the shear forces at the lumbosacral junction. This situation may be exacerbated by a low intercrestal line and small transverse processes of L5, resulting in muscular and ligamentous connections between the pelvis and the spine that are not robust enough to resist the forward slippage of the rostral vertebrae on the caudal vertebrae. Loder has demonstrated in children with higher grades of lumbosacral spondylolisthesis that the sacrum becomes more vertical as the slip worsens (45). When the sacrum becomes more vertical, there is an increase in the thoracic lordosis; this is likely an adaptive mechanism to maintain the normal upright posture.

Although mechanical considerations probably are the most significant factors in the development of lytic spondylolisthesis, genetic considerations have been discussed by some researchers (46). Familial studies have documented a high incidence (19% to 69%) of spondylolysis and spondylolisthesis in first-degree relatives of children with spondylolysis and dysplastic or isthmic spondylolisthesis (10, 47–50). Wynne-Davies and Scott noted an increased incidence of dysplastic lesions in affected relatives (50). First-degree relatives of patients with the dysplastic form of spondylolisthesis had a prevalence of

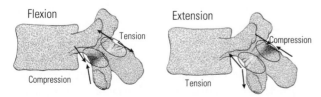

FIGURE 20-1. Compressive and tensile forces experienced in the region of the pars interarticularis during flexion and extension.

33%, compared to 15% for isthmic spondylolisthesis. These authors have suggested an autosomal dominant genetic predisposition, multifactorial and with reduced penetrance. Wiltse, on the other hand, suggested that a cartilaginous defect in the vertebral analogue may be an autosomal recessive characteristic with varying expressivity (32).

CLINICAL FEATURES

There are many possible causes for low back pain, and these must be distinguished from pain secondary to a spondylolisthesis. Although back pain is often a presenting symptom in spondylolisthesis, many asymptomatic spondylolytic defects are identified incidentally on spine or pelvic radiographs. Spondylolisthesis incidentally discovered during screening for low back pain after trauma is typically a stable, chronic entity, probably not a result of the trauma and presenting little, if any, risk of a catastrophic structural instability that would result in neurologic sequela (51). Mild-to-moderate spondylolisthesis does not necessarily predispose to low back pain (52).

Patients with symptomatic low back pain have a spondylolisthesis rate of 5.3% to 11%, whereas in asymptomatic patients occult spondylolisthesis may occur in 2.2% (53). Libson et al. (54) have documented a twofold increase in the incidence of spondylolisthesis in patients with symptomatic low back pain, compared to asymptomatic patients. Wiltse and Rothman (55) identified 11% of 1124 patients undergoing lumbosacral radiographic examination for back pain as having either unilateral or bilateral pars interarticularis defects. Saraste described radiographic features that correlated with low back symptoms: slip of <25%, L4 spondylolysis or spondylolisthesis, and early disc degeneration at the level of the slip (56). The most common period for the spondylolysis and spondylolisthesis to become symptomatic is during the adolescent growth spurt, between the ages of 10 and 15 years. However, the degree of the deformity does not always match the degree of pain (56).

The history of the patient is a crucial element in the diagnostic and therapeutic process; although radiographic investigations are important in defining the pathoanatomy, treatment is typically based on the patient's symptoms, history, and physical examination. The presence of a spondylolisthesis should not be presumed to be the cause of the patient's back and/or leg symptoms. Muscular strain induced by poor sagittal alignment and poor muscular tone could also be the cause (57). The pain is usually a dull, aching, low back discomfort and is localized to the low back with occasional radiation into the gluteal region and posterior thighs. This pain is most likely due to the instability caused by the pars interarticularis defect, and is generally exacerbated by participation in athletic or other physical activity, and relieved by rest or restriction of activities. In a few cases, the pain may also follow an acute traumatic episode, usually involving hyperextension during athletic participation.

The presenting symptoms may also include a change in the child's posture or gait, usually noted by his or her parents,

with or without accompanying pain. This can be present in mild degrees of spondylolisthesis, but is much more common in more marked degrees of slip. These patients may also present with scoliosis. As the degree of slip increases, the corresponding pain may cause a muscle-spasm–induced atypical scoliosis. Concomitant rotatory displacement of the spondylolisthetic segment can also create an olisthetic curve. Conversely, the presenting symptoms may be adolescent idiopathic scoliosis, with the spondylolysis or spondylolisthesis detected incidentally on the radiographic evaluation of the scoliosis.

It is important to clearly differentiate low back pain from radiculopathy. Radicular pain is atypical in the pediatric patient, being more common in the adolescent and adult (58, 59). If present, aggressive treatment of the radiculopathy should be undertaken along with management of the low back pain. The neurologic symptoms that accompany spondylolisthesis may be either unilateral or bilateral radiculopathy, and may be either intermittent or chronic. In patients with spondylolisthesis and significant degenerative disease, the resulting neuroforaminal compression may cause chronic radiculopathy or neurogenic claudication. In patients with low-grade slips that are hypermobile, intermittent radiculopathy may be a presenting complaint. In patients who have central stenosis with or without foraminal narrowing, neurogenic claudication or cauda equina syndrome may be the presenting symptom.

The mere presence of a spondylolisthesis does not implicate it in the patient's symptoms. Important physical examination parameters include body habitus, coronal and sagittal alignment, and spinal mobility. Pain with hyperextension is a common finding. The physical examination findings depend on whether pain is present, as well as on the degree of spondylolisthesis. In patients with spondylolysis and mild spondylolisthesis, the back and gait examinations may be completely normal, with no hamstring tightness. With increasing degrees of spondylolisthesis, there is usually some degree of hamstring tightness. This may significantly restrict straight-leg raising and forward bending, and may create postural and gait changes. The compensatory increased lumbar lordosis caused by the spondylolisthetic kyphosis creates a flattening of the buttocks ("heart-shaped"), shortening of the waistline, a protuberant abdomen, and a waddling-type gait pattern or Phalen-Dickson sign (5, 60, 61). The exact mechanism of the hamstring tightness remains unclear, but typically resolves after solid bony fusion (61, 62).

Palpation of the lumbosacral area may reveal a step-off with a prominent L5 spinous process. Palpation of the lumbosacral region may also elicit a localized area of tenderness. In addition, the child with a severe slip tends to stand with the hips and knees flexed because of the anterior rotation of the pelvis, with the gait examination demonstrating a shortened stride length caused by the patient's inability to extend the hips. Both static and dynamic examinations are important for eliciting pertinent symptoms. Pain on flexion and extension, with limitation of these motions, may suggest hypermobility as the cause of the pain. Neurologic examination is typically completely normal, but on occasion may reveal a diminished or absent ankle deep-tendon reflex or weakness of the extensor hallucis longus (EHL). Sphincter dysfunction is very rare (63). Provocation of neurologic symptoms during dynamic assessment may also imply the presence of hypermobility. Neurologic symptoms that correlate dermatome and myotome levels with the level of stenosis or lytic instability implicate the contribution of the spondylolisthesis to the development of symptoms. Scoliosis, which may be seen at the time of the presentation, is of the typical idiopathic type or, where there are more advanced grades of decompensation, may be caused by reflexive pain or spasm ("olisthetic scoliosis"). A thorough evaluation is essential to rule out other causations of the individual's pain and/or neurologic findings, such as tumors of bone, spinal cord, conus or cauda equina, disk herniation, and disk-space infection.

RADIOGRAPHIC FEATURES

Numerous imaging modalities are required in order to completely document the three-dimensional pathoanatomy of spondylolysis and spondylolisthesis (64). Each modality contributes a unique view of the various aspects of the pathology. Plain radiographs are obtained initially with the patient in an upright, preferably standing position (Fig. 20-3). Films of the patient supine may not show subtle instability (65). Initial plain radiographic imaging typically consists of anteroposterior and lateral projections. Left and right oblique projections can be helpful to visualize subtle defects. Ferguson anteroposterior and flexion-extension laterals can also be obtained but are not necessary for diagnosis.

Each of these radiographic views is useful in identifying certain aspects of the pathology. The routine posteroanterior and Ferguson anteroposterior projections may show spina bifida occulta, pars interarticularis defects, lumbar scoliosis, or dysplastic posterior elements (66). The lateral views show vertebral body alignment and often allow identification of a pars interarticularis defect even when a spondylolisthesis is not present. Oblique views will often better define the pars interarticularis defect, also known as the *collar* on the well-known "Scotty dog" (Fig. 20-4). The diagnosis of spondylolysis may be missed in 30% of symptomatic young patients if a lateral radiograph alone is obtained (67). The Ferguson anteroposterior provides an *en face* view of L5 that may improve the visualization of the transverse process and the sacrum and may more clearly identify a high-riding L5 vertebral body. Flexion–extension views may uncover subtle instabilities that are not apparent on static standing views. Other important anatomic features that can be identified on plain radiographs are rounding off of the anterior corner of the sacrum, wedging or erosion of L5 in higher grade spondylolisthesis, flexion at the S1-S2 disc, and bending of the sacrum (68). In cases of a unilateral defect, the only finding may be sclerosis of the facet, pedicle, lamina, or pars interarticularis on the intact side opposite the defect, secondary to increased bony stresses.

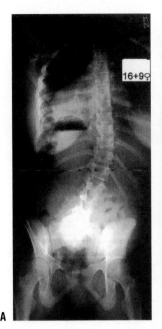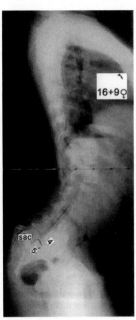

FIGURE 20-3. Long-cassette upright posteroanterior (**A**) and lateral (**B**) radiographs show olisthetic scoliosis and also marked forward sagittal vertical axis.

MEASUREMENT

The deformity in spondylolisthesis, usually at the lumbosacral junction, consists of anterior translation of L5 on S1, with obligatory forward rotation of L5 on S1 into lumbosacral kyphosis. The degree of slip can be quantified using the Meyerding classification, the percentage of slip described by Boxall et al. (Fig. 20-5), or the Newman classification that also describes angular slippage (Fig. 20-6A) (5, 27, 69–71). Sagittal rotation, slip angle, and sacral inclination are all direct measurements of the amount of lumbosacral kyphosis, and are assessed on spot lateral radiographs of the lumbosacral area taken with the patient in standing position (72).

Slip Percentage. The Meyerding classification, which grades the slip from grade 0 (spondylolysis) through grades I to IV (spondylolisthesis) and V (spondyloptosis), is probably the most functional and widely used technique (70) (Fig. 20-5). The amount of anterior translation of the olisthetic vertebra on the caudal level is measured at the posterior vertebral body line. This classifies the spondylolisthesis into five grades: grade I (slip of 1% to 25%), grade II (slip of 26% to 50%), grade III (slip of 51% to 75%), grade IV (slip of 76% to 100%), and grade V (spondyloptosis). Higher grade spondylolistheses have been shown to be predictive of spondylolisthetic progression (73). Boxall et al. describes a slip percentage that is more precise but requires exact measurements (74). On the radiograph, a line is drawn along the posterior border of the sacrum, and a perpendicular line is drawn at the upper end of the sacrum.

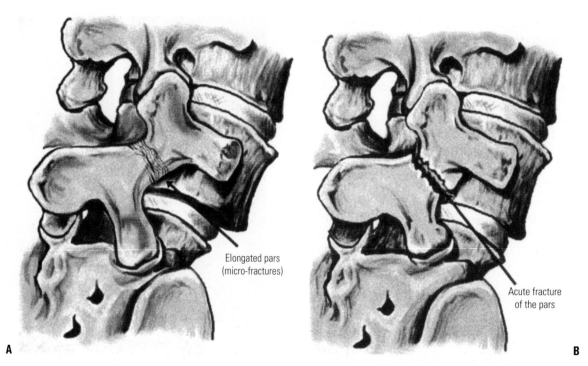

FIGURE 20-4. Sketches of an elongated pars interarticularis **(A)** and an acute fracture of the pars interarticularis **(B)** across the neck of the "Scotty dog."

The anterior displacement of the posteroinferior corner of L5 from the line along the posterior border of the sacrum is quantified as the numerator. The width of S1 forms the denominator, and the slip is expressed as a percentage. In the situation of a rounded superior end plate of S1, the anteroposterior width of L5 is used instead.

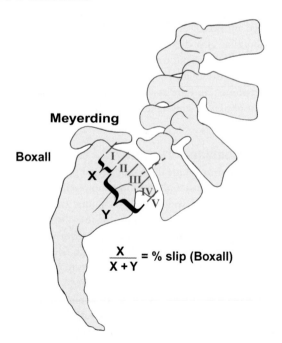

$$\frac{X}{X + Y} = \% \text{ slip (Boxall)}$$

FIGURE 20-5. Meyerding and Boxall measurement techniques for grading spondylolisthesis.

A limitation of the Meyerding classification is its inability to describe the rotational component in the sagittal plane of the subluxing rostral vertebrae. The modified Newman classification takes this into account (Fig. 20-6A). In this classification system, measurements are taken of both the anterior displacement (first number) and the vertical/downward displacement of the vertebral body in relation to the sacrum (second number). The superior end plate and the anterior face of the sacrum are divided into 10 equal segments. The first number is the position of the posteroinferior corner of the L5 vertebra with respect to the superior end plate of S1, and the second is the position of the anteroinferior corner of L5 relative to the anterior surface of S1. A score by this method utilizes both numbers, for example, 7 + 5, with the "7" indicating the amount of sagittal slip and the "5" indicating the amount of angular roll of L5 over the sacrum.

Although somewhat tedious, this classification allows a continuous scale of 0 to 20 to be applied to each spondylolisthesis, uniquely describing anterolisthesis and the degree of caudal migration of the rostral vertebrae (27, 69, 71).

Slip Angle. The slip angle is the most commonly described measurement of the lumbosacral kyphosis of L5 on S1 (Fig. 20-6B). On the radiograph, a perpendicular to the line drawn at the posterior cortex of the sacrum forms the sacral measuring line. A second line is drawn along the inferior end plate of L5, and the angle formed by these two lines is the slip angle that, in the normal condition, is in lordosis and is expressed by a negative number (72). Boxall et al. (5) have

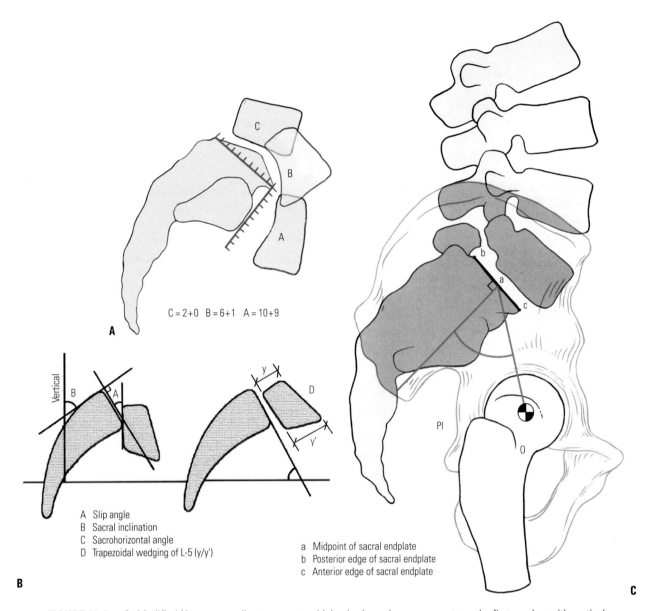

FIGURE 20-6. **A:** Modified Newman grading system, combining horizontal measurements as the first number with vertical measurements as the second number. **B:** Radiographic parameters for angular measurements in the description of spondylolisthesis. **C:** Radiographic parameters and pelvic incidence (posterior instrumentation).

used the line along the inferior edge of L5 for their measurement, but this edge is often difficult to visualize accurately, and when slippage is considerable, the vertebral body is often trapezoidal in shape. In such a situation, use of the inferior end plate as reference may increase the measured slip angle by erroneously adding the measurement of the kyphosis and the wedging of olisthetic vertebra. Slip angles of <+ 45 degrees (kyphosis) correlate with an increased risk of slip progression (5, 73, 75, 76).

Sagittal Rotation. The amount of sagittal rotation can also be measured, and is the angle between the posterior cortex

of the sacrum and the posterior cortex of the L5 vertebral body. This sagittal rotation angle should approximately equal the slip angle measured as described previously. In higher degrees of slip (translation or angulation), L4 may show retrolisthesis on L5. In severe slips of <50%, the slip angle of L4 in relation to the sacrum should also be measured, as this will be the new lumbosacral slip angle if surgical management is to be an L4 to S1 fusion.

Sacral Inclination. The inclination of the sacrum is determined by drawing a line along the posterior cortex of the sacrum and measuring the angle between that line and a vertical line from the floor (a line drawn parallel to the edge of the x-ray film) (Fig. 20-6B). Normal sacral inclination is <30 degrees; however, with higher degree slips, the sacrum usually becomes more vertical and sacral inclination decreases.

Pelvic Incidence.   This measurement assesses the relation between the sacropelvic and the hip joints. Pelvic incidence is the angle between a perpendicular-to-superior end plate of S1 and a line from the center of the superior end plate of S1 to the center of the femoral head (Fig. 20-6C). In normally aligned individuals, the gravity line should pass through the hip joints. Increased pelvic incidence has been shown to correlate with the degree of slippage (24, 74, 77).

OTHER IMAGING STUDIES

Computed Tomography Scan.   A computed tomography (CT) scan can be utilized in situations in which a pars interarticularis defect is strongly suspected on clinical evaluation but is not identifiable on the lateral or oblique radiographs. CT scans can delineate the pars interarticularis defects in the axial plane even when no spondylolisthesis is present. On the axial images, the spondylolytic defect is identified as a linear lesion of varying width with sclerotic osseous margins and hypertrophic osteophytes. The lytic defect is usually identified in the axial image either at, or immediately inferior to, the axial image containing the pedicles of the involved vertebrae. CT scans can also provide excellent visualization of complex anatomy in the coronal and sagittal planes when reformatted images are obtained.

Magnetic Resonance Imaging Scan.   Magnetic resonance imaging (MRI) is an excellent imaging modality for the evaluation of the soft-tissue component of the spondylolisthesis and can also help define the degree of associated degenerative disc disease (78, 79). Degenerative disc disease at, above, or below the slip level may be the cause of the patient's pain because of nuclear degeneration or annular injury. The MRI excels at visualizing the neural elements and the surrounding soft tissue, and it is the optimal modality when there is a neurologic deficit or the symptoms suggest a diagnosis other than spondylolysis or spondylolisthesis. MRI may not be as precise as CT myelography in distinguishing the soft tissues from the osseous elements of the pathology in high-grade slips; however, this small drawback is offset by the fact that MRI studies do not involve ionizing radiation, myelographic dye that could precipitate an anaphylactic reaction, or invasive techniques. MRI studies can identify both central and foraminal stenosis and provide a good indication of the degree of neural compression. A consistent finding on MRI, especially in moderate- to high-grade slips, is a large, bulging disc at the level of the spondylolisthesis causing neuroforaminal stenosis. In addition, the MRI can document the degree of encroachment

on the neural elements by the exuberant hypertrophic scar tissue that forms at the spondylolytic defect. The degeneration of adjacent discs can also be discerned by reviewing the MRI. The significance and the etiology of the degeneration of these adjacent discs are unclear. The MRI and the CT scans are also useful in identifying facet joint hypertrophy and degeneration at the level of the slip and adjacent levels, as these factors may also contribute to the patient's low back pain or discomfort.

Bone Scan.   In the context of recent onset of pain, or when there is a distinct history of trauma, a bone scan may be useful for detecting an acute fracture of the pars interarticularis or for excluding a bony tumor. Bone scans provide information about the metabolic activity of the bone and the capacity to form bony union. The most sensitive technique is a single-photon emission computed tomography (SPECT) scan because of the improved detail that it provides (80). An intensely "hot" SPECT scan suggests that the defect is metabolically active and could benefit from a period of immobilization or, failing this, direct osteosynthesis. A "cold" SPECT scan, on the other hand, implies that the lytic defect is chronic and metabolically inactive. These defects, when symptomatic, are not amenable to nonsurgical treatment such as immobilization. In patients with unilateral pars defects, the pedicle contralateral to the lesion often shows increased uptake as a result of the increased stress placed on it from the lysis. Symptomatic lytic lesions of the pars interarticularis that respond to local anesthetic injections may be amenable to fusion or repair (69).

OTHER DIAGNOSTIC STUDIES WHEN INDICATED

Discography.   Discography may be helpful when considering surgical intervention. When a pars interarticularis repair is contemplated and the health of the involved disc is not certain, discography may provide useful information about its functional quality. If a segmental fusion is required because of severe disc degeneration at the level of a pars interarticularis defect, and MRI shows degenerative changes at the adjacent level, discography may be helpful in deciding whether the fusion should include the adjacent degenerative level. Practically, however, we rarely carry out discography in pediatric patients.

Pathoanatomy.   In L5-S1 spondylolisthesis, the bony adaptive changes occur at both the superior end plate of S1 and at L5. At S1, the anterior lip typically undergoes resorption, thereby creating a rounded, dome-shaped surface. The rostral level, usually the fifth lumbar vertebra, becomes trapezoidal, specifically more narrow posteriorly and wider anteriorly. The amount of L5 wedging can be measured in terms of the lumbar index, with references to the height of the anterior aspect of the L5 vertebra expressed as a percentage of the height of the posterior aspect (Fig. 20-6B). Greater slip progressions tend to have lower lumbar indices (7, 56).

The pathoanatomy of neural element compression is complex. The fibrocartilaginous scar or hypertrophic callus that forms around the lytic defect may be responsible for the neuroforaminal compression posteriorly. Anterior to the nerve roots, annular bulging of the disc that results from the vertical collapse of the disc space and the anterior translation of the rostral vertebral body may cause a significant compression of the nerve root against the caudal surface of the pedicle. Although radiculopathy is usually caused by neuroforaminal stenosis at the level of the lytic defect with impingement of the exiting nerve roots, compression of traversing nerve roots by an anteriorly translated intact neural arch may cause radiculopathy in more distal roots/dermatomes, neurogenic claudication, or cauda equina syndrome.

Natural History. The natural history of spondylolisthesis was reported by Saraste in a 20-year follow-up study of 255 patients with spondylolysis and spondylolisthesis (56). In this study, 40% of adults showed no progression of the slip, and 40% showed an additional 1- to 5-mm slip. Spondylolisthesis was much more common than spondylolysis, with approximately 22% of patients initially presenting with only spondylolysis. Significant progression of the slip occurs in a low percentage of cases, occurring in 4% of patients in the series studied by Frennered et al., in 5% of the cases studied by Saraste, and in 3% of the 311 patients in the series studied by Danielson et al. (56, 75, 81). In the series of Fredrickson et al., progression was shown to be unlikely (1.4%) after adolescence (7), whereas other authors have reported progression, attributed to disc degeneration, during adolescence (17, 78, 82). Beutler reported a long-term follow-up of patients with spondylolisthesis and documented that the progression of the slippage declined with each decade (83). Various studies in the literature have reported that women are more likely to present at a younger age, and are at greater risk of slip progression in higher grade spondylolisthesis, and of having posterior element dysplasia and lumbosacral kyphosis of more than 45 degrees (5, 7, 51, 84, 85). In patients with preexisting lumbar spondylolisthesis, traumatic injuries usually do not aggravate the condition. Floman et al. (51) reported on 200 patients with thoracolumbar trauma and documented that major axial skeletal trauma had little or no effect on preexisting lumbar spondylolisthesis.

Several radiographic features have been associated with the likelihood of progression of the spondylolisthesis. Some researchers have associated the degree of slip at presentation with a greater chance of slip progression (60, 76, 86), but others have not (56, 75). In the growing child, the amount of spondylolisthetic kyphosis or of the slip angle, especially when severe, is associated with progression. Other morphologic changes found with high-grade slips, for example, dome-shaped sacrum and trapezoidal L5, are secondary or adaptive changes to the slip and have not been prognostic for slip progression (75).

TREATMENT RECOMMENDATIONS

Nonsurgical
Indications. The natural history of spondylolysis and mild spondylolisthesis is generally benign (7, 75, 87). All newly diagnosed patients with a symptomatic spondylolysis and/or spondylolisthesis are considered for nonoperative therapy. Nonsurgical management regimens generally include observation, activity modification, bracing, and physiotherapy (7, 10, 75, 58).

Options. As previously mentioned, most patients with spondylolysis are asymptomatic. In the patient with minimal to no symptoms, the follow-up will depend upon the child's age and growth potential. In the adolescent who has completed growth, no follow-up is necessary. In the growing child, however, lumbar radiographs should be obtained at the end of growth to monitor any potential for slip formation. The child with an asymptomatic spondylolysis can be allowed to participate in all sporting activities without restriction. In the long term, most young patients with spondylolysis managed nonoperatively, maintain good functional outcome up to 11 years after diagnosis (88). In fact, the unilateral defects can undergo bony healing, which may take up to 12 weeks; however, the bilateral defects may undergo degeneration, with mild slip over time (89). Beutler et al. (83) reported on a 45-year follow-up of patients with spondylosis and spondylolisthesis. Patients with unilateral pars interarticularis defects never experienced slippage over the 45-year period.

In general, when the child has a symptomatic spondylolysis, there is typically a long history of low back pain associated with activity. Restriction of activity is recommended along with physiotherapy emphasizing abdominal muscle and spinal extensor muscle strengthening, with short-term bed rest reserved for only the most exceptionally symptomatic patient. When the patient is asymptomatic, physical activities are gradually resumed.

A common dilemma that faces the spine surgeon is determining the duration of the child's symptoms. Patients with increased radiotracer uptake at the pars interarticularis during a SPECT bone scan are typically classified as having an acute injury or a fracture. In cases in which the scan is positive at the pars interarticularis in a patient with more acute onset of symptoms, immobilization in a cast or brace can be used for symptom abatement. The ideal method is to immobilize this area with a body cast including one thigh/leg in order to appropriately control the pelvis. Another less onerous option is to use a thoracolumbar sacral orthosis (TLSO) with thigh cuff extension. The use of a removable brace is better accepted by the patient and the family and will allow the individual to perform strengthening exercises out of the brace. The downside to a removable orthosis is the uncertainty of the patient's compliance with wearing the brace. Although bracing is a mainstay nonoperative therapy, Klein et al. (90) found that bracing does not influence the outcome of patients treated nonoperatively for spondylolysis or spondylolisthesis after pooling data from 15 observational studies. More prospective data are needed to truly answer the effectiveness of bracing in patients with spondylolysis.

Regarding healing of the pars interarticularis defect, varying levels of success have been described, with "healing" occurring in 3 to 4 months and typically being documented with oblique plain radiographic views or repeat bone scans (89, 91–93). In the patient with a cold SPECT scan, the use of a TLSO can be an option if the back pain is bothersome; however, the goal in this situation is not healing of the pars interarticularis defect, but rather, the elimination or the palliation of symptoms.

The nonsurgical options for treatment of spondylolisthesis consist primarily of observation, activity modification, bracing, and physiotherapy, and intervention in the form of medications or injections (94). An asymptomatic spondylolisthesis grade I or II in a skeletally immature child is kept under observation for progression with lateral lumbosacral radiographs taken with the patient in the standing position. A slip of <50% in an asymptomatic mature adolescent is also placed under close observation. If there is progression of the spondylolisthesis or persistent symptoms, surgical stabilization is indicated.

Activity modification involves the institution of proper bending and lifting activities and development of a sustained aerobic activities program. This program should aim at decreasing recumbent and sitting activities in favor of aerobic activities in order to facilitate achieving ideal body weight. A growing child who presents with low back pain and a spondylolisthesis grade I or II is advised to limit all physical activities that exacerbate the low back pain. Resumption of almost all activities is possible after symptoms have resolved.

If the pain does not resolve with restriction of activity, the use of a TLSO may be beneficial (92, 95, 96). This usually requires a period of 6 to 12 weeks in the brace. Once the symptoms are relieved, activities can gradually be resumed.

Physical therapy activities may be active or passive. Although passive modalities may be useful initially, when there is acute pain, active physical therapy techniques are probably more important in the long term. Examples of passive techniques are thermal therapy, massage, phonophoresis, ultrasound, immobilization, acupuncture, traction, and transcutaneous electrical nerve stimulation. These may facilitate the patient's acceptance of an active physical therapy program by ameliorating acute symptoms. Active physical therapy includes spinal flexibility exercises and muscle strengthening, especially abdominal and posterior lumbar muscles. Pelvic stabilization techniques are also important; these may involve isometric and isokinetic exercises as well as aerobic conditioning.

In the early phases of pain management, medications may be important. Nonsteroidal anti-inflammatory drugs should be instituted early and are the mainstay of drug therapy. Because the use of muscle relaxants and narcotics remains controversial, we tend to avoid prescription medication in children and teens, if at all possible. If medications are to be used, the patient must be informed that narcotics will not

be prescribed beyond a week or two, and their purpose is to facilitate the transition to physical therapy for managing the low back pain. Muscle relaxants may likewise be useful in the early, acute period to deal with muscle spasms secondary to injury.

Surgical

Indications. Indications for the surgical treatment of spondylolysis and spondylolisthesis can be generalized into two categories: slip progression or the presence of persistent symptoms. Surgery is indicated in any patient with a slip more than 50%, or with progression of a slip between 25% and 50%. This group of patients are surgical candidates even in the absence of symptoms given their increased risk for further slip progression (60, 85, 97, 98). Surgery can be considered for patients with progressive or persistent symptoms >6 months refractory to all nonsurgical modalities, such as rest, bracing, and physical therapy.

Options

Repair of Defect. Pars interarticularis repairs are particularly useful in young adults and adolescents. The ideal candidate has a spondylolysis of less than a full grade I slip, no degenerative disc disease at the olisthetic level, and has failed a full course of nonoperative treatment of the symptoms. Given such restrictive criteria of selection, this technique should be used cautiously in patients beyond the adolescent years. The use of pars interarticularis injections preoperatively can assist verifying that the defect is the sole cause of the back pain. An MRI is necessary to assess the involved intervertebral disk and vertebral end plate in order to identify any degree of disc degeneration or end-plate destruction that would preclude a successful outcome (17, 99).

In 1970, Buck described a translaminar screw osteosynthesis technique for direct repair (100, 101). He reported on 16 patients, out of whom 15 underwent fusion with this technique. One patient required salvage with a posterolateral fusion following failure of the pars interarticularis repair. Several other surgical techniques have also been described (102–105). Pedersen and Hagen (106) reviewed 18 patients treated with Buck's technique and reported 83% satisfactory results. Like Buck, they recommend pars interarticularis repair only in young patients with no degenerative disc disease. Bradford and Iza presented a technique of transverse process wiring bilaterally to fix the loose posterior element and to facilitate pars interarticularis osteosynthesis (107, 108). This technique has been modified with placement of pedicle screws as anchor points for the wiring, rather than the transverse processes. Of the 21 (of 22) cases available for follow-up, 90% obtained solid fusion of the pars interarticularis defect, and 80% had a good or an excellent result. Bradford and Iza (108) were also of the opinion that the technique is best suited for patients younger than 30 years without degenerative disc disease. This construct facilitates a compressive osteosynthesis across the laminar defect.

DIRECT REPAIR FOR SPONDYLOLYSIS AND SPONDYLOLISTHESIS

In young patients (younger than 25 years) with spondylolysis or grade I spondylolisthesis who have failed nonsurgical care, direct repair may provide an ideal alternative to standard posterolateral fusion (Figs. 20-7 and 20-8). The technique was originally described by Kimura in 1968 (109) and popularized by Buck in 1970 (100). In 1968, Scott, from Edinburgh, Scotland, first described a simple effective means of repairing spondylolysis or low-grade spondylolisthesis defects by the use of wiring and grafting (110). The Scott wiring technique functions as a tension band from the transverse process to the spinous process of the affected vertebrae. Many authors have described variations of this procedure with excellent results in approximately 90% of patients (108). A pedicle screw can be placed and used to secure the tension band wire. The technique as described by Scott and popularized by Bradford and Iza is described (108). The procedure can be used anywhere in the lumbar spine but is ideal for all defects above L5.

A sublaminar hook/pedicle screw technique has been demonstrated to achieve improved control over the fracture fragments, compared to the laminar or spinous process wiring technique. This improved technique includes replacing the posterior wire with bilateral, sublaminar hooks connected to the pedicle screws by a short rod. This facilitates direct compression across the lytic defect and provides improved control of the loose posterior element. In two small series of patients treated with sublaminar hook/pedicle screw constructs, 70% to 100% demonstrated clinical pain relief (102, 103, 111). The direct pars interarticularis repair is ideal for spondylolysis at the L4 level and above because it preserves lumbar motion segments.

A one-level L5 to S1 posterolateral fusion is performed in patients who are unresponsive to nonoperative treatment and who are not candidates for direct pars interarticularis repair. Traditionally, this has been performed through a midline skin incision with an intertransverse process to sacrum fusion, utilizing autologous iliac crest bone graft as described by Wiltse and Jackson (4). Postoperative immobilization is dependent upon the surgeon's preference and various parameters relating to the patient. Spica casting for 3 months has been advocated on the basis of reports documenting high levels of good and excellent outcomes (5, 95, 112–116). However, others report good results with no immobilization (93), or immobilization in a corset (117) or Boston brace (118). The use of posterior spinal instrumentation (i.e., pedicle screw) is gaining acceptance because it usually obviates the need for external immobilization and can rigidly maintain intraoperative correction. Overall, though, it is extremely rare for patients to require a fusion for a spondylolysis that fails conservative treatment.

Surgical intervention should be considered for persistently symptomatic spondylolisthesis that does not respond to nonoperative management, and that causes pain that prevents normal participation in daily and desirable physical activities. Additionally, the skeletally immature patient with slippage greater than grade II or the mature adolescent with

a slip of more than 75% should be treated surgically even in the absence of symptoms (60, 85, 97, 98). Surgical treatment options for symptomatic spondylolisthesis include decompression, fusion, or a combination of these techniques. In grade I and early grade II isthmic spondylolisthesis, the use of *in situ* posterolateral fusion is well established (Figs. 20-9 to 20-13). However, for higher grades of spondylolisthesis, the decision-making process becomes more complex, involving decisions about the number of levels that should be fused, whether to aim for partial or complete slip reduction, whether to include anterior fusion, and whether to use instrumentation and postoperative immobilization.

Decompression, alone or in combination with fusion, may be necessary if radicular or neurogenic claudication symptoms are present. Decompression alone may be a useful technique in patients with spondylolysis or a low-grade (grade II or less) spondylolisthesis when the symptoms are primarily neurologic and there is little evidence of instability. This situation is more common in adults than in children or adolescents. However, even patients with presumed stability and little back pain must be informed that decompression in the presence of a lytic defect or a low-grade spondylolisthesis may increase instability, causing low back pain. Intuitively, one would consider foraminotomies either unilaterally or bilaterally rather than a significant midline decompression in such a case. In 1955, Gill et al. reviewed 18 patients treated with complete removal of the loose posterior element (Gill laminectomy) and reported good results (119, 120). A long-term follow-up study of 43 patients, published in 1965, revealed an increased slip in 14% of patients, but a 90% satisfactory result in the group overall (121). These results, however, have not been universally observed. Osterman et al. reported on 75 patients with long-term follow-up averaging 12 years, and although the initial results at the end of 1 year showed fair, good, or excellent results in 83% of the patients, these results did not hold up over time (122). When these same patients were evaluated 5 years postoperatively, satisfaction ratings had dropped to 75%, and the spondylolisthesis had progressed in 27% of patients. Marmor and Bechtol described a patient who progressed from a grade II slip to a spondyloptosis after a Gill laminectomy (123). In a more dismal review of 33 patients with a 7-year follow-up, Amuso et al. reported 36% poor results following Gill laminectomy (124). These authors did not observe any significant progression of the spondylolisthesis and do not believe there is any correlation between the progression of spondylolisthesis and poor results.

With the currently available options for stabilization, the Gill laminectomy as a stand-alone intervention is not a reasonable procedure, especially in a growing child, and should always be accompanied by a spinal fusion (119, 120). However, decompression is often an important part of the surgical treatment of spondylolisthesis, and in patients with lytic defects, a Gill laminectomy is an efficient start for achieving a wide decompression. It also often results in sufficient autologous bone for fusion of that level. It should be noted that the Gill laminectomy alone does not decompress the involved

Text continued on page 808

Direct Repair for Spondylolysis and Spondylolisthesis (Figs. 20-7 and 20-8)

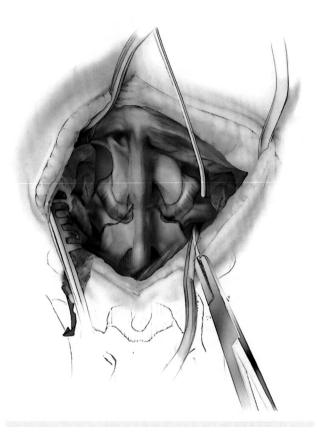

FIGURE 20-7. Direct Repair for Spondylolysis and Spondylolisthesis. The pars defect should be cleared of all soft tissues using fine curettes of varying sizes. The transverse process is carefully dissected with a Cobb elevator. Exposure of the anterior aspect of the transverse process may be aided by the use of a laminar elevator or a No. 4 Penfield dissector. Great care must be taken in exposing this area to avoid injury to the nerve root coursing anteriorly and also to the vessels coursing near the intervertebral foramen. A single strand of 18-gauge wire is passed anteriorly around the base of the transverse process on either side from the superior to the inferior direction and pulled as far medially as possible. The end of the wire is then passed superior to the base of the spinous process of the affected segment and back through the intraspinous ligaments.

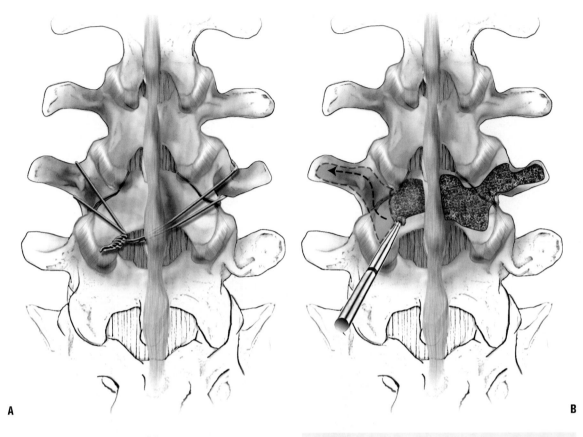

A

B

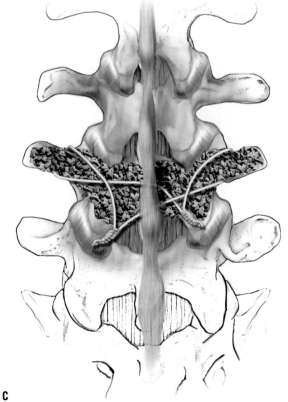

C

FIGURE 20-8.   Two alternatives can be used for fastening the wires. One involves passing the ends of the wires from one side of the spine, inferior to the spinous process of the loose elements, and then eventually securing the wires on one side of the spine **(A)**. The other alternative involves tying one knot on each side of the spinous process to assure stable fixation **(B)**. Bone graft from the iliac crest is harvested through the same skin incision. Prior to securing the wires, the spine should be decorticated and cancellous bone from the iliac crest taken and placed onto the surface of the defect and lamina in such a way as to be trapped by the wires as they are secured **(C)**. The wound is then closed in a standard fashion with or without a Hemovac drain.

Posterolateral Arthrodesis for Spondylolisthesis (Figs. 20-9 to 20-13)

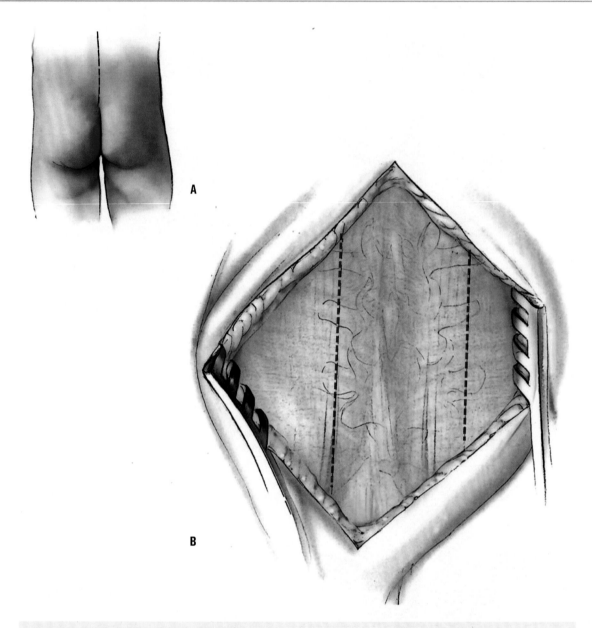

A

B

FIGURE 20-9.   Posterolateral Arthrodesis for Spondylolisthesis. The patient is placed prone on a Jackson table, so the abdomen remains free. We prefer a midline skin incision, as opposed to the two lateral incisions described by Wilste and colleagues (135). This incision should extend to the spinous process one level above the most cephalad vertebrae to be fused. Distally the incision can be made straight but extended slightly distally to be able to access the iliac crest for bone graft harvest. **A:** The skin is elevated in the interval between the deep investing fascia of the paraspinal muscles and the more superficial layer of fascia. The interval between this layer is easily identified in the midline. It is necessary to carry this dissection **(B)** laterally in each direction for about 4 to 5 cm.

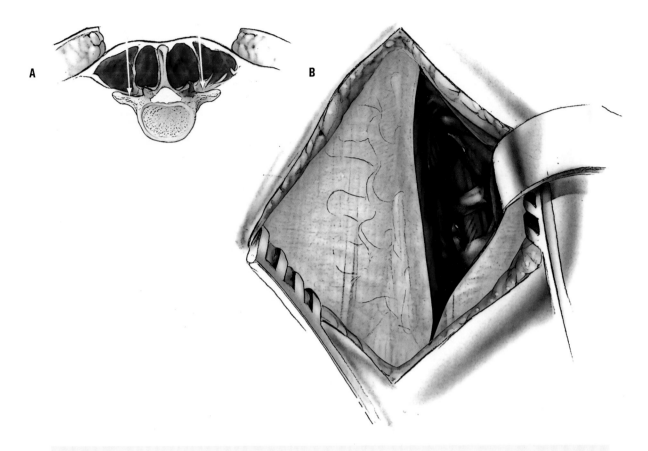

FIGURE 20-10. The sacrospinalis muscles **(A)** are now split about 3 to 4 cm from the midline over the transverse processes. The fascia is divided sharply **(B)** with a knife or an electrocautery; then, with a combination of blunt dissection and electrocautery, the muscle is split until the tips of the spinous processes are identified.

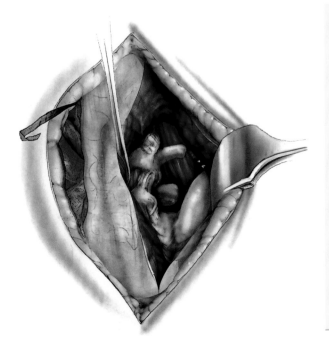

FIGURE 20-11. The subperiosteal dissection now proceeds toward the midline, staying on the transverse processes. As the lateral surface of the inferior facet is cleaned, the dissection proceeds to the facet capsule. In the L4 to sacral fusion, the capsule of the L4 to L5 facet is removed, as is the capsule of the L5 to S1 facet; however, the superior facet of L4 articulates with L3, which is not included in the fusion. Therefore, the dissection of the L4 transverse process should stop before removing the capsule of the L3 to L4 facet, which is encountered at the medial extent of the L4 transverse process. The dissection then may proceed onto the lamina, if desired, in an effort to broaden the fusion mass and incorporate the loose posterior elements in the fusion.

The transverse process of the L5 vertebra is the key to identifying the correct levels. In some patients, especially those with more severe slips, it may be difficult to identify because it lies directly anterior to the ala of the sacrum and may be small. Because of this, it is easy to mistake the L4 transverse process for the L5 process unless care is also taken to identify the lumbosacral facet and follow it down to the transverse process of L5. At the same time that the transverse process of L5 is exposed, the ala of the sacrum is exposed. Here, the periosteum is thick and adherent, and special effort is required to ensure that it is well exposed.

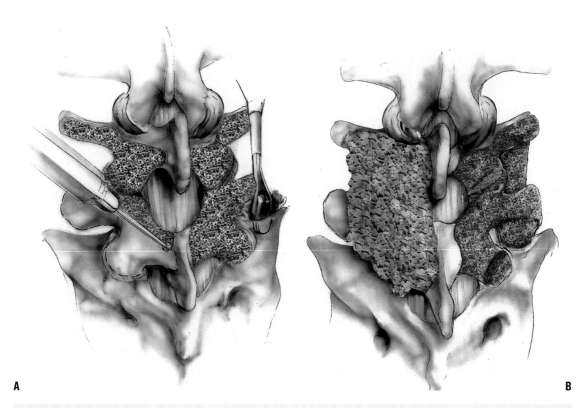

A   **B**

FIGURE 20-12.   We prefer to use a 5-mm burr for decortication because it gives excellent control and provides the ability to completely decorticate all of the transverse processes, the lateral side of the L4 superior facet, the lamina, and the facet joints. After this decortication is completed **(A)**, a gouge is used to create a hole in the ala of the sacrum. A piece of cortical bone **(B)** is placed in this hole and under the L5 transverse process. This can be difficult in severe slips because the transverse process of L5 lies adjacent to the ala and anterior to the hole in the ala. In these cases, a piece of cortical bone placed anterior to the transverse processes of L4 and into the hole in the ala will accomplish the same result. In mild slips (usually not the ones requiring fusion), the piece of cortical bone can extend from the ala to beneath both L5 and L4. This has the effect of preventing the muscles from displacing the cancellous bone graft, which is added next. After the bone graft is placed, the muscle layers are allowed to fall together. Care should be taken to be certain that the muscles do not dislodge the bone graft. If desired, the fascia can be closed to provide better hemostasis. Drains can be used beneath the flaps if it is believed necessary, and the midline incision is then closed.

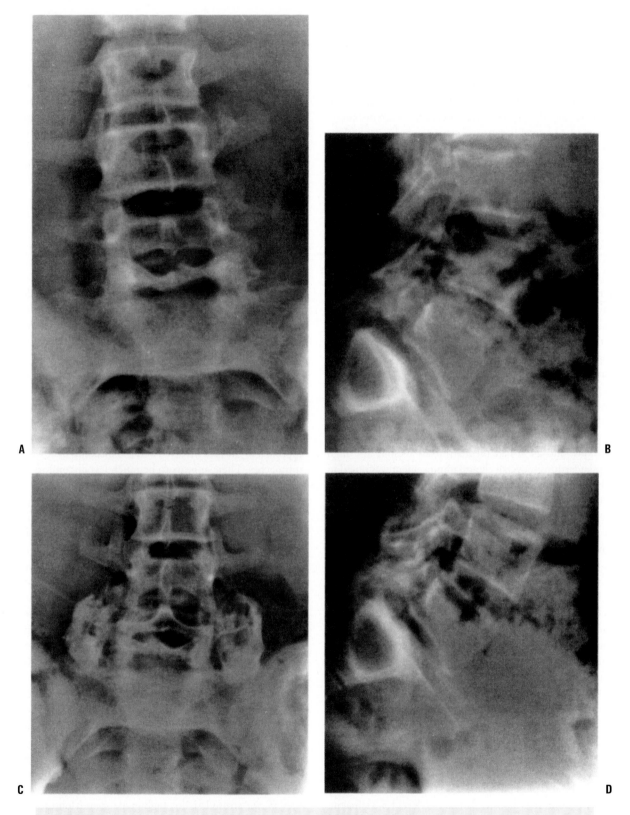

FIGURE 20-13. The anteroposterior and lateral radiographs **(A,B)** of a 13-year-old boy with a history of increasingly severe back pain over several years, made worse with activity. It was unresponsive to conservative measures during the past year. He underwent a posterolateral arthrodesis. Radiographs 6 months after surgery **(C,D)** demonstrate a consolidating arthrodesis.

foraminal nerve root; to achieve this, an additional dissection and a formal nerve root decompression is necessary. Wiltse and Jackson (4) proposed that root decompression is rarely necessary and that the tight hamstrings, abnormal reflexes, and motor weakness will recover after posterior fusion alone.

Fusion is the standard surgical technique for treatment of symptomatic spondylolisthesis and is necessary when instability (documented on lateral flexion and extension radiographs) and low back pain exist. Fusion is probably also reasonable when performing primarily decompressive surgery on patients whose main symptom is lower extremity radiculopathy, but whose spondylolisthesis is grade III or greater, especially in the presence of degenerative disc disease. Available techniques include anterior and posterior procedures, either alone or in combination. Posterior techniques include posterior lumbar interbody fusions (PLIF), transforaminal lumbar interbody fusion (TLIF), and posterolateral fusions with or without instrumentation.

Numerous historical studies extol the benefits of posterolateral uninstrumented fusions (Figs. 20-9 to 20-13). In these studies, fusion rates have ranged from 67% to 96%, with 60% to 100% of the patients showing good results (84, 118, 125–129). Although the outcomes of these multiple studies have been excellent, the actual pseudarthrosis rate may be much higher than reported. Lenke et al. (130) critically evaluated 56 patients with isthmic spondylolisthesis treated with *in situ* posterolateral fusions. When strict grading criteria were used, only 50% of the patients had bilateral solid fusions, 18% had unilateral solid fusions, and 21% had pseudarthrosis. Despite the high rate of pseudarthrosis, overall clinical improvement was noted in more than 80% of patients who had presented with preoperative symptoms of back or leg pain or hamstring tightness.

Recent studies by Bridwell et al. (131) highlight the benefit of instrumentation in achieving improved fusion rates and improved outcomes. Other groups have reported high fusion rates (90% to 95%) and 90% excellent or good outcomes with instrumented fusions for spondylolisthesis (132–134). External immobilization postoperatively is typically not necessary because the spinal fixation of transpedicular instrumentation provides sufficient rigidity; however, in cases with poor bone quality, an adjunctive postoperative cast or a brace may be helpful. *In situ* posterolateral fusion continues to offer satisfactory results for patients with grade I and some grade II spondylolistheses; the risks are within reasonable limits, and this technique remains a good approach for this category of patients. However, if the surgeon is comfortable placing pedicle screws in children, the procedure can provide definitive stabilization with less reliance on postoperative immobilization.

For the prototypical low-grade L5-S1 spondylolisthesis, the customary procedure is a posterolateral one-level L5-S1 fusion. Extension of the uninstrumented fusion to L4 may be indicated for greater degrees of slip (i.e., more than 50%) for two main reasons: (a) in high-grade slips the transverse process of L5 is displaced anterior to the sacral ala, making it difficult to expose the transverse process of L5 without exposing the L4-L5 facet and L4 transverse process; and (b) the fusion mass placed from L5 to the ala will be horizontal and under shear forces, whereas graft from the ala to the L4 transverse process will lie in a more biomechanically sound, vertical direction. A two-level uninstrumented arthrodesis may also be necessary in a slip of <50% if the transverse process of L5 is very small and provides an insufficient posterior bed for the fusion. With the advent of posterior instrumentation (i.e., pedicle screws) and anterior structural support (i.e., cages), the need for two-level fusion is decreasing, because of the high probability of creating a stable, solid bony union of the one-level fusion, even for high-grade slips. In addition, even a two-level L4-sacrum uninstrumented fusion is not guaranteed to heal in a grade III or IV spondylolisthesis. When pseudarthrosis and slip progression are noted postoperatively, revision fusion with instrumentation is indicated.

POSTEROLATERAL ARTHRODESIS FOR SPONDYLOLISTHESIS

The treatment of spondylolisthesis is complex and depends on the degree of slip, the slip angle, and the symptoms. Until recently, most children who required surgical treatment of spondylolisthesis were treated with an *in situ* arthrodesis without instrumentation. Because the posterior elements of the affected or slipping vertebrae are detached from the anterior body, the fusion is between the transverse processes lateral to the facets. Wiltse et al. (135) describe a paraspinal sacrospinalis muscle-splitting approach to the lower vertebrae of the lumbar spine. The advantages that the report cited were a more direct approach to the area involved and less bleeding than with other approaches. There appears to be much less discomfort postoperatively with this approach than with a midline approach.

Minor degrees of slip (<25%) usually do not have a pathologic slip angle; therefore, surgeons prefer to treat such patients with fusion *in situ*, unless there is demonstrable instability on flexion–extension lateral radiographs. However, with a more marked deformity in higher grade spondylolisthesis, especially in the presence of increased lumbosacral kyphosis and extreme spondyloptosis, some degree of reduction is necessary in order to realign the lumbar spine over the sacrum in a position that will permit a solid fusion with acceptable sagittal alignment. Studies on *in situ* fusions for higher grade slips have reported pseudarthrosis rates from 0% to 60% and slip progression rates of as much as 25%, gait disturbances, and persistent cosmetic deformity. These data have led many to advocate reduction of high-grade slips, not only to address these issues but also to save motion segments (8, 95, 117, 125, 133, 136–144). Although there is some concern regarding the neurologic risk at the time of reduction, *in situ* fusions for high-grade slips have also been associated with adverse neurologic outcomes (94). Schoenecker et al. reported on 12 patients who developed cauda equina syndrome after *in situ* arthrodesis for high-grade spondylolisthesis. Seven of the twelve patients had permanent neurologic injuries, which were attributed to the prone positioning during surgery and the postural reduction of the deformity during surgery (145).

In order to minimize complications associated with reduction procedures, a sound surgical technique and adherence to simple mechanical principles are important, including wide laminectomy and complete bilateral nerve root decompression. Often nerve root decompression must be performed beyond the vertebral column. This is because of soft-tissue constriction of the nerve roots within the paraspinal muscles and iliolumbar ligaments, which may result in neuropraxia caused by nerve root stretch during reduction of high-grade slips. Complete discectomy is necessary in order to release the olisthetic segment. Further release and mobilization of the olisthetic segment can be achieved by sacral dome osteotomy, which facilitates reduction without necessitating excessive vertebral distraction. Although excessive distraction may be dangerous, judicious distraction is a useful maneuver to help achieve reduction by lifting the L5 body out and away from the pelvis. Various techniques for achieving distraction have been reported since its initial description by Jenkins in 1936 (146). External traction, that is, halo-femoral (64, 127, 147), passive positional reduction (142), temporary casting (143), temporary intraoperative hook and rod constructs, and distraction using pedicle screw instrumentation as a staged part of the surgical procedure can all be useful (133, 141, 145, 148–151). If distraction is used across segments that are not to be included in the final levels to be instrumented and fused, careful attention must be given to the intervening soft tissue to make sure that the uninstrumented facet joints are not injured. Overdistraction may result in iatrogenic instability of those uninstrumented levels. If excessive distraction is placed across the final instrumentation, the pedicle screws may loosen, resulting in the loss of fixation postoperatively.

Posterior translation using reduction pedicle screws is a newly available technique. This instrumentation, used in conjunction with appropriate distraction, can constitute a powerful reduction method. However, it must be stressed that without first achieving appropriate soft-tissue release through a combination of sacral dome osteotomy, discectomy, and distraction to provide room to allow posterior translation of the olisthetic segment, any attempt at translation with reduction pedicle screws is likely to result only in the fracture of the pedicles and dislodgement of the pedicle screws. The possible complications associated with the reduction procedure, both intraoperatively and postoperatively (152, 153), raise questions about whether reduction is necessary or even desirable. Petraco et al. (154) have suggested that complete reduction causes excessive stretch of the L5 nerve root and should therefore not be performed. However, this study did not consider the effect that an adequate discectomy and sacral dome osteotomy have on shortening the spine, thereby making full reduction safer. Proponents for full but judicious and safe reduction point to the improved weight bearing, decreased shear stress, and the improved bed for fusion provided by a full reduction (133, 155–157). The improved biomechanical stability provided by full reduction with anterior column support may allow us to perform a shorter instrumentation and fusion because of the inherent stability found in the fully reduced construct. Once acceptable alignment is obtained after reduction, posterior instrumentation and anterior reconstruction with an intradisc graft or cage are typically necessary for maintaining the rigidity of the new lumbosacral alignment (127, 150, 155–158). As one would

expect with these complex spinal realignment or reduction techniques, there is a risk of iatrogenic radiculopathy, and this must be borne in mind during the decision-making process (90, 153, 157, 158). Perhaps a good compromise is a partial reduction of the translation and kyphotic angle component of the slip to an acceptable level, which usually entails less neurologic risk. As long as the L5-S1 disk space has been repositioned adequately to allow placement of an intradiscal support device, such as an allograft wedge or a cage, the new lumbosacral alignment should be biomechanically stable for fusion.

At present, the role of anterior fusion in the treatment of spondylolisthesis is reserved for cases in which it is necessary to reestablish segmental lordosis, to increase the size of the available fusion bed, or to increase the stability of the posterior instrumentation. Multiple studies on anterior fusion alone have reported overall good results when compared to posterior and circumferential fusions (159–162). Issues such as increased pseudarthrosis rate, and lesser correction of slip angle, slip grade, sacral inclination, and sacral rotation raise questions about the use of anterior fusion as a stand-alone procedure (159–162). Some authors have advocated combining anterior structural grafts with posterior pedicle screw constructs and posterolateral fusion; this approach would theoretically improve fusion rates while reducing and maintaining the spondylolisthesis in a more anatomic position (134, 157, 159, 163–166). La Rosa reported on 35 patients who underwent an instrumented posterolateral fusion, out of whom 17 had an additional PLIF. At 2-year follow-up, the PLIF group had better correction of subluxation, disc height, and maintenance of foraminal area; however, the clinical outcomes for patients in the two groups were statistically equivalent (167).

Bohlman and his associates have reported a single-stage technique for interbody fusion and posterior decompression for high-grade spondylolisthesis. Along with posterior decompression and fusion, this procedure additionally stabilizes the spondylolisthesis *in situ* by placing a fibular strut graft through the body of S1 and into the displaced body of L5 through a posterior approach (168, 169). This technique has been shown to be effective in primary and revision surgeries, and is associated with a low incidence of transient neurologic deficits (132, 157, 170). Hanson et al. reported on 17 patients who underwent combined partial slip reduction with dowel fibular strut grafts for high-grade dysplastic isthmic spondylolisthesis. Solid fusion was achieved in 16 of the 17 patients, and there were no cases of neurologic deficits (77) (Figs. 20-14 to 20-19).

PLIF and TLIF are attractive as surgical techniques for the treatment of high-grade spondylolisthesis. The wide exposure of the spinal canal at the time of decompression provides ideal access for performing a bilateral PLIF or unilateral TLIF, thereby permitting a biomechanically sound fusion of all three columns of the spine (157). The intervertebral structural grafts increase the surface area available for fusion, and permit compressive load sharing through normal spinal biomechanics while opening up the narrowed neuroforamen. Several series have reported excellent results on combining

One-Stage Decompression and Posterolateral and Anterior Interbody Fusion (Figs. 20-14 to 20-19)

FIGURE 20-14. **One-stage decompression and posterolateral and anterior interbody fusion.** The patient is placed prone on a standard operating room spinal table (e.g., spinal frame on a standard operating room table or on a special spinal table such as the Jackson table). Care should be exercised in turning the patient to the prone position because in unstable high-grade slips, particularly in type I spondylolisthesis, the cauda equina is at risk for injury (23). One limb should be prepared in a sterile fashion for later fibular bone graft harvest. A standard midline approach from L3 to S2 or S3 is made. The spine is carefully exposed subperiosteally from the tip of the transverse process of the fourth lumbar vertebra to the ala of the sacrum and down to S2 or S3. Care must be taken when dissecting the loose posterior element to avoid cauda equina injury.

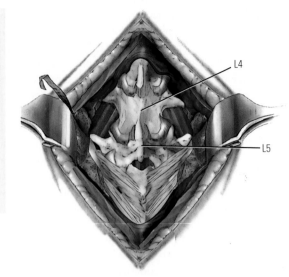

FIGURE 20-15. The loose posterior element of L5 is completely removed, taking great care not to injure underlying tissues. This is particularly important in patients who have had previous surgery. An additional laminectomy of the fourth lumbar to the first sacral segments is also performed. Extension of the laminectomy distally to S2 may later be necessary to allow for dural sac and sacral nerve root retraction later in the procedure. The fifth lumbar nerve roots are decompressed by foraminotomy, with excision of the inferior pedicle, disk, or both, as required. Occasionally, the pedicle can be drilled and hollowed out and the walls collapsed inward to allow for the L5 nerve root to be untethered. The L5 nerve roots are often scarred or compressed by the sacral dome. In these high-grade kyphotic deformities, the roots are coursing almost directly anteriorly. At this juncture, the exposed area should include the dural sac and all nerve roots from L4 to S2.

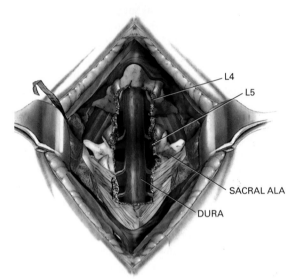

FIGURE 20-16. When preoperative MRI demonstrates a high-grade block because of posterior sacral obstruction, an osteotomy of the sacral prominence is accomplished to decompress the sacral dural sac. It may occasionally be necessary to remove a portion of the S2 or the S3 lamina to allow for adequate dural and nerve root retraction. This is also needed for safe placement of the cannulated drill for the interbody graft placement. The osteotomy of the sacral prominence is done with an osteotome, first from one side and then from the other, working underneath the dura. Care must be taken when retracting the dural sac and nerve roots. Any dural lacerations should be repaired with fine 6-0 suture at the time incurred, and/or with fascial grafting as necessary. Bone wax can be used to control sacral medullary bleeding after the osteotomy. When adequate bone has been removed, the dural sac will fall forward and therefore accomplish sacral root decompression.

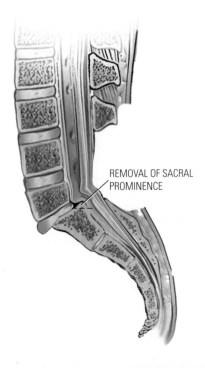

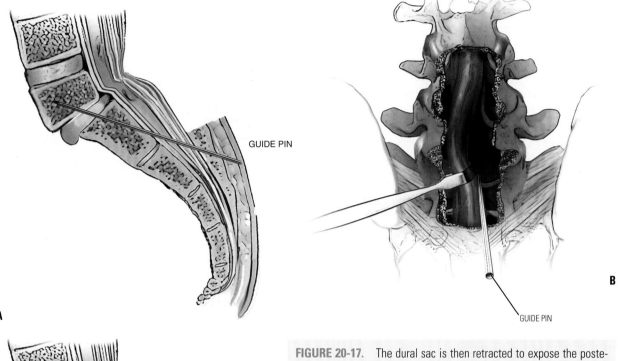

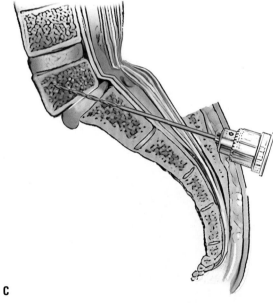

GUIDE PIN

A

B

GUIDE PIN

C

FIGURE 20-17. The dural sac is then retracted to expose the posterior aspect of S1. A 0.32-cm guide pin is inserted in the midline of the sacrum directed cranially into the dislocated and displaced body of the fifth lumbar vertebra. Fluoroscopic control is mandatory. A 1/2-inch or 10-mm cannulated drill is introduced over the guide pin, taking great care not to perforate the anterior cortex of the fifth lumbar vertebral body. The drilling can be done with a hand drill or a power drill as preferred by the surgeon. Cortical perforation of L5 could lead to serious complications, with vessel or organ injury.

FIGURE 20-18. A middiaphyseal fibular graft is harvested and is trimmed to fit (length; diameter is usually compatible with the 10-mm drill) into the drill hole when inserted. It is important to make certain that the fibular graft does not protrude into the spinal canal after insertion. The fibular graft is impacted up to the cortical edge of the cephalad surface of the L5 vertebral body. After this process is completed, a posterolateral fusion of L4 to S1 is completed in the standard fashion, with large amounts of allograft bone harvested from the iliac crest. The wound is closed over a suction drain. Prophylactic antibiotics are used preoperatively and perioperatively.

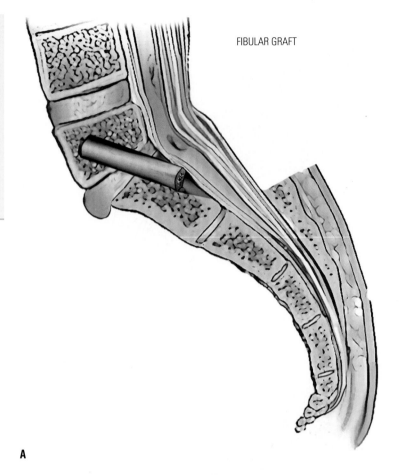

FIBULAR GRAFT

A

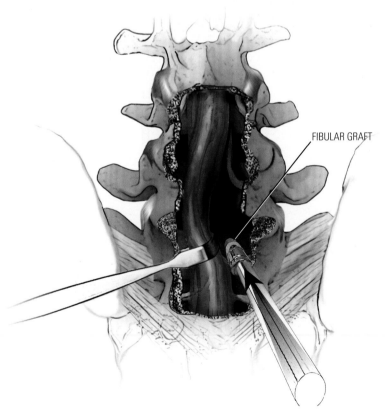

FIBULAR GRAFT

B

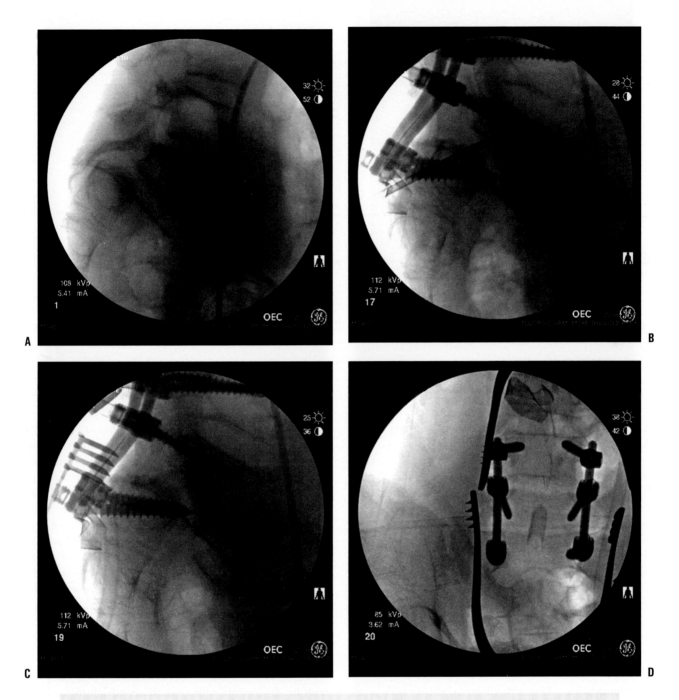

FIGURE 20-19. This is a 13-year-old male with a high-grade spondylolisthesis (dysplastic type) who had severe discomfort, an abnormal gait, and neurologic deficit. He had an L5 radiculopathy; weakness of the left EHL and could only lift his left leg 2 inches off of the exam table (right leg 5 inches); he had a short stride length gait; bowel and bladder control was normal. **A:** Cross table lateral radiograph with hips in extension on Jackson operating room table. **B:** and L4 to S2 decompression, L5 nerve root on left severely compressed. Pedicle screws placed L4,5 and S1. A 10-mm cannulated drill used to make channel from S1 to L5; suction tip in channel on x-ray. **C:** Intraoperative x-ray showing fibular dowel graft in place. **D:** Intraoperative AP x-ray showing fibular dowel graft in place. **E:** Lateral radiograph 6 months after surgery, demonstrating good graft in corporation. **F:** Ferguson AP view 6 months postsurgery. The patients EHL was now 5/5; radiculopathy had resolved and straight leg raising had improved to 60 degrees. (Case courtesy of Stuart L. Weinstein, MD.)

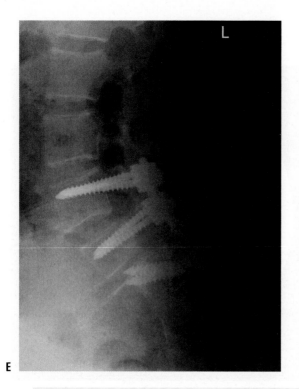

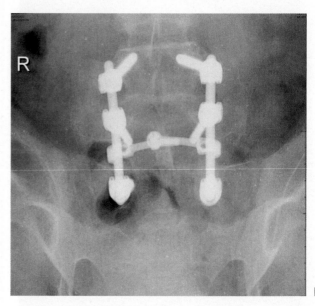

FIGURE 20-19. *(Continued)*

PLIF with an instrumented posterior reduction and fusion (134, 157, 167).

The kind of postoperative immobilization recommended after fusion varies from no immobilization at all (11, 171) or a brace to a single or bilateral spica cast (10, 95), with the patient ambulatory or in bed rest. The decision to use immobilization will depend upon several factors such as the patient's body habitus, likelihood of compliance, preoperative slip grade and angle, whether the surgery was primary or a revision, and the adequacy of reduction and instrumentation purchase. If a TLSO is used, the thigh must be included into the brace without a hinge joint, in order to adequately control the pelvis. Brace use is continued for 3 to 4 months postoperatively until solid fusion is noted radiographically.

Author's Preferred Recommendations

Grade I Spondylolysis. Direct pars interarticularis repair is an option in patients with spondylolysis or minimal spondylolisthesis, with L5 in a lordotic position, and no degenerative changes at the olisthetic level. A "hot" SPECT scan at the pars interarticularis implies a biologically active defect, making osteosynthesis a viable option. A "cold" SPECT scan is a relative contraindication to a direct pars interarticularis repair, because the lack of biologic activity indicates little inherent ability to create a bony union. In addition, the absence of neurologic findings is essential, because the technique of direct pars interarticularis repair is not amenable to a nerve root decompression.

For low-grade slips in patients requiring fusions, pedicle screw and rod constructs provide ample support, particularly when anterior interbody support is used. In the case of a mild or moderately degenerated disc without significant collapse, a posterolateral instrumented fusion alone may not be sufficient, even if a wide decompression is not necessary and a large posterolateral surface area exists for fusion. We prefer to always stabilize even grade I slips so as to enhance our fusion rates. Posterior instrumented fusions without anterior spinal fusion may be sufficient in patients with significant disk-space collapse at the olisthetic level. The inherent stability provided by the collapsed disc will decrease the stress on the construct and the interface between the screws and the vertebrae. However, in patients with a large or hypermobile disc, anterior column support may be necessary for an effective reconstruction.

Grade II. In patients with grade II spondylolisthesis, instrumentation and fusion along with decompression will likely be required. Anterior column support in the form of intradiscal cages or allograft wedges should be provided in order to ensure long-term stability of the construct and to allow for maximum correction of segmental sagittal alignment. The anterior column support can be achieved by either an anterior lumbar interbody fusion (ALIF) or a PLIF/TLIF technique. Another attractive option is to perform a transperitoneal approach, which permits quick and easy access to the disk space, allowing complete disc removal and placement of a large footprint interbody spacer while reestablishing lordosis. Reestablishing or maintaining segmental alignment of the olisthetic level will theoretically protect adjacent levels.

Grade III/IV. For slips of grade III or greater, the surgical technique can be extremely demanding. Because each high-grade slip presents with a unique combination of pathologic anatomy, biomechanics, and clinical symptoms, all surgical techniques should be considered and may be useful during any reduction and subsequent stabilization of the vertebral column (157, 164, 168). Slip angle reduction, anterior interbody support, and reconstruction of the anterior column are important components of the reconstruction for high-grade slips. With appropriate release, a complete discectomy, and possible sacral dome osteotomy, anterior column reconstruction may provide enough segmental stability to allow monosegmental fixation with a high degree of success. This has been advocated by Harms et al. (152) for many years. Wide nerve root decompression is an essential component in minimizing the development of iatrogenic nerve root injury at the time of reduction of the slip.

In patients with slips greater than or equal to grade III, in whom significant effort is required in order to achieve reduction of the olisthetic segment, fixation distal to S1 (i.e., iliac screws) should be provided for stability of the reconstruction. For these higher grade slips, a posterior approach for achieving an anterior column reconstruction (i.e., PLIF/TLIF technique) is more practical than an ALIF procedure, for several reasons. Because of the forward flexion of the rostral vertebra, access into the disk space anteriorly may be difficult or impossible. Because these higher grade slips often have significant posterior element dysplasia and neuroforaminal narrowing, the nerve roots should be identified and decompressed before vertebral reduction maneuvers are attempted. Failure to achieve an adequate decompression before reduction may result in severe irreversible nerve root injury. Usually by the time the wide laminectomy and the foraminal decompression are carried out for bilateral nerve root decompression, the posterior aspect of the disc is clearly exposed. This facilitates the PLIF/TLIF technique. Sacral dome osteotomy, which is another useful technique for achieving release of the deformity and facilitating reduction of high-grade slips, can be performed through the posterior approach. The posterior approach is also an advantage because of the expansive posterior decompression that is accomplished with the Gill laminectomy.

Grade V. In patients with grade V slips (i.e., spondyloptosis) options include L4-sacrum fusion *in situ*, augmented with fibular dowel grafts; posterior reduction as previously discussed; or an L5 spondylectomy. The posterior approach with sacral dome osteotomy can be used effectively in many of these cases (Fig. 20-11) However, we occasionally prefer to treat this pathology with a Gaines' procedure, which is a complete L5 vertebrectomy (172, 173). The first stage of this procedure is an anterior L5 corpectomy, followed by a posterior approach to resect the posterior elements. This technique is followed by the reduction of L4 to the sacrum and stabilization with pedicle screw instrumentation. Fusion is performed anteriorly

and posteriorly. The L5 nerve roots are in extreme jeopardy during anterior vertebral resection because they are usually trapped and tethered under the pedicles of L5, the posterior aspect of the vertebral body of L5, and the anterior cortex of the sacrum.

PEARLS AND PITFALLS

Spondylolysis Repairs. The midline approach permits direct access to both spondylolytic repair sites. Preparation of the bony bed of the lytic defect with the use of kerrison rongeurs and a high-speed burr permits removal of interposed fibrous tissue and removal of the avascular bone down to bleeding cancellous bone. If the defect is small, compression can be achieved across the defect with the construct of choice. However, occasionally the defect is large and compression across this may not achieve bony apposition without significantly altering the inferior facet joint. In this circumstance, the use of small Harms-style titanium mesh cages, compressed into an oval shape and filled with cancellous autograft, permits compression across the defect without significantly altering the position of the inferior articular facet of the lytic segment. The use of adjunctive biologics may improve the bony healing rate. Traditional constructs (i.e., wire constructs) in spondylolysis repairs have not utilized rigid fixation. The use of pedicle screws has permitted more rigid fixation of the repair site with the use of an infralaminar hook. Significant compression can be evenly obtained across both repair sites.

Spondylolisthesis. The operative treatment of spondylisthesis typically centers on grade III and IV deformities and involves some correction of the slip %-age and the slip angle. Greater amounts of reduction (angular and translation) of the spondylolisthesis place increasing tension on the L5 and S1 nerve roots and increase the risk of iatrogenic neurologic deficit. The use of direct nerve root stimulation can be helpful in monitoring nerve root function during nerve root decompression and deformity correction. This monitoring modality can be especially helpful in the presence of preoperative nerve root dysfunction. No absolute numerical value is indicative of nerve root dysfunction; however, increases of 2 or 3 mA can be concerning. To minimize the chance of iatrogenic neurologic deficit, wide decompression of the L5 and S1 nerve roots is recommended after performance of a Gill laminectomy.

Correction of the slip percentage is important to increase the surface area available for fusion, but correction of the slip angle is the most important biomechanically. This reestablishes more normal sagittal alignment of the sacropelvic unit and lumbar spine. The use of interbody devices increases the height of the pathologically shortened anterior column and permits more normal load sharing across the operative site. Placement of interbody devices has been typically performed from anterior approach; however, after the Gill laminectomy and nerve root decompressions, the disk space is easily accessible via a transforaminal (TLIF) or posterior (PLIF) approach. Many interbody devices are available and are surgeon-choice as none have proven superiority in spondylolisthesis correction and fusions. The other benefit of TLIF/PLIF is the creation of an anterior fusion. The surface area available for an isolated posterior fusion can be very small due to removal of the loose posterior elements (i.e., Gill procedure) and usually atrophic transverse processes.

Accessing the disk space can be accomplished via a unilateral or bilateral approach. The discectomy and end-plate preparation is easier, safer, and more complete when using bilateral approaches through the axilla of the nerve roots. Distraction across the disk space is possible by commercially available disk space distractors and when placed on one side permits better visualization of the disk space from the opposite side. Sacral dome osteotomy is performed when the superior end plate is domed, which permits evacuation of disc material anteriorly and better seating of interbody devices.

Current state-of-the-art spine fixation for spondylolisthesis are pedicle screws. Multiaxial pedicle screws can be used at each level; reduction screws placed at the slip level and any cephalad levels permit gradual dorsal reduction of the slip. Placement of pedicle screws is routine, except for the pedicle of the slip level (typically L5), which have a tendency to be more medially inclined than normal. For the routine L5-S1 grade I and II slips, fusion usually is only necessary from L5-S1. Higher grades of slip (III and IV) inclusion of L4 permits load-sharing fixation at four pedicle screws and additionally increases the fusion bed to include the L4 posterior elements and transverse processes.

Caudal fixation consists of bilateral S1 pedicle screws and another method of sacropelvic fixation to back up the S1 fixation. The strongest biomechanical construct uses bilateral iliac wing screws, which is the preferred technique for grade III and greater slips. For milder grade slips (i.e., grade I and II), the use of bilateral S2 alar screws is an option; however, it is recommended to place anterior body support placed via a TLIF or PLIF technique. Debate continues as to the necessity of including L4 into the construct, and some authors use L4 fixation but do not fuse from L4 to L5 and return at a later date to remove the L4 pedicle screws after bony union is assured.

- Asymptomatic grades I and II: If the child is <10 years old, follow up with radiographs every 6 months through 15 years, then annually until end of growth. No limitations on activity are necessary in grade I. Patients with grade II slips should avoid contact sports and activities requiring repetitive lumbar hyperextension.
- Symptomatic grades I and II: Nonoperative therapies should be tried. Contact sports and those calling for hyperextension should be avoided. Fusion is indicated for patients who are unresponsive to all nonoperative interventions.
- Grades III/IV: Surgical intervention is indicated regardless of symptoms.

COMPLICATIONS

The reported pseudarthrosis rate after fusion varies from 0% to 39% (5, 58, 95, 112, 113, 125, 164), with most of the sources reporting <15%. Higher pseudarthrosis rates have been associated with higher grade spondylolisthesis and fusion *in situ* of these deformities (5, 165).

The magnitude of the slip, as measured by the amount of displacement or kyphosis, can increase even in the presence of a solid fusion (4, 5, 17, 60, 132, 174, 175). However, it should be noted that the fusions reported on were uninstrumented and were assessed with plain radiographs. CT scans may have been able to demonstrate that some of the instances of increased slippage were actually caused by the lack of adequate fusion. Further slippage following an uninstrumented surgery is more common because the removal of midline-stabilizing structures at the time of decompression increases lumbosacral instability. This is also more common in higher grades of spondylolisthesis, in patients with a greater degree of anterior displacement, and in slip kyphosis.

Radiculopathy is the most common complication after reduction of spondylolisthesis; it is usually an L5 nerve root lesion and has varying recovery rates (90, 153, 157, 158). One series on partial slip reduction with the use of a dowel fibular strut graft for high-grade slips reported no permanent neurologic complications (77). In contrast, acute postoperative cauda equina syndrome has been reported after a simple posterolateral fusion without decompression or reduction (138, 145). This complication can occur through a midline or lateral muscle-splitting incision when the patient is prone or laterally positioned (112, 145). The cause of this significant complication is not definitely known. However, in high-grade slips, the MRI scan can demonstrate a cleaved intervertebral disk at the spondylolisthetic segment, with the posterior half indenting the dural sac. The development of cauda equina syndrome is likely secondary to acute neural compression caused by this posterior disc fragment in a patient with a marked slip, which partially reduces at the time of surgery, causing further compression of the already at-risk neural elements. Patients with high-grade slips and the congenital types of deformities are at an increased risk for neural compression at the time of surgery. MRI can be helpful in these situations by permitting visualization of the intervertebral disk pathology and neural compression, since such neurologic deficits can occur in the absence of any preoperative neurologic signs or symptoms (94, 145).

Prevention of postoperative neurologic deficits is optimal, because permanent neurologic deficits can occur postoperatively, even after immediate decompression of iatrogenic neurologic deficits. Patients with spondylolisthesis who experience postoperative neurologic deficits should undergo MRI or CT myelogram imaging of the neural elements in order to elucidate the causes of the deficits. Any preoperative nerve root compression, irrespective of the grade of the spondylolisthesis, should be decompressed. Adequate decompression typically destabilizes the spine, however, increasing the risk of slip progression, neurologic deficit, and pseudarthrosis and making posterior stabilization with pedicle screw constructs an ideal option. Intraoperative neuromonitoring can be useful at the time of decompression and, if necessary, reduction, so as to minimize iatrogenic neurologic deficits. However, somatosensory and elecromyographic monitoring may not predict L5 nerve root deficits, and therefore intraoperative wake-up test(s) are strongly recommended. Direct L5 and S1 nerve stimulation is another technique for monitoring nerve integrity more closely during various stages of the surgery. Careful neurologic follow-up postoperatively is essential in all cases.

REFERENCES

1. Herbiniaux G. *Traite sur divers accouchemens labprieux, et sur polypes de la matrice*. Bruxelles, Belgium: JL DeBoubers, 1782.

2. Kilian HF. *Schilderungen neuer beckenformen and ihres verhaltens im leben*. Mannheim, Germany: Verlag von Bassermann & Mathy, 1854.

3. Newman PH. Surgical treatment for spondylolisthesis in the adult. *Clin Orthop Relat Res* 1976;117:106–111.

4. Wiltse LL, Jackson DW. Treatment of spondylolisthesis and spondylolysis in children. *Clin Orthop Relat Res* 1976;117:92–100.

5. Boxall D, Bradford DS, Winter RB, et al. Management of severe spondylolisthesis in children and adolescents. *J Bone Joint Surg Am* 1979;61:479–495.

6. Borkow SE, Kleiger B. Spondylolisthesis in the newborn. A case report. *Clin Orthop Relat Res* 1971;81:73–76.

7. Fredrickson BE, Baker D, McHolick WJ, et al. The natural history of spondylolysis and spondylolisthesis. *J Bone Joint Surg Am* 1984;66:699–707.

8. Newnan PH. The etiology of spondylolisthesis. *J Bone Joint Surg Br* 1963;45:39.

9. Taillard WF. Etiology of spondylolisthesis. *Clin Orthop Relat Res* 1976;117:30–39.

10. Turner RH, Bianco AJ Jr. Spondylolysis and spondylolisthesis in children and teen-agers. *J Bone Joint Surg Am* 1971;53:1298–1306.

11. Wiltse LL. Spondylolisthesis in children. *Clin Orthop Relat Res* 1961;21:156.

12. Beguiristain JL, Diaz-de-Rada P. Spondylolisthesis in pre-school children. *J Pediatr Orthop B* 2004;13:225–230.

13. Wiltse LL. *Spondylolisthesis, classification and etiology: symposium on the spine*. American Academy of Orthopedic Surgeons. St. Louis, MO: CV Mosby, 1969:143–147.

14. Virta L, Ronnemaa T, Osterman K, et al. Prevalence of isthmic lumbar spondylolisthesis in middle-aged subjects from eastern and western Finland. *J Clin Epidemiol* 1992;45:917–922.

15. Stewart T. The age incidence of neural arch defects in Alaskan natives, considered from the standpoint of etiology. *J Bone Joint Surg Am* 1953;35:937.

16. Osterman K, Schlenzka D, Poussa M, et al. Isthmic spondylolisthesis in symptomatic and asymptomatic subjects, epidemiology, and natural history with special reference to disk abnormality and mode of treatment. *Clin Orthop Relat Res* 1993;297:65–70.

17. Henson J, McCall IW, Brien JPO. Disc damage above a spondylolisthesis. *Br J Radiol* 1987;60(709):69–72.

18. Roche M, Rowe C. The incidence of separate neural arch and coincident bone variations. *J Bone Joint Surg Am* 1952;34:491.

19. Rowe G, Roache M. Etiology of the separate neural arch. *J Bone Joint Surg Am* 1953;35:102.

20. Eisenstein S. Spondylolysis. A skeletal investigation of two population groups. *J Bone Joint Surg Br* 1978;60-B:488–494.

21. Jackson DW, Wiltse LL, Cirincoine RJ. Spondylolysis in the female gymnast. *Clin Orthop Relat Res* 1976;117:68–73.

22. Vaz G, Roussouly P, Berthonnaud E, et al. Sagittal morphology and balance of the spine and pelvis. *Eur Spine J* 2002;1:80–88.

23. Legaye J, Duval-Beaupere C, Hecquet J, et al. Pelvic incidence: a fundamental pelvic parameter for three-dimensional regulation of spinal sagittal curves. *Eur Spine J* 1998;7:99–103.

24. Labelle HH, Roussouly P, Berthonnaud E, et al. Spondylolisthesis, pelvic incidence, and spinopelvic balance: a correlation study. *Spine* 2004;29:2049–2054.

25. Ogilvie JW, Sherman J. Spondylolysis in Scheuermann's disease. *Spine* 1987;12:251–253.

26. Rosenberg NJ, Bargar WL, Friedman B. The incidence of spondylolysis and spondylolisthesis in nonambulatory patients. *Spine* 1981;6:35–38.

27. Newman PH, Stone KH. The etiology of spondylolisthesis: with a special investigation. *J Bone Joint Surg Br* 1963;45:39–59.

28. Troup JD. Mechanical factors in spondylolisthesis and spondylolysis. *Clin Orthop Relat Res* 1976;117:59–67.

29. Wiltse LL, Widell EH Jr, Jackson DW. Fatigue fracture: the basic lesion in isthmic spondylolisthesis. *J Bone Joint Surg Am* 1975;57:17–22.

30. Dietrich M, Kurowski P. The importance of mechanical factors in the etiology of spondylolysis: a model analysis of loads and stresses in human lumbar spine. *Spine* 1985;10:532–542.

31. Wiltse LL. Etiology of spondylolisthesis. *Clin Orthop Relat Res* 1957;10:4860.

32. Wiltse LL. The etiology of spondylolisthesis. *J Bone Joint Surg Am* 1962;44:539–560.

33. Chandler FA. Lesions of the isthmus (pars interarticularis) of the laminae of the lower lumbar vertebrae and their relation to spondylolisthesis. *Surg Gynecol Obstet* 1931;53:273–306.

34. Farfan HF, Osteria V, Lamy C. The mechanical etiology of spondylolysis and spondylolisthesis. *Clin Orthop Relat Res* 1976;117:40–55.

35. Lafferty JF, Winter WG, Gambaro SA. Fatigue characteristics of posterior elements of vertebrae. *J Bone Joint Surg Am* 1977;59:154–158.

36. Hutton WC, Stott JRR, Cyron BM. Is spondylolysis a fatigue fracture? *Spine* 1977;2:202–209.

37. Neill DBO, Micheli LJ. Postoperative radiographic evidence for fatigue fracture as the etiology in spondylolysis. *Spine* 1989;14:1342–1355.

38. Pennell RG, Maurer AH, Bonakdarpour A. Stress injuries of the pars interarticularis: radiologic classification and indications for scintigraphy. *AJR Am J Roentgenol* 1985;145:763–766.

39. Wiltse LL, Widell E Jr, Jackson DW. Fatigue fracture: the basic lesion is isthmic spondylolisthesis. *J Bone Joint Surg Am* 1975;57:17–22.

40. Cyron BM, Hutton WC. Variations in the amount and distribution of cortical bone across the partes interarticularis of L5: a predisposing factor in spondylolysis? *Spine* 1979;4:163–167.

41. Krenz J, Troup JD. The structure of the pars interarticularis of the lower lumbar vertebrae and its relation to the etiology of spondylolysis: with a report of a healing fracture in the neural arch of a fourth lumbar vertebra. *J Bone Joint Surg Br* 1973;55:735–741.

42. Sairyo K, Katoh S Sakamaki T, et al. Vertebral forward slippage in immature lumbar spine occurs following epiphyseal separation and its occurrence is unrelated to disc degeneration: is the pediatric spondylolisthesis a physis stress fracture of vertebral body? *Spine* 2004;29:524–527.

43. Hutton WC, Cyron BM. Spondylolysis: the role of the posterior elements in resisting the intervertebral compressive force. *Acta Orthop Scand* 1978;49:604–609.

44. Kajiura K, Katoh S, Sairyo K, et al. Slippage mechanism of pediatric spondylolysis: biomechanical study using immature calf spines. *Spine* 2001;26:2208–2212.

45. Loder RT. Profiles of the cervical, thoracic, and lumbosacral spine in children and adolescents with lumbosacral spondylolisthesis. *J Spinal Disord* 2001;14:465–471.

46. Miki T, Tamura T, Senzoku F, et al. Congenital laminar defect of the upper lumbar spine associated with pars interarticularis defect: a report of eleven cases. *Spine* 1991;16:353–355.

47. Albanese M, Pizzutillo PD. Family study of spondylolysis and spondylolisthesis. *J Pediatr Orthop* 1982;2:496–499.

48. Friberg S. Studies on spondylolisthesis. *Acta Chir Scand* 1939;82 (Suppl 55):56.

49. Laurent L, Einola S. Spondylolisthesis in children and adolescents. *Acta Orthop Scand* 1961;31:45.

50. Wynne-Davies R, Scott JH. Inheritance and spondylolisthesis: a radiographic family survey. *J Bone Joint Surg Br* 1979;61-B:301–305.

51. Floman Y, Margulies JY, Nyska M, et al. Effect of major axial skeleton trauma on preexisting lumbosacral spondylolisthesis. *J Spinal Disord* 1991;4:353–358.

52. Iwamoto J, Abe H, Tsukimura Y, et al. Relationships between radiographic abnormalities of the lumbar spine and incidence of low back pain in high school and college football players: a prospective study. *Am J Sports Med* 2004;32:781–786.

53. Stewart TD. The age incidence of neural-arch defects in Alaskan natives, considered from the standpoint of etiology. *J Bone Joint Surg Am* 1953;35:937–950.

54. Libson E, Bloom RA, Dinari G. Symptomatic and asymptomatic spondylolysis and spondylolisthesis in young adults. *Int Orthop* 1982;6:259–261.

55. Wiltse LL, Rothman SLG. Spondylolisthesis: classification, diagnosis, and natural history. *Semin Spine Surg* 1993;5:264–280.

56. Saraste H. Long-term clinical and radiological follow-up of spondylolysis and spondylolisthesis. *J Pediatr Orthop* 1987;7:631–638.

57. Virta L, Ronnemaa T. The association of mild-moderate isthmic lumbar spondylolisthesis and low back pain in middle-aged patients is weak and it only occurs in women. *Spine* 1993;18:1496–1503.

58. Sherman FC, Rosenthal RK, Hall JE. Spine fusion for spondylolysis and spondylolisthesis in children. *Spine* 1979;4:59–66.

59. Amundson G, Edwards C, Garfin S. Spondylolisthesis. In: Rothman R, Simeone EF, eds. *The spine*, 3rd ed. Philadelphia, PA: WB Saunders, 1992:913.

60. Hensinger RN. Spondylolysis and spondylolisthesis in children and adolescents (review). *J Bone Joint Surg Am* 1989;71:1098–1107.

61. Phalen G, Dickson J. Spondylolisthesis and tight hamstrings. *J Bone Joint Surg Am* 1961;43:505–512.

62. Barash H, Galante JO, Lambert CN, et al. Spondylolisthesis and tight hamstrings. *J Bone Joint Surg Am* 1970;52:1319–1328.

63. Harris R. Spondylolisthesis. *Ann R Coll Surg Engl* 1951;8:259–297.

64. Saraste H, Brostrom LA, Aparisi T. Prognostic radiographic aspects of spondylolisthesis. *Acta Radiol Diagn (Stockh)* 1984;25:427–432.

65. Lowe RW, Hayes TD, Kaye J, et al. Standing roentgenograms in spondylolisthesis. *Clin Orthop Relat Res* 1976;117:80–84.

66. Burkus JK. Unilateral spondylolysis associated with spina bifida occulta and nerve root compression. *Spine* 1990;15:555–559.

67. Libson E, Bloom RA, Dinari G, et al. Oblique lumbar spine radiographs: importance in young patients. *Radiology* 1984;151:89–90.

68. Antoniades SB, Hammerberg KW, DeWald RL. Sagittal plane configuration of the sacrum in spondylolisthesis. *Spine* 2000;25:1085–1091.

69. Suh PB, Esses SI, Kostuik JP. Repair of pars interarticularis defect: the prognostic value of pars interarticularis infiltration. *Spine* 1991;16 (Suppl 8):S445–S448.

70. Wiltse LL, Newman PH, Macnab I. Classification of spondylolysis and spondylolisthesis. *Clin Orthop Relat Res* 1976;117:23–29.

71. Newman PH. A clinical syndrome associated with severe lumbo-sacral subluxation. *J Bone Joint Surg Br* 1965;47:472–481.

72. Wiltse LL, Winter RB. Terminology and measurement of spondylolisthesis. *J Bone Joint Surg Am* 1983;65:768–772.

73. Huang RP, Bohlman HH, Thompson GH, et al. Predictive value of pelvic incidence in progression of spondylolisthesis. *Spine* 2003;28:2381–2385.

74. Rajnics P, Templier A, Skalli W, et al. The association of sagittal spinal and pelvic parameters with isthmic spondylolisthesis. *J Spinal Disord* 2002;15:24–30.

75. Frennered AK, Danielson BI, Nachemson AL. Natural history of symptomatic isthmic low-grade spondylolisthesis in children and adolescents: a seven-year follow-up study. *J Pediatr Orthop* 1991;11:209–213.

76. Seitsalo S, Osterman K, Hyvarinen H, et al. Progression of spondylolisthesis in children and adolescents. A long-term follow-up of 272 patients. *Spine* 1991;16:417–421.

77. Hanson DS, Bridwell KH, Rhee JM, et al. Dowel fibular strut grafts for high-grade dysplastic isthmic spondylolisthesis. *Spine* 2002;27:1982–1988.

78. Szypryt EP, Twining P, Mulholland RC, et al. The prevalence of disc degeneration associated with neural arch defects of the lumbar spine assessed by magnetic resonance imaging. *Spine* 1989;14:977–981.

79. Meyerding HW. Spondylolisthesis. *Surg Gynecol Obstet* 1932;54:371–377.

80. Bellah RD, Summerville DA, Treves ST, et al. Low back pain in adolescent athletes: detection of stress injury to the pars interarticularis with SPECT. *Radiology* 1991;180:509–512.

81. Danielson B, Frennered K, Selvik G, et al. Roentgenologic assessment of spondylolisthesis: an evaluation of progression. *Acta Radiol* 1989;30:65–68.

82. Schlenzka D, Poussa M, Seitsalo S, et al. Intervertebral disc changes in adolescents with isthmic spondylolisthesis. *J Spinal Disord* 1991;4:344–352.

83. Beutler WJ, Fredrickson BE, Murtland A, et al. The natural history of spondylolysis and spondylolisthesis: 45-year follow-up evaluation. *Spine* 2003;28:1027–1035.

84. Dandy DJ, Shannon MJ. Lumbo-sacral subluxation. (Group I spondylolisthesis). *J Bone Joint Surg Br* 1971;53:578–595.

85. Harris IE, Weinstein SL. Long-term follow-up of patients with grade-III and IV spondylolisthesis: treatment with and without posterior fusion. *J Bone Joint Surg Am* 1987;69:960–969.

86. Baker D, Hollick WM. Spondylolysis and spondylolisthesis in children. *J Bone Joint Surg Am* 1956;38:933.

87. Wiltse LL, Rothman LG. Spondylolisthesis: classification, diagnosis, and natural history. *Semin Spine Surg* 1989;1:78.

88. Miller SF, Congeni J, Swanson K. Long-term functional and anatomical follow-up of early detected spondylolysis in young athletes. *Am J Sports Med* 2004;32:928–933

89. Blanda J, Bethem D, Moats W, et al. Defects of pars interarticularis in athletes: a protocol for nonoperative treatment. *J Spinal Disord* 1993;6:406–411.

90. Klein G, Mehlman CT, McCarty M. Nonoperative treatment of spondylolysis and grade I spondylolisthesis in children and young adults: a meta-analysis of observational studies. *J Pediatr Orthop* 2009;29:146–156.

91. Morita T, Ikata T, Katoh S, et al. Lumbar spondylolysis in children and adolescents. *J Bone Joint Surg Br* 1985;77:620–625.

92. Steiner ME, Micheli LJ. Treatment of symptomatic spondylolysis and spondylolisthesis with the modified Boston brace. *Spine* 1985;10:937–943.

93. Wiltse LL. Proceedings: lumbar spine: posterolateral fusion. *J Bone Joint Surg Br* 1975;57:261.

94. Maurice HD, Morley TR. Cauda equina lesions following fusion in situ and decompressive laminectomy for severe spondylolisthesis. Four case reports. *Spine* 1989;14:214–216.

95. Hensinger RN, Lang LE, MacEwen GD. Surgical management of the spondylolisthesis in children and adolescents. *Spine* 1976;1:207–216.

96. Pizutillo PD, Hummer CD. Nonoperative treatment of pain adolescent spondylosis and spondylolisthesis. *J Pediatr Orthop* 1989;9:538–540.

97. Hensinger RN. Spondylolysis and spondylolisthesis in children. *Instr Course Lect* 1983;32:132–151.

98. Bell DF, Ehrlich MG, Zaleske DJ. Brace treatment for symptomatic spondylolisthesis. *Clin Orthop Relat Res* 1988;236:192–198.

99. Dam BV. Nonoperative treatment and surgical repair of lumbar spondylolisthesis. In: Bridwell KH, Rl DeWald E, eds. *The textbook of spinal surgery*, 2nd ed. Philadelphia, PA: Lippincott–Raven Publishers, 1997:1263–1269.

100. Buck JE. Direct repair of the defect in spondylolisthesis. Preliminary report. *J Bone Joint Surg Br* 1970;52:432–437.

101. Buck JE. Abstract: further thoughts on direct repair of the defect in spondylolysis. *J Bone Joint Surg Br* 1979;61:123.

102. Gillet P, Petit M. Direct repair of spondylolysis without spondylolisthesis, using a rod-screw construct and bone grafting of the pars interarticularis defect. *Spine* 1999;24:1252–1256.

103. Kakiuchi M. Repair of the defect in spondylolysis. Durable fixation with pedicle screws and laminar hooks. *J Bone Joint Surg Am* 1997;79:818–825.

104. Morscher E, Gerber B, Fasel J. Surgical treatment of spondylolisthesis by bone grafting and direct stabilization of spondylolysis by means of a hook screw. *Arch Orthop Trauma Surg* 1984;103:175–178.

105. Songer MN, Rovin R. Repair of the pars interarticularis defect with a cable-screw construct. A preliminary report. *Spine* 1998;23: 263–269.

106. Pedersen AK, Hagen R. Spondylolysis and spondylolisthesis: treatment by internal fixation and bone-grafting of the defect. *J Bone Joint Surg Am* 1988;70:15–24.

107. Bradford DS. Treatment of severe spondylolisthesis: a combined approach for reduction and stabilization. *Spine* 1979;4:423–429.

108. Bradford DS, Iza J. Repair of the defect in spondylolysis or minimal degrees of spondylolisthesis by segmental wire fixation and bone grafting. *Spine* 1985;10:673–679.

109. Kimura M. My method of filling the lesion with spongy bone in spondylolysis and spondylolisthesis (Jap). *Orthop Surg* 1968;19:285–295.

110. Nicol RO, Scott JH. Lytic spondylolysis: repair by wiring. *Spine* 1986;11:1027–1030.

111. Tokuhashi Y, Matsuzaki H. Repair of defects in spondylolysis by segmental pedicle screw hook fixation: a preliminary report. *Spine* 1996;21: 2041–2045.

112. Newton PO, Johnston CE II. Analysis and treatment of poor outcomes following in situ arthrodesis in adolescent spondylolisthesis. *J Pediatr Orthop* 1997;17:754–761.

113. Burkus JK, Lonstein JE, Winter RB, et al. Long-term evaluation of adolescents treated operatively for spondylolisthesis. A comparison of in situ arthrodesis only with in situ arthrodesis and reduction followed by immobilization in a cast. *J Bone Joint Surg Am* 1992;74:693–704.

114. Freeman BL III, Donati NL. Spinal arthrodesis for severe spondylolisthesis in children and adolescents. A long-term follow-up study. *J Bone Joint Surg Am* 1989;71:594–598.

115. Pizzutillo PD, Mirenda W, MacEwen GD. Posterolateral fusion for spondylolisthesis in adolescence. *J Pediatr Orthop* 1986;6:311–316.

116. Dubousset J. Treatment of spondylolysis in children and adolescents. *Clin Orthop Relat Res* 1997;337:77.

117. Bosworth D, Fielding J, Demarest L, et al. Spondylolisthesis: a critical review of a consecutive series of cases treated by arthrodesis. *J Bone Joint Surg Am* 1955;37:767.

118. Frennered AK, Danielson BI, Nachemson AL, et al. Midterm follow-up of young patients fused in situ for spondylolisthesis. *Spine* 1991;16:409–416.

119. Gill GG. Long-term follow-up evaluation of a few patients with spondylolisthesis treated by excision of the loose lamina with decompression of the nerve roots without spinal fusion. *Clin Orthop Relat Res* 1984;182:215–219.

120. Gill GG, Manning JG, White HL. Surgical treatment of spondylolisthesis without spine fusion: excision of the loose lamina with decompression of the nerve roots. *J Bone Joint Surg Am* 1955;37:493–520.

121. Gill GG, White HL. Surgical treatment of spondylolisthesis without spine fusion. A long-term follow-up of operated cases. *Acta Orthop Scand Suppl* 1965;85:5–99.

122. Osterman K, Lindholm TS, Laurent LE. Late results of removal of the loose posterior element (Gill's operation) in the treatment of lytic lumbar spondylolisthesis. *Clin Orthop Relat Res* 1976;117:121–128.

123. Marmor L, Bechtol CO. Spondylolisthesis: complete slip following the Gill procedure: a case report. *J Bone Joint Surg Am* 1961;43: 1068–1069.

124. Brien MO. Low and high grade spondylolisthesis in the pediatric and adult population. In: Lenke LG, Newton PO. *Semin Spine Surg* 2003;15(3): 291–314.

125. Velikas EP, Blackburne JS. Surgical treatment of spondylolisthesis in children and adolescents. *J Bone Joint Surg Br* 1981;63-B:67–70.

126. Johnson LP, Nasca RJ, Dunham WK. Surgical management of isthmic spondylolisthesis. *Spine* 1988;13:93–97.

127. Rombold C. Treatment of spondylolisthesis by posterolateral fusion, resection of the pars interarticularis, and prompt mobilization of the patient. An end-result study of seventy-three patients. *J Bone Joint Surg Am* 1966;48:1282–1300.

128. Stauffer RN, Coventry MB. Anterior interbody lumbar spine fusion. Analysis of Mayo Clinic series. *J Bone Joint Surg Am* 1972;54:756–768.

129. Hanley EN Jr, Levy JA. Surgical treatment of isthmic lumbosacral spondylolisthesis. Analysis of variables influencing results. *Spine* 1989;14:48–50.

130. Lenke LG, Bridwell KH, Bullis D, et al. Results of in situ fusion for isthmic spondylolisthesis. *J Spinal Disord* 1992;5:433–442.

131. Bridwell KH, Sedgewick TA, Brien MFO, et al. The role of fusion and instrumentation in the treatment of degenerative spondylolisthesis with spinal stenosis. *J Spinal Disord* 1993;6:461–472.

132. Roca J, Moretta D, Fuster S, et al. Direct repair of spondylolysis. *Clin Orthop Relat Res* 1989;246:86–91.

133. DeWald RL, Faut MM, Taddonio RF, et al. Severe lumbosacral spondylolisthesis in adolescents and children. Reduction and staged circumferential fusion. *J Bone Joint Surg Am* 1981;63:619–626.

134. Kai Y, Oyama M, Morooka M. Posterior lumbar interbody fusion using local facet joint autograft and pedicle screw fixation. *Spine* 2004;29: 41–46.

135. Wiltse LL, Bateman G, Hutchinson RH, et al. The paraspinal sacrospinalis-splitting approach to the lumbar spine. *J Bone Joint Surg Am* 1968; 50:919.

136. DeWald RL. Spondylolisthesis. In: Bridwell KH, DeWald RL, Hammerberg KW, et al., eds. *The textbook of spinal surgery*, 2nd ed. Philadelphia, PA: Lippincott–Raven Publishers, 1997;1201–1210.

137. Johnson JR, Kirwan EO. The long-term results of fusion in situ for severe spondylolisthesis. *J Bone Joint Surg Br* 1983;65:43–46.

138. Laurent LE, Osterman K. Operative treatment of spondylolisthesis in young patients. *Clin Orthop Relat Res* 1976;117:85–91.

139. Bradford D. Controversies: instrumented reduction of spondylolisthesis (con). *Spine* 1994;14:1536–1537.

140. Dick WT, Schnebel B. Severe spondylolisthesis: reduction and internal fixation. *Clin Orthop Relat Res* 1988;232:70–79.

141. Edwards C. Reduction of spondylolisthesis: biomechanics and fixation. *Orthop Trans* 1986;10:543.

142. Emans JB, Waters PM, Hall JE. Technique for maintenance of reduction of severe spondylolisthesis using L4-S4 posterior segmental hyperextension fixation. *Orthop Trans* 1987;11:113.

143. Scaglietti O, Frontino G, Bartolozzi P. Technique of anatomical reduction of lumbar spondylolisthesis and its surgical stabilization. *Clin Orthop Relat Res* 1976;117:165–175.

144. Shufflebarger HL. High grade isthmic spondylolisthesis: monosegmental surgical treatment. Scoliosis research society annual meeting, New York, 1998.

145. Schoenecker PL, Cole HO, Herring JA, et al. Cauda equina syndrome after in situ arthrodesis for severe spondylolisthesis at the lumbosacral junction. *J Bone Joint Surg Am* 1990;72:369–377.

146. Jenkins J. Spondylolisthesis. *Br J Surg* 1936;24:80.

147. Harrington PR, Dickson JH. Spinal instrumentation in the treatment of severe progressive spondylolisthesis. *Clin Orthop Relat Res* 1976;117: 157–163.

148. Bradford D. Management of spondylolysis and spondylolisthesis. In: Evarts EV, ed. *Instructional course lectures, American Academy of Orthopedic Surgeons*, Vol. 32. St. Louis, MO: CV Mosby, 1983:151.

149. Wiesel SW, Garfin SR, Boden SD, et al. Spondylolisthesis. *Semin Spine Surg* 1994:6.

150. Ohki I, Inoue S, Murata T, et al. Reduction and fusion of severe spondylolisthesis using halo-pelvic traction with a wire reduction device. *Int Orthop* 1980;4:107–113.

151. Sijbrandij S. Reduction and stabilization of severe spondylolisthesis. A report of three cases. *J Bone Joint Surg Br* 1983;65:40–42.

152. Harms J, Jeszenszky D, Stoltze D, et al. True spondylolisthesis reduction and monosegmental fusion in spondylolisthesis. In: Bridwell KH, DeWald RL, Hammerberg KW, et al., eds. *The textbook of spinal surgery*, 2nd ed., vol. 2. Philadelphia, PA: Lippincott–Raven Publishers, 1997;1337–1347.

153. Transfeldt EE, Dendrinos GK, Bradford DS. Paresis of proximal lumbar roots after reduction of L5-S1 spondylolisthesis. *Spine* 1989;14: 884–887.

154. Petraco DM, Spivak JM, Cappadona JG, et al. An anatomic evaluation of L5 nerve stretch in spondylolisthesis reduction. *Spine* 1996;21: 1133–1138; discussion 1139.

155. Balderston RA, Bradford DS. Technique for achievement and maintenance of reduction for severe spondylolisthesis using spinous process traction wiring and external fixation of the pelvis. *Spine* 1985;10:376–372.

156. Bradford DS, Boachie-Adjei O. Treatment of severe spondylolisthesis by anterior and posterior reduction and stabilization. A long-term follow-up study. *J Bone Joint Surg Am* 1990;72:1060–1066.

157. Molinari RW, Bridwell KH, Lenke LG, et al. Anterior column support in surgery for high-grade isthmic spondylolisthesis. *Clin Orthop Relat Res* 2002;394:109–120.

158. Matthiass HH, Heine J. The surgical reduction of spondylolisthesis. *Clin Orthop Relat Res* 1986;203:34–44.

159. Sevastikoglou JA, Spangfort E, Aaro S. Operative treatment of spondylolisthesis in children and adolescents with tight hamstrings syndrome. *Clin Orthop Relat Res* 1980;147:192–199.

160. Muschik M, Zippel H, Perka C. Surgical management of severe spondylolisthesis in children and adolescents. Anterior fusion in-situ versus anterior spondylodesis with posterior transpedicular instrumentation and reduction. *Spine* 1997;22:2036–2042.

161. Lindholm TS, Ragni P, Ylikoski M, et al. Lumbar isthmic spondylolisthesis in children and adolescents. Radiologic evaluation and results of operative treatment. *Spine* 1990;15:1350–1355.

162. van Rens TJ, van Horn JR. Long-term results in lumbosacral interbody fusion for spondylolisthesis. *Acta Orthop Scand* 1982;53:383–392.

163. Bradford DS, Treatment of severe spondylolisthesis. A combined approach for reduction and stabilization. *Spine* 1979;4:423–429.

164. Molinari RW, Bridwell KH, Lenke LG, et al. Complications in the surgical treatment of pediatric high-grade, isthmic dysplastic spondylolisthesis: a comparison of three surgical approaches. *Spine* 1999;24: 1701–1711.

165. Freebody D, Bendall R, Taylor RD. Anterior transperitoneal lumbar fusion. *J Bone Joint Surg Br* 1971;53:617–627.

166. Verbiest H. The treatment of lumbar spondyloptosis or impending lumbar spondyloptosis accompanied by neurologic deficit and/or neurogenic intermittent claudication. *Spine* 1979;4:68–77.

167. Rosa GL, Conti A, Cacciola F, et al. Pedicle screw fixation for isthmic spondylolisthesis: does posterior lumbar interbody fusion improve the outcome over posterolateral fusion? *J Neurosurg Spine* 2003;99: 143–150.

168. Bohlman HH, Cook SS. One-stage decompression and posterolateral and interbody fusion for lumbosacral spondyloptosis through a posterior approach. Report of two cases. *J Bone Joint Surg Am* 1982;64: 415–418.

169. Smith MD, Bohlman HH. Spondylolisthesis treated by a single-stage operation combining decompression with in situ posterolateral and anterior fusion. An analysis of eleven patients who had long-term follow-up. *J Bone Joint Surg Am* 1990;72:415–421.

170. Esses SI, Natout N, Kip P. Posterior interbody arthrodesis with a fibular strut graft in spondylolisthesis. *J Bone Joint Surg Am* 1995;77: 172–176.

171. Nachemson A. Repair of the spondylolisthetic defect and intertransverse fusion for young patients. *Clin Orthop Relat Res* 1976;117:101–105.

172. Gaines RW, Nichols WK. Treatment of spondyloptosis by two stage L5 vertebrectomy and reduction of L4 onto S1. *Spine* 1985;10: 680–686.

173. Huizenga B. Reduction of spondyloptosis with two-stage vertebrectomy. *Orthop Trans* 1983;7:21.

174. Seitsalo S, Osterman K, Poussa M. Scoliosis associated with lumbar spondylolisthesis. A clinical survey of 190 young patients. *Spine* 1988;13:899–904.

175. Lonstein JE. Spondylolisthesis in children. Cause, natural history, and management. *Spine* 1999;24:2640–2680.

The Cervical Spine

Many of the diseases and congenital anomalies affecting the pediatric cervical spine are simply a reflection of aberrant growth and developmental processes. This chapter discusses these diseases and anomalies in this framework. A basic knowledge of the normal embryology, growth, and development of the pediatric cervical spine is necessary to understand these conditions. Most of the anomalies and diseases involving the pediatric cervical spine are easily divided into those of the upper (occiput, C1, C2) and lower (C3-C7) segments.

NORMAL EMBRYOLOGY, GROWTH, AND DEVELOPMENT

Embryology

Occipitoaxioatlas Complex. The occiput is formed from at least four or five somites. All definitive vertebrae develop from the caudal sclerotome half of one segment and the cranial sclerotome half of the succeeding segment (1). These areas of primitive mesenchyme separate from each other during fetal growth and then undergo chondrification and subsequent ossification. This chondrification and ossification is a passive process, following the blueprint laid down by the mesenchymal anlage. Because of this sequencing, the cranial half of the first cervical sclerotome remains as a half segment between the occipital and the atlantal rudiments and is known as the proatlas. The primitive centrum of this proatlas becomes the tip of the odontoid process, whereas its arch rudiments assist in the formation of the occipital

condyles (2). The vertebral arch of the atlas separates from its respective centrum, becoming the ring of C1; the separated centrum fuses with the proatlas above and the centrum of C2 below, to become the odontoid process and body of C2. The axis forms from the second definitive cervical vertebral mesenchymal segment. The odontoid process is the fusion of the primitive centra of the atlas and the proatlas half segment. The posterior arches of C2 form from only the second definitive cervical segment.

Thus, the atlas is made up of three main components: the body and the two neural arches. The axis is made up of four main components: the body, two neural arches, and the odontoid (or five components if the proatlas rudiment is considered) (Figs. 21-1 and 21-2).

Vertebrae C3-C7. These vertebrae follow the normal formation schema of all vertebrae (3). A portion of the mesenchyme from the sclerotomal centrum creates two neural arches that migrate posteriorly and around the neural tube. This eventually forms the pedicles, the laminae, the spinous processes, and a very small portion of the body. The majority of the body is formed by the centrum. An ossification center develops in each of the two neural arches and one in the vertebral center, with a synchondrosis formed by the cartilage between the ossification centers.

Basic Science, Embryology, and Gene Expression. In the past decade, there has been an explosion of knowledge regarding the human genome and how it relates to normal developmental processes and pathologic conditions. Vertebral segmentation begins with clustering segments of the paraxial mesoderm, the somites. Segmentation of the mesoderm into somites is an important yet fundamental process that allows for spatial specialization in the organism and is under genetic control.

The homeobox is a highly conserved 160-base pair sequence found in the homeobox genes, termed *Hox* genes for short. These *Hox* genes encode a highly conserved family of transcription factors that play fundamental roles in morphogenesis during embryonic development. Vertebrate *Hox* genes help control developmental patterning in the embryo along the

FIGURE 21-1. **A:** Cross-sectional radiograph of C1 in a full-term neonate. The posterior ossification centers are present. No ossification is present in the anterior cartilage. The transverse ligament (*arrow*) separates the dens (D) from the spinal canal (S). **B:** AP radiograph of C1 in a term neonate. (From Ogden JA. Radiology of postnatal skeletal development. XI. The first cervical vertebrae. *Skeletal Radiol* 1984;12:12–20, with permission.)

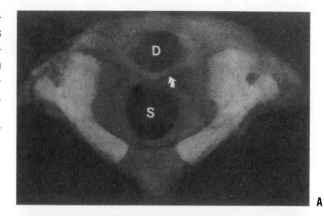

A

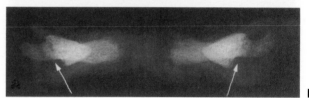

B

FIGURE 21-2. **A:** Cross-sectional radiograph of C2 in a neonate. The neurocentral (*solid arrows*) and posterior (*open arrows*) synchondroses are evident. A small area of accessory ossification is present in the right neurocentral synchondrosis anteriorly (*curved arrow*). Also note the central linear radiolucency (*black arrow*) indicating the synchondrosis between the dens ossificiation centers. The posterior ossification centers extend into the eventual vertebral body. **B:** The AP radiograph of C2 in a neonate. In this specimen, the dens ossification centers have not fused, leaving a midline synchondrosis (*arrows*) that extends from the chondrum terminale to the dentocentral synchondrosis. The superior margin of the eventual vertebral body is above the lower level of the dens. The neurocentral synchondroses are continuous with the "ring apophyseal" cartilage inferiorly, the facet cartilage inferiorly, and the dentocentral synchondrosis superiorly. (From Ogden JA. Radiology of postnatal skeletal development. XII. The second cervical vertebra. *Skeletal Radiol* 1984;12:169–177, with permission.)

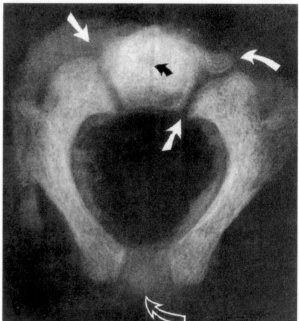

A

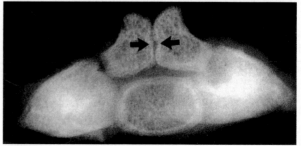

B

primary (head-to-tail) and secondary (genital and limb bud) axes. There are 39 *Hox* genes in vertebrates that are organized into four clusters located on different chromosomes. In the human, these clusters are named HOXA, HOXB, HOXC, and HOXD, located on chromosomes 7p14, 17q21, 12q13, and 2q31, respectively (4). In animals, they are written in lower case (e.g., *Hoxc*); in the human, they are written in upper case (e.g., HOXC). Each cluster contains 9 to 11 genes, all oriented in the same 5′ to 3′ direction of transcription. There are 13 possible subsets of genes; no single cluster contains a representative from all 13 known numbered subsets (paralogous groups). The numbering of the genes in each cluster is based on their sequence similarity and relative positions, starting from that end of the complex that is expressed most anteriorly (cranially). The equivalent genes in each complex are called a paralogous group.

The expression domains of the HOX clusters display a nested arrangement. Along the body axis, the *Hox* genes are generally expressed with discrete rostral cutoffs that coincide with either existing or emergent anatomic landmarks. *Hox* genes at the end of the 3′ cluster (e.g., HOXA1) are generally expressed early, in anterior and proximal regions; *Hox* genes at the 5′ end (e.g., HOXA13) are generally expressed later, in more posterior and distal regions. Thus, the lower numbered *Hox* genes are involved in the development of the axial skeleton, and the higher numbered *Hox* genes are involved in development of the limbs. There has been an explosion of knowledge regarding defects in the *Hox* genes and resultant congenital spinal anomalies in experimental animals, and to much lesser extent in humans (Table 21-1). The defect can be a distinct *Hox* gene mutation intentionally produced by the investigator or more random hits by teratogens (methanol, boric acid, retinoic acid, maternal hyperthermia) (13–17).

Another group of genes, the *Pax* genes, are also integrally involved in vertebral development. The *Pax* genes are a highly conserved family of developmental control genes that encode transcription factors containing a 128-amino acid DNA-binding domain (18, 19), called the paired box (20). To date, there are nine *PAX* genes (12, 21). The *Pax* gene family is broken down into four subgroups (*Pax1* and *Pax9*; *Pax2*, *Pax5*, and *Pax8*; *Pax3* and *Pax7*; *Pax4* and *Pax6*). *Pax1* and *Pax9* induce chondrogenic differentiation in the paraxial mesenchymal mesoderm of the sclerotome (19, 20, 22). *Pax1* expression is also seen in the posterior occiput, indicating that the basilar occiput from a developmental standpoint can be considered the uppermost vertebra (23). Thus, they are critically involved in vertebral formation. Abnormalities in the PAX1 sequence in humans have been associated in some patients with Klippel-Feil syndrome (12).

The Hedgehog family of proteins has also become increasingly recognized as crucial to axial skeletal development. The best known of these proteins is the sonic hedgehog (*shh*), which is expressed in the notochord (24, 25). *Shh* is believed to be the signal for induction of the ventral somite to differentiate into the sclerotome (25). In *shh* knockout mice, most sclerotomal derivatives are absent, in conjunction with reduced expression of *Pax1* (25). Thus, absence of *shh* leads to absence of *Pax1* expression and subsequent failure of the mesenchymal cells to chondrify. Defective *shh* signaling during embryogenesis in mice results in anomalies similar to those seen in the human VACTERL association (26).

Growth and Development

Atlas. Ossification is present only in the two neural arches at birth (27). These ossification centers extend posteriorly toward the rudimentary spinous process to form the posterior synchondrosis and anteriorly into the articular facet region to form all of the bone present in the facets. Anteromedial to each facet, the neurocentral synchondroses form, joining the neural arches and the body; this occurs on each side of the expanding anterior ossification center. The body starts to ossify between 6 months and 2 years, usually in a single center. By 4 to 6 years, the posterior synchondrosis fuses, followed by the anterior ones slightly thereafter. The final internal diameter of the pediatric C1 spinal canal is determined by 6 to 7 years of age. Further growth is obtained only by periosteal appositional growth on the external surface, which leads to thickening and an increased height, but without changing the size of the spinal canal. Thus, a spinal fusion after the age of 6 or 7 years has minimal impact on the internal canal diameter; when possible, surgical fusion should not be performed before this age due to the potential for later cervical stenosis.

TABLE 21.1	Axial Skeletal Malformations Due to Genetic Abnormalities			
Involved gene	**Gene abnormality**	**Phenotypic expression**	**Animal**	**Reference**
Hoxb-4	Knockout	C2 becomes C1	Mouse	(5)
Hoxd-3	Homozygous	Atlas fused to occiput, C2 becomes more like C1	Mouse	(6)
Hoxa-4	Homozygous	Development of ribs on C7	Mouse	(7)
Bapx1	Knockout	Malformed basioccipital bone. Absence of anterior arch of atlas	Mouse	(8)
Uncx4.1	Homozygous	Absence of pedicles and transverse processes, cervical vertebrae	Mouse	(9)
Cdx1	Homozygous	Cranial transformations of cervical spine: absence of anterior arch of C1 C2 becomes like C1 C3 becomes like C2 Development of ribs on C7	Mouse	(10, 11)
PAX1	Sequence changes	Klippel-Feil syndrome	Human	(12)

Axis.   The odontoid develops two primary ossification centers that usually coalesce within the first 3 months of life; these centers are separated from the C2 centrum by the dentocentral synchondrosis (28, 29). This synchondrosis is below the level of the C1-C2 facets and contributes to the overall height of the odontoid as well as to the body of C2. It is continuous with the vertebral body and facets, and it coalesces with the anterior neurocentral synchondroses and finally at the dentocentral synchondrosis. This closure occurs between 3 and 6 years of age. The tip of the dens comprises a cartilaginous region similar to an epiphysis, the chondrum terminale, which develops an ossification center between 5 and 8 years, becoming the ossiculum terminale. The ossiculum terminale fuses to the remainder of the odontoid between 10 and 13 years of age.

The posterior neural arches are partially ossified at birth, joined by the posterior synchondrosis. By 3 months of age, these arches, growing more posteriorly, form the rudimentary spinous process. By 1 year of age, ossification fills the spinous process, and by 3 years of age, the posterior synchondrosis has fused. Thus, both the posterior and the anterior synchondroses are closed by 6 years of age, and there is no further increase in spinal canal size after this age.

C3-C7.   At birth, all three ossification centers are present. The anterior synchondrosis (i.e., neurocentral synchondrosis) is slightly anterior to the base of the pedicles; it usually closes between 3 and 6 years of age. The posterior synchondrosis is at the junction of the two neural arches; it usually closes by 2 to 4 years of age. In the neonate and the young child, the articular facets are horizontal but become more vertically oriented as the child ages and reaches the normal adult configuration. They are also more horizontal in the upper cervical spine than in the lower cervical spine. The vertebral bodies enlarge circumferentially by periosteal appositional growth, whereas they grow vertically by endochondral ossification. Secondary ossification centers develop at the tips of the spinous processes and the cartilaginous ring apophyses of the bodies around the time of puberty. These ring apophyses are involved in the vertical growth of the body. These secondary ossification centers fuse with the vertebral body around age 25 years. There is an overall increase in pedicle axis width but not length as the child grows; thus, pedicle screw fixation of the cervical spine in children is not considered safe (30).

Vertebral Body and Canal Diameter Changes with Growth.   Due to the fact that the immature vertebrae are more cartilaginous compared to the mature adult vertebrae, there are significant differences between normal vertebral measurements in the child compared to the adult (31). As the child ages, the vertebral body height increases relative to the vertebral body depth. This is due to the activity of the apophyseal end plates that contribute proportionally more growth to the height of the vertebral body compared to the appositional growth that contributes to the depth of the vertebral body. The vertebral body height-to-depth ratio increases from approximately 0.5 in children <1 year of age to 0.8 to 0.9 in adults. This remains relatively constant for all vertebral bodies from C3 to C7. With these changes in the vertebral

body height relative to depth, there are also changes in the sagittal diameter of the canal relative to vertebral body depth. The ratio of the sagittal canal diameter to vertebral body depth is stable at 1.4 in children from birth to 7 to 8 years of age and then gradually decreases to the normal 1.0 adult value (31). Knowledge of these normal growth parameters is important when determining the possibility of platyspondyly or spinal stenosis.

Normal Radiographic Parameters.   Certain radiographic parameters that indicate pathology of the cervical spine in adults represent normal developmental processes in children (32). These parameters are the atlantooccipital motion and atlanto–dens interval (ADI), pseudosubluxation and pseudoinstability, variations in the curvature of the cervical spine that may resemble spasm and ligamentous injury, variations in the presence of skeletal growth and growth centers that may resemble fractures, and anterior soft-tissue widening. Normal cervical spine motion in children is also discussed.

Atlanto–Dens Interval and Atlantooccipital Motion.   These intervals are determined on lateral flexion and extension views, which should be performed voluntarily with the patient awake. The ADI is the space between the anterior aspect of the dens and the posterior aspect of the anterior ring of the atlas (Fig. 21-3). An ADI of more than 5 mm on flexion and extension lateral radiographs indicates instability (33, 34). This is more than the 3-mm adult value because of the increased cartilage content of the odontoid and ring of the atlas in children as well as the increased ligamentous laxity in children. In extension, overriding of the anterior arch of the atlas on top of the odontoid also can be seen in up to 20% of children (35) (see Fig. 21-6B).

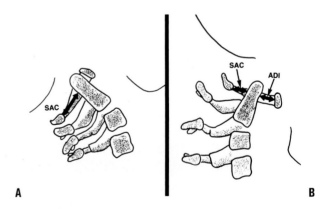

FIGURE 21-3.   Lateral view of the atlantoaxial joint. The ADI is the distance between the anterior aspect of the dens and the posterior aspect of the anterior portion of the ring of the atlas. The SAC is the distance between the posterior aspect of the dens and the anterior aspect of the posterior portion of the ring of the atlas. In children, an ADI of 5 mm or larger is abnormal. In teenagers and adults, a SAC of 13 mm or smaller can be associated with canal compromise. In younger children, spinal cord impingement is imminent if the SAC is equal to or less than the transverse diameter of the odontoid. **A:** The relations in extension. **B:** The relations in flexion.

A mild increase in the ADI may indicate a subtle disruption of the transverse atlantal ligament. In adults, an ADI > 5 mm indicates ligament rupture (36). In chronic atlanto-axial conditions (e.g., rheumatoid arthritis, Down syndrome, congenital anomalies), the ADI is less useful. In children with these disorders who are frequently hypermobile but do not have ruptured transverse atlantal ligaments, the ADI is increased beyond the 3- to 5-mm range. The complement of the ADI, the space available for the cord (SAC), is a more useful measure in this situation. This space is the distance between the posterior aspect of the dens and the anterior aspect of the posterior ring of the atlas or the foramen magnum. A SAC of <13 mm may be associated with neurologic problems (37).

In patients in whom there is an attenuation of the transverse atlantal ligament without rupture, the alar ligament provides some stability. It acts like a checkrein (38), first tightening up in rotation and then becoming completely taut as the odontoid process continues to move posteriorly for a distance equivalent to its full transverse diameter. This safety zone between the anterior wall of the spinal canal of the atlas, the axis, and the neural structures is an anatomic constant equal to the transverse diameter of the odontoid. This constant defines Steel's rule of thirds: one-third cord, one-third odontoid, and one-third space. This rule remains constant throughout the growth of the cervical spine (39). The cord can move into this space (safe zone) when the odontoid moves posteriorly because of an attenuated transverse atlantal ligament. It is here that the alar ligament becomes taut, acting as a checkrein and secondary restraint, preventing further movement of the odontoid into the cord. In the chronic situation, it is important to recognize when this safe zone has been exceeded and the child enters the region of impending spinal cord compression. In the case of trauma, the alar ligament is insufficient to prevent a fatal cord injury in the event of another neck injury similar to the one that caused the initial interruption of the transverse atlantal ligament.

Normal ranges of motion at the atlantooccipital joint are not well defined. In a series of 40 normal college freshman, the tip of the odontoid remained directly below the basion of the skull in both flexion and extension (40). Thus, the joint should not allow any horizontal translation during flexion and extension. Tredwell et al. (41) believe that a posterior subluxation of the atlantooccipital relation in extension of more than 4 mm indicates instability (Fig. 21-4). This can be measured

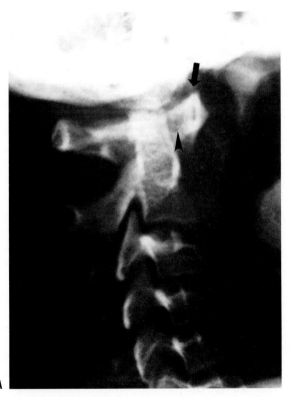 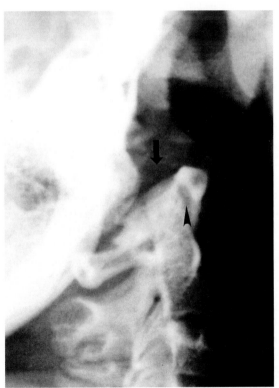

A **B**

FIGURE 21-4. Lateral (**A**) flexion and (**B**) extension radiographs of an 11-year-old boy with Down syndrome. The child presented with loss of hand control when flexing his neck. Using the method of Tredwell et al. (41), the atlantooccipital distance is measured as the distance between the anterior margin of the condyles at the base of the skull and the sharp contour of the anterior aspect of the concave joint of the atlas. More than 4 mm of posterior translation is abnormal. The atlantooccipital distance (*arrows*) measured 10 mm in extension and 1 mm in flexion. The ADI was 1 mm in extension and 6 mm in flexion, for a total of 5 mm of motion (*arrowheads*). The SAC was 17 mm in flexion and 20 mm in extension. Both occipitoatlantal instability (more than 4 mm posterior translation) and atlanto–dens hypermobility (5 mm ADI in flexion) were present.

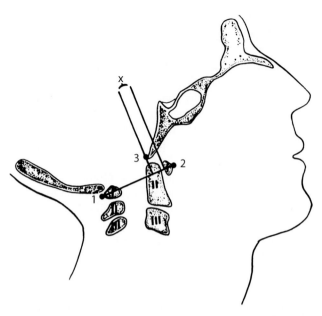

FIGURE 21-5. The method of measuring atlantooccipital instability according to Weisel and Rothman (42). The atlantal line joins points *1* and *2*. A perpendicular line to the atlantal line is made at the posterior margin of the anterior arch of the atlas. The distance (*x*) from the basion (*3*) to the perpendicular line is measured in flexion and extension. The difference between flexion and extension represents the AP translation at the occipitoatlantal joint; in normal adults, this translation should be no more than 1 mm. (From Gabriel KR, Mason DE, Carango P. Occipito-atlantal translation in Down's syndrome. *Spine* 1990;15:996–1002, with permission.)

as the distance between the anterior margin of the condyles at the base of the skull and the sharp contour of the anterior aspect of the concave joint of the atlas anteriorly, or as the distance between the occipital protuberance and the superior arch of the atlas posteriorly. Another method to measure posterior subluxation of the atlantooccipital joint is that of Wiesel and Rothman (42) (Fig. 21-5). With this technique, occiput-C1 translation from maximum flexion to maximum extension should be no more than 1 mm in normal adults. These norms in children have not yet been established.

Pseudosubluxation. The C2-C3, and to a lesser extent, the C3-C4 interspace in children, have a normal physiologic displacement. In a study of 161 children (35), marked anterior displacement of C2 on C3 was observed in 9% of children between 1 and 7 years old. In a more recent study, 22% of 108 polytrauma children demonstrated pseudosubluxation, and had no association with intubation status or injury severity (43). In some children, the anterior physiologic displacement of C2 on C3 is so pronounced that it appears pathologic (pseudosubluxation). To differentiate this from pathologic subluxation, Swischuk (44) has used the posterior cervical line (Fig. 21-6) drawn from the anterior cortex of the posterior arch of C1 to the anterior cortex of the posterior arch of C3. In physiologic displacement of C2 on C3, the posterior cervical line may pass

through the cortex of the posterior arch of C2, touch the anterior aspect of the cortex of the posterior arch of C2, or come within 1 mm of the anterior cortex of the posterior arch of C2. In pathologic dislocation of C2 on C3, the posterior cervical line misses the posterior arch of C2 by 2 mm or more.

The planes of the articular facets change with growth. The lower cervical spine facets change from 55 to 70 degrees, whereas the upper facets (i.e., C2-C4) may have initial angles as low as 30 degrees, which gradually increase to 60 to 70 degrees. This variation in facet angulation, along with normal looseness of the soft tissues, intervertebral discs, and the relative increase in size and weight of the skull compared with the trunk, are the major factors responsible for this pseudosubluxation. No treatment is needed for this normal physiologic subluxation.

Variations in the Curvature and Growth of the Cervical Spine That Can Resemble Injury. In the classic study of Cattell and Filtzer (35), 16% of normal children showed a marked angulation at a single interspace, suggestive of injury to the interspinous or posterior longitudinal ligament; 14% showed an absence of the normal lordosis in the neutral position; and 16% showed an absence of the flexion curvature between the second and the seventh cervical vertebrae, which could be erroneously interpreted as splinting secondary to injury. These findings may occur in children up to 16 years of age.

Spina bifida of the posterior arch, or multiple ossification centers of the ring of C1, may mimic fractures. They can be delineated from fractures by their smooth cortical margins. In some children, the posterior ring of C1 remains cartilaginous, which is usually of no clinical significance (45, 46). Spina bifida also may occur at other cervical levels, and the overlapping lucent areas on anteroposterior (AP) radiographs when crossing a vertebral body, may mimic a vertical fracture of the body. Defects in the posterior arch of the atlas are present in 3.7% of the normal population (47).

The dentocentral synchondrosis of C2 begins to close between 5 and 7 years of age (28). However, it may be visible in vestigial forms up to 11 years of age (35) and may be erroneously interpreted as an undisplaced fracture. Similarly, the apical odontoid epiphysis (i.e., ossiculum terminale) may appear by 5 years of age, although it most typically appears around 8 years of age. This also can be misinterpreted as an odontoid tip fracture.

Wedging of the C3 vertebral body is a normal radiographic finding in 7% of younger children (Fig. 21-6B); the wedging corrects as the child matures and is extremely rare after age 13 (48). If it is unclear whether the wedging is a normal variation or a true compression fracture in the face of a traumatic history, a computed tomography (CT) scan will demonstrate fracture lines through the body if a fracture is present. In the lower cervical levels, secondary centers of ossification of the spinous processes may resemble avulsion fractures (35).

Normal Lower Cervical Spine Motion. Generally, the interspinous distances increase with increasing age, being the smallest at C4-C5 and the largest at C6-C7, until 15 years

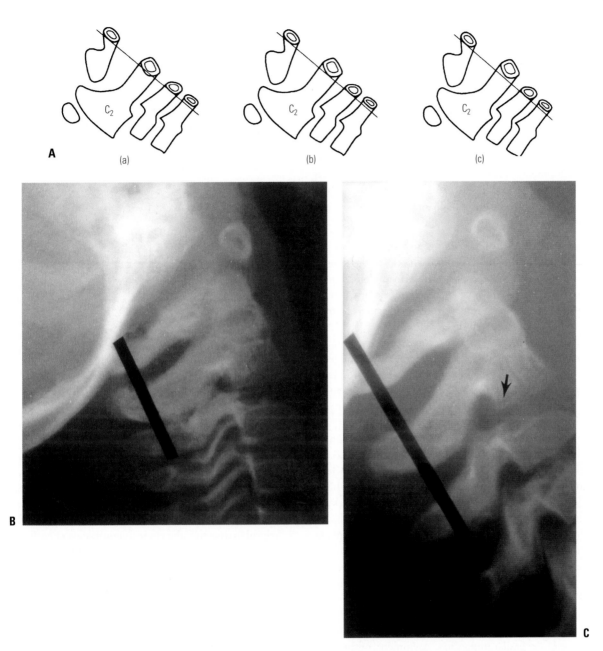

FIGURE 21-6.   A: The posterior cervical line of Swischuk. In C2-C3 pseudosubluxation, the posterior cervical line may pass through *(a)*, touch *(b)*, or lie 1 mm in front of the cortex of the posterior arch of C2. (From Shaw M, Burnett H, Wilson A, et al. Pseudosubluxation of C2 on C3 in polytraumatized children—prevalence and significance. *Clin Radiol* 1999;54:377–380, with permission). **B,C:** Lateral cervical radiograph of a 2-year, 6-month-old child with pseudosubluxation at C2-C3. The radiograph in extension (B) demonstrates no step-off at C2-C3, whereas the radiograph in flexion (C) demonstrates a step-off at C2-C3 *(arrow)*, but with a normal posterior cervical line *(solid line)*. Also note the anterior wedging of the C3 vertebral body. Similarly, note the overriding of the anterior arch of the atlas on the tip of the odontoid in extension.

of age, when this distance is largest at C5-C6 (34). The AP displacement, from hyperflexion to hyperextension, decreases from C2-C3 to C6-C7. The angular displacement is greatest (15 degrees) at C3-C4 and C4-C5 for children 3 to 8 years of age, is greatest (17 degrees) at C4-C5 for children 9 to 11 years of age, and is greatest (15 degrees) at C5-C6 for children 12 to 15 years of age.

CONGENITAL AND DEVELOPMENTAL PROBLEMS

Torticollis.   Torticollis is a combined head tilt and rotatory deformity. Torticollis indicates a problem at C1-C2 because 50% of the cervical spine rotation occurs at this joint. A head tilt alone indicates a more generalized problem in the cervical spine.

The differential diagnosis of torticollis is large and can be divided into osseous and nonosseous types. In a recent large series from a tertiary care pediatric orthopaedic center (49), a nonmuscular etiology of torticollis was found in 18% of patients, most frequently the Klippel-Feil syndrome or a neurologic disorder (ocular pathology, or central nervous system lesion).

Osseous Types.
Occipitocervical synostosis, basilar impression, and odontoid anomalies are the most common congenital/developmental malformations of the occipitovertebral junction, with an incidence of 1.4 to 2.5 per 100 children (50). These lesions arise from a malformation of the mesenchymal anlages at the occipitovertebral junction.

Basilar Impression. Basilar impression is an indentation of the skull floor by the upper cervical spine. The tip of the dens is more cephalad and sometimes protrudes into the opening of the foramen magnum. This may encroach on the brain stem, risking neurologic damage from direct injury, vascular compromise, or alterations in cerebrospinal fluid flow (51).

Basilar impression can be primary or secondary. Primary basilar impression, the most common type, is a congenital abnormality often associated with other vertebral defects (e.g., Klippel-Feil syndrome, odontoid abnormalities, atlanto-occipital fusion, and atlas hypoplasia). The incidence of primary basilar impression in the general population is 1% (52).

Secondary basilar impression is a developmental condition attributed to softening of the osseous structures at the base of the skull. Any disorder of osseous softening can lead to secondary basilar impression. These include metabolic bone diseases [e.g., Paget disease (53), renal osteodystrophy, rickets, osteomalacia (54, 55)] bone dysplasias and mesenchymal syndromes [e.g., osteogenesis imperfecta (56–62), achondroplasia (63), hypochondroplasia (64), neurofibromatosis (65), and rheumatologic disorders, e.g., rheumatoid arthritis, ankylosing spondylitis]. The softening allows the odontoid to migrate cephalad and into the foramen magnum.

These patients typically present with a short neck (78% in one series) (66). This shortening is only an apparent deformity because of the basilar impression. Asymmetry of the skull and face (68%), painful cervical motion (53%), and torticollis (15%) can also occur. Neurologic signs and symptoms are often present (67). Many children will have acute onset of symptoms precipitated by minor trauma (68). In cases of isolated basilar impression, the neurologic involvement is primarily a pyramidal syndrome associated with proprioceptive sensory disturbances (motor weakness, 85%; limb paresthesias, 85%). In cases of basilar impression associated with Arnold-Chiari malformations, the neurologic involvement is usually cerebellar, and symptoms include motor incoordination with ataxia, dizziness, and nystagmus. In both types, the patients may complain of neck pain and headache in the distribution of the greater occipital nerve and cranial nerve involvement, particularly those that emerge from the medulla oblongata (trigeminal [V], glossopharyngeal [IX], vagus [X], and hypoglossal [XII]). Ataxia is a very common finding in children with basilar impression (68). Hydrocephalus may develop as a

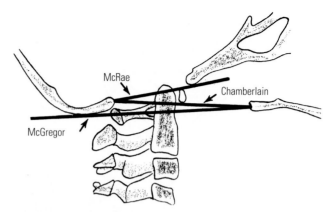

FIGURE 21-7. The landmarks on a lateral radiograph of the skull and the upper cervical spine used to assess basilar impression. McRae line defines the opening of the foramen magnum. Chamberlain line is drawn from the posterior lip of the foramen magnum to the dorsal margin of the hard palate. McGregor line is drawn from the upper surface of the posterior edge of the hard palate to the most caudal point of the occipital curve of the skull. McGregor line is the best line for screening because of the clarity of the radiographic landmarks in children of all ages.

result of obstruction of the cerebrospinal fluid flow by obstruction of the foramen magnum from the odontoid.

Basilar impression is difficult to assess radiographically. The most commonly used lines are Chamberlain (69), McRae (70), and McGregor (71) (Fig. 21-7). McGregor line is the best line for screening because the landmarks can be clearly defined at all ages on a routine lateral radiograph. McRae line is helpful in assessing the clinical significance of basilar impression because it defines the opening of the foramen magnum; in patients who are symptomatic, the odontoid projects above this line. At present, CT with sagittal plane reconstructions can show the osseous relations at the occipitocervical junction more clearly, and magnetic resonance imaging (MRI) clearly delineates the neural anatomy. MRI and CT norms have been recently established (72, 73). Occasionally, vertebral angiography or MR angiogram (MRA) is needed (74).

Treatment of basilar impression can be difficult and requires a multidisciplinary approach (orthopaedic, neurosurgical, and neuroradiologic) (59, 61, 75–78). The symptoms rarely can be relieved with customized orthoses (79); the primary treatment is surgical. If the symptoms are caused by a hypermobile odontoid, surgical stabilization in extension at the occipitocervical junction is needed. Anterior excision of the odontoid is needed if it cannot be reduced (80), but this should be preceded by posterior stabilization and fusion. In some cases, the anterior decompression can be performed endoscopically (81). If the symptoms are from posterior impingement, suboccipital decompression and often upper cervical laminectomy are needed. The dura often needs to be opened to look for a tight posterior band (66, 82). Posterior stabilization also should be performed (83). In a recent series of 190 cases, decompression of the foramen magnum was appropriate for those without an

Arnold-Chiari malformation; transoral anterior decompression was reserved for those with an associated Arnold-Chiari malformation (84). These are general statements, and each case must be considered individually. Secondary basilar impression tends to progress despite arthrodesis (61).

Atlantooccipital Anomalies. Children with congenital bony anomalies of the atlantooccipital junction present with a wide spectrum of deformities (85). The anterior arch of C1 is commonly assimilated to the occiput, usually in association with a hypoplastic ring posteriorly (Fig. 21-8), as well as condylar hypoplasia (86). The height of C1 is variably decreased, allowing the odontoid to project upward into the foramen magnum (i.e., primary basilar impression). More distal cervical anomalies can also occur in association with the atlantooccipital anomaly. The odontoid may be misshapen or directed posteriorly more than normal. Up to 70% of children with this condition have a congenital fusion of C2-C3 (see Fig. 21-8). (Posterior congenital fusion of C2-C3 is a clue that occiput-C1 anomalies, or other more distal cervical fusions, may be present. These may be cartilaginous initially, and not appear on plain radiographs until the child becomes more mature.) The fusion of C1 to the occiput is classified by zones (86); zone 1 is a fused anterior arch, zone 2 a fusion of the lateral masses, zone 3 a fused posterior arch, and zone 4 a combination of zones. Zone 4 fusions are most common, but the highest prevalence of spinal canal encroachment is in zone 2 patients.

Clinically, these children resemble those with the Klippel-Feil syndrome: short, broad necks; restricted neck motion; low hairline; high scapula; and torticollis (Fig. 21-9) (82, 87–89). Recently, hemifacial microsomia has been noted to have associated atlantooccipital anomalies (90), as well as children with the 22q11.2 deletion syndrome (91). The skull may demonstrate a positional deformational plagiocephaly. They also may have other associated anomalies, including dwarfism, funnel chest, jaw anomalies, cleft palate, congenital ear deformities, hypospadias, genitourinary tract defects, and syndactyly. They can present with neurologic symptoms during childhood, but more often present between 40 to 50 years of age. These symptoms can be initiated by traumatic or inflammatory processes, and they progress slowly and relentlessly. Rarely do they present suddenly or dramatically, although they have been reported as a cause of sudden death. The most common signs and symptoms, in decreasing order of frequency, are neck and

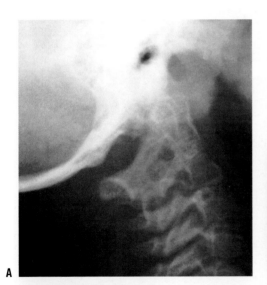

A

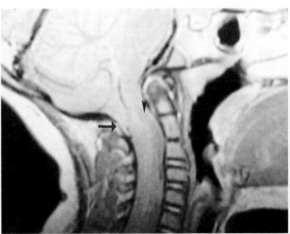

B

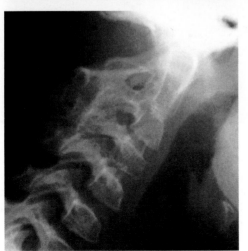

C

FIGURE 21-8. This 3-year, 9-month-old girl had a history of vertex headaches for 1 year. One month prior to presentation, she developed a painful, left-sided torticollis. **A:** Plain lateral radiograph shows fusion of C2-C3 and absence of the ring of C1 with occipitalization. **B:** The MRI shows an Arnold-Chiari malformation, with herniation of the cerebellar tonsils into the foramen magnum (*arrow*). Also note the cordal edema (*arrowhead*). **C:** The child underwent an occipital decompression and laminectomy to C3, posterior cervical fusion from the occiput to C4, and halo cast immobilization for 4 months. Flexion and extension lateral radiographs 1 year after treatment show solid incorporation of the fusion from C2-C4, with dissolution of the graft from the occiput to C2. However, there is no atlantooccipital instability. The child's symptoms resolved.

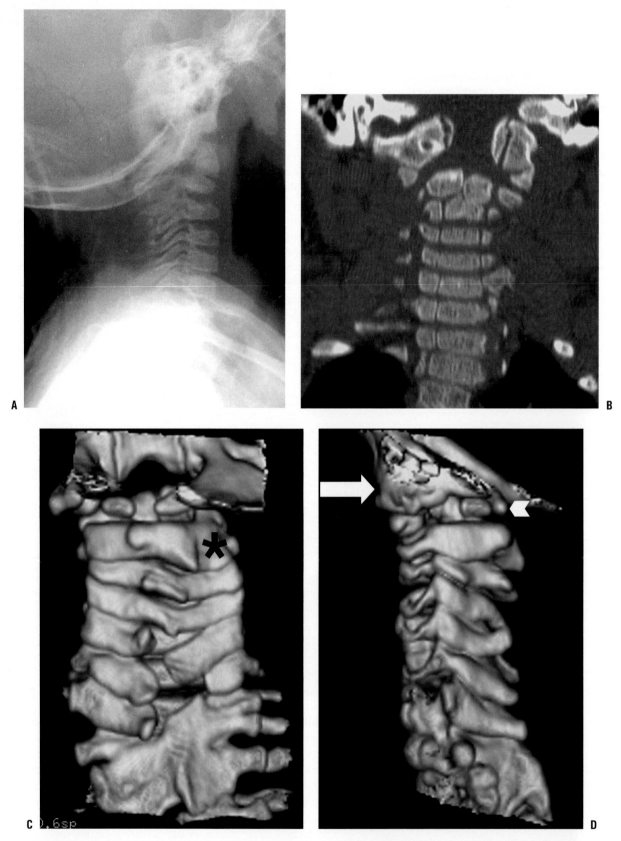

FIGURE 21-9. This 14-month-old girl presented with a history of torticollis since birth, with no response to physical therapy. Prenatal and birth history was unremarkable. Physical exam demonstrated a short neck with no sternocleidomastoid muscle contracture. **A:** A lateral cervical spine radiograph demonstrates overlap of the posterior elements and absence of the anterior portion of the C1 ring. **B:** A CT scan demonstrates multiple abnormal ossification centers of C2. **C:** A three-dimensional CT scan demonstrates fusion of the lateral masses and posterior elements of C2-C3 on the right (*asterisk*) and **D:** Fusion of the anterior atlas and skull base (*arrow*) with the posterior arch of C1 in a normal position (*arrowhead*).

occipital pain, vertigo, ataxia, limb paresis, paresthesias, speech disturbances, hoarseness, diplopia, syncope, auditory malfunction, and dysphagia (92, 93).

Standard radiographs are difficult to obtain because of fixed bony deformities and overlapping shadows from the mandible, occiput, and foramen magnum. An x-ray beam directed 90 degrees perpendicular to the skull (rather than the cervical spine) usually gives a satisfactory view of the occipitocervical junction. The anomaly usually is studied further with CT. In young children, the head-wag autotomography technique can be quite useful (94). This technique involves side-to-side rotation of the child's head, while a slow AP radiographic exposure of the upper cervical spine is performed. This rotation blurs the overlying head and mandibular structures, allowing for improved visualization of the occiput-C1-C2 complex.

The position of the odontoid relative to the opening of the foramen magnum has been described by measuring the distance from the posterior aspect of the odontoid to the posterior ring of C1 or the posterior lip of the foramen magnum, whichever is closer (87, 95). This should be determined in flexion because this position maximizes the reduction in the SAC. If this distance is <19 mm, a neurologic deficit is usually present. Lateral flexion and extension views of the upper cervical spine often show up to 12 mm of space between the odontoid and the C1 ring anteriorly (87); associated C1-C2 instability has been reported to develop eventually in 50% of these patients.

MRI is used to image the neural structures. Flexion-extension MRI is often necessary to fully evaluate the pathology (96). Compression of the brain stem or upper cervical cord anteriorly occurs from the backward-projecting odontoid. This produces a range of findings and symptoms, depending on the location and degree of compression. Pyramidal tract signs and symptoms (e.g., spasticity, hyperreflexia, muscle weakness, gait disturbances) are most common, although signs of cranial nerve involvement (e.g., diplopia, tinnitus, dysphagia, auditory disturbances) can be seen. Compression from the posterior lip of the foramen magnum or dural constricting band can disturb the posterior columns, with a loss of proprioception, vibration, and tactile senses. Nystagmus also occurs frequently as a result of posterior cerebellar compression. Vascular disturbances from vertebral artery involvement can result in brain stem ischemia, manifested by syncope, seizures, vertigo, and unsteady gait (97). Cerebellar tonsil herniation can occur. The altered mechanics of the cervical spine may result in a dull, aching pain in the posterior occiput and the neck with intermittent stiffness and torticollis. Irritation of the greater occipital nerve may cause tenderness in the posterior scalp.

The natural history of atlantooccipital anomalies is unknown. The neurologic symptoms may develop so late and progress so slowly because the frequently associated C1-C2 instability progresses with age, and the increased demands placed on the C1-C2 interval produce gradual spinal cord or vertebral artery compromise.

Treatment is difficult. Surgery for atlantooccipital anomalies is more risky than with isolated anomalies of the odontoid (82, 93). For this reason, nonoperative methods should be initially attempted. Cervical collars, braces, and traction often

help for persistent complaints of head and neck pain, especially after minor trauma or infection. Immobilization may achieve only temporary relief if neurologic deficits are present. Patients with evidence of a compromised upper cervical area should take precautions not to expose themselves to undue trauma.

When symptoms and signs of C1-C2 instability are present, a posterior C1-C2 fusion is indicated. Preliminary traction to attempt reduction is used if necessary. If a reduction is possible and there are no neurologic signs, surgery has an improved prognosis (82, 92, 93). Posterior signs and symptoms may be an indication for posterior decompression depending on the evidence of dural or osseous compression. Results vary from complete resolution to increased deficits and death (82, 98). In the instance of no instability but only compressive pathology, the role of concomitant posterior fusion has not yet been determined. However, if decompression, whether anterior or posterior, can destabilize the spine, then concomitant posterior fusion should be considered (86, 99, 100).

If occiput-C1 instability is present, then occiput–atlanto–cervical fusion is indicated (Figs. 21-10 to 21-16). These cases are often associated with posterior decompressions/laminectomies.

Occipitoatlantocervical instability requiring occipitocervical fusion is often complicated by the fact that decompression of the base of the skull and the upper two cervical vertebrae is either required or the cause of the instability. These circumstances compromise the ability to achieve fusion because of the lack of bone surface to form a bed for the grafts, the large gap that must be bridged, and the instability (101). In addition, it has been demonstrated that the conventional cervical orthoses do not provide much immobilization for the upper cervical spine (102).

To circumvent these problems and to provide stability to the fusion area, surgeons have developed methods of internal fixation (103, 104). Since these reports, fixation using screws and plates has become more popular in many centers, but these techniques require a considerable learning curve and are often not amenable to the very small child with small anatomy or the dysplastic anatomy secondary to dysplasia/dwarfisms. In the small child, a useful technique that has proved effective is the use of rib or other cortical-cancellous graft to provide an element of stability, as well as to serve as the graft for the fusion. This is supplemented by the use of a halo orthosis. A combined team approach with neurosurgery is often helpful in these complicated cases.

Unilateral Absence of C1. This congenital malformation of the first cervical vertebra is, in essence, a hemiatlas or a congenital scoliosis of C1. Doubousset (105) described 17 patients with this absence. No definite population incidence is known. The problem often is associated with other anomalies common to children with congenital spine deformities (e.g., tracheoesophageal fistula).

Two-thirds of the children present at birth; the others develop torticollis and are noticed later. A lateral translation of the head on the trunk, with variable degrees of lateral tilt and rotation (best appreciated from the back) is the typical finding.

Text continued on page 838

Occipitocervical Facet Fusion After Laminectomy (Figs. 21-10 to 21-16).

FIGURE 21-10. The patient is positioned in the prone position. If the halo has not been applied to the skull, it is done before the patient is turned prone. The halo may be attached to the operating table by use of a specially designed attachment, or it may be attached to a traction, depending on the needs of the case.

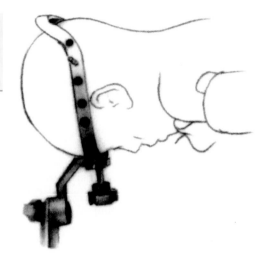

FIGURE 21-11. After the usual skin preparation and draping, a midline incision is used to expose the base of the skull and the cervical vertebrae to be fused. It is important to carry the subperiosteal dissection far enough laterally to have sufficient bone remaining after the laminectomy but not so far as to get into the venous plexus lateral to the facet joints or especially the vertebral artery at the C1 level. In the average-sized adult, the dissection should not proceed further than 1.5 cm lateral to the midline, to avoid the vertebral artery as it crosses the arch of C1. In the child, 1 cm is a safe limit to observe. The laminectomy and suboccipital decompressions are performed as indicated.

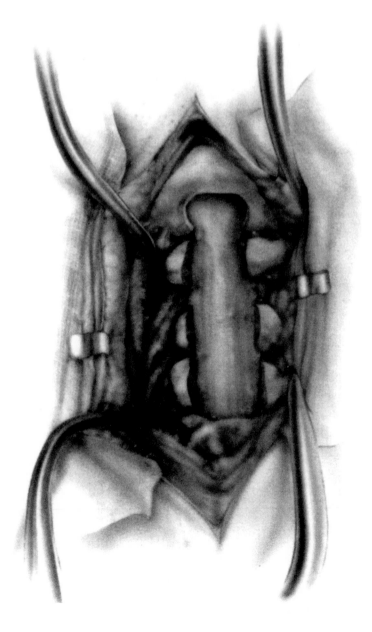

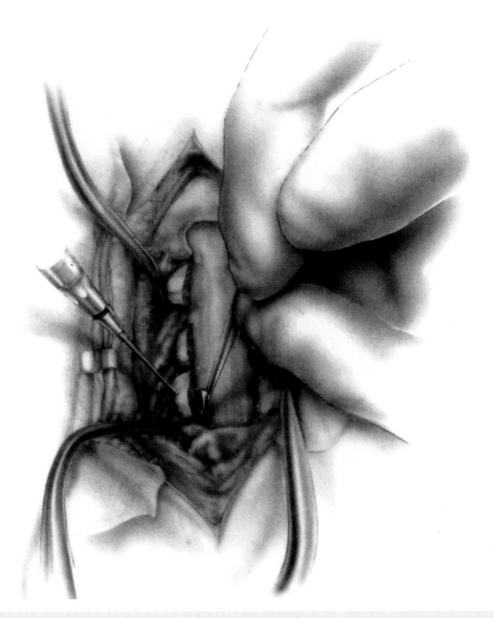

FIGURE 21-12.   After completion of the laminectomy, a small periosteal elevator is used to dissect the periosteum off the underside of the remaining portions of the lamina. A small thin elevator is then placed under the lamina to protect the dura. Using a high-speed drill, a small hole is made in each lamina through which a wire is passed. Care must be taken to be certain that the elevator is under the portion of the lamina that the drill will penetrate. If the occiput is included in the fusion, holes are made in the occiput. It is extremely important that this is done by someone with expertise in this field who is familiar with the anatomy of the base of the skull because the large venous sinuses in this area must be avoided.

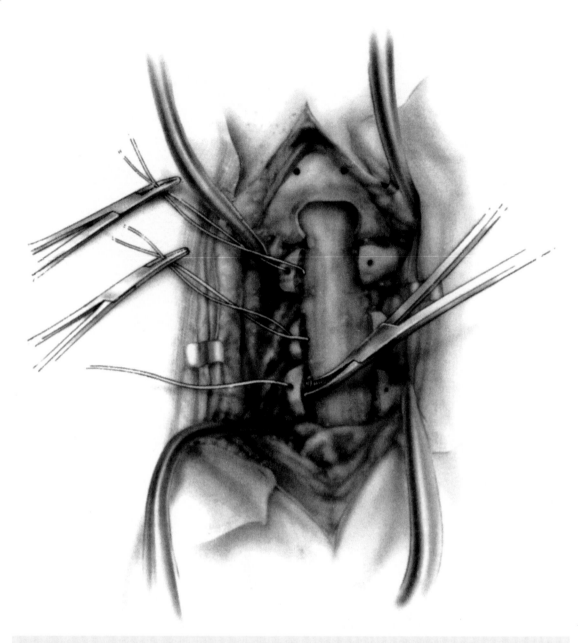

FIGURE 21-13. Depending on the size of the child and the lamina, a flexible wire (22-gauge), braided wire, or flexible cable is passed through each of the holes. If a wire is used, a small hemostat is used to reach under the lamina to grasp it as it comes through. After it is grasped, the wire is turned acutely so that it does not tear or puncture the dura, and it is then pulled through. If the child is large enough, braided cables are preferred because they are flexible and easier to use than wire.

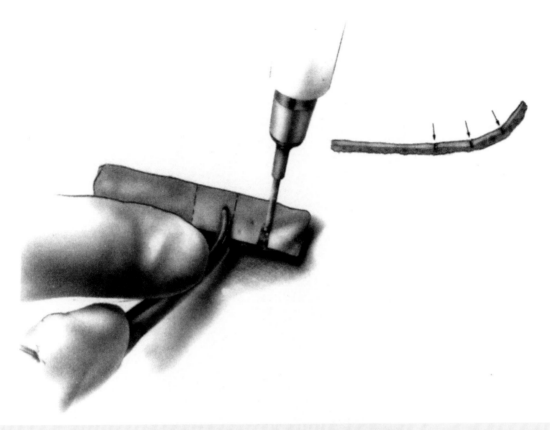

FIGURE 21-14.   The bone graft can be either rib or corticocancellous bone from the iliac crest. The advantage of corticocancellous bone is that the thick portion of cancellous bone can be placed directly against the lamina. Rib graft has the advantage of strength, which imparts additional stability to the spine. Although either the rib or a portion of the iliac crest may have the general contour desired for the cervical spine, it is usually necessary to bend the graft so that more curve is present to bring the graft in contact with the C1 lamina before it turns up onto the skull. This may be accomplished by kerfing the graft. A *kerf* is a cut or channel made by a saw. This can be accomplished by use of the high-speed drill to cut through the cortex on the concave side of the curve in the graft. After the graft has been harvested, cut, and bent to the desired shape, holes are placed in it to correspond to the holes in the lamina over which it will lie. This can be done by holding the graft over the operative site while estimating the correct placement of the hole or by marking the site with a marking pen and then removing the graft to the back table to cut the holes.

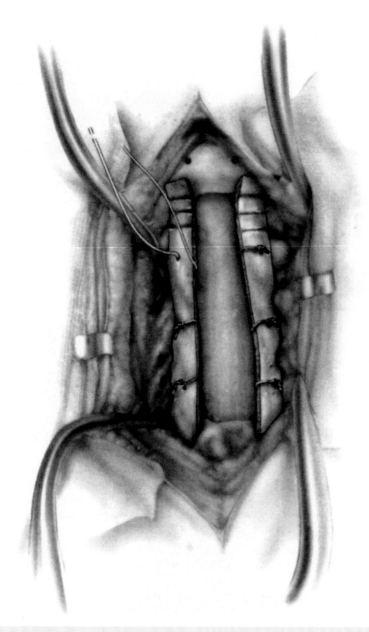

FIGURE 21-15.   The portion of the wire or cable coming through the surface of the lamina is drawn through the bone graft. The segment of the wire coming from under the lamina is brought around the graft. This pushes the graft laterally and prevents it from coming to lie over the dura. If there is no additional internal fixation, the graft is held firmly against the lamina while the wires or cables are tightened.

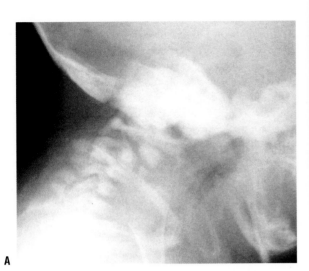

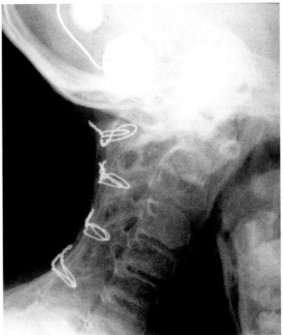

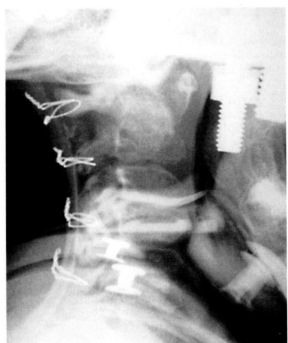

A

B

C

FIGURE 21-16.   A: The lateral radiograph of a 6-month-old child with Kniest syndrome, respiratory difficulty, cervical instability and narrow spinal canal. **B:** One month after extensive decompression and grafting, the ribs can be seen fixed to the remaining lamina. The patient is in a halo vest. She has had a cochlear implant. **C:** Seven years later, the incorporation of the graft and solid arthrodesis is seen. Although there is a small gap between the rib grafts and the base of the skull, no motion can be demonstrated at the craniocervical junction.

There also may be severe tilting of the eye line. The sterno-cleidomastoid muscle is not tight, although regional aplasia of the muscles in the nuchal concavity of the tilted side is noted. Neck flexibility is variable and decreases with age. The condition is not painful. Plagiocephaly can occur and increases as the deformity increases. Neurologic signs (e.g., headache, vertigo, myelopathy) are present in about one-fourth of the patients. The natural history is unknown.

Standard AP and lateral radiographs rarely give the diagnosis, although the open-mouth odontoid view may suggest it. Tomograms or CT scans usually are needed to see the anomaly (Fig. 21-17). The defect can range from a hypoplasia of the lateral mass to a complete hemiatlas with rotational instability and basilar impression. Occasionally, the atlas is occipitalized. There are three types of this disorder. Type I is an isolated hemiatlas. Type II is a partial or complete aplasia of one hemiatlas, with other associated anomalies of the cervical spine (e.g., fusion of C3-C4, congenital bars in the lower cervical vertebrae). Type III is a partial or complete atlantooccipital fusion and symmetric or asymmetric hemiatlas aplasia, with or without anomalies of the odontoid and the lower cervical vertebrae.

Once this malformation is diagnosed, entire spinal radiographs should be taken to rule out other congenital vertebral anomalies. Other imaging studies that may be needed are vertebral angiography and MRI. Angiography should be performed if operative intervention is undertaken, because arterial anomalies (e.g., multiple loops, vessels smaller than normal, abnormal routes between C1 and C2) often are found on the aplastic side. MRI also should be performed if operative intervention is undertaken, because many of these children will have stenosis of the foramen magnum, and occasionally an Arnold-Chiari malformation.

The deformity should be observed to document the presence or absence of progression. This observation is primarily clinical (e.g., photographs) because radiographic measurements are difficult if not impossible to obtain. Bracing does not halt progression of the deformity. Surgical intervention is recommended in those patients with severe deformities. A preoperative halo is used for gradual traction correction over 6 to 8 days. An ambulatory method of gradual cervical spine deformity correction has been described using the halo-Ilizarov technique (106). A posterior fusion from the occiput-C2 or -C3 is then performed, depending on the extent of the anomaly. Decompression of the spinal canal is necessary when the canal size is not ample, either at that time or if it is projected not to be able to fully accommodate the developed spinal cord. The ideal age for posterior fusion is between the ages of 5 and 8 years, corresponding to the age at which the canal size reaches adult proportions.

Familial Cervical Dysplasia. The epidemiology of this atlas deformity (107) is not known. Clinical presentation varies from an incidental finding to a passively correctable head tilt,

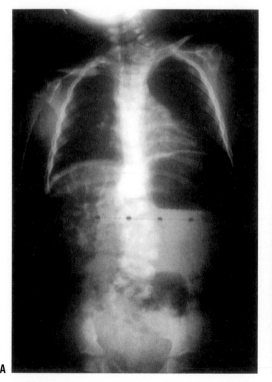

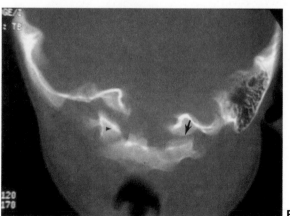

FIGURE 21-17. This 4-year, 10-month-old boy presented with a torticollis. **A:** The standing AP radiograph of his entire spine documents the head tilt to the left, along with left sided hemivertebrae in the left lower cervical spine. Also note the multiple hemivertebrae in the thoracic and lumbar spine. **B:** A CT scan with frontal reconstruction clearly demonstrates an absent lateral mass of C1 (*arrow*) with a normal right lateral mass (*arrowhead*). This thus represents a Doubosset-type II C1 unilateral absence.

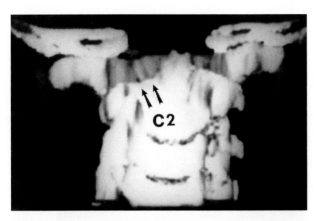

FIGURE 21-18.   A three-dimensional computed tomographic scan of the upper cervical cord in a child with familial cervical dysplasia. The left superior facet of C2 is shallow and hypoplastic (*arrows*). (From Saltzman CL, Hensinger RN, Blane CE, et al. Familial cervical dysplasia. *J Bone Joint Surg Am* 1991;73-A:163–171, with permission.)

suboccipital pain, decreased cervical motion, or a clunking of the upper cervical spine.

Plain radiographs are difficult to interpret. Various anomalies of C1, most commonly a partial absence of the posterior ring of C1, typically are seen. Various anomalies of C2 also commonly exist, for example, a shallow hypoplastic left facet. Other dysplasias of the lateral masses, facets, and posterior elements and occasionally spondylolisthesis are seen. Occiput-C1 instability is frequently seen; C1-C2 instability rarely is seen. The delineation of this complex anatomy often is seen best with a CT scan and a three-dimensional reconstruction (Fig. 21-18). When symptoms of instability are present, MRI in flexion and extension is recommended to assess the presence and magnitude of neural compression. Occipitocervical junction instability due to the malformation may lead to neural compromise.

Nonsurgical treatment consists of observation every 6 to 12 months to ensure that instability does not develop, either clinically (e.g., progressive weakness and fatigue or objective signs of myelopathy), or radiographically, with lateral flexion and extension radiographs. Surgical intervention is recommended for persistent pain, torticollis, and neurologic symptoms. A posterior fusion from the occiput to C2 usually is required, with gradual preoperative reduction using an adjustable halo cast (106).

Atlantoaxial Rotary Displacement.   Atlantoaxial rotary displacement is one of the most common causes of childhood torticollis. Rotary displacements are characteristically a pediatric problem, but they may occur in adults. There are several causes. Because the resultant radiographic findings and treatment regimens are the same for all pediatric causes, they are discussed as a unit and individual exceptions are noted where necessary.

The confusing terminology includes rotary dislocation, rotary deformity, rotational subluxation, rotary fixation, and spontaneous hyperemic dislocation (108, 109). "Atlantoaxial rotary subluxation" is probably the most accepted term used in describing the common childhood torticollis. "Subluxation" is misleading, however, because cases of "subluxation" usually present within the normal range of motion of the atlantoaxial joint. "Rotary displacement" is a more appropriate and descriptive term because it includes the entire range of pathology, from mild subluxation to complete dislocation. If the deformity persists, the children present with a resistant and unresolving torticollis that is best termed "atlantoaxial rotary fixation or fixed atlantoaxial displacement." Gradations exist between the very mild, easily correctable rotary displacement and the rigid fixation. Complete atlantoaxial rotary dislocation rarely has been reported in surviving patients.

The radiographic findings of rotary displacement are difficult to demonstrate (110). With rotary torticollis the lateral mass of C1 that has rotated anterior appears wider and closer to the midline (medial offset), whereas the opposite lateral mass is narrower and away from the midline (lateral offset). The facet joints may be obscured because of apparent overlapping. The lateral view shows the wedge-shaped lateral mass of the atlas lying anteriorly where the oval arch of the atlas normally lies, and the posterior arches fail to superimpose because of the head tilt (Fig. 21-19). These findings may suggest occipitalization of C1 because with the neck tilt the skull may obscure C1. The normal relation between the occiput and C1 is believed to be maintained in children with atlantoaxial rotary displacement. A lateral radiograph of the skull may demonstrate the relative positions of C1 and C2 more clearly than a lateral radiograph of the cervical spine. This is because tilting of the head also tilts C1, which creates overlapping shadows and makes interpretation of a lateral spinal radiograph difficult.

The difficulty with plain radiographs is differentiating the position of C1-C2 in a child with subluxation from that in a normal child whose head is rotated, since both give the same picture. Open-mouth views are difficult to obtain and interpret, and the lack of cooperation and the diminished motion on the part of the child often make it impossible to obtain these special views. Cineradiography has been recommended, but the radiation dose is high and patient cooperation may be difficult because of muscle spasms (110, 111). CT scans are helpful in this situation if it is done properly (112). A CT scan, when taken with the head in the torticollic position, may be interpreted by the casual observer as showing rotation of C1 on C2. If the rotation of C1 on C2 is within the normal range, as it usually is early on in this condition, the observer may attribute this rotation to patient positioning. A dynamic-rotation CT scan is helpful here. Views with the head maximally rotated to the right, and then to the left, will demonstrate atlantoaxial rotary fixation when there is a loss of normal rotation (Fig. 21-19). There are varying degrees of "locking" between the C1 and C2 vertebrae (113–115).

Rotary displacement can be classified into four types (Fig. 21-20) (108): type I is a simple rotary displacement without an anterior shift, type II is rotary displacement

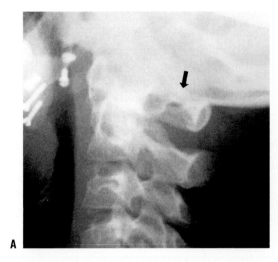

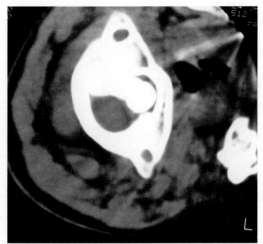

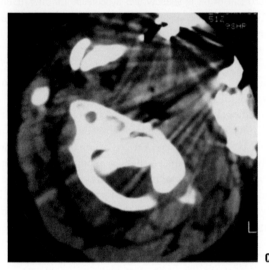

FIGURE 21-19. Radiographic findings in atlantoaxial rotary subluxation. **A:** The lateral cervical spinal radiograph. The posterior arches fail to superimpose because of the head tilt (*arrow*). Dynamic CT scans in a 9-year-old girl with a fixed atlantoaxial rotary displacement, with the head maximally rotated to the left (**B**), and the head maximally rotated to the right (**C**), which, in this case, does not reach the midline. The ring of C1 is still in the exact relation to the odontoid as in (**B**), indicating a fixed displacement.

FIGURE 21-20. The four types of atlantoaxial rotary displacement. (From Fielding JW, Hawkins RJ. Atlanto-axial rotatory fixation. *J Bone Joint Surg Am* 1977;59-A:37–44, with permission.)

with an anterior shift of 5 mm or less, type III is rotary displacement with an anterior shift >5 mm, and type IV is rotary displacement with a posterior shift. The amount of anterior displacement considered to be pathologic is >3 mm in older children and adults and >4 mm in younger children (33). Flexion and extension lateral-stress radiographs are suggested to rule out the possibility of anterior displacement.

Type I is the most common pediatric type. It is usually benign and frequently resolves by itself. Type II deformity is potentially more dangerous. Types III and IV are very rare, but because of the potential for neurologic involvement and even instant death, management must be approached with great caution.

The etiology and pathoanatomy is not known completely (116). Several causative mechanisms are possible. Cervical spine fracture is a rare etiology. More commonly, atlantoaxial rotary displacement occurs following minor trauma [e.g., clavicle fractures (117)], after head and neck surgery including simple central line insertion (118), or after an upper respiratory infection. The children present with a "cocked-robin" torticollis and resist any attempt to move the head because of pain. The associated muscle spasm is noted on the side of the long sternocleidomastoid muscle because the muscle is attempting to correct the deformity, unlike congenital muscular torticollis where the muscle causes the torticollis. If the deformity becomes fixed, the pain subsides but the torticollis persists, along with decreased neck motion. In long-standing cases, plagiocephaly and facial flattening may develop on the side of the tilt.

Spontaneous atlantoaxial subluxation with inflammation of adjacent neck tissues, also known as Grisel syndrome, is commonly seen in children after upper respiratory infections (Fig. 21-21). The children are frequently febrile (119). A direct connection exists between the pharyngovertebral veins and the periodontal venous plexus and suboccipital epidural sinuses (120). This may provide a route for hematogenous transport of peripharyngeal septic exudates to the upper cervical spine and an anatomic explanation for the atlantoaxial hyperemia of Grisel syndrome. In long-standing cases, soft-tissue abscesses or vertebral osteomyelitis may develop (121–123). Regional lymphadenitis is known to cause spastic contracture of the cervical muscles. This muscular spasm, in the presence of abnormally loose ligaments (hypothetically caused by the hyperemia of the pharyngovertebral vein drainage), could produce locking of the overlapping lateral joint edges of the articular facets. This prevents easy repositioning, resulting in atlantoaxial rotary displacement. The hyperemia after surgery of the oral pharynx, most frequently tonsillectomy and adenoidectomy,

enhances the passage of the inflammatory products into the pharyngovertebral veins. It is known that patients may develop Grisel syndrome after otolaryngologic procedures (124), especially with monopolar electrocautery (125). Kawabe and Tang (126, 127) have demonstrated meniscus-like synovial folds in the atlantooccipital and lateral atlantoaxial joints of children, but not in those of adults, and have found that the dens–facet angle of the axis is steeper in children than in adults. They postulate that excessive C1-C2 rotation, caused by the steeper angle, compounded by ligament laxity from an underlying hyperemia, allows the meniscus-like synovial folds to become impinged in the lateral atlantoaxial joint, leading to rotary fixation. The predominance of this syndrome in childhood correlates with the predilection for the adenoids to be maximally hypertrophied and inflamed at this same time, and located in the area drained by the pharyngo-vertebral veins.

Most atlantoaxial rotary displacements resolve spontaneously. Rarely, however, the pain subsides and the torticollis becomes fixed. The duration of symptoms and deformity dictates the recommended treatment (128).

Patients with rotary subluxation of <1 week can be treated with immobilization in a soft cervical collar and rest for about 1 week. Close follow-up is mandatory. If spontaneous reduction does not occur with this initial treatment, hospitalization and the use of halter traction, muscle relaxants (e.g., diazepam), and analgesics is recommended next. Patients with rotary subluxation of >1 week but <1 month should be hospitalized immediately for cervical traction, relaxants, and analgesics. Gentle halo traction is occasionally needed to achieve reduction. The reduction is noted clinically and confirmed with a dynamic CT scan. If no anterior displacement is noted after reduction, cervical support should be continued only as long as symptoms persist. If there is anterior displacement, immobilization should be continued for 6 weeks to allow ligamentous healing to occur. In patients with rotary subluxation for more than 1 month, cervical traction (usually halo skeletal) can be tried for up to 3 weeks, but the prognosis is guarded. These children usually fall into two groups: those whose rotary subluxation can be reduced with halo traction but, despite a prolonged period of immobilization, resubluxate when the immobilization is stopped and those whose subluxation cannot be reduced, and is fixed. It has been recently shown that those patients with recurrence of deformity have a larger difference in the lateral mass–dens interval on the initial AP radiograph (129).

When the deformity is fixed, especially when anterior C1 displacement is present, the transverse atlantal ligament is compromised with a potential for catastrophe. In this situation, posterior C1-C2 fusion should be performed. The indications for fusion are neurologic involvement, anterior displacement, failure to achieve and maintain correction, a deformity that has been present for more than 3 months, and recurrence of deformity following an adequate trial of conservative management (at least 6 weeks of immobilization after reduction). Before surgical fusion halo traction for several days is used to obtain as much straightening of the head and neck

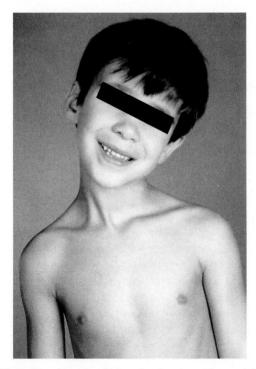

FIGURE 21-21. A 5-year-old boy developed an atlantoaxial rotary subluxation after an upper respiratory viral infection (Grisel syndrome). It rapidly resolved after treatment with a soft collar and mild doses of diazepam.

Text continued on page 845

Gallie Fusion (Figs. 21-22 to 21-30)

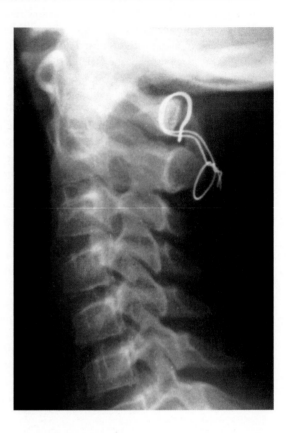

FIGURE 21-22. The child in Figure 21-19 had a fixed deformity that occurred 6 months earlier, immediately after reconstructive maxillofacial surgery for Goldenhar syndrome. It did not respond to traction, including halo traction. She underwent a posterior C1-C2 (Gallie-type) fusion. A solid fusion was present 9 months later; clinically, the patient achieved 80 degrees of rotation to the left and 45 degrees of rotation to the right.

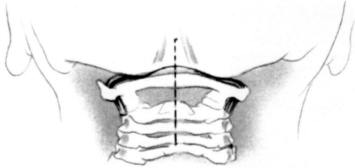

FIGURE 21-23. The most common arthrodesis of the cervical spine is between the axis and the atlas because of the numerous congenital and developmental problems that affect this region. Although several techniques have been advocated to achieve arthrodesis of these vertebrae, the technique attributed to Gallie (130) is the most reliable and the easiest to apply in children. In this technique, the wire not only helps to pull C1 back into position and hold it there but also holds the bone graft firmly in place (131, 132). Occasionally, the posterior arch of C1 is not formed completely, making this technique impossible; in these cases other techniques need to be used, such as only grafting with halo immobilization (104).

In cases in which there is a great deal of instability with chance for neurologic injury, it is preferred to place the patient in a halo vest or cast first. This can be done under local or general anesthesia, as needed. Reduction is achieved and confirmed by radiographs. If the halo was applied with the patient awake, anesthesia is then induced and the child turned prone for the posterior fusion. No head rest is necessary, and there is little danger of neurologic injury while carefully intubating and moving the patient with the halo vest in place.

The occipital region of the skull is shaved, and the posterocervical area and the posterior iliac crest are prepared and draped. The incision extends in the midline from the base of the skull to the spinous process of C4. Dissection is carried down to the tips of the spinous processes. At this point, a metal hub needle is placed in the spinous process of C2 and a lateral radiograph is taken. This is done to positively identify the correct vertebrae for exposure. In the young child, exposure of the base of the skull or any additional vertebrae may result in "creeping fusion."

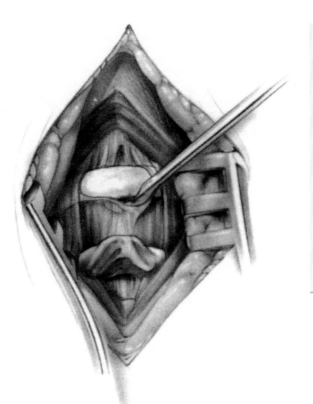

FIGURE 21-24. After correct identification of the levels involved, the posterior arch of C1 and the lamina of C2 are exposed subperiosteally by a combination of sharp and blunt dissection. It is important to remember that the vertebral arteries are unprotected by the bony foramen at the C1 level just lateral to the facets. In small children this is approximately 1 cm from the midline; in bigger children it is approximately 1.5 cm from the midline. In the child with an unreduced atlantoaxial rotatory fixation, the lamina of C1 will not be parallel with the floor, but one hemilamina will be angled upward and the other downward. It is extremely important to remember this pathologic anatomy when exposing C1.

To prepare the arch of C1 for the passage of the wire beneath it, the periosteum must be separated from its anterior surface. This can be accomplished with a small, angulated, neural elevator. The spinal canal does not need to be opened. After this, a dental burr can be used to decorticate the exposed lamina of C1 and C2. This does not have to be as deep a decortication as is performed in scoliosis cases.

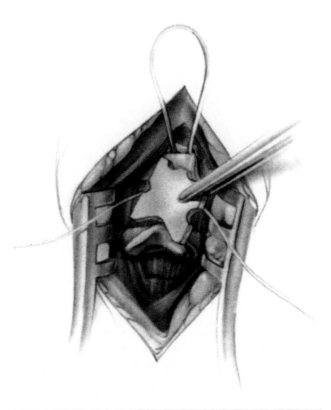

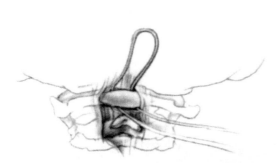

FIGURE 21-25. A double wire is passed under the arch of C1 from inferior to superior. The wire is bent back on itself, forming a smooth loop. Care should be taken not to introduce any sharp bends in the wire. The size of the wire depends on both the child's size and the surgeon's preference. Any size from 18- to 22-gauge can be used. Good-quality, fully annealed flexible wire allows a relatively larger size to be used because it pulls through easily without kinking.

FIGURE 21-26. The corticocancellous graft, which has previously been obtained and fashioned to fit over the lamina of C1 and C2, is now put in place. Small pieces of cancellous bone can be added beneath the corticocancellous graft. The loop of wire is pulled from under the arch of C1 over the graft and is placed around the spinous process of C2. A small notch cut in the base of the C2 spinous process helps to keep this in place.

FIGURE 21-27. The two ends of the wire that come out from under the arch of C1 inferiorly are pulled tight and brought around the sides and over the top of the graft. It is at this point, when the surgeon is pulling the wire tight, that the importance of a flexible wire that is not too large is realized. In working with the wire, it is best to keep it taut. This minimizes the possibility of the wire impinging on the spinal cord and makes tightening easier. After the wire is pulled tight, it can be secured with a wire twister.

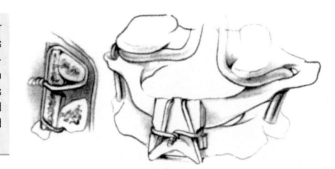

FIGURE 21-28. In children, the spinous process of C2 is often small and does not provide much strength for fixation of the wire. The spinous process K-wire technique is an alternative technique (133). A threaded K wire of appropriate size is passed through a small stab wound on the side of the neck and through the paravertebral muscles and is drilled through the spinous process of C2. It is cut so that approximately 1 cm is protruding on each side.

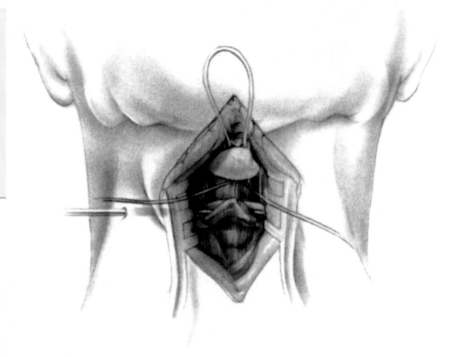

FIGURE 21-29. The corticocancellous graft is then put in place. It should fit under the K wire. The loop of wire that comes from under the arch of C1 is then drawn over the graft and looped around the spinous process of C2. The wire loop will be under the transverse Kirschner wire, however, which keeps it from slipping off the spinous process.

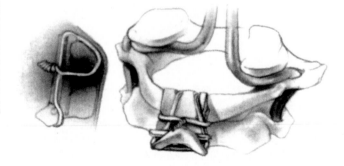

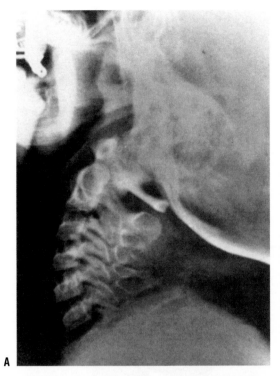

A

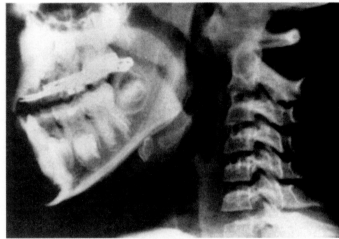

B

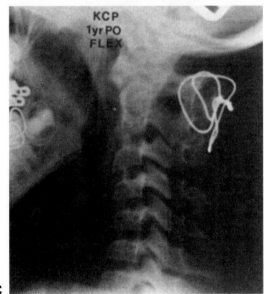

C

FIGURE 21-30. An 8-year-old child with a history of occipital headaches was observed by her orthodontist to have an absent odontoid. The extension lateral view of the cervical spine (**A**) demonstrates the os odontoideum. The flexion lateral radiograph (**B**) demonstrates the instability. One year after a posterior arthrodesis of C1 and C2 (**C**) with fixation by the Gallie technique, the spine is stable. Note the creeping fusion between the spinous processes of C2 and C3 where the interspinous ligament was cut.

(*Postoperative Care:* There should be radiographic evidence of solid arthrodesis in 10 to 12 weeks. The postoperative care concerns what type of immobilization should be used until that time. Our preference has been to leave the halo on for approximately 6 to 8 weeks in young and unreliable children, followed by some type of collar for an additional 4 weeks. In reliable adolescents, in whom the bone is stronger, a Philadelphia collar or similar device is usually adequate.)

as possible, a forceful or manipulative reduction should not be performed. Postoperatively, the child is simply positioned in a halo cast or vest in the straightened position obtained preoperatively; this usually obtains satisfactory alignment. A Gallie-type fusion with sublaminar wiring at the ring of C1 and through the spinous process of C2 is preferred to a Brooks-type fusion in which the wire is sublaminar at both C1 and C2. This is because of the decreased SAC at C2 with a higher risk of neurologic injury. This wiring does not reduce the displacement but simply provides some internal stability for the arthrodesis. The overall results for a Gallie fusion are very good (see Figs. 21-22 to 21-30) (131). Long-term results do not

indicate any significant abnormalities of the sagittal profile (134). In the nonreduced rotatory fixation, transarticular C1-C2 screw fixation is contraindicated due to the pathologic anatomy from the rotational deformity (Figs. 21-31 to 21-37). A few surgeons advocate reduction of the deformity (135, 136); if a fusion is later needed and the deformity reduced, then transarticular C1-C2 screw fixation can be used if appropriate size screws are available.

Author's Preferred Treatment. Patients with rotary subluxation of <1 week are treated with immobilization in a soft cervical collar and rest for about 1 week. If spontaneous reduction does

Text continued on page 853

Alternative to Gallie Fusion (Figs. 21-31 to 21-37)

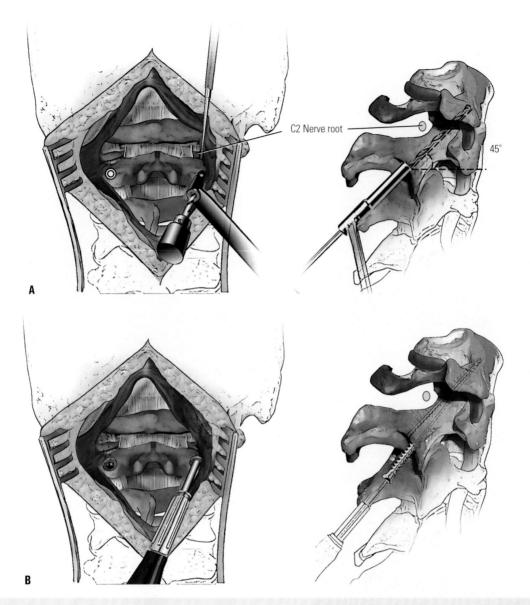

FIGURE 21-31. An alternative technique to the standard Gallie fusion uses either transarticular C1-C2 screws or lateral mass screws for both C1 and C2 with plate or rod connection. This technique can be used if there is an anatomic reduction of C1-C2 facets, but is not possible if there is atlantoaxial rotatory subluxation/fixation or anterior subluxation of the ring of C1 relative to the odontoid. The technique is the same through the exposure of the lamina of C1 and C2. The same precaution regarding the vertebral artery is necessary.

A: After exposure of the C1-C2 facet, transarticular screws may be placed. The C2-C3 facet capsule and upper portion of the C3 lamina needs to be clearly seen, and then the superior and medial aspect of the C2 lateral mass/pedicle is gently exposed with a Penfield dissector. The C2 nerve root exits laterally from the spinal canal overlying the C1-C2 joint ; it is undermined and mobilized with the Penfield dissector, and then the roof of the C2 pedicle is followed into the C1-C2 facet joint. The Penfield dissector is used to palpate the medial wall of the C2 pedicle. Under fluoroscopic guidance, the trajectory for the screw is confirmed. The typical trajectory is 15 degrees medial (to avoid the vertebral artery as the screw enters the C1 lateral mass) and 45 degrees cranial, crossing the C1-C2 facet and ending at the anterior arch of the atlas. The exact trajectory is confirmed with intraoperative fluoroscopy.

The C2 entry site is identified by first locating the inferomedial edge of the C2-C3 facet joint, without violating the joint or capsule. In an adult the entry site is ~3 mm superior and lateral to the inferomedial edge of the C2-C3 facet joint. This must be appropriately downsized in children. It is here that preoperative CT scans with sagittal and coronal reconstructions are necessary to determine appropriate trajectory, and screw diameter and length.

B: A high speed drill is used to pierce the outer cortex of the C2 lateral mass at this entry point, and then a guide wire from a cannulated screw set (if using cannulated screws) or an appropriate size drill (if using noncannulated screws) is directed up the C2 pedicle, across the C1-C2 facet joint, and into the lateral mass of C1, aiming for the anterior tubercle of C1.

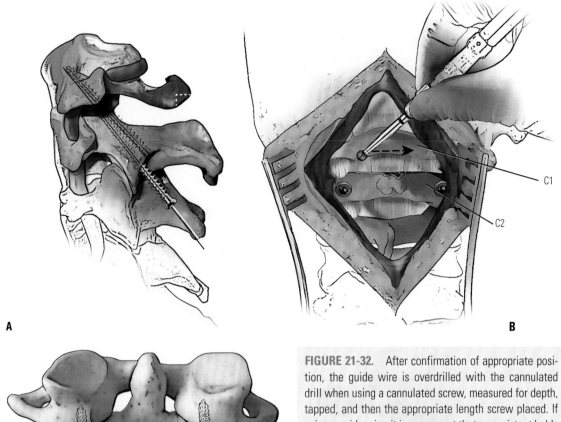

A

B

C1

C2

C

FIGURE 21-32. After confirmation of appropriate position, the guide wire is overdrilled with the cannulated drill when using a cannulated screw, measured for depth, tapped, and then the appropriate length screw placed. If using a guide wire, it is paramount that an assistant holds the wire with a needle driver while overdrilling, tapping, and placement of the screw to prevent it from advancing further anterior. This is performed bilaterally.

The posterior lamina of C1 and C2 are then decorticated and bone graft placed. Many authors also use a Gallie wiring to supplement this fixation, locking down the graft into the lamina of C1 and C2.

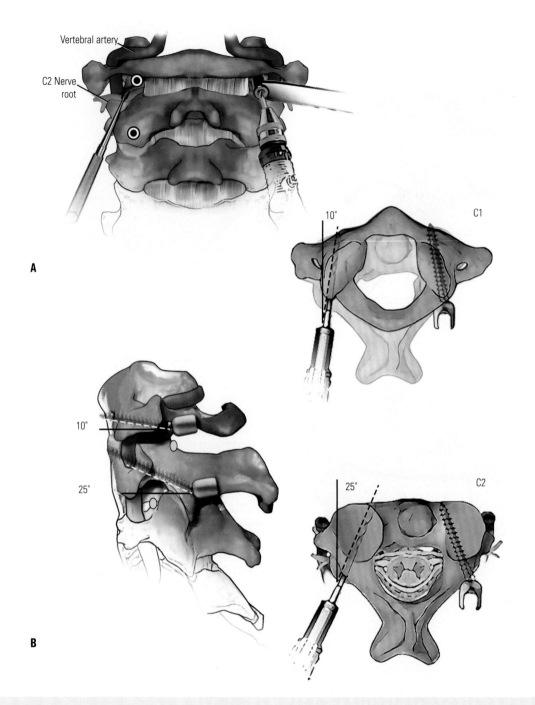

FIGURE 21-33. An alternative is to using lateral mass screws in both C1 and C2 linked with a rod. This entails the use of polyaxial screws. **A**: The entry point for the C1 lateral mass screw is at the midline of the lateral mass immediately inferior to the posterior arch of C1. Here again, the C2 nerve root exits laterally from the spinal canal overlying the C1-C2 joint and must be protected during screw placement. The high-speed drill is used to create the entry point, followed by placement of the screw after drilling. The trajectory for the drill is 0 to 10 degrees medial with intraoperative lateral fluoroscopy guiding the orientation of the drill into the lateral mass of C1 and engaging the anterior cortex. **B**: The hole is then tapped, measured, and a polyaxial screw placed, keeping the screw head above the C1 posterior arch. The C2 screw starting point is the same as for transarticular C1-C2 screw fixation, but the trajectory is more caudal and medial to avoid the transverse foramen.

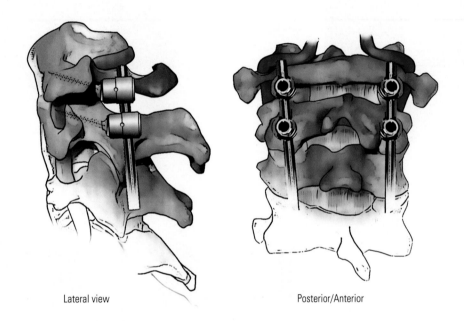

Lateral view   Posterior/Anterior

FIGURE 21-34.   After all the screws have been placed, contoured longitudinal rods are placed into the screw heads and tightened in position, followed by a crosslink construct. Arthrodesis is the same, decorticating the C1 and C2 lamina and placement of bone graft, typically before the crosslink is placed.

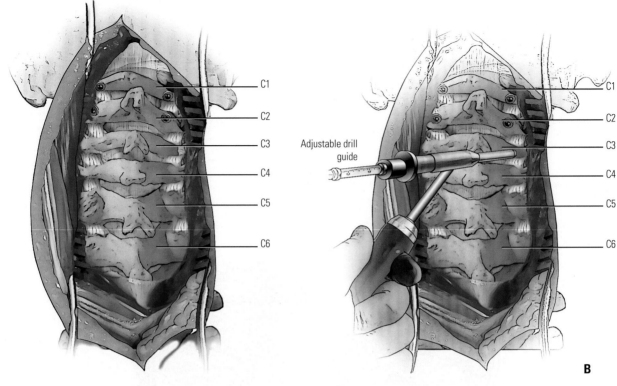

A

B

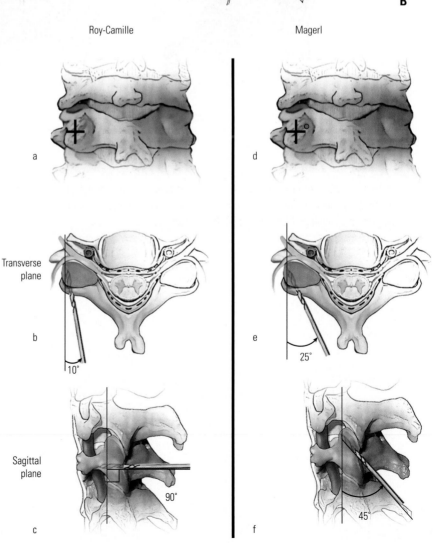

FIGURE 21-35. **A**: This technique can be extended into the subaxial spine, using polyaxial lateral mass screws or laminar hooks. **B,C**: There are two commonly used methods of lateral mass screw placement (Roy-Camille and Magerl). The Roy-Camille technique uses a starting point at the center of the lateral mass, with a trajectory directly perpendicular and 10 degrees lateral. The Magerl technique uses a starting point slightly medial and superior to the center of the lateral mass; in the sagittal plane the screw is oriented parallel to the surface of the superior articular facet (typically 15 to 30 degrees cranial) and 25 to 35 degrees lateral, with the screw tip engaging the superior and lateral portion of the ventral cortex of the superior facet. Fluoroscopic guidance is used to determine the exact trajectory in the sagittal plane.

C

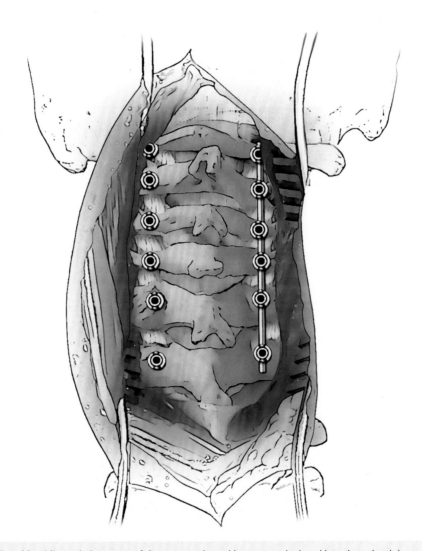

FIGURE 21-36. After bilateral placement of the screws, the rod is countered, placed into the polyaxial screws, and tightened in position. Standard decortication of the posterior elements and bone graft placement is performed for arthrodesis, followed by crosslink placement.

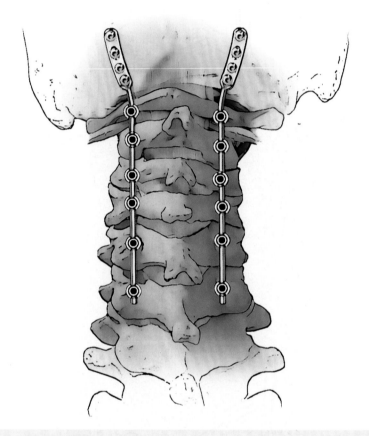

FIGURE 21-37. This technique can similarly be extended to the occiput. Many different manufacturers have occipital plates that change into rods for cervical spine fixation. When this technique is employed, it is typically best to place the C2 lateral mass screw first, followed by the subaxial lateral mass screws. Then the appropriate plate-rod construct is selected and contoured. The plate-rod construct is placed into the screw connectors. When the plate is against the occiput, drill holes in the outer cortex of the occiput are made, and appropriate-sized occipital screws are placed. A drill depth guide is strongly recommended to only drill the outer cortex. Again preoperative CT measurement of the occipital depth is useful. Standard arthrodesis is performed and then crosslinks placed.

not occur, halter traction, muscle relaxants (e.g., diazepam), and analgesics are prescribed. Patients with rotary subluxation of >1 week but <1 month should be hospitalized immediately for cervical traction, relaxants, and analgesics. Gentle halo traction is occasionally needed to achieve reduction. All reductions are confirmed with a dynamic CT scan. In patients with rotary subluxation for more than 1 month, cervical traction (usually halo skeletal) can be tried for up to 3 weeks, but the prognosis is guarded. If reduction cannot be achieved or maintained, then posterior C1-C2 arthrodesis is recommended (Fig. 21-23).

Nonosseous Types

Congenital Muscular Torticollis.   Congenital muscular torticollis, or congenital wry neck, is the most common cause of torticollis in the infant and young child, presenting at a median age of 2 months (137). The incidence of soft-tissues abnormalities in the neck as documented by ultrasound was approximately 4% in a series of 1021 newborn infants (138). The deformity is caused by contracture of the sternocleidomastoid muscle, with the head tilted toward the involved side and the chin rotated toward the opposite shoulder. A disproportionate number of these children have a history of a primiparous birth or a breech or difficult delivery. However, it has been reported in children with normal births and those born by cesarean section (137, 139, 140).

The exact cause is not known and there are several theories. Because of the birth history, one theory is that of a compartment syndrome occurring from soft-tissue compression of the neck at the time of delivery (141). Surgical histopathologic sections suggest venous occlusion of the sternocleidomastoid muscle (142). This occlusion may result in a compartment syndrome, as manifested by edema, degeneration of muscle fibers, and muscle fibrosis. This fibrosis is variable, ranging from small amounts to the entire muscle. It has been suggested that the clinical deformity is related to the ratio of fibrosis to remaining functional muscle. If ample muscle remains, the sternocleidomastoid will probably stretch with growth, and the child will not develop torticollis; if fibrosis predominates, there is little elastic potential, and torticollis will develop. Another theory is *in utero* crowding, since three of four children have the lesion on the right side (143) and up to 20% have developmental hip dysplasia (144). The fact that this condition can occur in children with normal birth histories or in children born by cesarean section challenges the perinatal compartment syndrome theory, and supports the *in utero* crowding theory. The fact that it can occur in families (145–147) (supporting a genetic predisposition) also questions the compartment syndrome theory. A third theory is primarily neurogenic (148), supported by histopathologic evidence of denervation and reinnervation. The primary myopathy initially may be due to trauma, ischemia, or both, and unequally involves the two heads of the sternocleidomastoid muscle. With continuing fibrosis of the sternal head, the branch of the spinal accessory nerve to the clavicular head of the muscle can be entrapped, leading to a later progressive deformity (148).

The final theory concerns mesenchymal cells remaining in the sternocleidomastoid from fetal embryogenesis. Recent histopathologic studies have demonstrated the presence of both myoblasts and fibroblasts in the sternocleidomastoid tumor in varying stages of differentiation and degeneration (149). The source of these myoblasts and fibroblasts is unknown. After birth, environmental changes stimulate these cells to differentiate, and the sternocleidomastoid tumor develops. Hemorrhagic and inflammatory reactions would be expected if the tumor was a result of perinatal birth trauma or intrauterine positioning, yet these cells were not seen in the sternocleidomastoid histopathologic studies. The occurrence of torticollis depends on the fate of the myoblasts in the mass. If the myoblasts undergo normal development and differentiation, then no persistent torticollis will occur and conservative treatment will likely succeed. If the myoblasts mainly undergo degeneration, then the remaining fibroblasts produce large amounts of collagen, with a scar-like contraction of the sternocleidomastoid muscle and the typical torticollis.

There are three clinical subgroups; those with sternocleidomastoid tumor (43% of cases), those with muscular torticollis (31% of cases), and postural torticollis (22% of cases) (150). The clinical features of congenital muscular torticollis depend on the age of the child. It is often discovered in the first 6 to 8 weeks of life. If the child is examined during the first 4 weeks of life, a mass or a "tumor" may be palpable in the neck (139). Although the mass may be palpable, it is unrecognized up to 80% of the time (151). Characteristically, it is a nontender, soft enlargement beneath the skin, and is located within the sternocleidomastoid muscle belly. This tumor reaches its maximum size within the first 4 weeks of life then gradually regresses. After 4 to 6 months of life, the contracture and the torticollis are the only clinical findings. In some children, the deformity is not noticed until after 1 year of age, which raises questions about both the congenital nature of this entity and the perinatal compartment syndrome theory. Recent studies (152) indicate that the rate of associated hip dysplasia in children with congenital muscular torticollis is 8%, lower than the previously cited 20% (144). The sternocleidomastoid tumor subgroup, the most severe group, presents at an earlier age, is associated with a higher incidence of breech presentation (19%), difficult labor (56%), and hip dysplasia (6.8%) (150).

If the deformity is progressive, skull and face deformities can develop (plagiocephaly) (153, 154), often within the first year of life. The facial flattening occurs on the side of the contracted muscle and is probably caused by the sleeping position of the child (155). In the United States, children usually sleep prone, and in this position, it is more comfortable for them to lie with the affected side down. The face therefore remodels to conform to the bed. If the child sleeps supine, reverse modeling of the contralateral skull occurs. In the child who is untreated for many years, the level of the eyes and ears becomes unequal and can result in considerable cosmetic deformity.

Ultrasound can be quite helpful in differentiating congenital muscular torticollis from other pathologies in the neck (138, 156). Radiographs of the cervical spine should be obtained to rule out associated congenital anomalies. Plain radiographs of the cervical spine in children with muscular torticollis are always normal, aside from the head tilt and rotation. If any suspicion exists about the status of the hips, appropriate imaging (e.g., ultrasonography, radiography) should be done, depending on the age of the child and the expertise of the ultrasonographer.

Research MRI studies demonstrate abnormal signals in the sternocleidomastoid muscle, but no discrete masses within the muscle (141, 157). The muscle diameter is increased two to four times that of the contralateral muscle. In older patients the signals are consistent with atrophy and fibrosis, similar to those encountered in compartment syndromes of the leg and forearm.

As the deficit in cervical rotation increases, the incidence of a previous sternocleidomastoid tumor, hip dysplasia, and the likelihood of needing surgery increases (158, 159). Treatment initially consists of conservative measures (139, 140, 151, 160, 161). Good results can be expected with stretching exercises alone, with one series reporting 90% success (160) and another 95% (159). Those children with a sternocleidomastoid tumor respond less favorably to conservative stretching exercises than those with a simple muscle torticollis; none of the children with postural torticollis need surgery (159). The extent of sternocleidomastoid fibrosis on ultrasound examination is also predictive of the need for surgery (162, 163). In those cases in which only the lower one-third of the muscle is involved with fibrosis, all responded to conservative therapy, and in those cases where the entire length of the muscle was involved with fibrosis, surgery was needed in 35% of the children (164).

The exercises are performed by the caregivers and guided by the physiotherapist. The ear opposite the contracted muscle should be positioned to the shoulder, and the chin should be positioned to touch the shoulder on the same side as the contracted muscle. When adequate stretching has occurred in the neutral position, the exercises should be graduated up to the extended position, which achieves maximum stretching and prevents residual contractures. Treatment measures to be used along with stretching consist of room modifications by modifying the child's toys and crib so that the neck is stretched when the infant is reaching for or looking at objects of interest. The exact role of the efficacy of these stretching measures, versus a natural history of spontaneous resolution, is not known (165); there are many anecdotal cases of spontaneous resolution. Occasionally, muscle stretching itself will result in partial or complete rupture of the sternocleidomastoid muscle (166). Recently, some have used botulinum toxin as an adjunct to assist in the stretching program, although dysphagia and neck weakness are significant side effects (167–169).

If stretching measures are unsuccessful after 1 year of age (159, 161, 165, 170), surgery is recommended. The child's neck and anatomic structures are larger, making surgery easier. Established facial deformity or a limitation of more than

30 degrees of motion usually precludes a good result, and surgery is required to prevent further facial flattening and further cosmetic deterioration (161). Asymmetry of the face and skull can improve as long as adequate growth potential remains after the deforming pull of the sternocleidomastoid is removed; good but not perfect results can be obtained as late as 12 years of life (151, 171, 172).

The best time for surgical release is between the ages of 1 and 4 years; (139, 173) for those treated surgically before the age of 3 years, excellent results can be expected in nearly all cases (171). Surgical treatments include a unipolar release (171) at the sternoclavicular or mastoid pole, bipolar release, middle third transection, and even complete resection. Although these surgical procedures are usually done open, endoscopic (174) and percutaneous (distal) approaches have been recently described (175). Bipolar release combined with a Z-plasty of the sternal attachment yielded 92% satisfactory results in one series, whereas only 15% satisfactory results were obtained with other procedures (170). Similar results, although not perfect, can even be achieved in older children with a bipolar release (172, 176). In a more recent series of surgical cases, excellent results were obtained with a unipolar release and aggressive postoperative stretching (171). Middle third transection has also been reported to give 90% satisfactory results (177). Z-plasty lengthening maintains the V-contour of the neck and cosmesis, which the middle third transection does not. Structures that can be injured from surgery are the spinal accessory nerve, the anterior and external jugular veins, the carotid vessels and sheath, and the facial nerve. Skin incisions should never be located directly over the clavicle because of cosmetically unacceptable scar spreading; rather, they should be made one finger breadth proximal to the medial end of the clavicle and sternal notch, and in line with the cervical skin creases. The postoperative protocol can vary from simple stretching exercises to cast immobilization. Some type of a bracing device to maintain alignment of the head and neck is probably a desirable part of the postoperative protocol (178).

Author's Preferred Treatment. For those children diagnosed before 1 year of age, a regimen of stretching exercises and room modifications is tried first. If this approach fails, or the child presents after 1 year of age, then a bipolar sternocleidomastoid release is performed (Figs. 21-38 to 21-41). Postoperative orthotic immobilization is employed along with frequent physiotherapy for at least 3 months after surgery.

Neurogenic Types. Although rare, these causes should be considered in the differential diagnosis of any atypical torticollis, especially when the condition is unresponsive or progressive in the face of therapy believed to be appropriate. The major neurogenic etiologies are central nervous system tumors (i.e., of the posterior fossa or the spinal cord), syringomyelia with or without cord tumor, Arnold-Chiari malformation, ocular dysfunction, and paroxysmal torticollis of infancy (179).

Text continued on page 862

Bipolar Sternocleidomastoid Release (Figs. 21-38 to 21-44)

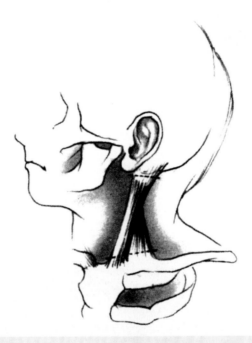

FIGURE 21-38.   Bipolar release of the sternocleidomastoid for congenital muscular torticollis maintains the V contour of the neck and is cosmetically more acceptable than transection or resection of the muscle. The mastoid release is performed first.

After induction of anesthesia, the head is tilted away from the side involved, which increases the visibility of the tight muscle. The scalp and hair in the mastoid area are trimmed as needed. Folding the ear over a sponge and gently taping it anterior to the field allows for an easier exposure. Adherent plastic drapes are attached with adhesive to the skin to keep the field clear as well as prevent prepping solution from draining into the ears and eyes. A transverse incision is made just distal to the tip of the mastoid.

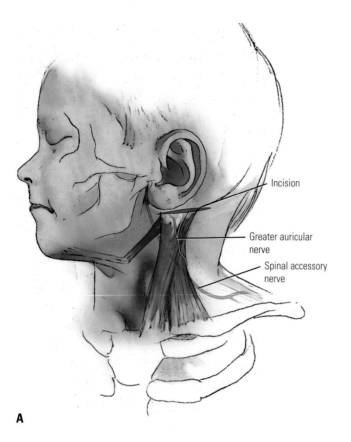

Incision

Greater auricular
nerve

Spinal accessory
nerve

A

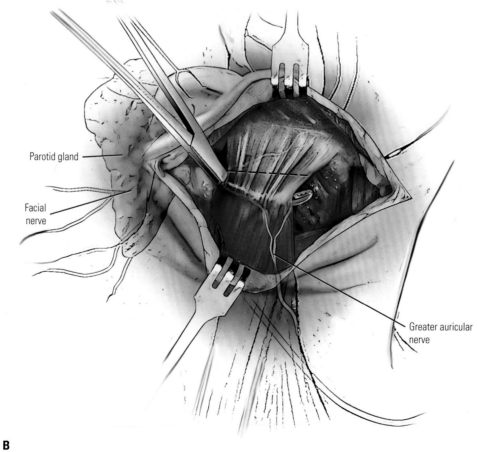

Parotid gland

Facial
nerve

Greater auricular
nerve

B

FIGURE 21-39. **A**: Dissection must not be too distal in order to avoid injury to the spinal accessory nerve. **B**: Similarly, dissecting too anterior places the facial nerve at risk where it exits from the parotid gland area. Once the mastoid origin is completely exposed, a careful transection is performed. Routine closure is performed.

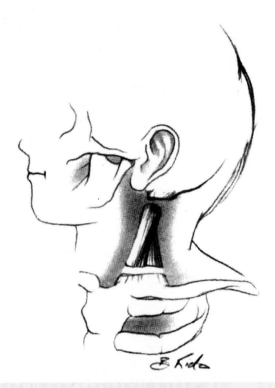

FIGURE 21-40.   Attention is then directed to the distal release. The incision should be placed in a skin crease a short distance above the clavicle. Because the skin is mobile and can be moved (not stretched) from a medial to a lateral position, the incision can be small, running from the lateral border of the sternal head to the midportion of the clavicular head.

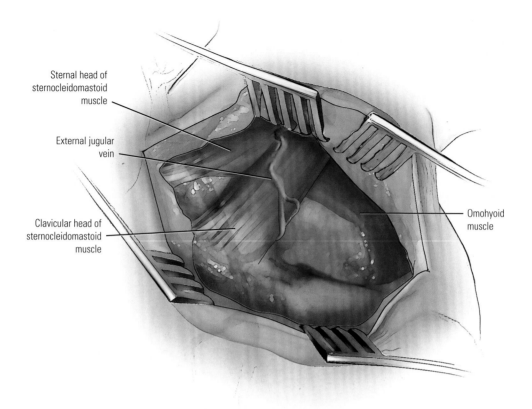

Sternal head of
sternocleidomastoid
muscle

External jugular
vein

Clavicular head of
sternocleidomastoid
muscle

Omohyoid
muscle

A

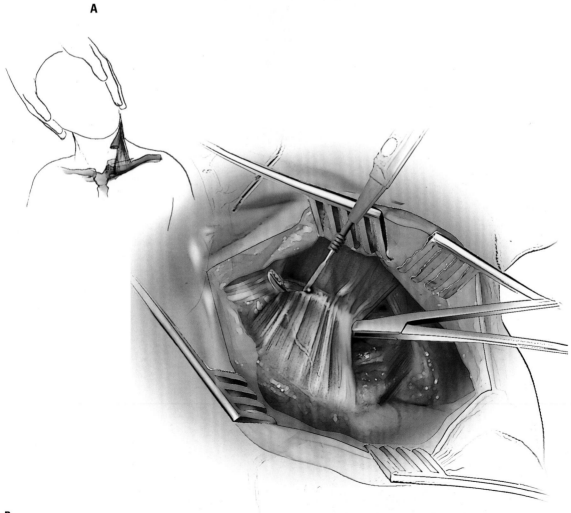

B

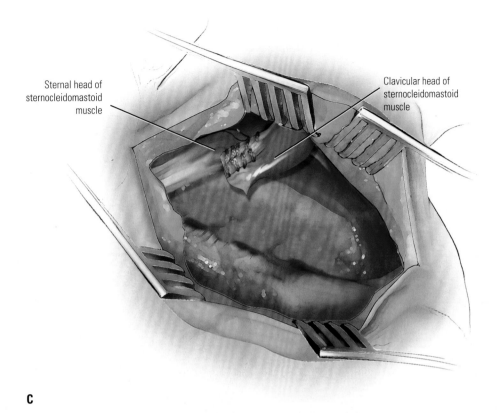

Sternal head of
sternocleidomastoid
muscle

Clavicular head of
sternocleidomastoid
muscle

C

FIGURE 21-41.   The platysma muscle should be identified as a separate and distinct layer so that it may be repaired at the time of closure. This helps preserve the contour of the neck and avoids an unsightly depression as a result of the released/lengthened muscle. **A**: Beneath the platysma muscle, the sternal and clavicular heads of the sternocleidomastoid muscle can usually be identified as distinct structures. In some cases, the clavicular head is thin and seems to be of little importance. Because the sternocleidomastoid muscle is adherent to the surrounding fascia, it should be dissected free for a distance of about 2 cm. In accomplishing this, the adherence of the muscle to the investing fascia is appreciated. If this dissection is not done, the muscular repairs lie in close proximity after the platysma muscle is repaired, and recurrence is likely. Although a fascial layer separates the sternocleidomastoid muscle from the deeper venous and arterial structures, the muscle is usually adherent and should be separated from this fascial layer with care. **B**: The clavicular head is first divided. After exposure, the muscle can be divided with a low cautery current close to the clavicle in its tendinous portion. If the anesthesiologist is asked to turn the head toward and away from the operative side, the tightness of this structure becomes apparent. Failure to divide the clavicular head usually produces disappointing results. **C**: Next, a z-plasty of the sternal head is performed, keeping the medial attachment of the sternal head preserved. After the z lengthening, the end-sand sutured together. The head is then moved and the operative area inspected and palpated for any remaining tight structures. Often deep fascial bands are identified; these should be divided. The wound is inspected for bleeding and irrigated; a small drain may be used if indicated. The wound is then closed in layers with particular attention to the platysma muscle.

(*Postoperative Care*: After 1 week, stretching exercises are resumed and continued for 3 months. Collars and orthotic devices are often helpful, especially in the older child in order to maintain correction during the healing phase.)

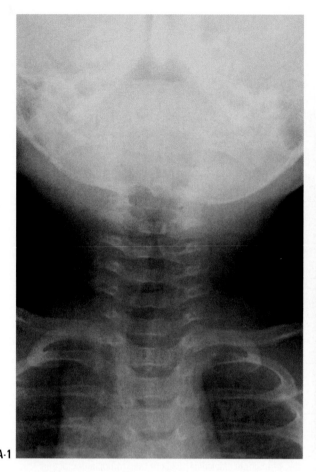

A-1

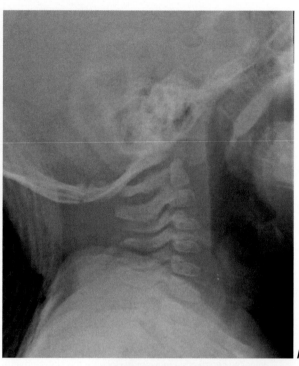

A-2

FIGURE 21-42.   A 3-month-old boy presented with a 2-month history of right-sided torticollis. His prenatal and delivery history were unremarkable. Cervical rotation to both the right and the left was full, and there was no tightness of the sternocleidomastoid muscle. **A:** Cervical spine radiographs (**A-1**) and lateral (**A-2**) demonstrated only the tilt with no congenital vertebral anomalies. **B:** An MRI was obtained that demonstrated an Arnold Chiari malformation; the inferior tip of the cerebellar tonsils is at the level of the odontoid neurocentral synchondrosis.

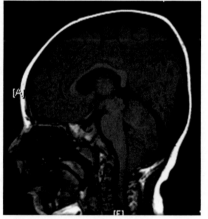

B

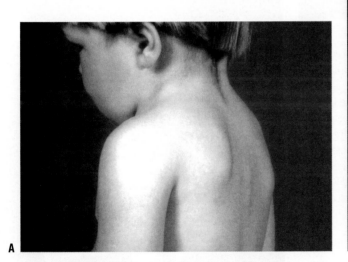
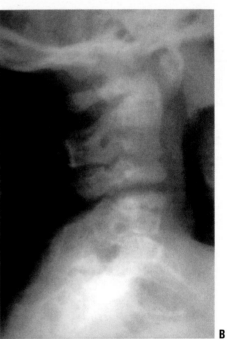

FIGURE 21-43.   This 3-year, 6-month-old boy presented with a short neck and reduced motion. **A:** Note the short neck and low posterior hair line. **B:** The lateral cervical spine radiograph demonstrates complete fusion of the posterior elements of C2-C3, with reduced disc height anteriorly at C2-C3. Note the reduced space between C3 and C4, which most likely represents a cartilage fusion between C3-C4 and will likely later become an osseous fusion.

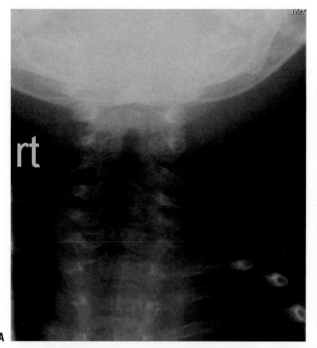

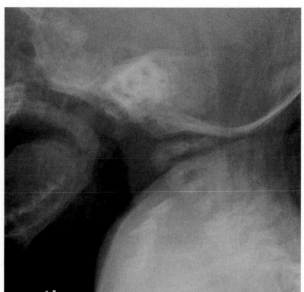

FIGURE 21-44.   A 3-month-old girl presented for concerns of shoulder asymmetry. Physical examination demonstrated a short neck with a hypoplastic right ear. **A:** The AP radiograph demonstrates incomplete closure of the posterior arches. **B:** The lateral radiograph is concerning for fusion of the posterior elements. **C:** The three-dimensional CT reconstruction (viewed from the right posterior to left anterior) demonstrates an omovertebral bar between the spinous processes of the cervical spine and the scapula, as well as fusion of the posterior elements of C2 and C3 and incomplete fusion of the neural arch C2-C4 (spina bifida occulta).

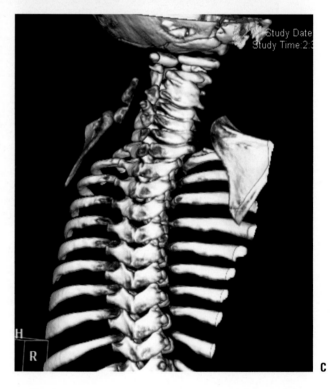

Posterior fossa tumors can present with torticollis (180–182). The ophthalmologic literature (183) has described three children with torticollis, photophobia, and epiphora (tearing). In all three children, the diagnosis was delayed with an initial diagnosis of a local ocular inflammatory condition. The age at presentation ranged from 1 to 23 months. The delay in diagnosis ranged from 5 months to 4 years. The neoplastic diagnosis was not considered initially by the ophthalmologists because the primary signs of poste-rior fossa tumors are extraocular muscle paresis, nystagmus, and papilledema.

Cervical cord tumors can present with torticollis, often early in their course (184–186). Frequently the initial diagnosis is congenital torticollis, obstetric birth palsy, muscular dystrophy, or cerebral palsy (184). The peculiar, often-overlooked signs of the tumor are spinal rigidity, early spinal deformity, and spontaneous or induced vertebral pain. In young children, pain may be expressed as irritability and restlessness (187).

Imaging of a child with a potential central nervous system tumor should consist of plain radiographs of the skull and the cervical spine followed by CT and MRI scans. Vertebral angiography also may be needed, both diagnostically and in neurosurgical planning.

The Arnold-Chiari malformation (Fig. 21-42) is caudal displacement of the hindbrain, often with other congenital deformities of the brain stem and the cerebellum (188, 189). It may be associated with myelomeningocele (i.e., type II malformation). The Chiari type I malformation is a downward displacement of the medulla oblongata with extrusion of the cerebellar tonsils through the foramen magnum and is encountered in older children. Dure et al. (188) described 11 children with Chiari type I malformations; torticollis was the presenting complaint at 5 years of age in 1 of the 11 children. It also was associated with headaches and paracervical muscle spasm; the torticollis was left sided. As with tumors, the workup of a child with the potential for a Chiari malformation consists of plain radiographs of the skull and the cervical spine followed by an MRI scan (188). The treatment is neurosurgical.

Ocular pathology accounts for up to one-third of children with no obvious orthopaedic cause of torticollis (190). The torticollis is usually atypical (191). These children typically present around 1 year of age. The face can be turned about a vertical axis, the head can be tilted to one shoulder with the frontal plane of the face remaining coronal, the chin can be elevated or depressed, or a combination of any of these positions can occur. These abnormal head positions optimize visual acuity and maintain binocularity. An ocular cause is likely if the head is tilted but not rotated or if the tilt changes when the child is lying versus sitting or standing up. Children with ocular torticollis have a full range of cervical motion without the fibrotic sternocleidomastoid muscle seen in congenital muscular torticollis. Ophthalmologic evaluation is usually positive for paralytic squint or nystagmus. Detailed tests conducted by an experienced ophthalmologist are diagnostic. Treatment of ocular torticollis is usually surgical.

Paroxysmal torticollis of infancy is a rare, unusual episodic torticollis lasting for minutes to days with spontaneous recovery (192–194). The attacks usually occur in the morning, last from minutes to days, with a frequency from less than one episode per month to three to four episodes per month. The attacks can be associated with lateral trunk curvature, eye movements or deviations, and alternating sides of torticollis. The children are usually girls (71%), the average age of onset is 3 months (1 week to 30 months), and the recovery period is 24 months (6 months to 5 years). It has been suggested that paroxysmal torticollis of infancy is equivalent to a migraine headache (195, 196) because of positive family histories for migraines in 29%, or it is a forerunner of benign paroxysmal vertigo of childhood (193). Whatever the cause, it is usually self-limiting and does not require therapy. It may be linked to a mutation in the CACNA1A gene (196), the gene associated with familial hemiplegic migraine.

Sandifer Syndrome. This is a syndrome of gastroesophageal reflux, often from a hiatal hernia, and abnormal posturing of the neck and trunk, usually torticollis (197, 198). The torticollis is likely an attempt of the child to decrease esophageal discomfort resulting from the reflux. The abnormal posturing also may present as opisthotonos or neural tics and often mimics central nervous system disorders. The majority of patients present in infancy. The incidence of gastroesophageal reflux is high (up to 40% of infants) (199), with the principal symptoms being vomiting, failure to thrive, recurrent respiratory disease, dysphagia, various neural signs, torticollis, and respiratory arrest. The diagnosis of symptom-causing gastroesophageal reflux frequently is overlooked. On careful examination of these infants, the tight and short sternocleidomastoid muscle or its tumor is not seen, eliminating congenital muscular torticollis. Further workup excludes dysplasias and congenital anomalies of the cervical spine, and central nervous system disorders. In these situations, the physician should consider Sandifer syndrome in the differential diagnosis.

Plain radiographs of the cervical spine eliminate congenital anomalies or dysplasias; contrast studies of the upper gastrointestinal tract usually demonstrate the hiatal hernia and gastroesophageal reflux (200). Esophageal pH studies may be necessary; many children, both asymptomatic and symptomatic, show evidence of gastroesophageal reflux (201). Treatment begins with medical therapy. When this fails fundoplication can be considered, which is usually curative (202).

Klippel-Feil Syndrome. Klippel-Feil syndrome consists of congenital fusions of the cervical vertebrae clinically exhibited by the triad of a low posterior hairline, a short neck, and variably limited neck motion (Fig. 21-43A,B) (203). Its incidence is approximately 0.7% (204). Other associated anomalies are often present both in the musculoskeletal and other organ systems. The congenital fusions result from abnormal embryologic formation of the cervical vertebral mesenchymal anlages. This unknown embryologic insult is not limited to the cervical vertebrae and explains the other anomalies associated with the Klippel-Feil syndrome. In some instances, the Klippel-Feil syndrome is familial, indicating a genetic transmission (205–207).

These children may have an associated Sprengel deformity and/or omovertebral bar (Fig. 21-44) (203, 208). Other anomalies associated with the syndrome are scoliosis (both congenital and idiopathic like) (203), congenital limb deficiency (209), renal anomalies (210), deafness (211), synkinesis (mirror movements) (212), small spinal cords but with increased SAC (213, 214), pulmonary dysfunction (215), and congenital heart and vascular disease (216–218). Radiographs demonstrate a wide range of deformity, ranging from simple block vertebrae to multiple and bizarre anomalies. The fusions become more apparent as the child ages, and posterior fusions are more common than anterior fusions when the fusions are incomplete (219). Klippel-Feil syndrome can be divided into three types depending upon the extent of vertebral involvement;

type I involves the cervical and upper thoracic vertebra, type II only the cervical vertebra alone, and type III the cervical vertebra as well as lower thoracic or upper lumbar vertebra (220). Superior odontoid migration may also occur (221). Associated scoliosis makes interpretation of the radiographs even more difficult. Flexion and extension lateral radiographs are used to assess for instability, and should always be done prior to any general anesthetic. If instability is noted on the flexion and extension radiographs, the anesthesiologist should be so informed. The anesthesiologist may elect to undertake intubation differently (e.g., awake nasotracheal, fiberoptic-guided). Any segment adjacent to unfused segments may develop hypermobility and neurologic symptoms (222, 223). A common pattern is fusion of C1-C2 and C3-C4, leading to a high risk of instability at the unfused C2-C3 level (224). If the flexion and extension radiographs are difficult to interpret, a flexion and extension CT or MRI scan can be useful. CT is especially helpful at the C1-C2 level in assessing the SAC; sagittal MRI is more helpful at other levels.

All children with Klippel-Feil syndrome should be further evaluated for other organ system problems. A general pediatric evaluation should be undertaken by a qualified pediatrician to ensure that no congenital cardiac or other neurologic abnormalities exist. Renal imaging should be done in all children; simple renal ultrasonography is usually adequate for the initial evaluation (225). MRI should be performed whenever any concern for neurologic involvement exists on a clinical basis in order to define the site and cause of neurologic pathology. An MRI should also be performed before any orthopaedic spinal procedure; this is to rule out any other intraspinal pathology that might not be present clinically or radiographically (e.g., Arnold-Chiari malformation, tethered cord, nonosseous diastematomyelia) (226).

The natural history depends on the presence of renal or cardiac problems with the potential for organ system failure and death. Cervical spine instability (227–229) can develop with neurologic involvement, especially in the upper segments or in those with iniencephaly (227, 230). The more numerous the occipitoatlantal anomalies, the higher the neurologic risk (231). Degenerative joint and disc disease develops in those patients with lower segment instabilities. In adulthood, many patients with Klippel-Feil syndrome will complain of headaches, upper extremity weakness, or numbness and tingling. Subtle findings on neurologic examination can be seen in up to half of these adults. Those with mirror movement disorders are likely to have cervicomedullary neuroschisis (232). Degenerative disc disease, as seen on MRI scans, occurs in nearly 100% of these patients (233).

Because children with large fusion areas (Fig. 21-45) are at high risk for developing instabilities, strenuous activities should be avoided, especially contact sports (229, 234). Other nonsurgical methods of treatment are cervical traction, collars, and analgesics when mechanical symptoms appear, usually in the adolescent or the adult patient. Arthrodesis is needed for neurologic symptoms because of instability. Asymptomatic hypermobile segments pose a dilemma regard-

ing stabilization. Unfortunately, no guidelines exist for this problem. The need for decompression at the time of stabilization depends on the exact anatomic circumstance, as will the need for combined anterior and posterior versus simple posterior fusions alone. Surgery for cosmesis alone is usually unwarranted and risky.

Author's Preferred Treatment. Once diagnosed, it is mandatory that imaging of the genitourinary system be performed if not already done. The patient is counseled against contact sports, especially collision sports (football, wrestling, ice hockey) and those sports that may place the cervical spine under stress (e.g., gymnastics, diving, basketball, soccer, volleyball). I typically ask the child what sports he/she likes to participate in, and then determine if that sport is likely to place the cervical spine under stress. If so, then that activity should be avoided. Arthrodesis is reserved for the very rare instance of symptomatic hypermobility.

Os Odontoideum. Os odontoideum is a rare anomaly where the tip of the odontoid process is divided by a wide transverse gap, leaving the apical segment without its basilar support (235). The exact incidence is not known. It most likely represents an unrecognized fracture at the base of the odontoid or damage to the epiphyseal plate during the first few years of life (235, 236). Either of these conditions can compromise the blood supply to the developing odontoid, resulting in the os odontoideum. MRI scans have further documented the presence nuchal cord changes consistent with trauma (237). A congenital etiology has also been proposed (238–241). It might represent an embryologic anomaly characterized by segmentation at the junction of the proximal 1½ somites of the 2½ somites from which the odontoid forms (242). Failure of segmentation of the dens from the anterior arch of the atlas (resulting in the so-called jig-saw sign) (240), with or without incomplete fusion of the atlas (the bipartite atlas) (239, 241). Sankar et al. (243) believe that the etiology is multifactorial and can be either congenital or posttraumatic.

Local neck pain is the usual presentation; transitory episodes of paresis, myelopathy, or cerebral brain stem ischemia due to vertebral artery compression from the upper cervical instability are less common. Sudden death rarely occurs.

Radiographs demonstrate an oval or a round ossicle with a smooth sclerotic border of variable size, located in the position of the normal odontoid tip. It is occasionally located near the basioccipital bone in the foramen magnum area. There are three radiographic types of os odontoideum; round, cone, and blunt tooth (244). The base of the dens is usually hypoplastic. The gap between the os and the hypoplastic dens is wider than in a fracture, usually well above the level of the facets. However, it may be difficult to differentiate an os odontoideum from nonunion following a fracture. Tomograms and CT scans are useful to further delineate the bony anatomy and flexion and extension lateral radiographs to assess instability. The instability index and the sagittal plane rotation angle can be measured (Fig. 21-46) (245). The presence of

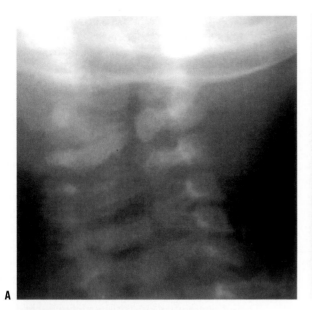

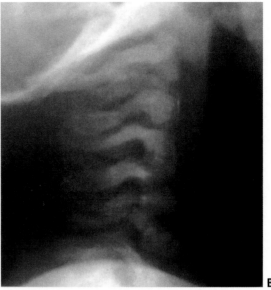

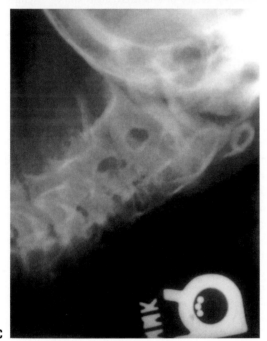

FIGURE 21-45. This 2-month-old girl presented with a left-sided torticollis. The AP (**A**) and lateral (**B**) cervical spine radiographs demonstrate congenital anomalies of the cervical spine at C1-C2. **C:** At age 7 years and 3 months, these have further ossified and matured, demonstrating massive congenital fusions of the cervical spine.

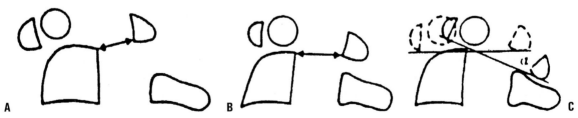

FIGURE 21-46. Radiographic parameters used to determine the instability index and sagittal plane rotation in os odontoideum. The minimum (**A**) and maximum (**B**) distances from the posterior border of the body of C2 to the posterior atlantal arch. The instability index = [(maximum distance – minimum distance)/maximum distance] × 100%. **C:** The change in the atlantoaxial angle between flexion and extension is the sagittal plane rotation. (From Watanabe M, Toyama Y, Fujimura Y. Atlantoaxial instability in os odontoideum with myelopathy. *Spine* 1996;21:1435–1439, with permission).

myelopathy is highly correlated with a sagittal plane rotation angle ≥ 20 degrees and an instability index ≥ 40%; it is also most common in the round type of os odontoideum (244). Myelopathy is also associated with cystic or fibrocartilaginous masses either behind the odontoid, within the transverse ligament, or at the level of the articulation between the os odontoideum and the remainder of the odontoid (238, 246–248); these typically regress after successful stabilization and arthrodesis (249).

The neurologic symptoms are due to cord compression from posterior translation of the os into the cord in extension or the odontoid into the cord in flexion. Hypermobility at the C1-C2 level may cause vertebral artery occlusion with ischemia of the brain stem and posterior fossa structures; this will result in seizures, syncope, vertigo, and visual disturbances.

Those with local pain or transient myelopathies often recover with immobilization. Subsequently, only nonstrenuous activities should be allowed, but curtailment of activities in the pediatric age group can be difficult. The risk of a small insult leading to catastrophic quadriplegia and death must be weighed. The long-term natural history is unknown.

Surgery is indicated when there is 10 mm or more of ADI, a SAC of 13 mm or less (37), neurologic involvement, progressive instability, or persistent neck pain. Surgery should also be strongly considered in asymptomatic patients with an instability index of >40% and/or a sagittal plane rotation angle of >20 degrees. A Gallie fusion is recommended. The surgeon must be careful when tightening the wire so that the os is not pulled back posteriorly into the canal and cord with disastrous consequences. In small children, the wire may be eliminated. In all children, a Minerva or a halo cast or vest also is used for at least 6 weeks, and often for 12 weeks. C1-C2 screw fixation has also been described in pediatric atlantoaxial instability (250) for those children older than 4 years of age. For all children undergoing C1-C2 posterior arthrodesis, care should be taken to avoid fixation of the C1-C2 segment in hyperlordosis, as that will lead to subaxial cervical kyphosis postoperatively (251).

Developmental and Acquired Stenoses and Instabilities

Down Syndrome.
Because of underlying collagen defects in these children, cervical instabilities can develop at both the occiput-C1 and C1-C2 levels. The instability may occur at more than one level and in more than one plane (e.g., sagittal and rotary planes). With the advent of the Special Olympics, there has been much concern regarding the participation of children with Down syndrome, and much confusion regarding the appropriate approach to the problem of upper cervical instability in these children. Outlined below are the most recent recommendations regarding this problem.

The incidence of occiput-C1 instability has been reported to be as high as 60% in children (41) and 69% in adults (252). The vast majority are asymptomatic (253, 254). Measurement reproducibility is poor (255), but a Power's ratio of <0.55 is more likely to be associated with neurologic symptoms (256).

Recent data also indicate that there are often underlying congenital differences in the shape of the occiput-C1 joint (lack of concavity of the superior surface of the lateral masses of C1) in Down children with occiput-C1 instability (257). No guidelines exist regarding the frequency of periodic screening or indications for surgery, with the exception of those for atlantooccipital fusion in the symptomatic child. Tredwell et al. (41) believe that treatment plans for these children should depend on the amount of room available for the cord rather than absolute values of displacement for both atlantoaxial and atlantooccipital instability.

Atlantoaxial instability in children with Down syndrome was first reported by Spitzer et al. in 1961 (252). Subsequently, there have been many reports on this instability. Despite these reports, there are none that document the true incidence of atlantoaxial dislocation (in contrast to instability), and there are no long-term studies regarding the natural history of this problem.

The incidence of atlantoaxial instability in children with Down syndrome has been estimated to range from 9% to 22% (41, 258–260). The incidence of symptomatic atlantoaxial instability is much less; it was reported to be 2.6% (258) in a series of 236 Down syndrome patients. Progressive instability and neurologic deficits are more likely to develop in boys older than 10 years (260). Children with Down syndrome have a significantly greater incidence of cervical skeletal anomalies, especially persistent synchondrosis and spina bifida occulta of C1, than do normal children (261). Also, children with both Down syndrome and atlantoaxial instability have an increased frequency of cervical spine anomalies, compared with other Down syndrome children without atlantoaxial instability (261). These spinal anomalies may be a contributing factor in the cause of atlantoaxial instability in these children.

The majority of children with atlantoaxial or occipitoatlantal hypermobility are asymptomatic. When symptoms occur, they are usually pyramidal tract symptoms, such as gait abnormalities, hyperreflexia, easy fatigability, and quadriparesis. Occasionally, local symptoms exist, such as head tilt, torticollis, neck pain, or limited neck mobility. The neurologic deficits are not necessarily attributable to hypermobility of the atlantoaxial or occipitoatlantal joints. Neurologic symptoms in one series of adult Down syndrome patients were equally as common in those with an increased ADI as those with a normal ADI (262). Further evaluation with flexion/extension CT or MRI scans to assess for cord compression is needed in this situation.

Rarely does sudden catastrophic death occur. Nearly all of the individuals who have experienced catastrophic injury to the spinal cord have had weeks to years of preceding, less severe neurologic abnormalities. In a review by the American Academy of Pediatrics, 41 cases of symptomatic atlantoaxial instability were compiled. In only 3 of these 41 children did the initiation or the worsening of symptoms of atlantoaxial instability occur after trauma during organized sports activities (259).

In the past, screening of Down syndrome patients with lateral flexion/extension radiographs had been recommended

(263). However, symptomatic atlantoaxial instability is very rare, and the chances of a sports-related catastrophic injury are even rarer. The reproducibility of radiographic screening for atlantoaxial and occipitoatlantal mobility is poor (254, 255, 264). Furthermore, the radiologic picture can change over time, most frequently from abnormal to normal (260). Because of all these factors, and the absence of any evidence that a screening program is effective in preventing symptomatic atlantoaxial and occipitoatlantal mobility (254), lateral cervical radiographs are of unproven value, and the previous recommendations for screening radiographs by the American Academy of Pediatrics have been retired (259).

The identification of patients with symptoms or signs consistent with symptomatic spinal cord injury is thus more important than radiographs. Neurologic examination is often difficult to perform and interpret in these children (41). Parental education as to the early signs of myelopathy is extremely important (e.g., increasing clumsiness and falling, worsening of upper extremity function). A thorough history and a neurologic examination are more important before participation in sports than are screening radiographs. However, further research is needed in this confusing matter, and because of persistent concerns, the Special Olympics does not plan to remove its requirement that all Down syndrome athletes have radiographs of the cervical spine before athletic participation.

Because of this requirement, spinal radiographs are often obtained without neurologic symptoms. When these are available, they should be reviewed to determine if there are any other associated anomalies, such as persistent synchondrosis of C2, spina bifida occulta of C1, ossiculum terminale, os odontoideum, or other less common anomalies. When the plain radiographs indicate atlantoaxial or atlantooccipital instability of 6 mm or more in an asymptomatic patient, CT and MRI scans in flexion and extension can determine the extent of neural encroachment and cord compression.

Once a Down syndrome patient presents with radiographic instability, what treatment should be instituted? Those with asymptomatic atlantoaxial or occipitoatlantal hypermobility should probably be followed up with repeat neurologic examinations; the role of repeat radiographs is more clouded as noted in the previous discussion. Because the risk of a catastrophic spinal cord injury is extremely low with organized sports in Down syndrome children without any neurologic findings, the avoidance of high-risk activities must be individualized. For those children with sudden-onset or recent progression of neurologic symptoms, immediate fusion should be undertaken if appropriate imaging confirms cord compromise. The most difficult question concerns the patient with upper cervical hypermobility with minimal or nonprogressive chronic symptoms. Before embarking upon arthrodesis, imaging with flexion/extension MRI (96) or CT should be undertaken to confirm cord compression from the hypermobility, and to eliminate other central nervous system causes of neurologic symptoms. CT is faster, reducing the need for sedation, which can be potentially dangerous in these children. CT also visualizes the C1-C2 relationships necessary to measure the

SAC. MRI is more useful for evaluating other central nervous system lesions. Even if successfully stabilized, patients with chronic symptoms often show little symptomatic improvement after arthrodesis (265).

Posterior cervical fusion at the levels involved is the recommended surgical treatment. The classic technique for posterior C1-C2 fusion uses autogenous iliac crest bone graft with wiring and postoperative halo cast immobilization. Internal fixation with wiring and/or transarticular (266) screws provides protection against displacement, shortens the time of postoperative immobilization, permits the consideration of using less rigid forms of external immobilization, and is reported to aid in obtaining fusion (267–270). However, internal fixation with sublaminar wiring poses added risk. If the instability does not reduce on routine extension films, the patient is at high risk for development of iatrogenic quadriplegia with sublaminar wiring and acute manipulative reduction (271, 272). For this reason, it has been recommended that preoperative traction be used to effect the reduction. If reduction does not occur with traction, then only an onlay bone grafting should be performed without sublaminar wiring (271). Sublaminar wiring at C2 is not recommended regardless of the success of reduction because sublaminar wiring at C2 was associated with the only death in one series (273). If wiring is to be performed, pliable, smaller-caliber wires should be used. Satisfactory results can be obtained with onlay bone grafts and rigid external immobilization without internal fixation (274).

The Down syndrome patient is at higher risk for postoperative complications (neurologic and other) after fusion (275–277). Neurologic complications can range from complete quadriplegia and death to Brown-Sequard syndrome (273). Another potential cause of neurologic impairment is over reduction if an unstable os odontoideum is present (273). A posterior translation of the ring of C1 and the os fragment into the SAC can occur from this over reduction. In a study of the results of surgical fusion in 35 symptomatic Down syndrome children, 8 made a complete recovery, 14 showed improvement, 7 did not improve, 4 died, and the outcome for 2 is unknown (258). Patients with long-standing symptoms and marked neural damage showed no or little postoperative improvement, whereas patients with a more recent onset of symptoms usually made an excellent recovery. Other complications are loss of reduction despite halo cast immobilization and resorption of the bone graft with a stable fibrous union or unstable nonunion (274, 275).

The long-term results after cervical fusion are not yet known. Individuals with Down syndrome who undergo short cervical fusions are at risk for developing instability above the level of fusion, such as occiput-C1 after a C1-C2 fusion or C1-C2 after lower level fusions (278, 279). This later instability occurred in four of five children between 6 months and 7 years after surgery (278).

Author's Preferred Treatment.   All children with Down syndrome should avoid collision sports (boxing, football, wrestling), even those with normal flexion/extension lateral radiographs. This seems prudent in view of the known underlying ligamentous laxity and potential for development of cervical instability. Also, all children with Down syndrome should avoid any sports or activities that do or potentially may stress the cervical spine (boxing, football, wrestling, ice hockey, basketball, diving, gymnastics). Certainly any child with progressive instability yet who is neurologically intact should also not participate in any cervical spine–stressing activities. These children should also be followed closely from a clinical perspective to observe for the development of any neurologic symptoms or signs. Those children with neurologic signs or symptoms and cervical instability should undergo arthrodesis, usually posterior. Most instabilities correct with simple positioning. Internal fixation is advised, except for sublaminar wires at C2. If instability is present and does not reduce on routine extension films, the patient is at high risk for development of iatrogenic quadriplegia with sublaminar wiring and acute manipulative reduction. Preoperative traction should be used in such a situation to effect reduction. If reduction does not occur, then only an onlay bone grafting should be performed without internal fixation. The high complication rate associated with these procedures should be remembered and parents counseled accordingly.

Marfan Syndrome.

Marfan syndrome affects ligamentous laxity and bone morphology. It is due to a mutation in the glycoprotein fibrillin, which has been mapped to the long arm of chromosome 15. Abnormalities regarding the cervical in this syndrome have only recently been described (280–282). These are primarily radiographic abnormalities but can be clinically significant instabilities (282). Focal cervical kyphosis involving at least three consecutive vertebrae occurs in 16%, with an average kyphosis of 22 degrees. The normal cervical lordosis is absent in 35%. Atlantoaxial hypermobility is common—54%. There is also an increased incidence of radiographic basilar impression (36%). Unlike Down syndrome, there is no increased incidence of cervical skeletal anomalies such as persistent synchondrosis and spina bifida occulta of C1. In spite of these radiographic abnormalities in those with Marfan syndrome, symptoms or neurologic compromise is rare. Neck pain is not increased compared to the general population. Patients with Marfan syndrome should be recommended to avoid sports with high-impact loading on the cervical spine; it does not appear necessary to routinely perform cervical spine radiographs for those undergoing general anesthesia. Atlantoaxial rotatory subluxation may be increased in those with Marfan syndrome, and this should be specially noted during surgical positioning.

Nontraumatic Occipitoatlantal Instability.

Nontraumatic occipitoatlantal instability is rare in the absence of any underlying syndrome (e.g., Down syndrome). Georgopoulos et al. (283) have described pediatric nontraumatic atlantooccipital instability. Congenital enlargement of the occipital condyles may have been the cause by increasing motion at this joint. The presenting symptoms were severe vertigo in one 14-year-old

boy and nausea with projectile vomiting in one 6-year-old girl. These symptoms are postulated to be a result of vertebrobasilar arterial insufficiency resulting from the hypermobility at the occiput-C1 junction. The diagnosis of instability is suggested by plain radiographs initially and confirmed by cineradiography. Both children were treated with a posterior occiput-C1 fusion with resolution of symptoms.

Cerebral Palsy.

Cervical radiculopathy and myelopathy in cerebral palsy (284–287) was first described in the athetoid types and subsequently in the spastic types. Athetoid cerebral palsy patients, when compared with the normal population, develop cervical disc degeneration at a younger age. This degeneration progresses more rapidly and involves more levels. Angular and listhetic instabilities also are more frequent and appear at a younger age (288). The combination of disc degeneration and listhetic instability predisposes these patients to a relatively rapid, progressive neurologic deficit.

The symptoms are brachialgia and weakness of the upper extremity with decreased functional use or increased paraparesis or tetraparesis (285–287). In ambulatory patients, a loss of ambulatory ability is often a sign of presentation. Occasional loss of bowel and bladder control also occurs. Atlantoaxial instability has been recently described in patients with severe spastic quadriplegia; the symptoms are usually apnea, opisthotonos, torticollis, respiratory problems, muscle tone abnormalities and hyperreflexia, and bradycardia (289).

Radiographic findings (Fig. 21-47) are narrowing of the spinal canal and premature development of cervical spondylosis; malalignment of the cervical spine with localized kyphosis, increased lordosis, or both; and instability of the cervical spine manifested as spondylolisthesis. Flattening of the anterosuperior margins of the vertebral bodies and beak-like projections of the anteroinferior margins are radiographic findings of the spondylosis. Myelography demonstrates stenosis, disc protrusion, osteophyte projection, and blocks in dye flow, most commonly at the C3-C4 and C4-C5 levels.

The kyphosis, herniated discs, and osteophytes result in nerve root and cord compression. It is believed that the exaggerated flexion and extension of the neck in these young adults with cerebral palsy causes accelerated cervical degeneration and cervical stenosis earlier than in unaffected people, who develop stenosis in the late fourth and fifth decades of life. Exaggerated flexion and extension occurs in patients with athetosis and writhing movements. Difficulty with head control also can cause exaggerated flexion and extension in the spastic cerebral palsy patient.

Treatment is primarily surgical. Anterior discectomy, resection of osteophytes, and interbody fusion have been the most effective methods. A halo is best and is well tolerated in some patients with athetosis (286). However, postoperative immobilization can be a problem for some patients, and thus some authors also recommend a posterior wiring of the facets as well to minimize the amount of time postoperative immobilization is needed (285). Posterior laminectomy alone (286) is contraindicated in cerebral palsy patients with developmental cervical stenosis because this will increase the instability. Long-term

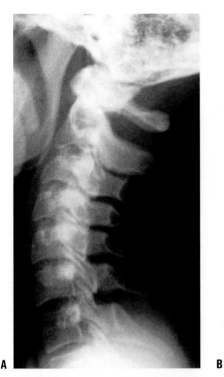 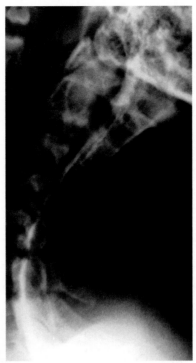 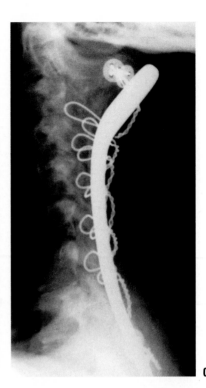

A   B   C

FIGURE 21-47.   A 14-year-old girl with spastic quadriparesis showed progressive loss of upper extremity function with loss of ability to control her wheelchair and feed herself. She also complained of some mild neck pain. **A:** The lateral radiograph shows marked stenosis from C3-C6, as evidenced by a spinal canal-to-vertebral body ratio (Torg ratio) of <0.8. **B:** The myelogram shows near complete block of the dye column from C3-C5. This stenosis was treated by posterior laminectomy from C3-C7 and posterior cervical fusion from C2-T1 using Luque rectangle fixation with spinous process and facet wiring. **C:** Eight months postoperatively, there is stable fixation and solid facet joint fusion. The girl's upper extremity strength is improved, and she is able to feed herself. (From Loder RT, Hensinger RN. Developmental abnormalities of the cervical spine. In: Weinstein SL, ed. *The Pediatric Spine: Principles and Practice*, 1st ed. New York, NY: Raven Press, 1994, with permission.)

follow-up of surgically treated patients demonstrates late disc degeneration and increased range of motion at adjacent segments in those who underwent anterior arthrodesis (290).

Postlaminectomy Deformity.   Cervical kyphosis is common after cervical laminectomy in children (291–299). This phenomenon is more likely in immature, growing children. It has been duplicated in animal models; a C3-C6 laminectomy in growing cats uniformly resulted in kyphosis; whereas normal cervical curves were maintained in adult cats (300). The natural history of postlaminectomy kyphosis is unknown; however, the incidence of kyphosis when extensive cervical laminectomies are performed in childhood varies from 33% to 100%, with an overall average of 70% (296). Postlaminectomy kyphosis is weakly age dependent (mean age at laminectomy of 10.5 years) and not dependent upon the total number of levels decompressed or the location of these levels (296) unless decompression spanning both the C1-C2 and C7-T1 levels is performed, which then increases the risk four fold (298). Postlaminectomy lordosis is less common and is strongly correlated with a peak age at decompression of 4 years (296). In one study, 12 of 15 children who had undergone a cervical or cervicothoracic

laminectomy prior to 15 years of age developed kyphosis (295). The normal posterior muscular attachments to the spinous processes and laminae, as well as facet capsules, the ligamentum nuchae, and the ligamentum flavum, are violated by the laminectomy. This loss of posterior supporting structures allows for a progressive deformity, which, if kyphotic in nature, can eventually result in neurologic symptoms and deficits. Early radiographic features are a simple kyphosis; later, vertebral body wedging and anterior translations of one vertebral body on another can develop. A late, severe deformity is the swan neck deformity (294). Neurologic problems result from cord stretch and compression from the anterior kyphotic vertebral bodies. MRI is useful to delineate the extent of cord attenuation and compression.

Nonsurgical treatment starts with frequent radiographic follow-up studies after a laminectomy; the role of prophylactic bracing is not yet known. If only instability becomes present, then posterior cervical facet fusion can be performed (Figs. 21-10 to 21-16). After kyphotic deformities develop, anterior vertebral body fusion with halo cast or vest; or Minerva cast immobilization is recommended (293) (Fig. 21-48). The role of a prophylactic posterior fusion at the time of laminectomy is

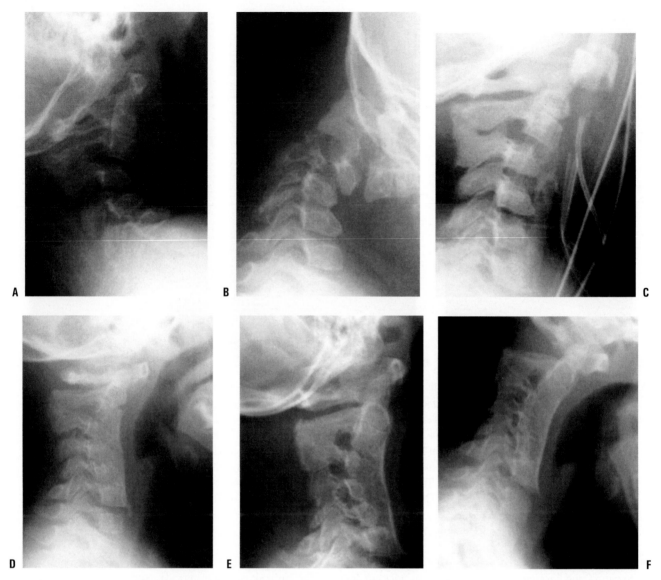

FIGURE 21-48. This girl underwent a cervical laminectomy from C2-C6 for a low-grade astrocytoma of the cervical cord. At 1 year and 7 months of age, she had a postlaminectomy kyphosis that was 45 degrees in extension (**A**) and 82 degrees in flexion (**B**). **C:** An anterior cervical discectomy and fusion from C2 to C6 was performed with autogenous iliac crest strut graft. Immediately postoperative, the kyphosis was corrected to 20 degrees. Halo-vest immobilization was used for 3 months. **D:** Solid incorporation of the fusion occurred by 6 months postoperatively. At 4-years and 7 months of age, flexion (**E**) and extension (**F**) lateral radiographs show maintenance of the correction, solid fusion, and no instability at the remaining levels.

not yet known (291), nor is the role of osteoplastic laminotomy instead of laminectomy (301), although this approach might not always be amenable to the primary pathology.

Other Syndromes

Fetal Alcohol Syndrome. Central nervous system dysfunctions, growth deficiencies, facial anomalies, and variable major and minor malformations are the characteristics of the fetal alcohol syndrome. The children present with developmental delay, especially in motor milestones, failure to thrive, mild-to-moderate retardation, mild microcephaly, distinct facies

(hypoplasia of the facial bones and circumoral tissues), and congenital cardiovascular anomalies. The cervical findings are similar to those in the Klippel-Feil syndrome. Radiographically congenital fusion of two or more cervical vertebrae occurs in approximately half of the children, resembling Klippel-Feil syndrome (302). The major visceral anomaly in the Klippel-Feil syndrome is the genitourinary system, whereas in fetal alcohol syndrome, it is in the cardiovascular system (302).

The natural history is not known. Radiographic imaging and treatment recommendations regarding the cervical spine are the same as those for the Klippel-Feil syndrome.

Craniofacial Syndromes. Cleft lip and palate is the most common craniofacial anomaly. It can be a solitary finding, but more often associated with other syndromes and anomalies. Children with cleft anomalies have a 13% to 18% incidence of cervical spinal anomalies compared with the 0.8% incidence of children undergoing orthodontia care for other reasons (303, 304). This incidence is highest in patients with soft palate and submucous clefts (45%). These anomalies, usually spina bifida and vertebral body hypoplasia, are predominantly in the upper cervical spine. The potential for instability is unknown, as is the natural history. No documented information regarding treatment is available; however, the clinician should be aware of this association and make sound clinical judgments as needed. They also demonstrate a reduced cervical lordosis compared to those without cleft lip and/or palate (304).

Craniosynostosis Syndromes. The craniosynostosis syndromes—Crouzon, Pfeiffer, Apert, Goldenhaar, and Saethre-Chotzen—exhibit cervical spine fusions, atlantooccipital fusions, and butterfly vertebrae (305–310). Fusions are more common in Apert syndrome (71%) than in Crouzon syndrome (38%) (305). Upper cervical fusions are most common in Crouzon and Pfeiffer syndromes (307), whereas in Apert syndrome the fusions are more likely to be complex and involve C5-C6 (305). However, this syndrome variation is not accurate enough for syndromic differentiation. Congenital cervicothoracic scoliosis with rib fusions is seen in Goldenhar syndrome, usually from hemivertebrae (307, 311). C1-C2 instability in Goldenhar syndrome may be as high as 33%, and these children should be monitored carefully for this potential problem (311).

The cervical fusions are progressive with age; in younger children the vertebrae appear to be separated by intervertebral discs, but as the children grow older the vertebrae fuse together. There are no specific, standard recommendations for treatment. The author recommends following the same principles as in Klippel-Feil syndrome. The main concern is the potential difficulty with intubation in these children. Odontoid anomalies are rare; however, if any question exists regarding the stability of the cervical spine, lateral flexion and extension radiographs should be obtained. Children with Goldenhar syndrome have a high incidence of C1-C2 instability (312) and failures of segmentation (313). Children with Goldenhar syndrome have a much higher incidence of their mothers being diabetic; it has recently been suggested that children with Goldenhar syndrome should be assessed for maternal diabetes exposure, which should aid in counseling concerning cause and recurrence risk (314).

Skeletal Dysplasias. Skeletal dysplasias are discussed in detail in Chapter 4.

Combined Soft-tissue and Skeletal Dysplasias.
Neurofibromatosis. Neurofibromatosis is the most common single gene disorder in humans. The proportion of patients with neurofibromatosis and cervical spine involvement is difficult to assess: 30% of patients in the series of Yong-Hing et al.

(315) and 44% of neurofibromatosis patients with scoliosis or kyphosis had cervical spine lesions. The cervical lesions are often asymptomatic (315). Symptoms, when they do occur, are diminished or painful neck motion, torticollis, dysphagia, deformity, and neurologic signs ranging from mild pain and weakness to paraparesis and quadriparesis (65, 316). Neck masses constituted 20% of presenting symptoms in one study of neurofibromatosis patients (317).

Radiographic features of neurofibromatosis in the cervical spine are vertebral body deficiencies and dysplasia or scalloping (Fig. 21-49) (315). This condition often is associated with kyphosis and foraminal enlargement (318). Lateral flexion and extension radiographs are recommended for all neurofibromatosis patients before general anesthesia or surgery (315). MRI is helpful for assessing the involvement of neural structures and dural ectasia. CT is useful for evaluating the upper cervical spine complex and bony definition of the neural foramen. The natural history regarding the cervical spine is unknown, but those with severe kyphosis often develop neurologic deterioration.

Surgical indications are cord or nerve root compression, C1-C2 rotary subluxation, pain, and neurofibroma removal (315, 316). Laminectomy alone without accompanying arthrodesis is contraindicated (319). A halo cast or vest is usually needed after fusion, with or without internal fixation, and is usually achieved with simple interspinous wiring. Kyphosis requires both anterior and posterior fusion. Pseudarthroses are frequent with isolated posterior fusions. Vascularized fibular grafts may be necessary to effect fusion in difficult cases (318, 320). If there are no indications for surgical treatment, then the patient should be followed closely.

Fibrodysplasia Ossificans Progressiva. Fibrodysplasia ossificans progressiva is an inherited, autosomal dominant disorder (321) of connective tissue with progressive soft-tissue ossification. The disorder itself is rare; most cases represent new spontaneous mutations. It likely represents overactivity of the BMP signaling pathway (322). Eventually all patients with this disorder develop cervical spine changes (323), often starting in childhood. These patients usually present with neck stiffness (324) within the first 5 years of life, and less commonly pain (325). No cases of neurologic compromise have been reported. Other general clinical features are big toe malformations, reduction defects of all digits, deafness, baldness, and mental retardation. Early in the course of the disease small, narrow vertebral bodies and large pedicles/posterior elements are seen radiographically. Occasionally, nuchal musculature ossification also is seen. Later, neural arch and facet fusions are seen (322). This factor reflects the progressive ossification of the cervical spinal musculature, ligament ossification, and spontaneous fusion of the cervical discs and apophyseal joints. No effective medical treatment is known. Surgical treatment of the cervical spine has not been necessary.

TRAUMA

Injuries to the cervical spine are rare in children and more common in boys than girls. In one study, the age- and gender-adjusted

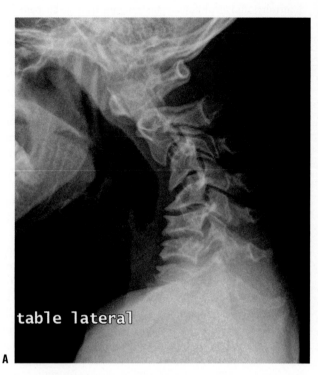

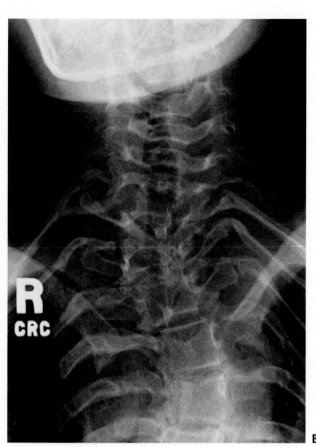

FIGURE 21-49. A 15-year-old girl with neurofibromatosis I has a painless deformity. **A:** Kyphosis on the lateral view. **B:** Notice the dysplastic changes in the vertebral bodies and the penciled ribs on the AP view.

incidence was 7.41 per 100,000 population per year (326); this incidence was much less in children (younger than 11 years of age, 1.19 per 100,000) compared with adolescents (older than 11 years of age, 13.24 per 100,00). The cause of the injury in children is frequently a fall, whereas in adolescents it is frequently sports, recreational activities, or motor vehicle crashes. Children involved in side impact crashes are more likely to have cervical spine injuries compared to those involved in frontal crashes (327). Unrestrained are more likely to sustain cervical spine injuries in motor vehicle crashes compared to restrained children (328, 329). In general, children (younger than 11 years of age) are more likely to sustain ligamentous injuries and injuries to the upper cervical spine, whereas adolescents are more likely to sustain fractures and injuries to the lower cervical spine (326). In a large series of 1098 children with cervical spine injury, upper spine injuries occurred in 52%, lower cervical spine injuries in 28%, and both upper and lower injuries in 7% (330). Upper cervical spine injuries carry a significantly higher mortality compared to lower cervical spine injuries (330, 331). By the age of 10 years, the bony cervical spine has reached adult configurations, and the injuries they sustain are essentially those of the adult. Therefore, the author will concentrate on those injuries sustained in the first decade of life.

Most children with potential cervical spine injuries have sustained polytrauma and frequently arrive immobilized on backboards and cervical collars. If the child is comatose or semiconscious, if there are external signs of head injury, or if the child complains of neck pain then cervical spine radiographs are needed. All children involved in motor vehicle crashes with head trauma and neck pain, or who have neurologic signs or symptoms, should have cervical spine radiographs (332, 333). The views recommended for this initial screening are the cross-table lateral and AP views. The need for an open-mouth odontoid is controversial, especially in children <5 years of age (334, 335). If the child is too critically ill to be positioned for all views, then the cross-table lateral view is adequate until a complete evaluation can be performed. Cervical spine precautions must be maintained until a complete evaluation has demonstrated no injury. Once a cervical injury has been identified, close scrutiny must be undertaken to ensure that there are no other injuries in the remainder of the axial skeleton.

The child arriving in the emergency suite is often on a standard backboard. Young children have a disproportionately large head, and positioning them on a standard backboard leads to a flexed posture of the neck (Fig. 21-50A) (336). This flexion can lead to further anterior angulation or translation of an unstable cervical spine injury and can also cause pseudosubluxation, which in itself in an injured child can be difficult to interpret. To prevent this undesirable cervical flexion in young children during emergency transport and radiography

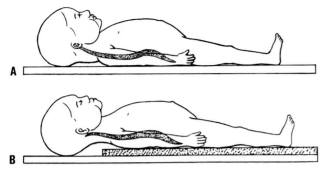

FIGURE 21-50. **A:** Positioning a young child on a standard back-board forces the neck into a kyphotic position because of the relatively large head. **B:** Positioning a young child on a double mattress, which raises the chest and torso and allows the head to translate posteriorly compensates for the relatively large head. This creates a normal alignment of the cervical spine. (From Herzenberg JE, Hensinger RN, Dedrick DK, et al. Emergency transport and positioning of young children who have an injury of the cervical spine. *J Bone Joint Surg Am* 1989;71-A:15–22, with permission).

modifications must be made by either creating a recess for the occiput of the larger head or using a double mattress to raise the chest (Fig. 21-50B). A simple clinical guideline is to align the external auditory meatus with the shoulder.

Flexion and extension lateral radiographs may be necessary to determine the stability of the cervical spine; hyperflexion ligamentous injuries may not be seen immediately, and flexion and extension views a few weeks later after the spasm has subsided may document instability. In one series of children with ligamentous injuries of the cervical spine, 8 of 11 children with lower cervical instability were diagnosed between 2 weeks and 4 months after the trauma (337).

Secondary signs of spinal injury in children often are seen before the actual injury or fracture itself. Malalignment of the spinous processes on the AP radiograph should be regarded as highly suspicious for a jumped facet. Widening of the posterior interspinous distances should be regarded as highly suspicious for a posterior ligamentous injury. In adults, an increase in the retropharyngeal soft-tissue space can indicate a hematoma in the setting of trauma and increase the suspicion on the part of the clinician that an upper cervical fracture exists. In children, however, the pharyngeal wall is close to the spine in inspiration, whereas there may be a large increase in this space with forced expiration, as in a crying child (338). This should be remembered when considering the significance of prevertebral pharyngeal soft tissue in the cervical spine radiographs of a frightened, crying child.

CT is useful to further assess the upper cervical spine, especially the occipital condyles, ring of the atlas, and occasionally the odontoid. As a rule, CT is not recommended for screening (339–342) but to further study suspicious areas on plain radiographs or for treatment planning (343). However, there is more interest in using CT as the initial screening study (344), but the concern for artifacts exists (345). It should be

used to study all fractures of C1. MRI scans are useful to assess the spinal cord, discs, and interspinous ligaments (346). In an injured child, an MRI is the exam of choice to assess the pediatric cervical spine when (a) the child is obtunded and/or nonverbal and a cervical spine injury is suspected, (b) there are equivocal plain radiograph findings, (c) neurologic symptoms without radiographic findings are present, or (d) inability to clear the cervical spine in a timely manner (347).

Fractures and Ligamentous Injuries of the Occipital Complex to the C1-C2 Complex

Atlantooccipital Dislocation. Atlantooccipital dislocation is rare (348), and most of the children do not survive (349). Deployment of air bags has been recently associated with this injury in children (350–353). With the present rapid response to trauma victims and more aggressive field care, more of these children now survive. These children are usually polytrauma victims with severe head injuries and present with a range of clinical neurologic pictures (348, 349). In the past, those who survived had incomplete lesions, often demonstrating cranial nerve dysfunctions and varying degrees of quadriplegia. Many of the children who presently survive have complete loss of neurologic function below the brain stem and live only because of outpatient ventilatory support. Other presentations may be a responsive child with hypotension or tachycardia to a complete cardiac arrest. Occasionally, some patients present with normal neurologic examinations. As of 2001, there have been 29 children with atlantooccipital dislocation who have survived (354).

In severe cases the diagnosis is evident; however, some of the cases do not demonstrate marked radiographic displacement. In the past, a Power's ratio >1.0 (Fig. 21-51A) was used to indicate the presence of atlantooccipital dislocation (355). This criterion can cause the practitioner to miss isolated distraction injuries, anterior atlantooccipital dislocations that have spontaneously reduced after injury, and posterior atlantooccipital injuries (348). For this reason, the distance between the tip of the dens and the basion (Fig. 21-51B) has been used, in which a distance of more than 12.5 mm indicates the potential for

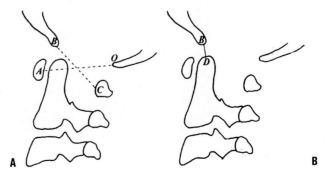

FIGURE 21-51. The *BC/OA* ratio (**A**) and the *DB* distance (**B**) are used to assess for traumatic atlantooccipital dislocation. (From Bulas DI, Fitz CR, Johnson DL. Traumatic atlanto-occipital dislocation in children. *Radiology* 1993;188:155–158, with permission.)

atlantooccipital dislocation. Recent studies have described the stabilizing nature of the tectorial membrane. When this membrane is disrupted, there is a high likelihood of atlantooccipital instability. If the C1-C2 to C2-C3 posterior interspinous ratio is >2.5, then there is a high chance of tectorial membrane disruption, and MRI evaluation is warranted (356).

The first obstacle in the treatment of this injury is its diagnosis. If the suspicion for craniocervical trauma is still present after inconclusive plain radiography, CT or MRI can be quite useful (Fig. 21-52). Subarachnoid hemorrhage at the craniocervical junction will be seen after atlantooccipital dislocation (357–359); CT can also assist in assessing osseous alignment

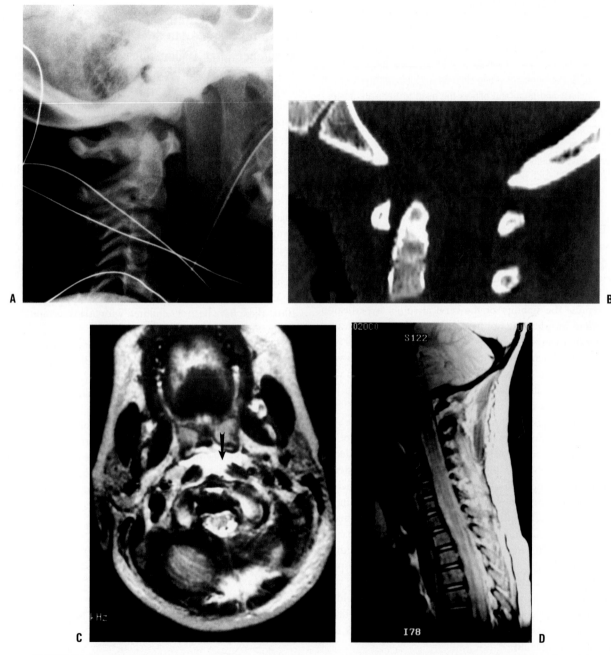

FIGURE 21-52. This 5-year, 6-month-old girl was hit by a van from behind and presented with bilateral palsies of cranial nerve VI. **A:** The lateral radiograph of the upper cervical spine demonstrates a rotational malalignment: the basion hemishadows fail to overlap while the C1 arches nearly superimpose upon each other, raising the concern for atlantooccipital dislocation. **B:** A CT scan with sagittal reconstruction demonstrates elevation of the periosteum at the caudal level of the clivus (*arrows*) and hemorrhage (*arrowheads*). **C:** An axial image from the MRI scan demonstrates abnormal fluid accumulation immediately anterior to the atlantooccipital junction (*arrow*). **D:** The MRI scan sagittal view demonstrates subarachnoid space narrowing at the level of the foramen magnum and atlantooccipital joint.

(360). Once diagnosed, standard respiratory and other supporting measures are given. Early definitive immobilization of the dislocation should be undertaken. The immobilization can be with a halo alone or with supplemental internal fixation and posterior fusion (357, 361, 362). Traction should be avoided because it can distract the joint and cause further neurologic injury (363). These children must be moved rapidly into an upright position to maximize pulmonary care. Late neurologic deterioration may indicate progressive hydrocephalus or retropharyngeal pseudomeningocele (364, 365).

Fractures of the Atlas.

The Jefferson fracture is rare in children (366–368). It is caused by an axial load from the head into the lateral masses. Unlike adults, a single fracture through the ring in children may be isolated, hinging on the synchondrosis (367, 369) instead of a double break in the ring. Alternatively, a bifocal posterior arch fracture can occur—a Jefferson fracture variant (370). A transverse atlantal ligament rupture may occur as the lateral masses separate, resulting in C1-C2 instability.

CT scans are useful in both the diagnosis of this injury and the assessment of healing. This injury in children is not commonly seen on plain radiographs, usually showing only an asymmetry between the odontoid and the lateral masses. If clearly seen on plain radiographs, CT should also be performed to confirm the diagnosis and to rule out a transverse alar ligament rupture. Treatment is usually simple immobilization with a Minerva or halo cast. In toddlers, limited ambula-

tion is recommended whenever a halo is applied (371). Rarely is surgery necessary unless rupture of the transverse alar ligament occurs, which renders the spine unstable. The timing of surgery needs to be individualized.

Transverse Atlantoaxial Ligament Ruptures.

Transverse atlantoaxial ligament ruptures may occur from either severe or mild trauma (337). Radiographically the ADI is increased, usually well beyond the normal 5 mm. Adequate ligamentous healing and stability does not occur from simple immobilization. The recommended treatment is reduction in extension, posterior cervical C1-C2 fusion with autogenous bone graft, and immobilization with a halo or Minerva cast. A solid arthrodesis is documented on flexion and extension lateral radiographs after 2 to 3 months of immobilization. If the ligament is avulsed from the lateral masses of C1 and the bony avulsion attached to the ligament is close to the lateral mass, simple immobilization may be adequate (372).

Odontoid Fractures.

Odontoid fractures are a common pediatric cervical spine injury (373). They are usually physeal fractures of the dentocentral synchondrosis, usually Salter-Harris type I fractures. These may occur after major or minor trauma. Neurologic deficits are rare. These fractures usually displace anteriorly with the dens posteriorly angulated (Fig. 21-53). This fracture usually is seen only on the lateral view. If there is confusion between the mild normal posterior

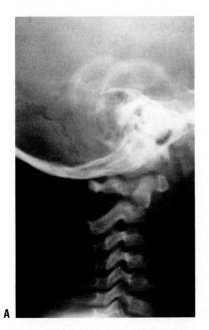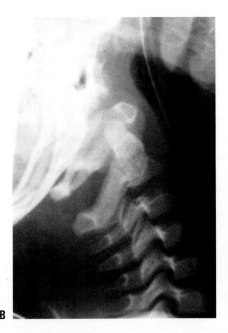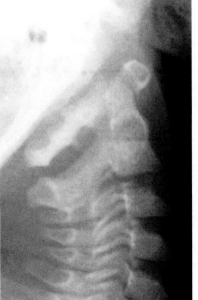

FIGURE 21-53. This 2-year, 9-month-old boy was brought to the emergency department unable to move his upper extremities and withdrew his lower extremities only in response to noxious stimuli. He had a history of falling off couches. On investigation, it became clear that the child had been battered. **A:** A lateral radiograph demonstrates the odontoid fracture through the dentocentral synchondrosis with anterior angulation and translation. A MRI scan did not reveal any abnormalities in the cord. **B:** Simple positioning with a double mattress allowed for reduction of the fracture; the child was maintained on a double mattress for several days to allow for subsidence of cord edema and early healing. He was then placed into a Minerva cast 10 days after the injury. The cast was removed 6 weeks after the injury, followed by immobilization with a soft collar. Flexion (**C**) and extension

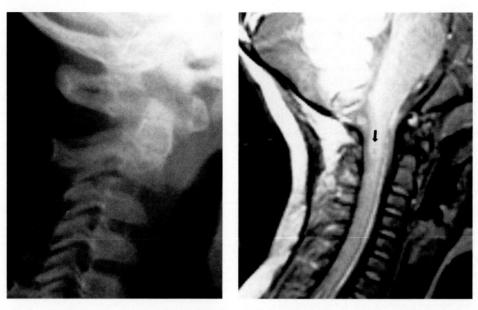

D

E

FIGURE 21-53. *(Continued)* (**D**) radiographs demonstrated no instability with the healed fracture. **E:** The child improved remarkably. By 2 months after injury, he was running and walking without difficulty. There were some subtle upper extremity changes, indicated by a change in hand dominance from right to left. MRI showed signal changes in the cord (*arrow*), which were interpreted as development of an early posttraumatic syrinx.

angulation of the dens, which occurs in up to 4% of normal children (374), dynamic flexion and extension CT scans with sagittal reconstructions can be performed to evaluate for any motion or instability.

Displaced odontoid fractures in children reduce easily with mild extension and posterior translation. In most circumstances, the simple double mattress technique is all that is needed to obtain a reduction. After a few days of recumbence and early healing, the fracture can be immobilized easily by the use of a Minerva or halo cast. As with all physeal fractures, healing is rapid, and immobilization usually can be stopped in 6 to 10 weeks. Flexion and extension lateral radiographs should be taken to confirm union with stability. These fractures, unlike those in adults, do not have a significant nonunion rate requiring subsequent C1-C2 fusion. The intact hinge of anterior periosteum most likely aids in the ease of reduction and accounts for the stability of reduction and rapid healing (375, 376).

Spondylolisthesis of C2. Spondylolisthesis of C2, also known as hangman fracture in adults, is rare in children. It most likely arises from hyperextension. Pizzutillo et al. (377) reported on a series of five cases in children. Care must be taken to not confuse this fracture with congenital anomalies that may mimic a Hangman fracture and lead to overtreatment (378–382). Similarly, they may be caused by child abuse (383). These fractures readily heal with immobilization in either a Minerva or a halo cast after gentle positioning to obtain a reduction. Traction alone, as with most cervical injuries in children, should be avoided because it overdistracts the spine with an increased potential for nonunion and more

serious neurologic injury. Posterior cervical fusion of C1-C3 is indicated for the rare case of nonunion or instability.

Fractures and Ligamentous Injuries of C3-C7. These injuries are more common in older children and adolescents than in young children (326, 384). The typical patterns of fracture usually are compression fractures of the vertebral body, or facet fractures and dislocations caused by hyperflexion. These injuries are adult patterns, and standard adult treatment should be used. Physeal fractures, usually of the inferior end plates, also can occur (385), which are caused by hyperextension. In older children, they are usually ring apophyseal fractures with minimal instability or neurologic damage. In younger children, they usually involve the entire end plate. Physeal fractures frequently are not recognized in severely injured children, or they may be noted for the first time at autopsy (385). They have a high incidence of neurologic injury (Fig. 21-54). In these children, simple positioning (e.g., double mattresses; rarely, traction), followed by immobilization, is all that is needed for treatment. Because these are physeal injuries, healing is rapid.

Traumatic ligamentous instability in children also can occur (337). The pivot point for younger children is in the upper cervical spine because of their large head size, weak cervical musculature, incompletely ossified wedge-shaped vertebrae, physiologic ligamentous laxity, and horizontal facet joints in this region. The upper cervical spine offers little resistance to traumatic shear forces, which often result in ligamentous instability. The goal is to differentiate this traumatic ligamentous instability from pseudosubluxation using the posterior cervical line.

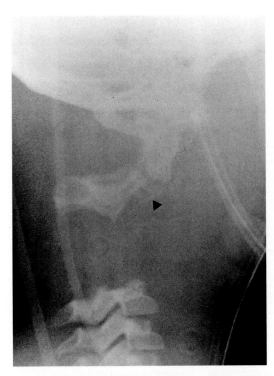

FIGURE 21-54. This 7-year, 2-month-old girl sustained polytrauma and presented in an agonal state. A lateral radiograph demonstrates complete separation at the C2-C3 level along with an associated C2 hangman fracture. Also note the small fleck of bone (*arrowhead*) attached to the base of the C2 body; this likely represents an avulsion of the superior aspect of the body of C3 with the C2-C3 disc.

Traumatic subluxation of the axis is a recently described true ligamentous instability at C2-C3, and not pseudosubluxation. The majority of the children sustain an injury with the head and neck in flexion, and are usually dues to falls or sports injuries (337, 386). The patients complain of severe neck pain. Immediately after injury, the instability may not be radiographically apparent and becomes noticeable only after progressive kyphosis is encountered. In younger children, avulsion of the cartilaginous tips of the C2 spinous process is not visible on plain radiographs or CT. Later on, the avulsion fragments become ossified. This late ossification along with the development of C2-C3 kyphosis leads to the diagnosis. In one study of ligamentous injuries of the cervical spine in children, 7 of 11 injuries occurred at the C2-C3 level. Treatment must be individualized; both simple immobilization and posterior cervical arthrodesis have been used with good results. When instability exists, treatment should consist of posterior cervical fusion with Minerva or halo immobilization (Fig. 21-55). Children undergoing cervical arthrodesis for cervical spine injury do demonstrate decreased mobility and increased osteoarthritis at long-term follow-up (387). Treatment for a mild sprain is immobilization for comfort followed by flexion and extension radiographs several weeks to a few months later to ensure that late instability does not occur.

Transient Quadriparesis. Transient quadriparesis is a neuropraxia of the cervical cord with transient quadriplegia. It is seen most often in collegiate and professional athletes (388, 389), although there are several cases in younger athletes (390). The incidence in the National Collegiate Athletic Association is 1.3 per 10,000 athletes per season (389).

The AP diameter of the spinal canal is decreased in these athletes. The spinal cord is compressed on forced hyperextension or hyperflexion, causing the transient quadriparesis. Sensory changes, such as burning pain, numbness, tingling, and loss of sensation and motor changes ranging from weakness to complete paralysis, are seen. These episodes are transient, and recovery occurs in 10 to 15 minutes; neck pain is not present at the time of injury. Transient quadriparesis needs to be differentiated from a brachial plexus stretch, or "burner." These present with a monoparesis of the upper extremity and often with neck pain.

No fractures or dislocations are present. The ratio of the spinal canal to the vertebral body is decreased, with a value of 0.8 used to indicate significant developmental cervical stenosis. Congenital fusions, cervical instability, and intervertebral disc disease also may exist. In children, this spinal canal to vertebral body ratio is not as accurate and is inconsistent in predicting spinal cord concussion (390). An MRI may be necessary to assess the presence or absence of a herniated nucleus pulposus.

Symptom resolution is universal. The only nonsurgical treatments that are needed are collars, analgesics, and antispasmodics. The role of fusions for coexistent instability, discectomy for herniated nucleus pulposus, or decompression for congenital cervical stenosis is not known.

The major concern is whether or not athletic participation should continue, and if so, the risk of a permanent quadriplegia developing with a later episode. Torg et al. (391) believe that those athletes with pure developmental spinal stenosis are not predisposed to more severe injuries if they do return to sports and that only those with instability or degenerative changes should be precluded from participation in contact sports. Odor et al. (392) found that one-third of professional and rookie football players have a spinal canal ratio of <0.8 and that it is difficult to make continued play decisions based on this ratio alone. Eismont et al. (393), however, have shown that smaller cervical canals are correlated with significant neurologic injury in routine trauma. Considering this finding, and the fact that narrowing of the spinal canal correlates even more poorly with spinal cord concussion in children (389), it is prudent to preclude any child who has had a cervical cord concussion from further contact sports until further epidemiologic data have been established.

Spinal Cord Injury without Radiographic Abnormality. Spinal cord injury without radiographic abnormality (SCIWORA) occurs in 5% to 55% of all pediatric spinal cord injuries in the neurosurgical literature (394); recent multicenter Spinal Cord Injury study databases suggest that it is much less (395). By definition, no disruption,

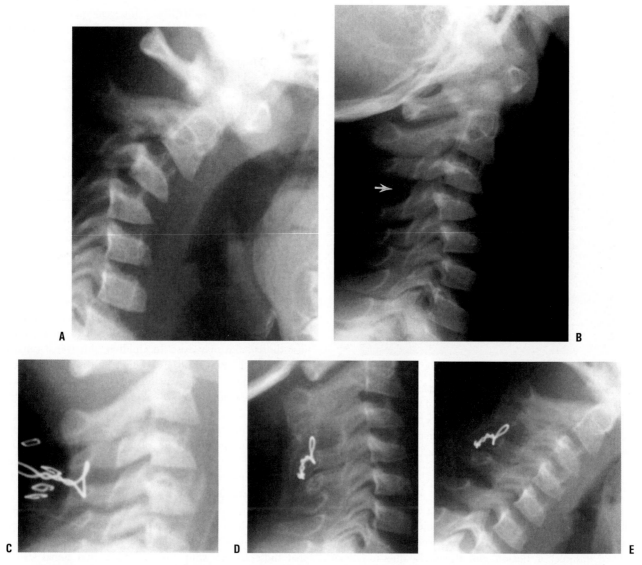

FIGURE 21-55. This 4-year, 9-month-old boy was run over by a snowmobile trailer 2 weeks before these radiographs were taken. He had complained of some neck pain and had been treated by chiropractic manipulation during these 2 weeks. The flexion (**A**) and extension (**B**) radiographs demonstrate marked instability at the C3-C4 interspace, which does not completely reduce, even with extension (*arrow*). **C:** He was treated by posterior fusion with iliac crest bone graft and interspinous wiring at C3-C4, as shown in this intraoperative radiograph. Halo-vest immobilization was used for 3 months (**D,E**). One year postoperatively, there was no instability at the C3-C4 level, and there was solid fusion, which had extended to C2 and C5, despite meticulous care not to expose the laminae of C2 and C5 or the interspinous ligaments of C2-C3 and C4-C5.

malalignment, or other abnormalities are seen on plain radiographs. The immature and elastic pediatric spine is more easily deformed than that of an adult. Momentary displacement from external forces endangers the spinal cord without disrupting bone or ligaments. The four major factors involved in this injury are hyperextension, flexion, distraction, and spinal cord ischemia. Ischemia may arise from cord contusion or direct vascular insult (396). Spinal stenosis is not a factor; the average Torg ratio was >1.0 in a recent study of 145 children with cervical SCIWORA (397).

The neurologic deficit may range from complete loss of spinal cord function to partial cord deficits. The physiologic disruption of the spinal cord is not necessarily associated with anatomic disruption. The majority of deficits (78%) are cervical; patients with upper cervical SCIWORA are more likely to have severe neurologic lesions than patients with lower cervical SCIWORA. An MRI is most useful to study the cord and disc/ligament complexes and correlates with clinical outcome (398). Positive MRI findings are typically seen only in children with very severe neurologic involvement at presentation (399). The outcome usually is determined by the presenting neurologic status. Approximately one-fourth of these children have a late deterioration in neurologic function.

Treatment is controversial. Immobilization in a Guilford brace for 3 months has been recommended by Pang and Pollack (394), with complete avoidance of all sports. However, in Pang's own series, no instability was noted in any of the children at initial evaluation, and only one child later developed instability on flexion and extension radiographs. Without documented radiographic instability, the biomechanical usefulness of brace immobilization is questionable. Pang however denotes this as treating "incipient instability" (394). More recent studies question both the existence of recurrence of a SCIWORA and the efficacy of bracing in the treatment of SCIWORA (397). Pang (400) has recently recommended that in children with transient neurologic deficits and who also have a normal MRI and somatosensory evoked potentials that bracing is not needed. Most ligamentous spine injuries, when allowed to heal with simple immobilization, do not return to the stability seen in the preinjury state; fusion usually is needed. It is atypical for SCIWORA to behave differently regarding instability, incipient or otherwise. Regardless of whether the child is braced, close follow-up of neurologic function is needed. Flexion and extension radiographs should be taken after 3 months of bracing; any late development of instability requires surgical stabilization.

Special Injury Mechanisms

Birth Injuries and Battered Children.
Birth trauma is a common cause of pediatric spinal cord injury and usually involves the cervical cord (401–403). Due to the increased incidence of Caesarean section, the number of these cases is fortunately decreasing (404). As in SCIWORA, the vertebral column is more elastic than the cord, and during delivery with prolonged distraction it may be tethered by nerve ends and blood vessels, injuring the cord but not the chondro-osseous structures. Damage to the vertebral artery with resultant ischemia of the cord also can occur (405). In battered children, the large head, poorly supported by the cervical musculature, makes the upper cervical spine vulnerable to repeated shaking with either SCIWORA (406) or a fracture (383, 407, 408). In a recent Canadian study, the incidence of cervical spine injury is 4% in the shaken baby syndrome (409).

The diagnosis is difficult, especially with incomplete neurologic injury (410). Pure transection of the cord itself is rare (411). Temperature regulation dysfunction can cause fevers, reflex movements may be mistaken for voluntary movements, and respiratory distress can occur from paralyzed intercostal muscles. They also may present with a cerebral palsy–like picture (412) or as sudden infant death syndrome (413). In one study, the diagnosis was delayed in three of four children, and the delay averaged 4.4 years from birth (414). Typically, no fractures are seen radiographically; MRI is often helpful in assessing cord damage. Anterior rupture of the lower cervical intervertebral discs is seen pathologically in children who are victims of shaking (415).

Some children without complete transection can improve neurologically. Treatment is usually nonsurgical because these are very young infants. Bed rest, respiratory support, and physical therapy, to prevent paralytic contractures should be instituted. Older children with bony injuries may need Minerva casts or halo immobilization. Surgical fusion with stabilization is rarely needed.

Car Seat Injuries.
Cervical fractures are described with the increased and recent use of infant car seats (416–419). When these devices, which clearly make automobile travel safer for children, are not adequately tightened, serious and potentially fatal injuries can occur. The harness must be adjusted periodically to account for normal growth and seasonal changes in clothing thickness. Car seat styles that allow the main lock to be attached to the crotch strap (Fig. 21-56) prevent forward sliding movements, which can apply hyperextension forces to the head, the neck, and the upper chest. Neurocentral synchondrosis separation between the body and the neural arches is a common pattern (417, 420). Adult three-point seatbelts also can cause a cervical spine injury (421).

Gunshot Wounds.
Spinal injuries from gunshot wounds (422) have been on the increase and accounted for one-half of adolescent spinal cord injuries (423). One-third of these injuries involve the cervical spine. Various degrees of neurologic loss are noted, with complete lesions in 75% in one series (422). Other body areas can be injured as well, which may cause more morbidity than the trauma to the neck itself.

Various degrees of fracture and intracanal bullets are seen radiographically. Other imaging studies, such as arteriography and esophagography, often are needed to look for other injuries (424). Panendoscopy is useful to assess injury to the trachea and esophagus. Spinal decompression is not indicated in

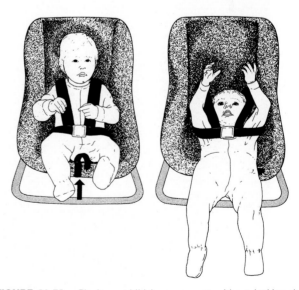

FIGURE 21-56. Placing a child in a car seat without locking the crotch strap (*arrow*) is a dangerous situation and can allow serious injury in a collision. (From Conry BG, Hall CM. Cervical spine fractures and rear car seat restraints. *Arch Dis Child* 1987;62:1267–1268, with permission.)

either complete or incomplete lesions (425). For patients with complete injuries, removal of retained bullet fragments from the canal does not improve neurologic outcome. Patients who undergo decompression have a higher risk of meningitis and spinal instability without any added benefit. Spinal instability is rare unless laminectomy is performed. Indications for neck exploration are a positive arteriogram, impending airway obstruction, tracheal deviation, widened mediastinum, expanding hematoma, and appropriate pathology on panendoscopy. Routine exploration of the neck and wound is not advised.

INFLAMMATORY AND SEPTIC CONDITIONS

Juvenile Rheumatoid Arthritis. Juvenile rheumatoid arthritis is a chronic synovitis that can affect the joints of the cervical spine as well. The subtypes that usually involve the cervical spine are the polyarticular- and systemic-onset types; only rarely does the pauciarticular type affect the cervical spine (426).

Cervical spine involvement usually occurs in the first 1 to 2 years from disease onset and presents with stiffness. Pain and torticollis are rare, and when they occur in a patient with juvenile rheumatoid arthritis, other causes should be examined, such as fracture, infection, or tumor. Torticollis was present in only 4 of 92 children in the series of Fried et al. (427) and in 1 of 121 children in the series of Hensinger et al. (426). Neurologic findings are also infrequent in these children.

The radiographic features consist of seven types (426):

1. Anterior erosion of the odontoid process
2. AP erosion of the odontoid process (apple-core odontoid)
3. Subluxation of C1 on C2
4. Focal soft-tissue calcification appearing adjacent to the ring of C1 anteriorly
5. Ankylosis of the apophyseal joints
6. Growth abnormalities
7. Subluxations between C2 and C7.

The most common radiographic features in children with neck stiffness are soft-tissue calcification at the leading edge of C1, anterior erosion of the odontoid process, and apophyseal joint ankylosis (Fig. 21-57). Although there may be mild hypermobility at C1-C2 with flexion and extension, true instability or myelopathy is rare. Basilar invagination, which often occurs in adult rheumatoid arthritis, also is rare in juvenile rheumatoid arthritis (427). The radiographic findings of juvenile rheumatoid arthritis that differ most from those of adult rheumatoid arthritis are late destruction of articular cartilage and bone, growth disturbances, spondylitis with associated vertebral subluxation and apophyseal joint ankylosis, and micrognathia (428, 429). In five patients who had long-standing disease (average age, 19 years), Hallah et al. (430) described a nonreducible head tilt due to collapse of an atlantoaxial lateral mass.

Other imaging studies are needed in the child with juvenile rheumatoid arthritis and neck pain. A bone scan is used to

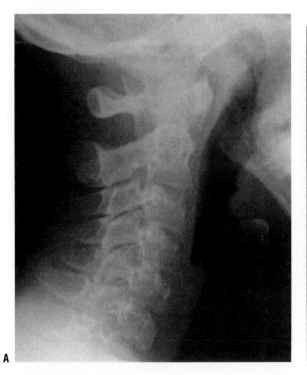
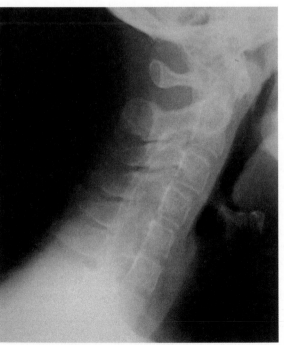

FIGURE 21-57. Cervical spine radiographs of a boy with systemic-onset juvenile rheumatoid arthritis. **A:** At age 10 years, note the facet joint narrowing posteriorly from C2 to C6. **B:** At age 17 years, the facet joints from C3 to C6 have totally fused, with complete bony ankylosis. Also note the apple core odontoid.

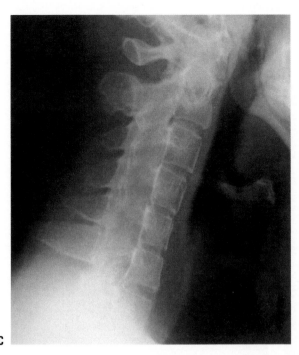

C

FIGURE 21-57. *(Continued)* **C**: By age 21 years, there has now been complete bony ankylosis between C2 and C3. The facet joint at C6-C7 is narrowed but not completely fused. Also note that the C4, C5, and C6 vertebral bodies are smaller in both height and depth.

pinpoint the exact anatomic location of activity and the anatomy further studied by a CT can. These studies can be helpful to look for occult fractures, infections, and bony tumors.

Odontoid erosion results from the inflammatory synovitis and the pannus of the synovial ring surrounding the odontoid process. The pannus erodes the odontoid anteriorly and posteriorly, but leaves the apical and alar ligament attachments free, creating the apple core lesion. This lesion is more susceptible to fracture, both from erosions and vascular compromise to the odontoid because the blood supply to the odontoid courses along its side (431), and may be disturbed by the invading pannus. Ankylosis of the apophyseal joints is most common in the systemic-onset subtype. In these young children, posterior ankylosis of the immature spine creates a tether, preventing further anterior growth. Decreased disc space height and smaller vertebral bodies, both longitudinally and circumferentially, result (428).

The treatment is generally nonsurgical, in conjunction with good rheumatologic care. Patients rarely develop flexion deformities; early in the course of the disease, a cervical collar may prevent this deformity (427). A cervical collar is recommended for patients with involvement of the odontoid process or subaxial subluxation whenever they are in an automobile or other mode of travel. If these patients need surgery for any reason, intubation can be difficult because of the micrognathia, flexion deformity, and neck stiffness. Cervical fusion rarely is needed and should be reserved for children with documented instability or progressive neurologic deterioration.

Intervertebral Disc Calcification. The first description of pediatric disc calcification was in 1924, and there are now more than 100 cases reported in the literature (432). It is slightly more common in boys than in girls (7:5 ratio), with an average age at presentation of 8 years (range, 8 days to 13 years). It occurs most often in the cervical spine and is especially symptomatic when located there. The etiology is unclear. Theories proposed are antecedent trauma (present in 30% of patients) and recent upper respiratory infections (present in 15% of patients, which may only reflect the normally high incidence of pediatric upper respiratory infections). There is no evidence to suggest metabolic disorders.

The most common clinical presentation is neck pain, which occurs in about one-half of the children (432). The onset of symptoms is abrupt: between 12 and 48 hours. Twenty-three percent of the children are febrile on presentation. Torticollis occurs in one-fourth of the children. Decreased cervical motion and spinal tenderness also can occur. Radicular signs and symptoms rarely may be seen, and they are never without local symptoms. Myelopathy is rare (3 of 127 cases).

Calcified deposits are seen delineating the nucleus pulposus. The number of calcified discs averages 1.7 per child (Fig. 21-58). No protrusions have been seen in the asymptomatic group; 38% of the symptomatic children have detectable protrusions. Recent reports have also shown signal changes in the vertebrae on MRI (433).

The natural history is very benign (434). Two-thirds of the children are free of symptoms within 3 weeks, and 95% are free of symptoms by 6 months. The radiographs show regression or disappearance of the calcific deposits in 90% of patients; about one-half of the radiographic improvement occurs within 6 months. Children who are asymptomatic may not show radiographic regression, even when followed for long periods. Children with multiple lesions show different rates of regression at the different disc levels. In some cases, persistent flattening of the vertebral bodies is noted into adulthood and may result in early degenerative changes (435).

Because of this natural history, treatment is symptomatic unless there is spinal cord compression, although a recent study demonstrated good results with nonoperative treatment even in the face of mild neurologic findings. Analgesics, sedation, and cervical traction can all be used depending on the severity of symptoms. A short trial of a soft cervical collar also may be helpful. Contact sports probably should be avoided. Surgical intervention rarely is needed. Two cases have been reported in which anterior discectomy was performed (436, 437).

Pyogenic Osteomyelitis and Discitis. Pyogenic osteomyelitis and discitis is a spectrum of disease defined as a symptomatic narrowing of the disc space, often associated with fever and infectious-like symptoms and signs. It affects all pediatric age ranges and is more common in boys than girls. The etiology is most likely infectious in nature; in about one-third of the children, an organism can be isolated, usually *Staphylococcus aureus* (438, 439).

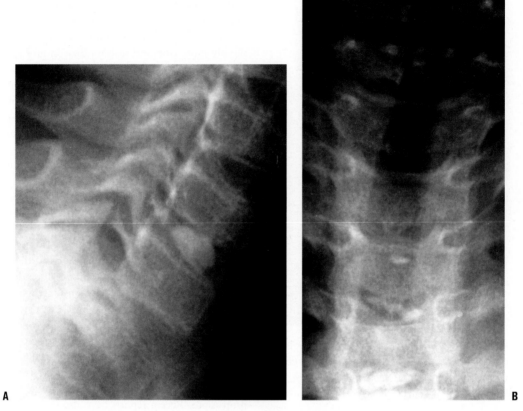

A

B

FIGURE 21-58. **A:** A 7-year-old boy with symptomatic intervertebral disc calcification at the C6-C7 level, as seen on a lateral radiograph. **B:** He also showed asymptomatic involvement at the T3-T4, T4-T5, and T5-T6 levels, as seen on an AP radiograph.

The children present with pain, difficulty in walking and standing, fever, and malaise. It usually involves the lumbar spine, with cervical involvement being rare. Early on, there is a loss of disc-space height; later, end-plate irregularities on both sides of the disc appear. Bone scans are very useful to identify the presence of discitis and osteomyelitis in a child with systemic symptoms when the anatomic location cannot be localized on clinical examination. The MRI findings are consistent with vertebral osteomyelitis (438, 440). Other helpful diagnostic studies are the erythrocyte sedimentation rate and blood cultures. Disc and bone cultures are necessary only if the child does not respond to an initial course of rest and antibiotic treatment.

Many of these children spontaneously improve without treatment. The intervertebral disc space reconstitutes to varying degrees but never to the normal height prior to illness. Sometimes, spontaneous vertebral body fusion occurs. Initially, nonsurgical treatment is given. This includes rest, immobilization, and intravenous antistaphylococcal antibiotics. Surgery is only necessary when there is no response to nonsurgical management; usually, biopsy and culture to isolate the infectious agent is all that is needed.

Tuberculosis. *Mycobacterium tuberculosis* infection in the cervical spine is rare, compared with other levels of the spine. There will likely be an increase in North America because of the increasing number of immigrants from Third World countries, the rise of human immunodeficiency virus infection, and the emergence of drug-resistant strains. There have been recent thorough reviews of this subject (441–443). In two studies, four of the six patients with upper cervical spine involvement and 24 of 40 with lower cervical spine involvement were children (441, 442). Involvement at the cervicodorsal junction is most frequent in children, followed by the C1-C2 level and then the midcervical spine (443, 444).

In cases of upper cervical spine involvement, the children present with neck pain and stiffness; torticollis, headaches, and constitutional symptoms may also be present. Neurologic symptoms vary from none to severe quadriparesis. In cases of lower cervical spine involvement, the children present with the same symptoms and also may have dysphagia, asphyxia, inspiratory stridor, and kyphosis. In children younger than 10 years of age, more diffuse and extensive involvement is seen, with large abscesses but with a decreased incidence of paraplegia and quadriplegia. The neurologic symptoms have a gradual onset over a period of 4 to 8 weeks. Sinus formation is not a prominent feature because of the thick cervical prevertebral fascia that contains the abscess. Cord compression occurs from the abscess and the kyphosis. Cultures and biopsies are not always positive. Because the infection is anterior, most cases will progress to spinal cord compression and paralysis if left untreated. Patients with involvement at the cervicodorsal junction have a very high incidence of neurologic loss (444).

Increased width of the retropharyngeal soft-tissue space is seen radiographically, as are osteolytic erosions. Instability at the C1-C2 level can be seen in some children; rarely is there a fixed C1-C2 rotatory subluxation. A kyphosis is present in one-fourth of patients with lower cervical spine involvement. Other useful imaging studies are chest radiography and renal studies.

Treatment involves antituberculous chemotherapy in all children. Surgery also is recommended for the cervical spine because it gives rapid resolution of the pain, upper respiratory obstruction, and spinal cord compression. This is in contrast to the thoracic and lumbar spine, in which chemotherapy alone is an established method of treating tuberculosis (445). Debridement is performed with or without grafting. For children younger than 2 years of age, grafting usually is not needed. For children with upper cervical spine involvement, consideration should be given to anterior transoral drainage and fusion across the lateral facet joints. Transarticular screw fixation can be used if permitted by the anatomy (446). Most children need halo traction with reduction prior to drainage, if possible. Cervicodorsal involvement typically needs anterior decompression via an extended lower cervical approach (444).

HEMATOLOGIC AND ONCOLOGIC CONDITIONS

The primary hematologic condition affecting the cervical spine is hemophilia (447). The involvement is usually asymptomatic, although mild neck discomfort may occur. Diminished lateral rotation can be noted on physical examination. Torticollis may be the initial presenting symptom due to cervicothoracic epidural hematoma (448). Radiographic findings, which begin to occur in adolescence and early adulthood, consist of cystic changes in the vertebral bodies or end-plate irregularities. Rarely is C1-C2 instability present. These radiographic changes can occur in patients with all degrees of severity of hemophilia. The pathoanatomy of these changes in the cervical spine is not known.

Many of these degenerative changes occur earlier than in the normal population; the natural history of these premature changes in the hemophiliac population is not known. There are no treatment recommendations at present, other than standard hemophiliac precautions.

Benign Tumors. The common benign tumors that involve the pediatric cervical spine (449, 450) are Langerhan cell histiocytosis, osteoid osteoma and osteoblastoma, osteochondroma, and aneurysmal bone cyst. All can be defined as neoplastic disorders without the propensity to metastasize. Although pathologically and physiologically benign, they can be clinically malignant if their surgical accessibility or risk of recurrence places the neural structures at high risk.

The majority of patients with benign cervical vertebral neoplasms are <20 years of age and present with local neck pain (450). Radicular pain may occur in up to one-third of the

patients (451); gross motor or sensory deficits are much less common. Neoplasms can cause torticollis. Probably the most common neoplasm causing childhood torticollis is osteoid osteoma. In one series, all four children with cervical osteoid osteomas presented with painful torticollis and decreased neck motion (452). The incidence in the literature of torticollis ranges from 10% to 100% in children with cervical osteoid osteomas (453–455). The pain of an osteoid osteoma classically responds to aspirin or other nonsteroidal anti-inflammatory medications. When basilar invagination is noted, Langerhan cell histiocytosis should be suspected (456), although it can also cause torticollis (457).

With osteoid osteoma the typical radiographic feature is sclerosis (Fig. 21-59), although it is not always evident. Bone scans are very helpful to locate the lesion; CT is then used to further delineate the anatomy. The osteoid osteoma causes a sclerotic reaction in the surrounding bone, but usually does not invade the epidural space. It is usually located in the laminae, followed by the pedicle and the body. An osteoblastoma is usually a mixture of lytic and blastic elements (458). Bone scans are also positive but usually are not needed to determine the presence or absence of disease because most tumors are seen on plain radiographs. CT is very helpful to further assess the anatomy, especially the presence or absence of epidural invasion, which is common in osteoblastoma. Typically, osteoid osteomas and osteoblastomas are located in the posterior elements or pedicles (459) and less commonly the vertebral body (460). Osteochondromas of the cervical spine (461–464) demonstrate the typical radiographic appearances as in any other parts of the body: expansile lesions with intact cortices and normal trabecular patterns, absence of calcification, and absence of soft-tissue masses. Half of patients have multiple osteochondromatosis. The majority are in the laminae or spinous processes and can be mistaken for osteoblastomas. Aneurysmal bone cysts are typically expansile lytic lesions with a thin rim of cortical bone and may involve contiguous vertebral elements (e.g., the posterior elements, pedicle, and body). CT is useful for determining the exact extent and potential involvement and proximity of the vertebral artery and neural elements. Angiography may be needed. Aneurysmal bone cysts usually arise in the posterior elements (465). Eosinophilic granuloma usually exhibits vertebra plana radiographically (466). The CT or MRI is useful for determining the potential encroachment on the neural structures. Eosinophilic granuloma usually arises in the vertebral body, with varying degrees of involvement and collapse.

In the cervical spine, the main concern is for vertebral artery and neural element involvement, which can lead to neurologic dysfunction. The intense inflammatory nature of the osteoid osteoma and osteoblastoma and its proximity to the neural elements causes nerve root irritation. This irritation, pain, and muscle spasm may result in torticollis. Compressive myelopathy also can occur, especially in patients with epidural compression, such as that seen with aneurysmal bone cysts (465, 467, 468) or osteochondroma (469).

The treatment of Langerhan cell histiocytosis of the cervical spine traditionally has been immobilization (e.g., collars, Minerva casts) and low-dose irradiation. Immobilization

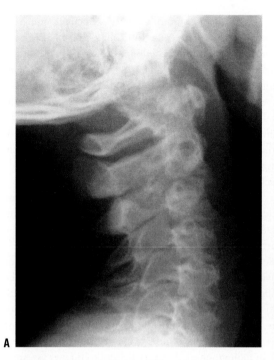
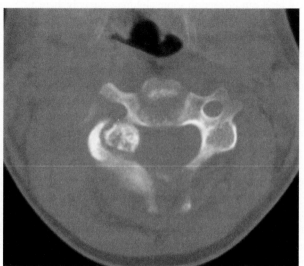

A   B

FIGURE 21-59. A 13-year-old boy had a 2-year history of neck pain that did not resolve with long-term chiropractic treatment. **A:** Plain radiographs show a sclerotic nidus with a surrounding lucency at the level of the C3 pedicle and C2-C3 foramen. **B:** CT scan confirms the typical appearance of an osteoid osteoma; note the proximity of the lesion to both the foramen and the nerve root as well as the vertebral artery.

is continued until early healing has appeared radiographically. Low-dose irradiation should be reserved only for those lesions with neurologic deficits that are not surgically accessible. Multiple laminectomies should be avoided. Rarely has immobilization alone been used, and one of these children presented with total collapse of the vertebral body (466). The overall natural history of Langerhan cell histiocytosis of the spine in the absence of systemic disease or spinal deformity is such that aggressive surgery or irradiation is not needed (470). Osteoid osteomas do not undergo malignant transformation. However, continued torticollis and pain may lead to fixed spinal deformities. For this reason, the author advocates surgical resection. Pain relief with complete resection is dramatic. Significant complaints of postoperative pain resembling the preoperative pain indicate either incomplete resection or recurrence. For osteoblastoma (471–473) and aneurysmal bone cysts (474), primary treatment is surgical, and nonsurgical treatment is used only as adjunctive therapy. The surgical goal is complete primary excision; however, this is often impossible because of the particular anatomic location of the cysts. In these situations, adjunctive therapy is useful (e.g., radiotherapy for eosinophilic granuloma, or embolization for aneurysmal bone cysts if the nondominant vertebral artery is involved) (475). Intralesional injection using both steroids and calcitonin may be useful in the difficult case of an aneurysmal bone cyst (476).

Prophylactic fusion should be performed if the resection renders the spine unstable. The amount of resection necessary to render the spine unstable is not known in children;

however, in adults, resection of more than 50% of one facet likely leads to segmental instability (477). Because the development of postlaminectomy cervical instability is even more likely in children than in adults, the author recommends an arthrodesis with any degree of facetectomy in children, and strong consideration should be given to an arthrodesis after any degree of laminectomy. Multiple laminectomies should be avoided if at all possible; if necessary, then fusion and stabilization also should be performed. Anterior fusion often is necessary because of insufficient posterior elements after surgical excision; supplemental halo cast/vest or Minerva cast immobilization usually is needed if fusion is required. The overall surgical management is individualized and multidisciplinary (e.g., orthopaedics, neurosurgery, radiotherapy, interventional radiology). Surgical complications include recurrence, pseudarthrosis of the fusion, neurologic deterioration, and vertebral artery injury (478).

Malignant Tumors. The majority of primary and metastatic malignant tumors involving the cervical spine occur in adults; rarely, the cervical spine in children can be involved by chordoma (479, 480), leukemia, Ewing sarcoma (481, 482), or metastatic neuroblastoma.

REFERENCES

1. O'Rahilly R, Meyer DB. The timing and sequence of events in the development of the human vertebral column during the embryonic period proper. *Anat Embryol* 1979;157:167–176.

2. Sensenig EC. The development of the occipital and cervical segments and their associated structures in human embryos. *Contrib Embryol Carnegie Inst Wash* 1957;36:141–156.

3. O'Rahilly R, Muller F, Meyer DB. The human vertebral column at the end of the embryonic period proper. 1. The column as a whole. *J Anat* 1980;131:565–575.

4. Goodman FR. Limb malformations and the human *HOX* genes. *Am J Med Genet* 2002;112:256–265.

5. Ramirez-Solis R, Zheng H, Whiting J, et al. Hoxb-4 mutant mice show homeotic transformation of a cervical vertebra and defects in the closure of the sternal rudiments. *Cell* 1993;73:279–295.

6. Condie BG, Capecchi MR. Mice homozygous for a targeted disruption of *Hoxd-3 (Hox-4.1)* exhibit anterior transformations of the first and second cervical vertebrae, the atlas and the axis. *Development* 1993;119:579–595.

7. Horan GSB, Wu K, Wolgemuth DJ, et al. Homeotic transformation of cervical vertebrae in *Hoxa-4* mutant mice. *Proc Nat Acad Sci U S A* 1994;91:12644–12648.

8. Tribioli C, Lufkin T. The murine *Bapx1* homeobox gene plays a critical role in embryonic development of the axial skeleton and spleen. *Development* 1999;126:5699–5711.

9. Leitges M, Neidhardt L, Haening B, et al. The paired homeobox gene Uncx4.1 specifies pedicles, transverse processes and proximal ribs of the vertebral column. *Development* 2000;127:2259–2267.

10. Subramanian V, Meyer BI, Gruss P. Disruption of the murine homeobox gene Cdx1 affects skeletal identities by altering the mesodermal expression domains of *Hox* genes. *Cell* 1995;83:641–653.

11. van den Akker E, Forlani S, Chawengsaksophak K, et al. Cdx1 and Cdx2 have overlapping functions in anteroposterior patterning and posterior axis elongation. *Development* 2002;129:2181–2193.

12. McGaughran JM, Oates A, Donnai D, et al. Mutations in *PAX1* may be associated with Klippel-Feil syndrome. *Eur J Hum Genet* 2003;11:468–474.

13. Connelly LE, Rogers JM. Methanol causes posteriorization of cervical vertebrae in mice. *Teratology* 1997;55:138–144.

14. Wéry N, Narotsky MG, Pacico N, et al. Defects in cervical vertebrae in boric acid-exposed rat embryos are associated with anterior shifts of *hox* gene expressed domains. *Birth Defects Res A Clin Mol Teratol* 2003;67:59–67.

15. Kessel M, Gruss P. Homeotic transformations of murine vertebrae and concomitant alteration of Hox codes induced by retinoic acid. *Cell* 1991;67:89–104.

16. Li Z-L, Shiota K. Stage-specific homeotic vertebral transformations in mouse fetuses induced by maternal hyperthermia during somitogenesis. *Dev Dyn* 1999;216:336–348.

17. Wellik DM. Hox patterning of the vertebral axial skeleton. *Dev Dyn* 2007;236:2454–2463.

18. Chi N, Epstein JA. Getting your Pax straight: Pax proteins in development and disease. *Trends Genet* 2002;18:41–47.

19. Wallin J, Wilting J, Koseki H, et al. The role of Pax-1 in axial skeletal development. *Development* 1994;120:1109–1121.

20. Rodrigo I, Hill RE, Balling R, et al. *Pax1* and *Pax9* activate *Bapx1* to induce chondrogenic differentiation in the sclerotome. *Development* 2003;130:473–482.

21. Smith CA, Tuan RS. Human *PAX* gene expression and development of the vertebral column. *Clin Orthop Relat Res* 1994;302:241–250.

22. Peters H, Wilm B, Sakai N, et al. Pax1 and Pax9 synergistically regulate vertebral column development. *Development* 1999;126:5399–5408.

23. Sonnesen L, Nolting D, Kjaer KW, et al. Association between the development of the body axis and the craniofacial skeleton studied by immunohistochemical analyses using collagen II, Pax9, Pax1, and Noggin antibodies. *Spine* 2008;33:1622–1626.

24. Villavicencio EH, Walterhouse DO, Iannaconne PM. The sonic hedgehog-patched-gli pathway in human development and disease. *Am J Hum Genet* 2000;67:1047–1054.

25. Weed M, Mundlos S, Olsen BR. The role of sonic hedgehog in vertebrate development. *Matrix Biol* 1997;16:53–58.

26. Kim JH, Kim PCW, Hui C-C. The VACTERL association: lessons from the Sonic hedgehog pathway. *Clin Genet* 2001;59:306–315.

27. Ogden JA. Radiology of postnatal skeletal development. XI. The first cervical vertebrae. *Skeletal Radiol* 1984;12:12–20.

28. Ogden JA. Radiology of postnatal skeletal development. XII. The second cervical vertebra. *Skeletal Radiol* 1984;12:169–177.

29. Ogden JA, Murphy MJ, Southwick WO, et al. Radiology of postnatal skeletal development. XIII. C1-2 interrelationships. *Skeletal Radiol* 1986;15:433–438.

30. Vara CS, Thompson GH. A cadaveric examination of pediatric cervical pedicle morphology. *Spine* 2006;31:1107–1112.

31. Remes VM, Heinänen MT, Kinnunen JS, et al. Reference values for radiological evaluation of cervical vertebral body shape and spinal canal. *Pediatr Radiol* 2000;30:190–195.

32. Avellino AM, Mann FA, Grady MS, et al. The misdiagnosis of acute cervical spine injuries and fractures in infants and children: the 12-year experience of a level 1 pediatric and adult trauma center. *Child Nerv Syst* 2005;21:122–127.

33. Locke GR, Gardner JI, van Epps EF. Atlas-dens interval (ADI) in children. A survey based on 200 normal cervical spines. *AJR Am J Roentgenol* 1966;97:135–140.

34. Pennecot GF, Gouraud D, Hardy JR, et al. Roentgenographical study of the stability of the cervical spine in children. *J Pediatr Orthop* 1984;4:346–352.

35. Cattell HS, Filtzer DL. Pseudosubluxation and other normal variations in the cervical spine in children. *J Bone Joint Surg Am* 1965;47-A:1295–1309.

36. Fielding JW, Cochran GVB, Lawsing JF III, et al. Tears of the transverse ligament of the atlas. A clinical and biomechanical study. *J Bone Joint Surg Am* 1974;56-A:1683–1691.

37. Spierings ELH, Braakman R. The management of os odontoideum. *J Bone Joint Surg Br* 1982;64-B:422–428.

38. Steel HH. Anatomical and mechanical considerations of the atlanto-axial articulations. *J Bone Joint Surg Am* 1968;50-A:1481–1482.

39. Jauregui N, Lincoln T, Mubarak S, et al. Surgically related upper cervical spine canal anatomy in children. *Spine* 1993;18:1939–1944.

40. El-Khoury GY, Clark CR, Dietz FR, et al. Posterior atlantooccipital subluxation in Down syndrome. *Radiology* 1986;159:507–509.

41. Tredwell SJ, Newman DE, Lockitch G. Instability of the upper cervical spine in Down syndrome. *J Pediatr Orthop* 1990;10:602–606.

42. Wiesel SW, Rothman RH. Occipitoatlantal hypermobility. *Spine* 1979;4:187–191.

43. Shaw M, Burnett H, Wilson A, et al. Pseudosubluxation of C2 on C3 in polytraumatized children—prevalence and significance. *Clin Radiol* 1999;54:377–380.

44. Swischuk LE. Anterior displacement of C2 in children: physiologic or pathologic. A helpful differentiating line. *Radiology* 1977;122:759–763.

45. Dolan KD. Developmental abnormalities of the cervical spine below the axis. *Radiol Clin North Am* 1977;25:167–175.

46. Caro FÁ, Prieto MP, Berciano FÁ. Congenital defect of the atlas and axis. A cause of misdiagnose when evaluating an acute neck trauma. *Am J Emerg Med* 2006;26:840.e1–e2.

47. Senoglu M, Safavi-Abbasi S, Theodore N, et al. The frequency and clinical significance of congenital defects of the posterior and anterior arch of the atlas. *J Neurosurg Spine* 2007;7:399–402.

48. Swischuk LE, Swischuk PN, John SD. Wedging of C-3 in infants and children: usually a normal finding and not a fracture. *Radiology* 1993;188:523–526.

49. Ballock RT, Song KM. The prevalence of nonmuscular causes of torticollis in children. *J Pediatr Orthop* 1996;16:500–504.

50. MacAlister A. Notes on the development and variations of the atlas. *J Anat Physiol* 1983;27:519–542.

51. Taylor AR, Chakravorty BC. Clinical syndromes associated with basilar impression. *Arch Neurol* 1964;10:475–484.

52. Burwood RJ, Watt I. Assimilation of the atlas and basilar impression. *Clin Radiol* 1974;25:327–333.

53. Epstein BS, Epstein JA. The association of cerebellar tonsillar herniation with basilar impression incident to Paget's disease. *AJR Am J Roentgenol* 1969;107:535–542.

54. Hurwitz LJ, Shepherd WHT. Basilar impression and disordered metabolism of bone. *Brain* 1966;89:223–234.
55. Tubbs RS, Webb D, Abdullatif H, et al. Posterior cranial fossa volume in patients with rickets: insights into the increased occurrence of Chiari I malformation in metabolic bone disease. *Neurosurgery* 2004;55:380–384.
56. Harkey HL, Crockard HA, Stevens JM, et al. The operative management of basilar impression in osteogenesis imperfecta. *Neurosurgery* 1990;27:782–786.
57. Pozo JL, Crockard HA, Ransford AO. Basilar impression in osteogenesis imperfecta. *J Bone Joint Surg Br* 1984;66-B:233–238.
58. Rush PJ, Berbrayer D, Reilly BJ. Basilar impression and osteogenesis imperfecta in a three-year-old girl: CT and MRI. *Pediatr Radiol* 1989;19:142–143.
59. Hayes M, Parker G, Ell J, et al. Basilar impression complicating osteogenesis imperfecta type IV: the clinical and neuroradiological findings in four cases. *J Neurol Neurosurg Psychiat* 1999;66:357–364.
60. Kovero O, Pynnönen S, Kuurila-Svahn K, et al. Skull base abnormalities in osteogenesis imperfecta: a cephalometric evaluation of 54 patients and 108 control volunteers. *J Neurosurg* 2006;105:361–370.
61. Sawin PD, Menezes AH. Basilar invagination in osteogenesis imperfecta and related osteochondrodysplasias: medical and surgical management. *J Neurosurg* 1997;86:950–960.
62. Ibrahim AG, Crockard HA. Basilar impression and osteogenesis imperfecta: a 21-year retrospective review of outcomes in 20 patients. *J Neurosurg Spine* 2007;7:594–600.
63. Yamada H, Nakamura S, Tajima M, et al. Neurological manifestations of pediatric achondroplasis. *J Neurosurg* 1981;54:49–57.
64. Wong VCN, Fung CF. Basilar impression in a child with hypochondroplasia. *Pediatr Neurol* 1991;7:62–64.
65. Isu T, Miyasaka K, Abe H, et al. Atlantoaxial dislocation associated with neurofibromatosis. *J Neurosurg* 1983;58:451–453.
66. de Barros MC, Farias W, Ataide L, et al. Basilar impression and Arnold-Chiari malformation. *J Neurol Neurosurg Psychiat* 1968;31:596–605.
67. Michie I, Clark M. Neurological syndromes associated with cervical and craniocervical anomalies. *Arch Neurol* 1968;18:241–247.
68. Teodori JB, Painter MJ. Basilar impression in children. *Pediatrics* 1984;74:1097–1099.
69. Chamberlain WE. Basilar impression (platybasia): bizarre developmental anomaly of occipital bone and upper cervical spine with striking and misleading neurologic manifestations. *Yale J Biol Med* 1939;11:487–496.
70. McRae DL. Bony abnormalities in the region of the foramen magnum: correlation of the anatomic and neurologic findings. *Acta Radiol* 1960;40:335–354.
71. McGregor M. Significance of certain measurements of skull in diagnosis of basilar impression. *Br J Radiol* 1948;21:171–181.
72. Cronin CG, Lohan DG, Mhuircheartigh JN, et al. MRI evaluation and measurement of the normal odontoid peg position. *Clin Radiol* 2007;62:897–903.
73. Kulkarni AG, Goel AH. Vertical atlantoaxial index. *J Spinal Disord Tech* 2008;21:4–10.
74. Pasztor E, Vajda J, Piffko P, et al. Transoral surgery for basilar impression. *Surg Neurol* 1980;14:473–476.
75. Menezes AH, van Gilder JC, Graf CJ, et al. Craniocervical abnormalities: a comprehensive surgical approach. *J Neurosurg* 1980;53:444–454.
76. Wood DE, Good TL, Hahn J, et al. Decompression of the brain stem and superior cervical spine for congenital/acquired craniovertebral invagination: an interdisciplinary approach. *Laryngoscope* 1990;100:926–931.
77. Goel A. Treatment of basilar invagination by atlantoaxial joint distraction and direct lateral mass fixation. *J Neurosurg Spine* 2004;1(3):281–286.
78. Goel A. Progressive basilar invagination after transoral odontoidectomy: treatment by atlantoaxial facet distraction and craniovertebral realignment. *Spine* 2005;30:e551–e555.
79. Hunt TE, Dekaban AS. Modified head-neck support for basilar impression with brain-stem compression. *Can Med Assoc J* 1982;126:947–948.
80. Menezes AH, VanGilder JC. Transoral-transpharyngeal approach to the anterior craniocervical junction. *J Neurosurg* 1988;69:895–903.
81. McGirt MJ, Attenello FJ, Sciubba DM, et al. Endoscopic transcervical odontoidectomy for pediatric basilar invagination and cranial settling. *J Neurosurg Pediatr* 2008;1:337–342.
82. Bharucha EP, Dastur HM. Craniovertebral anomalies (a report on 40 cases). *Brain* 1964;87:469–480.
83. Kim LJ, Rekate HL, Kloppenstein JD, et al. Treatment of basilar invagination associated with Chiari I malformations in the pediatric population: cervical reduction and posterior occipitocervical fusion. *J Neurosurg Pediatr* 2004;101(2):189–195.
84. Goel A, Bhatjiwale M, Desai K. Basilar invagination: a study based on 190 surgically treated patients. *J Neurosurg* 1998;88:962–968.
85. Hosalkar HS, Sankar WN, Wills BPD, et al. Congenital osseous anomalies of the upper cervical spine. *J Bone Joint Surg Am* 2008;90-A:337–348.
86. Gholve PA, Hosalkar HS, Ricchetti ET, et al. Occipitalization of the atlas in children. Morphologic classification, associations, and clinical relevance. *J Bone Joint Surg Am* 2007;89-A:571–578.
87. McRae DL, Barnum AS. Occipitalization of the atlas. *AJR Am J Roentgenol* 1953;70:23–46.
88. Al Kaissi A, Chehida FB, Safi H, et al. Progressive congenital torticollis in VATER association syndrome. *Spine* 2006;31:e376–e378.
89. Halanski MA, Iskandar B, Nemeth B, et al. The coconut condyle: occipital condylar dysplasia causing torticollis and leading to C1 fracture. *J Spinal Disord Tech* 2006;19:295–298.
90. Mesiwala AH, Shaffery CI, Gruss JS, et al. Atypical hemifacial microsomia associated with Chiari I malformation and syrinx: further evidence indicating that Chiari I malformation is a disorder of the paraxial mesoderm. *J Neurosurg* 2001;95:1034–1039.
91. Ricchetti ET, States L, Hosalkar HS, et al. Radiographic study of the upper cervical spine in the 22q11.2 deletion syndrome. *J Bone Joint Surg Am* 2004;86-A:1751–1760.
92. Greenberg AD. Atlantoaxial dislocation. *Brain* 1968;91:655–684.
93. Wadia NH. Myelopathy complicating congenital atlantoaxial dislocation (a study of 28 cases). *Brain* 1967;90:449–472.
94. Kuhns LR, Loder RT, Rogers E, et al. Head-wag autotomography of the upper cervical spine in infantile torticollis. *Pediatr Radiol* 1998;28:464–467.
95. McRae DL. The significance of abnormalities of the cervical spine. *AJR Am J Roentgenol* 1960;84:3–25.
96. Weng MS, Haynes RJ. Flexion and extension cervical MRI in a pediatric population. *J Pediatr Orthop* 1996;16:359–363.
97. Agrawal D, Gowda NK, Bal CS, et al. Have crani-vertebral anomalies been overlooked as a cause of vertebro-basilar insufficiency? *Spine* 2006;31:846–850.
98. Nicholson JT, Sherk HH. Anomalies of the occipitocervical articulation. *J Bone Joint Surg Am* 1968;50-A:295–304.
99. Fenoy AJ, Menezes AH, Fenoy KA. Craniocervical junction fusions in patients with hindbrain herniation and syringomyelia. *J Neurosurg Spine* 2008;9:1–9.
100. Menezes AH. Evaluation and treatment of congenital and developmental anomalies of the cervical spine. *J Neurosurg Spine* 2004;1:188–197.
101. Ransford AO, Crockard HA, Pozo JL. Craniocervical instability treated by contoured loop fixation. *J Bone Joint Surg Br* 1986;68-B:173–177.
102. Johnson RM, Hart DL, Simmons EF, et al. Cervical orthoses. A study comparing their effectiveness in restricting cervical motion in normal subjects. *J Bone Joint Surg Am* 1977;59-A:332–339.
103. Dormans JP, Drummond DS, Sutton LN, et al. Occipitocervical arthrodesis in children. *J Bone Joint Surg Am* 1995;77-A:1234–1240.
104. Koop SE, Winter RB, Lonstein JE. The surgical treatment of instability of the upper part of the cervical spine in children and adolescents. *J Bone Joint Surg Am* 1984;66-A:403–411.
105. Doubousset J. Torticollis in children caused by congenital anomalies of the axis. *J Bone Joint Surg Am* 1986;68-A:178–188.
106. Graziano GP, Herzenberg JE, Hensinger RN. The halo-Ilizarov distraction cast for correction of cervical deformity. *J Bone Joint Surg Am* 1993;75-A:996–1003.
107. Saltzman CL, Hensinger RN, Blane CE, et al. Familial cervical dysplasia. *J Bone Joint Surg Am* 1991;73-A:163–171.

108. Fielding JW, Hawkins RJ. Atlanto-axial rotatory fixation. *J Bone Joint Surg Am* 1977;59-A:37–44.

109. Jackson G, Adler DC. Examination of the atlantoaxial joint following injury with particular emphasis on rotational subluxation. *AJR Am J Roentgenol* 1956;76:1081–1094.

110. Fielding JW. Normal and selected abnormal motion of the cervical spine from the second cervical vertebra to the seventh cervical vertebra based on cineroentgenography. *J Bone Joint Surg Am* 1964;46-A: 1779–1781.

111. Fielding JW. Cineroentgenography of the normal cervical spine. *J Bone Joint Surg Am* 1957;37:1280–1288.

112. Fielding JW, Stillwell WT, Chynn KY, et al. Use of computed tomography for the diagnosis of atlanto-axial rotatory fixation. *J Bone Joint Surg Am* 1978;60-A:1102–1104.

113. Pang D, Li V. Atlantoaxial rotatory fixation: part 1-biomechanics of normal rotation at the atlantoaxial joint in children. *Neurosurgery* 2004;55:614–626.

114. Pang D, Li V. Atlantoaxial rotatory fixation: part 2-new diagnostic paradigm and a new classification based on motion analysis using computed tomographic imaging. *Neurosurgery* 2005;57:941–953.

115. Pang D, Li V. Atlantoaxial rotatory fixation: part 3-a prospective study of the clinical manifestation, diagnosis, management, and outcome of children with atlantoaxial rotatory fixation. *Neurosurgery* 2005;57:954–972.

116. Mathern GW, Batzdorf U. Grisel's syndrome. Cervical spine clinical, pathologic, and neurologic manifestations. *Clin Orthop Relat Res* 1989;244:131–146.

117. Bowen RE, Mah JY, Otsuka NY. Midshaft clavicle fractures associated with atlantoaxial rotatory displacement: a report of two cases. *J Orthop Trauma* 2003;17:444–447.

118. Brisson P, Patel H, Scorpio R, et al. Rotatory atlanto-axial subluxation with torticollis following central-venous catheter insertion. *Pediatr Surg Int* 2000;16:421–423.

119. Mezue WC, Taha ZM, Bashir EM. Fever and acquired torticollis in hospitalized children. *J Laryngol Otol* 2002;116:280–284.

120. Parke WW, Rothman RH, Brown MD. The pharyngovertebral veins: an anatomical rationale for Grisel's syndrome. *J Bone Joint Surg Am* 1984;66-A:568–574.

121. Dimaala J, Chaljub G, Oto A, et al. Odontoid osteomyelitis masquerading as a C2 fracture in an 18-month-old male with torticollis: CT and MRI features. *Emerg Radiol* 2006;12:234–236.

122. Simsek S, Yigitkanli K, Kazanci A, et al. Medically treated paravertebral *Brucella* abscess presenting with acute torticollis: case report. *Surg Neurol* 2007;67:207–210.

123. Wieringa JW, Wolfs TFW, van Houten MA. Grisel syndrome following meningitis and anaerobic bacteremia with *Bacteroides ureolyticus*. *Pediatr Infect Dis* 2007;26:970–971.

124. Yu KK, White DR, Weissler MC, et al. Nontraumatic atlantoaxial subluxation (Grisel syndrome): a rare complication of otolaryngological procedures. *Laryngoscope* 2003;113:1047–1049.

125. Tschopp K. Monopolar electrocautery in adenoidectomy as a possible risk factor for Grisel's syndrome. *Laryngoscope* 2002;112(8 Pt 1): 1445–1449.

126. Tang X-Y, Liu L-J, Yang H-J, et al. Anatomic study of the synovial folds of the occipito-atlanto-axial joints. *Clin Anat* 2007;20:376–381.

127. Kawabe N, Hirotani H, Tanaka O. Pathomechanism of atlantoaxial rotatory fixation in children. *J Pediatr Orthop* 1989;9:569–574.

128. Phillips WA, Hensinger RN. The management of rotary atlanto-axial subluxation in children. *J Bone Joint Surg Am* 1989;71-A:664–668.

129. Mihara H, Onari K, Hachiya M, et al. Follow-up study of conservative treatment for atlantoaxial rotatory displacement. *J Spinal Disord* 2001;14:494–499.

130. Gallie WE. Fractures and dislocations of the cervical spine. *Am J Surg* 1939;46:495–499.

131. Fielding JW, Hawkins RJ, Ratzan SA. Spine fusion for atlanto-axial instability. *J Bone Joint Surg Am* 1976;58-A:400–407.

132. McGraw RW, Rusch RM. Atlanto-axial arthrodesis. *J Bone Joint Surg Br* 1973;55-B:482–489.

133. Mah JY, Thometz J, Emans J, et al. Threaded K-wire spinous process fixation of the axis for modified Gallie fusion in children and adolescents. *J Pediatr Orthop* 1989;9:675–679.

134. Parisine P, Di Silvestre M, Greggi T, et al. C1-C2 posterior fusion in growing patients. *Spine* 2003;28:566–572.

135. Crossman JE, David K, Hayward R, et al. Open reduction of pediatric atlantoaxial rotatory fixation: long term outcome study with functional measurements. *J Neurosurg (Spine 3)* 2003;100:235–240.

136. Weibkopf M, Naeve D, Ruf M, et al. Therapeutic options and results following fixed atlantoaxial rotatory dislocations. *Eur Spine J* 2005; 14:61–68.

137. Ho BCS, Lee EH, Singh K. Epidemiology, presentation, and management of congenital muscular torticollis. *Singapore Med J* 1999;40: 675–679.

138. Chen M-M, Chang H-C, Hsieh C-F, et al. Predictive model for congenital muscular torticollis: analysis of 1021 infants with sonography. *Arch Phys Med Rehabil* 2005;86:2199–2023.

139. Ling CM. The influence of age on the results of open sternomastoid tenotomy in muscular torticollis. *Clin Orthop Relat Res* 1976;116:142–148.

140. MacDonald D. Sternomastoid tumor and muscular torticollis. *J Bone Joint Surg Br* 1969;51-B:432–443.

141. Davids JR, Wenger DR, Mubarak SJ. Congenital muscular torticollis: sequela of intrauterine or perinatal compartment syndrome. *J Pediatr Orthop* 1993;13:141–147.

142. Whyte AM, Lufkin RB, Bredenkamp J, et al. Sternocleidomastoid fibrosis in congenital muscular torticollis: MR appearance. *J Comput Assist Tomogr* 1989;13:163–166.

143. Ling CM, Low YS. Sternomastoid tumor and muscular torticollis. *Clin Orthop Relat Res* 1972;86:144–150.

144. Weiner DS. Congenital dislocation of the hip associated with congenital muscular torticollis. *Clin Orthop Relat Res* 1976;121:163–165.

145. Thompson F, McManus S, Colville J. Familial congenital muscular torticollis. *Clin Orthop Relat Res* 1986;202:193–196.

146. Hosalkar H, Gill IS, Gujar P, et al. Familial torticollis with polydactyly: manifestations in three generations. *Am J Orthop* 2001;30:656–658.

147. Engin C, Yavuz SS, Sahin FI. Congenital muscular torticollis: is heredity a possible factor in a family with five torticollis patients in three generations? *Plast Reconstr Surg* 1997;99:1147–1150.

148. Sarnat HB, Morrissy RT. Idiopathic torticollis: sternocleidomastoid myopathy and accessory neuropathy. *Muscle Nerve* 1981;4:374–380.

149. Tang S, Liu Z, Quan X, et al. Sternocleidomastoid pseudotumor of infants and congenital muscular torticollis: fine structure research. *J Pediatr Orthop* 1998;18:214–218.

150. Cheng JCY, Tang SP, Chen TMK, et al. The clinical presentation and outcome of treatment of congenital muscular torticollis in infants—a study of 1086 cases. *J Pediatr Surg* 2000;35:1091–1096.

151. Coventry MB, Harris LE. Congenital muscular torticollis in infancy. *J Bone Joint Surg Am* 1959;41-A:815–822.

152. Walsh JJ, Morrissy RT. Torticollis and hip dislocation. *J Pediatr Orthop* 1998;18:219–221.

153. van Vlimmeren LA, Helders PJM, van Adrichem LNA, et al. Torticollis and plagiocephaly in infancy: therapeutic strategies. *Pediatr Rehabil* 2006;9:40–46.

154. de Chalain TMB, Park S. Torticollis associated with positional plagiocephaly: a growing epidemic. *J Craniofac Surg* 2005;16:411–418.

155. Brackbill Y, Douthitt TC, West H. Psychophysiologic effects in the neonate of prone versus supine placement. *J Pediatr* 1973;81:82–84.

156. Dudkiewicz I, Ganel A, Blankstein A. Congenital muscular torticollis in infants: ultrasound-assisted diagnosis and evaluation. *J Pediatr Orthop* 2005;25:812–814.

157. Parikh SN, Crawford AH, Choudhury S. Magnetic resonance imaging in the evaluation of infantile torticollis. *Orthopedics* 2004;27:509–515.

158. Cheng JCY, Au AWY. Infantile torticollis: a review of 624 cases. *J Pediatr Orthop* 1994;14:802–808.

159. Cheng JCY, Wong MWN, Tang SP, et al. Clinical determinants of the outcome of manual stretching in the treatment of congenital muscular torticollis in infants. *J Bone Joint Surg Am* 2001;83-A:679–687.

160. Binder H, Eng GD, Gaiser JF, et al. Congenital muscular torticollis: results of conservative management with long-term follow-up in 85 cases. *Arch Phys Med Rehabil* 1987;68:222–225.

161. Canale ST, Griffin DW, Hubbard CN. Congenital muscular torticollis. A long-term follow-up. *J Bone Joint Surg Am* 1982;64-A:810–816.

162. Cheng JC-Y, Metrewell C, Chen TM-K, et al. Correlation of ultrasonographic imaging of congenital muscular torticollis with clinical assessment in infants. *Ultrasound Med Biol* 2000;26:1237–1241.

163. Hsu T-C, Wang C-L, Wong M-K, et al. Correlation of clinical and ultrasonographic features in congenital muscular torticollis. *Arch Phys Med Rehabil* 1999;80:637–641.

164. Lin J-N, Chou M-L. Ultrasonographic study of the sternocleidomastoid muscle in the management of congenital muscular torticollis. *J Pediatr Surg* 1997;32:1648–1651.

165. Wei JL, Schwartz KM, Weaver AL, et al. Pseudotumor of infancy and congenital muscular torticollis: 170 cases. *Laryngoscope* 2001;111:688–695.

166. Cheng JCY, Chen TMK, Tang SP, et al. Snapping during manual stretching in congenital muscular torticollis. *Clin Orthop Relat Res* 2001;384:237–244.

167. Collins A, Jankovic J. Botulinum toxin injection for congenital muscular torticollis presenting in children and adults. *Neurology* 2006;67:1083–1085.

168. Joyce MB, de Chalain TMB. Treatment of recalcitrant idiopathic muscular torticollis in infants with botulinum toxin type A. *J Craniofac Surg* 2005;16:321–327.

169. Oleszek JL, Chang N, Apkon SD, et al. Botulinum toxin type A in the treatment of children with congenital muscular torticollis. *Am J Phys Med Rehabil* 2005;84:813–816.

170. Ferkel RD, Westin GW, Dawson EG, et al. Muscular torticollis. A modified surgical approach. *J Bone Joint Surg Am* 1983;65-A:894–900.

171. Cheng JCY, Tang SP. Outcome of surgical treatment of congenital muscular torticollis. *Clin Orthop Relat Res* 1999;362:190–200.

172. Shim JS, Noh KC, Park SJ. Treatment of congenital muscular torticollis in patients older than 8 years. *J Pediatr Orthop* 2004;24:683–688.

173. Tse P, Cheng J, Chow Y, et al. Surgery for neglected congenital torticollis. *Acta Orthop Scand* 1987;58:270–272.

174. Burstein FD. Long-term experience with endoscopic surgical treatment for congenital muscular torticollis in infants and children: a review of 85 cases. *Plast Reconstr Surg* 2004;114:491–493.

175. Stassen LFA, Kerawal CJ. New surgical technique for the correction of congenital muscular torticollis (wry neck). *Br J Oral Maxillofac Surg* 2000;38:142–147.

176. Chen C-E, Ko J-Y. Surgical treatment of muscular torticollis for patients above 6 years of age. *Arch Orthop Trauma Surg* 2000;120:149–151.

177. Gürpinar A, Kiristioglu I, Balkan E, et al. Surgical correction of muscular torticollis in older children with Peter G. Jones technique. *J Pediatr Orthop* 1998;18:598–601.

178. Skaggs DL, Lerman LD, Albrektson J, et al. Use of a noninvasive halo in children. *Spine* 2008;33:1650–1654.

179. Nucci P, Kushner BJ, Serafino M, et al. A multi-disciplinary study of the ocular, orthopedic, and neurologic causes of abnormal head postures in children. *Am J Ophthalmol* 2005;140:65–68.

180. Taboas-Perez RA, Rivera-Reyes L. Head tilt: a revisit to an old sign of posterior fossa tumors. *Bol Asoc Med PR* 1984;76:62–65.

181. O'Brien DF, Allcutt D, Caird J, et al. Posterior fossa tumours in childhood: evaluation of presenting clinical features. *Ir Med J* 2001;94:52–53.

182. Dörner L, Fritsch MJ, Stark AM, et al. Posterior fossa tumors in children: how long does it take to establish the diagnosis? *Child Nerv Syst* 2007;23:887–890.

183. Marmor MA, Beauchamp GR, Maddox SF. Photophobia, epiphora, and torticollis: a masquerade syndrome. *J Pediatr Ophthalmol Strabismus* 1990;27:202–204.

184. Giuffrè R, di Lorenzo N, Fortuna A. Cervical tumors of infancy and childhood. *J Neurosurg Sci* 1981;25:259–264.

185. Visudhiphan P, Chiemchanya S, Somburanasin R, et al. Torticollis as the presenting sign in cervical spine infection and tumor. *Clin Pediatr* 1982;21:71–76.

186. Kumandas S, Per H, Gumus H, et al. Torticollis secondary to posterior fossa and cervical spinal cord tumors: report of five cases and literature review. *Neurosurg Rev* 2006;29:333–338.

187. Rauch R, Jungert J, Rupprecht T, et al. Torticollis revealing as a symptom of acute lymphoblastic leukemia in a fourteen-month-old girl. *Acta Paediatr* 2001;90(5):587–588.

188. Dure LS, Percy AK, Cheek WR, et al. Chiari type I malformation in children. *J Pediatr* 1989;115:573–576.

189. Wilkins RH, Brody IA. The Arnold-Chiari malformation. Neurological classics XXXVIII. *Arch Neurol* 1971;25:376–379.

190. Williams CRP, O'Flynn E, Clarke NMP, et al. Torticollis secondary to ocular pathology. *J Bone Joint Surg Br* 1996;78-B:620–624.

191. Rubin SE, Wagner RS. Ocular torticollis. *Surv Ophthalmol* 1986;30:366–376.

192. Parker W. Migraine and the vestibular system in childhood and adolescence. *Am J Otol* 1989;10:364–371.

193. Snyder CH. Paroxysmal torticollis in infancy. A possible form of labyrinthitis. *Am J Dis Child* 1969;117:458–460.

194. Drigo P, Carli G, Laverda AM. Benign paroxysmal torticollis of infancy. *Brain Dev* 2000;22:169–172.

195. Al-Twaijri WA, Shevell MI. Pediatric migraine equivalents: occurrence and clinical features in practice. *Pediatr Neurol* 2002;26:365–368.

196. Giffin NJ, Benton S, Goadsby PJ. Benign paroxysmal torticollis of infancy: four new cases and linkage to CACNA1A mutation. *Dev Med Child Neurol* 2002;44:490–493.

197. Murphy WJ Jr, Gellis SS. Torticollis with hiatus hernia in infancy. *Am J Dis Child* 1977;131:564–565.

198. Ramenofsky ML, Buyse M, Goldberg MJ, et al. Gastroesophageal reflux and torticollis. *J Bone Joint Surg Am* 1978;60-A:1140–1141.

199. Darling DB, Fisher JH, Gellis SS. Hiatal hernia and gastroesophageal reflux in infants and children: analysis of the incidence in North American children. *Pediatrics* 1974;54:450–455.

200. Darling DB. Hiatal hernia and gastroesophageal reflux in infancy and childhood. Analysis of the radiological findings. *AJR Am J Roentgenol* 1975;123:724–736.

201. Jolley SG, Johnson DG, Herbst JJ, et al. An assessment of gastroesophageal reflux in children by extended pH monitoring of the distal esophagus. *Surgery* 1978;84:16–24.

202. Johnson DG, Herbst JJ, Oliveros MA, et al. Evaluation of gastroesophageal reflux surgery in children. *Pediatrics* 1977;59:62–68.

203. Hensinger RN, Lang JE, MacEwen GD. Klippel-Feil syndrome. A constellation of associated anomalies. *J Bone Joint Surg Am* 1974;56-A:1246–1253.

204. Brown MW, Templeton AW, Hodges FJ III. The incidence of acquired and congenital fusions in the cervical spine. *AJR Am J Roentgenol* 1964;92:1255–1259.

205. Thompson E, Haan E, Sheffield L. Autosomal dominant Klippel-Feil anomaly with cleft palate. *Clin Dysmorphol* 1998;7:11–15.

206. Clarke RA, Kearsley JH, Walsh DA. Patterned expression in familial Klippel-Feil syndrome. *Teratology* 1996;53:152–157.

207. Clarke RA, Catalan G, Diwan AD, et al. Heterogeneity in Klippel-Feil syndrome: a new classification. *Pediatr Radiol* 1998;28:967–974.

208. Samartzis D, Herman J, Lubicky JP, et al. Sprengel's deformity in Klippel-Feil syndrome. *Spine* 2007;32:e512–e516.

209. Thomsen M, Krober M, Schneider U, et al. Congenital limb deficiencies associated with Klippel-Feil syndrome. A survey of 57 subjects. *Acta Orthop Scand* 2000;71:461–464.

210. Moore WB, Matthews TJ, Rabinowitz R. Genitourinary anomalies associated with Klippel-Feil syndrome. *J Bone Joint Surg Am* 1975;57-A:355–357.

211. Stark EW, Borton T. Klippel-Feil syndrome and associated hearing loss. *Arch Otolaryngol* 1973;97:415–419.

212. Gunderson CH, Solitare GB. Mirror movements in patients with the Klippel-Feil syndrome. *Arch Neurol* 1968;18:675–679.

213. Auerbach JD, Hosalkar HS, Kusuma SK, et al. Spinal cord dimensions in children with Klippel-Feil syndrome. *Spine* 2008;33:1366–1371.

214. Samartzis D, Kalluri P, Herman J, et al. 2008 Young Investigator Award: the role of congenitally fused cervical segments upon the space available for the cord and associated symptoms in Klippel-Feil patients. *Spine* 2008;33:1442–1450.

215. Baga N, Chusid EL, Miller A. Pulmonary disability in the Klippel-Feil syndrome. *Clin Orthop Relat Res* 1969;67:105–110.

216. Nora JJ, Cohen M, Maxwell GM. Klippel-Feil syndrome with congenital heart disease. *Am J Dis Child* 1961;102:110–116.

217. Abbas J, Nazzal N, Serrano P, et al. Aortic arch abnormality in a patient with Klippel-Feil syndrome. *Vascular* 2006;14:43–46.

218. Kawano Y, Tamura A, Abe Y, et al. Klippel-Feil syndrome accompanied by pulmonary artery sling. *Intern Med* 2008;47:327.

219. Samartzis D, Kalluri P, Herman J, et al. The extent of fusion within the congenital Klippel-Feil segment. *Spine* 2008;33:1637–1642.

220. Thomsen MN, Schneider U, Weber M, et al. Scoliosis and congenital anomalies associated with Klippel-Feil syndrome types I–III. *Spine* 1997;21:396–401.

221. Samartzis D, Kalluri P, Herman J, et al. Superior odontoid migration in the Klippel-Feil patient. *Eur Spine J* 2007;16:1489–1497.

222. Hall JE, Simmons ED, Danylchuk K, et al. Instability of the cervical spine and neurological involvement in Klippel-Feil syndrome. *J Bone Joint Surg Am* 1990;72-A:460–462.

223. Shen FH, Samartzis D, Herman J, et al. Radiographic assessment of segmental motion at the atlantoaxial junction in the Klippel-Feil patient. *Spine* 2006;31:171–177.

224. Epstein NE, Epstein JA, Zilkha A. Traumatic myelopathy in a seventeen-year-old child with cervical spinal stenosis (without fracture or dislocation) and a C2-3 Klippel-Feil fusion. *Spine* 1984;9:344–347.

225. Drvaric DM, Ruderman RJ, Conrad RW, et al. Congenital scoliosis and urinary tract abnormalities: are intravenous pyelograms necessary? *J Pediatr Orthop* 1987;7:441–443.

226. Ritterbusch JF, McGinty LD, Spar J, et al. Magnetic resonance imaging for stenosis and subluxation in Klippel-Feil syndrome. *Spine* 1991;16(Suppl):539–541.

227. Pizzutillo PD, Woods M, Nicholson L, et al. Risk factors in Klippel-Feil syndrome. *Spine* 1994;19:2110–2116.

228. Gupta SN, Piatt JH Jr, Belay B. Cervical spinal cord neurapraxia in the setting of Klippel-Feil anomaly: a diagnostic and therapeutic challenge. *Spinal Cord* 2007;45:637–640.

229. Samartzis D, Herman J, Lubicky JP, et al. Classification of congenitally fused cervical patterns in Klippel-Feil patients. Epidemiology and role in the development of cervical spine-related symptoms. *Spine* 2006;31:e798–e804.

230. Sherk HH, Shut L, Chung S. Iniencephalic deformity of the cervical spine with Klippel-Feil anomalies and congenital evaluation of the scapula. *J Bone Joint Surg Am* 1974;56-A:1254–1259.

231. Rouvreau P, Glorion C, Langlais J, et al. Assessment and neurologic involvement of patients with cervical spine congenital synostosis as in Klippel-Feil syndrome: study of 19 cases. *J Pediatr Orthop B* 1998;7:179–185.

232. Royal SA, Tubbs S, D'Antonio MG, et al. Investigations into the association between cervicomedullary neuroschisis and mirror movements in patients with Klippel-Feil syndrome. *AJNR Am J Neuroradiol* 2002;23:724–729.

233. Guille JT, Miller A, Bowen JR, et al. The natural history of Klippel-Feil syndrome: clinical, roentgenographic, and magnetic resonance imaging findings at adulthood. *J Pediatr Orthop* 1995;15:617–626.

234. Matsumoto K, Wakahara K, Sumi H, et al. Central cord syndrome in patients with Klippel-Feil syndrome resulting from winter sports: report of 3 cases. *Am J Sports Med* 2006;34:1685–1689.

235. Fielding JW, Hensinger RN, Hawkins RJ. Os odontoideum. *J Bone Joint Surg Am* 1980;62-A:376–383.

236. Verska JM, Anderson PA. Os odontoideum. A case report of one identical twin. *Spine* 1997;22:706–709.

237. Kuhns LR, Loder RT, Farley FA, et al. Nuchal cord changes in children with os odontoideum: evidence for associated trauma. *J Pediatr Orthop* 1998;18:815–819.

238. Sakaida H, Waga S, Kojima T, et al. Os odontoideum associated with hypertrophic ossiculum terminale. *J Neurosurg* 2001;94:140–144.

239. Garg A, Kaikwad SB, Gupta V, et al. Bipartite atlas with os odontoideum. Case report. *Spine* 2004;29:e35–38.

240. Fagan AB, Askin GN, Earwaker JWS. The jigsaw sign. A reliable indicator of congenital aetiology in os odontoideum. *Eur Spine J* 2004;13:295–300.

241. Osti M, Philipp H, Meusburger B, et al. Os odontoideum with bipartite atlas and segmental instability: a case report. *Eur Spine J* 2006;15(Suppl 5): S564–S567.

242. Currarino G. Segmentation defect in the midontoid process and its possible relationship to the congenital type of os odontoideum. *Pediatr Radiol* 2002;32:34–40.

243. Sankar WN, Wills BPD, Dormans JP, et al. Os odontoideum revisited: the case for a multifactorial etiology. *Spine* 2006;31:979–984.

244. Matsui H, Imada K, Tsuji H. Radiographic classification of os odontoideum and its clinical significance. *Spine* 1997;22:1706–1709.

245. Watanabe M, Toyama Y, Fujimura Y. Atlantoaxial instability in os odontoideum with myelopathy. *Spine* 1996;21:1435–1439.

246. Aksoy FG, Gomori JM. Symptomatic cervical synovial cyst associated with an os odontoideum diagnosed by magnetic resonance imaging. *Spine* 2000;25:1300–1302.

247. Chang H, Park J-B, Kim K-W. Synovial cyst of the transverse ligament of the atlas in a patient with os odontoideum and atlantoaxial instability. *Spine* 2000;25:741–744.

248. Chang H, Park J-B, Kim K-W, et al. Retro-dental reactive lesions related to development of myelopathy in patients with atlantoaxial instability secondary to os odontoideum. *Spine* 2000;25:2777–2783.

249. Jun B-Y. Complete reduction of retro-odontoid soft tissue mass in os odontoideum following the posterior C1-C2 transarticular screw fixation. *Spine* 1999;24:1961–1964.

250. Wang J, Vokshoor A, Kim S, et al. Pediatric atlantoaxial instability: management with screw fixation. *Pediatr Neurosurg* 1999;30:70–78.

251. Yoshimoto H, Ito M, Abumi K, et al. A retrospective radiographic analysis of subaxial sagittal alignment after posterior C1- C2 fusion. *Spine* 2004;29:175–181.

252. Spitzer R, Rabinowitch JY, Wybor KC. A study of the abnormalities of the skull, teeth, and lenses in Mongolism. *Can Med Assoc J* 1961;84: 567–568.

253. Matsuda Y, Sano N, Watanabe S, et al. Atlanto-occipital hypermobility in subjects with Down's syndrome. *Spine* 1995;20:2283–2286.

254. Selby KA, Newton RW, Gupta S, et al. Clinical predictors and radiological reliability in atlantoaxial subluxation in Down's syndrome. *Arch Dis Child* 1991;66:876–878.

255. Karol LA, Sheffield EG, Crawford K, et al. Reproducibility in the measurement of atlanto-occipital instability in children with Down syndrome. *Spine* 1996;21:2463–2468.

256. Parfenchuck TA, Bertrand SL, Powers MJ, et al. Posterior occipitoatlantal hypermobility in Down syndrome: an analysis of 199 patients. *J Pediatr Orthop* 1994;14:304–308.

257. Browd S, Healy LJ, Dopbie G, et al. Morphometric and qualitative analysis of congenital occipitocervical instability in children: implications for patients with Down syndrome. *J Neurosurg Pediatr* 2006;105 (1 Suppl):50–54.

258. Pueschel SM, Herndon JH, Gelch MM, et al. Symptomatic atlantoaxial subluxation in persons with Down syndrome. *J Pediatr Orthop* 1984;4:682–688.

259. Committee on Sports Medicine and Fitness of the American Academy of Pediatrics. Atlantoaxial instability in Down syndrome: subject review. *Pediatrics* 1995;96:151–154.

260. Burke SW, French HG, Roberts JM, et al. Chronic atlanto-axial instability in Down syndrome. *J Bone Joint Surg Am* 1985;67-A:1356–1360.

261. Pueschel SM, Scola FH, Tupper TB, et al. Skeletal anomalies of the upper cervical spine in children with Down syndrome. *J Pediatr Orthop* 1990;10:607–611.

262. Ferguson RL, Putney ME, Allen BL Jr. Comparison of neurologic deficits with atlanto-dens intervals in patients with Down syndrome. *J Spinal Disord* 1997;10:246–252.

263. Committee on Sports Medicine and Fitness of the American Academy of Pediatrics. Atlantoaxial instability in Down syndrome. *Pediatrics* 1984;74:152–154.

264. Wellborn CC, Sturm PF, Hatch RS, et al. Intraobserver reproducibility and interobserver reliability of cervical spine measurements. *J Pediatr Orthop* 2000;20:66–70.

265. Pueschel SM, Findley TW, Furia J, et al. Atlantoaxial instability in Down syndrome: roentgenographic, neurologic, and somatosensory evoked potential studies. *J Pediatr* 1987;110:515–521.

266. Brockmeyer DL, York JE, Apfelbaum RI. Anatomical suitability of C1-2 transarticular screw placement in pediatric patients. *J Neurosurg (Spine 1)* 2000;92:7–11.

267. Taggard DA, Menezes AH, Ryken TC. Treatment of Down syndrome-associated craniovertebral junction abnormalities. *J Neurosurg (Spine 2)* 2000;93:205–213.

268. Hedequist D, Hresko T, Proctor M. Modern cervical spine instrumentation in children. *Spine* 2008;33:379–383.

269. Reilly CW, Choit RL. Transarticular screws in the management of C1-C2 instability in children. *J Pediatr Orthop* 2006;26:582–588.

270. Gluf WM, Brockmeyer DL. Atlantoaxial transarticular screw fixation: a review of surgical indications, fusion rate, complications, and lessons learned in 67 pediatric patients. *J Neurosurg Spine* 2005;2:164–169.

271. Nordt JC, Stauffer ES. Sequelae of atlantoaxial stabilization in two patients with Down's syndrome. *Spine* 1981;6:437–440.

272. Lundy DW, Murrary HH. Neurological deterioration after posterior wiring of the cervical spine. *J Bone Joint Surg Br* 1997;79-B:948–951.

273. Smith MD, Phillips WA, Hensinger RN. Fusion of the upper cervical spine in children and adolescents. An analysis of 17 patients. *Spine* 1990;16:695–701.

274. Rizzolo S, Lemos MJ, Mason DE. Posterior spinal arthrodesis for atlanto-axial instability in Down syndrome. *J Pediatr Orthop* 1995;15:543–548.

275. Segal LS, Drummond DS, Zanotti RM, et al. Complications of posterior arthrodesis of the cervical spine in patients with have Down syndrome. *J Bone Joint Surg Am* 1991;73-A:1547–1554.

276. Smith MD, Phillips WA, Hensinger RN. Complications of fusion to the upper cervical spine. *Spine* 1991;16:702–705.

277. Doyle JS, Lauerman WC, Wood KB, et al. Complications and long-term outcome of upper cervical spine arthrodesis in patients with Down syndrome. *Spine* 1996;21:1223–1231.

278. Msall M, Rogers B, DiGaudio K, et al. Long-term complications of segmental cervical fusion in Down syndrome. *Dev Med Child Neurol* 1991;33(Suppl 64):5.

279. Tan GH, Tan KK, Afian MS, et al. Progressive supra-axial cervical instability in Down syndrome: a case report emphasising the role of extended short-segment fusion. *Med J Malaysia* 2005;60:111–113.

280. Hobbs WR, Sponseller PD, Weiss A-PC, et al. The cervical spine in Marfan syndrome. *Spine* 1997;22:983–989.

281. Herzka A, Sponseller PD, Pyeritz RE. Atlantoaxial rotatory subluxation in patients with Marfan syndrome. *Spine* 2000;25:524–526.

282. Place HM, Enzenauer RJ. Cervical spine subluxation in Marfan syndrome. A case report. *J Bone Joint Surg Am* 2006;88-A:2479–2482.

283. Georgopoulos G, Pizzutillo PD, Lee MS. Occipito-atlantal instability in children. *J Bone Joint Surg Am* 1987;69-A:429–436.

284. Ebara S, Harada T, Yamazaki Y, et al. Unstable cervical spine in athetoid cerebral palsy. *Spine* 1989;14:1154–1159.

285. Fuji T, Yonenobu K, Fujiwara K, et al. Cervical radiculopathy or myelopathy secondary to athetoid cerebral palsy. *J Bone Joint Surg Am* 1987;69-A:815–821.

286. Nishihara N, Tnabe G, Nakahara S, et al. Surgical treatment of cervical spondylotic myelopathy complicating athetoid cerebral palsy. *J Bone Joint Surg Br* 1984;66-B:504–508.

287. Reese ME, Msall ME, Owen S, et al. Acquired cervical impairment in young adults with cerebral palsy. *Dev Med Child Neurol* 1991;33:153–166.

288. Harada T, Ebara S, Anwar MM, et al. The cervical spine in athetoid cerebral palsy. *J Bone Joint Surg Br* 1996;78-B:613–619.

289. Tsirikos AI, Chang W-N, Shah SA, et al. Acquired atlantoaxial instability in children with spastic cerebral palsy. *J Pediatr Orthop* 2003;23:335–341.

290. Haro H, Komori H, Okawa A, et al. Surgical treatment of cervical spondylotic myelopathy associated with athetoid cerebral palsy. *J Orthop Sci* 2002;7:629–636.

291. Aronson DD, Kahn RH, Canady A, et al. Instability of the cervical spine after decompression in patients who have Arnold-Chiari malformation. *J Bone Joint Surg Am* 1991;73-A:898–906.

292. Cattell HS, Clark GL Jr. Cervical kyphosis and instability following multiple laminectomies in children. *J Bone Joint Surg Am* 1967;49-A:713–720.

293. Francis WR Jr, Noble DP. Treatment of cervical kyphosis in children. *Spine* 1988;13:883–887.

294. Sim FH, Svien HJ, Bickel WH, et al. Swan-neck deformity following extensive cervical laminectomy. *J Bone Joint Surg Am* 1974;56-A:564–580.

295. Yasuoka S, Peterson H, Laws ER Jr, et al. Pathogenesis and prophylaxis of postlaminectomy deformity of the spine after multiple level laminectomy: difference between children and adults. *Neurosurgery* 1981;9:145–152.

296. Bell DF, Walker JL, O'Connor B, et al. Spinal deformity after multiple-level cervical laminectomy in children. *Spine* 1994;19:406–411.

297. McLaughlin MR, Wahlig JB, Pollack IF. Incidence of postlaminectomy kyphosis after Chiari decompression. *Spine* 1997;22:613–617.

298. McGirt MJ, Chaichana KL, Attenello F, et al. Spinal deformity after resection of cervical intramedullary spinal cord tumors in children. *Child Nerv Syst* 2008;24:735–739.

299. Hwang SW, Riesenburger RI, Benzel EC. Pediatric iatrogenic spinal deformity. *Neurosurg Clin N Am* 2007;18:585–598.

300. Lee K-S, Moon M-S. The effect of multilevel laminectomy on the cervical spine of growing cats. *Spine* 1993;18:359–363.

301. Hirabayashi K, Satomi K. Operative procedure and results of expansive open-door laminoplasty. *Spine* 1988;13:870–875.

302. Tredwell SJ, Smith DF, Macleod PJ, et al. Cervical spine anomalies in fetal alcohol syndrome. *Spine* 1982;7:331–334.

303. Sandham A. Cervical vertebral anomalies in cleft lip and palate. *Cleft Palate J* 1986;23:206–214.

304. Ugar DA, Semb G. The prevalence of anomalies of the upper cervical vertebrae in subjects with cleft lip, cleft palate, or both. *Cleft Palate Craniofac J* 2001;38:498–503.

305. Hemmer KM, McAlister WH, Marsh JL. Cervical spine anomalies in the craniosynostosis syndromes. *Cleft Palate J* 1987;24:328–333.

306. Louis DS, Argenta LC. The orthopaedic manifestations of Goldenhar's syndrome. *Surg Rounds Orthop* 1987;July:43–46.

307. Sherk HH, Whitaker LA, Pasquariello PS. Facial malformations and spinal anomalies. A predictable relationship. *Spine* 1982;7:526–531.

308. Anderson PJ, Hall CM, Evans RD, et al. Cervical spine in Pfeiffer's syndrome. *J Craniofac Surg* 1996;7:275–279.

309. Moore MH, Lodge ML, Clark BE. Spinal anomalies in Pfeiffer syndrome. *Cleft Palate Craniofac J* 1995;32:251–254.

310. Anderson PJ, Hall CM, Evans RD, et al. The cervical spine in Saethre-Chotzen syndrome. *Cleft Palate Craniofac J* 1997;34:79–82.

311. Gibson JNA, Sillence DO, Taylor TKF. Abnormalities of the spine in Goldenhar's syndrome. *J Pediatr Orthop* 1996;16:344–349.

312. Healey D, Letts M, Jarvis JG. Cervical spine instability in children with Goldenhar's syndrome. *Can J Surg* 2002;45:341–344.

313. Tsirikos AI, McMaster MJ. Goldenhar-associated conditions (hemifacial microsomia) and congenital deformities of the spine. *Spine* 2006;31:e400–e407.

314. Ewart-Toland A, Yankowitz J, Winder A, et al. Oculoauriculovertebral abnormalities in children of diabetic mothers. *Am J Med Genet* 2000;90(4):303–309.

315. Yong-Hing K, Kalamchi A, MacEwen GD. Cervical spine abnormalities in neurofibromatosis. *J Bone Joint Surg Am* 1979;61-A:695–699.

316. Craig JB, Govender S. Neurofibromatosis of the cervical spine. *J Bone Joint Surg Br* 1992;74-B:575–578.

317. Adkins JC, Ravitch MM. The operative management of von Recklinghausen's neurofibromatosis in children, with special reference to lesions of the head and neck. *Surgery* 1977;82:342–348.

318. Nijland EA, van den Berg MP, Wuisman PIJM, et al. Correction of a dystrophic cervicothoracic spine deformity in Recklinghausen's disease. *Clin Orthop Relat Res* 1998;349:149–155.

319. Giaia G, Mandelli D, Capaccioni B, et al. Postlaminectomy cervical dislocation in von Recklinghausen's disease. *Spine* 1998;23:273–276.

320. Asazuma T, Yamagishi M, Nemoto K, et al. Spinal fusion using a vascularized fibular bone graft for a patient with cervical kyphosis due to neurofibromatosis. *J Spinal Disord* 1997;10:537–540.

321. Kaplan FS, McCluskey W, Hahn G, et al. Genetic transmission of fibrodysplasia ossificans progressiva. *J Bone Joint Surg Am* 1993;75-A: 1214–1220.

322. Schaffer AA, Kaplan FS, Tracy MR, et al. Developmental anomalies of the cervical spine in patients with fibrodysplasia ossificans progress are distinctly different from those in patients with Klippel-Feil syndrome. *Spine* 2005;30:1379–1385.

323. Hall CM, Sutcliffe J. Fibrodysplasia ossificans progressiva. *Ann Radiol* 1978;22:119–123.

324. Connor JM, Smith R. The cervical spine in fibrodysplasia ossificans progressiva. *Br J Radiol* 1982;55:492–496.

325. Falliner A, Drescher W, Brossman J. The spine in fibrodysplasia ossificans progressiva: a case report. *Spine* 2003;28:e519–e522.

326. McGrory BJ, Klassen RA, Chao EYS, et al. Acute fractures and dislocations of the cervical spine in children and adolescents. *J Bone Joint Surg Am* 1993;75-A:988–995.

327. Orzechowski KM, Edgerton EA, Bulas DI, et al. Patterns of injury to restrained children in side impact motor vehicle crashes: the side impact syndrome. *J Trauma* 2003;54:1094–1101.

328. Kokoska ER, Keller MS, Rallo MC, et al. Characteristics of pediatric cervical spine injuries. *J Pediatr Surg* 2001;36:100–105.

329. Brown RL, Brunn MA, Garcia VF. Cervical spine injuries in children: a review of 103 patients treated consecutively at a Level 1 Pediatric Trauma Center. *J Pediatr Surg* 2001;36:1107–1114.

330. Patel JC, Tepas JJ III, Mollitt DL, et al. Pediatric cervical spine injuries: defining the disease. *J Pediatr Surg* 2001;36:373–376.

331. Carreon LY, Glassman SD, Campbell MJ. Pediatric spine fractures. A review of 137 hospital admissions. *J Spinal Disord Tech* 2004;17:477–482.

332. Lally KP, Senac M, Hardin WD Jr, et al. Utility of the cervical spine radiograph in pediatric trauma. *Am J Surg* 1989;158:540–542.

333. Rachesky I, Boyce WT, Duncan B, et al. Clinical prediction of cervical spine injuries in children. Radiographic abnormalities. *Am J Dis Child* 1987;141:199–201.

334. Buhs C, Cullen M, Klein M, et al. The pediatric trauma c-spine: is the 'odontoid' view necessary? *J Pediatr Surg* 2000;35:994–997.

335. Swischuk LE, John SD, Hendrick EP. Is the open-mouth odontoid view necessary in children under 5 years? *Pediatr Radiol* 2000;30:186–189.

336. Herzenberg JE, Hensinger RN, Dedrick DK, et al. Emergency transport and positioning of young children who have an injury of the cervical spine. *J Bone Joint Surg Am* 1989;71-A:15–22.

337. Pennecot GF, Leonard P, Gachons SPD, et al. Traumatic ligamentous instability of the cervical spine in children. *J Pediatr Orthop* 1984;4: 339–345.

338. Ardraan GM, Kemp FH. The mechanism of changes in form of the cervical airway in infancy. *Med Radiogr Photogr* 1968;44:26–54.

339. Adelgais KM, Grossman DC, Langer SG, et al. Use of helical computed tomography for imaging the pediatric cervical spine. *Acad Emerg Med* 2004;11:228–236.

340. Jimenez RR, DeGuzman MA, Shiran S, et al. CT versus plain radiographs for evaluation of c-spine injury in young children: do benefits outweigh risks? *Pediatr Radiol* 2008;38:635–644.

341. Hernandez JA, Chuplk C, Swischuk LE. Cervical spine trauma in children under 5 years: productivity of CT. *Emerg Radiol* 2004;10:176–178.

342. Aulino JM, Tutt LK, Kaye JJ, et al. Occipital condyle fractures: clinical presentation and imaging findings in 76 patients. *Emerg Radiol* 2005;11:342–347.

343. Eubanks JD, Gilmore A, Bess S, et al. Clearing the pediatric cervical spine following injury. *J Am Acad Orthop Surg* 2006;14:552–564.

344. Van Goethem JWM, Maes M, Öxsarlak Ö, et al. Imaging in spinal trauma. *Eur Radiol* 2005;15:582–590.

345. Sciubba DM, Dorsi MJ, Kretzer R, et al. Computed tomography reconstruction artifact suggesting cervical spine subluxation. *J Neurosurg Spine* 2008;8:84–87.

346. Provenzale J. MR imaging of spinal trauma. *Emerg Radiol* 2007;13: 289–297.

347. Flynn JM, Closkey RF, Mahboubi S, et al. Role of magnetic resonance imaging in the assessment of pediatric cervical spine injuries. *J Pediatr Orthop* 2002;22:573–577.

348. Bulas DI, Fitz CR, Johnson DL. Traumatic atlanto-occipital dislocation in children. *Radiology* 1993;188:155–158.

349. Bucholz RW, Burkhead WZ. The pathological anatomy of fatal atlanto-occipital dislocations. *J Bone Joint Surg Am* 1979;61-A:248–250.

350. Giguere JF, St-Vil D, Turmel A, et al. Airbags and children: a spectrum of C-spine injuries. *J Pediatr Surg* 1998;33:811–816.

351. Angel CA, Ehlers RA. Atloido-occipital dislocation in a small child after air-bag deployment. *N Engl J Med* 2001;345:1256.

352. Bailey H, Perez N, Blank- Reid C, et al. Atlanto-occipital dislocation: an unusual lethal airbag injury. *J Emerg Med* 2000;18:215–219.

353. Okamoto K, Takemoto M, Okada Y. Airbag-mediated craniocervical injury in a child restrained with safety device. *J Trauma* 2002;52: 587–590.

354. Labbe J-L, Leclair O, Duparc B. Traumatic atlanto-occipital dislocation with survival in children. *J Pediatr Orthop B* 2001;10:319–327.

355. Powers B, Miller MD, Kramer RS, et al. Traumatic anterior atlanto-occipital dislocation. *Neurosurgery* 1979;4:12–17.

356. Sun PP, Poffenbarger GJ, Durham S, et al. Spectrum of occipitoatlanto-axial injury in young children. *J Neurosurg (Spine 1)* 2000;93:28–39.

357. Przybylski GJ, Clyde BL, Fitz CR. Craniocervical junction subarachnoid hemorrhage associated with atlanto-occipital dislocation. *Spine* 1996;21:1761–1768.

358. Farley FA, Gebarski SS, Garton HL. Tectorial membrane injuries in children. *J Spinal Disord Tech* 2005;18:136–138.

359. Guillaume D, Menezes AH. Retroclival hematoma in the pediatric population. *J Neurosurg (Pediatr)* 2006;105(4 Suppl):321–325.

360. Matava MJ, Whitesides TE Jr, Davis PC. Traumatic atlanto-occipital dislocation with survival. *Spine* 1993;18:1897–1903.

361. Sponseller PD, Cass JR. Atlanto-occipital fusion for dislocation in children with neurologic preservation. *Spine* 1997;22:344–347.

362. van d Pol GJ, Hanlo PW, Oner FC, et al. Redislocation in a halo vest of an atlanto-occipital dislocation in a child: recommendations for treatment. *Spine* 2005;30:e424–e428.

363. Botelho RV, Palma AMdS, Abgussen CMB, et al. Traumatic vertical atlantoaxial instability: the risk associated with skull traction. *Eur Spine J* 2000;9:430–433.

364. Naso WB, Cure J, Cuddy BG. Retropharyngeal pseudomeningocele after atlanto-occipital dislocation: report of two cases. *Neurosurgery* 1997;40:1288–1291.

365. Reed CM, Campbell SE, Beall DP, et al. Atlanto-occipital dislocation with traumatic pseudomeningocele formation and post-traumatic syringomyelia. *Spine* 2005;30:e128–e133.

366. Marlin AE, Williams GR, Lee JF. Jefferson fractures in children. *J Neurosurg* 1983;58:277–279.

367. Mikawa Y, Yamano Y, Ishii K. Fracture through a synchondrosis of the anterior arch of the atlas. *J Bone Joint Surg Br* 1987;69-B:483.

368. Judd DB, Liem LK, Petermann G. Pediatric atlas fracture: a case of fracture through a synchondrosis and review of the literature. *Neurosurgery* 2000;46:991–995.

369. Bayar MA, Erdem Y, Ozturk K, et al. Isolated anterior arch fracture of the atlas. Child case report. *Spine* 2002;27:E47–E49.

370. Abuamara S, Dacher J-N, Lechevallier J. Posterior arch bifocal fracture of the atlas vertebra: a variant of Jefferson fracture. *J Pediatr Orthop B* 2001;10:201–204.

371. Caird MS, Hensinger RN, Weiss N, et al. Complications and problems in halo treatment of toddlers. Limited ambulation is recommended. *J Pediatr Orthop* 2006;26:750–752.

372. Lo PA, Drake JM, Hedden D, et al. Avulsion transverse ligament injuries in children: successful treatment with nonoperative management. *J Neurosurg (Spine 3)* 2002;96:338–342.

373. Sherk HH, Nicholson JT, Chung SMK. Fractures of the odontoid process in young children. *J Bone Joint Surg Am* 1978;60-A:921–924.

374. Swischuk LE, Hayden CK Jr, Sarwar M. The posteriorly tilted dens. A normal variation mimicking a fractured dens. *Pediatr Radiol* 1979;8:27–28.

375. Fassett DR, McCall T, Brockmeyer DL. Odontoid synchondrosis fractures in children. *Neurosurg Focus* 2006;20:e7.

376. Tavares JO, Frankovitch KF. Odontoid process fracture in children: delayed diagnosis and successful conservative management with a halo cast. *J Bone Joint Surg Am* 2007;89-A:170–176.

377. Pizzutillo PD, Rocha EF, D'Astous J, et al. Bilateral fracture of the pedicle of the second cervical vertebra in the young child. *J Bone Joint Surg Am* 1986;68-A:892–896.

378. van Rijn RR, Kool DR, de Witt Hamer PC, et al. An abused five-month-old girl: hangman's fracture or congenital arch defect? *J Emerg Med* 2005;29:61–65.

379. Power DM, Cross JLL, Antoun NM, et al. Helical computed tomography and three-dimensional reconstruction of a bipedicular developmental anomaly of the C2 vertebra. *Spine* 1999;24:984–986.

380. Sheehan J, Kaptain G, Sheehan J, et al. Congenital absence of a cervical pedicle: report of two cases and review of the literature. *Neurosurgery* 2000;47:1439–1442.

381. Howard AW, Letts RM. Cervical spondylolysis in children: is it post-traumatic? *J Pediatr Orthop* 2000;20:677–681.

382. Grisoni NE, Ballock RT, Thompson GH. Second cervical vertebrae pedicle fractures versus synchondrosis in a child. *Clin Orthop Relat Res* 2003;413:238–242.

383. Ranjith RK, Mullett JH, Burke TE. Hangman's fracture caused by suspected child abuse. *J Pediatr Orthop B* 2002;11:329–332.

384. Evans DL, Bethem D. Cervical spine injuries in children. *J Pediatr Orthop* 1989;9:563–568.

385. Lawson JP, Ogden JA, Bucholz RW, et al. Physeal injuries of the cervical spine. *J Pediatr Orthop* 1987;7:428–435.

386. Matsumoto M, Toyama Y, Chiba K, et al. Traumatic subluxation of the axis after hyperflexion injury of the cervical spine in children. *J Spinal Disord* 2001;14:172–179.

387. McGrory BJ, Klassen RA. Arthrodesis of the cervical spine for fractures and dislocations in children and adolescents. *J Bone Joint Surg Am* 1994;76-A:1606–1616.

388. Ladd AL, Scranton PE. Congenital cervical stenosis presenting as transient quadriplegia in athletes. *J Bone Joint Surg Am* 1986;68-A:1371–1374.

389. Torg JS, Pavlov H, Genuario SE, et al. Neurapraxia of the cervical spinal cord with transient quadriplegia. *J Bone Joint Surg Am* 1986;68-A:1354–1370.

390. Rathbone D, Johnson G, Letts M. Spinal cord concussion in pediatric athletes. *J Pediatr Orthop* 1992;12:616–620.

391. Torg JH, Naranja RJ, Pavlov H, et al. The relationship of developmental narrowing of the cervical spinal canal to reversible and irreversible injury of the cervical spinal cord in football players. An epidemiological study. *J Bone Joint Surg Am* 1996;78-A:1308–1314.

392. Odor JM, Watkins RG, Dillin WH, et al. Incidence of cervical spinal stenosis in professional and rookie football players. *Am J Sports Med* 1990;18:507–509.

393. Eismont FJ, Clifford S, Goldberg M, et al. Cervical sagittal spinal canal size in spine injury. *Spine* 1984;9:663–666.

394. Pang D, Pollack IF. Spinal cord injury without radiographic abnormality in children—the SCIWORA syndrome. *J Trauma* 1989;29(5):654–664.

395. Hendey GW, Wolfson AB, Mower WR, et al. Spinal cord injury without radiographic abnormality: results of the national emergency x-radiography utilization study in blunt cervical trauma. *J Trauma* 2002;53:1–4.

396. Linssen WH, Praamstra P, Gabreels FJ, et al. Vascular insufficiency of the cervical cord due to hyperextension of the spine. *Pediatr Neurol* 1990;6:123–125.

397. Bosch PP, Vogt MT, Ward WT. Pediatric spinal cord injury without radiographic abnormality (SCIWORA). The absence of occult instability and lack of indication for bracing. *Spine* 2002;27:2788–2800.

398. Grabb PA, Pang D. Magnetic resonance imaging in the evaluation of spinal cord injury without radiographic abnormality in children. *Neurosurgery* 1994;35:406–414.

399. Dare AO, Dias MS, Li V. Magnetic resonance imaging correlation in pediatric spinal cord injury without radiographic abnormality. *J Neurosurg (Spine 1)* 2002;93:33–39.

400. Pang D. Spinal cord injury without radiographic abnormality in children, 2 decades later. *Neurosurgery* 2004;55:1325–1343.

401. Abroms IF, Bresnan MJ, Zuckerman JE, et al. Cervical cord injuries secondary to hyperextension of the head in breech presentations. *Obstet Gynecol* 1973;41:369–378.

402. Byers RK. Spinal-cord injuries during birth. *Dev Med Child Neurol* 1975;17:103–110.

403. Caird MS, Reddy S, Ganley TJ, et al. Cervical spine fracture-dislocation birth injury. Prevention, recognition, and implications for the orthopaedic surgeon. *J Pediatr Orthop* 2005;25:484–486.

404. Morgan C, Newell SJ. Cervical spinal cord injury following cephalic presentation and delivery by Caesarean section. *Dev Med Child Neurol* 2001;43:274–276.

405. Jones EL, Cameron AH, Smith WT. Birth trauma to the cervical spine and vertebral arteries. *J Pathol* 1970;100.

406. Feldman KW, Avellino AM, Sugar NF, et al. Cervical spinal cord injury in abused children. *Pediatr Emerg Care* 2008;24:222–227.

407. Lam FC, Mehta V, Fox R. Spondylolisthesis of C2 in an eight-week-old infant: long term followup. *Can J Neurol Sci* 2007;34:372–374.

408. Vialle R, Mary P, Schmider L, et al. Spinal fracture through the neurocentral synchondrosis in battered children. A report of three cases. *Spine* 2006;31:e345–e349.

409. King WJ, MacKay M, Sirnick A. Shaken baby syndrome in Canada: clinical characteristics and outcomes of hospital cases. *Can Med Assoc J* 2003;168:155–159.

410. Brand MC. Recognizing neonatal spinal cord injury. *Adv Neonatal Care* 2006;6:15–24.

411. Shulman ST, Madden JD, Esterly JR, et al. Transection of spinal cord. A rare obstetrical complication of cephalic delivery. *Arch Dis Child* 1971;46:291–294.

412. Hillman JW, Sprofkin BE, Parrish TF. Birth injury of the cervical spine producing a "cerebral palsy" syndrome. *Am Surg* 1954;20:900–906.

413. Towbin A. Central nervous system damage in the human fetus and newborn infant. *Am J Dis Child* 1970;119:529–542.

414. Farley FA, Hensinger RN, Herzenberg JE. Cervical spinal cord injury in children. *J Spinal Disord* 1992;5:410–416.

415. Saternus K-S, Wighton-Kernbach G, Oehmichen M. The shaking trauma in infants—kinetic chains. *Forensic Sci Int* 2000;109:203–213.

416. Conry BG, Hall CM. Cervical spine fractures and rear car seat restraints. *Arch Dis Child* 1987;62:1267–1268.

417. Mousny M, Saint-Martin C, Danse E, et al. Unusual upper cervical fracture in a 1-year-old girl. *J Pediatr Orthop* 2001;21:590–593.

418. Winter SCA, Quaghebeur G, Richards PG. Unusual cervical spine injury in a 1 year old. *Injury* 2003;34:316–319.

419. Howard A, McKeag AM, Rothman L, et al. Cervical spine injuries in children restrained in forward-facing child restraints: a report of two cases. *J Trauma* 2005;59:1504–1506.

420. Garton HJL, Park P, Papadopoulous SM. Fracture dislocation of the neurocentral synchondroses of the axis. *J Neurosurg (Spine 3)* 2002;96:350.

421. Deutsch RJ, Badawy MK. Pediatric cervical spine fracture caused by an adult 3-point seatbelt. *Pediatr Emerg Care* 2008;24:105–108.

422. Kupcha PC, An HS, Cotler JM. Gunshot wounds to the cervical spine. *Spine* 1990;15:1058–1063.

423. Haffner DL, Hoffer MM, Wiedbusch R. Etiology of children's spinal injuries at Rancho Los Amigos. *Spine* 1993;18:679–684.

424. Mohammed GS, Pillay WR, Robb JV. The role of clinical examination in excluding vascular injury in haemodynamically stable patients with gunshot wounds to the neck. A prospective study of 59 patients. *Eur J Vasc Endovasc Surg* 2004;28:425–430.

425. Aryan HE, Amar AP, Ozgur BM, et al. Gunshot wounds to the spine in adolescents. *Neurosurgery* 2005;57:748–752.

426. Hensinger RN, DeVito PD, Ragsdale CG. Changes in the cervical spine in juvenile rheumatoid arthritis. *J Bone Joint Surg Am* 1986;68-A:189–198.

427. Fried JA, Athreya B, Gregg JR, et al. The cervical spine in juvenile rheumatoid arthritis. *Clin Orthop Relat Res* 1983;103.

428. Laiho K, Savolainen A, Kautiainen H, et al. The cervical spine in juvenile chronic arthritis. *Spine J* 2002;2:89–94.

429. Martel W, Holt JF, Cassidy JT. Roentgenologic manifestations of juvenile rheumatoid arthritis. *AJR Am J Roentgenol* 1962;88:400–423.

430. Hallah JT, Fallahi S, Hardin JG. Nonreducible rotational head tilt and atlantoaxial lateral mass collapse. Clinical and roentgenographic features in patients with juvenile rheumatoid arthritis and ankylosing spondylitis. *Arch Intern Med* 1983;143:471–474.

431. Schiff DCM, Parke WW. The arterial supply of the odontoid process. *J Bone Joint Surg Am* 1973;55-A:1450–1456.

432. Sonnabend DH, Taylor TKF, Chapman GK. Intervertebral disc calcification syndromes in children. *J Bone Joint Surg Br* 1982;64-B:25–31.

433. Herring JA, Hensinger RN. Cervical disc calcification. Instructional case. *J Pediatr Orthop* 1988;8:613–616.

434. Dai L-Y, Ye H, Qian Q-R. The natural history of cervical disc calcification in children. *J Bone Joint Surg Am* 2004;86-A:1467–1472.

435. Wong CC, Pereira B, Pho RWH. Cervical disc calcification in children. A long term review. *Spine* 1992;17:139–144.

436. Smith RA, Vohman MD, Dimon JH III, et al. Calcified cervical intervertebral discs in children. *J Neurosurg* 1977;46:233–238.

437. Oga M, Terada K, Kikuchi N, et al. Herniation of calcified cervical intervertebral disc causes dissociated motor loss in a child. *Spine* 1993;18:2347–2350.

438. Ring D, II CEJ, Wenger DR. Pyogenic infectious spondylitis in children: the convergence of discitis and vertebral osteomyelitis. *J Pediatr Orthop* 1995;15:652–660.

439. Wenger DR, Bobechko WP, Gilday DL. The spectrum of intervertebral disc-space infection in children. *J Bone Joint Surg Am* 1978;60-A:100–108.

440. Ring D, Wenger DR. Magnetic resonance-imaging scans in discitis. *J Bone Joint Surg Am* 1994;76-A:596–601.

441. Fang D, Leong JCY, Fang HSY. Tuberculosis of the upper cervical spine. *J Bone Joint Surg Br* 1983;65-B:47–50.

442. Hsu LCS, Leong JCY. Tuberculosis of the lower cervical spine (C2-C7). *J Bone Joint Surg Br* 1984;66-B:1–5.

443. Govender S, Ramnarain A, Danaviah S. Cervical spine tuberculosis in children. *Clin Orthop Relat Res* 2007;460:78–85.

444. Govender S, Parbhoo AH, Kumar KPS. Tuberculosis of the cervicodorsal junction. *J Pediatr Orthop* 2001;21:285–287.

445. Eighth report of the Medical Research Council Working Party on Tuberculosis of the Spine. A 10-year assessment of a controlled trial comparing debridement and anterior spinal fusion in the management of tuberculosis of the spine in patients on standard chemotherapy in Hong Kong. *J Bone Joint Surg Br* 1982;64-B:393–398.

446. Bapat MR, Lahiri VJ, S. HN, et al. Role of transarticular screw fixation in tuberculous atlanto-axial instability. *Eur Spine J* 2007;16:187–197.

447. Romeyn RL, Herkowitz HN. The cervical spine in hemophilia. *Clin Orthop Relat Res* 1986;210:113–119.

448. Cuvelier GDE, Davis JH, Purves EC, et al. Torticollis as a sign of cervico-thoracic epidural haematoma in an infant with severe haemophilia A. *Haemophilia* 2006;12:683–686.

449. Bohlman HH, Sachs BL, Carter JR, et al. Primary neoplasms of the cervical spine. *J Bone Joint Surg Am* 1986;68-A:483–494.

450. Levine AM, Boriani S, Donati D, et al. Benign tumors of the cervical spine. *Spine* 1992;17:S399–S406.

451. Sherk HH, Nolan JP Jr, Mooar PA. Treatment of tumors of the cervical spine. *Clin Orthop Relat Res* 1988;233:163–167.

452. Raskas DS, Graziano GP, Herzenberg JE, et al. Osteoid osteoma and osteoblastoma of the spine. *J Spinal Disord* 1992;5:204–211.

453. Azouzi EM, Kozlowski K, Marton D, et al. Osteoid osteoma and osteoblastomas of the spine in children: report of 22 cases with brief literature review. *Pediatr Radiol* 1986;16:25–31.

454. Kirwan EOG, Hutton PAN, Pozo JL, et al. Osteoid osteoma and benign osteoblastoma of the spine: clinical presentation and treatment. *J Bone Joint Surg Br* 1984;66-B:159–167.

455. Nemoto O, Moser RP, van Dam BE, et al. Osteoblastoma of the spine: a review of 75 cases. *Spine* 1990;15:1272–1280.

456. Nanduri VR, Jarosz JM, Levitt G, et al. Basilar invagination as a sequela of multisystem Langerhan's cell histiocytosis. *J Pediatr* 2000;136:114–118.

457. Ngu BB, Khanna AJ, Pak SS, et al. Eosinophilic granuloma of the atlas presenting as torticollis in a child. *Spine* 2004;29:e98–e100.

458. Schwartz HS, Pinto M. Osteoblastomas of the cervical spine. *J Spinal Disord* 1990;3:179–182.

459. Ozaki T, Liljenqvist U, Hillmann A, et al. Osteoid osteoma and osteoblastoma of the spine: experiences with 22 patients. *Clin Orthop Relat Res* 2002;397:394–402.

460. Suttner NJ, Chandy KJ, Kellerman AJ. Osteoid osteomas of the body of the cervical spine. Case report and review of the literature. *Br J Neurosurg* 2002;16:69–71.

461. Cohn RS, Fielding JW. Osteochondroma of the cervical spine. *J Pediatr Surg* 1986;21:997–999.

462. Novick GS, Pavlov H, Bullough PG. Osteochondroma of the cervical spine: report of two cases in pre-adolescent males. *Skeletal Radiol* 1982;3:13–15.

463. Oga M, Nakatani F, Ikuta K, et al. Treatment of cervical cord compression, caused by hereditary multiple exostosis, with laminoplasty. *Spine* 2000;25:1290–1292.

464. Bess RS, Robbin MR, Bohlman HH, et al. Spinal exostoses. Analysis of twelve cases and review of the literature. *Spine* 2005;30:774–780.

465. Capanna R, Albisinni U, Picci P, et al. Aneurysmal bone cyst of the spine. *J Bone Joint Surg Am* 1985;67-A:527–531.

466. Sherk HH, Nicholson JT, Nixon JE. Vertebra plana and eosinophilic granuloma of the cervical spine in children. *Spine* 1978;3:116–121.

467. Stillwell WT, Fielding JW. Aneurysmal bone cyst of the cervicodorsal spine. *Clin Orthop Relat Res* 1984;187:144–146.

468. Garneti N, Dunn D, El Gamal E, et al. Cervical spondyloptosis caused by an aneurysmal bone cyst. *Spine* 2003;28:E68–E70.

469. Korinth MC, Ramaekers VT, Rohde V. Cervical cord exostosis compressing the axis in a boy with hereditary multiple exostoses. *J Neurosurg* 2004;100 (2 Suppl Ped):223.

470. Garg S, Mehta S, Dormans JP. Langerhans cell histiocytosis of the spine in children. Long-term follow-up. *J Bone Joint Surg Am* 2004;86-A:1740–1750.

471. Denaro V, Denaro L, Papalia R, et al. Surgical management of cervical spine osteoblastomas. *Clin Orthop Relat Res* 2006;455:190–195.

472. Bruneau M, Cornelius JF, George B. Osteoid osteomas and osteoblastomas of the occipitocervical junction. *Spine* 2005;30:979–984.

473. Zileli M, Cagli S, Basdemir G, et al. Osteoid osteomas and osteoblastomas of the spine. *Neurosurg Focus* 2003;15:Article 5, 1–7.

474. Liu JK, Brockmeyer DL, Dailey AT, et al. Surgical management of aneurysmal bone cysts of the spine. *Neurosurg Focus* 2003;15:4.1–4.7.

475. Disch SP, Grubb RL Jr, Gado MH, et al. Aneurysmal bone cyst of the cervicothoracic spine: computed tomographic evaluation of the value of preoperative embolization. *Neurosurgery* 1986;19:290–293.

476. Gladden ML Jr, Gillingham BL, Hennrikus W, et al. Aneurysmal bone cyst of the first cervical vertebrae in a child with percutaneous intralesional injection of calcitonin and methylprednisolone. *Spine* 2000;25:527–530.

477. Zdeblick TA, Warden KE, McCabe R, et al. Cervical stability after foraminotomy. *J Bone Joint Surg Am* 1992;74-A:22–27.

478. Smith MD, Emery SE, Dudley A, et al. Vertebral artery injury during anterior decompression of the cervical spine. *J Bone Joint Surg Br* 1993;75-B:410–415.

479. Sibley RK, Day DL, Dehner LP, et al. Metastasizing chordoma in early childhood: a pathological and immunohistochemical study with review of the literature. *Pediatr Pathol* 1987;7:287–301.

480. Barrenechea IJ, Perin NI, Triana A, et al. Surgical management of chordomas of the cervical spine. *J Neurosurg Spine* 2007;6:398–406.

481. Freiberg AA, Graziano GP, Loder RT, et al. Metastatic vertebral disease in children. *J Pediatr Orthop* 1993;13:148–153.

482. Ilaslan H, Sundaram M, Unni KK, et al. Primary Ewing's sarcoma of the vertebral column. *Skeletal Radiol* 2004;33:506–513.